T0175385

Contents in Brief

Introductory Maternity & Pediatric Nursing

EDITION 5

Nancy T. Hatfield, MAE, BSN, RN
Nursing Education Consultant
Former Program Director
Albuquerque Public Schools
Practical Nursing Program
Albuquerque, New Mexico

Cynthia A. Kincheloe, MSN, BSN, ADN, RN
RME Coordinator
New Mexico VA Health Care System
Albuquerque, New Mexico

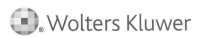. Wolters Kluwer

Philadelphia • Baltimore • New York • London
Buenos Aires • Hong Kong • Sydney • Tokyo

Vice President and Publisher: Julie K. Stegman
Senior Acquisitions Editor: Jonathan Joyce
Manager, Nursing Education and Practice Content: Jamie Blum
Associate Development Editor: Rebecca J. Rist
Editorial Coordinator: Vinoth Ezhumalai
Marketing Manager: Brittany Clements
Editorial Assistant: Molly Kennedy
Manager, Graphic Arts & Design: Stephen Druding
Art Director, Illustration: Jennifer Clements
Senior Production Project Manager: Alicia Jackson
Senior Manufacturing Coordinator: Margie Orzech-Zeranko
Prepress Vendor: TNQ Technologies

5th edition

Library of Congress Cataloging-in-Publication Data

ISBN-13: 978-1-975163-78-5

Cataloging in Publication data available on request from publisher.

Care has been taken to confirm the accuracy of the information presented and to describe generally accepted practices. However, the authors, editors, and publisher are not responsible for errors or omissions or for any consequences from application of the information in this book and make no warranty, expressed or implied, with respect to the currency, completeness, or accuracy of the contents of the publication. Application of this information in a particular situation remains the professional responsibility of the practitioner; the clinical treatments described and recommended may not be considered absolute and universal recommendations.

The authors, editors, and publisher have exerted every effort to ensure that drug selection and dosage set forth in this text are in accordance with the current recommendations and practice at the time of publication. However, in view of ongoing research, changes in government regulations, and the constant flow of information relating to drug therapy and drug reactions, the reader is urged to check the package insert for each drug for any change in indications and dosage and for added warnings and precautions. This is particularly important when the recommended agent is a new or infrequently employed drug.

Some drugs and medical devices presented in this publication have Food and Drug Administration (FDA) clearance for limited use in restricted research settings. It is the responsibility of the health care provider to ascertain the FDA status of each drug or device planned for use in his or her clinical practice.

shop.lww.com

To John
My partner, my best friend; you are the light and love of my life!

To Mikayla, Jeff, Greg, and Chelsea
You continue to show me that children bring happiness, joy, and love to a mother—even when those children are adults and parents themselves!

To Sierra, Jaymin, Riley, Hayley, Jettison, Jia, and Jagger
Being your Nana brings me new understanding, every single day, of the depth and meaning of love!

In Memory of my Dad, Edgar A. Thomas, and my Mother, Lucy L. Thomas
Dad and Mom, I miss you so much. I feel so fortunate to have the gift of being able to look at the beauty that surrounds me and see how much you both continue to bless me. Your unconditional love allowed me to be the child I was and the adult I am. My love for you is unending!

~Nancy

To Kinley
You are a true gift of grace and a beautiful example of peace. I love you!

To Margot and in Memory of Zern
You are a timeless illustration of love and friendship. Margot, your strength and courage is amazing and your love for my family is heart-warming. Zern, you are loved and missed.

To Flossie and Lester
You model faith and marriage daily. You "young pups" are a joy and a treasure and bless all who know you. Flossie you are an inspiration. Lester, thank you for your military service and laughter.

~Cynthia

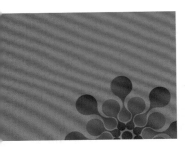

Preface

This fifth edition of *Introductory Maternity & Pediatric Nursing* reflects the underlying philosophy of love, caring, and support for childbearing women, their children, and their families. The content has been updated and revised according to the most current information available. Our goal in this text is to keep the readability of the text at a level with which the student can be comfortable because we recognize that the nursing student has limited time to study and learn maternity and pediatric nursing content. This fifth edition was carefully reviewed, edited, and developed in format to make what was a very readable text even more readable and easy to follow.

In this text, we recognize that cultural sensitivity and awareness are important aspects of caring for childbearing and child-rearing families. We also recognize that many children and pregnant people live in families other than two-parent family homes and therefore refer to reinforcing teaching and supporting childbearing clients and family caregivers of children in all situations and family structures.

Maternal–child healthcare has seen a shift from the hospital setting into community and home settings. More responsibility has fallen on the family and family caregivers to look after the pregnant client or ill child. We stress the importance of reinforcing teaching with the client, the family, and the child, with an emphasis on prevention.

We have attempted to identify all possible unfamiliar terms and define them within the text in recognition of the frustrations that can result from having to turn to a dictionary or glossary for words that are unfamiliar. This increases reading ease for students, decreases time necessary to complete assigned readings, and enhances understanding of the information.

The nursing process is used as the foundation for presenting nursing care. Nursing care plans are included that support the student in the clinical setting in recognizing potential concerns of their clients. Implementation information is presented in a narrative format to enable discussion of how planning, goal setting, and evaluation can be put into action. In the nursing process sections, nursing care focus is used instead of "nursing diagnosis" to more accurately reflect what the nurse is doing—that is, focusing on nursing care.

A full-color format, current photos, drawings, tables, and diagrams further aid students in using this text. Hundreds of drawings and photos are included in this fifth edition.

CLINICAL JUDGMENT

When caring for clients, the nurse uses their nursing knowledge and goes through a decision-making process to determine client needs. The nurse recognizes and prioritizes client concerns and takes action to help the client attain goals and have positive outcomes. The nurse uses clinical reasoning and clinical judgment throughout this process.

An important aspect of the National Council Licensing Exam (NCLEX) is to measure the ability of the nurse to use critical thinking skills and good clinical judgment to provide safe, effective, and quality care for every client. A goal in this text is to give the student opportunities and support to help in developing those clinical judgment skills.

RECURRING FEATURES

In an effort to provide the student opportunities to develop those clinical judgment skills and to offer the student and instructor a text that is informative, exciting, and easy to use, we have incorporated a number of special features throughout the text, many of which are included in each chapter.

Unfolding Case Studies

A short client-based clinical scenario is presented at the beginning of each chapter. The student is provided relevant information so they have the opportunity to critically evaluate the appropriate course of action. The student is challenged to think about the information introduced in the case study as they read the chapter. A mid-chapter scenario helps keep the student engaged and offers an opportunity to review content and again use critical thinking and clinical judgment skills. At the end of the chapter, the student is reminded of the clinical scenario from the beginning and mid-chapter and posed questions to promote critical thinking, review understanding of content material found in the chapter, and use clinical judgment to determine appropriate actions in caring for this client.

Learning Objectives

Measurable, student-oriented objectives are included at the beginning of each chapter. These help guide the student in recognizing what is important and why, and they provide the instructor with guidance for evaluating student understanding of the information presented in the chapter.

Key Terms

A list of terms that may be unfamiliar to students but essential to understanding the chapter's content are found at the beginning of each chapter. The first appearance of these terms in the chapter is in boldface type alongside the definition as part of the paragraph. All key terms can be found in the glossary at the end of the text.

Nursing Process and Care Plans

The nursing process serves as an organizing structure for the discussion of nursing care covered in the text. This feature provides the student with a foundation from which individualized nursing care plans can be developed. Throughout the text, Nursing Process and Care Plan sections provide students with a model to follow when using the information from the nursing process to develop specific nursing care plans for use in their clinical experiences. Each of these sections includes nursing assessment (data collection), outcome identification and planning, relevant nursing care focuses, implementations, and evaluation of the goals and desired outcomes. Emphasis is placed on the importance of involving the family and family caregivers in the assessment (data collection) process. In the Nursing Process and Care Plan sections, we have used terminology from Lippincott Advisor's Problem-based Care Plans. These are used to represent appropriate concerns for a particular condition, but we do not attempt to include all problems that could be identified. The student will find the goals specific, measurable, and realistic and will be able to relate the goals to client situations and care plan development. The evaluation of the goal and desired outcome provide a goal for each nursing care focus and criteria to measure the successful accomplishment of that goal.

Nursing Procedures

Nursing Procedures detail needed equipment and step-by-step instructions to help the students understand procedure they will encounter as nurses. These instructions can be easily used in a clinical setting to perform nursing procedures.

Concept Mastery Alerts

Concept Mastery Alerts are placed in select locations throughout the texts and highlight commonly misunderstood concepts. They also provide students with helpful explanations to clarify the concepts.

Tips for Reinforcing Family Teaching

Information that the student can use in reinforcing teaching with maternity clients, family caregivers, and children is presented in highlighted boxes ready for use.

Clinical Secrets

This is a recurring feature that shows a nurse who provides brief clinical pearls that students will find valuable in caring for clients in clinical settings. Examples of the types of important issues highlighted include safety, nutrition, and pharmacology concerns, as well as cultural and communication tips.

Personal Glimpse With Learning Opportunity

Personal Glimpses, included in every chapter, present actual first-person narratives that are unedited and just as the individual wrote them. Personal Glimpses offer the student an individual's view of an experience they had and expounds upon that person's feelings about or during the incident. These narratives are presented to enhance student understanding and appreciation for others' feelings. A Learning Opportunity at the end of each Personal Glimpse encourages students to think of how they might react or respond in the situation presented. These questions further enhance the student's critical thinking skills.

Cultural Snapshot

These boxes highlight issues and topics with cultural considerations. The student is encouraged to think about cultural differences and stress the importance of accepting the attitudes and beliefs of individuals from cultures other than their own.

Tables, Drawings, and Photographs

These important aspects of the text have been updated and developed in an effort to help the student visualize the covered content. Many color photographs in a variety of settings are included.

Key Points

Key Points listed at the end of each chapter help students focus on important aspects of the chapter. Key Points provide a quick review of essential content and address all Learning Objectives stated at the beginning of the chapter.

Internet Resources

Current websites are included at the end of each chapter as starting-point resources to help students gather information on certain conditions, diseases, and disorders. Websites that offer support and information for families are listed as well.

LEARNING OPPORTUNITIES

In order to offer students opportunities to check their understanding of material they have read and studied, we have included many learning opportunities throughout the text.

Test Yourself

These questions are interspersed throughout each chapter and are designed to test understanding and recall of the material presented. The student will quickly determine if a review of what was just read is needed.

Developing Clinical Judgment—Chapter Workbook

At the end of each chapter, the student will find a workbook section to help bolster development of clinical judgment and mastery of critical thinking needed to care for maternity and pediatric clients. This section includes:

- **NCLEX-Style Review Questions** written to test the student's ability to apply the material from the chapter. These questions use the client–nurse format to encourage the student to critically think about client situations as well as the nurse's response or action. Alternate format style questions, including multiple response questions, are included.
- **Study Activities** which are interactive activities that require the student to participate in the learning process. Important material from the chapter is incorporated into this section to help the student review and synthesize chapter content. Instructors will find many of the activities appropriate for individual or class assignments.
  - » Within the Study Activities, many chapters include an **Internet Activity** that guides students in exploring the internet. Each activity takes the student step-by-step into a website where they can access new and updated information as well as resources to share with clients and families. Some websites include fun activities to use with pediatric clients. These activities may require the use of Acrobat Reader, which can be downloaded free of charge.
- **Critical Thinking: What Would You Do?** which present real-life situations and encourage the student to think about the chapter content in practical terms. These situations require students

to incorporate knowledge gained from the chapter and apply it to real-life problems using clinical judgment skills. Questions provide the student with opportunities to problem solve, think critically, and discover their own ideas and feelings. The instructor can also use the questions as tools to stimulate class discussion.

» **Dosage Calculations** are found in the workbook section of each pediatric chapter where diseases and disorders are covered. These questions ask students to practice dosage calculations. This skill can be directly applied in a clinical setting.

ORGANIZATION

The text is divided into 10 units to provide content in an orderly approach. The first unit helps build a foundation for students who are beginning their study of maternity and pediatric nursing. This unit introduces the student to caring for childbearing women and children in various settings.

Maternity nursing content is covered in Units 2 to 6. Maternity topics that address low-risk women are covered first in Units 2 to 5. Unit 6 addresses issues related to at-risk pregnancy, childbirth, and newborn care. The instructor may choose to teach the normal content of pregnancy followed by the at-risk pregnancy chapters. The authors designed the content so that normal considerations would be covered first by instructors and then followed by discussion of the at-risk woman, fetus, and neonate with the hope that this grouping will ensure all normal content is covered before any at-risk topics are addressed, thereby reducing the need for parenthetical content in the at-risk chapters. It also encourages the student to review the normal chapters alongside studying at-risk content. This repetition of content is designed to help cement student understanding of the material. In Unit 6, the at-risk disorders are organized so that an explanation of the disorder is covered first and then followed by a discussion of medical treatment and nursing care.

Pediatric nursing content comprises Units 7 through 10. The basic approach to the study of caring for children is organized within a unit discussing health promotion for normal growth and development in each age group. Subsequent units discuss foundational pediatric nursing topics as well as special concerns. Finally, the specific health problems seen in children are covered using a body systems approach. This user-friendly approach to the study of nursing care of children is often used in nursing education curricula.

Unit 1, Overview of Maternal and Pediatric Healthcare
Unit 1 introduces the student to a brief history of maternity and pediatric nursing in Chapter 1 and discusses current trends in maternal–child healthcare in addition to maternal–child health status concerns. A discussion of the nursing process is also included. This edition uses Lippincott Advisor's Problem-based Care Plans as the foundation for developing and defining the nursing care focuses for each nursing care plan. Chapter 2 follows with a discussion of the family, its structure, and family factors that influence childbearing and child-rearing. The chapter introduces community-based healthcare and discusses various settings in the community through which healthcare is provided for maternity clients and children.

Unit 2, Foundations of Maternity Nursing
Unit 2 introduces the student in Chapter 3 to male and female reproductive anatomy, which is essential to the understanding of maternity nursing. The menstrual cycle and the sexual response cycle are also addressed. (Note: Pelvic anatomy is addressed in Chapter 8, and breast anatomy is addressed in Chapter 15.) Chapter 4 continues with a discussion of special reproductive issues to include family planning, elective termination of pregnancy, and issues of fertility.

Unit 3, Pregnancy
Unit 3 begins in Chapter 5 with a discussion of fetal development from fertilization through the fetal period. Chapter 6 introduces the student to how pregnancy is determined and physiologic and psychological adaptations of women during pregnancy; the chapter ends by outlining nutritional requirements of pregnancy. Chapter 7 covers the nurse's role in prenatal care and common fetal assessment tests. This chapter also discusses common discomforts of pregnancy women may experience, elements of self-care during pregnancy that the nurse needs to inform women about, substance use during pregnancy, and information to help women prepare for labor, birth, and parenthood.

Unit 4, Labor and Birth

Unit 4 begins with a discussion of the labor process in Chapter 8. The four components of birth, the process of labor, and maternal and fetal adaptations to labor are covered. Female pelvic anatomy is discussed here. Chapter 9 introduces the student to concepts of pain management during labor and birth. The chapter begins with an overview of the characteristics and nature of labor pain as well as general principles of labor pain management. Nonpharmacologic and pharmacologic methods of pain management are reviewed. Chapter 10 covers the nurse's role during labor and birth to include observation of uterine contractions and fetal heart rate. Chapter 11 discusses procedures the health care provider may utilize to assist in delivery of the fetus. Topics covered include induction and augmentation of labor, assisted delivery (episiotomy, vacuum, and forceps delivery), cesarean birth, and vaginal birth after cesarean.

Unit 5, Postpartum and Newborn

Unit 5 begins with a discussion of normal postpartum adaptation, nursing assessment, and nursing care in Chapter 12. Chapter 13 covers topics related to normal transition of the neonate to extrauterine life, general characteristics of the neonate, and the initial nursing assessment of the newborn. Chapter 14 presents the nurse's role in caring for the normal newborn and includes nursing care considerations in the stabilization and transition of the newborn, normal newborn care, assessment and facilitation of family interaction and adjustment, and discharge considerations. An emphasis is placed on teaching new parents how to care for their newborn. Chapter 15 explores issues related to infant nutrition. Breast-feeding and formula-feeding are presented, along with factors that affect a woman's selection of a feeding method. Advantages and disadvantages of each method are presented. Physiology of breast-feeding, including breast anatomy, is covered here. The nurse's role in assisting women who are breast-feeding and who are formula-feeding is discussed.

Unit 6, Childbearing at Risk

Unit 6 begins with Chapter 16 and focuses on the pregnancy that is placed at risk by preexisting and chronic medical conditions of the woman. This chapter covers the major medical conditions, such as diabetes and heart disease, as well as exposure to infectious agents harmful to the fetus, threats from intimate partner violence, and age-related concerns on either end of the age spectrum. Chapter 17 introduces the student to the pregnancy that becomes at-risk because of pregnancy-related complications and disorders. Threats from hyperemesis, blood incompatibilities, bleeding disorders of pregnancy, and hypertensive disorders are presented. Chapter 18 covers topics associated with the at-risk labor, such as dysfunctional labor, preterm labor, postterm labor, placental abnormalities, and emergencies associated with labor and birth. Chapter 19 looks at conditions that place the postpartum woman at risk. Postpartum hemorrhage, infection, venous thromboembolism, and postpartum mental health issues are addressed. In Chapter 20, gestational concerns and acquired disorders of the newborn are discussed. Chapter 21 addresses congenital disorders of the newborn, including congenital malformations, inborn errors of metabolism, and chromosomal abnormalities.

Unit 7, Health Promotion for Normal Growth and Development

Unit 7 begins with Chapter 22, Principles of Growth and Development, which provides a foundation for discussion of growth and development in later chapters. The issues of children of divorce, latchkey children, runaway children, and homeless children and families are examined. Influences on and theories of growth and development are presented. The rest of this unit is organized by developmental stages from infancy through adolescence. It includes aspects of normal growth and development.

Unit 8, Foundations of Pediatric Nursing

Unit 8 presents Chapter 28, which covers collecting subjective and objective data from children and families. The chapter also includes interviewing and obtaining a history, general physical assessments and examinations, and assisting with diagnostic tests. Chapter 29 presents the pediatric unit, infection control in the pediatric setting, admission and discharge, children undergoing surgery, pain management, the hospital play program, and safety in the hospital. Chapter 30 covers specific procedures for pediatric clients as well as the role of the nurse in assisting with procedures and treatments. Chapter 31 includes dosage calculation, administration of medications by various routes, and intravenous therapy.

Unit 9, Special Concerns of Pediatric Nursing

Unit 9 begins with Chapter 32, which presents concerns that face the family of a child with a chronic condition. The chapter discusses the impact on families caring for a child with a chronic condition and the nurse's role in assisting and supporting them. Chapter 33 explores the serious issue of child abuse in its many forms. It addresses the problems of domestic violence and parental substance abuse and the impact that they have on children. This chapter also includes issues surrounding children who are the victim of bullying. Chapter 34 concludes this unit with the dying child. A teaching aid is included in this chapter to help the nurse perform a self-examination to help reflect on their personal attitudes about death and dying, as well as concrete guidelines to use when interacting with a grieving child or adult.

Unit 10, The Child With a Health Disorder

Unit 10 is structured according to a body systems approach as the basis for discussion of diseases and disorders seen in children. Each chapter begins with a brief review of basic anatomy and physiology of the discussed body system. Throughout the text, family-centered care is stressed. Nursing process and care plans are integrated throughout this unit. Developmental enrichment and stimulation are stressed in sections on nursing process. The basic premise of each child's self-worth is fundamental in all of the nursing care presented.

Appendices, Glossary, and References

Seven appendices are included at the back of the text and contain important information for the nursing student in maternity and pediatrics courses. **Appendices** include:

- Appendix A: Standard and Transmission-Based Precautions
- Appendix B: Good Sources of Essential Nutrients
- Appendix C: Breast-Feeding and Medication Use
- Appendix D: Cervical Dilation Chart
- Appendix E: Growth Charts
- Appendix F: Pulse, Respiration, and Blood Pressure Values for Children
- Appendix G: Temperature and Weight Conversion Charts

The text concludes with a **Glossary** of key terms, an **English–Spanish Glossary** of maternity and pediatric phrases, and a listing of **References and Selected Readings.**

TEACHING AND LEARNING RESOURCES

Resources for Instructors

Tools to assist you with teaching your course are available on the Instructor Resources on thePoint at https://thePoint.lww.com/Hatfield5e. Resources include:
- A **Test Generator** that lets you put together exclusive new tests from a bank containing over 1,200 questions that span the text's topics in both maternity and pediatrics and is meant to help you assess student understanding of the material.
- An extensive collection of materials is provided for each book chapter.
  1. **Pre-lecture Quizzes** (and answers) are quick, knowledge-based assessments that allow you to check student reading.
  2. **PowerPoint Presentations** provide an easy way for you to integrate the textbook into the classroom experience, either via slide shows or handouts.
  3. **Guided Lecture Notes** walk you through the chapters, objective by objective, and provide you with corresponding PowerPoint slide numbers.
  4. **Discussion Topics** (and suggested answers) can be used as conversation starters or in online discussion boards.
  5. **Assignments** (and suggested answers) include group, written, clinical, and web assignments.
  6. **Case Studies** with related questions (and suggested answers) give students an opportunity to apply their knowledge to a client case similar to one they might encounter in practice.

- An **Image Bank** lets you use the photographs and illustrations from this textbook in your own presentation materials for your course.
- **Answers to Workbook Questions** from the book are provided and may be given to students.
- A sample **syllabus** provides guidance for structuring your maternity and pediatric nursing course.

Resources for Students

Valuable learning tools for students are available on thePoint at https://thePoint.lww.com/Hatfield5e. Resources include:

- **NCLEX-style Review Questions** that correspond with each book chapter help students review important concepts and practice for the NCLEX.
- **Watch and Learn Videos** demonstrate important concepts related to the developmental tasks of pregnancy, cesarean delivery, breast-feeding, care of the hospitalized child, medication administration, and developmental considerations in caring for children. Icons appear in the text to direct students to relevant video clips.
- A **Spanish–English Audio Glossary** provides helpful terms and phrases for communicating with clients who speak Spanish.
- **Learning Objectives** from each chapter, **Heart & Breath Sounds**, and **CDC Immunization Schedule** for children are also included.

Lippincott CoursePoint+

Lippincott® *CoursePoint* is an integrated, digital curriculum solution for nursing education that provides a completely interactive and adaptive experience geared to help students understand, retain, and apply their course knowledge and be prepared for practice. The time-tested, easy-to-use, and trusted solution includes engaging learning tools, evidence-based practice, case studies, and in-depth reporting to meet students where they are in their learning, combined with the most trusted nursing education content on the market to help prepare students for practice. This easy-to-use digital learning solution of *Lippincott*® *CoursePoint,* combined with unmatched support, gives instructors and students everything they need for course and curriculum success!

Lippincott® *CoursePoint* includes:

- Engaging course content with a variety of learning tools to engage students of all learning styles.
- Adaptive and personalized learning helps students learn the critical thinking and clinical judgment skills needed to help them become practice-ready nurses.
- Immediate, evidence-based, online nursing clinical-decision support with Lippincott Advisor for Education.
- Unparalleled reporting provides in-depth dashboards with several data points to track student progress and help identify strengths and weaknesses.
- Unmatched support includes training coaches, product trainers, and nursing education consultants to help educators and students implement *Lippincott*® *CoursePoint* with ease.

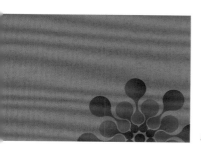

Acknowledgments

As we began the exciting process of revising and updating this fifth edition of ***Introductory Maternity & Pediatric Nursing,*** thinking of the students who will use this text was always our top priority. Our goal was to continue to provide the student with an accessible, user-friendly textbook in order to easily read, comprehend, and enjoy learning about childbearing women, children, and their families. Many people were involved in the creation of this project. With gratitude and appreciation, we would like to express our thanks to all of the Wolters Kluwer team whether they had a small or a large part in the process of publishing this textbook:

- Beck Rist, Associate Content Editor, Development, for overseeing this project with skill and expertise.
- Vinoth Ezhumalai, Editorial Coordinator, for helping us with the many little details involved in completing this project.
- Jonathan D. Joyce, Senior Acquisitions Editor, for his support of this project and his behind the scenes managing the business aspect of this text.
- Jennifer Clements, Director of Art, for her detailed eye and helping to breathe life into the art of this text.
- Alicia Jackson, Senior Production Project Manager, for helping guide us through the production stages of this text.
- Stephen Druding, Manager, Graphic Arts & Design, who helped us realize the intricacies in the design and beautiful cover of this text.
    Our thanks to each of you!

Nancy T. Hatfield
Cynthia A. Kincheloe

When we began this project, little did we know the challenges and hurdles that were ahead of us. Who would have ever guessed what life would bring during those many months of working on this revision!! Cynthia, I can't imagine getting through these challenges and this project without you! Your dedication, hard work, and many late hours are so appreciated. Thank you. My heartfelt thanks and gratitude go to my husband, John, for his never ending love, confidence, patience, and encouragement, and his sincere support of this project. I thank my children Mikayla and Jeff, their spouses Greg and Chelsea, for their love, phone calls, and positive words of encouragement—always just when I needed them. A special thanks to my grandchildren Sierra, Jaymin, Riley, Hayley, Jettison, Jia, and Jagger, for reminding me every day just how much I love and adore children. My extended family and special friends offered support, gave me insight and advice—always affirming this project could be accomplished. Star, a special thanks to you for being my rock and stabilizer through this entire process. You listened, you heard me, and were always there to put me back together when things feel apart!! Holly, thank you for being my cheerleader, your encouragement has meant so much!
    Thank you all.

Nancy

I am so very thankful for everyone who has supported and encouraged me as a person, nurse, and writer. First, to God, for giving me the passion and opportunity to write and share the privilege of maternity nursing with others. Nancy, I am so thankful that God placed me in your path first as my teacher and now as a friend and writing partner. You are the voice of this book! Thank you for all of your encouragement. Your attention to detail and care for the nursing student's learning is ever present in this textbook. Jay, you continue to support, encourage, and make me laugh. I love you and daily thank God for you! Deanna and Kathryn; you bless me daily with your faith, love, and respect for others. You each are half of my heart. God graced me with the gift of the two of you! Kinley, thank you for reaffirming my love in maternity and newborn nursing. You are treasured and priceless! God blessed me with three amazing life-long friends. Mary, Sally, and Paula, I treasure your friendship and love you dearly. No words can capture the depth of love and admiration I have for each of you. You three are the strongest, smartest, and most self-less people I have been privileged to know and the world is a better place because of you. Mom, you are an example of a strong woman and demonstrate this in your faith and life. Your life experiences are a legacy to your daughters, granddaughters, and great-granddaughter. In memory of my Dad, Leland R. Alhorn. Dad, you are missed, remembered, and loved. Your love of Christ, your family, and your country is a testimony to everyone who knew you. Lastly, to the patients I have been entrusted to care for—each one of you has shaped me into the nurse I am today.

From the bottom of my heart, thank you to each and every one of you!

Cynthia

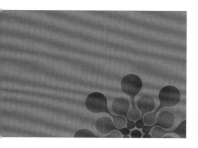

Contents

UNIT 6
Childbearing at Risk **327**

UNIT 7

Health Promotion for Normal Growth and Development **491**

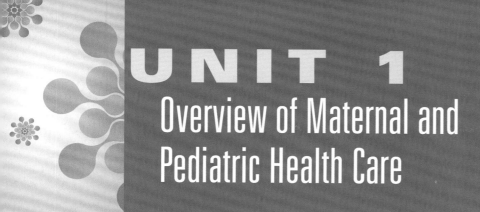

UNIT 1
Overview of Maternal and Pediatric Health Care

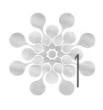

The Nurse's Role in a Changing Maternal–Child Healthcare Environment

1

Learning Objectives

At the conclusion of this chapter, you will:

1. Discuss factors influencing the development of maternity and pediatric care in the United States.
2. Describe how current trends in maternal–child care have affected the delivery of care to mothers, infants, and children in the United States.
3. Name three ways that nurses contribute to cost containment in the United States.
4. Discuss maternal–child health status in the United States.
5. Discuss two possible reasons the United States lags behind other developed countries in terms of infant mortality rate.
6. Discuss major objectives of Healthy People 2020 as they relate to maternal and pediatric nursing.
7. List new roles of nurses providing maternal and pediatric nursing care.
8. Discuss how nurses use critical thinking skills in maternal and pediatric nursing.
9. List the five steps of the nursing process.
10. Explain the importance of complete and accurate documentation.

After doing a home pregnancy test, **Carmin**, age 26, and **Wesley Buronski**, age 28, have discovered that Carmin is pregnant with their third child. They have a 2-year-old girl and a 6-year-old boy. Wesley has just been laid off from his job and no longer has health insurance. Carmin has a part-time job with no benefits. As you read this chapter, consider what issues and concerns will likely affect this couple in relationship to the pregnancy and to the health concerns of their family.

As a nurse preparing to care for childbearing and child-rearing families, you face vastly different responsibilities and challenges than did earlier maternal and pediatric nurses. Nurses, and other healthcare professionals, are becoming increasingly concerned with much more than the care of pregnancies and sick children. Health teaching, preventing illness, and promoting optimal (most desirable or satisfactory) physical, developmental, and emotional health have become a significant part of contemporary nursing.

Scientific and technologic advances have reduced the incidence of communicable disease while also helping control medical disorders such as diabetes. As a result, health care providers increasingly provide care outside the hospital. Clients now receive healthcare not only from their primary care providers but also in the home, at schools, clinics, and at mobile clinic sites such as at a homeless shelter. Prenatal diagnosis of birth defects, transfusions and other treatments for the unborn fetus, and improved life support systems for premature infants are but a few examples of the rapid progress in fetal and neonatal care.

Ethical discussions exist in maternal–child health surrounding issues such as abortion, infertility treatments, treating cancer in pregnant women, research on umbilical cord blood, and treatment of extremely premature infants. Maternal–child nurses are faced with caring for their clients while also facing some of these ethical issues.

Tremendous sociologic changes have also affected concepts in maternal–child health. American society is largely suburban with a population of highly mobile persons and families. The structure of families has changed because of factors such as single-parent families, mothers working outside the home, divorce, changes in attitudes toward gender roles, and artificial insemination or adoption by single adults. Consumers of healthcare expect to receive quality care for their medical dollars spent or their insurance payments. In addition, the demand for financial responsibility in healthcare has contributed to shortened hospital stays and alternative methods of healthcare delivery.

The reduction in the incidence of communicable and infectious diseases has made it possible to devote more attention to such critical problems as preterm birth, congenital anomalies, child abuse, learning and behavior disorders, developmental disabilities, and chronic illness. Research in these areas continues. As these findings become available, nurses will be among the individuals who will help translate this research into improved healthcare for pregnant women, children, and families.

However, in order to translate relevant research into nursing practice, you must understand the predictable but variable phases of pregnancy and of a child's growth and development. It is also necessary to be understanding of and sensitive to the importance of family interactions.

CHANGING CONCEPTS IN MATERNAL–CHILD HEALTHCARE

Maternity care has changed dramatically throughout the years as attitudes and opinions have altered. Historically, maternity care was a function of lay midwives, and most births occurred in the home setting. As knowledge increased about birth interventions, the family physician became the provider of choice for prenatal care and delivery, whereas hospitals, instead of homes, became the accepted place to give birth.

In today's society two different trends have emerged. On one hand, maternity care has become increasingly specialized. Obstetricians often provide routine prenatal and delivery care while a perinatologist, a physician who specializes in the care of women with high-risk pregnancies, follows the

at-risk client and neonatologists provide expert specialized care to at-risk newborns. On the other hand, there is the view that birth is a natural process in which little intervention is required. Therefore, some women choose midwives to provide maternity care, and some elect to deliver at home or in birth centers, which provide a homelike atmosphere.

Pediatrics has evolved from a subset of internal medicine to a specialty that focuses on the child in health and illness through all phases of development. Technologic advances account for many changes in pediatrics in the last 50 years, but sociologic changes, particularly society's view of the child and the child's needs, have been just as important.

The U.S. Department of Health & Human Services website has a timeline that highlights important events and developments in maternal–child health. The timeline can be found at http://mchb.hrsa.gov/about/timeline/index.asp.

Development of Maternity Care

Historically most births occurred at home. The lay midwife, who had no formal education, attended the woman throughout labor and birth. Women of the community shared experience and knowledge about childbirth. Childbirth was truly a woman's affair.

As physicians became educated in maternity practices and began to use instruments such as forceps, to which the midwives had no access, physicians began to replace lay midwives as the attendant at deliveries. Few women at that time became physicians because of the cultural pressures for a woman to fulfill the roles of housewife and mother.

Physicians began to rely increasingly on interventions to assist the natural process of labor and hasten delivery. Lay midwives mainly provided support and encouragement to a woman during her labor and relied on nature to take its course. Therefore, as more physicians began to attend deliveries, labor came to be viewed as an illness, or at the very least, a condition that required the skillful intervention of a physician. Two major developments greatly influenced the way maternity care was practiced in the United States— acceptance of the germ theory and development of anesthesia to decrease the pain of childbirth.

Acceptance of the Germ Theory

Before scientists knew the principles of infection transmission, it was common for a woman to develop **puerperal fever**, an illness marked by high fever caused by infection of the reproductive tract after the birth of a child. Puerperal fever was often fatal. Although rates of infection and mortality (deaths) were much higher in hospitals, women who delivered at home were also susceptible to puerperal fever.

In the late 1700s, Alexander Gordon, a Scottish physician, was the first to recognize that puerperal fever was an infection transmitted to clients by physicians and nurses as they moved between treating clients with puerperal fever and attending births or caring for women who had already delivered. The work of two other men confirmed Gordon's infection theory.

In 1842, Oliver Wendell Holmes, wrote an essay on puerperal fever based on conclusions he made after observing physicians in clinical practice. He strongly advocated that a physician who performed autopsies on individuals who died of infection should not attend women during childbirth. In 1848, Ignaz Philipp Semmelweis made similar observations in his practice. He noticed a dramatic difference in rates of puerperal fever between two maternity wards, one in which medical students practiced, the other run by midwives. The death rate in the ward attended by medical students was two to three times higher than that of the ward in which the midwives delivered. He noticed that the only difference between the two wards was that the medical students would dissect cadavers and then go immediately to the maternity ward to examine clients. The midwives, of course, did not dissect cadavers. Also at this time, a physician from the hospital died from an infected hand wound received from examining a woman who died of puerperal fever. These observations convinced Semmelweis that the puerperal fever was spread by the hands of the physicians. He began requiring medical students to wash their hands in a chlorinated lime solution between examinations. Immediately, the mortality rate fell from approximately 18% to 1%, equivalent to the death rate in midwife wards.

The topic of "infection" did not become important to the medical community until Louis Pasteur, a French chemist and microbiologist, proved that microorganisms cause infection. Joseph Lister, a British surgeon, embraced Pasteur's theory and used carbolic acid as an antiseptic during surgery which greatly improved the survival rates of his surgical clients. This led to general acceptance of the germ theory by physicians in Europe and the United States. As physicians began to use antiseptic techniques during the childbirth process, maternal mortality rates fell.

Easing the Pain of Childbirth

The development and use of anesthesia during childbirth was a change that influenced wealthy and middle class women to begin delivering their children in hospitals, rather than at home. In the 1920s and 1930s, a method called "twilight sleep" greatly increased the number of women who chose to deliver in hospitals. Physicians administered morphine and scopolamine at the beginning of labor to induce twilight sleep. Morphine eased the pain of labor, and scopolamine, an amnesiac, induced a hypnoticlike state that caused the woman to be unable to recall the pain of labor. This development allowed women to experience painless childbirth and gave the physician more control over the birth process. Therefore, the public came to view the hospital as the safest and most humane place in which to deliver a baby.

Development of Pediatric Care

Prior to the development of antibiotics and immunizations, epidemics were common, and many children died in infancy or childhood. In some cases, disease wiped out entire families. Families were large to compensate for the children who did not live to adulthood. Society viewed children as additional hands to help with the family farm chores or as contributors to family income. Sick children were often cared for by the adults in the family or by a neighbor with a reputation of being able to care for the sick.

Physicians treated hospitalized children as small adults. Often, children were treated on the same hospital units with adults. Unfortunately, early institutions for children were notorious for their unsanitary conditions, neglect, and lack of proper infant nutrition. Well into the 19th century, mortality rates were very high among institutionalized children in asylums or hospitals.

Many view the physician Arthur Jacobi as the father of pediatrics. Under his direction, several New York hospitals opened pediatric units. He helped found the American Pediatric Society in 1888. During the early 1900s, diarrhea was a primary cause of death in children's institutions. Initiation of the simple practices of boiling milk and isolating children with septic conditions lowered the incidence of diarrhea. The practice of pasteurizing milk was instrumental in decreasing the rate of death in children.

After World War I, a period of strict asepsis for newborns and pediatrics began. Institutions provided individual cubicles for babies and strictly forbade nurses to pick up the children, except when necessary. Nurses draped clean sheets over the crib sides, leaving infants with nothing to do but stare at the ceiling. These practices did not consider the now recognized importance of toys in a child's environment; as the prevailing thought was that such objects could transmit infection. Also lacking was stimulation from human interactions. Parents could only visit for brief time periods and were often prevented from picking up and holding their child.

Despite these precautions, high infant mortality rates continued. One of the first people to suspect the cause was Joseph Brennaman. In 1932, he suggested that the infants suffered from a lack of stimulation. Other researchers and physicians studied this and concluded that a lack of maternal interaction or institutionalized care was harmful to infants both physically and psychologically.

In 1951, John Bowlby received worldwide attention, with his study that revealed the negative results of the separation of child and mother because of hospitalization. His work led to a reevaluation and liberalization of hospital visiting policies for children.

In the 1970s and 1980s, physicians Marshall Klaus and John Kennell carried out important studies on the effect of the separation of newborns and parents. They established that early separation may have long-term effects on family relationships and that offering the new family an opportunity to be together at birth and for a significant period after birth may provide benefits that last well into early childhood (Fig. 1-1). These findings have also helped to modify hospital policies. Hospital regulations changed slowly, but they gradually began to reflect the needs of children and their families. Isolation practices have been relaxed for children who do not have infectious diseases; children are encouraged to ambulate as early as possible and to visit the

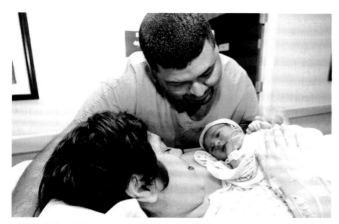

FIGURE 1-1 The mother, father, and infant son soon after birth. (Photo by Joe Mitchell.)

playroom, where they can be with other children. Nurses at all levels who work with children are prepared to understand, value, and use play as a therapeutic tool in the daily care of children.

CURRENT TRENDS IN MATERNAL–CHILD HEALTHCARE

Family-Centered Care

Society began to view childbirth as a safe and natural process as maternal and infant mortality rates began to fall. Women questioned the need for intense intervention in every birth. Also in question were the effects that medications and anesthesia had on the fetus and the newborn. Many women began to insist on natural childbirth methods that allowed nature to take its course with minimal medical involvement. Some women voiced the desire for increased control over decisions about the timing and extent of interventions during labor and birth.

These efforts led to family-centered maternity care, which has now become the norm for American hospitals. Physicians and other health care providers began to respect the rights of women to participate in planning the type of care given to them during labor and birth. Fathers were at first allowed, and later encouraged, to participate in the birth process. Hospitals allowed siblings greater access to the mother and the newborn. Birthing rooms and later, labor-delivery-recovery rooms (LDRs) replaced the old assembly-line system of moving the woman in labor from a labor room, to a delivery room, to a recovery room then to the postpartum unit. Many hospitals provide couplet care where mothers and newborns remain together in the same room and receive care from one nurse. This type of postpartum care takes the place of the older model, in which a nursery nurse cared for the newborn in the nursery and a postpartum nurse took care of the mother on a separate unit.

Family-centered pediatric nursing is a new and broadened concept in the healthcare system of the United States. It is no longer acceptable to treat children with attention given exclusively to their medical problems. Instead, health care providers recognize that children belong to a family, a

External factors
Physical variables
Biologic variables
Social variables
Cultural variables

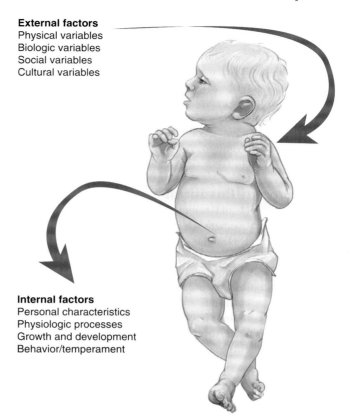

Internal factors
Personal characteristics
Physiologic processes
Growth and development
Behavior/temperament

FIGURE 1-2 Internal and external factors that influence the health and illness patterns of the child.

community, and a particular way of life or culture and that these factors influence the child's health (Fig. 1-2). Even if nursing care is delivered entirely inside the hospital, family-centered care pays attention to each child's unique emotional, developmental, social, scholastic, and physical needs. Family-centered nursing care also strives to help family members to cope, function normally, understand the child's condition and their role in the healing process, and also to alleviate their fears and anxieties (see Chapter 2).

Centralized Care

During the past several decades, there has been a definite trend toward centralization of maternity and pediatric services. Providing high-quality medical care for the at-risk client necessitates transporting the pregnant woman or the child to large medical centers with the best resources for diagnosis and treatment. The centralized location includes such specialists as maternal–fetal medicine specialists, neonatologists, pediatric neurologists, geneticists, pediatric oncologists, play therapists, child psychiatrists, neonatal nurse practitioners (NNPs), pediatric nurse practitioners (PNPs), and clinical nurse specialists (CNSs). These large regional centers have specialized units such as at-risk antenatal units, neonatal intensive care units (NICUs), burn care units, and also have highly specialized equipment such as computed tomography (CT) and MRI scanners.

Centralized care often takes the maternity, neonatal, and pediatric client far from home. Family caregivers must travel a longer distance to visit than if the client were at a local suburban hospital. Family-centered care becomes even more important under these circumstances. Measures are taken to keep the hospitalization as brief as possible and the family close and directly involved in the client's care. For the child in particular, separation from the family is traumatic and may actually slow recovery. Many of these centralized medical centers have accommodations where families may stay during the hospitalization of the pregnant woman, the neonate, or the child.

Advances in Research

Huge technologic and scientific advances emerged at the same time the movement for family-centered care was gaining momentum. Researchers and health care providers have made much progress in understanding and treating infertility. Diagnostic techniques have been perfected to detect congenital and acquired diseases. Surgical procedures to correct life-threatening deformities (e.g., diaphragmatic hernia) on the fetus while in utero have been developed. New research and techniques make it possible to treat children born with congenital problems and disorders almost immediately after birth. Pediatric specialists and specialty units have the ability to treat childhood disorders.

Two areas of intense scientific inquiry are the prediction and prevention of preterm labor and the causes, prevention, and treatment of preeclampsia, a condition exclusively found in pregnancy marked by high blood pressure, edema, and high levels of protein in the urine. Progress in the prevention and treatment of these disorders would help to further decrease maternal and infant mortality rates.

Scientists are studying ways to prevent and treat genetic disorders with gene therapy. Many animal, human, and stem cell studies are underway to better understand and treat a variety of obstetric and congenital disorders.

Bioethical Issues

An ethical issue is one in which there is no one "right" solution that applies to all instances of the issue. Ethical decision-making is a complex process that should involve many groups of individuals with varying experiences and perspectives. Recent scientific and medical advances have raised bioethical issues that previously did not exist. Examples of bioethical issues that are present in our world today include the Human Genome Project (HGP), prenatal genetic testing, surrogate motherhood, and the treatment of extremely premature infants.

The HGP began in 1990 with the purpose of studying all of the human genes and how they function. New concepts and ideas regarding many aspects of health and disease emerge as research continues. Identification of gene mutations in people who may be carriers of genetic disorders or who may be at risk for developing inherited disorders later in life has been a big part of the research findings in the project. Genetic testing and counseling is one area greatly affected by the HGP. Another focus of the HGP is to detect predisposition to certain diseases that do not become evident until adulthood. The ability to study the human genes and

factors related to the inheritance of disease and disorders has an impact on the future health of all individuals.

Today it is possible to know many factors about a child before birth. Ultrasound can reveal the gender of the fetus and certain abnormalities early in pregnancy. Genetic testing of the fetus, done via amniocentesis or chorionic villus sampling, can allow for diagnosis of many chromosomal abnormalities during the pregnancy. This knowledge allows the parents to make decisions about continuing the pregnancy or preparing to cope with a child who has a genetic disorder. Some parents want to know everything possible before the child is born, whereas others do not wish to interfere with the natural order of things and decline any type of prenatal testing.

Many ethical questions surround prenatal testing. Is it right to end a pregnancy because a child has a mild genetic abnormality or even the probability of a genetic abnormality? Will we become a society in which parents can choose or reject an unborn child based on their genetic code or sex? Is it right to bring a child into the world with a severe defect, which may cause them and their family caregivers untold pain and suffering? Is it OK to make life and death decisions based on quality of life? Or is any form of life sacred regardless of someone else's definition of quality of life? Because of technology that makes prenatal diagnosis possible, these and other ethical questions abound.

Surrogacy is an arrangement whereby a woman or a couple who is infertile contract with a fertile woman to carry a child. The fetus may result from in vitro fertilization techniques; then the embryos created from such techniques are implanted in the surrogate woman's womb. At other times, the surrogate mother becomes pregnant by artificial insemination with the sperm of the man or with the sperm of an unknown donor. Surrogate motherhood is a situation filled with ethical dilemmas. Questions that surround this issue include the following: Who has the right to make decisions about the pregnancy? Who is legally obligated to the unborn child? What if one or the other of the parties changes their minds before the end of the pregnancy? What happens if the infant is born with a genetic disorder that leaves them physically or mentally disabled?

Advances in neonatal care have made it possible for premature infants to survive outside the womb at younger gestational ages. With advanced technological care, these very premature infants are able to survive, but some have severe conditions because of the medical interventions that saved their lives. Some of these conditions, such as blindness and shortened intestinal tracts, will last a lifetime. Questions that surround this issue include: Is it right to spend enormous amounts of finances and money on saving the life of a child who will continue to need

Did You Know?

Many professional organizations have developed guiding principles for making certain ethical decisions. For example, the American Academy of Pediatrics (AAP) recommends that the rules surrounding adoption be used to guide decision-making in surrogacy cases. This principle helps safeguard the rights of the child in this unusual situation.

lifelong and expensive medical care? Who will pay for the medical and nursing care of this child throughout their lifetime? At what cost is it worth to save a life?

Demographic Trends

Several demographic trends are influencing the delivery of maternal–child healthcare in the United States. The aging of society and the tendency of American families to have fewer children have caused a shift in focus from the needs of women and children to those of older adults. Relocating to different parts of a city, or to a different state, or even a change in insurance plans can lead to choosing different health care providers, which can cause an interruption in or lack of healthcare services such as immunizations or screenings.

Nurses and other health care providers need to provide culturally appropriate care. Health care providers must assess the use of nontraditional methods of healing and traditional remedies and integrate these methods into the plan of care as appropriate.

Poverty

One social issue that greatly influences maternity and pediatric care is that of poverty. A woman who lives in poverty is less likely to have access to adequate prenatal care. Poverty also has a negative impact on the ability of a woman and her children to be adequately nourished and sheltered and increases the risk for substance abuse and exposure to diseases such as tuberculosis, human immunodeficiency virus/acquired immunodeficiency syndrome (HIV/AIDS), and other sexually transmitted infections. Each of these factors increases the chance of adverse outcomes for childbearing women and their children.

Cost Containment

Cost containment refers to strategies developed to reduce inefficiencies in the healthcare system. Inefficiencies can occur in the way consumers use healthcare. For example, taking a child to the emergency department (ED) for treatment of a cold is an inefficient use of resources and finances. It would be more efficient to treat the child's cold at a clinic.

Inefficiencies can also relate to the setting in which healthcare is given. For example, in the past, physicians admitted all surgical clients to the hospital the night or sometimes even several days before the scheduled procedure. This practice demonstrates an inefficient use of the hospital setting. Preparation of the client for surgery takes place more efficiently on an outpatient basis without reducing quality.

Inefficiencies can also exist in the delivery of health services. For example, a NICU is a highly specialized, costly unit to operate. If every hospital in a large city were to operate a NICU, this would be an inefficient delivery of health services. It is more cost effective to have one large centralized NICU.

Costs can also be controlled by providing alternative delivery systems. Many hospitals found that it is cost efficient to send a client home earlier and provide follow-up care using a home health agency. Skilled and intermediate nursing and rehabilitation facilities and hospice programs are other examples of alternative delivery systems.

Nurses are instrumental in providing care via several specific cost-containment strategies. These include health promotion and screenings, case management, and the use of critical care paths. Nurses have long advocated health promotion activities as a valuable way to control healthcare costs. Health promotion involves helping people make lifestyle changes to move them to higher levels of wellness. Health promotion includes all aspects of health: physical, mental, emotional, social, and spiritual. Many nurses and nursing organizations lobby for increased spending on health promotion and illness prevention activities. For example, nurses may testify at a public hearing that it is more cost effective to provide comprehensive prenatal care for low-income women than to pay the high cost of highly specialized care in a NICU for a preterm newborn. Nurses may also lobby for low-cost programs to provide periodic screening examinations in schools. The belief is that it is cheaper to screen for illness and provide early treatment than to provide care when a disease is well advanced and harder to treat.

Although nurses are not the only licensed professionals qualified to provide case management, many case managers are nurses. **Case management** involves monitoring and coordinating care for individuals who need high-cost or extensive healthcare services. An at-risk pregnant woman with diabetes is a good candidate for case management because she requires frequent monitoring of her blood sugar and the coordination of several health care providers. Case management is used to prevent overlapping of services or diagnostic tests from different health care providers who are medically managing the client.

Concerns about cost containment, quality improvement, and managed care have led many facilities to use a system of standard guidelines, termed critical pathways. **Critical pathways** are standard care plans used by the entire multidisciplinary team to organize and monitor the care provided. It provides outcome-based guidelines within a designated length of stay. A critical pathway includes all aspects of care such as diagnostic tests, consultations, treatments, activities, procedures, teaching, and discharge planning (Table 1-1). Other names for critical pathways are care maps, collaborative care plans, case management plans, clinical paths, and multidisciplinary plans. To ensure success, the critical pathways must be a collaborative effort of all disciplines involved, and all members of the health team must follow them. The nursing process is part of the underlying framework of critical pathways. Documentation of nursing interventions and outcomes is essential to the overall process.

TEST YOURSELF

✔ Name two major developments that contributed to the modernization of maternity care in the United States.

✔ Describe what is meant by family centered care.

✔ Identify two bioethical issues facing maternal–child nurses.

TABLE 1-1 Critical Path for School-Age Child With Long-Leg Cast After Fracture

	DAY 1	DAY 2
Diagnostic Tests	CBC. X-ray left leg.	
Assessments	Establish baseline neurovascular status, then neurovascular checks every 2 hours. Inspect cast. Assess head, chest, and abdomen for other injuries. Assess skin integrity.	Perform neurovascular checks every 4 hours. Demonstrate to family how to perform neurovascular checks. Inspect cast. Show family how to do cast inspection. Assess skin integrity. Observe family perform skin integrity assessment.
Diet	Diet as tolerated.	Diet as tolerated. Provide instruction on adding foods rich in protein.
Activity	Elevate leg when lying or sitting. Start non–weight-bearing crutch walking. Initiate safety precautions.	Elevate leg when lying or sitting. Assess ability to use non–weight-bearing crutch walking for discharge. Maintain safety precautions.
Medications	Tylenol with codeine for pain as ordered.	Tylenol with codeine for pain as ordered. Tylenol for pain as ordered.
Psychosocial	Assess developmental status. Promote self-care (bathing, dressing, grooming, etc.). Provide diversional activities. Assist in continuing school work. Reinforce safety.	Provide instruction on diversional activities for home. Instruct family on how to promote self-care. Reinforce safety information.
Discharge Planning	Reinforce cast care. Demonstrate and observe crutch walking. Arrange for home tutoring.	Provide written instructions and obtain feedback on cast care. Provide written instructions and obtain feedback on crutch walking. Provide written instructions for home tutoring. Include family and child in activities and instructions. Arrange for follow-up appointment.

PAYMENT FOR HEALTH SERVICES

Healthcare insurance often facilitates access to and use of healthcare services. Typically, families with healthcare insurance are more likely to have a primary health care provider and to participate in appropriate preventive care.

Most employers provide some form of medical insurance for employees and their families; or families may elect to purchase their own insurance apart from an employer. In either situation, this type of insurance is called private insurance. For those who are uninsured, the federal and state governments provide means to access healthcare services. In addition, specialized services, often funded by local, state, or federal governments or administered by private organizations, are available.

Federally Funded Sources
Medicaid
Medicaid was founded in 1965 under Title XIX of the Social Security Act. This federal program supplies grants to states to provide healthcare for individuals who have low incomes and meet other eligibility criteria. Under broad federal guidelines, each state develops and administers its own Medicaid program; therefore, eligibility requirements and application processes vary from state to state. Pregnant women and children who meet the income guidelines qualify for this program.

State Child Health Insurance Program
Many families make too much money to qualify for Medicaid; however, health insurance is not available or affordable to them. Because of this, many pregnant women and children are not able to get preventive care such as prenatal care, well-child visits, and immunizations. In response to this need, the federal government instituted another grant program to states under Title XXI of the Social Security Act. The State Child Health Insurance Program, first known by its acronym "SCHIP" now referred to as "CHIP," was enacted in 1997. CHIP provides health insurance to newborns and children in low-income families who do not otherwise qualify for Medicaid and are uninsured.

Special Supplemental Nutrition Program for Women, Infants, and Children
One federally funded program that continues to successfully meet its goal to enhance the nutritional status for women and children is the Special Supplemental Nutrition Program for Women, Infants, and Children (WIC). WIC began serving low-income, nutritionally at-risk pregnant, breast-feeding, and postpartum women and their children (as old as 5 years)

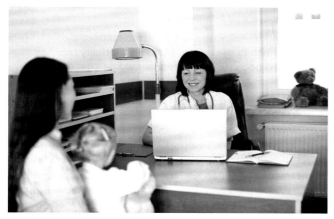

FIGURE 1-3 A trained registered nurse screens a woman and her child at a WIC clinic.

in 1974 (Fig. 1-3). Nutritional risk factors are categorized as medically based risk and diet-based risk. Examples of medical risk factors include conditions such as young maternal age, anemia, poor pregnancy outcomes, and being underweight. Diet-based risk includes diets with deficiencies in any of the major food groups, vitamins, or minerals.

Eligible women and their children receive food vouchers to redeem at participating grocery stores. The vouchers allow the woman to purchase foods that are high in at least one of the following nutrients: protein, iron, calcium, and vitamins A and C. Fortified cereals, milk, eggs, cheese, peanut butter, and legumes are examples of eligible foods. Breast-feeding is encouraged; however if a participant chooses to bottle-feed, the WIC program provides some formula assistance.

Specialized Services

Other institutions and organizations across the United States provide healthcare services to children for special conditions. Examples include the Shriners Hospital for Children, Easterseals, and St. Jude Children's Research Hospital. The Shriners Hospital provides a wide variety of services to children with orthopedic disorders, burns, spinal cord injuries, and cleft lip and palate. Easterseals is a healthcare organization that focuses on the needs of people with disabilities, and other diagnosis, throughout the lifespan and includes helping veterans. St. Jude Children's Research Hospital focuses on treating children with cancer. There are national support networks, online or in-person, for many specific conditions. Examples of these include the National Down Syndrome Society (NDSS), The Compassionate Friends (support for family after a child's death), and the Substance Abuse and Mental Health Services Administration (SAMHSA). In addition, there are local support groups based out of community groups or hospitals.

Here's How You Can Help!
Provide the client and family with a list of available resources. This information can be of great help, especially if the family needs financial assistance to afford adequate medical treatment.

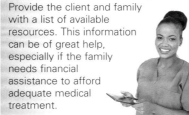

| BOX 1-1 | Selected Vital Statistics Definitions |

Birth rate: The number of live births per 1,000 population (in a calendar year).

Neonatal mortality rate: The number of infant deaths during the first 28 days of life for every 1,000 live births.

Infant death: Death of a live-born child before their first birthday (includes neonatal death).

Infant mortality rate: The number of infant deaths per 1,000 live births within a calendar year (includes neonatal mortality rate).

Maternal mortality rate: The number of maternal deaths per 100,000 live births caused by a pregnancy-related complication that occurs during pregnancy or during the 42 days after pregnancy.

Remember **Carmin** and **Wesley Buronski** from the beginning of the chapter. What are some resources you might suggest to this couple to help them investigate what is available for their family?

MATERNAL–CHILD HEALTH TODAY

The Centers for Disease Control (CDC) and the National Centers for Health Statistics track statistics that are measures of our nation's health. Birth and death rates, life expectancy, and morbidity rates are examples of health statistics that are tracked. The statistics of particular interest to the maternity and pediatric nurse include maternal, infant, and child mortality rates. In addition to tracking statistics, the CDC develops and supports programs and interventions to improve maternal–child health.

Maternal–Infant Health Status

Mortality (death) rates are statistics recorded as the ratio of deaths in a given category to the number of individuals in that category of the population. The CDC reports all mortality rates relating to the fetus, neonate, and infant as the number of deaths for every 1,000 live births. Maternal deaths are reported per 100,000 live births. Box 1-1 defines selected terms used in vital statistics. Box 1-2 lists the leading causes of infant and maternal deaths.

Both infant and maternal mortality rates have fallen dramatically since the early 1900s. At that time, for every 1,000 live births, approximately 100 infants died before they reached their first birthdays. In 1940, that number had dropped to a little less than 50 deaths per 1,000 live births. Between 1940 and 2009 the **infant mortality rate** (the number of infant deaths per 1,000 live births within a calendar year) steadily decreased and in 2018 it was at 5.79 deaths per 1,000 live births (Centers for Disease Control and Prevention, 2020) (Fig. 1-4).

Maternal mortality rates (the number of maternal deaths per 100,000 live births caused by a pregnancy-related complication that occurs during pregnancy or anytime within the 42 days after pregnancy) at the turn of the century ranged between 600 and 900 deaths per 100,000 live births, and in 2016, there were approximately 16.9 deaths

Infant Mortality[a]

1. Congenital malformations, deformations, and chromosomal abnormalities
2. Disorders related to short gestation and low birth weight
3. Newborns affected by maternal complications of pregnancy

Maternal Mortality[b]

1. Hemorrhage
2. Sepsis
3. Hypertensive disorders

[a]Kochanek, K. D., Murphy, S. L., Xu, J., & Arias, E. (2019). Deaths: Final data for 2017. *National Vital Statistics Reports*, 68(9):1–77. https://www.cdc.gov/nchs/data/nvsr/nvsr68/nvsr68_09-508.pdf.
[b]World Health Organization (2019). Maternal Mortality. https://www.who.int/news-room/fact-sheets/detail/maternal-mortality

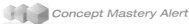

Concept Mastery Alert

The infant mortality rate is a good indicator of the overall health of the nation. Maternal mortality rate has decreased because more pregnant women get good prenatal care. Rates go up when this care is not available.

per 100,000 live births (CDC, 2019). A number of factors, including variables in the way causes of death are reported and recorded and increasing numbers of woman who have chronic health conditions which make them higher pregnancy risks, contribute to making maternal deaths related to pregnancy difficult to trend.

The United States lags behind other industrialized nations with regard to infant mortality. Two factors which contribute to these rates include the large number of preterm births in the United States—1 in 8 births compared to 1 in 18 births in other countries—and the differences in reporting of live births in various countries.

Many factors may be associated with high infant mortality rates and poor health. Low birth weight and late or nonexistent prenatal care are factors in the poor rankings in infant mortality. Other major factors that compromise infant health include congenital anomalies, sudden infant death syndrome (SIDS), respiratory distress syndrome, and increasing rates of HIV. Low birth weight and other causes of infant death and chronic illness are often linked to maternal factors, such as lack of prenatal care, smoking, use of alcohol and illicit drugs, pregnancy before age 18 or after age 40, poor nutrition, lower socioeconomic status, lower educational levels, and environmental hazards.

Child and Adolescent Health Status

In the first half of the 20th century, many children died during or after childbirth or in early childhood because of disease, infections, or injuries. Infectious diseases such as polio, diphtheria, scarlet fever, measles, and whooping cough once posed the greatest threat to children. Technologic and socioeconomic changes have influenced both the health problems today's children face and the healthcare they receive. Communicable diseases of childhood and their complications are no longer a serious threat to the health of

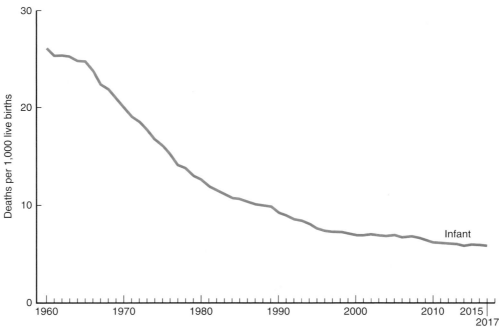

FIGURE 1-4 U.S. infant mortality rates from 1960 to 2017. (Redrawn from Kochanek, K. D., Murphy, S. L., Xu, J., & Arias, E. (2019). Deaths: Final data for 2017. *National Vital Statistics Reports*, 68(9):1–77. https://www.cdc.gov/nchs/data/nvsr/nvsr68/nvsr68_09-508.pdf. Xu J., Murphy S.L., Kochanek K.D., & Arias E. (2020 January). Mortality on the United States, 2018. *NCHS Data Brief No. 355*. https://www.cdc.gov/nchs/products/databriefs/db355.htm)

children. However, today, the largest risk to all children and adolescents is unintentional (accidental) injury, frequently the result of motor vehicle accidents. Other unintentional injuries include drowning, falls, poisonings, and fires. Currently, health problems for children focus more on social concerns including substance abuse, violence, abuse, and mental health issues. Families, communities, and government agencies minimize the risks of injury-related death through protection and safety measures. Children who are uninsured often lack preventative healthcare such as routine check-ups, immunizations, and hearing and vision screenings. These children may not have a regular health care provider. Healthcare for children is provided by clinics, school nurses, and EDs. Additionally, parents may rely on culturally based remedies, procedures, or the use of traditional healers before ever seeking care from medical personnel. **Morbidity** refers to the number of persons afflicted with the same disease condition per a certain population. Morbidity rates among children are often associated with environmental and socioeconomic issues. Increasing complexity in the environment seems to have created new morbidities that greatly affect the child's psychosocial development. These include the following:

• School problems, including learning disabilities and attention difficulties
• Child and adolescent mood and anxiety disorders
• Increasing rates of adolescent suicide and homicide
• Firearms in home
• School violence
• Drug and alcohol abuse
• HIV and AIDS
• Effects of media on violence, obesity, and sexual activity

Historically, disease conditions affecting children were very different from those affecting adults. Today, an increasing number of health conditions that used to be seen only in adults are occurring in children. For example, hyperlipidemia and hypercholesterolemia are appearing more frequently in children. There is an increase in the number of children older than 12 years identified with hypertension (elevated blood pressure). Obesity is another major health concern in children. In addition, children are now included in the statistics for clients experiencing depression.

Developmental problems related to socioeconomic factors are on the rise, including intellectual disability (formerly called mental retardation), learning disorders, emotional and behavioral problems, and speech and vision impairments. Lead poisoning appears to be a major threat to the child's developmental well-being. Although strict laws have minimized the amount of lead in gas, air, food, and industrial emissions, many children live and play in substandard housing areas where exposure to old, chipped, lead-based paint, dust, and soil often occurs.

Other prevalent factors that affect children's health include respiratory illness, violence toward children in the form of child abuse and neglect, homicide, suicide, cigarette smoking, alcohol and illicit drug use, risky sexual behavior, obesity, and lack of exercise.

Establishment of healthy living habits takes place in early childhood. Many schools educate students about the hazards of tobacco, drugs, and the importance of exercise, nutrition, and safe sex. Many also provide immunization and screening programs.

Campaigns to Improve Maternal–Child Health Status

The United States has successfully improved the health of women and their children in many areas. Examples include the Newborn Hearing Screening program to reduce preventable complications of early hearing loss. Another success is the 50% reduction in cases of SIDS after initiation of the Back to Sleep campaign. Breast-feeding Friendly Workplace initiatives and the U.S. Surgeon General's Call to Action to Support Breast-feeding further support breast-feeding mothers. Immunization against infectious diseases was one of the most significant public health achievements of the 20th century. The CDC sponsors National Immunization Awareness Month (NIAM), with the goal of increasing awareness about immunizations across the lifespan and promoting the benefits of immunization.

Prevention measures to reduce maternal and infant mortality and to promote the health of all childbearing-aged women and their newborns should start before conception and continue through the postpartum period. Box 1-3 lists ways to continue to decrease maternal and infant mortality.

Healthy People 2030

In 1990, the U.S. government developed Healthy People, a national initiative with goals related to preventing illness, promoting health, increasing quality of life, and eliminating health disparities so that people live long, healthy lives. Healthy People 2000 was the initial document published. The current document is Healthy People 2030.

Prevention of illness, or health promotion, is the underlying theme of the goals. Each goal was further broken down into focus areas with specific objectives. The objective was a measurable component to evaluate if the goal was met or not. Many of the focus areas and goals directly relate to pregnant women and children and their healthcare. Box 1-4 identifies some of the maternal–child specific focus areas and goals from Healthy People 2030. Nurses caring for pregnant women and children use these objectives as underlying guidelines in planning care. The complete list of topics and objectives can be found at https://health.gov/healthypeople/objectives-and-data/browse-objectives.

TEST YOURSELF

✔ Name some of the causes of maternal mortality in the United States.
✔ Name one healthcare milestone related to women or children for each decade of the 20th century.
✔ What is the vision for the Healthy People 2030 initiative?

BOX 1-3 Opportunities to Reduce Maternal and Infant Mortality

Before Conception
- Screen women for health risks and preexisting chronic conditions, such as diabetes, hypertension, and sexually transmitted diseases.
- Counsel women about contraception and provide access to effective family planning services (to prevent unintended pregnancies and unnecessary abortions).
- Counsel women about the benefits of good nutrition; encourage women, especially, to consume adequate amounts of folic acid supplements (to prevent neural tube defects) and iron.
- Advise women to avoid alcohol, tobacco, and illicit drugs.
- Advise women about the value of regular physical exercise.

During Pregnancy
- Provide women with early access to high-quality care throughout pregnancy, labor, and delivery. Such care includes risk-appropriate care, treatment for complications, and the use of antenatal corticosteroids when appropriate.
- Monitor and when appropriate, treat preexisting chronic conditions.

- Screen for and when appropriate, treat reproductive tract infections including bacterial vaginosis, group B streptococcus infections, and human immunodeficiency virus.
- Vaccinate women against influenza, if appropriate.
- Continue counseling against use of tobacco, alcohol, and illicit drugs.
- Continue counseling about nutrition and physical exercise.
- Educate women about the early signs of pregnancy-related problems.

During Postpartum Period
- Vaccinate newborns at age-appropriate times.
- Provide information about well-baby care and benefits of breast feeding.
- Warn parents about exposing infants to second-hand smoke.
- Counsel parents about placing infants to sleep on their backs.
- Educate parents about how to protect their infants from exposure to infectious diseases and harmful substances.

BOX 1-4 Excerpt from: Healthy People 2030 Topics Related to Childbearing Women and Children

Topic: Family Planning
Goal: Improve pregnancy planning and prevent unintended pregnancy
- Reduce the proportion of unintended pregnancies
- Increase the proportion of adolescents who have never had sex
- Reduce the proportion of pregnancies conceived within 18 months of a previous birth
- Reduce pregnancies in adolescents
- Increase the proportion of adolescent males who used a condom the last time they had sex

Topic: Vaccination
Goal: Increase vaccination rates
- Maintain the elimination of measles, rubella, congenital rubella syndrome, and polio
- Maintain the vaccination coverage level of one dose of the measles-mumps-rubella (MMR) vaccine in children by age 2 years
- Increase the proportion of people who get the flu vaccine every year
- Increase the proportion of adolescents who get recommended doses of the HPV vaccine

Topic: Injury Prevention
Goal: Prevent injuries
- Reduce unintentional injury deaths
- Reduce emergency department visits for medication overdoses in children under 5 years
- Reduce deaths from motor vehicle crashes

Topic: Violence Prevention
Goal: Prevent violence and related injuries and deaths
- Reduce intimate partner violence
- Reduce child abuse and neglect deaths
- Reduce firearm-related deaths

Topic: Pregnancy and Childbirth
Goal: Prevent pregnancy complications and maternal deaths and improve women's health before, during, and after pregnancy
- Reduce preterm births
- Increase the proportion of women who get screened for postpartum depression
- Increase the proportion of women of childbearing age who get enough folic acid

Note: This is not a comprehensive list.
Adapted from Office of Disease Prevention and Health Promotion. (January 16, 2020). *Topics and objectives.* https://health.gov/healthypeople/objectives-and-data/browse-objectives

A Personal Glimpse

My grandpa's eyes gave me my first vision of nursing. An LPN, he filled my head with hospital stories and my belly with chocolate milk. He saw people hurt by pain and fear, and he made them feel better. I wasn't much bigger than the children he saw, but I knew I wanted to make them feel better too. So I went to nursing school in the same hospital where I shared chocolate milk with Grandpa.

My pediatric nursing career started at graduation 35 years ago. Back then, the community pediatric unit was always filled to capacity. Outpatient and critical care services for children were minimal, so disorders ranged from the mild to the severe. Newborns through teens were treated for everything from mild diarrhea to significant trauma. But two things remained constant regardless of age or diagnosis: the pain and the fear.

Soon, helping sick children feel better was no longer enough. I realized early in my career that the best way to help was to prevent children from getting sick in the first place. So I went back to school to get baccalaureate and master's degrees to become a PNP. Twenty years later, I still practice as a PNP in a rural community.

Changes in healthcare have put more emphasis on various nonhospital settings, where most children receive care. Healthy children are less likely to become ill and more likely to become healthy adults. Prevention and health promotion are essential. They should be part of the care of all children (and adults!), including those who are hospitalized. I always take the time to teach the importance of immunizations, proper nutrition, growth, and development. A little goes a long way, and there is tremendous satisfaction in knowing that I've helped to ease pain and fear before they've had a chance to get started.

Mary

Learning Opportunity: What are the challenges for the nurse caring for the child in a community health setting? Describe the priorities of the pediatric nurse in health promotion and disease prevention.

CRITICAL THINKING

In all nursing roles it is important to use clinical judgment and purposeful thought and reasoning to make decisions; doing so leads to positive outcomes for the client. This process is called critical thinking. The nurse collects data and uses skills and knowledge to make a conscious plan to care for the client and family. As the plan is carried out, the care of the client is continually evaluated, always keeping the desired outcomes in mind. By using critical thinking, the nurse is more effective at meeting the needs of the client. Critical thinking involves a systematic process and is refined through experience. A critical thinker realizes there is often more than one solution to a problem and that the client's needs are ever changing.

THE NURSING PROCESS

The **nursing process** is a proven form of problem solving based on the scientific method. The nursing process consists of five components:

- Assessment (data collection)
- Nursing care focus (sometimes called nursing diagnosis)
- Outcome identification and planning
- Implementation
- Evaluation

Based on the data collected during the assessment, nurses determine the nursing care focuses (nursing diagnoses), plan and implement nursing care, and evaluate the results. The process does not end here but continues through reassessment, establishment of new nursing care focuses, additional plans, implementation, and evaluation. The goal is to identify and deal with all the client's nursing problems (Fig. 1-5).

Assessment (Data Collection)

Nursing assessment is a skill that is practiced and perfected through study and experience. The licensed practical–vocational (LPN/LVN) nurse collects data that contribute to the client's assessment. It is important to be skilled in understanding the concepts of verbal and nonverbal communication; concepts of growth and development; anatomy, physiology, and pathophysiology; and the influence of cultural heritage and family social structure. Data collected form the basis of all nursing care for the client.

Data collection begins with the admission interview and physical examination. During this phase, a relationship

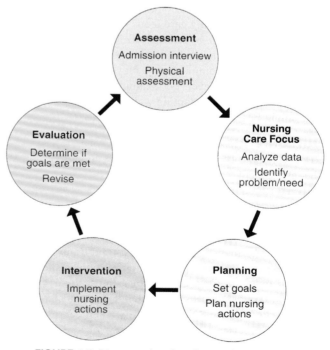
FIGURE 1-5 Diagram showing the nursing process.

of trust begins to build between the nurse, the client, and the family. This relationship forms more quickly when the nurse is sensitive to the client's cultural background. Careful listening and recording of **subjective data** (data spoken by the client or family) and careful observation and recording of **objective data** (data the nurse observes) are essential to obtaining a complete picture of the client.

Nursing Care Focus (Nursing Diagnosis)

The process of determining a nursing care focus begins with analysis of information (data) gathered. Along with the RN, the LPN/LVN participates in the development of a nursing care focus based on actual or potential health problems that fall within the range of nursing practice. These nursing care focuses are not medical diagnoses; rather, nursing care focuses describe the client's response to a disease process, condition, or situation. Nursing care focuses change as the client's responses change; therefore, nursing care focuses are in a continual state of reevaluation and modification.

Nursing care focuses can relate to actual, risk, and wellness concerns for the client. **Actual nursing focuses** identify existing health problems. For example, a child who has asthma may have an actual nursing care focus stated as *ineffective airway clearance related to increased mucus production as evidenced by dyspnea and wheezing.* This statement identifies a health problem the child actually has (ineffective airway clearance); the etiology which is the factor that contributes to its cause (increased mucus production); and the signs and symptoms. This is an actual nursing care focus because of the presence of signs and symptoms and the child's inability to clear the airway effectively.

Risk nursing focuses identify health problems to which the client is especially vulnerable. These identify clients at high risk for a particular problem or problems. An example of a risk nursing care focus is *injury risk related to repeated falls secondary to crutch walking.*

Wellness nursing focuses identify the potential of a person, family, or community to move from one level of wellness to a higher level. For example, a wellness nursing care focus for a family adapting well to the birth of a second child might be *appropriate psychosocial adaptation.*

Outcome Identification and Planning

To plan nursing care for the client, data must be collected (the assessment component of the nursing process) and analyzed (the nursing care focus component of the nursing process) and outcomes identified in cooperation with the child and family caregiver. These **outcomes** (goals) should be client-focused (specific), stated in measurable terms, attainable, and realistic and include a time frame in which the goal should be accomplished. For example, a short-term expected outcome for a child with asthma could be "The child will demonstrate use of metered-dose inhaler within 2 days." Although the RN may identify a number of possible nursing care focuses and outcomes, they must review them, rank them by urgency and client input, and select those that require immediate attention. If the client does not have input

into their plan of care, they are less likely to follow with the plan.

To accomplish the goals, the nurse must propose nursing interventions to achieve them. This is the planning component of the nursing process. These nursing interventions may be based on evidence-based nursing research, clinical experience, knowledge of the health problem, standards of care, standard care plans, or other resources. Interventions must be discussed with the client and family to determine if they are practical and workable. Interventions are modified to fit the individual client. If standardized care plans are used, they must be individualized to reflect the client's developmental and cognitive levels and family, economic, and cultural influences.

Implementation

Implementation is the process of putting the nursing care plan into action. This is when the nurse is performing the planned interventions for and with the client. The interventions may be independent, dependent, or interdependent. **Independent nursing actions** are actions that may be performed based on the nurse's own clinical judgment, for example, initiating protective skin care for an area that might break down. **Dependent nursing actions**, such as administering analgesics for pain, are actions that the nurse performs as a result of a health care provider's order. **Interdependent nursing actions** are actions that the nurse must accomplish in conjunction with other health team members, such as meal planning with the dietary therapist and reinforcing breathing exercises with the respiratory therapist.

Evaluation

Evaluation is a vital part of the nursing process. The LPN/LVN participates with other members of the healthcare team in the client's evaluation. Evaluation measures if the nursing plan of care was successful or not. Success is determined if the client met the identified outcomes or not. Like assessment, evaluation is an ongoing process. If the goals have not been met in the specified time, or if implementation is unsuccessful, the nurse needs to reevaluate and revise part of the care plan. Possibly the outcome is unrealistic and needs to be discarded or adjusted. Both objective data (measurable) and subjective data (based on responses from the client and family) are used in the evaluation and the nursing process continues.

DOCUMENTATION

One of the most important parts of nursing care is recording information about the client on the permanent record. This record, the client's chart, is a legal document and must be accurate and complete. In it are nurse observations and findings. Nursing care is provided and documented and then the client's responses to care are also documented. This helps explain and justify the nurse's actions. In maternity and pediatric settings, documentation is extremely important because records can be used in legal situations many years after the fact.

You may complete various forms of documentation, including admission assessments, nurse's or progress notes, graphic sheets, checklists, medication records, and discharge checklists or summaries. Many healthcare settings use computerized or bedside documentation records. Whatever the system or form used, it is important to document concise and factual information. Everything handwritten must be legible and clear and include the date and time. Document nursing actions, such as medication administration, as soon as possible after the intervention to ensure the action is communicated to all members of the healthcare team, especially in the care of childbearing women and children.

TEST YOURSELF

✔ During the nursing process, analysis of information (data) gathered during the assessment is done in order to determine the _____ _____ (two words).

✔ In which part of the nursing process is it determined whether or not identified outcomes have been met?

✔ Name at least one important criterion the nurse must meet when documenting health information.

Think back to **Carmin** and **Wesley Buronski** from the beginning of the chapter. What are some of the issues and concerns you think might affect this family in relationship to their health and well-being?

KEY POINTS

- Two major developments that changed maternity care in the United States were acceptance of the germ theory that led to decreased deaths from infection and the development of obstetric anesthesia to ease the pain of childbirth.

- Many changes have taken place in the care of children in the past century. Until the early part of the 20th century, society viewed children as miniature adults and expected them to behave that way.

- The concept of family-centered care developed in conjunction with the consumer movement that led childbirth to be viewed as a safe and natural process. Family-centered pediatric care recognizes that children should receive care within the context of their families and cultural norms.

- Centralization of care contributes to economic responsibility by avoiding duplication of services and expensive equipment.

- Ethical dilemmas are by definition difficult to decide and involve complex choices and conflicts. Ethical decision-making requires careful consideration and input from a variety of sources.

- Recent advances in research have led to new ethical dilemmas that must be addressed by health care providers. Examples include the Human Genome Project, prenatal genetic testing, surrogate motherhood, and the treatment of very premature newborns.

- The increase in the number of older Americans, the tendency for American families to limit the number of children, and changes in government funding have influenced a shift in focus away from programs for childbearing women and their infants.

- Poverty has negative impacts on the health of childbearing women and children and increases the chance that complications will occur.

- Nurses have been especially helpful with the cost-containment strategies of health promotion activities, use of critical care pathways, and case management.

- Payment for health services for pregnant women and children may be provided through private insurance; federally funded programs such as Medicaid, CHIP, or WIC; and specialized programs that offer services to children with special conditions.

- One way in which the health status of a nation is measured is through morbidity (illness) and mortality (death) rates. Measures particularly useful to maternity and pediatric health include maternal and pediatric mortality rates.

- The three leading causes of infant mortality are congenital disorders, prematurity and low birth weight, and maternal complications from pregnancy. The three leading causes of maternal mortality are hemorrhage, hypertensive disorders, and sepsis.

- Although its infant mortality rate is improving, the United States still remains behind other industrialized countries. Low birth weight and lack of or inadequate prenatal care are two major causes of this problem.

- Technologic and socioeconomic changes have influenced child health status. Many previous health concerns, such as communicable diseases of childhood have been eliminated. Health problems for children today focus more on social concerns.

- *Healthy People 2030* set goals for healthcare with a focus on health promotion and prevention of illness.

- The role of the nurse has changed to include the responsibilities of educator, adviser, resource person, advocate, and researcher, as well as care provider.

- Critical thinking skills must be used to take data collected and use them to develop a plan to meet the desired outcomes for the client.

- The nursing process is essential in the problem-solving process necessary to plan nursing care. The five steps of the nursing process include assessment (data collection), nursing care focus, outcome identification and planning, implementation, and evaluation.

- Accurate and timely documentation is essential for providing a legal record of care given. This is particularly important to the maternity and pediatric nurse because legal action can occur many years after an event.

INTERNET RESOURCES

U.S. Statistics on Health
http://www.cdc.gov/nchs/fastats/Default.htm
www.childstats.gov

USDA Food and Nutrition Service
www.fns.usda.gov/wic

Healthy People 2020
https://www.healthypeople.gov/

Shriners Hospitals for Children
http://www.shrinershospitalsforchildren.org/shc

Easterseals
https://www.easterseals.com/

National Down Syndrome Society
https://www.ndss.org/

The Compassionate Friends
https://www.compassionatefriends.org/

Substance Abuse and Mental Health Services Administration (SAMHSA)
https://www.samhsa.gov/

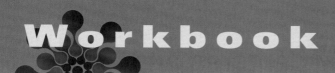
NCLEX-STYLE REVIEW QUESTIONS

1. Preventing and treating infections during childbirth have reduced maternal and infant mortality rates. Of the following, which scientific advancement has done the *most* to improve neonatal mortality statistics?
   a. Control of puerperal fever
   b. Use of anesthesia during labor
   c. Enforcement of strict rules in hospitals
   d. Treatment advances for preterm infants

2. Which of the following are ethical dilemmas? (Select all that apply)
   a. Using a surrogate for a pregnancy
   b. Being part of a stepfamily
   c. Research on umbilical cord blood
   d. Treating a very premature infant
   e. Testing for infections

3. The nurse collects data and begins to develop a trust relationship with the client in which component of the nursing process?
   a. Assessment
   b. Planning
   c. Implementation
   d. Evaluation

4. The nurse gives the client a bed bath and assists the client to eat his breakfast. This is which component of the nursing process?
   a. Assessment
   b. Planning
   c. Implementation
   d. Evaluation

5. In caring for clients, a healthcare team often uses critical pathways. Which of the following are reasons critical pathways are used? (Select all that apply.) The critical pathway:
   a. decreases cost for the client and hospital.
   b. helps establish a trusting relationship with clients.
   c. is followed by all members of the health team.
   d. provides organization for the care of the client.
   e. includes all treatments and procedures.

STUDY ACTIVITIES

1. Choose the three social issues you think have the highest impact on healthcare concerns of children. Thinking of these issues, complete the following table.

	How Does This Issue Affect Children's Healthcare?	What is the Nurse's Role in Dealing With This Issue?
Social issue:		
Social issue:		
Social issue:		

2. Go to http://mchb.hrsa.gov/about/timeline/index.asp
   a. Identify three of the events you feel have made the greatest impact on maternal–child care.
   b. Describe your rationale for choosing these events.
   c. How do you think these events will affect you as a nurse?

3. Compare and contrast the care delivered to children in institutions in the 19th and early 20th centuries, the hospital care of infants and children in the period immediately after World War I, and the hospital care of infants and children today.

CRITICAL THINKING: WHAT WOULD YOU DO?

1. A new mother tells you that her husband makes a few dollars an hour over the minimum wage, so her newborn is not eligible for Medicaid. She sighs and wonders aloud how she is going to pay the medical bills. What would you say to the new mother? Does she have any options? If so, what are they?

2. A staff member says to you, "Things were better the way we cared for infants in the old days." How would you respond?

3. While working, you overhear an older nurse complaining about family caregivers "being underfoot so much and interfering with client care." Describe how you would defend open visiting for family caregivers to this person.

Family-Centered and Community-Based Maternal and Pediatric Nursing

Key Terms

blended family
client advocacy
cohabitation family
communal family
community-based nursing
couplet care
cultural competency
extended family
immediate family
primary prevention
secondary prevention
single-parent family
socialization
stepfamily
tertiary prevention

Learning Objectives

At the conclusion of this chapter, you will:

1. Identify the primary purpose of the family in society.
2. Describe the five functions of the family.
3. Discuss the types of family structure.
4. List factors that have contributed to the growing number of single-parent families.
5. Describe how family size and sibling order affect children.
6. Explain the trend of families spending less time together.
7. Identify the focus of community-based healthcare.
8. Describe the advantages of community-based healthcare for the pregnant woman, child, and family.
9. Differentiate between primary, secondary, and tertiary prevention, and give one example of each.
10. Discuss community care settings for maternity and pediatric clients.
11. List the skills needed by a community health nurse.
12. Explain the information a nurse needs to successfully lead an information session for a group of individuals.
13. Describe how client advocacy helps clients in community-based healthcare.
14. Discuss the challenges and issues of community-based nursing.

Omar and Aman Khan, their three children, ages 15, 10, and 8, and Omar's senior parents have recently moved to your community. Their teenage daughter, Niza, is 4 months pregnant and has not had any prenatal care. As you read this chapter, consider the family structure and needs of the Khan family. Think about what community resources might be important for you to share with this family.

Each person is a member of a family and a member of many social groups, such as church, school, and work. Families and social groups together make up the fabric of the larger society. When caring for maternity and pediatric clients, it is critical for you to recognize the context of the client's needs within the client's family and community.

THE FAMILY AS A SOCIAL UNIT

The arrival of a child forever changes the primary social unit—a family—in which all members influence and are influenced by each other.

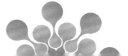

Each subsequent child joining that family continues to reshape both the individual members and the family unit. In addition, the community affects family members as individuals and as a family unit.

Nursing care of women and children demands a solid understanding of normal patterns of growth and development—physical, psychological, social, and intellectual (cognitive)—and an awareness of the many factors that influence those patterns. It also demands a respect for the uniqueness of each individual and each family. For nursing care to be complete and as effective as possible, you must consider the identified client as a member of a family and a larger community.

Throughout history, family structure and member roles have changed in response to social and economic events. In the nuclear families of 40 or 50 years ago, the father worked outside the home, and the mother cared for the children. Today, many American women with children work outside the home. Also, many children live in single-parent homes. Changes such as these place bigger demands on parents and the family unit. Blended families, also known as stepfamilies, have created other major changes in family structure and interpersonal interactions within the family. Divorce, abandonment, and delayed childbearing are some of the factors that affect the composition of families.

Family Function

The family is civilization's oldest and most basic social unit. The family's primary purposes are to ensure survival of the unit and its individual members and also to continue its knowledge, customs, values, and beliefs. It establishes a primary connection to a group responsible for a person until that person becomes independent. After the person becomes independent, the family may continue to provide a connection and resources for the individual.

Although family structure varies among different cultures, its functions are similar. For each family member, the family functions to provide sustenance and support in the five areas of wholeness: physical, emotional, intellectual, social, and spiritual.

Physical Sustenance

The family is responsible for meeting each member's basic needs for food, clothing, shelter, and protection from harm, including illness. Sometimes families need help fulfilling these needs and reach outside the family for resources to help. For instance, a community program might partially fulfill a pregnant woman's nutritional needs. While another family composed of very young parents may benefit from parenting classes to learn infant and child care.

Traditionally, division of labor between the mother and the father was very clear. The mother provided total care for the children, and the father provided the resources to make care possible. These attitudes have changed so that in a two-parent family, each parent has an opportunity to share in child care and other aspects of family living.

Emotional Support

The process of parental attachment to a child begins before birth and continues throughout life. Encouragement of early interaction between the new parents and the newborn enhances this process. Research studies continue to support the importance of early parent–child relationships to emotional adjustment in later life.

Don't Be Quick to Judge!
A single parent has many responsibilities. The Big Brother or Big Sister program (bbs.org) might be able to help single parents provide their children with another role model. Big Brothers Big Sisters of America is a program in which an older adolescent or young adult "adopts" a child and provides special social opportunities for them; for instance, going to a ballgame, museum, or simply playing videogames together.

Within the family, children learn who they are and how their behavior affects other family members. Children observe and imitate the behavior of family members. They quickly learn which behaviors the parents reward and which behaviors bring punishment. Participation in a family is a child's primary rehearsal for parenthood. How parents treat the child has a powerful influence on how the child will treat future children. Studies show that abused children often grow up to abuse their own children and that children exposed to violence against a parent often have relationships as an adult that mimic that intimate partner violence pattern, either by abusing their partner or being the victim of the abuse.

Intellectual Stimulation

The need for intellectual development continues throughout life. The newborn needs to have input through the five senses to develop optimally. Brightly colored toys and playing frequently with the infant facilitate stimulation of the senses. Talking and reading to the infant and small child is another way parents contribute to cognitive development. Many experts suggest that parents read to their unborn child and play music to provide early cognitive stimulation. The newborn recognizes and finds comfort in parent voices.

As the child grows, the need for intellectual stimulation continues. Young children enjoy being read to and playing with toys and games. Learning through schoolwork also facilitates this need.

Socialization

Within the family, a child learns a process called **socialization** whereby the child learns the rules of the society and culture in which the family lives including language, values, ethics, and acceptable behaviors. The family accomplishes this process by training, education, and role modeling. For example, the family teaches children acceptable ways of meeting physical needs, such as eating and elimination, and certain skills, such as dressing oneself. The child learns about relationships with other people inside and outside the family through observing and imitating interactions with others. Children learn what their society permits and approves and what it forbids.

Each family determines how to accomplish goals based on its principles and values. Family patterns of communication, methods of conflict resolution, coping strategies, and disciplinary methods develop over time and contribute to a family's sense of order.

Spirituality

Spirituality addresses meaning in life. Each family bases its values and principles in large part on its spiritual foundation. Religion is one way a family may express spirituality, but religion is not the only way to define spirituality. Cultivating an appreciation in children for the arts (literature, music, theater, dance, and visual art) gives them the basis from which to begin their own spiritual journey in addition to providing intellectual stimulation.

Family Structure

Various family structures exist. The structures that occur in many cultures are the immediate family and the extended family. There are many variations of the immediate family: a single-parent family, a communal family, a stepfamily, and same-sex marriage family. The adoptive family can have any of these variations in structure. Each family is unique and has its own set of challenges and advantages. It is important to note that the children from any family structure that experiences a change, or frequent changes, in the adult relationships or makeup of the family unit may feel a sense of insecurity.

 Concept Mastery Alert

Roles have more to do with how a family functions. *Family structure* relates to who makes up a family.

Immediate Family

The **immediate family** is composed of one or two parent figures and their children (either biologic or adopted) who share a common household (Fig. 2-1). The immediate family is a more mobile and independent unit than an extended family, but it is often part of a network of related immediate families within close geographic proximity.

Extended Family

The **extended family** consists of one or more immediate families plus other relatives, often crossing generations to include grandparents, aunts, uncles, and cousins. This is a typical structure in agricultural societies. The needs of individual members are subordinate to the needs of the group, and the family considers children an economic

Here's an Important Tip

In some cultures, the extended family plays an important role in everyday life. It may be challenging if there are large numbers of visitors when the extended family comes to visit the new mother and newborn or the hospitalized child. It is important to be sensitive to the needs of the family.

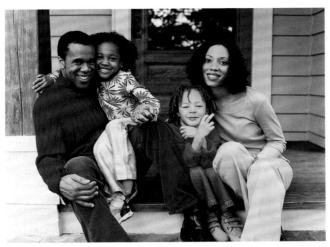

FIGURE 2-1 The immediate family is an important and prominent type of family structure in American society.

asset. Grandparents aid in child-rearing, and children learn respect for their elders by observing their parent's behavior toward the older generations.

 A Personal Glimpse

Living with both my mother and grandmother definitely has its advantages. Even though I had a male figure around me while I was growing up, it wasn't really the same as having a father who would always be there. I lived with my aunt and her family along with my mother and my grandmother. I had my uncle or cousin to turn to if I needed advice that my mother or my grandmother couldn't give me. However, my uncle wasn't always around, and neither was my cousin, so a lot of my questions were left unanswered. Questions that I didn't think anybody else other than a man could answer. I learned a lot of things on my own, whether it was by experience or by asking somebody else.

Things are different now. It's only my mother, my grandmother, and myself. As I grow older, I'm finding that I can open up to both of them a lot more. There is no reason to keep secrets. I can tell them anything, and they understand. Actually, they are a lot more understanding than I thought they would be about certain things. Every day I'm realizing that I can tell them anything.

People often ask me what it is like not knowing about my father. They ask me if I'm curious about my father. And I say, "Of course I'm curious. Who wouldn't be?" I also tell them that love is a lot stronger than curiosity. I love and care about my mother and grandmother more than anything in this world. No one father could ever give me as much love and devotion as the two of them give me. And I wouldn't give that up for anything.

Juan, age 15 years.

Learning Opportunity: *Where would you direct Juan's mother to go to find opportunities for her son to interact with adult men who could be positive role models for him? What are the reasons it would be important to have appropriate adult male role models for this child? What are some of the reasons these individuals seek their biologic parents if someone other than the biologic parent has raised them?*

Single-Parent Family

Rising divorce rates, the women's movement, increasing acceptance of children born out of wedlock, and changes in adoption laws have resulted in a growing number of **single-parent families**, those families that are headed by one adult and one or more children. The percentage of single-parent households has increased significantly from the 1980s, with women heading most of these households. This family situation places a heavy emotional and economic burden on the parent.

Communal Family

A **communal family** is a large group of various couples and children, including single friends and senior adults. In a communal family, the members share responsibility for homemaking and child-rearing; all children are the collective responsibility of adult members. The communal family is a variation of the extended family and is not actually a new family structure. This structure occurs in many settings and times throughout modern and primitive history. Communal families are seen in various cultures throughout the world.

Same-Sex Marriage Family

In the same-sex family, two people of the same sex live together, bound by a formal or informal commitment, with or without children. Children may be the result of a prior relationship, the foster child system, adoption, artificial insemination, or surrogacy. These families often face complex issues: discrimination; legal complexities regarding who is able to give consent for procedures, who may receive information, or who becomes the custodial parent if the relationship ends; and harassment for their lifestyle that can trickle down to their children.

Stepfamily and Blended Family

The **stepfamily** consists of a custodial parent and children and a new spouse. If both partners in the marriage bring children from previous marriages into the household, then the family is usually referred to as a **blended family**. The stress that remarriage of the custodial parent places on a child seems to depend in part on the child's age. The children have to adjust and learn to live not only with a new parent but often also with step-siblings. Second marriages may produce children of that union and contribute to blended family adjustment. Remarriage may provide the stability of a two-parent family and may offer additional resources for the child.

Cohabitation Family

In the immediate family, the parents are married by law; in the **cohabitation family**, couples live together but are not married by law. The children in this family may be children of earlier relationships, or they may be a result of the cohabitation family.

Adoptive Family

The adoptive family falls into a category of its own, regardless of family structure. The parents, child, and siblings in the adoptive family all have challenges that differ from other family structures. A variety of methods of adoption are available: the use of agencies, international sources, private adoptions, etc. A family who decides to adopt a child faces several potential sources of stress and anxiety from paperwork, interviews, home visits, long periods of waiting, and often large sums of money. Sometimes the adopted child has health, developmental, or emotional concerns. Some have been in a series of foster homes or have come from abusive situations. The family who adopts a child from another culture may experience prejudice and discrimination from friends and family. These factors add to the challenges the adoptive family faces.

TEST YOURSELF

✔ What are the five areas of wholeness?

✔ What can be a consequence of a child who is exposed to violence against a parent?

✔ Name two family structures and a challenge that each one faces.

Family Factors That Influence Childbearing and Child-Rearing

Family Size

The number of children in the family has a significant impact on family interactions. The smaller the family, the more time there is for individual attention to each child. Children in small families, particularly only children, often spend more time with adults and typically relate better to adults than to peers. Only children tend to have more advanced language development and intellectual achievement. A large family emphasizes the group more than the child. Less time is available for parental attention to each child. There is greater interdependence among the children and less dependence on the parents (Fig. 2-2).

Sibling Order and Gender

Whether a child is the first-born, a middle child, or the youngest also makes a difference in the child's relationships and behavior. First-born children receive a great deal of attention from parents and grandparents. Parent inexperience, anxieties, and uncertainties also affect first-born children. Often parent expectation for the oldest child are greater than that for subsequent children. Generally, first-born children are greater achievers than their siblings are. Parents tend to be more relaxed and permissive with second and subsequent children. These children are likely to be more relaxed and are slower to develop language skills. They often identify more with peers than with parents.

Gender identity in relation to siblings also affects a child's development. Girls raised with older brothers tend to have more male-associated interests than girls raised with older sisters. Boys raised with older brothers tend to be more aggressive than are boys raised with older sisters.

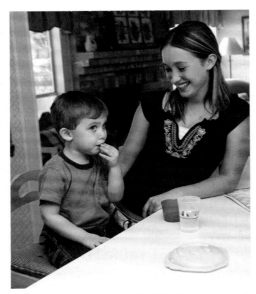

FIGURE 2-2 Children from large families learn to care for one another. Many older children are expected to help with homework and prepare after-school snacks. (Photo by Joe Mitchell.)

Parental Behavior

Many factors have contributed to the change in the older family structure model of mother-at-home, father-at-work image of the American family (Fig. 2-3). A majority of American mothers of children younger than age 18 years work outside the home. Some mothers work because they are the family's only source of income. Others work because the family's economic status demands a second income. Still, others work because their career is highly valued. More than half of all children between the ages of 3 and 5 years spend part of their day being cared for by someone other than their parents.

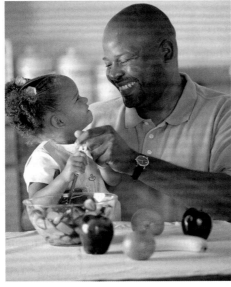

FIGURE 2-3 In some American families, roles embraced by older generations are being reversed: The father cares for the children while the mother is at work.

There is a trend for families to spend less time together. Many factors contribute to this trend which may include two working parents; the children participate in many extracurricular activities; family members watch television, rather than talking together at mealtime, or eat fast food or individual meals without sitting down together as a family; or an emphasis on the acquisition of material goods, rather than the development of relationships. New technology like mobile devices or gaming engines can bolster social relationships virtually, but they can also offer impulsive escapism that a younger person might not understand how to balance with face-to-face personal interactions in order to develop relationship building skills. All these factors impact a family's communication and interpersonal relationships.

Divorce

The number of divorces increased from 1970 to 1990 every year with recent years showing a slight decrease. Although these children are obviously affected, it is difficult to determine the exact extent of divorce on a child and what effect the divorce has on the child later on in life. Children whose lives were seriously disrupted before a divorce may feel relieved, at least initially, when the situation is resolved. Others who were unaware of parental conflict and felt that their lives were happy may feel frightened and abandoned. All these emotions depend on the children involved, their ages, and the kind of care and relationships they experience with their parents after the divorce.

Children may go through many emotions when a divorce occurs. Feelings of grief, anger, rejection, and self-worthlessness are common. These emotions may follow the children for years, even into adulthood, even though children may understand the true reasons for the divorce. In addition, the parents, either custodial or noncustodial, may try to influence the child's thinking about the other parent, placing the child in an emotional trap. If the noncustodial parent does not keep in regular contact with the child, feelings of rejection may be overwhelming. The child often desperately wants a sign of that parent's continuing love.

Culture

Each person is the product of a family, a culture, and a community. In some cultures, family life is gentle and permissive; other cultures demand unquestioning obedience of children and expect children to endure pain and hardship stoically. The child may be from a cultural group that places a high value on children, in which relatives and friends give children lots of attention, or the child may be from a group that has taught the child from early childhood to fend for oneself (Fig. 2-4). Additionally, the culture may place a high value on the family unit as a whole with little emphasis on the individual, or conversely, the culture may place an emphasis on the individual and not the family unit.

Culture influences the timing and number of children desired by the childbearing family. Cultural values and beliefs about birth control, abortion, and sexual practices influence the choices individuals and couples make about childbearing.

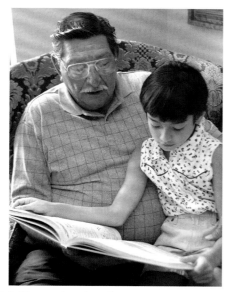

FIGURE 2-4 Many cultural preferences are seen in families. In some cultures, extended family members such as grandparents participate in raising children. (Photo by Joe Mitchell.)

Culture also determines the family's health beliefs and practices. Respect for a person's cultural heritage and individuality is an essential part of nursing care. To plan culturally appropriate and acceptable care, it is important to understand the health practices and lifestyle of families from various cultures. Rather than memorizing a list of generalized facts regarding different cultures, it is more useful to develop **cultural competency**, the capacity to work effectively with people by integrating the elements of their culture into nursing care (Betancourt, Green, & Carrillo, 2020).

To develop cultural competency, you must first do a self-assessment to understand cultural influences on your own life. These include factors that are easy to identify such as language, food, and clothing, but also influences that are not as obvious including communication styles, beliefs, attitudes, values, and perceptions. Only after recognizing these influences and any biases present in your own life is it possible to recognize and accept the different attitudes, behaviors, and values of another person's culture.

Integrating cultural attitudes toward food, cleanliness, respect, and freedom into nursing care is of the utmost importance in providing client-centered care. The nurse should be especially sensitive to the concerns of the client who is separated from their culture and may find the food, language, people, and surroundings of the healthcare facility different and also possibly frightening. Cultural competency enhances cooperation from the client and family, minimizing frustration. These factors are essential in restoring health so that the client may once again be a functioning part of the family and the community.

TEST YOURSELF

✔ Name one way that family size affects a child's development.

✔ What are two factors that contribute to American families spending less time together?

✔ Define cultural competency.

Remember the Khan family. How would you describe their family structure? What benefits and needs would you want to identify when providing nursing care to this family?

HEALTHCARE SHIFT: FROM HOSPITAL TO COMMUNITY

Over the last century, healthcare has gone through a number of changes. The sophisticated healthcare currently available is extremely expensive and has strained healthcare funding to a point where other healthcare approaches have become necessary. This need for change has led to the emergence of community-based healthcare and an emphasis on wellness and preventive healthcare instead of illness and hospital-based care.

The shift to community-based healthcare has influenced maternity and pediatric care. For example, a pregnant woman who develops complications can sometimes receive care at home with the assistance of a nurse case manager who helps coordinate her care. This allows the woman to receive high-quality care at a lower cost than if she were to require hospitalization and in an environment that is familiar to her. In the community, the child can also receive preventive care and wellness information from various sources such as schools and mobile clinics.

Community-Based Nursing

Community-based nursing focuses on prevention and is directed toward the individuals and families within a community and delivered outside the traditional hospital system. The goals are to help people meet their healthcare needs and to maintain continuity of care as they move through the various healthcare settings available to them. Nurses often made home visits in the early days of public health nursing. Through the years, the setting for healthcare gradually shifted to clinic and physician offices. Recently, in an effort to meet the challenges of cost containment and decreased or limited access to care, home visits by nurses and at home care for the client has increased.

The role of the nurse who works in the community is different from that of the hospital nurse. Generally, the nurse in the community focuses on **primary prevention**, which includes health-promoting activities to prevent the development of illness or injury. This level of prevention includes giving information regarding safety, diet, rest, exercise, and disease prevention through immunizations and emphasizes the nursing roles of educator and client advocate. Some examples of primary prevention are:

- The school nurse giving a drug education program to a fourth-grade class.
- A nurse in a maternity clinic giving tips on proper nutrition during pregnancy.

In some community settings, the nurse's role focuses on **secondary prevention**, which is health-screening activities that aid in early diagnosis and encourage prompt treatment before long-term negative effects arise. Secondary prevention is provided in such settings as clinics, home care nursing, or schools. The nurse participates in data collection measures such as height, weight, hearing, and vision screening. During well-child visits and follow-up, the nurse compiles a health history and collects data, including vital signs, blood work, and other diagnostic tests as ordered by the health care provider. Some examples of secondary prevention are:

- A school nurse identifies a child with pediculosis (head lice). The school nurse contacts the child's caregivers and provides instructions on the care of the child and other family members to eliminate the infestation.
- A community clinic nurse identifies a pregnant adolescent who is gaining insufficient weight and is possibly anemic. The nurse works with the adolescent to review the family's dietary habits and nutritional state. This would help determine if the problem is limited to the pregnancy or if other family members are also malnourished or if there is lack of knowledge or inadequate means for a healthy diet. After finding these answers, the nurse can help the family provide better nutrition for the entire family and focus on nutritional issues unique to the pregnant adolescent.

Tertiary prevention is health-promoting activities that focus on rehabilitation and providing information to prevent further injury or illness. Tertiary prevention occurs in special settings. For example, community-based healthcare interventions might help the at-risk infant or child through special intervention programs, group homes, or selected outpatient settings focusing on rehabilitation, such as an orthopedic clinic. An example of tertiary prevention would be:

- A young rural family with a child who has spina bifida who needs urinary catheterization several times a day. The family brings the child regularly to a specialized clinic at a major medical center. The family has no insurance, and the cost of catheters is such that the family caregivers feel they can no longer afford them. The nurse collaborates with a social worker to help the family with exploring additional resources for financial help, such as an organization that will help fund their trips to the clinic for regular appointments or to find a source to help cover the costs of catheters and other incidental expenses.

An advantage of community-based healthcare is that pregnant women and children receive care in settings familiar to them—homes, schools, or community centers. In the community setting, the child's caregivers are encouraged to participate in and provide the child's care. Although involved in direct care, the nurse in the community spends a great part of their time as a communicator, educator, advocate, administrator, and manager.

Community Care Settings for the Maternity Client

Prenatal and Postpartum Home Healthcare

While the majority of prenatal care occurs at a clinic or physician's office, evidence shows that mothers and infants experience positive health outcomes when nurses go to the home for visits throughout pregnancy and the first year of the child's life. Positive outcomes include increases in maternal-infant interactions and the father's impact and decreases in preterm births and substance use. In many countries a community health worker is the one who makes these visits.

Settings for Birth

Cultural beliefs, personal preferences, and an increase in options (settings and providers) guide the woman's choice of a birth setting. The choices of birth settings are primarily the home, birth centers, and hospitals (Fig. 2-5).

Home

In the early 20th century, home births were the norm before the availability of anesthesia and pain medication in the hospital setting. Today, home births account for a small percentage of births. A woman may choose to deliver at home for a variety of reasons. She may desire a more comfortable setting or more control over birthing conditions and positions. In addition, a woman may prefer to give birth at home so that she can take care of her healthy newborn, rather than experiencing periods of separation while the newborn is cared for in a hospital nursery.

The attendant for home births is usually a midwife. Some are lay midwives, often trained through apprenticeships with experienced lay midwives. Others are formally trained certified nurse-midwives (CNMs) who practice independently in home settings and clinics with physician backup for consultation and referral. Laws in individual states regulate the practice of midwifery. There remains an ongoing debate in the medical community over the safety of giving birth at home.

Birth Centers

Since the early 1980s, birth centers have increased in popularity and availability as a birth site choice. The environment is usually comfortable with furnishings and lighting designed to make the laboring woman and her family feel welcome. There are often family areas (e.g., kitchens and sitting rooms) and bathrooms with showers and whirlpool tubs. Birth centers employ a variety of healthcare professionals, including registered nurses (RNs), CNMs, licensed practical or vocational nurses, and doulas (specialized birth attendants). Medical interventions occur rarely, so physicians are seldom present. However, birth centers are often affiliated with a hospital and obstetricians and pediatricians as consultants.

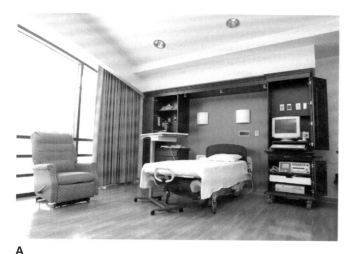

A

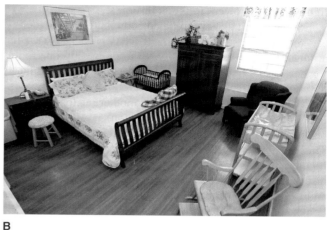

B

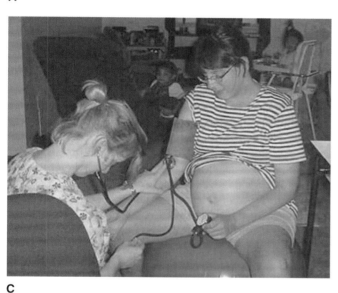

C

FIGURE 2-5 There are many different settings in which a woman can choose to give birth. These decisions are influenced by preferences regarding methods of pain control and general beliefs about how a birth should be managed. **A.** Hospital LDRP. **B.** Birth center. **C.** Home setting. (Photos **A** and **C** by Joe Mitchell. Photo **B** by Gus Freedman.)

Midwives at birth centers screen prospective clients prenatally and only accept low-risk women as clients. Most birth centers have medical equipment such as intravenous lines and fluids, oxygen, newborn resuscitation equipment, infant warmers, and local anesthesia for repair of perineal tears or infrequently performed episiotomies. If a laboring woman decides she wants an epidural anesthesia, or if she presents with complications that put her or the fetus at risk, the woman is transported to a hospital for the remainder of her labor and delivery. It has been shown that homelike birth settings are associated with increased maternal satisfaction, fewer medical interventions, and lower costs (Stapleton, 2019).

Hospitals

Americans accepted childbirth in a hospital setting by the 1920s. By 1950, the vast majority of births in the United States took place in hospitals. Today, most of births in the United States are in hospitals, with a majority of these births attended by medical doctors.

Until the 1970s, giving birth in a hospital required the woman to endure uncomfortable procedures (e.g., enemas, shaving); to labor, deliver, and recover in at least three separate rooms; and to be separated from her newborn until several hours after birth. In the mid-1970s, clients began to desire a more natural and family-centered childbirth approach. Family-centered maternity care included more time with the newborn and less time moving from room to room. Hospital administrators, health care providers, and nurses began to listen to client needs and desires, and hospital policies began to change. As a result, the trend in many hospitals is to promote family-centered maternity care in more homelike settings. Most hospitals today offer combination labor–delivery–recovery rooms (LDRs), which minimize the number of rooms the woman is in during her hospital stay. The rooms are larger to accommodate family support and to allow healthcare professionals enough room to attend the birth. In addition, LDRs are aesthetically appealing, with homelike furnishings, wallpaper, softer lighting, and showers in the bathrooms.

Some hospitals have initiated combination labor–delivery–recovery–postpartum rooms (LDRPs) (Fig. 2-5A). This arrangement allows for the woman to be in only one room for her hospital stay. Another concept that some hospitals have embraced is **couplet care** where the healthy newborn remains in the same room with the mother (as long as there is no medical indication for separation) and one nurse is responsible for the care of both the newborn and the mother. This practice encourages early bonding and provides time for new parents to learn to care for their newborn before discharge. Parents learn to recognize their newborn's cues and therefore are better prepared to care for the newborn at home.

TEST YOURSELF

✔ Define primary prevention.

✔ Give one example of tertiary prevention.

✔ Name two childbirth settings and an advantage of each.

Community Care Settings for the Child

Care for a child occurs in a wide variety of community settings. Some settings primarily provide wellness care, whereas others provide specialized care for children with particular diagnoses or conditions. These include outpatient settings, home care, schools, camps, community centers, parishes, intervention programs, and group homes.

Outpatient Settings

There are a variety of outpatient settings for children. As the healthcare delivery system continues to move into the community, more settings will emerge. Outpatient clinics may be privately owned, an extension of a hospital, or may be part of a regional, county, or city health department. Clinics provide services including education, anticipatory guidance, immunizations, diagnosis, treatment, and rehabilitation. Clinics may treat a variety of clients, or be specialized and treat a specific population such as at-risk infants born to drug-addicted mothers or clients with sickle cell anemia.

 A Personal Glimpse

The clinic is where you go when you're on the public access card and cannot afford real insurance. You hardly see the same doctor twice. A lot are interns working out their internships.

My baby was about 2 months old when he developed a bumpy rash on the crown of his head. I took him to the clinic because it was spreading, and I didn't know what it could be. A doctor who I could hardly understand was on duty. This was the same doctor that told me I had

chickenpox when I was pregnant (I didn't). He looked at the rash and looked at me very strange, then said, "This looks similar to a rash connected to HIV." He requested a test for AIDS! You cannot know the thoughts that go through your head. How? Where? Who? Why? Then, I remembered that I had been tested when I first found out I was pregnant, and it was negative. Since Jack, the baby's father, and I had not been with anyone else, I knew there must be another reason for this rash.

That doctor never took a sample to test or asked another doctor to come in and look at the rash. I took little Tommy home and started to use an ointment I'd heard about on his head every day for about a month. The rash went away, and I've changed clinics since—they're not all really the same. You get what you pay for.

Michelle

Learning Opportunity: What feelings do you think this mother might have been experiencing in this situation? What specific things could the nurse do to be of support and help to this mother?

Home Healthcare

Shortened acute care stays in the hospital have contributed to the increasing number of children cared for by home nurses. Children are often more comfortable in familiar home surroundings (Fig. 2-6). Children and infants can be successfully treated for many conditions at home, where they and their caregivers are more comfortable, and they can receive the love and attention of family members. Common conditions for which an infant or child may receive home care services include the following:

• Phototherapy for elevated bilirubin levels
• Intravenous antibiotic therapy for systemic infections
• Postoperative care
• Chronic conditions, such as asthma, sickle cell anemia, cystic fibrosis, HIV/AIDS, and leukemia
• Respirator (ventilator) dependence

Other home healthcare team members may include a physical therapist, respiratory therapist, speech therapist,

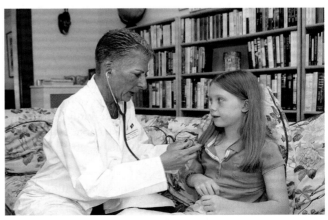

FIGURE 2-6 During a visit by the nurse, the child is comforted by the familiar surroundings of her home.

occupational therapist, home schooling teacher, home health aide, primary health care provider (physician or nurse practitioner), and social worker. Members of the team vary with the child's health needs.

Schools and Camps

Schools and camps have been the sites for provision of healthcare for many years, but the role of healthcare professionals in these settings has expanded (Fig. 2-7). The school nurse may be responsible for classroom health information sessions, health screenings, immunizations, first aid for injured children, care of ill children, administering medication, assisting with sports physicals, and identifying children with problems and recommending programs for them. Health information geared for each grade level can cover personal hygiene, sex education, substance abuse, safety, and emotional health.

Many school-aged children have chronic health problems that need daily supervision or care; for example, a child with spina bifida who needs to be catheterized several times each day or a child with diabetes who needs to perform glucose monitoring and administer insulin during school hours. The school maintains health records on each child. Some schools have clinics that provide routine dental care, physicals, screening for vision, hearing, scoliosis, tuberculosis, and follow-up on immunizations.

Camp nurses provide first aid for campers and staff, maintain health records, giving first aid and cardiopulmonary resuscitation classes, offer relevant health education, maintain an infirmary for ill campers, and provide care to homesick children.

At camps for children with special needs, camper healthcare needs determine the type of nursing care required. For example, the nurse may discuss self-administration of insulin and the many aspects of diabetic care at a camp for diabetic children. Other camps may specialize in children with developmental delays, physical challenges, or chronic illness such as asthma or cystic fibrosis. Others have specific purposes, such as weight control or behavior management. In each of these settings, the nurse provides basic healthcare with health information sessions geared toward the camper needs.

Community Centers and Parishes

Community centers and parishes provide care relevant to a particular community. Parish centers may sponsor outreach programs in a church, synagogue, or other religious setting. These centers design services to meet community needs. For example, in an area with many homeless people or a high rate of poverty, centers may provide basic healthcare, food, shelter, clothing, vouchers, health classes, addiction services, or other resources. Some communities offer walk-in or residential clinics for special purposes such as teen pregnancy or mental health; or they may offer day care services for children or senior adults.

Residential Programs

Residential programs, often called group homes, provide services for a number of individuals and their health needs. Residential programs geared primarily toward children include chemical dependency treatment centers or homes for children with mental or emotional health needs. These homes vary in size and setup according to the needs of the children at the home.

The nurse may work for the local health department or for a corporation that owns several group homes or may be part of a healthcare agency that serves the residential program. For example, in a home with six children with minimal disabilities, the nurse may visit every 2 weeks to meet with and educate the staff, update health records, and provide immunizations. Homes that serve many children or that serve children with complex needs may need to have nurses present 24 hours a day. Some group homes have on staff a multidisciplinary team of health care providers that may include nurses, medical social workers, counselors, therapists (physical, speech, or occupational), teachers, home health aides, and health care providers. Not all the team members provide services to group homes on a full-time basis.

Skills of the Community-Based Nurse

The nursing process serves as the foundation of nursing care in the community, just as it does in a healthcare facility. Data collection and communication with the client and family is essential. Education is a fundamental part of community-based care because of the emphasis on health promotion and preventive healthcare. An important role of the nurse in the community is that of advocacy.

The Nursing Process

The focus of the community-based nurse is the client within the context of the family. The initial family data collection interview provides information about how various family members interact and affect the pregnant woman or the

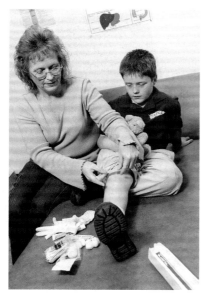

FIGURE 2-7 The school nurse cares for a young boy who injured his knee. In addition to first aid, the school nurse's duties include counseling, health education, and health promotion.

child and their condition. Noticing cues in the environment provides additional information. Upon completion of data collection, the RN and healthcare team focus on identifying the nursing care focuses based on the family's strengths, weaknesses, and needs. Family interaction and cooperation leads to collaborative goal setting and proposed interventions. The ongoing nursing process requires that the nurse evaluates these interventions as the cycle continues.

Communication

Positive, effective communication is fundamental to the nursing process and the care of childbearing and child-rearing families in the community. Establishing rapport with the client and the family, understanding and appropriately responding to cultural practices, and being sensitive to the needs of the client and family all require good communication skills. (See Chapter 22 for further discussion of communicating with children and family caregivers.)

Education

Health education is a key component of community-based nursing care. The nurse provides information to families or caregivers, small groups of children or adults, or large groups (Fig. 2-8). A successful group experience relies on the nurse being prepared before the session in addition to providing factual, unbiased information. It is important to know the needs of the target population to provide information to a group successfully. Important information about the group includes age, educational level, ethnic and gender mix, language barriers, cultural attitudes regarding receiving and acknowledging information, and any previous education the group has already had on the subject. Knowledge of growth and developmental principles will help identify the appropriate level of information, content, learning activities, and average attention span. Additional information includes any available resources, group size, seating arrangements, and other advantages or restrictions of the environment. For instance:

- Are the chairs movable for small-group discussions?
- Is there a DVD player or computer available to show a video?

- Can the group members leave the session early?
- Will a lot of noise disturb others in the building?
- Will the classroom teacher or teacher's aide attend?

> **Here's an Idea**
>
> When working with a group with which you are unfamiliar, ask the group leader prior to the session for group demographics and dynamics to help develop an appropriate education plan.

Client Advocacy

Client advocacy is speaking or acting on behalf of clients. This helps them gain greater independence and to make the healthcare delivery system more responsive and relevant to their needs. The nurse working in a community setting often develops a long-standing relationship with the family because of the ongoing nature of client contact. This type of relationship may allow the nurse to discover broader health and welfare issues (Fig. 2-9). Examples of advocacy interventions include the following:

- Identifying a need of the family and assisting with referrals and acquisition of needed resources
- Providing information on inexpensive or free transportation services to medical appointments
- Making telephone calls to coordinate special equipment needed by a physically challenged child
- Listening to the family's wishes about their preferred type of care and relaying this information to their health care provider

Aspects of Community-Based Nursing

For care to be effective, it is important for the nurse to first understand the family's resources, priorities, and cultural

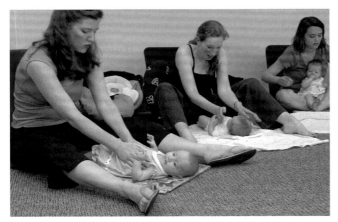

FIGURE 2-8 The nurse takes the opportunity to provide client education regarding normal growth and development to these mothers attending a mom and baby class with their infants.

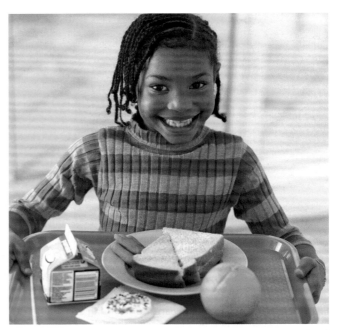

FIGURE 2-9 A nurse advocate can help the child enter a school lunch program so that nutritional needs are met.

influences. The nurse must be unbiased when the family's priorities seem different than the nurse's or the mainstream healthcare environment. For example, if the pregnant woman delays prenatal care, then consider if there were financial, transportation, child care, lack of knowledge, or cultural reasons for the delay. While exploring these issues with the client and family, it is important that the nurse remain neutral during the data collection and avoid statements or gestures that would imply blame or dissatisfaction with the client's choices.

Unlike the hospital setting, community-based nursing practice is autonomous and the nurse is often called on to be self-reliant. There may not be many other health care providers with whom to consult and those available may be physically distant from the nurse and client. Providing childbearing and child-rearing families with high-quality care requires well-developed data collection and decision-making skills. Implementation of nursing care often requires creative approaches.

Community practice tends to be more holistic. A holistic philosophy views the individual as an integrated whole where mind, body, and spirit interact with the environment, family, and community. The community nurse must consider the effects of the client's health on family functioning, the child's educational progress, and the multiple services the family and client need.

Another difference in the community-based setting is the focus on wellness rather than illness. Women and children are well but may be going through growth and developmental crises. The nurse intervenes to ease the transition from one developmental stage to another. The nurse provides anticipatory guidance to family caregivers and emphasizes health promotion and preventive health practices. With a focus on wellness, the community nurse provides a service that eventually improves the health of the entire community.

Community nurses work in many ways to prevent unnecessary hospitalization. Examples of health problems that the community nurse seeks to prevent include injuries to a child not appropriately secured in a car seat, severe burns to the face of a toddler from grabbing a tablecloth and spilling a cup of coffee, a near-drowning in a backyard pool, an infant who fails to thrive because the parents do not know that infants need specific amounts of formula, or a pregnant adolescent who contracts HIV because of unsafe sex practices.

The nurse in a community-based setting sees the client over time. This allows the nurse to have a broader understanding of the context which the individual and family lives. The clinic nurse may see the same family for different problems over a period of many years. The school nurse watches children grow and gets to know siblings and families over time. A group home nurse works intensely with a group of developmentally disabled children and gets to know each one and rejoice in their successes.

TEST YOURSELF

✔ Name two conditions for which a child or infant could receive home healthcare.

✔ Define client advocacy.

✔ Name three unique aspects of community-based nursing.

Think back to the Khan family. What do you think are the highest priority healthcare needs and concerns for the members of this family? What community resources do you think would be helpful to suggest to this family?

KEY POINTS

- The family is the basic social unit. It provides for survival and teaches the knowledge, customs, values, and beliefs of the family's culture.

- To meet the needs of individual members, the family functions to provide support in the five areas of wholeness: physical, emotional, intellectual, social, and spiritual.

- The immediate family and the extended family are two types of family structures that exist in most cultures. The single-parent family, communal family, and cohabitation family are examples of other types of family structures.

- Changing attitudes about children born out of wedlock, divorce, women working outside the home, and changes in adoption laws have all contributed to an increase in single-parent families.

- Family size affects the child's development. Children from small families receive more individual attention and tend to relate better to adults. Children from large families develop interdependency skills.

- Birth order also influences development. First-born children tend to be high achievers. Subsequent children are often more relaxed and are slower to develop language skills.

- Families tend to spend less time together than in the past. Some reasons for this include that both parents may work, the children participate in many school activities, families often do not eat together, and there is an emphasis on acquisition of material goods rather than the development of relationships.

- Community-based healthcare focuses on wellness and prevention and on helping people and families meet their healthcare needs.

- Community-based healthcare is advantageous for the pregnant woman, child, and family because it allows the individual to receive care within the context of the community and culture. Identifying and meeting needs within the community may also allow for less costly care than that provided in a hospital setting.

- Primary prevention focuses on preventing illness and injury. An example is a nurse in a maternity clinic giving tips on proper nutrition during pregnancy.
- Secondary prevention involves health-screening activities that aid in early diagnosis and encourage prompt treatment before long-term negative effects occur. An example is a school nurse who identifies a child with head lice, then contacts the family caregivers with instructions on how to rid the child and family members of infestation.
- Tertiary prevention involves health-promoting activities that focus on rehabilitation and providing information to prevent additional injury or illness. An example is a child with spina bifida who requires frequent catheterizations and trips to a specialized clinic. The nurse assists the family in finding resources so that proper care and medical monitoring can continue to prevent the development of additional problems.
- Prenatal and postpartum home healthcare can help decrease the cost of care as well as increase access to care, especially for at-risk populations. Settings for birth include the home, birth centers, and hospitals.
- Community-based care for pediatric clients occurs in outpatient settings and through home healthcare. Children's healthcare needs may be addressed and met in school and in specialized camp settings. Many communities have centers and programs that children and families can access for healthcare services.
- The community-based nurse uses the nursing process to plan and provide care to families and groups, communicates effectively, gives information to individuals and groups, and practices client advocacy.
- An effective community nurse educator must identify and gather data on the target population by determining the age, educational level, ethnic and gender mix, cultural influences, language barriers, and any previous education the group may have had. The nurse must observe each audience and gear the information session appropriately using appropriate materials.
- The community nurse functions as a child advocate by taking actions to improve the child's health or quality of life. One example of child advocacy is a nurse assisting with the referral process to help the child and family obtain the services and resources needed to maintain health.
- Community-based nursing provides the nurse an opportunity to function autonomously in a holistic, wellness-focused environment. Seeing positive outcomes and improved health statuses, often over a period of time, is rewarding for the community-based nurse.

INTERNET RESOURCES

Transcultural Nursing
https://tcns.org/

Minority Health
http://www.minorityhealth.hhs.gov/

Kids Health
https://kidshealth.org/en/kids/

Parish Nursing
https://www.parishnurse.org/

Public Health Nursing
https://phnurse.org/

Workbook

NCLEX-STYLE REVIEW QUESTIONS

1. In working with families, the nurse recognizes that different family structures exist. Which example best describes a blended family? A family in which:
   a. the adult members share in homemaking as well as in child-rearing.
   b. both partners in the marriage bring children from previous marriages into the household.
   c. grandparents live in the same house with the grandchildren and their parents.
   d. partners of the same sex share a household and raise children together.

2. One role of the nurse in a community-based setting focuses on primary prevention. An example of primary prevention would be:
   a. screening children for vision in a preschool.
   b. giving an information session on bicycle safety in an after-school program.
   c. identifying head lice in a child in elementary school.
   d. exploring financial help for a client in a home setting.

3. Which of the following would be an intervention made by the community health nurse? Select all that apply.
   a. Arranging for parents whose infant is in the NICU to attend a parenting class
   b. Helping the family purchase a car to attend medical appointments at the clinic
   c. Leading a class at a local church about normal infant development
   d. Calling parents of children discharged from the emergency department to see if they filled their child's prescriptions
   e. Screening children at a homeless shelter for head lice

4. A mother of a child being cared for in a home setting makes the following statements. Which statement **best** illustrates one of the positive aspects of home healthcare?
   a. "My family gets to visit once a week when my child is in the hospital."
   b. "I can do my child's care since you taught the procedure to me."
   c. "Our insurance pays for us to go to the well-child clinic."
   d. "The neighbor's child likes being in the group home."

5. When a nurse is providing information in a community-based setting, it is **most** important for the nurse to:
   a. ask questions about the histories of those present.
   b. use posters that everyone in the group can read.
   c. tell the participants about the nurse's background.
   d. know the needs of the audience.

STUDY ACTIVITIES

1. Survey your community to discover the community-based health care providers available. Use the information you found to complete the following table.

Community-based health care providers	How are they funded?	What types of health-care for children do they provide?

2. Using the information you obtained above, evaluate your community's healthcare services by answering the following:
   a. Does your community have adequate healthcare services for childbearing and child-rearing families?
   b. Are funding concerns an issue for your community? In what ways?
   c. What other services do you think are needed to care for the childbearing and child-rearing families in your community?

3. Go to http://www.culture-advantage.com/awarenesspage1.html.
   a. Read through the information. At the bottom of the page, click on "Go to next page."
   b. Read through the information and complete exercises 1 to 7 (you will need to "click on next page" to finish exercise 7.)
   c. Which exercise was the easiest and which was the hardest for you to complete? Which exercise made you think about yourself the most?
   d. Which client did you find it hardest to "take care of" and why?

4. Go to http://www.lehman.cuny.edu/faculty/jfleitas/bandaides. At "Bandaides & Blackboards," click on "Kids." Go to "Lots of Stories" and click on the star.
   a. In working with school-age children, what are some of the stories in this site you would encourage the children to read?
   b. List the topics and diseases included in the stories that you could share with school-age children.

CRITICAL THINKING:
WHAT WOULD YOU DO?

Apply your knowledge of the family and the nurse's role in the community to the following situations.

1. Nine-year-old Shawn has become withdrawn, his school grades have fallen, and he complains of having headaches and stomachaches since his parents divorced 3 months ago. He lives with his mother during the week and visits his father, who lives with a girlfriend, on weekends.

   a. What concerns do you think Shawn's parents would have about his changes in behavior and his physical complaints?

   b. What advice would you offer Shawn's parents regarding these concerns?

   c. What could these parents do to help Shawn better adjust to the divorce?

2. You are making a home visit to the Andrews family because their newborn needs home phototherapy treatment for 3 to 5 days. You find the newborn's sibling, 6-year-old Samantha, ill with bronchitis. Both parents smoke. Outline an education plan for these caregivers regarding the health of their family.

3. Mrs. Perez, a second-grade teacher, asks you to teach a unit on personal hygiene to her class.

   a. Identify the information you will need from Mrs. Perez.

   b. Describe how you will present the lesson to these children.

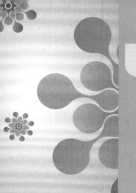

UNIT 2
Foundations of Maternity Nursing

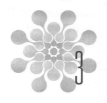

3

Structure and Function of the Reproductive System

Learning Objectives

At the conclusion of this chapter, you will:

1. Discuss major functions of each reproductive structure, gland, and organ for both men and women.
2. Describe the path of sperm through a man's reproductive system from the site of formation to ejaculation from the body.
3. Describe the process of semen production.
4. Compare hormonal regulation of reproductive functions in men and women.
5. Illustrate the interrelationships of the ovarian and uterine cycles and the overall menstrual cycle.
6. Describe and compare the sexual response cycles of women and men.

Sandra Dickinson, 23 years old, has come to the clinic for her annual examination. She has been having periods since she was 13 years old. She tells you, "I don't really know how my body works." As you read this chapter, think about what you would tell Sandra about her reproductive organs and the way they function.

The obstetric nurse interacts with prospective parents before and throughout pregnancy and childbirth. Also, many health care providers provide gynecologic services to their clients. The nurse working with clients of childbearing age requires a working knowledge of reproductive anatomy and physiology and the menstrual cycle. This knowledge guides the selection of appropriate interventions for the childbearing woman and her family.

The main purpose of the reproductive systems for men and women is to produce offspring. **Gametes**, or sex cells, are produced by men in the testes and by women in the ovaries. The gamete for men is spermatozoa (sperm) and the gamete for women is ova (egg). Each gamete contains one half of the genetic material needed to produce a human baby. Some of the structures in the reproductive tract serve dual purposes. Most often, these alternate functions have to do with urinary elimination because the urinary and reproductive systems are closely connected.

You will notice that most structures in the reproductive tract are paired (e.g., the testes, ovaries, labia majora, labia minora) and that reproductive systems for men and women are complementary: testes in men and ovaries in women; scrotum in men and labia majora in women; and glans penis in men and clitoris in women. It is important to know

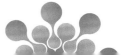

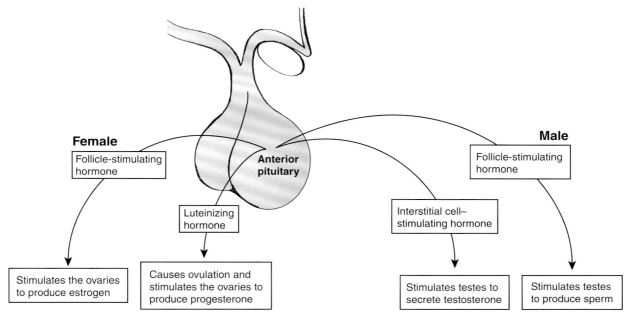

FIGURE 3-1 Hormones of the anterior pituitary stimulate the reproductive system in men and women.

that the pituitary gland governs reproductive hormone production and function (Fig. 3-1).

REPRODUCTIVE SYSTEM OF MEN

Sometimes the man's contribution to childbirth may be overlooked because of the focus on the pregnant woman and her growing fetus. However, the man's role is crucial to this process. His genetic material not only determines the sex of the unborn child, but also influences numerous other inherited traits. The reproductive anatomy of men consists of external and internal reproductive organs. The purpose of the reproductive tract of men is to allow for sexual intimacy and reproduction of offspring and provide a conduit for urinary elimination.

External Genitalia

The man's external reproductive organs, the external genitalia, consist of the penis and scrotum (Fig. 3-2).

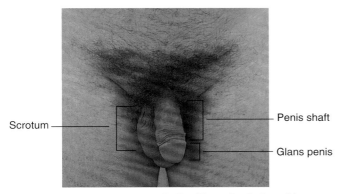

Scrotum ———

——— Penis shaft

——— Glans penis

FIGURE 3-2 Male external genitalia. (Photo by B. Proud.)

Penis

The penis serves a dual role as the organ of reproduction for men and as the external organ of urinary elimination. The penis is composed of a bulbous head, commonly called the glans penis or glans, and a shaft. The glans is the most sensitive area on the penis because it contains the greatest concentration of nerve endings. At birth, a layer of tissue called the **prepuce**, or foreskin, covers the glans (Fig. 3-3).

Three columns of erectile tissue compose the shaft of the penis (Fig. 3-4): the paired cavernous bodies (corpus cavernosa) and the spongy body (corpus spongiosum). The cavernous bodies are parallel, and the spongy body lies ventral and midline. The spongy body is cradled in the channel formed at the junction of the cavernous bodies. A thick sheath called the tunica albuginea encases each column. Two layers of fascia encircle all three columns along the length of the shaft. The fascia gives the penis support, allowing it to become a firm structure during sexual stimulation.

> **Make a Note of This!**
> The prepuce is removed in the surgical procedure called circumcision. If the parents choose to do this optional procedure, it is usually done within the first few days of life. Although an adult man can undergo circumcision (usually for medical reasons), this procedure is not frequently done in adulthood.

The erectile tissue is well supplied with blood vessels and nerves. When the penis is stimulated sexually, parasympathetic nerves cause the veins in the shaft to dilate. The sinuses within the erectile tissue fill up with blood causing an erection. The erect penis is capable of penetrating a woman's vagina during sexual intercourse. If the erect penis is stimulated to ejaculation within the vagina, it deposits sperm in the woman's reproductive tract.

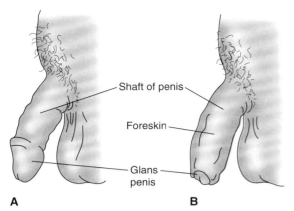

FIGURE 3-3 Circumcised (**A**) and uncircumcised (**B**) penis. (From Carter P. J. (2020). *Lippincott textbook for nursing assistants: A humanistic approach to caregiving.* Wolters Kluwer.)

The urethra passes through the shaft of the penis within the spongy body. It functions to eliminate urine from the bladder and to transport semen out of the man's body.

Scrotum

The scrotum is an external sac that houses the testes, each in its own internal compartment. The main functions of the scrotum are to protect the testes from trauma and to regulate the temperature within the testes; a process that is extremely important to the production of healthy gametes (sperm). The ideal temperature within the scrotum is approximately 96°F (35.6°C), just slightly lower than normal body temperature. When either the environmental or the body temperature is increased, the cremaster muscle within the scrotal sac remains relaxed, which lowers the scrotum, so that the testes are not close to the man's body. This helps to keep the temperature in the testicles lower than body temperature. If the temperature is cold, the cremaster muscle contracts, pulling the scrotum in toward the man's body, thereby increasing the temperature in the testicles. The skin of the scrotum is greatly pigmented and folded into grooves called rugae.

Internal Reproductive Organs

Internal reproductive organs of men include the testes and a system of glands and ducts that are involved in the formation of a fluid that nourishes and provides for the transport of the sperm out of the man's body (Fig. 3-5).

Testes

The testes are two oval shaped organs, one within each scrotal sac (Fig. 3-6). The testes serve two important functions: production of androgens (i.e., sex hormones for men) and formation and maturation of spermatozoa. Each testis is about 4 cm long by 2.5 cm wide and is divided into lobes. The lobes contain **seminiferous tubules**, tiny coils

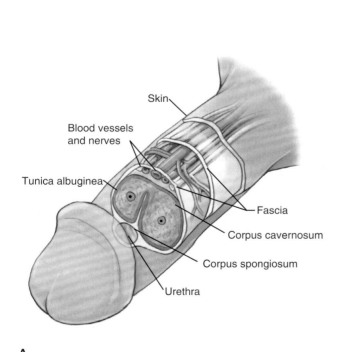

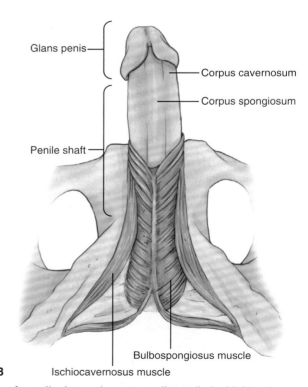

FIGURE 3-4 Internal structure of the penis. **A.** Notice the three columns of erectile tissue; these are well supplied with blood and nerve tissue. The cavernous bodies (corpus cavernosa) contain sinuses that fill with blood during an erection. The urethra traverses the shaft encased within the spongy body (corpus spongiosum). **B.** This view of the ventral aspect shows how the spongy body lies in relation to the cavernous bodies. Notice how the root of the penis is anchored to the pelvis by the tough connective tissue and muscle.

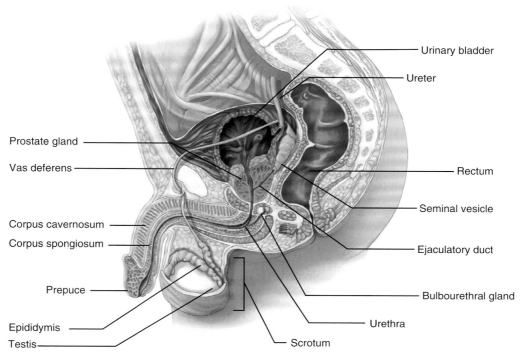

Urinary bladder

Ureter

Prostate gland

Vas deferens

Rectum

Corpus cavernosum

Seminal vesicle

Corpus spongiosum

Ejaculatory duct

Prepuce

Bulbourethral gland

Epididymis

Urethra

Testis

Scrotum

FIGURE 3-5 Internal reproductive anatomy of men. (From The Anatomical Chart Company. (2001). *Atlas of human anatomy.* Springhouse.)

of tissue in which **spermatogenesis** (production of sperm) occurs. Interstitial cells surround the seminiferous tubules and produce the androgen testosterone, which is necessary for the maturation of sperm. A system of tiny tubes called

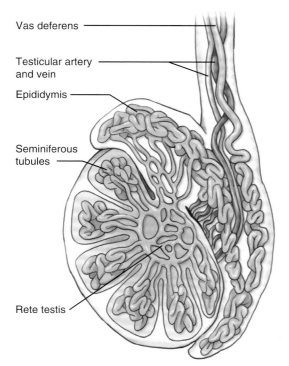

Vas deferens

Testicular artery and vein

Epididymis

Seminiferous tubules

Rete testis

FIGURE 3-6 Internal structure of a testis.

the rete testis lead from the seminiferous tubules to the **epididymis**, an intricate network of coiled ducts on the posterior portion of each testis that is approximately 6 m (20 ft) in length. It is here that sperm mature. Table 3-1 provides a summary of the hormones that influence reproduction in men.

Many health care providers recommend that men (ages 15 years and older) perform a testicular self-examination (TSE) monthly to detect early changes associated with the testicular cancer. Refer to Chapter 27 for how to perform the TSE.

Share This Tip With Your Client!

Sperm production is most efficient when the temperature within the testes is slightly lower than core body temperature. Constrictive clothing (e.g., tight jeans) holds scrotal contents close to the body. The resultant transfer of heat can reduce sperm production and possibly lead to infertility in men.

Ductal System

The **vas deferens** is the muscular tube in which sperm begin their journey out of the man's body. It connects the epididymis with the ejaculatory duct. The vas deferens is sheathed in the spermatic cord, which also contains the blood vessels, nerves, and lymphatics that serve the testes. The left spermatic cord is usually longer than the right so that the left testis hangs lower than the right.

The spermatic cord (and vas deferens contained within it) leads into the abdominal cavity through the inguinal

TABLE 3-1 Hormonal Control of Reproductive Functions in Men

HORMONE	SOURCE	REPRODUCTIVE FUNCTIONS
Follicle-stimulating hormone	Anterior pituitary	• Stimulates production of sperm in the seminiferous tubules
Interstitial cell–stimulating hormone	Anterior pituitary	• Stimulates the interstitial cells to secrete testosterone
Testosterone	Interstitial cells	• Assists sperm in maturing • Influences the development of secondary sex characteristics (facial and pubic hair growth, deepening of the voice, growth of the penis)

canal, arches over the urinary bladder, and then curves downward on the posterior side of the bladder. It is at this point that the vas deferens joins with the ejaculatory duct. The paired ejaculatory ducts then connect with the urethra, which transports the sperm out of the man's penis during ejaculation.

Accessory Glands and Semen

The seminal vesicles are paired glands that empty an alkaline, fructose-rich fluid into the ejaculatory ducts during ejaculation. The prostate is a muscular gland, approximately the size of a chestnut, which surrounds the first part of the urethra as it exits the urinary bladder. The gland contracts during ejaculation, secreting alkaline prostatic fluid. The bulbourethral (Cowper) glands also secrete an alkaline fluid that coats the last part of the urethra during ejaculation.

The alkaline fluids secreted by these glands serve several key functions, including:

• Enhancement of sperm motility (i.e., ability to move)
• Nourishment of sperm (i.e., provides a ready source of energy with the simple sugar fructose)
• Protection of sperm (i.e., sperm are maintained in an alkaline environment to protect them from the acidic environment of the vagina)

The alkaline fluids and sperm combine to form a thick, whitish secretion termed semen or seminal fluid. An average human ejaculate has a volume of 1 to 5 mL and contains several hundred million sperm.

TEST YOURSELF

✔ What is the general term that refers to sex cells for women and men?

✔ Name two important functions of the testes.

✔ Describe the path sperm travel through a man's reproductive tract to outside of the body beginning at the seminiferous tubules. Name all the ducts and glands along the way.

REPRODUCTIVE SYSTEM OF WOMEN

A woman's reproductive tract consists of external genitalia, or the vulva, and internal reproductive organs. The purpose of female woman's reproductive tract is to allow for sexual intimacy and fulfillment and to produce children through the processes of conception, pregnancy, and childbirth. Each part of the women's reproductive tract contributes in some way to these purposes.

The bony pelvis and mammary glands are also part of the reproductive system of women. Chapter 8 describes the bony pelvis, and Chapter 15 discusses breast anatomy in conjunction with infant nutrition and lactation. Chapter 27 explains how to do a breast self- examination, an important procedure to detect breast cancer in the early stages.

External Genitalia (Vulva)

The external genitalia consist of the mons pubis, labia majora and minora, clitoris, vestibule, and perineum. Figure 3-7 illustrates these structures.

Mons Pubis

The mons pubis, or mons, is a rounded fatty pad located atop the symphysis pubis. Coarse pubic hair and skin cover the mons. The function of the mons is to protect the pelvic bones during sexual intercourse.

Labia

The labia majora (singular: labium majus) are paired fatty tissue folds that extend anteriorly from the mons pubis and then join posteriorly to the true perineum. Labia majora are covered with pubic hair, are vascular, and contain oil and sweat glands. Inside the labia majora are the labia minora (singular: labium minus). The labia minora are thinner than

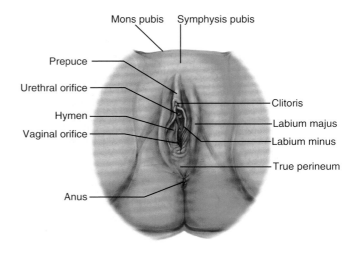

FIGURE 3-7 External genitalia of women.

the labia majora, are hairless, contain sebaceous glands, and are sensitive to stimulation.

Clitoris

The clitoris is a hooded body composed of erectile tissue located at the apex of the labia minora. The clitoris, similar to the glans penis, is highly sensitive and allows the woman to experience sexual pleasure and orgasm during sexual stimulation. The prepuce is the hooded structure over the clitoris.

 Cultural Snapshot

Female genital mutilation (FGM), also known as female circumcision, involves the removal of part or all of a woman's external genitalia. It is done in countries in Africa, Asia, and the Middle East, and is also seen in migrants from these areas. Reasons for performing FGM vary, but often cited reasons include as a measure to preserve virginity and marital fidelity, a cultural norm or tradition, or a rite of passage. FGM is done on young girls but in some cultures may be done on infant girls or adolescent girls. Immediate complications from FGM include common surgical complications such as pain, bleeding, and infections. Long-term complications include scarring, urinary or vaginal issues, risk for childbirth complications, decreased sexual satisfaction, and self-esteem issues (WHO, 2020).

Vestibule

The vestibule is the area between the labia minora. The urethral meatus (opening to the urethra), paraurethral (Skene) glands, vaginal opening or introitus, and Bartholin glands are located within the vestibule. The paraurethral and Bartholin glands are each paired glands whose secretions moisten the delicate vaginal mucosa and raise the pH of vaginal fluid during sexual intercourse to enhance the sperm motility.

The hymen is an avascular fold of tissue located around or partially around the introitus. It varies in shape from woman to woman and throughout an individual woman's reproductive life span. In the past, people believed that an intact hymen was evidence of a woman's virginity. However, activities other than sexual intercourse, such as heavy physical exertion or the use of tampons, can tear the hymen, so the appearance of this tissue is not a reliable method of determining virginity.

Perineum

The **perineum** is a band of fibrous, muscular tissue that extends from the posterior portion of the labia majora to the anus. Several sets of superficial and deep muscle groups meet at the perineum to provide support for pelvic structures. The perineum and muscles of the pelvic floor are capable of great stretching during childbirth to allow for delivery of the fetus. These structures are also subject to the stresses and trauma of childbirth. The birth attendant sometimes cuts an episiotomy (see Chapter 11) into the perineum to aid the delivery of the infant during the birth process. Lacerations can also occur to the perineum during delivery. If lacerations are not repaired properly, or if they do not heal appropriately and the pelvic floor is weakened, the woman may experience stress incontinence or prolapse of pelvic organs later in life. Stress incontinence may have other causes including multiple vaginal births, forceps use during delivery, obesity, and pelvic surgery.

Be Careful!

It is easy to confuse the clitoris with the urethral meatus. When preparing to insert a urinary catheter, carefully locate the urethral meatus between the labia minora below the clitoris. If you touch the sensitive tissue of the clitoris with the catheter, you may cause the woman discomfort.

Internal Reproductive Organs

The internal reproductive organs include the vagina, uterus, fallopian tubes, and ovaries. Figure 3-8 illustrates the internal reproductive structures.

Vagina

The **vagina**, also called the birth canal, is a muscular tube that leads from the vulva to the uterus. From the opening within the vestibule, it slopes up and backward to the cervix. Because the walls of the vagina extend beyond the uterine cervix, the cervix dips into the vagina and forms fornices, which are archlike structures or pockets. The posterior fornix is largest because the posterior vaginal wall is longer than the anterior wall (approximately 9 and 7 cm long, respectively).

The vagina serves several important functions. The inner folds, or rugae, allow the vagina to stretch during birth to accommodate a full-term infant. In addition, the vagina normally maintains an acidic pH of 4 to 5, which protects the vagina from infection. The vagina receives the penis during sexual intercourse and serves as the exit point for menstrual flow.

Share This Information!

The acidic environment of the vagina is protective. Any change that alters the pH multiplies the risk for irritation and infection. Examples of substances that can alter the pH of the vagina include antibiotics, douches, tampons, or sanitary pads that contain deodorant. Explain to the woman that the vagina is self-cleansing and douching is not necessary.

Uterus

The **uterus**, also called the womb, is a hollow, pear-shaped, muscular structure located within the pelvic cavity between the bladder and the rectum. In the nonpregnant woman, the uterus is approximately 7.5 cm long by 5 cm wide (at the widest portion) and weighs approximately 40 g. The uterus normally tips forward and rests just above the urinary bladder (Fig. 3-8). The functions of the uterus are to prepare for pregnancy each month, protect and nourish the growing fetus when pregnancy occurs, and aid in childbirth. The uterus (Fig. 3-9) is divided into four sections:

- cervix
- uterine isthmus
- corpus
- fundus

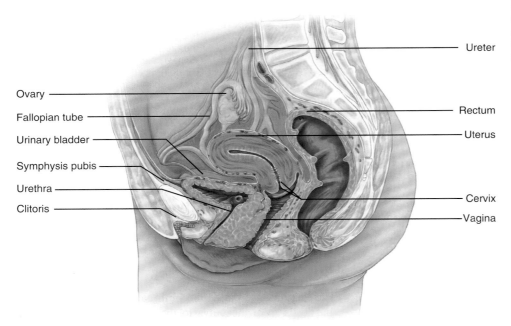

FIGURE 3-8 Internal reproductive anatomy of women. (From The Anatomical Chart Company. (2001). *Atlas of human anatomy.* Springhouse.)

The **cervix** is a tubular structure that connects the vagina and uterus. The external os (opening) dips into the vagina, and the internal os opens into the uterine isthmus, the lower portion of the uterus. The cervix normally has a tiny slit that allows sperm to enter and the menstrual flow to exit. During childbirth, the cervix must be thin and open fully so that the baby can be born. The ciliated epithelium that lines the inner walls of the cervix produces mucus that lubricates the vaginal canal and protects the uterus from ascending infectious agents.

The uterine isthmus is a narrow opening that connects the cervix to the main body of the uterus. During pregnancy and childbirth, the uterine isthmus is referred to as the lower uterine segment. This is the thinnest portion of the uterus and does not participate in the muscular contractions of labor. Because the tissue is so thin, the lower uterine segment is the area that is most likely to rupture during childbirth.

The corpus is the main body of the uterus, and the fundus is the top-most section resembling a dome. The walls of the corpus and fundus have three layers. The perimetrium is the tough outer layer of connective tissue that supports the uterus. The middle layer is the **myometrium**, a muscular layer that is responsible for the contractions of labor. The muscle fibers of the myometrium wrap around the uterus in three directions: obliquely, laterally, and longitudinally. This muscle configuration allows for the strong contractions and expulsion of the fetus during labor and birth. The **endometrium** is the vascular mucosal inner layer. This layer changes under hormonal influence every month in preparation for possible conception and pregnancy.

Four ligaments provide support and hold the uterus in position (Fig. 3-9). These ligaments anchor the uterus at the base (cervical region), leaving the upper portion (corpus) free in the pelvic cavity. The broad ligament attaches the lower sides of the uterus to the sidewalls of the pelvis. The right and left cardinal ligaments anchor the walls of the cervix and vagina to the lateral pelvic walls. The round ligaments are paired fibromuscular bands that tip the uterus forward and hold it in an anteflexed position. They extend from the anterior/lateral portions of the uterus to the labia majora. The uterosacral ligaments anchor the lower posterior portion of the uterus to the sacrum.

Fallopian Tubes

The paired **fallopian tubes** (also known as oviducts) are tiny, muscular corridors that arise from the superior surface of the uterus near the fundus and extend laterally on either side toward the ovaries. They are 8 to 14 cm in length. Each fallopian tube has three sections: isthmus, the medial third of the tube that connects to the uterus; ampulla, the middle portion of the tube; and infundibulum, the outer portion that opens into the lower abdominal cavity. At the outer edges of the infundibulum are fimbriae, fingerlike projections that make gentle wavelike motions over the ovaries.

The fallopian tubes have a critical role in conception. When the ovary releases an egg, the fimbriae make wavelike movements that attract the egg toward the fallopian tube. Once the egg is within the tube, muscular contractions and beating of tiny cilia within the tube propel the egg toward the uterus. If sperm are present, fertilization of the egg is possible. Fertilization most frequently occurs in the ampulla section of the tube. The tubes secrete lipids and glycogen to provide nourishment to the fertilized egg as it makes its way to the uterus. The functions of the fallopian

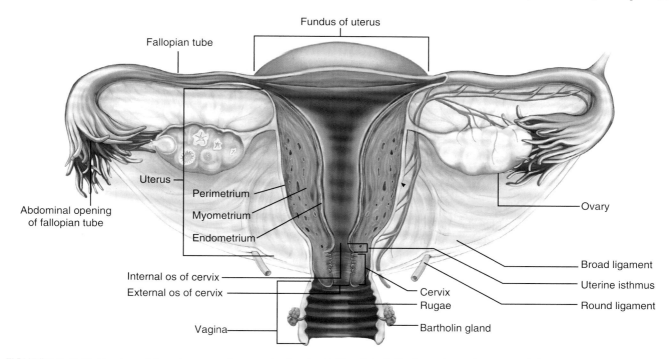

FIGURE 3-9 Anterior view of female woman's reproductive tract. The right fallopian tube and ovary and the entire uterus, and vagina are shown in a cross-sectional view to demonstrate the internal structure of these organs.

tubes are to provide a site for fertilization, a passageway, and a nourishing, warm environment for the fertilized egg to travel to the uterus.

Ovaries

The **ovaries** are glands located on either side of the uterus. They are similar to almonds in size and shape. The broad and ovarian ligaments provide support to the ovaries. The functions of the ovaries are to store ova and help them mature and also to produce the hormones estrogen and progesterone in women. Estrogen and progesterone are responsible for a woman's secondary sex characteristics and also the regulation of the menstrual cycle in response to anterior pituitary hormones (see the "Menstrual Cycle" section for description of their functions).

Every woman is born with all the ova (eggs) that she will ever have. Typically, women are born with approximately 2 million eggs, many of which will deteriorate during childhood. The ovaries normally release the remaining ova at a rate of 1 per month until the woman's reproductive years are over.

More Than Enough

If one ovum matures every month during the childbearing years (from age 12 through 50), a woman would only use 456 ova. On average, a baby girl is born with 2 million immature ova; therefore, there are significantly more ova available than will ever be used.

Blood Supply for the Pelvic Organs

The pelvic organs have a rich blood supply (Fig. 3-10). The blood supply comes from the abdominal aorta and the

internal iliac artery, which is a branch of the common iliac artery. Venous return from the pelvic organ empties into the renal, femoral, great saphenous, and internal iliac veins, and also into the inferior vena cava.

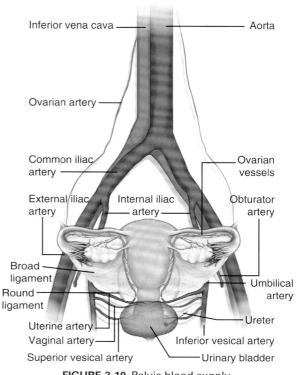

FIGURE 3-10 Pelvic blood supply.

REGULATION OF REPRODUCTIVE FUNCTION

Puberty

Puberty is the time of life in which the individual becomes capable of sexual reproduction. Puberty occurs on average between the ages of 10 and 14 years. This phase is marked by maturation of the reproductive organs and development of secondary sex characteristics. Secondary sex characteristics are external physical evidence of sexual maturity but are not essential to reproduction. Secondary sex characteristics include growth of pubic and axillary hair, growth of external genitals (labia and penis), breast development in women, and in men, appearance of facial hair and deepening of the voice.

The changes associated with puberty happen in response to hypothalamic and pituitary hormones. Secondary sex characteristics develop in an orderly sequence, although the timing varies between individuals. Breast budding in a young woman is usually the first physical sign noted and occurs between the ages of 10 and 12 years on average. Appearance of pubic hair usually occurs just before **menarche**, the first menstrual period. Menarche occurs most frequently between the ages of 12 and 14 years.

Cultural Snapshot

Some cultures have a special ceremony or phrases to celebrate the onset of a girl's menstruation. In the Navajo culture, a 4-day ceremony is held to celebrate the girl's passage into womanhood. In India, when a girl first menstruates she is said to have "borne the flower." In some cultures or religions, a menstruating woman may be prohibited from cooking, bathing, or touching others, or may be secluded during this time.

Menstrual Cycle

The **menstrual cycle** refers to the recurring changes that take place in a woman's reproductive tract associated with menstruation and the events that surround menstruation. **Menstruation**, the casting away of blood, tissue, and debris from the uterus as the endometrium sheds, is variable in amount and duration. On average, menstrual flow lasts 4 to 6 days, with a total blood loss of 25 to

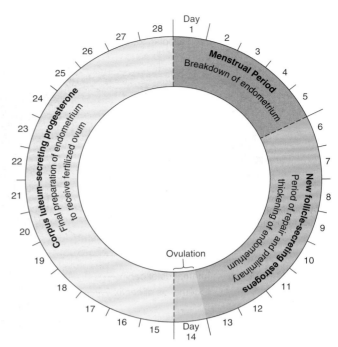

FIGURE 3-11 When one menstrual cycle ends, another one immediately begins. (Reprinted from Cohen B. J., & Wood D. L. *Memmler's the human body in health and disease* (11th ed.). Lippincott Williams & Wilkins, 2009, with permission.)

60 mL. Although this loss is seemingly negligible, with time it can contribute to low iron stores and anemia.

The menstrual cycle encompasses the events that transpire in the woman's reproductive organs between the beginnings of two menstrual periods (Fig. 3-11). Hormones from the ovaries and the pituitary gland regulate these cyclical changes. The average cycle lasts 28 days, approximately 1 month; however, there are great variations between women, and also an individual woman's cycle may vary in duration from cycle to cycle. For ease of understanding, the following discussion of the menstrual cycle is based on the average 28-day cycle.

Knowledge is Important!
When you understand the menstrual cycle, you will then be able to understand the process of conception, and you will be better prepared to counsel families on how to prevent pregnancy or how to increase the probability that pregnancy will occur.

There are two main components of the menstrual cycle: the ovarian cycle and the uterine cycle. Although each cycle is discussed separately below, it is important to remember that both cycles work together simultaneously to produce the menstrual cycle (Fig. 3-12). Changes in cervical mucus take place during the course of the menstrual cycle and these changes are also discussed.

Ovarian Cycle

Cyclical changes in the ovaries occur in response to two anterior pituitary hormones: follicle-stimulating hormone

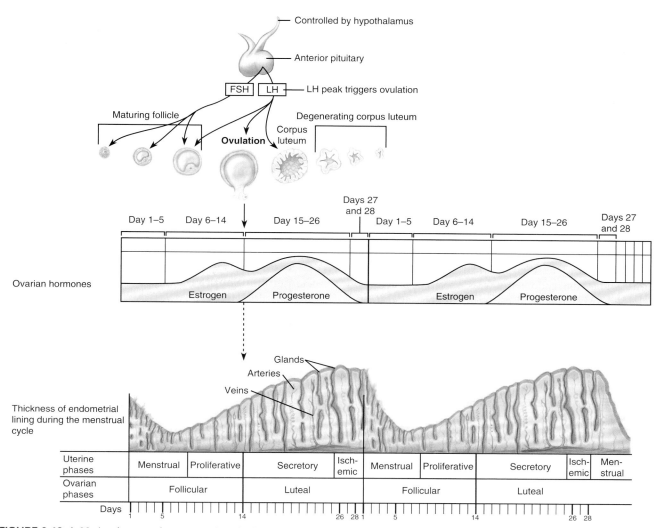

FIGURE 3-12 A 28-day (average) menstrual cycle. Two complete cycles are shown. The anterior pituitary hormones control the ovarian cycle. The ovaries produce hormones that control the uterine cycle.

(FSH) and luteinizing hormone (LH). There are two phases of the ovarian cycle, each named for the hormone that has the most control over that particular phase. The follicular phase, controlled by FSH, encompasses days 1 through 14 of a 28-day cycle. LH controls the luteal phase, which includes days 15 through 28.

Follicular Phase

The ovary has follicles on it, which are depressions that contain an ovum that has started to develop, but not completed maturation. At the beginning of each menstrual cycle, a follicle on one of the ovaries begins to develop in response to rising levels of FSH. The follicle produces estrogen, which causes the ovum contained within the follicle to mature. As the follicle grows, it fills with estrogen-rich fluid and begins to resemble a tiny blister on the surface of the ovary.

When the pituitary gland detects high levels of estrogen from the mature follicle, it releases a surge of LH. This sudden increase in LH causes the follicle to burst open, releasing the mature ovum into the abdominal cavity, a process

called **ovulation**. Ovulation typically occurs on day 14 of a 28-day cycle. As the ovum floats along the surface of the ovary, the gentle beating of the fimbriae draws it toward the fallopian tube.

Luteal Phase

After ovulation, LH levels remain elevated and cause the remnants of the follicle to develop into a yellow body called the **corpus luteum**. In addition to producing estrogen, the corpus luteum secretes a hormone called progesterone. If fertilization does not take place, the corpus luteum begins to degenerate, and estrogen and progesterone levels fall. This process leads back to day 1 of the cycle, and the follicular phase begins anew.

Remember!

All of the ova already exist within the ovaries in an immature state. In order to ripen, or mature, an ovum needs a stimulus. FSH is the messenger from the pituitary that provides the required stimulus.

Uterine Cycle

The uterine cycle refers to the changes that occur in the inner lining of the uterus. These changes happen in response to the ovarian hormones estrogen and progesterone. There are four phases to this cycle: menstrual, proliferative, secretory, and ischemic.

Menstrual Phase

The onset of menstruation begins day 1 of the menstrual cycle. During the menstrual phase of the uterine cycle, the uterine lining, the endometrium, is shed because of low levels of progesterone and estrogen. At the same time, a follicle begins to develop and starts producing estrogen. The menstrual phase ends when the menstrual period stops on approximately day 5 of the cycle.

Proliferative Phase

When estrogen levels are high enough, the endometrium begins to regenerate. Estrogen stimulates blood vessels to develop. The blood vessels in turn bring nutrients and oxygen to the uterine lining, which begins to grow and become thicker. The proliferative phase ends with ovulation on day 14.

Secretory Phase

After ovulation, the corpus luteum begins to produce progesterone. This hormone causes the uterine lining to become rich in nutrients in preparation for pregnancy. Estrogen levels also remain high to maintain the lining. If pregnancy does not transpire, the corpus luteum gradually degenerates, and the woman enters the ischemic phase of the menstrual cycle.

Ischemic Phase

On days 27 and 28, estrogen and progesterone levels fall because the corpus luteum is no longer producing them. Without these hormones to maintain the blood vessel network, the uterine lining becomes ischemic. When the lining starts to shed, the woman has come full cycle and is once again at day 1 of the menstrual cycle.

Cervical Mucus Changes

Changes in cervical mucus take place over the course of the menstrual cycle. Some women use these characteristics to help determine when ovulation is likely to happen. During the menstrual phase, the cervix does not produce mucus. Gradually, as hormonal changes transpire and the proliferative phase begins, the cervix begins to produce a yellow or white mucus that is tacky and crumbles when dried. As the time of ovulation draws near, the mucus becomes progressively clear and thin with lubricating properties. At the peak of fertility (i.e., during ovulation), the mucus has a distensible, stretchable quality called *spinnbarkeit* (see Chapter 4, for further discussion of cervical mucus changes that indicate ovulation). After ovulation, the mucus again becomes scanty, thick, and opaque.

Remember Sandra Dickinson from the beginning of the chapter. How would you describe the menstrual cycle to her in regard to frequency, length, and body changes that occur during the cycle?

Menopause

Menopause refers to the time in a woman's life when reproductive capability ends. Gradually the ovaries cease to function, and hormone levels fall. The woman begins to experience irregular menstrual cycles until they finally end. Menopause is defined as 1 year without a menstrual cycle. The average age at which menopause occurs is between 47 and 55 years. The postmenopausal time is after the woman has gone for 1 year without a period.

Prior to menopause, the woman's body goes through gradual hormonal changes which cause physical symptoms. The woman may state that she has mood swings, sweating, or trouble sleeping during this time. The time leading up to menopause is called **perimenopause**, also known as the climacteric.

SEXUAL RESPONSE CYCLE

Sexuality is part of our human nature. It is a normal and important part of an individual's well-being. Human beings have the capacity to give and receive pleasure through the process of sexual stimulation. Therefore, a discussion of reproduction would be incomplete without mention of the physiology of sexual response.

There are two underlying physiologic responses to sexual stimulation in both men and women: vasocongestion and myotonia (muscular tension). These two processes are fundamental to almost all physiologic responses that take place during sexual arousal.

Vasocongestion occurs in the pelvic organs during sexual excitement because the arteries dilate, allowing inflow of blood that is greater than venous capacity to drain the area. The result is widespread congestion of the pelvic tissues. Vasocongestion leads to erection of the penis and clitoris, vaginal lubrication, and engorgement of the labia and testicles. Other tissues, such as the nipples and earlobes, may also be affected.

Myotonia is present throughout the body during sexual arousal and orgasm. It is evident in voluntary and involuntary contractions. Facial grimacing, spasmodic contractions of the hands and feet, and the involuntary muscular contractions during orgasm are the most notable examples of myotonia.

There are four phases of the sexual response: excitement, plateau, orgasm, and resolution. These phases occur in both sexes and follow the same general patterns, regardless of the method of sexual stimulation.

During the excitement phase, the woman's clitoris engorges and enlarges, the labia majora separate, and the labia minora increase in size. The uterus increases in size and begins to elevate. For the man, excitement leads to erection of the penis, thickening of the scrotal sac, and testicular elevation. In both sexes, increases in heart rate, blood pressure, and respirations mark the onset of the excitement phase. Some individuals experience a "sex flush," a reddening of the skin on the chest and neck. Duration of the excitement phase is from several minutes to several hours.

No set event marks the beginning of the plateau phase. Vasocongestion and myotonia continue, and the heart rate and blood pressure remain elevated. For women, the outer third of the vagina engorges, the clitoris retracts behind its hood, and the labia minora deepen in color. The uterus is fully elevated in the pelvic cavity. The head of a man's penis engorges further, and the testes remain engorged and elevated. The plateau phase is typically a few seconds to several minutes in duration.

A series of muscular contractions marks orgasm, the climax of sexual response. The clitoris remains retracted behind the hood, and the outer third of the vagina, rectal sphincter, and uterus undergo rhythmic contractions. A man experiences contractions of the urethra, base of the penis, and rectal muscles, as well as emission and expulsion of semen.

During resolution, the muscles gradually relax, and there is a reversal of vasocongestion. The heart rate, blood pressure, and breathing return to normal. The clitoris descends, and the labia and internal organs return to their pre-arousal positions and color. A man loses his erection, the testes descend, and the scrotum thins.

 A   P e r s o n a l   G l i m p s e

For the first 12 years of my marriage, I never experienced an orgasm. My husband and I married very young, just out of high school. In the early years of marriage, sex was OK but never great for me. Then, after three kids and no sleep, I really did not enjoy sex. I began to think there was something wrong with me. Why couldn't I enjoy sex when everyone else seemed to enjoy it? I began to speak confidentially with my nurse practitioner at my obstetrician's office. She had delivered two of my kids, and I trusted her completely. I explained my concerns to her. She said that this is a very normal concern and that I was right to come see her. She said she would perform a physical examination to rule out any physical reasons for my lack of interest in and enjoyment of sex. A few days after the examination, we sat in her office and talked. She told me that I was in great physical shape, my laboratory work looked fine, and my reproductive tract was healthy. She asked what kind of stimulation my husband provided before intercourse. I said none. She explained that this could be the reason I did not enjoy sex. She explained in detail how the clitoris was designed and how it functions to bring sexual pleasure and orgasm during sexual stimulation. She showed me drawings of where it is located on my body and described how it changes during sexual stimulation. She encouraged me to locate it on my own body and ask my husband to stimulate that area during sexual intercourse. I took her advice and now I really enjoy sex with my husband. I wish someone had explained female reproductive anatomy to me earlier in my marriage.

Donna

Learning Opportunity: *What message might be conveyed if the nurse avoids discussing sexual matters with the client?*

Think back to Sandra Dickinson from the beginning of the chapter. What would be the most important information to give her, keeping in mind the time allotted for her visit? How would you evaluate her understanding of the information you gave her?

KEY POINTS

- Two major functions of the reproductive system are to produce offspring and to provide the experience of pleasure through physical intimacy.
- The testes and ovaries are responsible for the production of sex cells or gametes.
- External genitalia in men include the penis and scrotum. The penis serves to eliminate urine from the bladder and functions to deposit sperm in woman's reproductive tract for the purposes of reproduction. The scrotum regulates the temperature and protects the testes from trauma.
- The testes and ductal system compose the man's internal reproductive tract. Spermatogenesis occurs in the testes, and the ductal system serves as the exit route for sperm from the man's body.
- Sperm are formed in the seminiferous tubules and mature in the epididymis. During ejaculation, sperm travel from the epididymis through the paired vas deferens and ejaculatory ducts to the urethra and out of the body.
- Sperm need an alkaline environment and an energy source to be motile. The seminal vesicles, prostate gland, and the bulbourethral glands contribute alkaline

secretions to semen. The seminal vesicles also contribute fructose, an energy source for sperm.

- Testosterone, FSH, and interstitial cell-stimulating hormone (ICSH) are the hormones in men responsible for production of sperm and the development of secondary sex characteristics.
- A woman's external genitalia, or vulva, includes the mons pubis, labia majora, labia minora, clitoris, urethral meatus, vaginal opening, and Bartholin glands. The vestibule is the area within the boundaries of the labia minora and includes the urethral meatus, vaginal opening, and Bartholin glands.
- The vagina is an internal reproductive organ that functions as a woman's organ for sexual intercourse, exit point for the menstrual flow, and as the birth canal. Rugae, or folds, allow for stretching during the birth process.
- The main divisions of the uterus are the cervix, isthmus, corpus, and fundus. The walls of the uterus have three layers: perimetrium (protective cover), myometrium (muscle), and endometrium (lining).
- The fallopian tubes lead from the uterus toward the ovaries. The isthmus is the narrow portion near the uterus. The ampulla is the middle portion, and the infundibulum is the outer portion close to the ovaries. Fimbriae on the infundibulum make wavelike motions over the ovary to guide the released ovum toward the fallopian tube.

- The ovarian hormones, estrogen and progesterone, play a major role in the menstrual cycle and in the development of secondary sex characteristics in women.
- The menstrual cycle begins with day 1 being the start of menstrual flow. The cycle encompasses the ovarian cycle and the uterine cycle. FSH and LH from the pituitary govern the ovarian cycle, and estrogen and progesterone from the ovaries guide the uterine cycle.
- The sexual response cycle is divided into four phases: excitement, plateau, orgasm, and resolution. Vasocongestion and myotonia are the primary physiologic processes that contribute to sexual response in both the women and men.

INTERNET RESOURCES

Men
www.nlm.nih.gov/medlineplus/malereproductivesystem.html

Women
www.nlm.nih.gov/medlineplus/femalereproductivesystem.html

Menstrual Cycle
https://www.nlm.nih.gov/medlineplus/menstruation.html

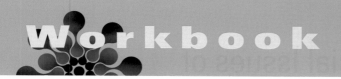

NCLEX-STYLE REVIEW QUESTIONS

1. Which of the following are true regarding the menstrual cycle? (*Select all that apply*)
   a. The menstrual cycle encompasses the events between the beginnings of two menstrual periods.
   b. The menstrual cycle keeps the woman's cervical mucus the same throughout the cycle.
   c. The menstrual cycle phases are menstrual, proliferative, ovulatory, and ischemic.
   d. The menstrual cycle can be divided into two phases: the follicular phase and the luteal phase.
   e. The menstrual cycle is controlled by both the posterior pituitary and the ovaries.

2. The vagina is a unfavorable environment for sperm. What characteristic of semen protects sperm from the vaginal environment?
   a. Acidic fluid
   b. Alkaline fluid
   c. Presence of testosterone
   d. Secretions from seminiferous tubules

3. You are preparing to perform a urinary catheterization on a woman client. In which location will you expect to find the urinary meatus?
   a. Above the clitoris
   b. Below the vaginal opening
   c. On the true perineum
   d. Within the vestibule

4. You are caring for a woman in labor. The health care provider is concerned that the uterus might rupture. Which part of the uterus requires the closest assessment because it is the thinnest part of the uterus?
   a. Corpus
   b. Fundus
   c. Inner cervical os
   d. Lower uterine segment

5. Which ovarian hormone regulates the proliferative phase of the uterine cycle?
   a. FSH
   b. LH
   c. Estrogen
   d. Progesterone

STUDY ACTIVITIES

1. In each row of the table, you will find a reproductive organ for either women or men listed. In the column that is missing information, fill in the name of the homologous reproductive organ.

Men's Reproductive Organ	Women's Reproductive Organ
Glans penis	
	Round ligaments
	Ovaries
Foreskin or prepuce	

2. In your clinical group, have a discussion as to why it is important for a nurse to understand the menstrual cycle.

CRITICAL THINKING: WHAT WOULD YOU DO?

Apply your knowledge of reproductive anatomy and physiology to the following situation.

1. Doug and Nancy, a young married couple, ages 26 and 22 years, respectively, have not been using any contraception for the past year, but Nancy has not become pregnant. Doug is a rancher and dresses in cowboy gear, including tight jeans. He works in a hot, humid environment for 10 to 12 hours almost every day.
   a. Using your knowledge about reproductive anatomy in men, what is one possible reason pregnancy has not occurred?
   b. What advice might be helpful for Doug to increase the likelihood that pregnancy will occur?

2. Nancy complains of frequent vaginal infections. During an office interview, Nancy tells you that she douches at least once per week.
   a. What other questions should you ask regarding Nancy's hygiene habits?
   b. What advice might be helpful for Nancy to decrease her risk for vaginal infections?

Special Issues of Women's Healthcare and Reproduction

4

Key Terms

abstinence
amenorrhea
coitus interruptus
dysmenorrhea
dyspareunia
endometriosis
gestational surrogate
induced abortion
infertility
menorrhagia
metrorrhagia
perimenopause
postcoital test
spontaneous abortion

Learning Objectives

At the conclusion of this chapter, you will:

1. Describe health screening recommendations for women.
2. Differentiate between dysmenorrhea and premenstrual syndrome (PMS).
3. Explain the clinical manifestations, treatment, and nursing care for endometriosis.
4. Discuss risk factors for pelvic inflammatory disease (PID).
5. Explain causes and risk factors for pelvic support disorders.
6. Discuss the significance of preconception care.
7. Compare and contrast methods of contraception.
8. Explain advantages and disadvantages for each method of contraception.
9. List possible causes and treatments for fertility problems.
10. Identify major considerations for the peri- and postmenopausal client.

Sondra Simone comes into the health care provider's office with complaints of heavy, painful menstrual periods. During her intake assessment, she states, "My husband and I had hoped that I would be pregnant by now." As you read the chapter, consider what additional information you would need to collect from Sondra. What factors may be contributing to Sondra's nonpregnant state?

This chapter examines issues related to women's health and reproduction. Women's health issues include preventive healthcare, menstrual disorders, pelvic infections, disorders of the uterus and ovaries, and pelvic support disorders. Issues related to the reproductive life cycle include family planning and contraception, elective termination of pregnancy, infertility, and menopause.

Several *Healthy People 2030* (U.S. Department of Health & Human Services, 2020) objectives relate to the topics in this chapter. Selected goals include the following:

- Increase the proportion of females who receive a breast cancer screening.
- Increase the proportion of women who receive a cervical cancer screening based on the most recent guidelines.

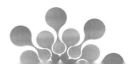

- Reduce the proportion of pregnancies that are unintended.
- Reduce pelvic inflammatory disease (PID) in adolescent and young females (aged 15 to 24 years).

WOMEN'S HEALTH ISSUES

Women's health issues encompass a broad variety of topics. Current research is highlighting the unique needs of women in relation to medical–surgical conditions, such as diabetes, heart disease, and stroke. Although these topics are critical to the overall health of women, this chapter focuses on conditions that occur universally, or nearly universally, in women.

HEALTH SCREENING FOR WOMEN

Health promotion is a broad concept that involves educating and assisting individuals to make behavior and lifestyle modifications for the prevention or early detection and treatment of disease. Because nurses are trusted healthcare professionals, individuals and families often turn to them for information and advice on health-related matters. As a result, health promotion for women is an area in which nurses can have great influence.

Health screening is a component of health promotion. Screening tests do not diagnose disease. Instead, a positive result indicates the need for more thorough testing. The following discussion encompasses screening procedures that promote the early detection of disorders that are unique to, or commonly occur in, women.

Breast Cancer Screening

In the United States, breast cancer is the second most common leading cause of cancer death in women, exceeded only by lung cancer (American Cancer Society, 2020a). In the United States from 2013 to 2017, out of every 100,000 women, 128 were diagnosed with breast cancer; for the same time period, out of every 100,000 women, 20 died from breast cancer (National Cancer Institute, 2020a). Detection of breast cancer before axillary node involvement increases the woman's chance for survival. For early identification of breast cancer, the American Cancer Society (ACS) recommends breast self-awareness by the woman and mammography. For women with average risk for breast cancer, yearly mammograms should start at age 45 and can change to having mammograms every 2 years beginning at age 55. Women who are at a higher risk for breast cancer due to family history or another reason may need to begin screening earlier and more often

Bare Is Best

Instruct the woman going for a mammogram to avoid applying deodorant, powder, and lotions prior to the mammogram. These substances, especially those with aluminum, may cause areas that look like calcifications to appear, which can impact the test results.

(ACS, 2020b). Reinforce to the woman the importance of mammography and how to perform a breast self-examination (BSE).

A BSE is a self-scheduled, systematic approach the woman uses to check her breasts. In the past, monthly BSEs were recommended for all women. The ACS now presents BSE as optional because current research indicates that performing BSE does not decrease mortality associated with breast cancer. However, the ACS recommends that each woman know how her breasts normally look and feel; if she finds changes, she should immediately report them to a health care provider (ACS, 2020c). (Refer to Chapter 27 for instructions on how to perform BSE.) Clinical breast examination involves inspection and palpation of the breasts by a health care provider.

Mammography is a screening tool that uses very low-dose x-ray for examination of breast tissue. It is useful in the early detection of cancer because a mammogram can detect a breast tumor or abnormality 2 years before the woman or the health care provider can palpate it. For the mammogram procedure, the breast is placed on a platform and compressed firmly between the platform and a plastic paddle (Fig. 4-1). Routine views include a top-to-bottom and a side view. The compression can be uncomfortable for some women. The most common recommendation is to schedule the examination for the week after the menstrual period when the breasts are less tender to minimize discomfort.

Pelvic Examination and Pap Smear

Every woman should have a yearly physical examination. A pelvic examination should be part of the total physical examination. A pelvic examination detects changes associated with certain gynecologic conditions such as infection, inflammation, pelvic pain, and cancer. Cervical cancer screening is one part of the pelvic examination but is not necessarily done with every examination.

The pelvic examination begins with the woman in the lithotomy position. The health care provider palpates and examines the appearances of the structures of the vulva, and then inserts a speculum to examine the walls of the vagina and the cervix. When the cervix is clearly visible, the health care provider swabs the cervix to obtain cell samples for cervical cancer screening and secretions to culture for pelvic infection. Following the speculum examination, a bimanual examination is done by inserting two lubricated fingers into the vagina with one hand and using the other hand to palpate uterine and ovarian structures through the abdominal wall. Frequently, a rectal examination to test for fecal occult blood and to palpate the rectovaginal wall completes the examination. See Nursing Procedure 4-1 for guidance in assisting the health care provider with collecting a Pap smear.

Cervical cancer screening includes samples sent from the cervical swab for the Papanicolaou test (Pap smear) and for the human papillomavirus (HPV). The

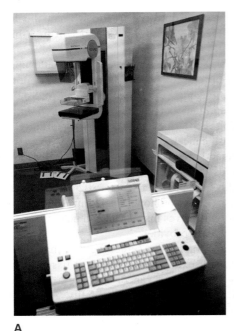

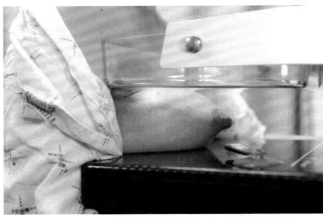

B

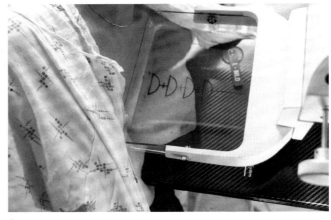

C

FIGURE 4-1 Mammography. **A.** Mammography equipment. **B.** A top-to-bottom view of the breast. **C.** A side view of the breast.

NURSING PROCEDURE 4-1 Assisting With Collection of a Pap Smear

EQUIPMENT
Examination table with stirrups or foot pedals
Drapes
Sterile gloves for the examiner
Speculum
Swab for the Pap test
Glass slide
Fixative
Sterile lubricant (water soluble)

PROCEDURE
1. Explain procedure to the client (Fig. A).

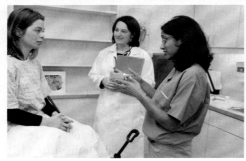

A

2. Instruct the client to empty her bladder. (A full bladder inter-feres with the pelvic examination and causes discomfort for the woman.)
3. Wash hands thoroughly.
4. Assemble equipment, maintaining sterility as indicated (Fig. B).

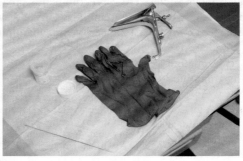

B

5. Position client on stirrups or foot pedals so that her knees fall outward.
6. Drape the client with a sheet or other draping for privacy, covering the abdomen but leaving the perineal area exposed.
7. Open packages as needed.

8. Encourage the client to relax.
9. Provide support to the client as the health care provider obtains a sample by spreading the labia (Fig. C), inserting the speculum (Fig. D) with the aid of lubricating jelly, inserting the cytobrush (Fig. E) to swab the endocervix, and inserting the plastic spatula (Fig. F) to swab the cervix.

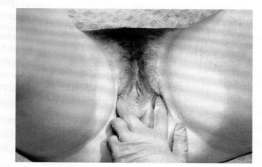

C

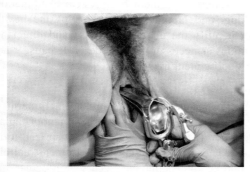

D

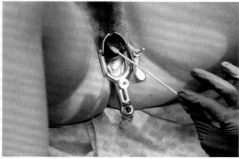

E

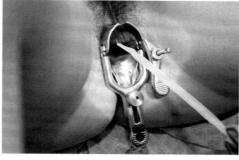

F

10. Transfer specimen to container (Fig. G) or slide. If a slide is used, spray fixative on the slide.

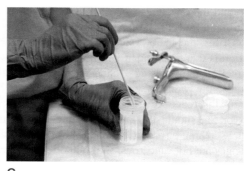

G

11. Wash hands thoroughly.
12. Label specimen according to facility policy.
13. After the health care provider removes the speculum and finishes the pelvic examination, assist the woman to a sitting position, and offer her tissues or a washcloth to clean her perineal area of excess lubricant.
14. Rinse reusable instruments and dispose of waste appropriately (Fig. H).

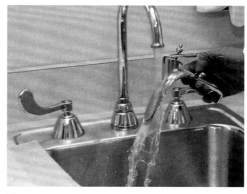

H

15. Wash hands thoroughly.

overall rates of cervical cancer have decreased by 60% over the last 50 years due to the routine performance of Pap smears (leading to early detection and prompt treatment of precancerous cervical changes) and also because of the HPV vaccine. Most cases of cervical cancer are caused by HPV. In parts of the world where Pap smears are not done routinely, cervical cancer is a leading cause of death for women.

The health care provider may screen for HPV, may combine the HPV screen with a Pap smear, or do a Pap smear only. A woman who has a negative screen for HPV has a very low risk for developing cervical cancer (National

Cancer Institute, 2020b). Current guidelines recommend that the woman obtain the initial Pap smear at 21 years of age, regardless of when she first has sexual intercourse, then every 3 years thereafter from age 21 to 29, and then every 5 years after age 30 if HPV screening is done or every 3 years if a Pap smear alone is done (National Cancer Institute, 2020c). The woman's health care provider may advise more frequent examinations for the woman who has abnormal Pap smears, has human immunodeficiency virus (HIV), has HPV, or is immunocompromised. Women should still have an annual examination even if cervical cancer screening is not done each time.

Vulvar Self-Examination

Some health care providers recommend that women older than 18 years (and those younger who are sexually active) should perform a monthly self-examination of the external genitalia. As with a BSE, the major value of the monthly vulvar self-examination is that the woman will become familiar with her own normal anatomy. Using a hand mirror and an adequate light source, the woman should inspect her vulva for any lesions, growths, reddened areas, unusual discharge, or changes in skin color. She should also take note of any changes in sensation, such as itching or pain. Caution the woman that although most changes are not cancerous, she should report all changes to her health care provider for evaluation.

COMMON DISORDERS OF WOMEN'S REPRODUCTIVE TRACT

There are several commonly occurring reproductive tract disorders in women. Many involve disorders of menstruation. Others are related to or caused by infections or decreased support of the pelvic floor.

Menstrual Disturbances

Disturbances of the menstrual cycle include increased or decreased frequency; absent, excessive, or irregular bleeding; or pain. Nursing interventions depend on the cause and treatment of the disorder, but also include providing information about recommended treatments or prescribed medications, caring for the woman before and after a procedure, and providing emotional support and reassurance.

Amenorrhea

Amenorrhea refers to the absence of menstruation and is classified as either primary or secondary amenorrhea. Primary amenorrhea is the absence of menarche (the first menstrual period) by 15 years of age. Secondary amenorrhea is the absence of three menstrual cycles or 6 months in a woman who was previously menstruating (Welt & Barbieri, 2020).

The presence of regular menstrual periods is a sign of overall health. Regular menses signals that the pituitary and ovaries are working together properly and that appropriate amounts of sex hormones are present.

Because pregnancy is the most common cause of amenorrhea in women of reproductive age, a pregnancy test is often the first test performed when a woman presents with amenorrhea.

Once the health care provider rules out pregnancy as a cause of amenorrhea, the next step is a thorough review of systems.

Amenorrhea associated with endocrine symptoms, such as hot flashes, night sweats, and vaginal dryness, often indicates ovarian dysfunction. Several factors can cause the ovaries to stop working. These include a history of radiation, chemotherapy, or menopause. Amenorrhea without endocrine symptoms may indicate disorders of the hypothalamus and pituitary glands or may indicate a problem with the outflow tract. Factors that can interfere with normal hypothalamic function include excessive exercise; endocrine disorders, such as hyperthyroidism or hypothyroidism; HIV/acquired immunodeficiency syndrome (AIDS); malnutrition; and major psychiatric disorders.

There are several conditions involving the outflow tract that can cause amenorrhea. Adhesions that have scarred the endometrium will prevent it from responding to ovarian stimulation. An imperforate hymen, underdevelopment of the lower reproductive tract, or scarring from female circumcision will also prevent the menstrual flow from exiting the body normally.

A thorough assessment by physical examination, history taking, and laboratory testing helps the health care provider identify the underlying cause and direct medical interventions as necessary. The underlying cause guides the woman's subsequent treatment.

Atypical Uterine Bleeding

There are several types of atypical (abnormal) uterine bleeding. Heavy or prolonged bleeding, called **menorrhagia**, is the most common menstrual complaint and can lead to anemia if left untreated. **Metrorrhagia** refers to menstrual bleeding that is normal in amount but occurs at irregular intervals between menstrual periods. Metrorrhagia that occurs with hormonal contraceptive drugs is called breakthrough bleeding. This type of bleeding frequently decreases over time.

Many of the factors that contribute to amenorrhea can also cause menorrhagia. Menorrhagia can also be caused by ovarian dysfunction, polyps, and fibroids (leiomyomas). A thorough history and physical examination can rule out systemic causes. If there are no readily apparent causative factors, the practitioner may initiate a trial of oral progestin therapy to alleviate the menorrhagia. If this therapy does not work, the health care provider might insert an intrauterine device (IUD) that releases progestin into the uterine cavity. The advantage of this therapy is that systemic hormone levels remain low because the hormones discharge directly into the uterine cavity. If traditional measures do not work, another therapy option is endometrial ablation, removal of the uterine lining (Sharp, 2020). Hysterectomy, the surgical removal of the uterus, remains a treatment alternative when all other measures fail.

This Is Worth Noting

Pregnancy is the most common cause of abnormal bleeding during the reproductive years. Bear in mind that any woman of childbearing age who presents with atypical or irregular bleeding may be pregnant and a pregnancy test should be done.

Dysmenorrhea

Dysmenorrhea is painful or difficult menses. Primary dysmenorrhea refers to painful menstrual periods that are not associated with a disease process. Secondary dysmenorrhea is painful menses secondary to a pelvic condition such as endometriosis or uterine fibroids. Primary dysmenorrhea is the more common of the two conditions and results from the action of prostaglandins on the uterus. Prostaglandins contribute to dysmenorrhea in two ways. They cause the uterus to contract, which leads to painful cramping, and they decrease blood flow to the myometrium, which contributes to lactic acid buildup and additional pain.

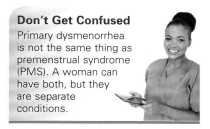

Don't Get Confused

Primary dysmenorrhea is not the same thing as premenstrual syndrome (PMS). A woman can have both, but they are separate conditions.

Primary dysmenorrhea affects many women during their childbearing years. It occurs at a higher rate in younger women who have not born children. As age and number of children delivered increase, the incidence of primary dysmenorrhea decreases. Risk factors that increase the severity of symptoms include earlier age at menarche, long and heavy menstrual flow, smoking, and a family history of the condition (Smith & Kaunitz, 2020).

Clinical Manifestations

Primary dysmenorrhea typically begins within 6 months to 2 years after menarche. Major symptoms consist of severe intermittent cramping in association with constant pain in the lower abdomen, which may radiate to the lower back or upper thighs. Common symptoms that occur with dysmenorrhea include nausea, diarrhea, fatigue, and headache. Symptoms usually begin shortly before or with the onset of menstrual flow.

Treatment

The most effective treatments have been acetaminophen, nonsteroidal anti-inflammatory drugs (NSAIDs), and oral contraceptive drugs (birth control pills) given alone or in combination. NSAIDs, such as ibuprofen or naproxen, reduce symptoms by lowering prostaglandin levels and relieving pain. NSAIDs are most effective when taken around the clock as soon as menstrual flow begins. They are less effective when taken on an as-needed basis. Oral contraceptive drugs relieve symptoms by inhibiting ovulation, thinning the endometrial lining, and decreasing prostaglandin production. Nonpharmacologic therapies that may help decrease the discomfort related to dysmenorrhea include heat application, relaxation, massage, yoga, acupuncture, and herbal or homeopathic remedies.

Nursing Care

Nursing care of the woman with primary dysmenorrhea involves education about the condition, its treatment, and interventions to relieve discomfort. Explain medication actions, common side effects, measures to reduce side effects, and timing of administration. Reassure the woman that sometimes medication changes occur several times before the best therapy for her symptoms is determined. Reinforce that she should take her NSAIDs on a schedule, rather than waiting until the pain begins or becomes severe and that they should be taken with food to avoid gastrointestinal side effects.

There are several nonpharmacologic interventions that can help relieve the pain associated with dysmenorrhea. Heat can be soothing. Suggest the use of hot baths or applying heating pads to the abdomen or lower back. Sometimes changing positions can be helpful. Some women report relief when they assume a knee-chest position. Pain is usually less severe when the woman is in good general health. Encourage adequate exercise, diet, rest, and hygiene, and discourage smoking. Many women who have dysmenorrhea become upset and discouraged; reassure the woman that the pain has a physiologic, not emotional, cause.

> **TEST YOURSELF**
> ✔ Define amenorrhea.
> ✔ What is the medical term for heavy menstrual flow?
> ✔ What is the difference between primary and secondary dysmenorrhea?

Premenstrual Syndrome (PMS)

Most women experience some discomfort just before the menstrual period, most commonly breast tenderness, food cravings, and pelvic heaviness or bloating. PMS is defined as physiologic and emotional symptoms that occur during the second half of the menstrual cycle over repeated menstrual cycles and impact the woman's daily activities. These symptoms include headaches, weight gain, changes in activity and appetite, anxiety, and sadness. Symptoms of PMS usually resolve with the onset of the woman's menses. It is unclear why some women experience PMS while others do not.

It is also unclear the exact percentage of women who experience PMS. Some studies inquire about symptoms but do not investigate the severity of the symptoms or the impact they have upon the woman's daily activities. Worldwide, women report similar symptoms that occur with PMS, but in some countries women do not report having PMS as that term does not exist in their language (Yonkers & Casper, 2020).

Although the exact causes of PMS remain unknown, research shows that PMS symptoms are very complex and do not arise from one single causal factor. In fact, PMS results from the interplay between the central nervous system, the endocrine system, and other factors, such as genetics.

Premenstrual dysphoric disorder (PMDD) is a more severe form of PMS and is seen in a small percentage of women. PMDD includes all of the physical symptoms of PMS with additional and more debilitating emotional symptoms.

Clinical Manifestations

PMS presents with a wide variety of symptoms, which may be physical, behavioral, or both. The symptoms can be highly distressing for the woman and her family. In making a diagnosis of PMS, the crucial component is the cyclical nature of the symptoms. Box 4-1 lists the common physical and behavioral symptoms seen in PMS. Typically, the severity of symptoms progresses over time. In the early stages of PMS, women describe symptoms beginning a few days before their period and stopping when bleeding begins. With time, symptoms begin to appear 1 to 2 weeks before the onset of menses. Some women describe a cluster of symptoms occurring at the time of ovulation, followed by a symptom-free week, then a recurrence of symptoms a week before menses. PMS does not necessarily indicate dysmenorrhea will occur. Many women with symptoms of PMS do not have pain with menses.

Treatment

Pregnancy and menopause are the only two events that eliminate PMS. Treatment of PMS aims to alleviate specific signs and symptoms. Some studies show that supplementation with vitamin B$_6$, calcium, and magnesium is beneficial. Medications may be used to help relieve the symptoms of PMS. These include diuretics to reduce bloating, NSAIDs or acetaminophen to reduce pain and cramping, and antianxiety drugs or antidepressant drugs. Stress reduction, relaxation therapy, and exercise may also provide the woman with some relief. Some women report relief of PMS after starting contraceptive drugs.

PMDD responds to treatments similar to those used for PMS. In addition, the use of selective serotonin reuptake inhibitors (SSRIs) during the last half of the cycle has been effective in treating the severe mood swings and other emotional symptoms that are seen in PMDD.

BOX 4-1 **Common Symptoms Seen in Premenstrual Syndrome (PMS)**

Physical Symptoms
- Breast tenderness
- Abdominal bloating
- Headache, migraine
- Edema of the extremities

Behavioral Symptoms
- Angry outbursts
- Confusion
- Depression
- Withdrawal from others
- Anxiety
- Irritable mood
- Feelings of edginess

Nursing Care

Assist the woman in finding ways to decrease stress. A healthy lifestyle contributes to a general sense of well-being. Encourage regular exercise, even when she is experiencing symptoms. Encourage reduction or elimination of caffeine and alcohol. Explain that limiting salt intake and carbonated beverages may decrease symptoms of bloating. Additional relief measures are described in Tips for Reinforcing Family Teaching: Relief Measures for Premenstrual Syndrome (PMS).

TIPS FOR REINFORCING FAMILY TEACHING

Relief Measures for Premenstrual Syndrome (PMS)

Diet
- Reduce or eliminate caffeine intake (including coffee, tea, colas, and chocolate).
- Avoid simple sugars (as in candy, cakes, and cookies).
- Reduce salt intake (pickles, fast foods, and chips).
- Eat a diet rich in complex carbohydrates and low in fat, particularly in the 2 weeks before the menstrual period.
- Eat six small meals per day (to stabilize blood glucose levels).

Exercise
- Do aerobic exercise, such as walking or jogging, several times each week.

Stress Management
- Keep a diary of symptoms, and alter your schedule to minimize stressors when symptoms are most severe.
- Use interventions such as relaxation techniques, massage, and warm baths.
- Consider cognitive behavioral therapy, a short-term structured psychotherapeutic approach that focuses on the interplay of current thinking patterns with behavior choices.

Sleep and Rest
- Maintain a regular sleep schedule.
- Drink a glass of warm milk before bedtime.
- Schedule exercise for early morning or early afternoon.
- Give yourself a quiet time to relax just before going to bed.

Endometriosis

Endometriosis is a painful reproductive disorder in which endometrial tissue grows outside of the uterus, usually in the pelvic cavity. These tissue implants respond to the cyclic hormonal changes of the menstrual cycle and cause menstrual-like internal bleeding that leads to inflammation, scarring, and adhesions in the pelvic cavity. The exact number of women who experience endometriosis is hard to define as some women have severe symptoms and others are without symptoms. Endometriosis is a common finding in women having a laparoscopy to determine cause of pelvic pain.

Clinical Manifestations

Some women with advanced endometriosis are without symptoms and are unaware of the disease until the condition presents during abdominal or pelvic surgery. Other women may experience debilitating, almost continuous pelvic pain, with only minimal abnormal tissue growth. The woman typically experiences the most pronounced symptoms right before the onset of the menstrual period.

Cyclic pelvic pain that occurs in conjunction with menses is a classic symptom of endometriosis. Menorrhagia, dysmenorrhea, and **dyspareunia** (painful intercourse) are other common symptoms. Depending on where the extra endometrial tissue is located, the pain and bleeding can involve the bladder, leading to hematuria, or it can affect the bowel, leading to blood in the stools and painful defecation. Although endometriosis appears to play a role in infertility for some women, others experience no apparent difficulty with conception.

Endometriosis is difficult to diagnose due to the varied symptoms. In addition, the health care provider can easily attribute the symptoms to other conditions. Physical examination reveals pelvic tenderness, particularly during menses. Laparoscopy is the primary diagnostic tool for endometriosis because the surgeon can directly visualize the characteristic endometrial lesions and take biopsy samples. The disadvantage to this diagnostic tool is that it is an invasive surgical technique.

Treatment

Treatment for endometriosis depends on the severity of the woman's symptoms, extent of the disease, desire for fertility, and the woman's treatment goals. The woman with mild pain may respond well to NSAIDs and contraceptive drugs. Medication therapy for severe symptoms aims to suppress ovulation and induce an artificial menopause, which in turn results in suppression of abnormal tissue and relief of pain. Side effects include symptoms associated with menopause, such as labile emotions, hot flashes, and vaginal dryness. Bone density should be monitored in artificially induced menopausal clients.

Surgical intervention can be conservative, destroying the abnormal tissue while preserving reproductive ability. Surgical intervention can also be semiconservative, destroying reproductive function but maintaining ovarian function, or radical, involving removal of the uterus and ovaries.

Nursing Care

Chronic pain is a common symptom for the woman with endometriosis. Evaluate the characteristics and severity of pain. Assist the woman in finding ways to cope with and decrease pain. Nonpharmacologic measures used to relieve PMS discomfort can also be used for the woman experiencing pain from endometriosis. Encourage the use of analgesic medications, as ordered.

Provide emotional support. Frequently the woman has suffered years of pain before the health care provider makes a diagnosis of endometriosis. Allow the woman a chance to discuss her feelings. She may particularly have this need if the endometriosis is causing infertility problems. Encourage the woman to ask questions. Assist the woman in making treatment decisions by providing information regarding the advantages, disadvantages, possible risks, and likely outcomes of each treatment option.

Infectious Disorders

Infections of the reproductive tract can have long-term consequences such as infertility and chronic pelvic pain. Sexually transmitted organisms cause many of these infections. Chapters 16 and 41 discuss sexually transmitted infections (STIs). This section covers toxic shock syndrome (TSS) and pelvic inflammatory disease (PID).

Toxic Shock Syndrome (TSS)

TSS is an illness typically caused by an exotoxin produced by the bacteria *Staphylococcus aureus* although TSS can be caused by other pathogens. TSS was first recognized in 1978; authorities quickly noticed that the majority of cases occurred in women who were using certain types of high-absorbency tampons. Shortly thereafter, manufacturers made changes to the composition and absorbency of tampons, and TSS cases declined dramatically. However, women who use tampons, diaphragms, or contraceptive sponges are still at risk for the illness.

TSS starts suddenly with a high fever (higher than 102°F/38.9°C), nausea, vomiting, abdominal pain, a rapid drop in blood pressure, watery diarrhea, headache, sore throat, and muscle aches. Within 24 hours, a sunburnlike rash develops. The skin, particularly on the palms and soles, may peel approximately 1 to 2 weeks later. Treatment requires hospitalization, often in an intensive care setting, intravenous fluids, and antibiotic drugs.

Nurses can be helpful in the prevention of TSS. Explain to the woman who uses tampons to wash her hands thoroughly before and after inserting or removing a tampon. She should use the lowest absorbency that will handle her menstrual flow, change tampons frequently (at least every 2 to 3 hours), or alternate tampons with sanitary napkins and never use more than one tampon at once. Between periods, tampons should be stored away from heat and moisture to help prevent bacterial growth. The woman should frequently remove and clean any vaginal device (e.g., a diaphragm) that she is using.

Pelvic Inflammatory Disease (PID)

PID is a broad term used to refer to inflammation of any portion of a woman's reproductive tract, such as the uterus, fallopian tubes, or ovaries. PID occurs most commonly in association with untreated STIs, in particular gonorrhea and chlamydia (CDC, 2020a), but other organisms have been found to cause PID. Untreated PID can lead to scarring, ectopic (tubal) pregnancy, and chronic pelvic pain. Peritonitis and sepsis are other life-threatening complications. Women at risk for PID include those younger than 25 years, who have multiple sex partners, and who douche. IUDs for contraception have been linked to PID if the woman is not tested for infections prior to the IUD insertion.

Clinical Manifestations

Major symptoms of PID include lower abdominal pain and abnormal vaginal discharge. Other symptoms include chills, fever, vomiting, dyspareunia, menorrhagia, dysmenorrhea, fatigue, loss of appetite, backache, and painful or frequent urination. Some women are without symptoms but can still experience permanent damage to the reproductive tract.

Diagnosis is made by a complete history and physical examination to include a pelvic examination. Generally, specimens are collected and cultured for STIs. Other tests that may be ordered include ultrasound, endometrial biopsy, or laparoscopy.

Treatment

Frequently it is impossible to identify the causative organism, so current guidelines suggest that the health care provider prescribe at least two wide-spectrum antibiotic drugs. Sometimes two courses of antibiotic drugs are necessary. Occasionally, hospitalization is required for intravenous antibiotic therapy. Sex partners of the woman with PID must also receive antibiotic treatment, even if they do not have symptoms.

Nursing Care

Client education is an important nursing function for the woman with PID. Reinforce information that was given regarding the transmission, treatment, and prevention of infection. Encourage the woman to take all of her antibiotic drugs, even after she starts to feel better. Explain the use of any prescribed pain medications. Explain the importance of treatment of her partner to prevent reinfection. Instruct the woman to avoid sexual intercourse until she finishes the full course of antibiotic drugs and her partner is treated. Douching can force bacteria into the reproductive tract and should be avoided.

Instruct the woman on ways to prevent STIs and PID because the more frequently she experiences these infections, the more likely the infection will lead to scarring and infertility. The best way to prevent PID is to avoid sexual intercourse or to remain in a monogamous relationship, one in which both partners are sexually faithful to the other. The next best way is for the woman's partner to use latex condoms for all sexual acts. Diaphragms and other barrier methods afford some protection but are not as reliable as condoms.

Disorders of the Uterus and Ovaries

Cervical Polyps

Cervical polyps are benign tumors that hang on a stemlike pedicle and protrude through the cervical os. Cervical polyps are associated with infection and chronic inflammation. Postcoital (after intercourse) bleeding, metrorrhagia, menorrhagia, and leukorrhea (white or yellow vaginal discharge) are associated symptoms. The health care provider can visualize cervical polyps during a speculum examination of the cervix and may remove them during the procedure. Tissue is sent to pathology for microscopic examination.

The health care provider usually prescribes prophylactic antibiotic drugs after removal of the polyps.

Uterine Fibroids

Uterine fibroids are benign estrogen-responsive tumors of the uterine wall that often regress with menopause. Fibroids (leiomyomas) may first be diagnosed in women in their 20s, occur in approximately 70% of women by the age of 50, and are much more common in Black women than in white women (Stewart and Laughlin-Tommaso, 2020). Many uterine fibroids do not cause any symptoms; however, the tumors can enlarge and cause pelvic pressure, pain, and menstrual irregularities. They can be particularly problematic during pregnancy. Fibroids (leiomyomas) tend to shrink in the postmenopausal period due to a decrease in hormone levels. Diagnosis is made via bimanual pelvic examination; transvaginal or abdominal ultrasound; or hysteroscopy (insertion of a scope through the cervical canal into the uterine cavity).

Therapy depends on the symptoms and whether the woman wishes to retain fertility. The presence of uterine fibroids is the most common reason cited for hysterectomy and may be the treatment of choice if the woman does not want a future pregnancy. A less-radical procedure, myomectomy (removal of the fibroid), is the traditional option for the woman who wishes to maintain fertility. The surgeon sometimes chooses laparoscopy to remove multiple fibroids.

Another procedure, uterine artery embolization, uses a technique similar to heart catheterization. A catheter is introduced into the uterine artery and then a substance is injected that flows to the arteries supplying the fibroids and blocks the blood flow to them. The fibroids shrink after the procedure because of decreased blood supply. Uterine artery embolization is not recommended for women who desire to become pregnant.

Pharmacologic treatment options are also available. Hormonal regulation with GnRH (gonadotropin-releasing hormone) agonists can shrink fibroids. Treatment with mifepristone can also be effective.

Ovarian Cysts

Ovarian cysts are fluid-filled sacs that develop in or on the ovary. Ovarian cysts are common during the childbearing years, and the woman may or may not have symptoms. Common symptoms are lower abdominal pain or pressure, usually on one side. Women describe the pain as sharp or dull, and it varies in duration from constant to intermittent. Ovarian cysts do not interfere with the woman's menstrual cycle.

One condition, polycystic ovary syndrome (PCOS), is the presence of multiple small cysts on the ovaries. In PCOS, the menstrual cycles are irregular and may interfere with fertility. Women with PCOS have other symptoms such as obesity, abnormal body hair, and acne.

Ovarian cysts are usually benign but can lead to complications, such as hemorrhage (which can be life-threatening), ovarian torsion (twisting), inflammation, rupture, necrosis, and bacterial infection leading to septic shock. Pelvic adhesions, infertility, and chronic pelvic pain syndrome are chronic complications that can occur.

Diagnosis of ovarian cysts is made based upon the woman's symptoms. Transvaginal and abdominal ultrasounds are effective methods for diagnosing an ovarian cyst. Laparoscopy can be done to diagnose and remove cysts, although many do not require surgical intervention and will resolve spontaneously. Some health care providers adopt a "wait and see" approach, which normally results in regression of the cyst. The mainstay of medical therapy is oral contraceptive drugs, which regulate the menstrual cycle and may cause regression of a cyst or prevention of additional cyst formation.

Pelvic Support Disorders

Muscle, ligaments, and fascia provide support to hold the pelvic organs in place. These support structures function like a hammock to support the urethra, bladder, small intestine, rectum, uterus, and vagina. Problems occur when the support structures relax or weaken, allowing the organs to drop down or protrude through the vaginal wall.

The names of pelvic support disorders correspond to the affected organs.

- Cystocele occurs when the bladder bulges into the front wall of the vagina.
- Rectocele occurs when the rectum protrudes into the back wall of the vagina.
- Enterocele occurs when the small intestine and peritoneum jut downward between the uterus and rectum.
- Uterine prolapse occurs when the uterus drops down into the vagina.

Figure 4-2 illustrates pelvic support disorders.

The most common causes of pelvic support disorders are pregnancy, vaginal birth, and aging. Women with histories of multiple vaginal births are at the highest risk for pelvic support disorders. Other causes include obesity, chronic coughing, frequent constipation, and hysterectomy.

Clinical Manifestations

Pelvic support disorders are hernias in which organs prolapse (abnormally protrude) through the weakened tissues of the support structure. Common symptoms are a feeling of heaviness or pressure in the vaginal area or a feeling that "something is dropping out of the vagina." Symptoms tend to occur when the woman is upright and may be relieved when she is in the recumbent position. Dyspareunia is sometimes present. In mild cases, the woman may be without

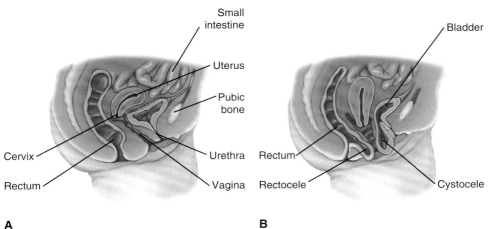

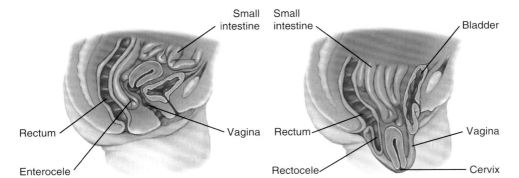

FIGURE 4-2 Types of pelvic support disorders. **A.** Normal. **B.** Rectocele and cystocele. **C.** Enterocele. **D.** Uterine prolapse.

symptoms. Some symptoms are specific to a certain type of prolapse. A cystocele may lead to urinary incontinence, whereas a rectocele may cause constipation.

Diagnosis of pelvic floor disorders is made during a pelvic examination. The health care provider asks the woman to cough or bear down during the examination. Then the examination is repeated with the woman in a standing position. Other tests may be done to test bladder or bowel functioning.

Treatment

Treatment options depend upon the type of pelvic floor dysfunction, severity of the dysfunction, and symptoms the woman is experiencing. For mild cases that are without symptoms, no treatment may be necessary. If treatment is recommended, it is helpful to start with less invasive techniques and then progress toward invasive techniques as needed.

Kegel exercises can strengthen pelvic floor muscles and improve tone. The woman can wear support garments that relieve some of the pressure. Another option is a pessary, which is a device that holds pelvic organs in place when inserted into the vagina. Pessaries are available in various shapes and sizes. The health care provider measures and fits the pessary to the woman, who must take it out periodically, clean it with soap and water, and then reinsert the device. Some women benefit from physical therapy and biofeedback, which help them with relaxing and coordination of the pelvic floor muscles.

Surgical techniques are often necessary to treat pelvic support disorders. Hysterectomy is the classic treatment option for uterine prolapse. During a hysterectomy procedure, the surgeon can repair other pelvic support disorders. Pelvic floor prolapse can be treated by surgical reconstructive measures. The repair can be either through the abdomen or through the vagina. Surgical repair sometimes requires a repeat surgery for an effective repair.

Nursing Care

Instruct the woman to do Kegel exercises regularly. To do a Kegel exercise, instruct the woman to tightly squeeze the muscles used to stop the stream of urine. She then holds the squeeze tightly while she counts to 10. The woman repeats the exercise 10 to 20 times in a row several times per day. A woman can perform Kegel exercises discreetly while sitting, standing, or lying down.

Anything that increases intra-abdominal pressure can worsen the prolapse. Counsel the woman to lose weight, if needed. She should avoid lifting heavy objects, and chronic coughing. Smoking causes coughing, so advise her to quit smoking. Constipation and straining with bowel movements can also worsen the prolapse. Measures to prevent constipation include increased fluid intake, a high-fiber diet, and regular exercise.

Instruct the woman to recognize signs of urinary tract infection (UTI): pain or burning upon urination, urinary frequency and urgency, and cloudy urine. The woman with a cystocele is at higher risk for UTIs. Other measures to prevent infection are to drink plenty of fluids, including fruit juices, to wipe from front to back after using the toilet, and to get enough rest.

Age-Specific Considerations

Older women may not feel comfortable talking about subjects that involve private body parts, such as pelvic organ prolapse. They may avoid asking pertinent questions or they may not report important symptoms. Women raised in a culture that values modesty may find it difficult to openly discuss these issues. Be patient and ask specific questions. Clarify any vague terminology the woman uses, such as "it" or "down there."

TEST YOURSELF

✔ Name five symptoms of PMS.
✔ How would you describe endometriosis to a client?
✔ Identify three ways to prevent PID.

REPRODUCTIVE LIFE CYCLE ISSUES

Life cycle issues related to reproduction are present throughout the life span. Major milestones include prenatal differentiation of reproductive organs, growth and development of reproductive organs during childhood, maturation of the reproductive system in adolescence, reproductive capability during early and middle adulthood, declining reproductive capability during middle adulthood, and the end of reproductive capability in late-middle to older adulthood. This section addresses issues directly related to reproductive functioning.

FAMILY PLANNING

Family planning consists of two complementary parts: planning pregnancy and preventing pregnancy. Family planning gives the client control over the number of children desired and allows determination of when births will occur in relation to each other and when reproduction can stop. The client can avoid unwanted pregnancies, bring about wanted births, and control the intervals between births. Family planning may be a component of the nurse's role for the nurse employed in a family planning clinic; a health care provider or nurse-midwife practice; or the acute care setting, such as in the postpartum or gynecology units.

Planning Pregnancy

For many women of childbearing age, a planned pregnancy occurs simply by discontinuing the use of contraception. However, pregnancy planning should include "prepregnancy" planning called preconception care. The condition of the woman before pregnancy affects the outcome of the pregnancy. Therefore, a healthy pregnancy begins well in advance of conception.

Good health and avoiding exposure to harmful substances are significant contributing factors for a successful pregnancy and a healthy baby. If the woman waits until she is pregnant to remedy factors that can put her or an unborn child at risk, it may be too late to prevent complications. Box 4-2 describes components of preconception care. Preconception care is especially important for the woman with a history of problems with a previous pregnancy, such as miscarriage or preterm labor or birth. In many cases, identification and treatment of causative factors can reduce the risk for problems in subsequent pregnancies. Preconception care is equally important for the woman with a predisposing condition such as a chronic medical condition or a family history of genetic disorders.

Areas of Focus for Preconception Care

Because a woman may not realize she is pregnant during the early and vulnerable weeks of fetal development, any woman of childbearing age should be aware of health problems or medication regimens that may adversely affect pregnancy and the birth of a healthy baby. There are several key areas of focus while planning for a pregnancy. These areas include nutrition and exercise, lifestyle changes, chronic illness and genetic disorders, and medications.

Nutrition and Exercise

The woman should optimize her intake of folic acid several months before becoming pregnant. Folate occurs naturally in foods such as dark green leafy vegetables and legumes. If needed, the woman can take folic acid supplements to meet daily requirements. Folic acid has been shown to decrease the incidence of neural tube defects such as spina bifida. Since folic acid fortification was required in 1998, there has been a 35% decrease in the rate of neural tube defects in the United States (CDC, 2020b).

Research has shown that although there is mandatory fortification, neural tube defects remain higher in some populations. Neural tube defects are more likely to be seen in infants born to women who are Hispanic/Latina (CDC, 2020d). Several reasons have been identified for this including lower folate levels, genetics, and lower likelihood to consume foods that are fortified or take a multivitamin (CDC, 2020d). To help increase folate levels for this population, the U.S. Food and Drug Administration allows for the voluntary fortification of folic acid to corn masa flour, a common food staple in the diet of many Hispanic/Latina people.

Regular aerobic exercise conditions the heart, lungs, muscles, and other organs in preparation for the increased demands of pregnancy. Exercise can also be helpful in building up strength in the low back and abdomen—two areas that can cause discomfort throughout pregnancy.

Lifestyle Changes

Smoking cessation is an important consideration when planning for pregnancy. Women who smoke are at higher risk for miscarriage, and their infants are at risk for lower birth weight, sudden infant death syndrome, and infant respiratory illnesses.

Alcohol intake can affect the developing child. Fetal alcohol spectrum disorder is a cause of serious and irreversible birth defects, particularly mental underdevelopment. The level of alcohol intake that causes birth defects to occur is unknown, so women of childbearing age should abstain from alcohol before as well as during pregnancy.

Chronic Illness and Genetic Disorders

A woman with a chronic illness, such as diabetes, asthma, heart disease, seizures, or high blood pressure, is at higher

---

> **BOX 4-2** **What Is Preconception Care?**
>
> Preconception care is not simply one prepregnancy visit to a health care provider before becoming pregnant. Preconception care involves almost every encounter with a woman of childbearing age. The Centers for Disease Control (CDC) has identified steps and goals for women desiring to become pregnant to help increase the health of the woman and the future pregnancy. The following is a summary of recommendations from the CDC for preconception health.
> - **Plan pregnancies:** This includes using contraception correctly and at all times until pregnancy is desired. It also includes planning when to start attempting to conceive.
> - **Eat healthy.**
> - **Be active.**
> - **Take 400 micrograms (µg) of folic acid daily:** Folic acid intake has been shown to decrease birth defects of the brain and spinal cord. Folic acid is found in foods and in vitamin supplements.
> - **Protect against sexually transmitted infections (STIs):** This includes getting checked for any infections, as some may not have any symptoms.
> - **Protect against other infections**: This includes washing hands frequently and having someone else change cat litter.
> - **Avoid harmful chemicals, metal, or other toxic substances at home or in the workplace.**
> - **Make sure vaccinations are up-to-date:** This includes flu and booster vaccines (some booster vaccines, such as rubella, need to be given when the woman is not pregnant).
> - **Manage and reduce stress.**
> - **Stop smoking.**
> - **Stop using street drugs or prescription medications that are not prescribed for the woman before becoming pregnant and during pregnancy.**
> - **Reduce alcohol intake before becoming pregnant and stop drinking while pregnant.**
> - **Stop partner violence.**
> - **Manage any preexisting health conditions:** Any medication regime should balance the risk to an unborn child, and any chronic condition should be well under control before pregnancy occurs.
> - **Learn about the family's health history.**
> - **Get regular checkups**.
>
> Adapted from CDC. (2020, April 16). *Planning for Pregnancy*. Before Pregnancy. https://www.cdc.gov/preconception/planning.html

risk for poor pregnancy outcome. Therefore, the woman with a chronic disorder will need to consult with her health care provider about possible risks related to medications or therapies. Adjustment of medication regimens before pregnancy can decrease the risk to the woman and her fetus. The woman should not abruptly stop any current medical regime without talking to her health care provider first. Some medication therapies can cause harm if abruptly stopped.

Some women may need genetic counseling. Genetic counseling is recommended when:

- The woman or her partner has a genetic disorder
- Either partner is a known carrier for a genetic condition
- A previous child was born with a genetic syndrome
- There is a strong family history of a genetically transmitted disorder

Medications

Many medications cross the placenta easily and can cause birth defects. Preconception care includes assessment of medications the woman is taking, including prescription, over-the-counter, and herbal remedies. This assessment allows for timely adjustments in dosage or alterations in choice of medication.

Nursing Care

Nurses, especially those working in settings such as clinics or a health care provider's office or in public health, play an important role in pregnancy planning and preconception care. A major nursing focus of preconception care is education and counseling, which the nurse may offer individually or in group settings. Nurses are also be responsible for data collection regarding the woman's and her partner's health histories, including current health status and lifestyle practices. Nursing interventions include anticipatory guidance or reinforcing information given, discussing issues such as lifestyle, risk behaviors or risk factors, and corrective or preventative measures. Encourage the woman who is trying to become pregnant to follow the recommendations in Tips for Reinforcing Family Teaching: Pregnancy Planning.

Be Very Careful!
A woman should never stop taking her prescribed medications before discussing it with her health care provider, even if she suspects she is pregnant. In some conditions, the risk to the baby or mother of an uncontrolled medical condition outweighs the risk of harm from medications.

TIPS FOR REINFORCING FAMILY TEACHING

Pregnancy Planning

At least 3 months before attempting to conceive:

- Stop or considerably reduce smoking.
- Stop or considerably reduce alcohol consumption.
- Stop use of recreational drugs.
- Eat a healthy diet that is rich in protein, calcium, iron, and zinc.
- Avoid raw meats. Be sure to thoroughly wash your hands before and after handling raw meat.
- Take folic acid tablets (400 µg/day) to supplement the folate in a diet that includes leafy green vegetables, beans, and whole wheat breads. Vitamin B complex is also beneficial.

- Begin a regular exercise program that includes aerobic conditioning.
- Share with your health care provider any family history of genetic disorders or history of recurrent pregnancy loss.
- Know your rubella and varicella (chickenpox) immunity status and get vaccinated at least 3 months in advance of conception if nonimmune to either disease.
- Avoid exposure to x-rays.
- Consult your health care provider about existing medical conditions or medications.

Preventing Pregnancy

Part of preconception care includes the individual taking steps to prevent pregnancy until desired. Almost half of all pregnancies in the United States are unplanned at the time of conception.

The client who wishes to avoid or delay pregnancy has a wide variety of contraceptive options. An ideal method of contraception is one that is effective, easy for the client to understand and use, and acceptable to both partners. There should be minimal side effects and low risk of long-term consequences. The best contraceptive method does not directly interfere with intercourse or sexual pleasure. It should be inexpensive and easy to maintain. Protection from STIs is an additional consideration. Reversible methods should allow the couple to conceive readily after discontinuing use of the method. Table 4-1 compares major contraceptive methods.

Natural Methods

A natural contraceptive method refers to any method that does not use hormones, pharmaceutical compounds, or physical barriers that block sperm from entering the uterus. Natural methods of birth control include abstinence, coitus interruptus, and natural family planning or fertility awareness methods.

Abstinence

Abstinence as related to birth control means refraining from vaginal sexual intercourse. Abstinence can include other means of sexual stimulation, such as oral sex. Complete, or strict, abstinence refers to the avoidance of all sexual contact. Abstinence is a normal and acceptable alternative to sexual intercourse, especially for teens and singles in noncommittal relationships. The use of

TABLE 4-1 Comparison of Common Contraceptive Methods

	ADVANTAGES	DISADVANTAGES	PREVENTS STIS	HORMONAL	PERCENT EFFECTIVE (WHEN USED REGULARLY AND AS INDICATED)
Oral contraceptive drugs	Eases menstrual cramps	Must be taken daily	No	Yes	99%
Hormonal implants	No daily pills No interference with sexual activity	Requires incision and local anesthesia for implanting Weight gain common Irregular bleeding patterns may occur	No	Yes	99%
Condoms for men	Effective in preventing STIs	May decrease sensation, may break	Yes	No	85%
IUD	Lasts for several years	Can fall out	No	No for copper Yes for others	99%
Diaphragm	Does not interfere with sensation	Needs to be inserted prior to intercourse	No	No	84% (when combined with a spermicide)
Sterilization	Permanent	Surgically invasive	No	No	99%
Spermicides	No need for prescription	Irritating for some people, may increase risk of STI transmission	No	No	71%

IUD, intrauterine device; STI, sexually transmitted infections.

complete abstinence as a method of birth control has no cost, is readily available, and is the only 100% effective method for preventing pregnancy and sexually transmitted infections (STIs). A major drawback is that it can be difficult to maintain abstinence. A couple may make a rash decision during the heat of passion, which may leave them without a means of preventing pregnancy.

Coitus Interruptus

Coitus interruptus, also called withdrawal, requires the man to pull the penis out of the vagina before ejaculation to avoid depositing sperm in or near the vagina. However, the pre-ejaculate fluid may contain sperm, so pregnancy can still occur. Effectiveness is dependent on the man's ability to withdraw his penis before ejaculation.

One advantage of coitus interruptus is that it provides some level of pregnancy protection when no other method is available. However, the disadvantages are many. This is an unreliable method of birth control, and it offers little, if any, protection from STIs. This method requires a great deal of self-control on the part of a man and is not effective if the man ejaculates prematurely. Ejaculate that is present at the vaginal introitus (opening) can still cause pregnancy.

Lactational Amenorrhea Method

Breast-feeding offers some level of contraceptive protection because elevated prolactin levels help suppress ovulation. The method works best during the first 6 months after childbirth. The woman must breastfeed frequently, every 2 to 3 hours without fail. Advantages of breast-feeding include promotion of weight loss, suppression of menses, and a more

rapid return of the uterus to its prepregnant state. A major disadvantage is that the woman will not know for sure when fertility returns and pregnancy can occur even prior to the onset of her first menstrual cycle after childbirth.

Fertility Awareness Methods

Fertility awareness methods, also known as the rhythm method, refer to all methods that use the identification of fertile and infertile phases of a woman's menstrual cycle to plan or prevent pregnancy. Such methods involve observing and charting the signs and symptoms of the menstrual cycle (e.g., menstrual bleeding, cervical mucus changes, and variations in basal body temperature) to determine the woman's fertile period. The woman then uses abstinence or a barrier contraceptive method during days identified as fertile to reduce the risk of pregnancy. Fertility awareness methods are also effective in planning pregnancy.

Fertility awareness methods require the cooperation of both partners. Advantages of these methods are that they are inexpensive, do not require the use of artificial devices or drugs, and have no harmful side effects. Disadvantages include that the method requires discipline to use and can seem cumbersome for a woman or couple with a busy lifestyle. It also has a high failure rate during the first year with typical use.

A foundational component for practicing fertility awareness methods is knowledge about the menstrual cycle. Guidelines derive from the assumption that ovulation occurs exactly 14 days before the onset of the next menstrual cycle and that the fertile window extends 3 to 4 days before and after ovulation, or in other words, between days 10 and 17 of the menstrual cycle. Five methods used to anticipate the fertile window are as follows:

1. Calendar method
2. Basal body temperature method
3. Cervical mucus method
4. Symptothermal method
5. Standard days method (SDM)

In addition to these five methods, some couples use an ovulation predictor test to determine ovulation and thus the fertile period.

Calendar Method. With the calendar method, fertile days are determined by an accurate charting of the length of the menstrual cycle over a period of 6 months. The woman counts the number of days per cycle, beginning on the first day of menses. The beginning of the fertile period is determined by subtracting 18 days from the length of the shortest cycle. The end of the fertile days is determined by subtracting 11 days from the length of the longest cycle. Box 4-3 gives an example of how to calculate the fertile period using this method. To avoid pregnancy, the couple abstains from sexual intercourse or uses a barrier method during the identified fertile period.

The major drawbacks of this method are that the couple is using data about past cycles to predict what will happen in the future, and they are counting on the regularity of what can be an unpredictable event. In reality, the timing of the fertile period can be highly variable, even for women who think that they have regular cycles. The method is contraindicated for women who do not have regular cycles, such as women who are anovulatory (absence of ovulation), adolescents, women approaching menopause, and women who have recently given birth.

Basal Body Temperature Method. The basal body temperature (BBT) is the lowest normal temperature of a

---

BOX 4-3 **Calculation of Fertile Window Using the Calendar Method**

A woman keeps track of the length of her menstrual cycles for at least 6 months. Then she calculates her fertile window by subtracting 18 days from her shortest cycle and 11 days from her longest cycle. For example, for a woman whose shortest cycle is 24 days and longest cycle is 28 days, the calculation would be as follows.

Shortest Cycle	Longest Cycle
24	28
−18	−11
6	17

Therefore, the woman's fertile window would be days 6 to 17 of her menstrual cycle. She and her partner would then use abstinence or a barrier method to prevent pregnancy during the fertile window.

---

healthy person, taken immediately after waking and before getting out of bed. The BBT method relies on identifying the shift in body temperature that occurs normally around the time of ovulation.

The BBT averages 97.2°F (36.2°C) during menses and for about 5 to 7 days after. At about the time of ovulation, a slight drop in temperature may occur, followed by a slight rise (approximately 0.4°F to 0.7°F or 0.2°C to 0.4°C) after ovulation, in response to increasing progesterone levels. This temperature elevation persists until 2 to 4 days before menstruation. The BBT then drops to the lower levels recorded during the previous cycle, unless pregnancy occurs.

To prevent conception, the couple avoids unprotected intercourse from the day the BBT drops through the fourth day of temperature elevation. The woman must chart the BBT daily on a graph for an entire month to accurately determine a pattern. Confounding factors such as fatigue, infection, anxiety, awakening late, getting fewer than 3 hours sleep, jet lag, alcohol consumption, and sleeping in a heated waterbed or using an electric heating blanket may all cause temperature fluctuation, altering the expected pattern. Because so many factors can interfere, BBT alone is not a reliable method for predicting ovulation. Using BBT along with the calendar or cervical mucus methods increases the effectiveness.

Cervical Mucus Method. The cervical mucus method requires recognition and interpretation of characteristic changes in the amount and consistency of cervical mucus through the menstrual cycle. Accurate assessment of cervical mucus requires that the mucus be free of contraceptive gel or foam, semen, blood, or abnormal vaginal discharge for at least one full cycle.

Before ovulation, cervical mucus is thick and does not stretch easily. This quality inhibits sperm from entering the cervix. Just before ovulation, changes occur that facilitate the viability and motility of sperm, allowing the sperm to survive in a woman's reproductive tract until ovulation. Cervical mucus becomes more abundant and thinner with an elastic quality. It feels somewhat slippery and stretches 5 cm or more between the thumb and forefinger, a quality referred to as spinnbarkeit (Fig. 4-3). These cervical mucus changes indicate the period of maximum fertility.

Observation begins on the last day of menses and repeats several times a day for several cycles. The woman obtains mucus samples at the vaginal introitus, so there is no need to attempt to reach into the vagina to the cervix. Factors that can affect the cervical mucus appearance include the presence of sperm, contraceptive gels or foam, vaginal discharge, use of douches or vaginal deodorants, sexual arousal, and medications, such as antihistamines. Although self-evaluation of cervical mucus can help the woman predict ovulation, this method is more effective when used in combination with the calendar and BBT methods. This method may be unacceptable for the woman who is uncomfortable touching her genitals.

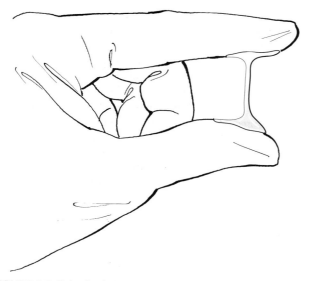

FIGURE 4-3 Spinnbarkeit refers to the stretchable, distensible quality of cervical mucus around the time of ovulation. Some fertility awareness methods (fertility awareness methods) rely on this quality to help determine when ovulation has occurred.

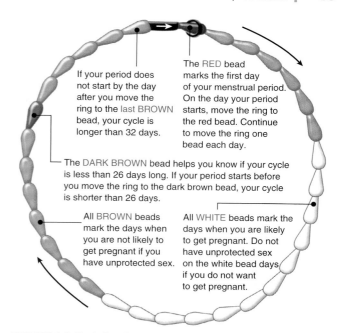

If your period does not start by the day after you move the ring to the last BROWN bead, your cycle is longer than 32 days.

The RED bead marks the first day of your menstrual period. On the day your period starts, move the ring to the red bead. Continue to move the ring one bead each day.

The DARK BROWN bead helps you know if your cycle is less than 26 days long. If your period starts before you move the ring to the dark brown bead, your cycle is shorter than 26 days.

All BROWN beads mark the days when you are not likely to get pregnant if you have unprotected sex.

All WHITE beads mark the days when you are likely to get pregnant. Do not have unprotected sex on the white bead days if you do not want to get pregnant.

FIGURE 4-4 CycleBeads help women use the standard days method.

Symptothermal Method. The symptothermal method is a combination of the calendar, BBT, and cervical mucus methods, along with an awareness of other signs of fertility. The woman acquires fertility awareness as she begins to understand the secondary physiologic and psychological symptoms marking the phases of her cycle. These secondary symptoms include increased libido, mid-cycle spotting, mittelschmerz (unilateral lower abdominal pain in the ovary region associated with ovulation), pelvic fullness or tenderness, and vulvar fullness. The woman may palpate the cervix to assess for changes that normally occur with ovulation. The cervical os dilates slightly, the cervix softens and rises in the vagina, and cervical mucus becomes abundant with a slippery consistency. Calendar calculations and cervical mucus changes are useful to approximate the beginning of the fertile period. Changes in cervical mucus and BBT may predict the end of the fertile period. Some studies have demonstrated a lower failure rate when the woman uses multiple indicators to predict the fertile window.

Standard Days Method. Another fertility awareness method, standard days method (SDM) does not require detailed record keeping or complicated ways to keep track of fertile days. Most women who practice SDM use a special ring of beads to track their cycles (Fig. 4-4). There are 32 beads, each representing a day in the menstrual cycle. The woman moves a rubber ring onto one bead each day. The red bead marks the first day of her period. Brown beads correspond to days when she is likely *not* to get pregnant. These are "safe" days in which to have sexual intercourse. White beads stand for days when she is likely to get pregnant. These are "unsafe" times to have unprotected vaginal intercourse.

For successful use of SDM, the woman must have regular menstrual cycles. Her cycles must never be shorter than 26 days and never longer than 32 days. The beads help her determine if she meets the cycle length criteria.

Ovulation Predictor Test. The ovulation predictor test is a handheld device that detects metabolites of Luteinizing hormone (LH) and estrogen in the urine. LH levels surge during the 12 to 24 hours before ovulation, and the test detects the increase. The home kit supplies testing materials for testing the urine over several days during a cycle. An easily read color change indicates a positive reaction for LH. Currently women use the device to determine ovulation to increase their chance of becoming pregnant. However, research is ongoing to determine the usefulness of the device as a contraceptive method.

Barrier Methods

Barrier methods of contraception provide a physical and/or chemical barrier to prevent sperm from entering the cervical os. Types of barrier methods of contraception include spermicidal gels or foams, condoms, diaphragms, and cervical caps. Spermicidal gels or foams used in conjunction with condoms, diaphragms, or cervical caps increase the effectiveness of barrier methods. Many barrier methods of contraception have the added benefit of providing at least some protection against STIs.

Spermicidal Agents

Vaginal spermicides provide a physical barrier that prevents sperm penetration and a chemical barrier that kills the sperm. The most commonly used chemical spermicide in the United States is nonoxynol-9 (N-9). Spermicides are available as aerosol foams, foaming tablets, suppositories, films, creams, gels, and the contraceptive sponge. Most of these products are designed to be inserted vaginally immediately before or within a few hours before engaging in vaginal sexual intercourse.

Advantages include that this method is readily available without a prescription. Because spermicides can be inserted several hours before vaginal sexual intercourse, the woman can use them discreetly. Some disadvantages are that effectiveness rates are highly variable and spermicides do not protect against the transmission of STIs. The effectiveness of spermicides greatly increases when combined with other physical barrier methods, such as the condom, diaphragm, or cervical cap.

Condoms for Men

Condoms for men are thin, stretchable sheaths that cover the erect penis during sexual intercourse. A condom functions as a contraceptive by collecting semen before, during, and after ejaculation to prevent sperm from entering the vagina and causing pregnancy. The majority of condoms are made of latex rubber, although a small percentage is composed of other substances, such as natural membrane or polyurethane. Some condoms manufactured include different shapes and the addition of lubricants and spermicides. One feature related to shape is the presence or absence of a sperm reservoir tip. Some condoms are contoured, are rippled, or have a roughened surface to enhance vaginal stimulation. A thinner sheath increases heat transmission and penile sensitivity. Some condoms provide lubrication with a wet jelly or a dry powder and some have spermicide added to the interior or exterior surface. Effectiveness is dependent upon correct and consistent application and usage. Tips for Reinforcing Family Teaching: Safe Condom Use provides guidelines for use.

TIPS FOR REINFORCING FAMILY TEACHING

Safe Condom Use

Putting on a Condom

Following these steps, put the condom on as soon as the penis is erect and before any genital contact is made.

- Retract the foreskin if not circumcised.
- Press out the tip of the condom to remove air bubbles and to leave a 1/2-in space at the end (Fig. A).

- Holding the tip of the condom, carefully roll it down the shaft of the erect penis (Fig. B).
- Be certain that the condom covers the full length of the penis, with the rim of the condom at the base of the penis (Fig. C).

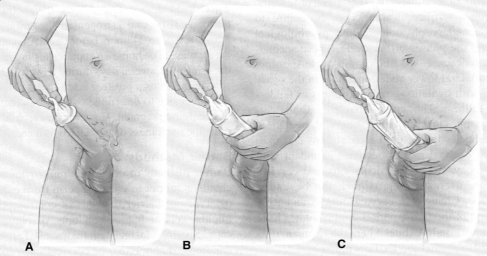

A   B   C

Instructions for Condom Usage

- Use a new condom each time.
- Heat can damage condoms. Store them in a cool, dry place out of direct sunlight.
- Handle condoms carefully to avoid damaging them with fingernails, teeth, or other sharp objects.
- Do not use a condom after its expiration date. Condoms in damaged packages or condoms that show obvious signs of deterioration (e.g., brittleness, stickiness, or discoloration) should not be used, regardless of the expiration date.
- The most effective type of condom for birth control is prelubricated latex with a tip or reservoir pretreated with nonoxynol-9 spermicide.
- If the condom is not pretreated, you may lubricate the inside by placing a few drops of water or water-based lubricant such as K-Y Jelly and a spermicidal jelly or foam containing nonoxynol-9 into the condom.

- Lubricate the outside of the condom as much as desired with a water-soluble lubricant.
- Do not use oil-based products such as mineral oil, massage oil, body lotions, cooking oil, shortening, or petroleum jelly for lubrication; they weaken the latex and decrease the effectiveness of the condom.
- If the condom starts to slip during intercourse, hold it on. Do not let it slip off. Condoms come in sizes, so if there is a problem with slipping, look for a different size.
- After ejaculation, hold the rim of the condom at the base of the penis and withdraw before losing the erection.
- Remove the condom and tie a knot in the open end. Dispose of it so that no one can come in contact with semen.
- Immediately after intercourse, both partners should wash off any semen or vaginal secretions with soap and water.

One significant advantage of condom use is the protection provided against STIs. Individuals may use condoms as an additional protective measure against the transmission of HIV and other STIs in conjunction with another method of contraception (such as oral contraceptive drugs or barrier methods). Other advantages include low cost, easy availability (over-the-counter), no need for a visit to a health care provider, and that application of condoms can be part of sexual play. Some men find condom use helpful in preventing premature ejaculation or maintaining an erection for a longer period.

There are also disadvantages. The condom can break, which decreases its effectiveness. Some couples find that condoms decrease sexual sensation. Some individuals perceive the use of condoms as inhibiting spontaneity, or the man may feel self-conscious. Another potential disadvantage is latex allergy; however, polyurethane condoms can be used instead.

Condoms for Women

Condoms for women, or vaginal sheaths, are thin tubes made of polyurethane, with flexible rings at both ends (Fig. 4-5). The closed end is inserted into the vagina and anchored around the cervix. The open end covers the labia. Like condoms for men, condoms for women collect sperm before, during, and after ejaculation to protect against pregnancy and STIs. The woman can apply the condom before intercourse, a feature that may increase spontaneity. She can also add a spermicide, if not already present. Condoms for women come in one size and, like condoms for men, are available without a prescription.

Advantages of condoms for women are that they can be inserted before intercourse, an erection is not necessary to keep the condom in place, individuals who are allergic to latex can use them, and the external ring may supply clitoral stimulation. Reported disadvantages are that the condom may be difficult to apply, make noise, or cause vaginal or penile irritation. Another disadvantage is that it may slip into the vagina during vigorous intercourse, which will decrease its effectiveness.

Diaphragm and Cervical Cap

The diaphragm is a shallow dome-shaped latex rubber device with a flexible, circular wire rim that fits over the cervix. A diaphragm works by mechanically blocking sperm from entering the cervix.

Diaphragms are available by prescription in a wide range of diameters. They require special fitting by a trained health care provider. The woman must apply spermicidal jelly or cream to the rim and center of the diaphragm before inserting and positioning the diaphragm over the cervix (Fig. 4-6). A diaphragm may be inserted several hours before intercourse, and it must be left in place over the cervix for at least 6 hours afterward to allow the spermicide time to destroy the sperm. If the device is inserted and more than 6 hours pass before sexual intercourse, or if intercourse is repeated, the woman should leave the diaphragm in place

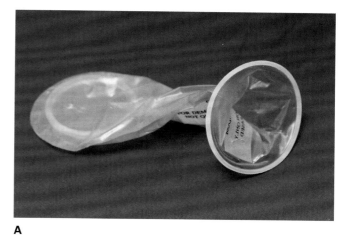

A

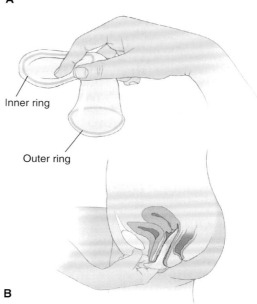

Inner ring

Outer ring

B

FIGURE 4-5 **A.** Condom for women. **B.** Insertion technique.

and insert another application of spermicidal cream, jelly, or foam into the vagina. The woman should not leave a diaphragm in place for longer than 24 hours.

The cervical cap is much smaller than the diaphragm and is available in four sizes. Its rubber dome has a firm, pliable rim that fits snugly around the base of the cervix, close to the junction of the cervix and the vaginal fornices. The device should remain in place 6 to 8 hours after the last act of intercourse, but no longer than 48 hours. The seal of the cap provides a mechanical barrier. Spermicide applied in the center of the cap provides an additional chemical barrier.

Another Application Is Necessary

The woman must insert additional spermicidal jelly, cream, or foam into the vagina if she has intercourse again within 6 hours. With the cervical cap, using additional spermicide for repeated episodes of intercourse is optional.

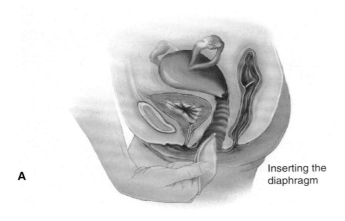

A — Inserting the diaphragm

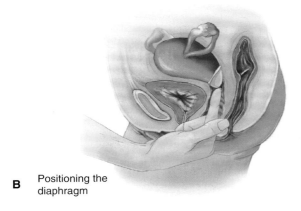

B — Positioning the diaphragm

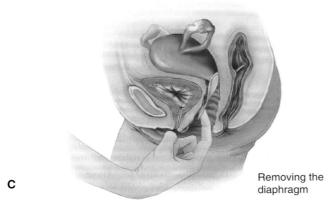

C — Removing the diaphragm

FIGURE 4-6 Application of a diaphragm. **A.** To insert, fold the diaphragm in half, separate the labia with one hand, and then insert upward and back into the vagina. **B.** To position, make certain the diaphragm securely covers the cervix. **C.** To remove, hook a finger over the top of the rim and bring the diaphragm down and out.

The typical failure rates for both devices are similar for the woman who has never had a vaginal delivery. However, the failure rate of the cervical cap in the woman who has delivered children vaginally is quite high, even with perfect use. A health care provider must specifically fit the diaphragm or cervical cap to each woman. Both devices require refitting after pregnancy (whether it ends in miscarriage, abortion, or delivery), abdominal or pelvic surgery, or weight gain or loss of 10 lb (4.5 kg) or more. The woman must learn how to insert and remove the cap or diaphragm correctly and to verify proper placement. Before insertion, the woman should check either device for pinholes or weakened areas by holding it up to the light.

Typical advantages for the use of diaphragms and cervical caps are that both devices offer some protection against STIs and PID. Both may be inserted ahead of time and are not easily felt by either partner. Both methods are safe for use during breast-feeding and are immediately reversible.

Disadvantages unique to the diaphragm are that some sexual positions, penis sizes, and vigorous thrusting techniques can dislodge the device during intercourse, which decreases its effectiveness. Some women develop frequent bladder infections or cannot use the diaphragm because of poor vaginal tone. Disadvantages of both methods are that they can be difficult to insert, the woman must feel comfortable touching her genitals, and she must have the device on hand for all instances of vaginal intercourse. Also, there is a risk for infection if the woman leaves either of these devices in for longer than recommended periods of time.

Hormonal Methods

Hormonal methods of contraception include oral contraceptive drugs, implants, injections, vaginal estrogen/progestin (contraceptive) ring, and transdermal patches. Oral contraceptive drugs, also known as "the pill," are the most commonly used reversible method of contraception (Daniels and Abma, 2018). Depending on their hormonal composition, hormonal methods may prevent or suppress ovulation and may thicken cervical mucus, making it resistant to sperm penetration.

Advantages of hormonal contraceptive drugs are that they are highly effective in preventing pregnancy when used consistently and correctly. In addition, hormonal methods may provide noncontraceptive health benefits, such as menstrual cycle improvements, management of dysmenorrhea, and protection against certain cancers, ovarian cysts, and acne.

Although efficacious in preventing pregnancy, there are disadvantages to the use of hormonal methods of contraception. Many new users discontinue hormonal methods during the first year of use because of experienced or perceived side effects. In addition, hormonal contraceptive drugs do not offer protection from STIs, including HIV, for either partner. Therefore, the couple must use condoms if they desire STI protection.

Oral Contraceptive Pills

Oral contraceptive pills (OCPs) can be monophasic or phasic. Monophasic pills provide fixed doses of estrogen and progestin, whereas phasic pills (biphasic, triphasic, and multiphasic) are formulated to alter the amount of progestin, and in some cases, estrogen, within each cycle. Phasic preparations reduce the total dosage of hormones in a cycle without sacrificing effectiveness. Typically, a pill is taken daily throughout the cycle (Fig. 4-7A). The last 7 pills of the 28-pill pack are inert but help maintain the habit of taking the daily pill. Menstruation occurs during the time the woman takes the inert pills. Some health care providers prescribe longer regimens of OCPs to suppress menstruation while also providing birth control. The woman must take the pill at the same time each day for it to be effective.

If taken daily as prescribed, OCPs provide a high contraception effectiveness rate. In addition, OCP therapy offers many noncontraceptive benefits, in particular menstrual cycle improvements, including a decrease in menstrual blood loss, reduction in the occurrence of iron-deficiency anemia, regulation of irregular cycles, lessening of the symptoms of dysmenorrhea (painful menstrual periods), and lower incidence of PMS. OCPs offer protection against endometrial and ovarian cancer. They are associated with a reduced incidence of benign breast disease, protection against the development of functional ovarian cysts and some types of PID, and a decreased risk for ectopic pregnancy (Kaunitz, 2020).

Disadvantages of OCPs include that they do not offer any protection from HIV and other STIs. In addition, the woman must remember to take the pill at the same time every day. A large percentage of women stop using OCPs because of side effects. Common side effects include nausea, headache, breast tenderness, weight gain, breakthrough spotting or bleeding, and amenorrhea. These side effects usually decrease over time and are less common with lower dose preparations. OCPs may promote growth of estrogen-dependent breast cancer, although they probably do not cause breast cancer. Another disadvantage is the expense. Oral contraceptive drugs require a visit to the health care provider and are available by prescription only.

Some women should not use OCPs, or should use them only with great caution. Box 4-4 outlines contraindications for their use. Instruct the woman to report any preexisting health problems, any change in health that may affect her use of OCPs, and the occurrence of any warning signs, including severe abdominal or chest pain, dyspnea, headache, weakness, numbness, blurred or double vision, speech disturbances, or severe leg pain and edema (Box 4-5).

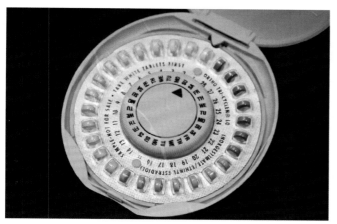

A

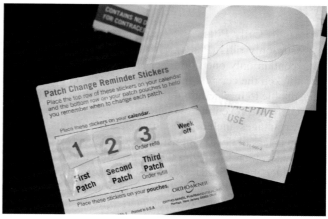

B

C

FIGURE 4-7 Hormonal contraceptive agents. **A.** Oral contraceptive drugs. **B.** Transdermal contraceptive patch. **C.** Vaginal contraceptive ring.

Progestin-Only Pills

Progestin-only pills (POPs), also referred to as the "mini-pill," contain only one hormone, progestin. Its major effect is to thicken the cervical mucus and make the endometrium inhospitable to implantation. POPs are slightly less effective than OCPs in preventing ovulation.

Advantages include no estrogen side effects, so the woman is less likely to quit using the contraceptive drugs. In addition, women for whom OCPs are contraindicated (e.g., those older than 35 years who also smoke and those who have a history of thrombophlebitis) may take POPs. There are no "hormone-free" days or inert pills to take, so the woman can maintain a daily routine of taking the same pill every day. The woman who is lactating can take POPs after the newborn is 6 weeks old. POPs decrease dysmenorrhea and the pain sometimes associated with ovulation.

Menstrual irregularities are one disadvantage of POPs, although periods are usually very short and scanty, which some women find desirable. The woman must take POPs every day at the same time of day without fail because their main action (thickening cervical mucus) lasts only 22 to 24 hours. As with OCPs, POPs do not provide STI protection and require a health care provider visit and a prescription.

Hormonal Injections

One type of injectable hormonal contraceptive is available in the United States. Depot medroxyprogesterone acetate (DMPA) is a progestin-only agent. It provides a level of contraceptive protection similar to that of POPs. As with other hormonal contraceptive methods, DMPA does not provide protection against STIs.

DMPA consists of a slow-release form of progestin that prevents ovulation. Intramuscular injections provide 3 months of protection. The health care provider administers the first injection within 7 days of the onset of menses. After that, the woman must schedule appointments every 13 weeks for an injection. A lower dose subcutaneous form of DMPA is available.

Take It Easy!
When administering an injection of DMPA, do not massage the site. This could hasten absorption of the hormone and cause a shorter period of effective contraception.

Advantages are that the woman does not have to remember to take a pill on a daily basis, and she does not have to use a product at the time of sexual intercourse. DMPA provides the woman with a high level of privacy. No one has to know she is using this method of birth control, unless she chooses to share this information. Lactating mothers and women who cannot take estrogen products can use DMPA. Other advantages include decreased risk of endometrial cancer and improvement of PMS and the pain associated with endometriosis.

Disadvantages include prolonged amenorrhea. Many women stop menstruating after the third DMPA injection. This effect is not harmful, and some women may even consider it an advantage. In addition to menstrual irregularities, the most common side effects are weight gain, headache, and nervousness. Sometimes depression and premenstrual symptoms worsen. Another potential disadvantage is the length of time it takes (an average of 10 months) before fertility returns after discontinuing the method. DMPA may lower the woman's estrogen levels, leading to loss of bone mineral density and increased risk of fractures. Contraindications for using DMPA include pregnancy, history of breast cancer, stroke, and liver disease.

Hormonal Implant

The hormonal implant currently available in the United States is the etonogestrel or single-rod progestin implant. The implant is a progestin-only, flexible plastic rod about the size of a matchstick. The health care provider inserts the rod using local anesthesia just under the skin on the inside of the upper arm. Insertion takes approximately 1 minute. Removal requires a small incision and takes about 3 minutes. Contraceptive protection is evident for 3 years.

The implant is an extremely effective method of birth control. Advantages include having no daily pills to remember and no interference with sexual activity to use the method. Fertility returns quickly (within a month) after the implant is removed. The implant frequently improves symptoms of dysmenorrhea, does not have an effect on bone density like DMPA does, and appears to be safe for lactating women.

Disadvantages include unscheduled bleeding, which is the most common reason women stop using this method of birth control; headache; weight gain; and acne. The implant does not provide protection from STIs.

Transdermal Patch

The transdermal contraceptive patch supplies continuous levels of estrogen and progestin (see Fig. 4-7B). It is available only as a prescription. The woman places the patch on the lower abdomen, upper outer arm, buttock, or upper torso (excluding the breasts) on the first day of her menstrual period. She then applies a new patch every week for 3 weeks and then removes it for 1 week to allow menses to occur. The woman should apply each new patch on the same day of the week and should not wear more than one patch at a time.

Individuals who use the patch are more likely to be compliant with the method than with oral contraceptive drugs because there is no daily requirement. It is a highly effective form of birth control. Disadvantages include decreased effectiveness in women who weigh more than 198 lb (89.8 kg). The most common side effects include breast symptoms, application site reactions, and headache. Women are at increased risk for venous thromboembolism and cardiovascular risks. Women who smoke and women who are breast-feeding should not use the transdermal patch. The transdermal patch does not protect the woman from STIs.

Vaginal Estrogen/Progestin (Contraceptive) Ring

The vaginal estrogen/progestin (contraceptive) ring is a soft, flexible ring, approximately 5 cm in diameter, that contains estrogen and progestin (see Fig. 4-7C). The woman places the ring into the vagina once a month, during which time it releases low levels of hormones. Lower dosing is possible because of the location of the ring in the vagina. After 21 days (3 weeks), the woman removes the ring to allow menstruation.

Advantages include low estrogen exposure with high effectiveness. There is a low incidence of hormone-related side effects such as headaches, nausea, and breast tenderness. It is easy to insert and generally discreet to use. Disadvantages include that a woman must feel comfortable touching her genitals, some women or their partners may be able to sense the ring during intercourse, the ring may slip out during intercourse, and the device may cause increased vaginal discharge. The vaginal estrogen/progestin (contraceptive) ring does not protect the woman from STIs.

Intrauterine Device

The intrauterine device (IUD) is a small T-shaped device that the health care provider inserts into the uterine cavity (Fig. 4-8). There are two types of IUDs. The first is a nonhormonal copper device and the other type contains the hormone progestin, which is slowly released over a long period of time. The copper-bearing device is effective for up to 10 years, and the progestin-releasing devices for 5 years. As a safety measure, IUDs are radiopaque (can be seen on x-ray). Each month, the woman must check for presence of the string in the vagina to confirm continued placement of

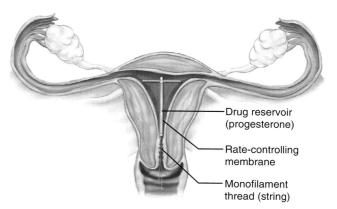

FIGURE 4-8 An intrauterine device in place in the uterus.

the device. The device must be removed by the health care provider and not by the woman.

The copper-bearing IUD acts by damaging sperm in transit through the uterus. Few viable sperm are able to reach the ovum, thus preventing fertilization. The progestin-bearing device makes the cervical mucus inhospitable to sperm and also prevents development of the endometrial lining. The IUD typically causes no disruption of ovulation. The absence of estrogen makes the copper IUD a more appropriate contraceptive for women older than 35 years; for heavy smokers; and for women with hypertension, vascular disease, or familial diabetes.

> **You Can Help Inform the Woman**
>
> The copper in the IUD decreases the effectiveness of sperm. The progestin in the hormonal IUD makes it hard for the sperm to penetrate the cervical mucus and also prevents the endometrial lining from developing each month.

The IUD offers continuous protection from unwanted pregnancy without the need to remember a daily pill or to interrupt sex for contraception use. Placement of the IUD can occur at any time during the menstrual cycle after obtaining a negative pregnancy test. It is effective for use immediately after childbirth or after an abortion. When the woman wants to become pregnant, the health care provider removes the device, and fertility returns. The progestin-bearing device offers the added benefits of decreasing dysmenorrhea and is useful for decreasing bleeding in women with menorrhagia (abnormally long or heavy menstrual periods).

Side effects include cramping and bleeding upon insertion of the device. Common reasons for removal of the copper device include dysmenorrhea and increased menstrual flow. Headache, breast tenderness, and acne are common side effects of the progestin-releasing device. Risks include uterine perforation and accidental device expulsion. The IUD offers no protection against STIs. Box 4-6 outlines signs of complications with IUD use.

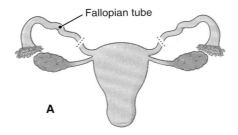

A

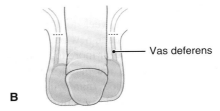

B

FIGURE 4-9 **A.** Tubal ligation. **B.** Vasectomy.

Sterilization

Sterilization is a permanent method of birth control performed via a surgical procedure. Although in some instances reversal may be accomplished, the procedure to do so is expensive and often not successful. Therefore, those who choose surgical sterilization procedures should consider them permanent methods of birth control.

Sterilization in Women

Sterilization in women is accomplished by tubal ligation or tubal occlusion. Tubal ligation involves tying the fallopian tubes and then cutting the tubes into two parts. Tubal occlusion involves application of bands or clips via laparoscopy (Fig. 4-9A). The surgeon makes a small vertical incision in the abdominal wall near the umbilicus, brings each tube through the incision, and then performs ligation, clip application, or cauterization of the tube. Regional or general anesthesia is required. Oral analgesic medications are usually sufficient to relieve postoperative discomfort. Sterilization of women is a minor surgical procedure, and the postoperative recovery period is about 1 to 2 days. The woman should report bleeding or signs of infection. The procedure may be done immediately after giving birth (within 24 to 48 hours), at the time of an abortion, or during any phase of the menstrual cycle.

Sterilization in Men

Sterilization in men, called vasectomy, can be performed using local anesthesia in an outpatient setting. The procedure takes about 20 minutes to perform. The health care provider makes a small incision on each side of the scrotum over the spermatic cord. The next step is ligation and cutting of each vas deferens (Fig. 4-9B). The cut ends of the vas deferens may be cauterized and then buried in the scrotal fascia to reduce the chance of spontaneous re-anastomosis. Closure of the skin incisions completes the procedure, and a dressing may be applied.

The man should expect some pain, bruising, and swelling of the scrotum after the procedure. Effective comfort measures include rest, application of an ice pack, scrotal support, and a mild oral analgesic medication. The health care provider usually recommends moderate inactivity for 1 to 2 days because of scrotal tenderness. The man should report any signs of bleeding or infection.

The man may resume sexual intercourse as desired; however, with vasectomy, loss of fertility is not immediate because sperm remain in the system distal to the ligation. It takes approximately 1 month for the remaining sperm to be eliminated from the man's system. Therefore, it is necessary

for the couple to use another method of birth control until a negative sperm count verifies sterility. Vasectomy has no effect on the man's ability to achieve or maintain erection or on the volume of ejaculate. In addition, there is no interference with the production of testosterone, so secondary sexual characteristics are not affected.

Remember Sondra Simone. What information would you want to know about her past contraceptive choices and use that may help in understanding her concerns about not being pregnant at this time?

Emergency Contraception

Emergency contraception (EC) refers to methods used to reduce the risk of pregnancy in the event of unprotected sexual intercourse or if the birth control being used failed (e.g., the condom breaks, the man did not pull out in time). The sooner the woman uses EC after the unprotected intercourse, the more effective it is at preventing pregnancy. EC should not be the only method of birth control a woman uses. It is much more effective to use a consistent form of birth control. EC does not protect against STIs.

There are several oral medications approved for EC. Levonorgestrel is a one-dose over-the-counter treatment that the woman takes within the first 72 hours after the unprotected intercourse. The other medications are available with a prescription from a health care provider, are either a one- or two-dose treatment, and must be started between 72 and 120 hours after the unprotected intercourse. EC medications work to prevent pregnancy by either delaying or inhibiting ovulation or by preventing implantation in the endometrium.

Regardless of the EC medication used, the woman should also restart her initial birth control right away or use another form of birth control, as her fertility can return rapidly and she can get pregnant with subsequent unprotected acts of intercourse.

Another form of EC is the insertion of a copper IUD, which can be inserted up to 5 days after unprotected intercourse. One advantage of this method is that it is very effective at preventing pregnancy and it provides long-term protection. A woman who has an active STI or who is at high risk for STIs should not use this form of EC.

Nursing Process and Care Plan
for Assisting the Client With Choosing a Contraceptive Method

Providing care related to contraception is a collaborative process, involving a variety of healthcare personnel. The nurse often works alongside a physician, certified nurse-midwife, nurse practitioner, family planning counselor, or social worker. Roles for each team member may vary across settings and may overlap within a specific setting. The nurse may be involved in history taking, reinforcing teaching, counseling, and/or assisting during the physical examination. Components essential to providing quality care include clear communication among team members and clear protocols for data collection, counseling, and information to be given.

Steps toward developing excellence in nursing practice include clarifying personal feelings about family planning, maintaining a current knowledge base through independent study and continuing education activities, awareness of current standards of practice, and striving to avoid allowing personal prejudices to influence nursing care. Application of the nursing process provides a framework for working with clients desiring a method of contraception.

Assessment (Data Collection)

Assessment is an essential initial step for identifying the needs and desires of the client regarding contraception. Data collection should be done in an unhurried and accepting atmosphere with adequate privacy to make the client feel comfortable. It is important to treat the client with respect even when their feelings and beliefs differ from your personal perspective. This step of the nursing process includes gathering physiologic, psychoemotional, sociocultural, and cognitive data related to the issue of preventing pregnancy.

The health care provider takes the client's medical, reproductive, and contraceptive history. Examples of contraception-related questions include the following:

- What types of contraception were used in the past?
- What, if any, problems occurred?
- What did the couple like or dislike about the method?
- What factors contributed to discontinuing the previous method?

The health care provider also performs a physical examination, which includes a general medical examination, a complete gynecologic examination, and routine diagnostic laboratory testing. This information assists in identifying any contraindications to a specific birth control method.

Psychoemotional data include information about the client's feelings regarding sexuality, family planning needs in general, and specific methods of contraception. To develop a long-range plan of care, it is important to discuss goals for family planning and how they align with her partner's goals. Family planning includes the number of children the couple wants and the preferred spacing of those children. The client's perception of her partner's support is a major predictor of her use, or nonuse, of any particular method and therefore should be evaluated. Other important issues helpful in identifying the optimal contraceptive method include the client's self-image, level of comfort with her body, and willingness to touch her genitals.

Sociocultural issues such as family background, religious beliefs, or culture may influence the couple's compliance with a particular method for contraception. It is important to identify myths regarding contraception and also cultural views on contraception and childbearing. Information about the nature of the client's sexual activity, such as the number of partners and her desire for partner involvement in contraception should be identified. In some cultures, discussion of sexual matters is taboo or may be a source of embarrassment, which may impede the data gathering process. The relationship between the client and her partner, and their communication, also influences the choice and subsequent use of contraception. Financial issues may also influence the choice of contraceptive method.

Data gathering related to emotional or sociocultural needs should take place in a private area. This allows the client to freely express feelings, opinions, and concerns related to contraception. It also allows for privacy to answer questions about intimate, personal aspects of her life. It is important for the nurse to establish a trusting relationship with the client, provide an accepting atmosphere, and remain sensitive to the client's needs and concerns. It is appropriate to explore religious, cultural, social, and financial concerns. This knowledge enables the nurse to assist the client with choosing a contraceptive method.

 Cultural Snapshot

It is important to identify the client's cultural views related to contraception, pregnancy, and childbirth. If their culture places a high value on fertility and views lack of fertility as shameful, such as in the Swazi culture, then the client most likely will not seek out or utilize contraception. If the main decision maker about the spacing of children is the man, then the woman will be less likely to seek contraception. In some cultures, such as the Navajo people, and religions, such as Members of the Church of Jesus Christ for Latter-Day Saints, children are highly valued and importance is placed on having many children. Women who choose contraception in these cases may choose a method that is not apparent to men, such as IUD or injections. However, the client who chooses contraception against the will of their significant other may be at increased risk for intimate partner violence and should be screened.

Cognitive issues include the client's level of understanding about the reproductive cycle and knowledge of the different types of birth control available. The client's knowledge base regarding contraception is often based upon various nonmedical sources including friends, popular magazines, television, or the internet. Some of their information may be incomplete or incorrect. Identifying educational needs can be done as part of an interview or by using assessment questionnaires. This helps the nurse to understand the client's knowledge about contraception and personal preferences and identify any misconceptions that need to be clarified.

Nursing Care Focus

When selecting a nursing care focus for the client seeking contraception, consideration should be given to the client's existing knowledge about different contraceptive options. It is also important to recognize the client may have internal conflict related to their choice of contraception. This conflict may be related to the different view of their contraceptive choice and their religion and culture, or the unwillingness of their partner to agree with the choice of contraception, or possible side effects of contraceptive choice. This internal conflict can lead to nonadherence with the contraception.

Outcome Identification and Planning

Major goals for the client seeking contraception include that the client will verbalize adequate knowledge of the reproductive cycle and contraceptive method of choice. Goals also include that the client will choose a method of contraception they are comfortable with using and will use. The ideal contraception will be one that is acceptable to the client, that is effective, and that will be used consistently and correctly. Plan other goals and interventions according to the individual needs of the client.

Nursing Care Focus

- Knowledge deficiency related to contraception choice and use

Goal

- The client will demonstrate knowledge retention related to available contraceptive methods and use of chosen method.

Implementations for Knowledge Deficiency

Nursing implementations to address knowledge deficiency are initially focused on reinforcing teaching. Having the client teach-back the information to the nurse is an effective way to measure the client's understanding of the information.

Reinforcing Teaching

Reinforce teaching in an unbiased manner, dispelling myths and misinformation and providing needed information. Some individuals may not be comfortable discussing sexual matters in group settings; therefore, individual discussions

are more effective. It is most important to provide complete and accurate information. Any reinforcement of teaching related to contraceptive methods should include the following information:

- A description of the method, including an example or illustration
- The mode of action, showing how the method acts to prevent pregnancy
- The effectiveness or failure rate of the method and causes for method failure
- Requirements for use, such as how to obtain and use the method, any precautions to take, and if any follow-up appointments are needed
- Possible effects on sexual intercourse, such as when the method should be implemented in relation to coitus, and possible effects on coitus
- Advantages and disadvantages of the method
- Risks, contraindications, side effects, drug interactions, warning signs, and any factors related to safe use
- Effectiveness of the method to protect against STIs and HIV
- Reversibility of the method, including how to discontinue the method and the length of time until the return of fertility

Assisting With Follow-Up

After the client has chosen a method, follow-up is important to determine satisfaction with the method and ability to use the method correctly. Often a follow-up telephone call is appropriate. Ask the client if they are satisfied with the chosen method. Inquire about any adverse effects or any problems they are having that might cause them to quit using the method. Have the client explain the steps of the chosen method and correct any misperceptions the client may have or misuse of the method. Future office visits provide opportunities to reinforce teaching.

Evaluation of Goal/Desired Outcome

- The client identifies different methods of contraception available for use.
- The client verbalizes the steps in using chosen method of contraception.
- The client utilizes contraception correctly.

Nursing Care Focus

- Nonadherance to contraceptive therapy related to knowledge deficiency and internal conflict.

Goal

- The client will use the chosen contraception consistently.

Implementations for Nonadherance

It is important for the nurse to be nonjudgmental when the client is not adhering to the method of contraception that was chosen. To assist the client in adhering to the method, the nurse must first explore factors leading to the method of contraception not being used or being used incorrectly or inconsistently. Questions to ask include:

- What was the main factor that led to not using the method?
- Did client experience any side effects from the method?
- Was the client's partner unsatisfied with or unwilling to participate in, the method?

Reinforcement of teaching should continue. This includes answering any questions the client has about the contraceptive choice. To reinforce teaching it may be necessary to provide appropriate education materials such as pamphlets, educational sheets, or written step-by-step instructions for contraceptive use. It is also important to ask the client how they learn best. It may be that the client initially was given written information but does not learn from written materials, or is illiterate. In this case, the written materials provided were ineffective for the client's learning needs.

Ask the client if they received additional information on the contraception from friends or relatives. If so, clarify any misconceptions or myths regarding the contraception and pregnancy. Determine if another method of contraception might be more desirable for the client to use.

Determine any barriers the client might have for using the contraception, and develop methods to reduce barriers. For example, if a barrier is financial reasons, refer to appropriate community resources to assist with obtaining the contraception. Or if a barrier is their partner's cooperation or acceptance of the method, it would be important to meet with the couple to discuss contraception.

Evaluation of Goal/Desired Outcome

- The client states they will use contraception.
- The client utilizes chosen contraception consistently.

TEST YOURSELF

✔ Describe the difference between barrier and hormonal methods of birth control.

✔ List one advantage and one disadvantage to the use of coitus interruptus as a birth control method.

✔ List one fertility awareness method, two barrier, and two hormonal methods of birth control.

ABORTION

An **induced abortion** (medical abortion) is the purposeful termination of a pregnancy. A **spontaneous abortion** is another medical term for early pregnancy loss (miscarriage) and is a pregnancy that ends before the fetus reaches the limit (age) of viability at 20 weeks' gestation.

The type of abortion procedure used depends on the length of the pregnancy. Within 8 weeks from conception, a woman may opt for medical or surgical procedures to terminate pregnancy (Table 4-2). Between the 8th and 12th weeks, the health care provider may elect to use dilatation and curettage (D&C). The procedure used for abortions after 12 weeks is dilatation and evacuation. After 20 weeks' gestation, there are other techniques used including methods to induce labor.

Nursing care roles and responsibilities vary, depending upon the setting, method of abortion used, and the woman's needs. In some settings, the nurse and physician may be the only health care providers involved. In others, care providers may include social workers or counselors. In either situation, the nurse's role is central to achieving optimal client care outcomes. It is important to examine your personal beliefs and values related to abortion before assuming responsibility for the care of women choosing to have an abortion. You must be able to provide compassionate and nonjudgmental care.

Document the amount and characteristics of bleeding after the abortion procedure. Save anything that appears to be tissue or clots. A pad count with an estimation of pad saturation provides a more accurate record of blood loss. Assess the woman's vital signs frequently, as for other postoperative care, observing for signs and symptoms of hypovolemic shock. The physician usually orders hematocrit testing before discharge. The woman who is Rh-negative needs a dose of Rh-immune globulin.

Postabortion information should include information about signs and symptoms of possible complications, including elevated temperature, continued/excessive vaginal bleeding, malodorous vaginal discharge, and back or abdominal pain. The woman should report any of these symptoms immediately to the health care provider. Advise the woman to delay sexual intercourse for 1 to 2 weeks. Contraception information and instructions about follow-up care and appointments are important.

INFERTILITY

Infertility is the inability to conceive after a year or more of regular and unprotected intercourse or the inability to carry a pregnancy to term. Infertility affects approximately 10% of women in the United States (Office on Women's Health). There are two main types of infertility: primary and secondary. A couple who has never been able to conceive has primary infertility, whereas a couple who has been able to conceive in the past but is currently unable to do so has secondary infertility.

Causes of Infertility

For conception to occur, many factors have to work together perfectly. Viable sperm must enter a woman's reproductive tract. The passageway through the woman's cervix, uterus, and fallopian tubes has to be clear for sperm to negotiate the journey toward the egg. Ovulation has to occur. The egg must enter a fallopian tube. Fertilization of the egg must occur within 12 to 24 hours after ovulation before it begins

TABLE 4-2 Selected Induced Abortion (Medical Abortion) Techniques

METHOD	PROCEDURE	SPECIAL CONSIDERATIONS
Surgical Techniques		
Menstrual aspiration	Aspiration of the endometrial cavity with a flexible cannula and syringe	• Possible complications include missing the implanted zygote (pregnancy continues), unrecognized ectopic pregnancy, and uterine perforation (rare)
Dilatation and curettage (D&C)	1. Dilation (dilatation) of the cervix with a blunt instrument or laminaria 2. Scraping of the endometrium and removal of uterine contents with a sharp instrument called a curette 3. Suction to aspirate uterine contents, as needed	• Primary procedure used in the United States • Possible complications include uterine perforation, cervical laceration, hemorrhage, incomplete removal of products of conception, and infection
Dilatation and evacuation (D&E)	Procedure is similar to D&C; however, D&E requires wider dilation (dilatation) of the cervix to facilitate removal	• Complications are the same as for D&C
Medical Technique		
Medications taken orally and vaginally		For all medical procedures the woman will experience vaginal bleeding and cramping. Other physical symptoms the woman may experience include nausea, fever, diarrhea, or headache.
	Oral dose of mifepristone and misoprostol Oral dose of mifepristone and vaginal misoprostol	• Used for terminations under 8 weeks • Complications include hemorrhage secondary to incomplete expulsion of pregnancy or rupture of an unrecognized tubal pregnancy
	Vaginal misoprostol	• Effective if used before 9 weeks • Used alone is less effective than if used in combination with other medical abortion medications
	Methotrexate and vaginal misoprostol	• More often used for ectopic pregnancies than induced abortions • May take up to a month to complete the abortion

to disintegrate. After fertilization, the egg must travel down the fallopian tube to the uterus and implant. Any factor that prevents the sperm and egg from meeting or interferes with the fertilized egg traveling to or implanting in the uterine lining can result in infertility.

If a couple is having trouble conceiving, it is helpful for them to review their health histories to identify risk factors for infertility (Box 4-7). Risk factors specific to women include any condition or situation that interferes with ovulation, patency of the cervix or fallopian tubes, or ability of the fertilized ovum to implant in the uterine lining. Risk factors specific to men include anything that can cause decreased or abnormal sperm production or any factor that prevents sperm from being deposited in the woman's reproductive tract.

 Concept Mastery Alert

Surgical repair of cryptorchidism before puberty does not affect fertility in men. There is more risk associated with men who work at a desk job since their sedentary work raises the risk of becoming overweight. It also raises the risk of raising the temperature of the scrotum and of having constricting clothing around the scrotum. These factors can reduce sperm production.

Initial Evaluation of Infertility

Frequently, the client presents when the woman has been unable to conceive. The health care provider performs the initial evaluation. If complex problems exist, or the problem is not readily identifiable, the health care provider refers the client to a reproductive endocrinologist for additional evaluation and treatment.

 A Personal Glimpse

My husband and I had been married 5 years when we decided to start a family. I tried to get pregnant for 8 months without success. My aunt advised me to get a physical examination. Reluctantly, I called to make an appointment. The physician couldn't see me for several months, so I booked the appointment with the women's health nurse practitioner. She performed a thorough physical examination. She told me that nothing appeared to be wrong with my reproductive tract. She said that many couples don't get pregnant right away. She instructed me that healthy living habits were good not only for a healthy heart, but also for a healthy reproductive tract. She advised me to start a regular program of exercise and to eat a well-balanced diet. She told me that stress can interfere with getting pregnant, and she referred me for yoga lessons after I indicated to her that I had always wanted to learn yoga. I followed her advice, and 6 months later I was pregnant.

Sylvia

Learning Opportunity: *What advice can nurses give to couples who want to start a family? What information would you want to gather for a woman who followed the advice and still was not pregnant after 6 months?*

Because of the high incidence of multiple contributing factors, evaluation of infertility should include both partners. Evaluation begins with a thorough history and physical examination for both partners to identify evidence of conditions that may be affecting fertility. Important health history information includes the following:

- The woman's menstrual pattern
- Number of pregnancies with the current partner or any other partner, and the pregnancy outcomes
- Identification of any sexual dysfunction for both partners
- History of STIs or genital tract surgery or trauma for both partners
- Lifestyle issues, such as alcohol consumption, tobacco use, recreational drug use, occupation, and patterns of physical activity for both partners
- Chronic medical conditions and treatment for both partners
- The couple's pattern of intercourse as related to the woman's ovulatory cycle
- Length of time the couple has had unprotected intercourse
- Natural techniques or home tests the couple has already used

In addition to the health history, the health care provider will do a complete review of systems to help identify any endocrinologic or immunologic issues that might contribute to infertility. The health care provider then completes a thorough physical examination. A gynecologist may evaluate the woman, whereas a urologist often performs the initial evaluation of a man.

BOX 4-7 Risk Factors for Infertility

Risk Factors That Affect Both Women and Men

Behavioral Factors
- Cigarette or marijuana smoking
- Alcohol use (even in moderation)
- Excessive exercise
- Being 10% to 15% over or under ideal body weight
- Multiple sexual partners (increases risk for sexually transmitted infection [STIs])

Occupational and Environmental Factors
Exposure to the following:
- High environmental temperatures
- Certain chemicals
- Radiation
- Heavy electromagnetic or microwave emissions

Emotional Factors
- High stress levels
- Depression

Risk Factors Specific to Women

Factors That May Interfere With Ovulation
- Advancing age (fertility declines with advancing age for women)
- Polycystic ovarian syndrome
- Chronic medical conditions and associated treatments, examples include the following:
  - Diabetes
  - Thyroid dysfunction
  - Systemic lupus erythematosus (SLE)
  - Rheumatoid arthritis
  - Hypertension
- Hormonal imbalance, signaled by any of the following:
  - Menstrual irregularities
  - Menorrhagia (prolonged or excessive bleeding)
  - Hirsutism
  - Acne
  - Ovarian cysts

Factors That May Interfere With Gamete Transport
- Surgical or invasive procedures involving the cervix or uterus, such as the following:
  - Cone biopsy or cryosurgery
  - Dilatation and curettage (D&C)
  - Myomectomy
- Uterine fibroids
- In utero diethylstilbestrol (DES) exposure
- Any surgical procedure directly involving the fallopian tubes
- Any pelvic surgery
- Endometriosis
- Ectopic pregnancy
- History of STIs or pelvic inflammatory disease (PID)

Factors That May Interfere With Implantation
- More than one induced abortion (medical abortion)
- Hormonal imbalance

Specific Risk Factors for Men

Factors That May Interfere With Sperm Viability
- Prescription medications for ulcers or psoriasis
- DES exposure in utero
- Exposure of the genitals to hot temperatures
  - Hot tubs
  - Steam rooms
  - Tight clothing
- Cryptorchidism
- Prostatitis
- Varicocele
- Genital tract infection
- Mumps after puberty

Factors That May Interfere With Sperm Deposition
- Erectile dysfunction
- Retrograde ejaculation
- History of hernia repair
- Hypospadias
- Vasectomy

The woman's physical examination includes a pelvic examination, Pap smear, cultures for STIs, and a bimanual examination. A pelvic ultrasound may also be performed. A man's examination includes determining if any genital tract abnormalities are present in addition to a sperm count. The health care provider discusses results of the initial evaluation with the couple and explains plans for a more comprehensive evaluation if needed.

Comprehensive Evaluation and Diagnostic Testing

Diagnostic testing for infertility usually begins with the simplest testing methods and moves toward the more complex and invasive methods. The timing of diagnostic testing is in relation to the woman's menstrual cycle.

Frequently, evaluation of infertility in men is performed first because the testing is often simpler than that for testing of women. The first diagnostic test is usually a semen analysis. For this procedure, the man must collect semen via masturbation or in a special condom during intercourse if masturbation is unacceptable to the couple. The man must abstain from ejaculation for 3 to 5 days before the test to obtain optimal results. The man must deliver the entire ejaculate in a sterile container to the laboratory no later than 30 minutes after collection. The laboratory examines the sample for semen volume and quality and for number, shape, motility, and viability of the sperm. If the semen analysis is normal, diagnostic testing then focuses on the woman partner.

If the semen analysis results are abnormal, additional analysis 1 month later can rule out short-term causes or inadequate specimen collection. Additional tests of fertility in men include hormonal analysis, genital structure assessment, and sperm analysis. Follicle-stimulating hormone (FSH), LH, testosterone, and prolactin include hormones found in men that are tested. Scrotal ultrasonography can help identify structural abnormalities that could interfere with fertility. In some cases, a testicular biopsy may be performed. Sperm function tests can determine the ability of the sperm to penetrate and fertilize the egg.

Comprehensive fertility evaluation of the client often begins with the least invasive techniques. The **postcoital test** evaluates the interaction of the man's sperm with the woman's cervical mucus. The timing of the test is critical for accurate results. The woman uses a urine LH predictor kit to predict ovulation. When she determines that ovulation is near, the couple performs vaginal intercourse without lubricants. Several hours later, the health care provider collects a sample of cervical mucus and evaluates it for mucus characteristics, a sperm count, and evaluation of sperm motility. Endocrine testing is also useful. The health care provider orders serum hormone levels of estrogen, progesterone, thyroid-stimulating hormone, prolactin, and androgen to determine if endocrine abnormalities are present.

More invasive techniques include hysterosalpingogram, hysteroscopy, and laparoscopy. A hysterosalpingogram allows for the identification of an obstruction anywhere along the tract. A hysteroscopy facilitates direct visualization of the endometrial cavity. This method can diagnose and treat some endometrial conditions. Laparoscopy is usually the last test performed because it involves surgical and anesthetic risk and cost. This procedure provides for direct visualization of the pelvic cavity.

Management of Infertility

The health care provider chooses appropriate therapy based on the underlying causes identified during diagnostic testing, duration of infertility, and the woman's age. As with testing, therapies begin with the simplest and least invasive and progress toward the more complex, as needed. Possible interventions include medication administration, hormonal replacements, surgical procedures, insemination techniques, advanced reproductive techniques, and alternative parenting/childbirth options.

Treatment of Cervical Factors

The easiest, most successful therapy for cervical abnormalities is intrauterine insemination. Near the time of ovulation, the health care provider passes a thin flexible catheter through the cervix and inserts sperm directly into the uterus. Frequently, more than one insemination is required to ensure that insemination coincides with ovulation. Sperm can be from the woman's partner or from a donor. After the insemination, the woman should remain supine for at least 10 minutes.

Treatment of Endometrial and Tubal Factors

Most endometrial and tubal causes of infertility require various surgical techniques. Options include hysteroscopy, laparoscopy, or laparotomy, followed by a hysterosalpingogram to evaluate effectiveness of treatment. Discussion of treatment for endometriosis, a common cause of infertility, occurs earlier in this chapter.

Treatment of Ovarian Factors

Medications to stimulate ovulation, also known as fertility drugs, are the treatment of choice when lack of ovulation is the cause of infertility. All have side effects and potential complications, which can be severe. Multifetal pregnancy is common with these medications. Clomiphene citrate, human menopause gonadotropins, and pure FSH are examples of fertility drugs used to treat ovarian dysfunction.

Treatment of Factors in Men

If a varicocele is the cause of low sperm production, surgery is required. If the cause of a low sperm count is unknown and FSH, LH, and testosterone levels are normal, then the health care provider may prescribe clomiphene citrate to increase sperm production.

Assisted Reproduction Technologies

The first assisted reproduction technology to be successful in humans was in vitro fertilization (IVF) and occurred in 1978. Since that time, researchers have developed additional assisted reproduction technologies. The five leading assisted reproduction technologies are IVF, gamete intrafallopian transfer, zygote intrafallopian transfer, tubal embryo transfer, and intracytoplasmic sperm injection. The nurse's role

BOX 4-8 **Ethical and Legal Issues Related to Assisted Reproduction Technologies (ARTs)**

Research in the area of ARTs has resulted in additional technologies that, while giving new hope to couples who once considered their infertility irreversible, are also creating ethical and legal dilemmas for all concerned. Common ethical and legal questions include the following:
- Who should have the right to reproduce?
- Should ARTs be limited to married couples?
- Who owns the embryos produced?
- Should embryos be frozen for later use?
- Who are the parents?
- Do the biologic donors or surrogates have custodial rights?
- Should donors only be anonymous?
- Should fetal reduction techniques be done when ARTs result in multifetal gestation?

with the client undergoing assisted reproduction technology includes providing emotional support, assisting the health care provider with data collection, assisting with procedures as appropriate, and reinforcing teaching related to the risks and benefits to facilitate the client's decision-making process. Box 4-8 lists some ethical and legal questions associated with assisted reproduction technologies.

Surrogate Parenting

Surrogate parenting is a process by which a woman carries the fetus of an infertile couple to term. A **gestational surrogate**, or surrogate mother, may donate only the use of her uterus, or she may also donate her ovum and agree to insemination with the man's sperm. Surrogate parenting has raised legal and ethical issues that require counseling for both the infertile couple and the surrogate and possibly the surrogate mother's spouse and family.

Psychological Aspects of Infertility

Psychosocial consequences related to infertility include shock, guilt, isolation, depression, and stress. The partner who has the identified problem is at most risk for feelings of guilt. It is important to avoid using words that imply blame when discussing the problem of infertility.

The client who is having difficulty conceiving may feel isolated and different from others who are able to conceive. Separation from others, either physically or emotionally, in an attempt to avoid emotional pain is common. Infertility will challenge the client's self-image, self-worth, and sense of command over events in their life. A "roller coaster" of emotions, ranging from hope to despair with each ovulatory cycle, is a common experience described by the infertile client.

Infertility places stress on the client's relationship. Common feelings include low self-esteem and feelings of being unworthy or unlovable. A man may find it difficult to perform sexually or provide semen specimens on demand. Intimacy, love, and support, essential components of a couple's sexual relationship, may be lost because intercourse takes on a clinical and mechanical tone.

Inability to achieve pregnancy may lead the client to consider adoption. Adoption is a viable option for parenting. Honest and open communication between the adoptive parents is essential. The client must examine their feelings regarding adoption and take into consideration questions such as:

- What are their preferences regarding health status, race, and possibly other characteristics desired in an infant?
- Are they willing to adopt an older child, a child of another race, or a child with special needs?
- How will they feel about having minimal information about the child's background?
- How would they feel about knowing the child's birth mother or father?

The client must consider these and other questions before deciding to adopt. The nurse will be instrumental in listening to the client and supporting the client's feelings and decisions. The nurse should use positive language when discussing the client's options.

Some clients who experience infertility may opt to remain childless instead of choosing adoption or surrogacy. These clients may need support with their decision. Well-meaning friends or family members may offer statements to the client such as "You can always adopt" that may cause unintentional emotional distress. Also, family or friends may not understand the pain the client may experience when hearing of other pregnancies or being invited to a child's birthday party.

Nursing Care

The major focus of nursing care related to infertility involves providing support for the client as they undergo diagnosis and their chosen treatment option. Therapeutic communication skills are an essential component in nursing care. It is important to facilitate the client's and partner's ability to communicate with each other and to encourage each partner to discuss his or her own feelings and be accepting of the other's. Reinforce the client's coping strategies or assist with exploring new coping strategies. This helps them to increase their sense of control in this situation.

After the health care provider has informed the client about the diagnosis and potential treatment options, the major role of the nurse is to reinforce teaching and offer emotional support. The client needs support throughout the decision-making process. The client will need support either with the grief process related to infertility or with pregnancy if treatment options are successful. Providing emotional support is an essential component of care, especially when a treatment has been unsuccessful.

TEST YOURSELF

✔ Define common causes of infertility.

✔ Which test of infertility is normally the first to be done?

✔ Describe nursing care for the infertile client.

MENOPAUSE

Menopause, the cessation of menses, signals the end of the woman's reproductive capability. The climacteric, as defined in Chapter 3, refers to the gradual changes associated with declining ovarian function. **Perimenopause** refers to the time before menopause when vasomotor symptoms (hot flashes, night sweats) and irregular menses begin. Menopause is a normal part of the life cycle and is not a disease, although associated symptoms may be distressing to the woman and require interventions.

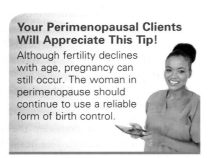

Your Perimenopausal Clients Will Appreciate This Tip!

Although fertility declines with age, pregnancy can still occur. The woman in perimenopause should continue to use a reliable form of birth control.

Menopause occurs when the ovaries no longer respond to stimulation from the pituitary. During the perimenopausal period, the woman begins to experience variable menstrual cycles and irregular bleeding. Although these changes occur normally in response to hormonal changes, the woman should report all irregular bleeding to her health care provider for evaluation.

Clinical Manifestations

The perimenopausal woman typically experiences a set of symptoms known as climacteric syndrome. These symptoms include hot flashes, insomnia, weight gain, bloating, emotional lability, irregular menses, and headache.

A hot flash is a sudden feeling of warmth or intense heat sometimes accompanied by reddening of the skin on the upper body. The average length of symptoms in the perimenopausal woman is 2 years; however, some women experience hot flashes for 5 or more years. A hot flash corresponds to low estrogen levels and periodic surges of LH.

Physical changes associated with hormone depletion include changes to the reproductive organs. The vaginal mucosa thins and becomes pale and dry. Vaginal rugae disappear, and the vaginal walls become smooth. The uterus and ovaries decrease in size. Pelvic support muscles can lose tone.

Decreased bone mineral density is one of the changes that can have life-threatening effects on the menopausal woman. The overall effect of decreased bone mineral density is loss of bone mass with resulting reduction of bone strength and increased risk for fracture. This systemic condition is osteoporosis. Box 4-9 lists common risk factors for osteoporosis. It is important to know the risk factors for osteoporosis because this disease often has no symptoms until a serious bone fracture occurs.

Treatment

Hormone replacement therapy (HRT) was the traditional approach for the prevention and treatment of perimenopausal symptoms as a whole. However, recent research is showing

---

BOX 4-9   Risk Factors for Osteoporosis

- Having the biologic sex of a woman
- Being of White (non-Hispanic) or Asian origin
- Slender build
- Advanced age
- Estrogen deficiency because of menopause (especially if early or surgically induced)
- Low bone mass density
- Family history of osteoporosis
- Personal history of fracture as an adult
- Smoking
- Excessive alcohol intake
- Low dietary intake of calcium
- Vitamin D deficiency
- Inactive lifestyle
- Use of glucocorticoids
- Use of anticonvulsants

HRT may not be the best option for many women. HRT was associated with an increased risk for coronary heart disease, stroke, venous thromboembolism, and pulmonary embolism without a decrease in cardiovascular disease. Current recommendations for the use of HRT include control (not prevention) of perimenopausal symptoms. The health care provider should prescribe the lowest dose to control symptoms for the shortest time possible. Benefits of HRT include decreased risk for colorectal cancer and osteoporotic fractures.

Treatment for Hot Flashes and Sweats

Hot flashes and sweats are the most common reasons that the perimenopausal woman seeks medical treatment. To date, the most effective therapy for hot flashes continues to be HRT. Hormonal alternatives to HRT include progestins alone, which are beneficial in treating hot flashes. Nonhormonal options include the anticonvulsant gabapentin and SSRI antidepressant drugs, such as paroxetine.

Treatment for Osteoporosis

HRT continues to be beneficial for reducing the risk of osteoporosis and fractures in the peri- and postmenopausal woman. However, other treatment options also lower the risk for fractures. These options include parathyroid hormone, raloxifene, calcitonin, and bisphosphonates. Calcium with vitamin D supplementation and regular weight-bearing exercise are preventive measures.

Treatment for Vaginal Atrophy and Dryness

HRT continues to be an effective treatment, although the use of local applications of estrogen-containing vaginal creams, tablets, or suppositories brings relief of symptoms with minimal systemic absorption. If estrogen use is contraindicated, the woman may benefit from nonestrogenic vaginal lubricants.

Nursing Care

Nurses have a large role to play in health promotion for the peri- and postmenopausal woman. It is important to develop a rapport with the woman and to let her know that you are available to talk about her concerns. Reassure the woman of the normality of menopause.

Reinforce teaching on HRT and other therapies. Some women are reluctant to discuss menopausal symptoms, and for those clients it may be helpful to give pamphlets or handouts that can be read at home. It is important that the woman understand the risks and benefits of any therapy so that she can make an informed decision.

Suggest lifestyle modifications to decrease the discomfort of hot flashes. These include dressing in lightweight clothing and dressing in layers. Regular exercise and setting the thermostat to a lower temperature may also be helpful. Suggest that she avoid spicy foods, caffeine, and alcohol.

Give the woman information on strategies to prevent osteoporosis. Encourage regular weight-bearing activity, such as walking and stair climbing, at least three to four times per week. The postmenopausal woman should continue to take calcium and vitamin D supplements. She should take her calcium supplements with orange juice (or another vitamin C source) and avoid caffeine, which tends to interfere with the absorption of calcium.

Safety instructions can help prevent fractures from falls inside the house. Encourage the postmenopausal woman to have her bed lowered, if possible; to eliminate throw rugs and clutter from the floors; and to use night-lights throughout the house. In the bathroom, it is helpful to install safety tread and safety rails. All of her slippers and shoes should have tread and should provide traction and stability. To reduce falls outside the home, instruct the woman to take extra precautions after dark. Advise her to use railings whenever possible. She should clear walkways of debris and avoid walking on ice.

Review medications with the woman. She should understand how to take her medications and what side effects to report. She should also understand how often she should see her health care provider and have required routine screening examinations, such as yearly mammograms and bone density measurements. Tips for Reinforcing Family Teaching: Reducing the Discomfort of Menopause lists helpful information to share with the woman and her family.

TIPS FOR REINFORCING FAMILY TEACHING

Reducing the Discomfort of Menopause

- Wear cotton clothes in layers.
- Avoid caffeine intake (e.g., soft drinks, black tea, coffee).
- Explore relaxation activities because stress exacerbates vasomotor symptoms.
- Discuss hormone replacement therapy with your health care provider.
- Consider nutritional supplements as recommended by your health care provider to help reduce vasomotor symptoms.

- Use a water-soluble lubricant before intercourse.
- Nonprescription, long-lasting vaginal moisturizers are effective for the relief of vaginal dryness.
- If using an estrogen vaginal cream, apply it at bedtime.
- Perform Kegel exercises to improve pelvic muscle tone.
- Drink at least five glasses of water per day. Do not count caffeine-containing drinks as part of this water intake.
- Urinate regularly; do not allow the bladder to become over-distended.
- Practice good hygiene, such as wiping from front to back after toileting.

TEST YOURSELF

✔ Define perimenopause.

✔ Name five symptoms that are part of the climacteric syndrome.

✔ Describe three nonpharmacologic suggestions that you can offer the perimenopausal woman to help with symptom relief.

Recall Sondra Simone from the beginning of the chapter. What do you think the possible causes of her dysmenorrhea could be? What might be potential causes of Sondra's delay in getting pregnant?

KEY POINTS

- Self-awareness of breast characteristics and yearly clinical breast examinations are appropriate for women of all ages. Women older than 45 years should have yearly mammograms.

- The woman's first Pap smear should be at age 21, regardless of when she first had sexual intercourse, and then every 3 years from age 21 to 29 and every 5 years after age 30.

- Dysmenorrhea is painful or difficult menses. Premenstrual syndrome encompasses a group of symptoms that are cyclical in nature and progress with time.

- A classic symptom of endometriosis is cyclic pelvic pain that occurs in conjunction with menses. Therapy aims to suppress ovulation and induce an artificial menopause to curb growth of abnormal tissue and relieve symptoms. The nurse's role is to help the woman find pain relief and provide support.

- The major risk factor for development of pelvic inflammatory disease is untreated sexually transmitted infections (STIs). The woman and her partner should be treated with antibiotic drugs.

- Weakening of the structures that support the pelvic organs causes pelvic support disorders including cystoceles, rectoceles, and prolapse of the uterus. Major risk factors for pelvic support disorders include pregnancy, vaginal delivery, and poor muscle tone.

- Family planning involves the two components of planning pregnancy and preventing pregnancy. Family planning should include preconception care, which involves focusing on nutrition and exercise, lifestyle changes, counseling and treatment for chronic illness and genetic disorders, and evaluation of medications.
- Preconception care is important as the health of the mother, including any medications she is taking or preexisting health conditions, affects the health of the fetus and the outcome of the pregnancy.
- Natural methods of contraception do not use hormones or other physical barriers to prevent conception. These methods include abstinence, coitus interruptus, and fertility awareness methods. Natural methods do not require the use of artificial devices or hormones but require a great deal of education and discipline to be effective.
- Barrier methods of contraception provide a physical and chemical barrier to prevent pregnancy. These include spermicides, condoms for women and men, the diaphragm, and cervical cap. Many barrier methods have the advantage of decreasing the risk for STIs.
- Hormonal methods of contraception include oral contraceptive pills, progestin-only pills, hormonal injections, hormonal implants, the transdermal patch, and the vaginal estrogen/progestin (contraceptive) ring. Hormonal contraceptive drugs are highly effective but do not provide reliable protection against STIs.
- IUDs provide long-term pregnancy protection. They must be inserted by a health care provider and require removal every 5 to 10 years. They do not provide protection against STIs.
- Sterilization techniques of men and women are highly effective, permanent methods of contraception.
- Emergency contraception refers to methods used to prevent pregnancy after unprotected intercourse. It can be medication or the insertion of a copper IUD.
- Infertility is the inability to conceive after a year of unprotected intercourse. Multiple factors contribute to infertility.
- Evaluation of infertility begins with the least invasive and complex and progresses to the more invasive and complex techniques. All infertility evaluations begin with a thorough history and physical examination of both partners. Usually the first test is a sperm analysis, and the second test is a postcoital examination.
- Treatment of infertility depends on the identified cause. Surgical techniques to correct structural problems, medication to stimulate ovulation, and assisted reproduction technology may all be used in the treatment of infertility.
- A couple undergoing evaluation and treatment for infertility may feel guilt, shock, isolation, depression, and stress. It is stressful on a relationship to sexually perform on demand, and intercourse often takes on a clinical and mechanical tone, rather than the desired traits of intimacy, love, and support.
- Menopause is a natural part of the life cycle. It is not a disease; however, the associated symptoms may need medication or other interventions.
- Hormone replacement therapy used to be the gold standard of treatment for major menopausal symptoms; however, recent research has highlighted serious adverse effects that may be associated with hormone replacement therapy.
- Hot flashes, osteoporosis, and vaginal atrophy and dryness are the major symptoms for which women need and desire treatment and nursing care during menopause.

INTERNET RESOURCES

Endometriosis
https://www.endometriosis.org

Family Planning
https://www.cdc.gov/reproductivehealth/contraception/index.htm

Infertility
https://resolve.org/

Osteoporosis
https://www.nof.org/

Mammogram
https://www.cancer.org/cancer/breast-cancer/screening-tests-and-early detection/mammograms.html

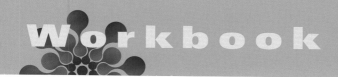

NCLEX-STYLE REVIEW QUESTIONS

1. An adolescent girl asks the nurse when she should have her first "Pap test." How should the nurse reply?

   a. "I don't know. Ask your health care provider."
   b. "When you first start having sex."
   c. "As soon as possible and every year thereafter."
   d. "It is recommended you have your first Pap smear when you turn 21."

2. A 35-year-old woman reports very heavy menstrual periods. How does the nurse chart this in the medical record?

   a. "Chief complaint: dysmenorrhea."
   b. "Complains of metrorrhagia."
   c. "Reports amenorrhea."
   d. "Reports menorrhagia."

3. A woman is having severe symptoms of PMS. She asks the nurse what she can do to obtain relief from these symptoms. What reply by the nurse is most likely to be helpful?

   a. "Antibiotic drugs are necessary to treat the underlying infection."
   b. "Diuretic medications tend to be the most helpful medications for PMS treatment."
   c. "Don't worry. The medication your health care provider has prescribed will take care of your symptoms."
   d. "In addition to taking medications, stress reduction and regular exercise are beneficial."

4. Which statement by a woman with a pelvic support disorder should alert the nurse to instruct the woman to come in immediately for examination by a health care provider?

   a. "My urine is cloudy."
   b. "I forgot to do my Kegel exercises today."
   c. "Every time I cough, a little bit of urine comes out."
   d. "I took my pessary out to wash it and forgot to put it back in."

5. Which of the following statements made by the nurse are true regarding preconception care? Select all that apply.

   a. "The woman should increase her intake of folic acid."
   b. "The woman should stop rigorous exercise."
   c. "The woman should discontinue all her medications."
   d. "The woman should be up to date on her vaccines."
   e. "The woman should stop smoking."

STUDY ACTIVITIES

1. Develop a 10-minute presentation on considerations a couple should make before deciding on a method of birth control.

2. Go to www.arhp.org/hormonalcontraception. What methods of contraception are mentioned? Which methods do they list as highly effective? How does the menstrual cycle differ for a woman who is not taking any hormonal contraception as compared to a woman who is taking oral contraceptive drugs?

3. Using the table below, compare natural methods of contraception.

Method	How It Works to Prevent Pregnancy	Special Nursing Considerations

CRITICAL THINKING: WHAT WOULD YOU DO?

Apply your knowledge of infertility and its treatments to the following situation.

1. Amanda Rodriguez is a 37-year-old woman who has never before been pregnant. She put off pregnancy to pursue her career as an attorney. Now she and her husband have been trying to conceive for 2 years without success. She has come to the clinic for initial evaluation.

   a. Explain to Amanda what she can expect from today's visit.
   b. The health care provider asks you to assist her during the physical examination. What equipment and supplies will you gather?
   c. If Amanda is experiencing infertility, what type is it?
   d. Amanda confides in you that she thinks God is punishing her for waiting to start a family. She says that she should have tried to have children several years ago when all her friends were having babies. How would you reply to Amanda?

2. The health care provider tells Amanda that her husband will need to have a semen analysis and then a postcoital test will be done.

   a. Explain both of these procedures to Amanda.
   b. The semen analysis reveals a low sperm count. What additional tests might be ordered to evaluate male causes of infertility?

3. Apply your knowledge of menopause to the following situation: Cindy McFarland, a 52-year-old woman, comes to the clinic because she has been experiencing hot flashes. She tells you that the hot flashes are very intense and seem to last "forever." She says that her sweat drenches her clothes, and she is embarrassed to go out in public.

   a. Explain the physiology of hot flashes to Cindy.
   b. What treatments will the health care provider likely recommend for Cindy?
   c. What other advice do you have for Cindy during this time of her life?

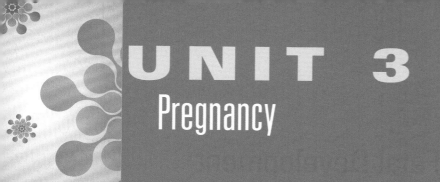

UNIT 3
Pregnancy

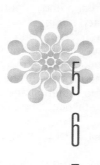

5 Fetal Development

Learning Objectives

At the conclusion of this chapter, you will:

1. Explain mitosis and meiosis and differentiate between the two.
2. Describe the processes of spermatogenesis and oogenesis and how they differ.
3. Explain how the sex of the conceptus is determined.
4. Describe the three developmental stages of pregnancy with regard to beginning and ending periods and major events occurring during each stage.
5. Describe the difference between the amnion and the chorion.
6. Name four major functions of amniotic fluid.
7. Discuss three functions of the placenta.
8. List the steps in the process of the exchange of nutrients and wastes between the maternal and fetal bloodstreams.
9. Trace the path of fetal circulation, including the three fetal shunts.
10. Name three categories of teratogens, and list examples of each kind.
11. Discuss the threat to pregnancy that occurs with ectopic pregnancy.
12. Differentiate between the types of multifetal pregnancies.

Bethany Sanders, a 17-year-old client, comes to the health care provider's office for a prenatal visit. She asks you, "How does the baby breathe underwater while inside me?" She also asks, "How does the baby eat?" As you read the chapter, think of how you would answer Bethany's questions. How would you phrase your answers if Bethany was 30 years old instead of 17?

INTRODUCTION

Every human being starts out as two separate germ cells, or gametes. The woman's gamete is the ovum, and the man's gamete is the spermatozoon, or sperm for short. At conception, the gametes unite to form the cell that eventually becomes the developing fetus. Human development is an ongoing process that begins at fertilization and continues even after birth. Many factors affect development. Some of these factors can cause abnormalities and birth defects. Others are part of the normal process of human development, such as sex determination. This chapter discusses the major processes involved in human fertilization and development.

CELLULAR PROCESSES

There are two major categories of cells and two major types of cellular division involved in the reproduction of human life.

Types of Cells

Cells are the building blocks of all organs. There are two major types of cells—soma cells, which make up the organs and tissues of the human body, and gametes, also known as germ cells or sex cells. The gametes are only found in the reproductive glands (testes in men and ovaries in women).

The nucleus of each soma cell contains 46 chromosomes, which are arranged in 23 pairs. Each chromosome is composed of genes, which are segments of DNA that control hereditary traits. At conception, each parent donates one chromosome from every pair. Of the 23 pairs of chromosomes, 22 are autosomes which determine all genetic traits such as eye and hair color. The remaining pair, the sex chromosomes, determines an individual's sex.

The ovum is a woman's gamete and the sperm is a man's gamete. Each gamete has 23 chromosomes, exactly half of the 46 required chromosomes needed for human development.

Cellular Division

There are two types of cellular division involved in the creation of human life: mitosis and meiosis.

Mitosis

Mitosis is the process by which somatic (body) cells divide to create new cells. Each new cell contains the same number of chromosomes as the original cell. The body grows and replaces somatic cells through the process of mitosis (Fig. 5-1).

Meiosis

Meiosis is the process by which gametes undergo two sequential cellular divisions of the nucleus. This process reduces the number of chromosomes in the gametes by half. Remember, each gamete has only 23 chromosomes, which is half (also known as the haploid number) of the total number of chromosomes required for human cells (Fig. 5-2). The woman's gamete, the ovum, undergoes meiosis in the ovaries just before ovulation. The man's germ cells, the spermatozoon, divide in the seminiferous tubules of the testes.

The formation and development of gametes by this process of meiosis is called **gametogenesis**. More specifically, the formation of the man's gamete is called spermatogenesis and the formation of the woman's gamete is called oogenesis.

Spermatogenesis

From Human genetics: Spermatogenesis begins at puberty in young men. In the testes, primary spermatocytes, each containing 46 chromosomes, undergo the first meiotic division, which results in two secondary spermatocytes, each with 23 chromosomes. These spermatocytes then undergo a second meiotic division, resulting in a final number of four spermatids that contain the haploid number of chromosomes (23). The spermatids undergo a change in form to become mature spermatozoa but undergo no further meiotic divisions (Fig. 5-3A).

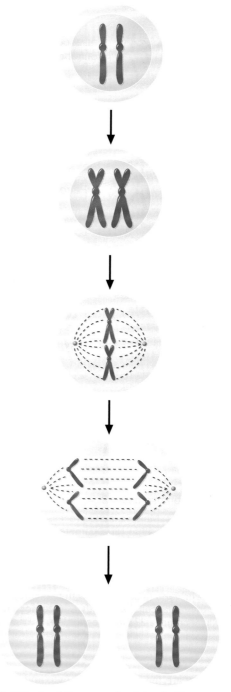

FIGURE 5-1 Mitosis of the soma (body) cell. (From Zschocke, J. (2018). Molekulare Grundlagen. In: *Basiswissen Humangenetik*, 978-3-662-56146-1, © Springer-Verlag.)

Oogenesis

Oogenesis begins in the ovaries before birth but is not fully complete until the childbearing years. At birth, the ovaries contain primary oocytes, which have completed the prophase stage of the first meiotic division. The completion of the first meiotic division occurs before ovulation. The two cells that result from this division are not

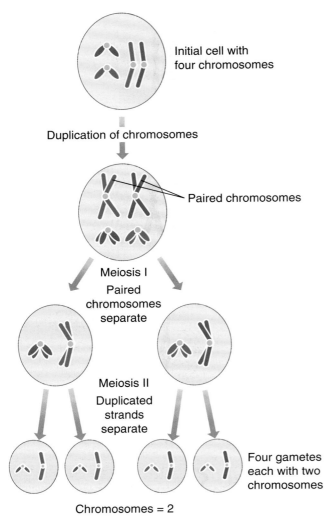

Initial cell with four chromosomes

Duplication of chromosomes

Paired chromosomes

Meiosis I
Paired chromosomes separate

Meiosis II
Duplicated strands separate

Four gametes each with two chromosomes

Chromosomes = 2

FIGURE 5-2 Meiosis. Meiosis is the process that reduces the chromosomes in half to form gametes (the sex cells, spermatozoa and ovum). The first step of the process is the replication of chromosomes (meiosis I) and the second step is the separation of the duplicate strands (meiosis II). In the diagram, the initial cell has four beginning chromosomes and the result is four gamete cells each with two chromosomes. In the human, the initial cell starts with 46 chromosomes and the gamete cells each have 23 chromosomes.

identical. They are the secondary oocyte and the first polar body. The secondary oocyte contains the haploid number of chromosomes. The first polar body divides and becomes the polar bodies which soon disintegrate because they contain almost no cytoplasm. The secondary oocyte begins its second meiotic division at ovulation and is a mature ovum (Fig. 5-3B) but does not complete the process unless a sperm fertilizes it.

STAGES OF FETAL DEVELOPMENT

The three stages of human development during pregnancy are the pre-embryonic, embryonic, and fetal stages (Fig. 5-4).

The pre-embryonic stage begins at fertilization and lasts through the end of the second week after fertilization. The embryonic stage begins approximately 2 weeks after fertilization and ends at the conclusion of the eighth week after fertilization. By the end of the embryonic stage, all of the organ systems have begun development, and the conceptus is distinctly human in form. The fetal stage begins at 9 weeks after fertilization and ends at birth. However, birth is not the end of human development. Human development is an ongoing process of transformation that begins with fertilization and continues through the teenage years and beyond.

In this chapter, fertilization age (number of weeks after fertilization) will be used rather than gestational age (number of weeks after the last menstrual period) when discussing development during pregnancy. Table 5-1 compares postfertilization and gestational dates.

Pre-Embryonic Stage

The pre-embryonic stage begins with fertilization and lasts for 2 weeks. Cellular division and implantation occur during this stage of development.

Fertilization

Fertilization, also called conception, occurs when the sperm penetrates the ovum. The ovum is receptive to fertilization for approximately 24 to 48 hours after ovulation and the sperm are viable for 24 to 72 hours after ejaculation into the woman's reproductive system. During ejaculation the man releases approximately 300 to 600 million sperm. However, only one sperm will fertilize the mature ovum. After the sperm are ejaculated into the vagina, they travel through the cervix, into the uterus, and then into the fallopian tube. Prostaglandins in the semen increase smooth muscle contractions of the uterus that facilitate transport of sperm. Conception usually occurs when the ovum is in the ampulla (the outermost half) of the fallopian tube.

Once a single sperm has penetrated the thick membrane that surrounds the ovum, called the zona pellucida, a chemical reaction occurs that causes the ovum to become impenetrable to other sperm. A **zygote**, or conceptus, results when an ovum and a sperm unite. Because the chromosomes of the sperm merge with those of the ovum, the zygote has the full complement of 46 chromosomes (also called the diploid number), arranged in 23 pairs.

You Do the Math!

Sperm are able to fertilize the ovum for up to 72 hours after ejaculation, and the ovum remains fertile for a maximum of 48 hours after ovulation. Thus, the window of opportunity for conception to occur is approximately 3 days before until 2 days after ovulation.

Sex Determination

Sex determination occurs at the time of fertilization based on the inheritance of X or Y chromosomes. The ovum contains

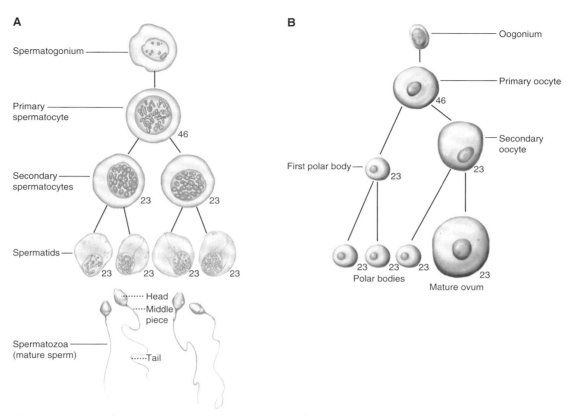

FIGURE 5-3 In gametogenesis (both spermatogenesis and oogenesis) the chromosomes are reduced to one half the number characteristic for the general body cells of the species. In humans, the number in the somatic (body) cells is 46 chromosomes, while in each mature spermatozoa and mature ovum, the number is 23 chromosomes. **A.** Spermatogenesis. One spermatogonium gives rise to four spermatozoa. **B.** Oogenesis. From each oogonium, one mature ovum and three polar bodies are produced.

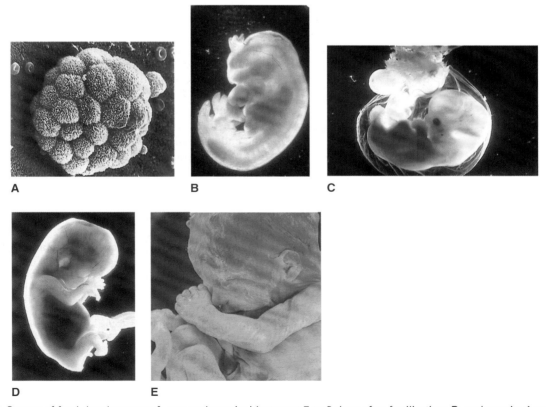

FIGURE 5-4 Stages of fetal development: **A.** pre-embryonic: blastocyst 7 to 8 days after fertilization; **B.** embryonic: 4-week embryo; **C.** embryonic: 5-week embryo; **D.** embryonic: 6-week embryo; **E.** fetal: 15-week fetus.

TABLE 5-1 Comparison of Gestational Age to Fertilization Age

STAGE OF DEVELOPMENT	WEEKS AFTER FERTILIZATION	GESTATIONAL AGE
Pre-embryonic	0–2	3–4 weeks' gestation
Embryonic	3–8	5–10 weeks' gestation
Fetal	9–38	11–40 weeks' gestation

two X chromosomes, and the sperm contains either an X or Y chromosome. Because the sperm can have either an X or a Y chromosome, a man's gamete is responsible for fetal sex determination. A female zygote (XX) develops when the ovum (X) unites with a sperm with an X chromosome. Conversely, fertilization with a sperm that contains a Y chromosome will produce a male zygote (XY) (Fig. 5-5). Research indicates that there is an approximately 50–50 chance of either occurrence.

A Specialist Can Spot the Difference!

Some genetic diseases are sex specific. A fertility specialist can separate the semen into X and Y sperm to help the couple prevent such diseases if they are known carriers.

This is Worth Noting

Some couples mistakenly believe that they can influence sex determination by using certain sexual positions, ingesting particular foods before intercourse, or timing sex to occur at specific times during the menstrual cycle. These beliefs are often rooted in folklore and are not based on scientific principles.

Cellular Reproduction

After fertilization, the zygote begins the process of mitotic division known as **cleavage**. As the cells divide, the zygote transforms from one cell into two cells, and then each cell further divides to form four cells. Each of these cells in turn divides to form eight cells and so on. Each new cell contains the diploid number of chromosomes (46), beginning with the first mitotic division. The fallopian tube is lined with cilia (tiny, hairlike structures) that move the zygote toward the uterus.

At about 3 days after fertilization, the total cell count reaches 32. The solid cell cluster is now called a **morula** (a Latin word for mulberry, which is what the morula resembles). The morula continues its journey toward the uterine cavity while cleavage and transformation of the cells continue. By about 5 days after fertilization, the cell mass is now called a **blastocyst**. The blastocyst has three parts: an outer layer of cells called the trophoblast, a fluid-filled hollow core, and an inner cell mass. The trophoblast will go on to become the structures that nourish and protect the developing conceptus. By the end of the pre-embryonic period, the inner cell mass becomes the embryonic disk, which will eventually become the fetus.

Implantation

On about the sixth day after fertilization, the trophoblast develops fingerlike projections that help the blastocyst burrow into the nutrient-rich endometrium. By the 10th day after fertilization, the blastocyst has completely buried itself in the uterine lining. During the process of implantation, small cavities, called lacunae, develop around the blastocyst. Maternal blood pools in the lacunae, which allows the exchange of nutrients from the woman's blood for metabolic wastes from the blastocyst. The lacunae eventually become the intervillous spaces of the placenta. The tiny blastocyst begins to produce human chorionic gonadotropin (hCG), which signals the corpus luteum to continue producing progesterone to maintain the endometrial lining and the pregnancy.

At this point in the woman's menstrual cycle, the endometrium is ready to support the pregnancy. From this point through the end of pregnancy, the endometrium is called the **decidua**. The woman has not yet missed her menstrual period and is unaware of her pregnancy. Figure 5-6 illustrates the transport of the ovum from ovulation to fertilization and the transport of the zygote from fertilization to implantation.

Here is a Teaching Opportunity

Some women have a small amount of bleeding during the time of implantation, which is known as implantation bleeding. This bleeding can be mistaken for a scanty menstrual period and can lead to miscalculation of fetal age.

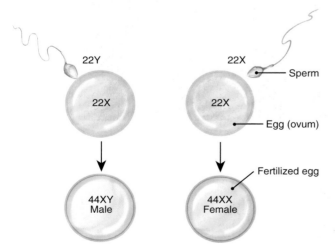

FIGURE 5-5 Inheritance of sex. Each ovum contains 22 autosomes and an X chromosome. Each spermatozoon (sperm) contains 22 autosomes and either an X chromosome or a Y chromosome. The sex of the zygote is determined at the time of fertilization by the combination of the sex chromosomes of the sperm (either X or Y) and the ovum (X).

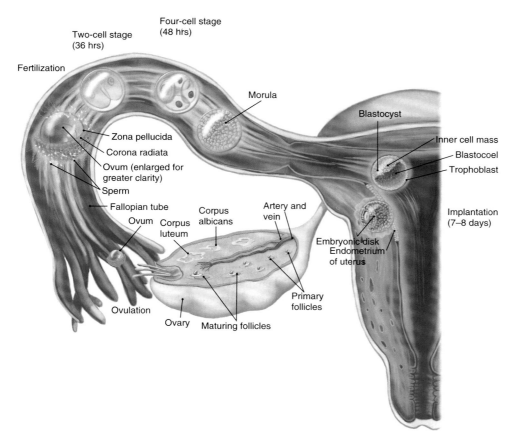

Two-cell stage
(36 hrs)

Four-cell stage
(48 hrs)

Fertilization

Morula

Blastocyst

Zona pellucida
Corona radiata
Ovum (enlarged for
greater clarity)
Sperm

Inner cell mass
Blastocoel
Trophoblast

Fallopian tube

Corpus
albicans

Artery and
vein

Implantation
(7–8 days)

Ovum   Corpus
luteum

Embryonic disk
Endometrium
of uterus

Ovulation

Primary
follicles

Ovary   Maturing follicles

FIGURE 5-6 Fertilization and tubal transport of the zygote. From fertilization to implantation, the zygote travels through the fallopian tube, experiencing rapid mitotic division (cleavage). During the journey toward the uterus, the zygote evolves through several stages, including morula and blastocyst.

TEST YOURSELF

✔ Gametogenesis occurs by which type of cellular division: mitosis or meiosis?

✔ A male fetus carries which two sex chromosomes?

✔ What is the name of the single cell that results from fertilization?

Embryonic Stage

The embryonic stage lasts from the end of the second week after fertilization until the end of the eighth week. During this stage, the woman misses her first menstrual period. The developing conceptus is now called the **embryo**. By the end of the embryonic stage, all of the organ systems and major structures are present, and the embryo is fully recognizable as human in form.

During the embryonic period, the cells of the embryo multiply, and tissues begin to assume specific functions, a process known as differentiation. It is through differentiation that tissues form the beginning of organs and organ systems.

In the third week after fertilization, three germ layers develop in the embryo. These layers are the ectoderm, mesoderm, and endoderm. The germ layers will become the different organs and tissues of the developing embryo. The ectoderm, which is the outer layer of cells, develops to form skin, hair, nails, and the nervous system. The mesoderm is the middle layer, which will form the skeletal, muscular, and circulatory systems. Lastly, the endoderm, which is the inner layer, will form the glands, lungs, and urinary and digestive tracts (Table 5-2).

Advise the Woman Who is Trying to Become Pregnant to be Very Careful

Exposure to a teratogen (any substance or process that can lead to birth defects) during the embryonic stage produces the greatest damaging effects because cells are rapidly dividing and differentiating into specific body structures.

Fetal Stage

The fetal stage begins in the ninth week after fertilization and continues until birth. At this time, the developing human is called the **fetus**. During the fetal stage, there is additional growth and maturation of the organs and body systems. At the beginning of this stage, the fetus is about 50 mm long and weighs about 8 g. By the end of the fetal stage, the fetus will be about 36 cm long and weigh approximately 3,400 g. Box 5-1 summarizes and illustrates the highlights of growth during the embryonic and fetal stages.

TABLE 5-2 Body Structures Developing From the Primary Germ Cells

GERM LAYER	STRUCTURE FORMATION
Ectoderm	Skin Nervous system Nasal passages Crystalline lens of the eye Pharynx Mammary glands Salivary glands
Mesoderm	Muscles Circulatory system Bones Reproductive system Connective tissue Kidneys Ureters
Endoderm	Gastrointestinal tract Respiratory tract Bladder Pancreas Liver

TEST YOURSELF

✔ What is the name of the stage of development that occurs during weeks 3 to 8 postconception?

✔ List the three germ layers in the embryo.

✔ Describe the events that occur from fertilization to implantation.

DEVELOPMENT OF SUPPORTIVE STRUCTURES

Several structures support the nourishment and protection of the fetus. These structures are the fetal membranes, the amniotic fluid, and the placenta. Fetal membranes surround the fetus in a protective sac filled with fluid that allows for protection and unrestricted growth. The woman's blood delivers nutrients to the fetus and also removes the metabolic wastes created by the fetus. This exchange now happens at the placenta. The umbilical cord connects the fetus and the placenta. Table 5-3 summarizes characteristics of the supportive structures.

Fetal Membranes

A small space begins to form between the inner cell mass—which will become the embryo—and the tissue that has embedded into the endometrial lining. This space will become the amniotic cavity in which the fetus will grow. The amniotic cavity begins to develop around 9 days after conception. The amnion surrounds the amniotic cavity. The **amnion** is a thick fibrous membrane made up of several layers that helps protect the fetus and forms the inner part of the sac in which the fetus grows. Amniotic fluid

fills this sac. Lying next to the amnion, toward the exterior of the blastocyst, is the chorion. The **chorion** is a second layer of thick fibrous tissue that surrounds the amnion. The amnion and chorion are not fused but lie in close contact with each other and together they make up the fetal membranes (Fig. 5-7).

At the end of the second week after fertilization, chorionic villi begin to appear on the chorion. **Chorionic villi** are fingerlike projections that extend out from the chorion, giving it a rough appearance. Around 15 to 20 days after fertilization, cells in the chorionic villi form arterial–capillary–venous networks, which become fetal blood vessels. These fetal blood vessels pick up oxygen and nutrients from maternal blood that enters the intervillous spaces and also exchange waste products and carbon dioxide to the maternal blood from the developing embryo.

Around the eighth week, some of the chorionic villi disintegrate, leaving a large area of the chorion that is smooth. The remaining chorionic villi increase in number and size and continue to branch out. The chorionic villi eventually become the fetal part of the placenta, where the exchange of nutrients and wastes occurs.

Amniotic Fluid

A specialized fluid called **amniotic fluid** fills the amniotic cavity. Amniotic fluid serves four main functions for the fetus: physical protection, temperature regulation, space for unrestricted movement, and allowance for symmetrical growth. Amniotic fluid can provide information for fetal evaluation because it collects substances from the fetal gastrointestinal, renal, and respiratory tracts. The fetal membranes produce amniotic fluid throughout pregnancy. The fluid is produced from maternal blood, fetal urine, and secretions from the fetal respiratory tract. The fluid is composed mostly of water (98% to 99%). Electrolytes, creatinine, urea, glucose, hormones, fetal cells, lanugo (fine downy hair), and vernix caseosa (a cheesy substance that protects fetal skin) make up the remaining 1% to 2% of the fluid.

Amniotic fluid acts as a cushion around the fetus. It protects the fetus from injury if the woman falls or if her abdomen is bumped. It helps maintain a constant temperature around the fetus because the fetus is not mature enough and does not have enough body fat to regulate its own temperature. Amniotic fluid allows the fetus to move freely, which helps the muscles to develop and aids in symmetric growth by providing an unrestricted environment early on in the pregnancy. Lastly, it is a fluid source that the fetus drinks and then urinates. The fetal intestines absorb the swallowed amniotic fluid, and then the fetus urinates the fluid back into the amniotic sac.

The fetus also takes in and then releases amniotic fluid when it practices fetal breathing movements. During fetal exhalation, the lungs release surfactant into the amniotic fluid. The fetal lungs produce surfactant around 22 to 28 weeks. Surfactant helps decrease the surface tension in

BOX 5-1 **Embryonic and Fetal Development**

End of 4 Weeks
Chorionic villi form.
The embryo is C shaped.
Length: 0.75–1 cm
Weight: 400 mg
Arms and legs are budlike structures.
Rudimentary eyes, ears, and nose are discernible.
Foundations for nervous system, genitourinary system, skin, bones, and lungs are formed.

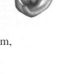

End of 8 Weeks
Length: 2.5–3 cm
Weight: 8 grams
The head is disproportionately large as a result of brain development.
The heart, with a septum and valves, is beating rhythmically.
The fingers and toes are distinct and separated.
Sex differentiation begins.
Organogenesis is complete.

End of 12 Weeks
Length: 8 cm
Weight: 25 grams
Placenta is complete.
Divisions of the brain begin to develop.
The face is well formed.
The eyes are widely spaced and fused.
Heartbeat is audible by Doppler.
Kidney secretion has begun.
Spontaneous movements occur (may not yet be discernible by the woman).
Sex is discernible by outward appearance.

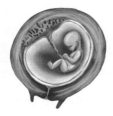

End of 16 Weeks
Length: 10–17 cm
Weight: 55–120 grams
Lungs are fully shaped.
Fetus swallows amniotic fluid.
Skeletal structure is identifiable.
Downy lanugo hair present on body.
Liver and pancreas are functioning.
Sex can be determined by ultrasound.

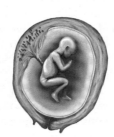

End of 20 Weeks
Length: 25 cm
Weight: 220 grams
Eyebrows and scalp hair are present.
Lanugo covers the entire body.
Vernix caseosa begins to form.
Heart sounds can be heard with a fetoscope.
Fetal movements are felt by the woman.

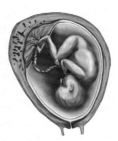

End of 24 Weeks
Length: 28–36 cm
Weight: 550 grams
Eyelids are now open.
Pupils are capable of reacting to light.
Active production of lung surfactant begins.
Exhibits a startle reflex.
Skin is red and wrinkled, with little subcutaneous fat.
Vernix caseosa covers the skin.
May survive if born in a facility with a fully equipped neonatal intensive care unit (NICU).

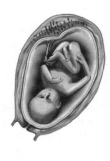

End of 28 Weeks
Length: 35–38 cm
Weight: 1,200 grams
Respiratory system is developed enough to provide gaseous exchange; however, the fetus needs care in a NICU in order to survive.
Adipose tissue begins to accumulate.
Male: The testes begin to descend into the scrotal sac.
Female: Clitoris is prominent and labia majora are small and do not cover the labia minora.

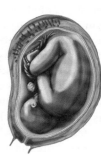

End of 32 Weeks
Length: 38–43 cm
Weight: 1,600 grams
The lungs are not yet fully developed, but the fetus usually does well if born at this time.
Active Moro reflex is present.
Steady weight gain occurs.
Male: Testes descend into the scrotum. The scrotal sac has few rugae.

End of 36 Weeks
Length: 42–48 cm
Weight: 1,800–2,700 grams
Lanugo begins to thin.
Sole of the foot has few creases.
Birth position is usually assumed (vertex, head down).

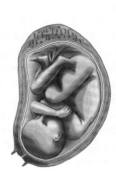

End of 40 Weeks (Full Term)
Length: 48–52 cm
Weight: 3,000 grams
Vernix caseosa is evident in body folds.
Lanugo remains on the shoulders and upper back only.
Creases cover at least two thirds of the surface of the sole of the foot.
Female: The labia majora are well developed.

TABLE 5-3   Characteristics of Supportive Structures

SUPPORTIVE STRUCTURE	CHARACTERISTICS
Placenta	2–3 cm thick, thickness established by 20 weeks 15–20 cm in diameter 500–600 grams in weight Made up of 15–20 lobes called cotyledons
Amniotic fluid	About 1 L at term Filtered and replaced every 3 hours Pale yellow to straw-colored
Umbilical cord	50 cm long and 2 cm wide Blood flow through cord is about 400 mL/min Two arteries, which carry deoxygenated blood to placenta from fetus One vein, which carries oxygen and nourishment from placenta to fetus Formed from the amnion

the alveoli. Sampling of the amniotic fluid can help to determine if the fetal lungs are mature enough for birth.

The fetus swallows its shed hair, epithelial cells, and sebaceous secretions. These substances form meconium as they gather in the fetal intestinal system. Meconium is the first bowel movement the infant has after birth. If the fetus is stressed during pregnancy or labor, the anal sphincter may relax and release meconium into the amniotic fluid. This action stains the normally colorless fluid a green color. This meconium stained amniotic fluid will be noticed at delivery when the fetal membranes rupture (also known as the "waters breaking"). During the normal fetal process of swallowing and inhaling amniotic fluid in utero, the thick meconium particles can lodge in the fetal lungs. The newborn is then at risk for meconium aspiration syndrome which can be potentially fatal (see Chapter 20).

Did You Know?

You can learn a lot from amniotic fluid! During pregnancy, through a procedure called amniocentesis, the health care provider obtains a sample of amniotic fluid. The fluid is analyzed to determine whether the fetal lungs are mature enough to support respiration outside the womb. The fluid can also be used for genetic testing because the fluid contains fetal cells with fetal DNA.

Placenta

The placenta is the organ that sustains and nourishes the growing pregnancy. The placenta has three main functions: to provide for the transfer and exchange of substances, to act as a barrier to certain substances, and to function as an endocrine gland by producing hormones. The placenta begins to develop during the fifth week after

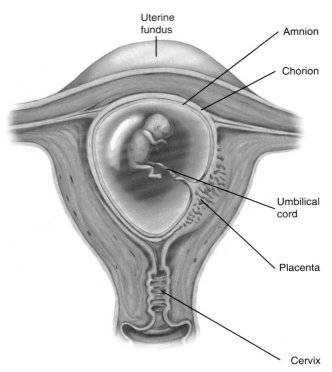

FIGURE 5-7 The embryo is surrounded by amniotic fluid in the amniotic sac, which is made up of the protective fetal membranes (amnion and chorion).

fertilization at the site of implantation. Most of the placenta is of embryonic origin, but about 20% is maternal in origin.

Many lobes, or sections, called cotyledons, comprise the placenta. Each cotyledon consists of two or more main stem villi and their branches. A main stem villus consists of a branch of the umbilical vein and umbilical artery that branches out into the intervillous space. Maternal blood from endometrial arteries pools in the intervillous spaces (Fig. 5-8).

The placenta is the exchange site for nutrients and wastes between the fetal and maternal circulatory systems. The maternal blood supply brings nutrients such as oxygen, water, electrolytes, vitamins, and glucose to the placenta. These nutrients cross to the fetal circulatory system for use by the fetus. The fetal circulatory system brings wastes such as carbon dioxide, carbon monoxide, urea, and uric acid to the placenta for removal by the maternal circulatory system. The nutrients and wastes cross at the level of the placenta by diffusion and active transport at the chorionic villi sites.

The fetus receives passive immunity from the woman by transfer of maternal antibodies. Maternal antibodies to diphtheria, smallpox, and measles travel across the placenta to the fetus. The fetus does not receive immunity to rubella, cytomegalovirus (CMV), varicella, or measles. If the woman encounters these pathogens during her pregnancy, fetal infection may occur. Some pathogens can cause birth defects. For this reason it is important for the

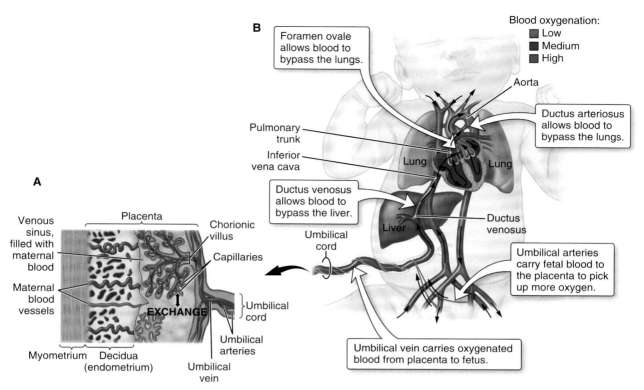

FIGURE 5-8 A. Chorionic villus and intervillous space in the placenta. Exchange of nutrients and wastes occurs in the intervillous space. **B.** Overview of fetal circulation. (From Zschocke, J. (2018). Molekulare Grundlagen. In: *Basiswissen Humangenetik*, 978-3-662-56146-1, © Springer-Verlag.)

woman to be up to date on her vaccines before becoming pregnant and to avoid infectious people or potentially infectious agents (e.g., cat feces or raw meats) during pregnancy.

The placenta acts as a barrier to some medications and hormones that are in the maternal blood supply. However, not all medications and substances are stopped by the placental barrier, and many of these substances cross over to the fetus. Some therapeutic medications are known to cause birth defects. For this reason the woman should discuss with her health care provider her medications before she becomes pregnant.

The placenta also secretes hormones that help to sustain the pregnancy. These include progesterone, estrogen, and hCG. Progesterone is necessary to maintain the nutrient-rich endometrial lining, the decidua. It also functions to keep the myometrium from having premature contractions. Estrogen functions to provide a rich blood supply to the decidua and placenta. The main function of

hCG is to sustain the corpus luteum at the beginning of the pregnancy.

The well-being of the fetus is dependent upon free access to nutrients from the woman. Any anomaly of the placenta or of the maternal–placental circulation that impedes fetal nourishment may lead to fetal growth restriction, fetal stress, or death. Intrauterine growth restriction (IUGR), also referred to as fetal growth restriction, indicates that fetal growth has slowed for some reason, resulting in a fetus that is smaller than expected for gestational age. IUGR can have many causes. Box 5-2 summarizes some of these common causes.

Don't Pass Up This Teaching Opportunity

The woman should consider that everything she takes in will pass to the fetus. Teach her to check with her health care provider before taking any substance, including over-the-counter medications and herbal preparations that are not specifically ordered for her. This warning extends to immunizations as well.

> **BOX 5-2 Common Causes of IUGR**

- Chromosomal abnormalities
- Fetal infection
- Placental infarcts
- Maternal nutritional deficiencies
- Maternal hypertension
- Preeclampsia
- Maternal renal disease
- Maternal smoking
- Maternal illegal drug use
- Toxin/teratogen exposure
- Multifetal pregnancy

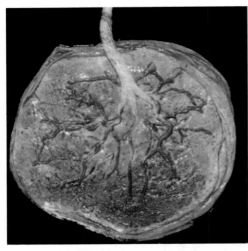

FIGURE 5-9 Placenta and umbilical cord. The fetal side of the placenta, from where the umbilical cord arises, is shown and the vascular nature of the placenta is evident. The fetal side of the placenta has a shiny appearance. Note that the amnion and chorion remain attached to the placenta (in the photo it appears as the pink membranous rim that is surrounding the placenta).

Maternal hypertension or infectious agents can cause areas of infarction and subsequent calcification in the placenta. These areas lead to a decreased surface area, which decreases the amount of nutrients that travel to the fetus at a given time. Vasoconstriction caused by hypertension, smoking, or illicit drug use also decreases the flow of blood to the fetus.

Umbilical Cord

The umbilical cord extends from the umbilicus of the fetus to the fetal surface of the placenta (Fig. 5-9). In the cord are two arteries that bring deoxygenated blood from the fetus to the placenta and one vein that carries oxygenated and nourished blood from the placenta to the fetus. The three vessels are surrounded by **Wharton jelly**, which is a clear gelatinous substance that gives support to the cord and helps prevent compression of the cord. Unrestricted blood flow through the cord is essential to the growth and health of the fetus.

> **Don't Get Confused**
>
> In the umbilical cord the two umbilical arteries carry deoxygenated blood and the one umbilical vein carries oxygenated blood. This is different than in the majority of human circulation.

Cultural Snapshot

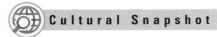

Certain ethnic groups, such as people from Asia, commonly produce offspring that are smaller than those from other ethnic groups. The fetuses of these ethnic groups are not growth-restricted (IUGR). It is important to take into account the country of origin and stature of both the mother and the father when evaluating an infant for IUGR.

> **TEST YOURSELF**
>
> ✔ Describe how nutrients and wastes are exchanged between the woman and the fetus.
> ✔ Name the four functions of amniotic fluid.
> ✔ List three hormones produced by the placenta.

Remember Bethany from the beginning of the chapter. As the nurse taking care of her, what information do you think is important to reinforce to her regarding fetal development? What information should she be encouraged to share with her health care provider?

FETAL AND PLACENTAL CIRCULATION

Fetal Circulation

Fetal circulation differs from the pattern of human circulation that is present after birth. While in utero, the fetus is dependent upon the maternal circulation for its oxygenation, and the fetus does not use its lungs to oxygenate blood. Because the level of oxygen that is in the fetus's bloodstream is lower than maternal levels, fetal circulation aids in carrying oxygenated blood from the placenta to the major organs, especially the brain, liver, and kidneys. Fetal circulation is possible because of three major shunts that are present in the fetus, but these shunts close shortly after birth. These shunts are the ductus venosus, foramen ovale, and the ductus arteriosus.

Fetal blood that is deoxygenated and contains metabolic waste products flows away from the fetus to the placenta via the two umbilical arteries located in the umbilical cord. Each umbilical artery serves one half of the placenta. The arteries branch off into main stem chorionic villi that then branch down toward the intervillous spaces. The exchange of oxygen and nutrients from the woman's bloodstream for waste products from the fetus occurs at this level.

Oxygenated and nourished fetal blood flows to the fetus from the placenta via the umbilical vein located in the umbilical cord. In the umbilical vein, the saturation of fetal blood with oxygen is about 80%. The umbilical cord enters the fetus at the site that will be the umbilicus after birth. Approximately half of the oxygenated blood circulates from the umbilical vein to the liver, and the other half of oxygen-rich blood shunts past the liver and flows directly into the inferior vena cava by way of the **ductus venosus**. In the inferior vena cava, the oxygenated blood mixes with deoxygenated blood that is returning to the heart from the lower limbs, abdomen, and pelvis, making the oxygen saturation of the blood entering the right atrium about 67%.

The majority of the blood in the right atrium flows into the left atrium via the foramen ovale. The **foramen ovale** is a hole that connects the right and left atria so the majority of oxygenated blood can quickly pass into the left side of the fetal heart and go to the brain and the rest of the fetal body. Blood entering the right atrium from the superior vena cava is mostly deoxygenated. In the right atrium, this blood mixes with some of the more oxygenated blood from the inferior vena cava. This mixed blood then enters the right ventricle, which pumps it to the fetal lungs via the pulmonary trunk.

In utero, the fetus does not oxygenate its own blood in the lungs; therefore, blood supplied to the fetal lungs is for nourishment of the lung tissues only. The fetal lungs are collapsed and filled with fluid, which leads to high resistance. Because of this resistance, only 5% to 10% of the blood in the pulmonary artery enters the fetal lungs. The remainder of blood coming from the right ventricle enters the ductus arteriosus. The **ductus arteriosus** is a fetal shunt that links the pulmonary artery with the aorta and allows the oxygenated blood to flow to the body without having to reenter the heart.

In the left atrium, the oxygenated blood mixes with some deoxygenated blood that is returning to the heart from the lungs. The blood then travels to the left ventricle, which pumps the blood to the aorta. The higher oxygenated blood from the ascending aorta flows to the heart, head, and upper limbs by way of the aortic arch branch.

Blood in the abdominal aorta divides so that half of the blood supply returns to the placenta for reoxygenation, whereas the other half goes to nourish the viscera and lower half of the body. The internal iliac arteries branch off to form the two umbilical arteries. The umbilical arteries then carry deoxygenated blood and waste products back to the placenta, which completes the fetal circulation circuit (Fig. 5-10).

At birth, when the umbilical cord is clamped, fetal blood no longer flows to the placenta for oxygenation. Rapid physiologic changes occur to allow the newborn to oxygenate their own blood by their lungs. After birth, the ductus venosus, ductus arteriosus, and umbilical vein and arteries constrict and eventually form ligaments, which remain present for the rest of the infant's life. It is possible for the ductus arteriosus to remain open, especially in premature infants or infants with hypoxia. When this shunt remains open, it is called patent ductus arteriosus, and medications or surgery may be required to close the duct. Refer to Chapter 13 for a discussion of the circulatory changes that occur in the newborn and Chapter 21 for a discussion of patent ductus arteriosus.

Placental Circulation

The uterine arteries supply the uterus with maternal blood. The endometrial, or spiral, arteries then carry the blood to the intervillous spaces. In the intervillous spaces, maternal blood flows around the chorionic villi, where nutrients and oxygen from the maternal circulation are transferred by diffusion and active transport across a layer of cells into the fetal circulation. Likewise, fetal wastes diffuse into the maternal bloodstream. Blood leaves the intervillous spaces by the endometrial veins and returns to the maternal circulatory system.

TEST YOURSELF

✔ Name the three fetal shunts.
✔ Describe the path of fetal circulation.
✔ Explain how the ductus arteriosus and foramen ovale aid the fetus in quickly getting oxygen-enriched blood to the tissues.

SPECIAL CONSIDERATIONS OF FETAL DEVELOPMENT

Teratogens and the Fetus

A **teratogen** is a substance that causes birth defects. The severity of the defect depends on when during development the conceptus is exposed to the teratogen (i.e., which body systems are developing at the time of exposure) and the particular teratogenic agent to which the fetus is exposed.

Effects of Teratogens on the Developing Fetus

During the pre-embryonic stage, exposure to a teratogen has an all-or-nothing effect. Either the exposure will cause death of the zygote or there will be no effect because there is no connection between the maternal blood supply and the zygote.

Exposure to a teratogen during the embryonic stage produces the greatest damaging effects. It is during this time that development of the primary structure and function of organs and tissues occurs. Developing organs and body systems are highly susceptible to teratogens, and major abnormalities can result. Table 5-4 lists structures commonly affected by teratogen exposure during the embryonic period. Because the central nervous system (CNS) develops continuously throughout pregnancy, these structures are always vulnerable to teratogens.

Exposure to a teratogen during the fetal stage will have less of an effect on the fetus than exposure during the embryonic period. The effect of a teratogen during the fetal stage may cause physiologic defects and minor structural abnormalities. The CNS and brain continue to be susceptible to damage from teratogens during the fetal period.

Types of Teratogenic Agents

Teratogens usually fall into one of three categories: an ingested, infectious, or environmental substance. Table 5-5 summarizes some of the common teratogens and their effects.

Ingested Teratogens

Most substances ingested by the pregnant woman pass to the fetus from the maternal bloodstream through

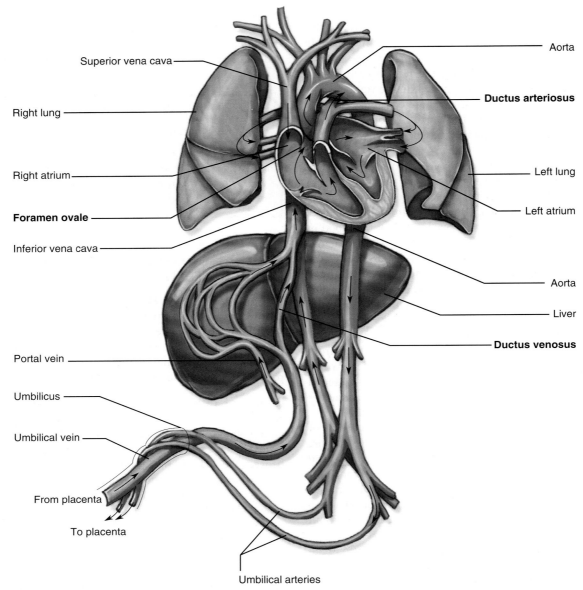

FIGURE 5-10 Fetal circulation. *Arrows* indicate the path of blood. Names in **bold** are the three fetal shunts. The umbilical vein carries oxygen-rich blood from the placenta to the liver and through the ductus venosus. From there the blood is carried to the inferior vena cava to the right atrium of the heart. Some of the blood is shunted through the foramen ovale to the left side of the heart where it is routed to the brain and upper extremities. The rest of the blood travels down to the right ventricle and through the pulmonary artery. A small portion of the blood travels to the nonfunctioning lungs, while the remaining blood is shunted through the ductus arteriosus into the aorta to supply the rest of the body.

the placenta and then into fetal circulation. Commonly ingested teratogens include prescription medications, illicit drugs, and alcohol. Some medications may be therapeutic for the woman but also have teratogenic properties. For example, phenytoin is therapeutic for preventing seizures in the woman but can cause cleft palate and other abnormalities in the fetus. In such a circumstance, the health care provider weighs the risk to the woman against the risk to the developing fetus before prescribing a potential teratogen. An alternative nonteratogenic medication may be prescribed instead. Not all medications are teratogenic.

Acetaminophen is an example of a medication that, when taken as directed, is non-teratogenic. Some medications, such as heparin, are unable to cross the placental barrier and are therefore safe to use during pregnancy.

Your Sensitivity Can Make a Big Difference

Guilt is a common feeling for the mother of an infant with a birth defect. Many defects happen before the woman knows she is pregnant. Avoid statements that imply blame. For example, do not say, "You shouldn't have been around x-rays while you were pregnant."

TABLE 5-4 Structures Commonly Affected by Teratogens During the Embryonic Period

WEEK OF DEVELOPMENT (NO. OF WEEKS AFTER FERTILIZATION) IN WHICH EXPOSURE OCCURS	STRUCTURES COMMONLY AFFECTED
3	Heart and central nervous system (CNS)
4	Lip, heart, arm, leg, CNS
5	Heart, eye, arm, leg, CNS
6	CNS, heart, ear, teeth
7	CNS, ear, teeth, palate, heart
8	CNS, ear, palate, heart, external genitalia

TABLE 5-5 Common Teratogens and Associated Effects

TERATOGEN	POSSIBLE EFFECT
Ingested Agents	
Phenytoin	Cleft palate
Chemotherapy agents	Major congenital malformations, especially of the central nervous system
Tetracycline	Damage to developing dental and osseous tissue
Alcohol	Fetal alcohol spectrum disorder with facial defects, low birth weight, effects on brain
Infectious Agents	
Varicella	Fetal varicella syndrome, which ranges in severity from generalized multiorgan damage to isolated defects, such as incomplete limb development or skin scarring
Rubella (German measles)	Cataracts, deafness, and cardiac malformations
CMV	Hearing loss, microcephaly
Environmental Agents	
Mercury	Neurologic damage, blindness
Radiation	Congenital malformations, intellectual disability (seen in large amounts of ionizing radiation)

One of the fetus's main body systems affected throughout the embryonic and fetal period is the CNS, including the brain. Alcohol and illicit drugs such as marijuana, cocaine, and heroin negatively affect the developing CNS. Infants exposed to these substances during pregnancy may be born with a physical dependence on the substance to which they were exposed. In addition, these substances can lead to decreased mental capacity and cause other defects and pregnancy complications. Therefore, ingestion of these substances should be avoided during pregnancy.

Infectious Teratogens

If the pregnant woman develops an infection during her pregnancy, the infection can pass to the fetus and affect fetal development. Some common infections that have teratogenic effects include varicella, CMV, and rubella. The Zika virus, when contracted during pregnancy, has been shown to cause birth defects including microcephaly.

Prevention is the woman's best protection against an infectious teratogen. The woman should take precautions to avoid sick individuals during her pregnancy. Thoroughly cooking foods, including meats, and frequent hand washing are ways the woman can help protect herself. Mosquitos have been identified in the transmission of the Zika virus, so the woman should take precautions with avoiding mosquitos by using preventative measures and avoiding travel to areas known to have large mosquito infestations. She should also avoid cleaning cat litter boxes and bird cages. Cat feces are known to carry the parasite that causes toxoplasmosis, whereas histoplasmosis is a disease caused by fungus that thrives in bird droppings. Both toxoplasmosis and histoplasmosis can be teratogenic.

Environmental Teratogens

Substances in the environment can have a teratogenic effect. X-rays, radioactive substances, and certain chemicals can cause birth defects. The pregnant woman should take precautions to avoid these substances during her pregnancy. Avoiding unnecessary x-rays, or using a lead shield for unavoidable x-rays, and using gloves and masks when handling chemicals are two ways the woman can help protect her developing fetus.

 A Personal Glimpse

The worrying began when I found out I was pregnant with my oldest child. We hadn't been officially trying to get pregnant, and so right away I started thinking about all the things I had ingested while already pregnant. I was a three-cup-a-day coffee drinker; I had taken several doses of Tylenol for headaches; and I remembered celebrating my birthday with a few glasses of wine. To top it all off, I hadn't been taking prenatal vitamins. I started panicking about the harm I had caused my developing baby. I immediately stopped drinking caffeine completely (which gave me very bad headaches); swore off wine for the duration; avoided taking any kind of medication for pain; never missed a day taking prenatal vitamins; and avoided eating fish, hot dogs, and lunch meat (I had heard that these foods were bad to eat during pregnancy). I was also concerned about microwave rays (and stopped using the microwave completely), cats and cat litter, gardening, being around my friends' children (they might have some lurking virus), and mold in the house. I was starting to drive my husband and myself crazy.

At my first prenatal appointment, I talked with the staff at my primary care provider's office. They gave me a brochure that listed things to avoid completely during pregnancy; things to limit during pregnancy; and things that were OK during pregnancy. It also contained practical advice for maintaining a healthy home environment during pregnancy and childrearing. I remained careful during my pregnancy, but I learned to relax a bit more and just use common sense.

Allison

Learning Opportunity: *How can the nurse help the woman of childbearing age be aware of possible teratogens without unduly scaring her? How should the nurse advise the woman who is very worried that she may have done something to harm her unborn child before she was aware of the pregnancy?*

Ectopic Pregnancy

There are instances when the zygote implants in places other than the uterus. When the zygote implants outside the uterus, an **ectopic pregnancy** is the result. Of the implantations that occur outside of the uterine cavity, most occur in the fallopian tube. An ectopic pregnancy that occurs in a fallopian tube is called a tubal pregnancy. Usually tubal pregnancies are caused by blockage or scarring of the fallopian tubes, from either infection or trauma (e.g., abdominal surgery or tubal ligation reversal). Ectopic pregnancy is the leading cause of maternal death in the first trimester (Tulandi, 2020).

As the embryo grows in the confined space of the fallopian tube, it causes the tube to dilate. The tube will eventually rupture if the condition remains undetected. If the tube ruptures, hemorrhage into the peritoneal cavity can lead to maternal death. Surgical removal of the affected tube and the products of conception is the most common treatment. Because there is no way to transplant the embryo into the uterine cavity and continue the pregnancy, tubal pregnancies always result in the death of the embryo. Chapter 17 also discusses ectopic pregnancy.

Multifetal Pregnancy

When a woman is carrying more than one fetus at the same time, it is called a multifetal pregnancy. Multifetal pregnancies can result in twins, triplets, or more. The overall prevalence of naturally occurring twin pregnancies in the United States is once in 250 deliveries, with triplets occurring once in 8,000 deliveries, and quadruplets occurring once in 600,000 pregnancies (Fletcher, 2019). The overall rates of multifetal pregnancies have changed during the last few decades because of the increasing number of assisted reproductive procedures and the use of fertility medications.

Twins can be either identical or fraternal. Identical twins derive from one zygote (one egg and one sperm which divides into two zygotes shortly after fertilization), so identical twins are **monozygotic** twins. They share the same genetic material and are always the same sex. Fraternal twins develop from separate egg and sperm fertilizations and are **dizygotic** twins. Fraternal twins may or may not be the same sex, and their genetic material is not identical (Fig. 5-11). In pregnancies that have more than two fetuses, they may have all developed from a single fertilized egg, also referred to as monozygotic; or they may have developed from separate eggs; or they may be a combination of both types.

Twins are classified one of three ways—diamniotic–dichorionic, diamniotic–monochorionic, and monoamniotic–monochorionic. Diamniotic–dichorionic twins each develop in their own amniotic sac. Their placentas do not share any vessels. Diamniotic–monochorionic twins each have their own amniotic sac but share a common chorionic sac. They each have a separate placenta, but the placentas share some vessels. These types of twins are at risk for developing a condition referred to as twin-to-twin transfusion syndrome. In this syndrome, one fetus gives the other fetus part of its blood volume but does not receive any in return. Lastly, twins can be monoamniotic–monochorionic. These types of twins have one amniotic cavity that they both share. The greatest risk to these twins is

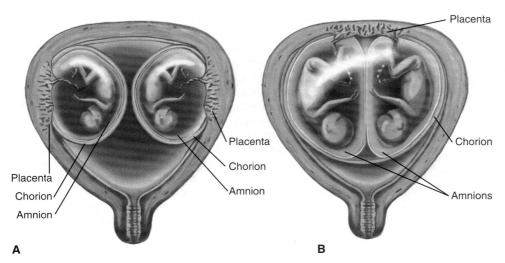

A

B

FIGURE 5-11 Twin pregnancy. **A.** Fraternal (dizygotic) twins with two placentas, two amnions, and two chorions (diamniotic–dichorionic). **B.** Identical (monozygotic) twins with one placenta, two amnions, and one chorion (diamniotic–monochorionic).

Placenta
Chorion
Amnion

Placenta
Chorion
Amnion

Placenta
Chorion
Amnions

cord entanglement. They are also at risk for twin-to-twin transfusion syndrome.

Certain factors increase a woman's chance of becoming pregnant with dizygotic twins. She is more likely to have dizygotic twins if she is herself a twin or has twin siblings, if she recently stopped using oral contraceptives, if she is tall or has a large stature, or if she is of African American heritage. The use of fertility medications, such as clomiphene citrate or menotropins, increases a woman's chance of carrying a multifetal pregnancy. Multifetal pregnancies are at higher risk and require close monitoring (see Chapter 17).

TEST YOURSELF

✔ Which organ system is susceptible throughout the pregnancy to teratogenic effects?

✔ Describe the risks associated with an ectopic pregnancy.

✔ Why are fraternal twins called dizygotic twins?

Remember Bethany Sanders from the beginning of the chapter. She had some questions about her pregnancy. How would you answer her question about the "baby breathing underwater"? How does the fetus "breathe"? How would you explain to Bethany how her fetus gets the nutrients it needs to grow and develop?

KEY POINTS

- Mitosis is the process of cell division by which two daughter cells are produced that have the diploid number of chromosomes (46). Meiosis is a special type of cell division that results in the formation of cells with the haploid number of chromosomes (23).

- Spermatogenesis begins at puberty, whereas oogenesis starts during the fetal stage in the female and then stays in an arrested state until puberty. Spermatogenesis ends with four spermatids, each with 23 chromosomes. Oogenesis ends with one ovum containing 23 chromosomes.

- Sex determination occurs when the ovum and the sperm unite. The ovum always contributes an X chromosome, whereas the sperm contributes either an X or a Y chromosome. Two X chromosomes (XX) is female. An X and a Y chromosome (XY) is male.

- The pre-embryonic stage lasts from fertilization until the end of the second week after conception. During this time, the two sets of chromosomes combine, implantation occurs, and the beginning of maternal–fetal circulation occurs.

- The embryonic stage lasts from the end of the second week until the end of the eighth week. During this time, the organs and tissues begin to differentiate and assume specific functions. By the end of this stage, all organs are developed, and the embryo is distinctly human in appearance.

- The fetal stage lasts from the end of the eighth week until birth. During this time, there is additional maturation and growth of already existing tissues and organ systems.

- The amnion and chorion form the fetal membranes. The amnion makes up the inner part of the membrane and is in contact with amniotic fluid and the fetus. The chorion is adjacent to (but not fused with) the amnion and has no contact with the fetus.

- Amniotic fluid serves as a cushion to protect the fetus from injury, a temperature control mechanism, and a medium that allows free movement and unrestricted growth.

- The placenta transfers nutrients, such as oxygen and glucose, to the fetus while removing waste products, such as carbon dioxide and urea. The placenta acts as a barrier to some harmful substances but does not prevent most substances from passing to the fetus. The placenta has an endocrine function in that it secretes hormones that help sustain the pregnancy. These hormones include hCG, estrogen, and progesterone.

- Maternal blood rich in oxygen and nutrients reaches the placenta at the level of the intervillous spaces that are surrounded by the chorionic villi. The chorionic villi contain the fetal blood vessels. Exchange of nutrients for wastes occurs by simple diffusion or active transport across a thin membrane that separates the fetal and maternal bloodstreams.

- Fetal blood that contains newly oxygenated blood and nutrients leaves the placenta via the umbilical vein and enters the fetal inferior vena cava via the ductus venosus. From there it travels to the right atrium, where most of the blood crosses the foramen ovale into the left atrium. The blood then travels through the aortic arch to the brain and the upper body. Some of the blood enters the right ventricle and goes to the lungs to nourish the tissues. Most of the blood that leaves the right ventricle is shunted to the aorta via the ductus arteriosus. Deoxygenated fetal blood returns to the placenta via the two umbilical arteries.

- Teratogens are classified as ingested, infectious, or environmental. Ingested teratogens include medications and illegal substances. Infectious teratogens include diseases such as CMV, and rubella. Environmental teratogens include x-rays and chemicals.

- An ectopic pregnancy is one that develops outside of the uterus. Most ectopic pregnancies occur in a fallopian tube, which can rupture and lead to maternal hemorrhage and death. A tubal pregnancy always leads to death of the embryo, whether from tubal rupture or from removal during surgery.

- Identical twins are monozygotic because they arise from one zygote and therefore share identical chromosomes. Fraternal twins are dizygotic because they arise from two separate zygotes and therefore do not share the same chromosomes.

INTERNET RESOURCES

Fetal Development
https://www.parents.com/pregnancy/week-by-week/baby-development/

IUGR
http://kidshealth.org/parent/medical/endocrine/iugr.html

Teratogens
https://www.stanfordchildrens.org/en/topic/
default?id=medical-genetics-teratogens-90-P09519&sid=

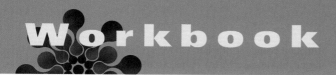

NCLEX-STYLE REVIEW QUESTIONS

1. How long does the embryonic stage last?
   a. Ovulation to conception
   b. 1 to 14 days after conception
   c. 3 through 8 weeks after conception
   d. 9 through 38 weeks after conception

2. What is the main purpose of the chorionic villi?
   a. To adhere the blastocyst to the endometrial lining
   b. To form the tissues that will become the placenta
   c. To produce amniotic fluid
   d. To provide an exchange site for nutrients and wastes

3. Which of the following is a shunt that aids in fetal circulation? (Select all that apply)
   a. Foramen primum
   b. Septum secundum
   c. Foramen ovale
   d. Ductus deferens
   e. Ductus venosus
   f. Ductus arteriosus

4. What is the classification of twins who share the same chromosomal material?
   a. Monozygotic
   b. Dizygotic
   c. Fraternal
   d. Trizygotic

5. A client with epilepsy was on phenytoin when she became pregnant. She is worried that her baby will have a birth defect. Which is the most therapeutic reply from the nurse?
   a. "All substances and medications increase the risk of birth defects when you are pregnant. It is important for you to discontinue any medications or over-the-counter medications immediately. This is the best way you can protect your baby."
   b. "Please don't worry, phenytoin is a very safe medication and unlikely to cause a birth defect."
   c. "Yes, phenytoin increases the risk of certain defects in the fetus; however, overall the risk is low that your baby will be affected. Your health care provider weighs the risk of untreated epilepsy with the risk of the medication when making decisions about your treatment plan."
   d. "Yes, there is a very high risk that your fetus will have major birth defects. Your health care provider will most likely switch you to a safer medication. Are you on any other medications?"

STUDY ACTIVITIES

Use the following table to compare major developmental milestones at each of the indicated gestational ages. Refer to this textbook and to https://www.parents.com/pregnancy/week-by-week/baby-development/

Gestational Age (in Weeks)	Major Developmental Milestones
4	
8	
12	
16	
20	
28	
32	
36	

1. Talk to the following individuals in your community about teratogens. Have each person discuss several substances or processes that might be damaging to the fetus and how a pregnant woman can best protect her fetus from harm.
   a. Pharmacist
   b. Obstetrician
   c. Chemist
   d. Radiologist

2. Develop a teaching plan for a pregnant adolescent. Explain the processes of fertilization and development in language she will likely understand. Prepare the answers to three to four questions you anticipate she may ask you.

CRITICAL THINKING: WHAT WOULD YOU DO?

Apply your knowledge of fetal development to the following situation.

1. Rebecca, a 25-year-old woman, has just discovered she is pregnant for the first time. She missed her first menstrual period 4 weeks ago and came to the office for a pregnancy test, which was positive.
   a. Rebecca asks you what her baby looks like right now. What will you tell her?
   b. Rebecca is worried because she has taken acetaminophen several times during the past week for tension headaches. How will you advise her?

2. Rebecca comes in for her 12-week checkup. She measures larger than expected for dates, so the health care provider orders a sonogram.
   a. Rebecca asks you to tell her what her baby looks like at this stage. How will you answer?
   b. The sonogram shows that Rebecca is carrying twins. She wants to know whether they are identical or fraternal. How will you answer her?

Maternal Adaptation During Pregnancy

Key Terms

ballottement
Braxton Hicks contractions
Chadwick sign
colostrum
couvade syndrome
diastasis recti
glycosuria
Goodell sign
Hegar sign
linea nigra
lordosis
melasma (chloasma)
pica
pyrosis
striae gravidarum
supine hypotensive syndrome

Learning Objectives

At the conclusion of this chapter, you will:

1. Differentiate among presumptive, probable, and positive signs of pregnancy.
2. Relate normal anatomy and physiology of the nonpregnant woman to that of the pregnant woman.
3. Explain expected changes in the major body systems during pregnancy.
4. Discuss maternal psychological adaptation to pregnancy.
5. Describe changing nutritional requirements during pregnancy.

Samantha Chavez and her significant other have come to the prenatal clinic after she had a positive home pregnancy test. Samantha is most concerned about what will happen to her body while she is pregnant. Her partner asks you what foods Samantha should eat to have a healthy baby. As you read the chapter, think of how you can answer the two questions.

Pregnancy is a time of adaptation and change not only physically, but also psychologically as the woman and her partner prepare for parenthood. The woman's body must adapt to accommodate the needs of the growing fetus. This chapter explores the signs of pregnancy, the physiologic and psychological changes associated with pregnancy, and the changing nutritional requirements of pregnancy.

SIGNS OF PREGNANCY

A woman wants confirmation of pregnancy whether she is trying to get pregnant or thinks she might be pregnant when she was not planning a pregnancy. The health care provider uses a combination of signs to diagnose pregnancy (Box 6-1). These signs can be categorized as presumptive, probable, and positive. The presumptive, or subjective, signs are the symptoms the woman experiences and reports to the health care provider. Each of these signs, taken alone, can have causes other than pregnancy. The same is true for probable or objective signs. The positive signs are objective data noted by the examiner and are the only signs that are 100% diagnostic of pregnancy.

Presumptive (Possible) Signs

Presumptive signs of pregnancy are subjective data that the woman reports. The most common presumptive sign of pregnancy is a

BOX 6-1 **Signs of Pregnancy**

Presumptive (Possible) Signs

After each symptom, a cause other than pregnancy (if any) is listed. The presence of symptoms may vary in individual women:

- Amenorrhea (missed period). May be caused by irregular menstrual cycles, emotional stress, illness or disorders, intense exercise
- Nausea or morning sickness. May be related to gastrointestinal disorders, emotional distress
- Fatigue. May be related to anemia, lack of sleep, infection
- Breast changes. May be because of hormonal changes, oral contraceptives
- Frequent urination. Can be associated with urinary tract infection, nervousness

Probable Signs

After each sign, a cause other than pregnancy (if any) is suggested:

- 4 to 12 weeks: Presence of hCG in blood. May be caused by a hydatidiform mole
- 6 to 12 weeks: Presence of hCG in urine. May be caused by choriocarcinoma
- 8+ weeks: Uterine growth. May be caused by a tumor
- 16 weeks: Braxton Hicks (painless contractions). Could be gastrointestinal (GI) upset
- 16 to 28 weeks: Ballottement of fetus. Could be uterine polyps

Positive Signs

- 6+ weeks: Visualization of fetus by ultrasound
- 9 to 10+ weeks: Fetal heart sounds by Doppler
- 18 to 20+ weeks: Fetal heart sounds by fetal stethoscope (fetoscope)
- 22+ weeks: Fetal movements palpable by a trained practitioner
- Late pregnancy: Fetal movements visible

missed menstrual period or amenorrhea. There are many causes of amenorrhea. Some women have irregular periods. Emotional distress can cause a woman to skip a menstrual period. Some disorders, such as anorexia nervosa, can lead to amenorrhea. Women who perform intense exercise, such as marathon running, may experience amenorrhea. Because so many factors, other than pregnancy, can cause a woman to miss a menstrual period, amenorrhea is classified as a presumptive or subjective sign of pregnancy.

Other presumptive signs include nausea; fatigue; swollen, tender breasts; and frequent urination. Nausea can be caused by emotional distress, a viral infection, gastritis, or many other problems. Anemia, lack of sleep, overexertion, or infection can lead to fatigue. Breast tissue can become swollen and tender in response to hormonal changes just before a woman starts her menstrual period. Frequent urination can result from a urinary tract infection, nervousness, or from taking in substances, such as caffeine, that have diuretic properties.

Probable Signs

Probable signs of pregnancy are those detected by a trained examiner. These include objective data, such as the **Chadwick sign,** a bluish-purplish color of the cervix, vagina, and perineum. The examiner identifies **Hegar sign**, softening of the uterine isthmus, and **Goodell sign**, softening of the cervix, during the speculum and digital pelvic examinations. Other objective signs include a change in the shape of the uterus, an enlarging uterus, and Braxton Hicks contractions. **Ballottement** occurs when the examiner pushes up on the uterine wall during a pelvic examination, then feels the fetus bounce back against the examiner's fingers. The reason these signs are considered probable, rather than positive, is that pelvic tumors and some types of cancers can cause similar signs.

Another probable sign is the pregnancy test. Although pregnancy tests performed in a laboratory are highly reliable (from 97% to 99%), there is still the small possibility for error. Pregnancy tests measure the presence of human chorionic gonadotropin (hCG) in the urine or the blood. These levels can be elevated in conditions other than pregnancy, such as hydatidiform mole and choriocarcinoma.

Many women use home pregnancy tests to determine whether they are pregnant. These home pregnancy tests are approximately 95% reliable when they are performed correctly and done within the time frame specified by the test. Some tests can detect the presence of hCG within 1 day of the woman's missed period. It is important for the woman to know that the home pregnancy test is more likely to be correct when it reveals a positive result than when a negative result is obtained. In other words, if the home pregnancy test is negative, she should still monitor for signs of pregnancy and repeat the test or schedule an appointment with her health care provider.

Testing for hCG can be done in approximately 10 minutes, is reliable within 7 or 8 days after ovulation, and can be done on urine or the woman's serum. If urine is used, it is best to have the first voided specimen of the morning because this urine is highly concentrated, making detection of hCG easier.

Positive Signs

Positive signs are diagnostic of pregnancy because no other condition can cause the sign. The positive sign that can be elicited earliest in the pregnancy is visualization of the gestational sac or fetus. With transvaginal ultrasound, the gestational sac can be seen as early as 10 days after implantation. The fetal outline and cardiac activity are visible by abdominal ultrasound at 7 to 8 weeks of gestation.

The fetal heartbeat, heard at 9 to 10 weeks of gestation with Doppler technology and by 18 to 20 weeks with a fetoscope, is a positive sign of pregnancy. Palpation of fetal movements by a trained examiner is a positive sign of pregnancy.

PHYSIOLOGIC ADAPTATION TO PREGNANCY

The woman's body must make tremendous changes to accommodate a pregnancy (Table 6-1). While she is pregnant, her body must maintain all her vital functions and those of the growing fetus. Some changes are structural and occur because of pressure exerted by the growing fetus and expanding uterus. Other changes are hormone related. The next section discusses the physiologic changes that occur during pregnancy by body system.

Reproductive Changes

Obviously, the reproductive system changes during pregnancy. Instead of shedding endometrial tissue every month, the uterus must maintain the decidua (the name for the endometrium during pregnancy). The myometrium (uterine muscle) must stay relatively relaxed. If it contracts too forcefully, the pregnancy will be lost. The uterus undergoes changes immediately after conception and continues to grow and change throughout the pregnancy. The cervix, vagina, perineum, and breasts also undergo changes.

Uterus

During the first weeks after conception, the uterine muscle cells begin to hypertrophy, causing the uterus to expand. It is thought that estrogen stimulates this muscle cell hypertrophy. At first, the uterine walls become thicker, but as the pregnancy progresses, the growing fetus and accessory

TABLE 6-1 Anatomy and Physiology Changes in the Pregnant Woman

SYSTEM OR STRUCTURE	CHARACTERISTICS DURING PREGNANCY (AT TERM, UNLESS OTHERWISE INDICATED)
Uterus	• Uterine weight increases 1.5–2 times from prepregnancy weight • Uterine cavity capacity increases • Structure and shape changes (becomes a round shaped, thin, muscular sac) • Enlarges to fill the abdominal cavity
Breasts	• Initially tender • Enlarged • Darkened areola with increased projections of Montgomery glands (Montgomery tubercles)

Blood	• Blood volume increases to 100 mL/kg
	• Red blood cell volume increases
	• Plasma volume increases by 30%–50%
	• Hematocrit decreases, particularly in the third trimester as plasma volume increases
	• White blood cell (WBC) count becomes as great as 16,000 mm^3
	• Physiologic anemia present due to:
	  • Increase in plasma volume that is greater than the RBC increase
	  • Hemoglobin: 12.5 g/dL
	  (Note: A hemoglobin level of <11.0 g/dL in late pregnancy is abnormal; this may indicate iron deficiency anemia and needs evaluation.)

Coagulation	• Procoagulant factors such as fibrinogen, factors II, VII, VIII, X, XII, and XIII increase • Decrease in natural anticoagulant factors (e.g., anticoagulant protein S) • In general, pregnancy is considered to be a state of hypercoagulability
Heart	• Blood pressure decreases slightly, particularly in the second trimester • Heart rate increases by 10–30 bpm • Cardiac output increases • Systemic vascular resistance decreases
Respiratory	• Nasal stuffiness and epistaxis • Increased oxygen requirement • Gradual onset of dyspnea throughout pregnancy (known as physiologic dyspnea) (Note: Dyspnea that has a sudden onset or adventitious breath sounds (e.g., wheezing or crackles) or dyspnea accompanied by a cough or pain is NOT physiologic dyspnea and requires immediate evaluation by the healthcare practitioner.)

Renal	• Increase in kidney size
	• Increased renal plasma flow and perfusion
	• Increase in glomerular filtration rate (GFR)
	• Dilation (dilatation) of renal pelvises leading to urinary stasis
	  • This urinary stasis predisposes the woman to pyelonephritis
	• In late gestation, left lateral positioning increases GFR and sodium excretion
	• Half of pregnant women experience glycosuria via dipstick testing that is not related to gestational diabetes but rather is due to decreased glucose reabsorption
	• Decrease in bladder volume due to enlarging uterus
	  • This can cause urinary frequency, nocturia, dysuria, urgency, and stress incontinence

Adapted from: Bauer (2020); Foley (2020); Thadhani and Maynard (2020); and Weinberger (2019).

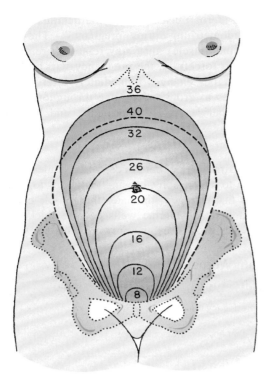

FIGURE 6-1 Height of the fundus throughout pregnancy.

structures begin to exert pressure so that the uterus enlarges and the uterine walls become thinner. By the end of the 12th week, the uterus expands upward into the abdominal cavity. At 16 weeks, the fundus can be palpated approximately halfway between the symphysis pubis and the umbilicus. At 20 weeks, the fundus reaches the level of the umbilicus. By the end of the pregnancy, the uterus occupies much of the abdominal cavity (Fig. 6-1).

Beginning in the first trimester, the uterus begins to contract sporadically. These contractions are usually painless and do not cause cervical changes. By the second trimester, these contractions are palpable. **Braxton Hicks contractions**, the painless, intermittent, "practice" contractions of pregnancy, are named after the physician who first wrote about them, Braxton Hicks. During the third trimester, as the pregnancy approaches term, Braxton Hicks contractions become more frequent and can sometimes cause discomfort. As the time for labor draws near, the contractions can become somewhat regular, causing the woman to think that she is in labor.

> **You Can Help**
> Encourage women who are fewer than 37 weeks pregnant to report contractions that do not go away with rest or if they are accompanied by cramping, pain, or low backache. These are signs of preterm labor.

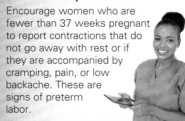

Blood supply to the uterus increases dramatically throughout pregnancy. Under the influence of estrogen, new blood vessels grow in the placenta and uterine walls, and vasodilation occurs in maternal vessels to allow increased blood flow to the uterus and placenta. The diameter of the uterine artery increases during pregnancy. By 20 weeks, it doubles in diameter from the nonpregnant state.

Cervix and Ovaries

The cervix undergoes characteristic changes under the influence of estrogen and progesterone. Vascularity is increased, and glandular tissue multiplies during pregnancy. The vascular congestion and increase in glandular tissue is responsible for Goodell, Hegar, and Chadwick signs. Shortly after conception, a thick mucous plug develops in the opening of the cervix, which helps protect the uterine cavity from infection. The mucous plug is expelled shortly before or at the beginning of labor. Small capillaries break when the plug is expelled, causing a bloody show.

> **This Will Reassure Your Client**
> Because the cervix increases in vascularity during pregnancy, a pelvic examination can rupture capillaries and cause spotting. After a pelvic examination, inform the woman that she can expect some spotting, particularly when she wipes after voiding.

Follicles in the ovaries do not mature during pregnancy, and ovulation stops. The corpus luteum continues to function and produces progesterone for approximately 6 to 7 weeks. If the corpus luteum stops functioning before that time, an early pregnancy loss (miscarriage) will occur. After 7 weeks, the placenta produces enough progesterone to maintain the pregnancy.

Vagina and Perineum

The vagina and perineum are affected by hormonal changes and increased blood supply to the area. The vagina takes on a bluish-purplish hue (Chadwick sign) because of vascular congestion. The vagina and cervix produce copious secretions because of the increased blood flow to the area.

Breasts

In the first few weeks of pregnancy, the breasts become tender, and the woman may feel tingling sensations. As pregnancy progresses, the breasts increase in size under the influence of estrogen. Prolactin, an anterior pituitary hormone, stimulates glandular production, causing the breast tissue to feel nodular. The areolas darken. Montgomery glands (Montgomery tubercles), sebaceous glands on the areolas, produce secretions that lubricate the nipple. They become more prominent during pregnancy. Tiny veins become visible on the surface of the breasts. **Striae gravidarum**, more commonly known as stretch marks, sometimes appear. Striae gravidarum appear reddish at first, then gradually fade to a light silvery color after childbirth.

As the mammary glands develop, the breasts begin to produce and secrete **colostrum**, a thick, yellow fluid that precedes milk production. During the first 3 days of breast-feeding, colostrum is the nourishment the baby receives. It is rich in antibodies, calories, and protein.

CHANGES TO BODY SYSTEMS DURING PREGNANCY

Endocrine Changes

The hormonal changes that occur in pregnancy are tremendous. Rising levels of certain pregnancy hormones cause changes in almost every body system. The placental hormones are discussed in Chapter 5. Changes in the endocrine system itself occur during pregnancy. The pituitary and thyroid glands enlarge. In fact, pregnancy could not occur without the interaction of the pituitary hormones, follicle-stimulating hormone, and luteinizing hormone.

Prolactin levels increase progressively during pregnancy. Although this hormone is not necessary for the successful completion of pregnancy, it is crucial for lactogenesis (production of breast milk). Oxytocin, a posterior pituitary hormone, is responsible for the rhythmic uterine contractions of labor. Oxytocin stimulates the letdown reflex during breast-feeding and stimulates the uterus to continue contracting after delivery to control maternal bleeding.

Hyperplasia of glandular tissue and increased vascularity cause the thyroid gland to increase in size. The need for insulin is increased. Some women have borderline pancreatic activity when they are not pregnant. During pregnancy, these women may develop gestational diabetes because the borderline pancreas cannot handle the increased demands placed upon it.

TEST YOURSELF

- ✔ List three positive signs of pregnancy.
- ✔ Describe three changes that occur in breast tissue during pregnancy.
- ✔ What is the purpose of the hormone prolactin?

Hematologic Changes

Blood volume increases by approximately 40% to 45% above prepregnancy levels by the end of the third trimester. Blood plasma and red blood cells (RBCs) both increase in volume, although plasma volumes increase at a higher percentage (50%) than do RBCs (30%). This physiologic hemodilution causes a slight decrease in hemoglobin and hematocrit levels. The average hemoglobin level at term is 12.5 g/dL. The hemoglobin level is considered normal until it falls below 11 g/dL. It is important to note that in the absence of sufficient iron, RBC volume increases by only 18%, rather than 30%.

Some blood clotting factors, such as fibrinogen and others, increase during pregnancy, making pregnancy a hypercoagulable state. However, clotting times and bleeding times remain within normal limits. The enlarging uterus inhibits blood return from the lower extremities, a situation that can cause venous stasis. A combination of venous stasis and hypercoagulability places the pregnant woman at risk for venous thrombosis (clot formation in veins).

The increased blood volume and hypercoagulability of the blood serve protective functions during pregnancy. The expanded blood volume helps meet the needs of the enlarging uterus. It helps protect the woman and the fetus from harmful effects of decreased venous return when the woman is standing or lying supine, and it enhances the exchange of nutrients and respiratory gases between the pregnant woman and fetus. The increased blood volume and hypercoagulable state serve to protect the woman from the blood loss that normally occurs during delivery.

Cardiovascular Changes

Pregnancy places tremendous demands upon the cardiovascular system. The heart has to handle the increased load of an expanded blood volume. It must also adjust to the demands of organ systems with increased workloads, such as the kidneys and uterus. In addition, the heart is physically pushed upward and to the left by the enlarging uterus; this may cause systolic murmurs.

Hormonal changes cause the woman's blood vessels to relax and dilate. This systemic decrease in vascular resistance along with blood flow to the placenta causes the woman's blood pressure to lower slightly during pregnancy, about 5 to 10 mm Hg systolic and up to 15 mm Hg diastolic. This decrease is greatest during the second trimester but returns to near prepregnancy levels by term. The heart rate rises by 10 to 30 beats per minute on average. Cardiac output increases, beginning in the early weeks of pregnancy and continuing throughout pregnancy.

When the woman lies flat on her back in the latter half of pregnancy, the uterus and its contents compress the aorta and vena cava against the spine (Fig. 6-2). This compression decreases the amount of blood returned to the heart; therefore, the cardiac output and the blood pressure fall, leading to **supine hypotensive syndrome**. The woman may feel light-headed and dizzy; her skin may exhibit pallor and clamminess. The cure (and prevention) is for the woman to rest on her side. The traditional position for a pregnant woman at rest is left side-lying. This position has been shown to increase cardiac output (Foley, 2020) by keeping pressure from the uterus off of the major abdominal blood vessels.

An Ounce of Prevention

Advise the woman not to lie on her back in late pregnancy to prevent supine hypotension. If she wishes to lie on her back, instruct her to place a pillow under her right hip to enhance blood flow through the great vessels.

Respiratory Changes

The respiratory system must accommodate the changing needs and demands of pregnancy. Vasocongestion of the upper respiratory tract lining causes symptoms similar to that of the common cold. Nasal congestion and voice changes may persist throughout pregnancy. The nasal lining is more fragile, increasing the likelihood of nosebleeds. It is thought that estrogen influences these characteristic changes.

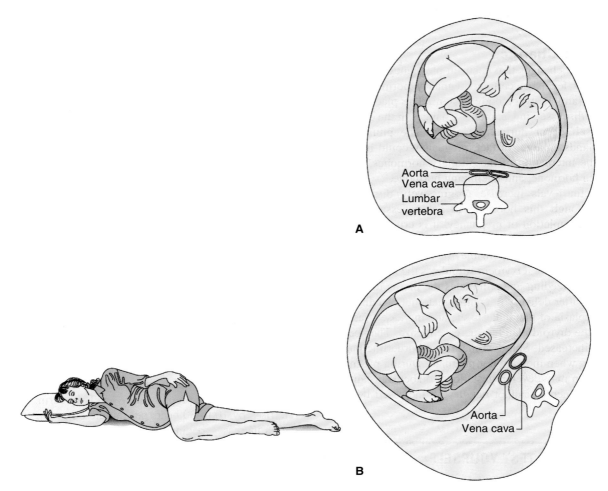

Aorta
Vena cava
Lumbar
vertebra

A

Aorta
Vena cava

B

FIGURE 6-2 Supine hypotension can occur if a pregnant woman lies on her back (not shown). **A.** The weight of the uterus compresses the vena cava, trapping blood in the lower extremities. **B.** If a woman turns on her side, pressure is lifted off the vena cava (shown).

As the uterus enlarges, it pushes up on the diaphragm. The body compensates for this crowding of the thoracic cavity by increasing the anteroposterior and transverse diameters of the chest so that total lung capacity stays approximately the same as it was before pregnancy. Ligaments loosened under the influence of hormones allow for the increased thoracic diameters.

The woman becomes more aware of the need to breathe and may feel short of breath even when she is not. In the third trimester, pressure exerted on the diaphragm from the expanding uterus can also cause the woman to feel dyspneic.

Musculoskeletal Changes

Lordosis, an increased curvature of the spine, becomes more pronounced in the later weeks of pregnancy (Fig. 6-3), as the expanding uterus alters the woman's center of gravity. Lordosis helps counterbalance the effect of the protruding abdomen and keeps the center of balance over the lower extremities. The increased curvature can result in low backache. Hormonal influences on pelvic joints cause them to increase in mobility, which contributes to lower back discomfort and causes the characteristic waddling gait of pregnancy.

The enlarging uterus puts pressure on the broad and round ligaments that support it. Prolonged pressure can lead to round ligament pain. This type of pain has been described as either a sharp stabbing, a dull ache, or a burning sensation which is felt internally and follows the path of a high bikini-cut outline. A woman who has been pregnant several times or who is carrying twins is more likely to experience **diastasis recti**, separation of the rectus abdominis muscle that supports the abdomen.

TEST YOURSELF

✔ Explain why blood volume increases during pregnancy.

✔ Describe the changes to the respiratory system during pregnancy.

✔ Describe the cause of lordosis during pregnancy.

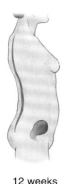
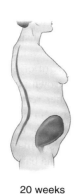
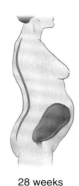
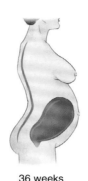
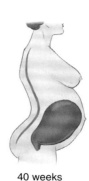

| 12 weeks | 20 weeks | 28 weeks | 36 weeks | 40 weeks |

FIGURE 6-3 Postural changes during pregnancy. Notice how the lumbar and thoracic curves become more pronounced as pregnancy progresses.

Gastrointestinal Changes

Nausea and vomiting are common in the first trimester under the influence of rising hCG levels. Occasionally, a large increase in saliva production (ptyalism) occurs. The gums may become tender and bleed easily.

As the uterus expands upward into the abdominal cavity, the intestines are displaced to the sides and upward. The stomach is pushed upward and compressed (Fig. 6-4).

The lower esophageal sphincter relaxes under the influence of hormones. Pressures in the esophagus are lower than in the nonpregnant state, whereas pressures within the stomach increase. These changes lead to an increased incidence of **pyrosis** (heartburn) caused by acid reflux through the relaxed lower esophageal sphincter.

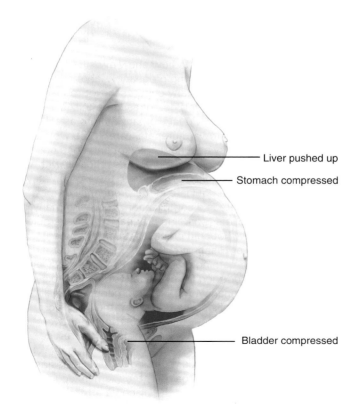

Liver pushed up

Stomach compressed

Bladder compressed

FIGURE 6-4 A full-term pregnancy. Note how the uterus displaces the organs in the abdomen.

Displacement of the intestines, and possible slowed motility of the gastrointestinal tract under the influence of progesterone, may lead to delayed gastric emptying and decreased peristalsis. As a result of these changes, the pregnant woman is predisposed to constipation. Constipation and elevated pressures in the veins below the uterus contribute to hemorrhoid development.

Progesterone interferes with normal gallbladder contraction, leading to stasis of bile. Cholestasis and increased cholesterol levels increase the risk of gallstone formation. Cholestasis can occur within the liver and lead to pruritus (itching).

Urinary Changes

Renal and ureteral dilation occur as a result of hormonal changes and mechanical pressure of the growing uterus on the ureters. The dilation causes an increase in kidney size, particularly on the right side. Peristalsis decreases in the urinary tract, leading to urinary stasis with a resultant increased risk for pyelonephritis.

The glomerular filtration rate rises because of increased cardiac output and decreased renal vascular resistance. The rise in glomerular filtration rate occurs as early as the 10th week and is largely responsible for the increased urinary frequency noted in the first trimester. Urinary frequency is not a common complaint in the second trimester but occurs again in the third trimester because of the pressure of the expanding uterus on the bladder (Fig. 6-4).

Glycosuria, glucose in the urine, may occur normally because the kidney tubules are not able to reabsorb as much glucose as they were before pregnancy. However, if the woman is spilling glucose in her urine, additional testing is warranted to rule out gestational diabetes. Protein is not normally found in the urine of a pregnant woman.

Integumentary Changes

Many skin changes in pregnancy result from hyperpigmentation. The so-called mask of pregnancy, **melasma (chloasma)**, can appear as brown blotchy areas on the forehead, cheeks, and nose of the pregnant woman. This condition may be permanent or it may regress between pregnancies. The skin in the middle of the abdomen may develop a darkened line called the **linea nigra** (Fig. 6-5). Striae gravidarum (stretch marks) may appear on the abdomen in response to

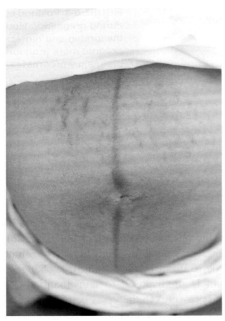

FIGURE 6-5 Linea nigra.

elevated glucocorticoid levels. As discussed in the section on breast tissue, the striae gravidarum appear reddish and are more noticeable during pregnancy. After pregnancy, they tend to fade and become silvery white in color.

TEST YOURSELF

✔ List two reasons the pregnant woman is predisposed to pyrosis.

✔ Name two urinary changes normally experienced during pregnancy.

✔ List two conditions that result from hyperpigmentation during pregnancy.

Remember Samantha Chavez from the start of this chapter. She was concerned about how her body would change during pregnancy. What changes would you want to tell her about? How can you present this information without overwhelming her?

PSYCHOLOGICAL ADAPTATION TO PREGNANCY

While adapting to rapid changes in physiology, the pregnant woman must also come to terms with her new role as parent. No matter how many children the woman has, each new pregnancy brings with it a role change. Adjusting to the role of parenting is a process that occurs throughout pregnancy and beyond.

Many factors influence how a woman adjusts to her role as parent. Societal expectations and cultural values may dictate the way a woman responds to pregnancy and the idea of parenthood. Family influences are usually very strong. The way the woman was raised and the values surrounding children and parenthood in her family of origin impact the way a woman adapts to pregnancy. Her own personality and ability to adapt to change influences her response. Even her past experiences with pregnancy have an effect on the way she deals with the current pregnancy. For example, if she has a history of infertility or a stillbirth, she may not fully accept the pregnancy or begin to bond with the baby until they are born.

Social support is critical during pregnancy. If the woman is in a long-term relationship and feels supported, she will be much better prepared to handle the demands of pregnancy than if she feels alone and isolated without support. If the woman does not have a supportive partner, it is important for her to identify someone with whom she can share the experience of pregnancy. Often this will be a friend or perhaps the woman's own mother.

The pregnant woman should be screened for depression. Depression is the most common mental health issue and can be present in the woman prior to pregnancy or can develop during pregnancy. Because of the stigma of depression and the common belief that "pregnancy is a happy time," the woman may not disclose feelings and symptoms related to depression. It is more valuable to use a screening tool for depression instead of asking a single question such as, "Are you feeling depressed?"

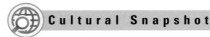

Cultural Snapshot

The woman's culture impacts how she views the pregnancy and her behaviors during pregnancy, labor and delivery, and postpartum. Many cultures view pregnancy as a positive event; however, do not assume this is a positive event for the individual woman. Culture affects the woman's attitude toward prenatal care. If the woman's culture sees pregnancy as a natural event and does not participate in many preventative practices, such as with some Americans of Arabic descent, then the woman may not seek prenatal care until late in the pregnancy or may seek care only if there is a complication. There are many specific cultural beliefs regarding pregnancy. For example, women who follow hot/cold practices, such as some East Indians, Chinese, or Hispanic cultures, may avoid certain foods or alter their bathing practices during pregnancy and postpartum. It is common for Chinese women to avoid funerals during pregnancy. Mexican women traditionally avoid watching a lunar eclipse to prevent the baby from having a cleft lip or palate. Culture also affects the woman's behavior during labor. Korean women often refuse pain medication during labor, and women from Sri Lanka and Taiwan are often very quiet during labor, expressing little or no pain. During postpartum, the woman's culture may dictate what is done with the placenta after delivery. Native Americans or women from Cambodia may want to bury the placenta instead of allowing the birth facility to dispose of it.

First-Trimester Task: Accept the Pregnancy

Pregnancy is a development stage; as such, psychological tasks of pregnancy have been identified. The first task of pregnancy is to accept the pregnancy. This task is usually met during the first trimester, although some women have difficulty fully accepting the pregnancy until they can feel the baby move.

 A Personal Glimpse

When I first found out that I was pregnant, I started shaking. I couldn't believe that I was pregnant. My husband and I didn't plan for this to happen so soon. We had wanted to wait about 8 more months before beginning our family. We weren't ready; we had only been married 5 months. We still had some financial debt to pay off, and we had certain goals we wanted to meet.

We both wanted and loved children very much. In fact, we both wanted and planned to have three children. However, it was the timing that was wrong. I couldn't even tell my husband the news because he was away for several weeks. This added to my anxiety. Not only was I worried about my ability to be a mother, but I was worried that I may have eaten or been exposed to something harmful to my baby before knowing I was pregnant. I ended up confiding in my mother and best friends, who truly helped me to calm down and get a grip.

I started to relax and accept the fact that although the timing was off, this was pretty exciting. When I was finally able to tell my husband, he just beamed with joy. I knew in that moment that everything would be all right.

Sandra

Learning Opportunity: How would you advise this mother-to-be regarding her feelings when she found out that she was pregnant? How can the nurse help the woman and her family deal with the emotions that surround finding out about a pregnancy?

Initially the woman may be shocked that she is pregnant. Or she may be ecstatic or excited. There are a myriad of emotions that a woman may experience when she first hears the news that she is pregnant. Even if the pregnancy is intensely desired, a certain amount of ambivalence is a normal initial response to pregnancy. Ambivalence refers to the feelings of uncertainty most women must deal with in the early weeks of pregnancy. The woman may have tried to get pregnant for a while before conceiving, and now that the pregnancy has occurred, she may have second thoughts or doubts about her ability to be

Acceptance Can Be Healing

Listen to your client. If she wishes to talk, encourage her and use active listening skills. Reassure her it is normal to experience a wide array of feelings during pregnancy.

a good parent. Or the pregnancy may have been unplanned, so she must sort through her feelings about this unexpected event. It may be helpful for her to hear that ambivalence is a healthy response because she may feel guilty about her uncertainty.

As the woman experiences the early physiologic changes of pregnancy, she gradually comes to accept that she is pregnant. She is usually introverted and focused on herself during the first trimester. The nausea associated with early pregnancy may leave her feeling sick and irritable. She may be fatigued. Often, she is moody and sensitive.

It is important to be supportive of the woman's partner during this time. The partner might also have feelings of ambivalence. In addition to accepting the pregnancy, the partner must learn to accept the pregnant woman as she changes with pregnancy. The mood swings, sensitivity, and irritability can make it difficult to cope. Jealousy of the unborn child can occur. It can be difficult to adjust to the introversion and self-focus of the woman. Often, the partner is relieved to learn that the changes the pregnant woman is going through are normal responses to pregnancy.

Second-Trimester Task: Accept the Baby

Generally, during the first trimester, the woman is focused on the pregnancy and on accepting this new reality as being part of her identity. Gradually, as the pregnancy progresses, she comes to have a sense of the child as their own separate entity. This acceptance may be enhanced when she first hears the fetal heartbeat, when she feels the baby move inside her, or when she sees the fetal image during a sonogram.

As she comes to accept the uniqueness of her baby, she may begin to shop for baby clothes or prepare the nursery. When an ultrasound is done in the second trimester, it is generally possible to detect the sex of the child. The couple may name the baby once they know if it is a boy or a girl.

🌐 **Cultural Snapshot**

Do not make the mistake of thinking that the woman has not yet accepted the baby if she does not name the baby during pregnancy. It is common in the Chinese culture to give the unborn child a "milk name" that is unattractive and prevents attention by evil spirits. The "milk name" may even be an animal or something unappealing as "mud face." Some parents do not decide on a name until several days after the baby is born. Some cultures, such as Native Americans, Jewish people, and Africans, may not call the child by name until after a naming ceremony occurs. The family may refer to the infant as "it," "he," or "the baby" until after the official naming ceremony.

During the second trimester, the woman may become more extroverted. She often feels much better once the nausea and fatigue of the first trimester have passed. The fetus has begun to grow large enough that the pregnancy becomes apparent to those around her. Frequently, the second trimester is a happy time. The woman may enjoy the extra attention and deference society gives to pregnant women.

It is important to remember that the partner is experiencing the pregnancy along with the woman. Some partners actually experience some of the physical symptoms of pregnancy, such as nausea and vomiting, along with their partners; a phenomenon called **couvade syndrome**. It may be easier for the woman's partner to accept her now that she is feeling better and is less introverted. In any event, it is important to encourage the couple to communicate their needs effectively to each other. Each needs the support of the other.

Third-Trimester Task: Prepare for Parenthood

Nesting instincts often begin in the third trimester. The couple may prepare the nursery and shop for baby furniture and clothes. A name may be chosen. The woman usually has a heightened interest in safe passage for herself and the baby during labor.

Toward the end of pregnancy, most women begin to feel tired of being pregnant. Many discomforts of pregnancy arise during the third trimester. It may be difficult to get comfortable at night, so it may be hard to get a good night's sleep. Backache and round ligament pain may be bothersome. Urinary frequency often returns as the gravid uterus presses down against the bladder. Braxton Hicks contractions may become uncomfortable and more frequent. It is important to be supportive of the woman and listen to her concerns.

It is helpful for the couple to attend childbirth preparation classes, which are often offered in the third trimester. Not only does the couple learn techniques to help them prepare for labor, but they are also able to interact with other couples who are facing issues similar to their own. The social aspect of childbirth preparation can be a powerful source of support to the woman and her partner.

> ### TEST YOURSELF
> ✔ Describe two psychological characteristics normally associated with a woman in the first trimester of pregnancy.
> ✔ Describe two common reactions the partner of the pregnant woman may experience.
> ✔ List two activities many women perform in the third trimester.

CHANGING NUTRITIONAL REQUIREMENTS OF PREGNANCY

Nutrition is an area that requires special attention during pregnancy. The fetus needs nutrients and energy to build new tissue, and the woman needs nutrients to build her blood volume and maternal stores. There is an increased demand for energy and for almost every nutrient type. Most nutrient requirements can be met through careful attention to diet, although there are several nutrients that require supplementation during pregnancy. The U.S. Department of Agriculture and U.S. Department of Health and Human Services provide an interactive website, www.choosemyplate.gov, where an individual can enter their statistics and receive an individualized nutrition plan. Figure 6-6 shows general dietary suggestions for the pregnant woman.

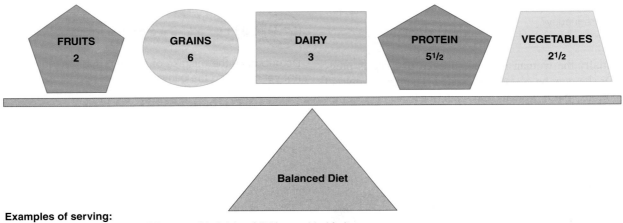

Examples of serving:
Fruit: 1 cup of raw fruit OR 1 cup of fruit juice OR 1/2 cup dried fruit
Grain: 1 slice of bread OR 1/2 cup cooked pasta or rice OR 1 oz ready-to-eat cereal
Dairy: 1 cup of milk OR 8 oz yogurt OR 1 1/2 oz cheese
Protein: 1 oz lean meat or poultry or fish OR 1 egg OR 1/2 oz nuts OR 1 tbsp peanut butter OR 1/4 cup cooked dried beans
Vegetable: 1 cup of vegetables (raw or cooked) OR 1 cup vegetable juice OR 2 cups raw leafy vegetables

FIGURE 6-6 Dietary Suggestions During Pregnancy. Servings are shown for first trimester. Second and third trimester suggestions are as follows: fruits 2 servings, grains 8 servings, dairy 3 servings, protein 6½ servings, vegetables 3 servings. (Based upon information from the U.S. Department of Agriculture.)

Energy Requirements and Weight Gain

Energy requirements increase during pregnancy because of fetal tissue development and increased maternal stores. During the first trimester, the recommended weight gain is 1 to 4 lb (0.5 to 2 kg) total. Subsequently, for the remainder of pregnancy, the recommendation is roughly 1 lb (0.5 kg) per week, for a total weight gain of 25 to 35 lb (11.5 to 16.0 kg) for a woman who begins pregnancy with a normal body mass index (BMI).[1] Total weight gain recommendations vary depending upon the woman's prepregnancy BMI. A woman who is underweight when she enters pregnancy (low BMI) should gain 28 to 40 lb (12.5 to 18.0 kg), whereas a woman who has a high BMI (overweight) is recommended to gain 15 to 25 lb (7.0 to 11.5 kg) during the pregnancy (Garner, 2020).

Failure to gain enough weight, and in particular gaining less than 16 lb (7.25 kg) during pregnancy, has been associated with an increased risk of delivering a low-birth-weight baby (less than 2,500 g or 5.5 lb). Low birth weight has consistently been associated with poor neonatal outcomes. Conversely, a woman who gains too much weight is at increased risk for delivering a macrosomic (4,000 g or 8.5 lb or more) baby. High-birth-weight babies experience complications and poor outcomes more frequently than do babies with normal birth weights. A woman who gains too much weight is also at greater risk of requiring cesarean section.

Many women falsely assume that "eating for two" requires a significantly increased caloric intake. In fact, the required caloric increase during the first trimester is negligible. During the second and third trimesters, approximately 300 kcal/day is required above the woman's prepregnancy needs. It is important that the diet supply enough calories to meet energy needs; otherwise, protein will be broken down to supply energy, rather than to build fetal and maternal tissues.

Protein Requirements

Protein needs are increased during pregnancy because of growth and repair of the fetal tissue, placenta, uterus, breasts, and maternal blood volume. It is recommended that the pregnant woman obtain adequate protein from animal sources, including milk and milk products. Milk is an excellent source of protein and calcium for the pregnant or breast-feeding woman. As stated previously, it is important for the woman to have adequate caloric intake to preserve protein stores for tissue building and repair. When protein is used to supply energy, there is less protein available for fetal, placental, and maternal tissue growth needs.

During the average pregnancy, the fetus and placenta account for approximately half of the added protein needs. The remaining protein is distributed among uterine muscle cells, mammary glandular tissue, and maternal blood in the form of hemoglobin and plasma proteins.

Mineral Requirements

The woman can obtain most minerals from a varied diet without supplementation, even during pregnancy. However, it is important for a pregnant woman to get sufficient amounts of minerals to prevent deficiencies in the growing fetus and maternal stores.

Iron

Iron is necessary for the formation of hemoglobin; therefore, it is essential to the oxygen-carrying capacity of the blood. If a woman's diet is iron deficient during pregnancy, her RBC volume will increase by only 18%. The woman who receives an adequate supplementation of iron has a 30% increase in RBC volume. This extra "cushion" of RBC volume increases the amount of oxygen available at the placenta for the fetus and helps protect the woman from the effects of blood loss after delivery.

Almost all of the additional iron requirements are necessary during the second half of pregnancy, so the need for iron increases dramatically after 20 weeks. If the woman is iron-deficient, she will develop anemia. However, the fetus will get the iron needed to manufacture its RBCs. This is one instance in which nature robs from the woman to adequately supply the fetus.

It is almost impossible for the woman to receive an adequate amount of iron from her diet alone. Therefore, it is recommended that the pregnant woman take iron supplementation. The health care provider may choose to omit iron supplement during the first trimester because it often intensifies the nausea and vomiting of early pregnancy. The dose varies depending on the individual needs of the woman. If she enters pregnancy with normal hemoglobin and hematocrit values, she will require lower doses of iron than if she is anemic when she becomes pregnant. A woman carrying twins or an obese woman will both require higher doses of supplemental iron.

Iron + Vitamin C = Best Practice

Iron is best absorbed by the body if taken with vitamin C. Encourage the woman to take her iron supplement with either a vitamin-C–rich food or with her vitamin C supplement. Orange juice or oranges are often recommended.

Calcium

Calcium needs are not increased above prepregnancy levels mainly because pregnancy enhances calcium absorption. However, it is important for the pregnant woman to obtain sufficient amounts of calcium. Calcium is needed for a variety of bodily processes, including nerve cell transmission, muscle contraction, bone building, and blood clotting. Recent research has demonstrated that calcium supplementation during pregnancy may reduce the risk of preeclampsia (see Chapter 17) in women who have a preexisting low dietary calcium intake (August, 2020).

---

[1]BMI refers to body weight corrected for height of the person. Normal BMI is 18.5 to 24.9. An individual can calculate their BMI online at https://www.nhlbi.nih.gov/health/educational/lose_wt/BMI/bmicalc.htm.

Calcium continuously moves between bone and blood because a precise amount is needed in the blood to maintain normal muscle contraction (including cardiac muscle contraction). Normally the movement of calcium in and out of bones is balanced—there is neither a net gain nor a net loss. However, if insufficient amounts are ingested or if calcium is not absorbed from the gastrointestinal tract, the body will take calcium from the bones to maintain blood levels. This process will also occur to meet the calcium needs of the growing fetus.

Vitamin D is necessary for adequate absorption of calcium. The amount of vitamin D obtained from 10 to 20 minutes of exposure to sunlight per day is normally sufficient. If this source is not readily available, vitamin D is also present in fortified milk products.

Zinc

Zinc is needed during pregnancy to provide for fetal growth and during lactation for milk production. Because zinc is needed for nucleic acid synthesis and protein metabolism, adequate amounts are particularly important during early pregnancy when fetal body systems are developing. Milk production requires higher levels of zinc than the fetus demands during pregnancy; therefore, the RDA for zinc during lactation is higher than that for pregnancy. Foods that contain zinc include meat, seafood, and, to a lesser extent, whole grains.

Iodine

Iodine is needed for normal thyroid activity. Women with severe iodine deficiencies deliver infants with congenital hypothyroidism, which is marked by stunted growth and intellectual disability. Recent studies have linked subclinical hypothyroidism with increased rates of cognitive deficits.

Most women in the United States get sufficient amounts of iodine, but during pregnancy, a woman loses larger amounts of iodine in the urine than when she is not pregnant. The current recommendation is for all pregnant women to use iodized salt.

Vitamin Requirements

Vitamins are known catalysts for many chemical reactions in the body. A varied diet that includes adequate servings from each of the food groups (fruits, grains, vegetables, proteins, and dairy) should supply sufficient amounts of most vitamins during pregnancy. A brief description of the function and selected food sources for each vitamin are highlighted.

Folic Acid (Vitamin B9)

Folic acid is a B vitamin that can prevent up to 70% of birth defects of the central nervous system, called neural tube defects, such as spina bifida. Because formation of the nervous system occurs during the first few weeks of pregnancy, usually before a woman knows she is pregnant, all women of childbearing age should take a daily 400 μg supplement of folic acid in addition to a nutritious diet. Recent studies suggest that intake of adequate folic acid can prevent other birth defects, such as cleft lip and palate. Folic acid can be found in some fortified foods such as rice, pasta, bread, some breakfast cereals, and corn masa flour.

Vitamin A

Vitamin A is usually found in sufficient amounts in the diets of women who live in the United States. One concern is when a pregnant woman consumes too much vitamin A. In very large amounts, levels at or above 10,000 IU or 3,000 μg, vitamin A can cause birth defects. For this reason, pregnant women are encouraged to get the majority of their vitamin A intake from beta-carotene, a substance found in fruits and vegetables with yellow, orange, and red coloration, such as carrots and sweet potatoes. The body converts beta-carotene to vitamin A and is much less toxic than preformed vitamin A. The key is balanced intake of this nutrient. Too much can be toxic to the fetus, but too little can stunt fetal growth and cause impaired dark adaptation and night blindness.

Vitamin C

Vitamin C is essential in the formation of collagen, a necessary component of wound healing. Scurvy, a disease characterized by spongy gums, loosened teeth, and bleeding into the skin and mucous membranes, results from severe vitamin C deficiency. Less severe deficiencies lead to easy bruising. Vitamin C is necessary for normal fetal growth and bone formation. This vitamin also helps the body to absorb iron. Vitamin C is found in most fresh fruits and vegetables. The best sources include citrus fruits, papaya, and strawberries. Broccoli and tomatoes are also good sources of vitamin C.

Vitamin B6

Vitamin B6, or pyridoxine, assists in the metabolism of the macronutrients (proteins, fats, and carbohydrates), helps convert amino acids to proteins, and forms new RBCs. This vitamin is necessary for the healthy development of the fetus's nervous system. Although increased amounts of the vitamin are needed during pregnancy, a varied diet should supply all that is needed.

Vitamin B12

Vitamin B12, or cobalamine, is needed to maintain healthy nerve cells and RBCs. It is also needed to form DNA. Vitamin B12 only occurs naturally in animal sources, such as fish, milk, dairy products, eggs, meat, and poultry. This vitamin can also be found in fortified breakfast cereals. The two instances in which vitamin B12 deficiency generally occurs are when a person lacks intrinsic factor or she is vegan (see discussion of vegetarianism that follows). Persons who lack intrinsic factor cannot absorb vitamin B12. Without intramuscular injections of the vitamin, these individuals experience pernicious anemia.

Dietary Supplementation

It is thought that a diet that includes a variety of food types is sufficient to meet the needs of the pregnant woman. There are several exceptions. The woman who has nutritional risk factors requires a daily prenatal multivitamin supplement. Nutritional risk factors include multiple gestation, substance abuse, vegetarianism, and problems with hemoglobin formation. Some health care providers still recommend a daily vitamin supplement for all pregnant women.

Iron supplementation is recommended for all pregnant women after 28 weeks' gestation. If the woman has low hemoglobin, is obese, or is carrying twins, higher doses of iron are necessary. Folic acid supplementation is recommended prenatally and during pregnancy to prevent neural tube defects.

Dietary Restrictions During Pregnancy

There are several nutrition-related practices that the pregnant woman should avoid. It is not helpful for the pregnant woman to limit her intake to try to avoid weight gain. Often, this practice results in too few nutrients ingested to meet the increased demands of pregnancy. In addition, consumption of unwashed fruits and vegetables, unpasteurized dairy products, raw eggs, or undercooked meats can be harmful to the growing fetus.

Although seafood has many nutritional benefits, many types are contaminated with methylmercury, a metal that can irreversibly harm the developing fetal brain. Therefore, the Food and Drug Administration (FDA) gives specific recommendations regarding the type and amount of seafood a pregnant woman should consume. Tips for Reinforcing Family Teaching: Food Safety During Pregnancy outlines the major points to cover when educating the pregnant woman about food safety.

 TIPS FOR REINFORCING FAMILY TEACHING

Food Safety During Pregnancy

Food Preparation Guidelines

Follow the FDA guidelines to clean, separate, cook, and chill food.

Clean
- Wash hands thoroughly with warm water and soap before and after handling food and after using the bathroom, changing diapers, or handling pets.
- Wash cutting boards, dishes, utensils, and countertops with hot water and soap.
- Rinse raw fruits and vegetables thoroughly under running water.

Separate
- Separate raw meat, poultry, and seafood from ready-to-eat foods.
- If possible, use one cutting board for raw meat, poultry, and seafood and another one for fresh fruits and vegetables.
- Place cooked food on a clean plate. If cooked food is placed on an unwashed plate that held raw meat, poultry, or seafood, bacteria from the raw food could contaminate the cooked food.

Cook
- Cook foods thoroughly. Use a food thermometer to check the temperature.
- Keep foods out of the danger zone: the range of temperatures at which bacteria can grow, usually between 40°F and 140°F (4°C and 60°C).
- 2-hour rule: Discard foods left out at room temperature for more than 2 hours.

Chill
- Place an appliance thermometer in the refrigerator and check the temperature periodically. The refrigerator should register at or below 40°F (4°C) and the freezer at or below 0°F (−18°C).
- Refrigerate or freeze perishables (foods that can spoil or become contaminated by bacteria if left unrefrigerated).

Listeria Precautions

Take precautions to avoid *Listeria*, a harmful bacterium that can grow at refrigerated temperatures.

- Do not eat hot dogs and luncheon meats, unless they are reheated until steaming hot.
- Do not eat soft cheese, such as feta, brie, camembert, blue-veined cheeses, queso blanco, queso fresco, and panela, unless it is labeled as made with pasteurized milk.
- Do not eat refrigerated pâtés or meat spreads.
- Do not eat refrigerated smoked seafood unless it is in a cooked dish, such as a casserole. (Refrigerated smoked seafood, such as salmon, trout, whitefish, cod, tuna, or mackerel, is most often labeled as nova-style, lox, kippered, smoked, or jerky.)
- Do not drink raw (unpasteurized) milk or eat foods that contain unpasteurized milk.

Seafood Recommendations

Follow the FDA recommendations about appropriate fish consumption to avoid mercury poisoning.

- Do not eat any shark, swordfish, king mackerel, or tilefish during pregnancy.
- Limit intake of other fish to no more than 12 oz (about two to three servings) per week.
- Limit consumption of fish caught in local waters to 6 oz (one serving) per week.
- Do not eat more than one 6-oz can of white tuna or two 6-oz cans of light tuna.
- It is probably best to avoid tuna steaks because they often have high mercury levels. If you decide to eat tuna steak, do not eat more than 6 oz per week.

Reference

The FDA has information on food safety during pregnancy; this can be found at https://www.fda.gov/media/83740/download.

Special Nutritional Considerations

Several situations require unique nutritional considerations. These include vegetarianism, lactose intolerance, and pica.

Vegetarianism

There are different categories of vegetarians. The lacto-ovo-vegetarian does not eat any flesh meats, but does include milk, eggs, and dairy products in the diet. The vegan is a strict vegetarian who does not eat milk, eggs, or any dairy product. A fruitarian only consumes fruits and nuts.

A lacto-ovo-vegetarian can easily get all of the required nutrients for pregnancy by careful attention to a few basic principles. Protein has always been an area of concern for vegetarian diets. Fortunately, a lacto-ovo-vegetarian can get sufficient protein by drinking milk; by eating eggs, cheese, yogurt, and other dairy products; and by combining foods. Although vegetables and grains do not contain all of the essential amino acids, when they are skillfully combined, all of the essential amino acids can be obtained. The general rule is to combine a grain and a legume. For instance, a corn tortilla (grain) eaten with pinto beans (legume) provides all of the essential amino acids and qualifies as a complete protein. Other combinations include lentils and whole grain rice, peanut butter on whole wheat bread, and whole grain cereal with milk.

A vegan will need to take extra care to get enough protein because she does not use milk or dairy products. Food combining, as discussed in the previous paragraph, is an important nutritional strategy for the vegan. It can also help to suggest adding fortified soy milk and rice milk to the diet. Larger amounts of nuts and seeds can help offset the protein requirements. Vitamin B_{12} must be supplemented for the pregnant vegan.

A fruitarian will need intensive support from her health care provider and a dietitian to meet the nutritional requirements of a healthy pregnancy. Multivitamin supplementation is necessary in this situation.

Iron and zinc requirements are also of concern for the vegetarian. Nonmeat sources of iron are generally not absorbed as efficiently as meat sources. Therefore, the iron requirement for the vegetarian is higher. The same is true for zinc absorption and requirements.

Lactose Intolerance

Individuals with lactose intolerance lack the enzyme lactace, which is necessary to break down and digest milk and milk products. Symptoms of lactase deficiency include abdominal distention, flatulence, nausea, vomiting, diarrhea, and cramps after consuming milk.

Don't Get Confused!

A vegan can take oral forms of vitamin B_{12}. Only the woman who lacks intrinsic factor needs vitamin B_{12} injections. Without intrinsic factor, the woman cannot absorb vitamin B_{12} through the gastrointestinal system; therefore, she needs intramuscular injections.

Calcium deficiency is a major concern for the pregnant woman who is lactose intolerant. There are several ways to address this concern. Some lactose-intolerant individuals are able to tolerate cooked forms of milk, such as pudding or custard. Cultured or fermented dairy products, such as buttermilk, yogurt, and some cheeses, may also be tolerated. A chewable lactase tablet may be taken with milk. Lactase-treated milk is available in most supermarkets and may be helpful. Other options are to drink calcium-enriched orange juice or soy milk or to take a calcium supplement. If the woman is infrequently exposed to sunlight, she will need a vitamin D supplement to aid in the absorption of calcium.

Pica

Pica is the persistent ingestion of nonfood substances such as clay, laundry starch, freezer frost, or dirt. It results from a craving for these substances that some women develop during pregnancy. These cravings disappear when the woman is no longer pregnant. Pica may be accompanied by iron deficiency anemia (Young and Cox, 2019). If you suspect or discover that a pregnant woman is practicing pica, tell the registered nurse or the practitioner immediately. Special counseling is indicated in this situation.

Cultural Snapshot

The practice of pica is found in many cultures worldwide. It is important to approach the woman who reveals pica behavior in a culturally sensitive manner. It would be inappropriate to abruptly tell her to stop the practice without first assessing for cultural implications.

TEST YOURSELF

✔ What is the recommended weight gain for the woman with a normal BMI?

✔ What are the two important reasons for the pregnant woman to get adequate amounts of protein?

✔ State three vitamins/minerals that are important for the pregnant woman to ingest daily and possible consequences if the woman is deficient in these vitamins/minerals.

Remember Samantha Chavez and her significant other from the beginning of the chapter. Her partner was concerned about her diet. What foods should Samantha eat and what should she avoid? Where could you guide her to on the Internet for dietary information during pregnancy?

KEY POINTS

- Presumptive signs of pregnancy, such as nausea and vomiting, can have causes other than pregnancy and are noticed only by the mother.

- Probable signs of pregnancy are objective signs the examiner detects that point to pregnancy; however, they are not 100% indicative of pregnancy. Pregnancy tests and changes in the reproductive organs, such as Chadwick and Hegar signs, are probable signs of pregnancy.

- A positive sign of pregnancy is diagnostic because no other condition except pregnancy can cause the sign. Positive signs include visualization of the gestational sac or fetus with ultrasound, hearing the fetal heartbeat with Doppler or fetoscope, and palpation of fetal movements by a trained examiner.

- Changes in maternal anatomy and physiology during pregnancy include the change of the uterus from a solid, pear-shaped, pelvic organ to a thin, globular-shaped, muscular sac that fills the abdominal cavity. Blood volume increases by 40% to 45%. Coagulation factors increase. Cardiac output increases by as much as 50%.

- The woman's reproductive system undergoes significant changes during pregnancy. The uterus enlarges, and the endometrial lining (decidua) is maintained. Blood supply to the uterus increases significantly. Increased vascularity to the reproductive tract is responsible for Goodell, Hegar, and Chadwick signs.

- Endocrine system changes include enlargement of the pituitary gland, an increase in prolactin levels, and an increased need for insulin. The thyroid gland increases in volume.

- Hematologic changes enhance the exchange of nutrients and gases between the woman and the fetus and protect the woman against blood loss during childbirth but predispose the woman to venous thrombosis.

- The heart must adapt to the increased demands of the greatly expanded blood volume. The woman should lie on her side and not lie on her back for prolonged periods late in pregnancy to avoid supine hypotensive syndrome, which taxes the cardiovascular system and decreases blood flow to the placenta.

- Respiratory system changes lead to nasal stuffiness and shortness of breath.

- Increasing lordosis (increased curvature of the spine) shifts the center of gravity and leads to a waddling gait in the last half of pregnancy.

- Gastrointestinal changes include nausea and vomiting in early pregnancy, pyrosis (heartburn) in middle and late pregnancy, constipation, and hemorrhoid formation.

- Changes in the urinary tract lead to an increased risk for pyelonephritis during pregnancy. Urinary frequency is common in the first trimester because of an increased glomerular filtration rate and again in the third trimester because of pressure of the gravid uterus on the bladder.

- Increased pigmentation, such as that seen in chloasma, and the linea nigra, along with striae gravidarum, are common integumentary changes.

- Psychological tasks of pregnancy include accepting the pregnancy (first trimester), accepting the baby (second trimester), and preparing for parenthood (third trimester). Ambivalence is a normal feeling when pregnancy is first diagnosed. Couvade syndrome occurs when the partner experiences some of the physical discomforts of pregnancy along with the pregnant partner.

- Nutritional requirements change during pregnancy. The woman needs nutrients to build extra blood volume and tissue, and the fetus needs nutrients to grow. Energy requirements are increased. A woman who enters pregnancy at normal weight should gain 25 to 35 lb (11.5 to 16.0 kg) during pregnancy. A woman who is underweight should gain more, whereas a woman who is overweight should gain less. In no instance is it recommended for a woman to gain less than 15 lb (6.8 kg) during pregnancy.

- Protein requirements increase during pregnancy. Most vitamins and minerals can be obtained without supplementation if the diet is adequate.

- After the first trimester, it is generally recommended for a woman to take an iron supplement because it is difficult to get adequate amounts of this mineral from diet alone.

- Although calcium needs do not increase, it is important for the pregnant woman to get sufficient amounts of this mineral.

- Folic acid supplementation is recommended to help prevent neural tube defects. Vitamin A can be toxic in large amounts. It is best to use beta-carotene (plant) sources to meet vitamin A needs during pregnancy.

- Vitamin C deficiency can lead to scurvy (severe), easy bruising, and possibly gestational hypertension.

- The woman who lacks intrinsic factor must take intramuscular injections of vitamin B_{12}, and the vegan must supplement this vitamin orally.

- Iron and folic acid supplementation is generally recommended for all pregnant women.

- Vegetarians can receive an adequate diet with close attention to combining foods. The lacto-ovo-vegetarian can use milk and dairy products to obtain sufficient protein. The vegan can carefully combine foods (legumes and grains) to supply all of the essential amino acids and should take vitamin B_{12} supplements. The fruitarian needs to be followed closely by a dietitian and must take multivitamin supplements.

- When individuals lack the enzyme lactase, they are lactose intolerant. To consume a sufficient number of dairy products, these individuals can try taking lactase when they consume dairy products or may tolerate cooked forms of milk.

- Pica is ingestion of nonfood substances. It can lead to iron-deficiency anemia and other nutritional deficiencies and requires follow-up.

INTERNET RESOURCES

Pregnancy Signs

https://www.webmd.com/baby/guide/pregnancy-am-i-pregnant#1

https://www.medicinenet.com/pregnancy_symptoms_am_i_pregnant/
article.htm

Nutrition During Pregnancy

https://www.womenshealth.gov/pregnancy/youre-pregnant-now-what/
staying-healthy-and-safe

https://www.ncbi.nlm.nih.gov/pmc/articles/PMC6470702/

https://www.choosemyplate.gov/browse-by-audience/view-
all-audiences/adults/moms-pregnancy-breastfeeding/
moms-daily-food-plan

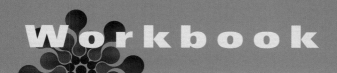

NCLEX-STYLE REVIEW QUESTIONS

1. The client who is 38 weeks pregnant tells the nurse that sometimes during her nap she feels light-headed and starts to sweat but feels better when she gets up. What is the client most likely experiencing?

   a. Decrease in oxygenation
   b. Supine hypotensive syndrome
   c. Vasocongestion of the lower extremities
   d. Hypoglycemic episode

2. During the obstetric pelvic examination, the health care provider documents several findings. Identify the finding with its correct classification.

a. Chadwick sign	1 = Positive
b. Fetal heart tones via Doppler	2 = Presumptive
c. Goodell sign	3 = Probable
d. Positive pregnancy (hCG) test	
e. Quickening	
f. Morning sickness	

3. The client is 16 weeks pregnant. If the pregnancy is progressing as expected, where would the health care provider be able to palpate the uterine fundus?

   a. Just above the pubic bone
   b. Halfway between the pubic bone and the umbilicus
   c. At the umbilicus
   d. The uterine fundus would not be palpable at 16 weeks

4. The nurse is reinforcing teaching with a pregnant client about a proper diet during pregnancy. Which statement shows the client understands approximately how many calories per day she needs over her normal prepregnant needs?

   a. "I will need about 300 more calories."
   b. "I will need approximately 500 more calories."
   c. "I need to double my calories because I'm eating for two."
   d. "I should not increase my calories while I'm pregnant."

5. The pregnant client states at her 36-week prenatal visit, "My back is really hurting and no position really seems to help it." When examining the client, you notice that the curve of her lower spine is more pronounced toward her abdomen. What is the client most likely experiencing?

   a. Kyphosis
   b. Pyrosis
   c. Lordosis
   d. Thrombosis

STUDY ACTIVITIES

1. Devise a 3-day meal plan for a vegan who is pregnant. How will you meet her needs for protein, iron, calcium, and vitamin B$_{12}$?

2. Perform an Internet search using the key terms "pica" and "pregnancy." Share your findings with your clinical group.

3. Develop a teaching plan on the importance of folic acid for a group of women who wish to become pregnant. Be sure to address why women of childbearing age should get enough of this nutrient, how much is required, and examples of food sources.

CRITICAL THINKING: WHAT WOULD YOU DO?

Apply your knowledge of maternal physiologic and psychological adaptation to pregnancy to the following situations:

1. Carla is 20 weeks pregnant. You are assisting the midwife during this prenatal visit.

   a. Where do you expect to find Carla's uterine fundus?
   b. You attempt to listen to the fetal heartbeat with a Doppler. Do you expect to be able to hear the heartbeat?
   c. Carla reports that she is excited about the pregnancy and that she and her husband have been shopping for the nursery. What do you chart regarding Carla's psychological adaptation? Is she showing evidence that she is completing the appropriate task for the trimester?

2. Carla is in the office for her 32-week checkup. She has gained a total of 20 lb so far during her pregnancy. When you enter the room to check her vital signs, you notice that she is lying on her back and she looks pale. Her blood pressure is 70/40 mm Hg.

   a. What is the likely cause of Carla's symptoms?
   b. What action do you take first, and why?
   c. How should you advise Carla regarding her weight gain?

3. Monica has just found out that she is pregnant. She is a vegan.

   a. How would you advise Monica to get enough protein in her diet?
   b. Monica complains that the iron pills her health care provider prescribed are causing constipation. She asks you why she needs to take iron. How do you reply?
   c. Monica loves carrot juice, but she has heard that too much vitamin A could be unhealthy for the baby. How would you advise her?

7

Prenatal Care

Learning Objectives

At the conclusion of this chapter, you will:

1. Describe the information included in the history that is taken at the first prenatal visit.
2. Describe the physical examination performed at the first prenatal visit.
3. List the laboratory tests completed during the first prenatal visit.
4. Describe methods for estimating the due date, and use Naegele rule to calculate the due date.
5. Identify factors that put the pregnancy at risk.
6. Describe components of subsequent prenatal visits.
7. For each fetal assessment test, outline the nursing care and implications of the test results.
8. Identify symptoms that require immediate follow-up during pregnancy.
9. Describe information that should be given to the pregnant woman regarding common discomforts of pregnancy, self-care during pregnancy, and labor and delivery.

Stefani Mueller comes in for a prenatal visit after she has missed two menstrual periods. This is the third time she is pregnant. Her last pregnancy ended in a miscarriage, and she is worried that she could miscarry again. As you read the chapter, think about what diagnostic tests the health care provider may order to observe the well-being of Stefani's pregnancy. Also, think about what signs you should monitor her for and what signs she should report immediately to the health care provider.

Early prenatal care is crucial to the health of the woman and her unborn baby. The best strategy is for the woman to seek care before she conceives. One of the Healthy People 2030 objectives is to increase the proportion of pregnant women who receive early and adequate prenatal care (HealthyPeople.gov, 2030).

The goal of early prenatal care is to optimize the health of the woman and the fetus and to increase the odds that the fetus will be born healthy to a healthy mother. Early prenatal care allows for the initiation of strategies to promote good health and for early intervention in the event a complication develops. As a nurse, you play a large role in

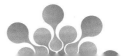

educating women about the importance of early and continued prenatal care.

Assessment of maternal and fetal well-being is the focus of prenatal care. Nursing responsibilities include a heavy emphasis on providing information throughout the pregnancy. At each prenatal visit, it is the role of the nurse to screen the woman, monitor vital signs, perform other data collection and procedures as ordered by the health care provider, answer questions, and provide appropriate information.

ASSESSMENT OF MATERNAL WELL-BEING DURING PREGNANCY

First Prenatal Visit

Ideally, the first prenatal visit occurs as soon as the woman thinks she might be pregnant. Often, the event that signals the woman to seek care is a missed or late menstrual period. She also may be experiencing some of the signs associated with pregnancy, such as nausea, fatigue, frequent urination, or tingling and fullness of the breasts. The utmost question on the woman's mind, regardless of whether the pregnancy was planned or not, is, "Am I pregnant?" If the woman obtained a positive pregnancy test at home, she will want to confirm the results. If she did not, then she may feel anxious, nervous, excited, or any number of emotions until the health care provider confirms the diagnosis of pregnancy.

The first prenatal visit is usually the longest because the baseline data are obtained at this visit. All subsequent assessments are compared to these baseline data. The major objectives of this visit are to confirm or rule out a diagnosis of pregnancy, ascertain risk factors, determine the due date, and answer questions. These objectives are met through history taking, a physical examination, laboratory work, and providing information on maintaining a healthy pregnancy. The woman may not be mentally prepared for all the questions and tests that are usually done at this time, particularly because her main goal at the first visit is to determine whether she is pregnant.

History

The history is one of the most important elements of the first prenatal visit. The woman may fill out a written questionnaire or the history may be obtained exclusively during a face-to-face interview by the health care provider. Whatever method is chosen, review the history thoroughly, and report any abnormal or unusual details. There are several parts to the history, including chief complaint, reproductive history, medical–surgical history, family history, and social history.

Chief Complaint

The chief complaint is the reason a client seeks care from the health care provider. For the woman seeking prenatal care, the chief complaint is usually a missed menstrual period. Ask the woman about any presumptive and probable signs of pregnancy she is experiencing.

Reproductive History

Note the age of menarche, as well as a summary of the characteristics of the woman's normal menstrual cycles. Common questions include, "Are your periods regular?" and "How frequently do your periods occur?" Note the first day of the last menstrual period (LMP).

The obstetric history is a part of the reproductive history. Review details of each pregnancy, including history of miscarriages or abortions and the outcome of each pregnancy (e.g., how many weeks the pregnancy lasted and whether the pregnancy ended with a living child).

There are specific medical terms that relate to the obstetrical history. The word "gravid" means pregnant. **Gravida** refers to the number of pregnancies the woman has had, including the present pregnancy, regardless of the outcome. For example, a woman who has had one pregnancy is a gravida 1, whereas a woman who has had five pregnancies is a gravida 5. A woman who has never been pregnant is a **nulligravida** (gravida 0), a woman who is pregnant for the first time is a primigravida, and a woman who has had more than one pregnancy is a **multigravida**.

> **Here's a Tip**
>
> If another person accompanies the woman, find a tactful way to separate them for at least part of the history collection. There may be details in the woman's reproductive history that she will not be willing to reveal in the presence of others, such as a previous abortion. Ensuring privacy will increase the accuracy of the history.

Parity, or para, refers to the number of pregnancies (not fetuses) carried past the age of viability (20 or more weeks). Each pregnancy is counted as one, even if the woman delivers twins or triplets. The current pregnancy is not counted in parity. Nonviable fetuses that deliver before the end of 20 weeks' gestation are termed spontaneous abortions. Abortions, either spontaneous or therapeutic, are not counted in the parity total. The term *primipara* is used for the woman delivering for the first time and *multipara* denotes a woman who has delivered more than once.

One of the most common methods of recording the obstetric history is to use the acronym GTPAL (Box 7-1). Some health care providers further divide abortions into therapeutic (induced) and spontaneous and note multiple births and ectopic pregnancies.

It is important to obtain information regarding complications that may have occurred with other pregnancies. A problem the woman had in a previous pregnancy may develop again in the current pregnancy or increase the chance that she will develop another type of complication. For example, if a woman hemorrhaged after a previous delivery, she has a higher risk of hemorrhaging after subsequent deliveries. This is also true for a previous history of gestational diabetes and preterm deliveries. Any finding that presented in a previous pregnancy is an important part of the obstetric history.

Gravida: Total number of pregnancies

Term deliveries: Number of pregnancies that went to term (at or beyond 38 weeks' gestation)

Preterm deliveries: the number of pregnancies that delivered 20 weeks and before the end of 37 weeks' gestation

Abortions: the number of pregnancies that ended before 20 weeks' gestation

Living children: the number of children delivered who are alive at the time of history collection

Susie is 38 weeks pregnant. This is her second pregnancy. She delivered a healthy baby boy at 39 weeks with her first pregnancy. What is this woman's GTPAL?

- Right now, her GTPAL is G2, T1, P0, A0, L1 because she has not yet delivered her second baby. Once she does, she will be at G2, T2, P0, A0, L2.

Use What You Know!

A pregnant woman comes into the office for prenatal care. When taking her history, she reports that her first pregnancy was a baby girl born at 29 weeks, a miscarriage at 17 weeks, and her third child was a term girl born at 40 weeks. All of her children are living. How would you describe her history in the GTPAL format?

Medical–Surgical History

After eliciting a thorough reproductive history, the health care provider must obtain a detailed medical–surgical history. If the woman has any major medical problems, such as heart disease or diabetes, she will require closer surveillance throughout the pregnancy. The prenatal record should list all medications the woman is taking, including vitamins, over-the-counter medications, and herbal remedies.

Part of the medical history involves determining if there are risk factors for infectious diseases. If the woman has been exposed to anyone with tuberculosis, she needs additional screening to rule out the disease. Determine the woman's immunization status. The woman who is nonimmune for a particular infection is at risk to contract that infection. Although most immunizations are contraindicated during pregnancy, the woman who is nonimmune can take precautions to decrease the chance she will contract infection during pregnancy. Determine risk factors for human immunodeficiency virus/acquired immunodeficiency syndrome (HIV/AIDS) and other sexually transmitted infections (Box 7-2).

Family History

A family history is important because it may highlight the need for genetic testing or counseling. Verify the health status of the father of the baby and any close relatives of the couple. If there is a family history for cystic fibrosis or other genetically linked disorders, the health care provider may recommend genetic screening. The ethnic background

- Sex with multiple partners
- Sex with a partner who has risk factors
- Intravenous drug use (needle sharing)
- Anal intercourse
- Vaginal intercourse with a partner who also engages in anal intercourse
- Unprotected (no condom) intercourse

TABLE 7-1 Genetic Disorder Screening Criteria

ORIGIN	GENETIC DISORDERS FOR WHICH SCREENING MAY BE RECOMMENDED
People of African, Indian, or Middle Eastern origin	Sickle cell anemia; thalassemia
People of European origin with Jewish ancestry or people of French Canadian origin	Tay–Sachs disease
People of Mediterranean or Southeast Asian origin	Thalassemia
People of White or European origin	Cystic fibrosis

of the woman, the father, and relatives of the unborn child is an important factor to consider. See Table 7-1 for examples of genetic diseases that may be present in people.

Social History

The social history focuses on environmental factors that may influence the pregnancy. A woman who has strong social support, adequate housing and nutrition, and greater than a high school education is less likely to develop complications of pregnancy than is a woman who lives with inadequate resources. The type of employment may influence the health of the pregnancy. A job that requires exposure to harmful chemicals is less safe for the woman and fetus than is a job that does not involve this type of exposure. Employment that requires the woman to stand for long periods of time, such as sales clerks, waitresses, and nurses, can increase her risk for preterm labor. Intimate partner violence can also threaten the pregnancy; therefore, it is important to screen every woman for intimate partner violence. Intimate partner violence affects women and men of all socioeconomic, religious, and cultural backgrounds (see Chapter 16 for detailed discussion of intimate partner violence).

Smoking, alcohol, and drug use (including illicit drugs, prescription, or over-the-counter medications) can all potentially harm a growing fetus. Therefore, it is important to determine the woman's use of these substances, particularly since conception. If the woman owns a cat or likes to garden, she is at increased risk for contracting toxoplasmosis. Toxoplasmosis is caused by a protozoan that is passed from animals to humans, usually

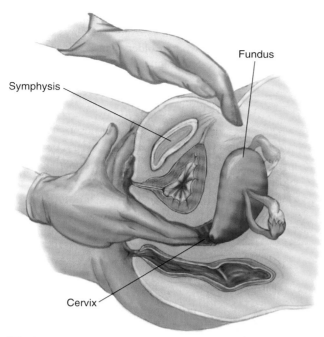

FIGURE 7-1 Bimanual examination. The examiner palpates the fundus (*top portion*) of the uterus through the abdominal wall while the hand in the vagina holds the cervix in place. This examination can determine the size of the uterus, which helps date the pregnancy.

in contaminated soil or by animal feces. If the woman contracts toxoplasmosis while she is pregnant, it can cause the woman to miscarry or can result in severe abnormalities in the fetus. It can also cause visual or hearing problems in the infant later on after birth.

Physical Examination

The health care provider performs a complete physical examination. As the nurse, you may be asked to provide assistance as needed. The head-to-toe physical is done first. The examiner looks for signs of disease that may need treatment and for any evidence of previously undetected maternal disease or other signs of ill health. A breast examination is part of the physical. Although it is rare, breast cancer in a pregnant woman is a possibility.

A vaginal speculum examination and a bimanual examination of the uterus follow the head-to-toe physical. During the speculum examination, a Papanicolaou test (Pap test) is performed (see Nursing Procedure 4-1 in Chapter 4). Signs of pregnancy, such as Chadwick sign, may be noted by the health care provider. The bimanual examination (Fig. 7-1) allows the provider to feel the size of the uterus and to elicit Hegar sign.

Laboratory Assessment

Many laboratory tests are done during the course of the pregnancy. A complete blood count gives information about the overall health status of the woman. Anemia is evaluated by checking for a low hemoglobin and hematocrit. Anemia can be caused by the pregnancy, or it can be an indicator of decreased nutritional status in the woman. A woman who is

at risk for sickle cell anemia or thalassemia is given a hemoglobin electrophoresis test.

Other laboratory tests routinely ordered include a blood type and antibody screen. This test helps identify women who are at risk of developing antigen incompatibility with fetal blood cells. Blood type incompatibilities (A, B, and O) as well as Rho(D) incompatibilities can develop. If the woman develops an antigen incompatibility, the fetus in a subsequent pregnancy may suffer from hemolytic anemia, as the mother's antibodies cross the placenta and attack the fetus's red blood cells (see Chapter 20 for further discussion of antigen incompatibilities).

Other tests screen for the presence of infection. The woman will undergo tests for hepatitis B, HIV, syphilis, gonorrhea, and chlamydia. Each of these infections can cause serious fetal problems unless they are treated. A rubella titer determines if the woman is immune to rubella. If she is not, she will need a rubella immunization immediately after delivery because the rubella vaccine cannot be given safely during pregnancy. A urine culture screens for bacteria in the urine, a situation that can lead to urinary tract infection and premature labor if it is not treated. The Pap test screens for cervical cancer. Vaginal and anal cultures, as well as urine testing, for group B streptococcus are obtained usually at 35 to 37 weeks. If the woman is positive for this bacterium, she is at an increased risk for premature delivery and may require antibiotic drugs at the time of delivery to avoid causing an infection in the newborn.

Traditionally, screening for hypothyroidism is done only when the woman has risk factors or symptoms of hypothyroidism. However, some women may have subclinical hypothyroidism, and may not experience symptoms and therefore may not be screened. Because of the negative effects on the fetus's developing nervous system from hypothyroidism, many health care providers will include thyroid screening for the pregnant woman.

A glucose tolerance test (GTT) is done to evaluate the woman for gestational diabetes. The GTT is usually done between 24 and 28 weeks' gestation if the woman does not have any prior history of gestational diabetes or risk factors for this condition. Women who are at risk may be screened as early as the first prenatal visit (Durnwald, 2020). See Chapter 16 for a discussion of the GTT and gestational diabetes.

Due Date Estimation

One important aspect of the first visit is to calculate the **estimated date of delivery** (EDD), also called the woman's due date. An older term that is sometimes used is estimated date of confinement (EDC). Both terms refer to the estimated date that the baby will be born. This is critical information for the health care provider because problems that may arise during the pregnancy are managed differently, depending on the gestational age of the fetus. Therefore, it is essential to have an accurate due date.

There are several ways to date a pregnancy. A common way to calculate the EDD is to use **Naegele rule**. To determine the due date using Naegele rule, add 7 days to the date of the first day of the LMP, then subtract 3 months. This is a simple way to estimate the due date, but it is dependent upon the woman knowing when the first day of her LMP was and is also based upon the woman having a 28-day menstrual cycle. Sometimes the EDD is impossible to determine based upon Naegele rule, particularly if the woman experiences irregular menstrual cycles, or if she cannot remember the date.

During the pelvic examination, the health care provider feels the size of the uterus to get an idea of how far along the pregnancy is. For instance, a uterus that is the size of a small pear is approximately 7 weeks. If the uterus feels to be the size of an orange, the pregnancy is approximately 10 weeks along, and at 12 weeks the uterus is the size of a grapefruit.

Other ways to validate the gestational age are to note landmarks during the pregnancy. Initial detection of the fetal heartbeat by Doppler ultrasound takes place between 10 and 12 weeks. **Quickening**, when the woman feels the fetus move for the first time, typically occurs around 16 weeks for multigravidas and 20 weeks for primigravidas. At 20 weeks, the uterus reaches the level of the umbilicus.

One of the most common and reliable ways to date the pregnancy is through an obstetric **sonogram**, a picture obtained with ultrasound. High-frequency sound waves reflect off fetal and maternal pelvic structures, allowing the sonographer to visualize the structures in real time. The sonographer measures fetal structures, such as the head and the femur. These measurements allow the health care provider to estimate the gestational age of the fetus and thereby determine a due date. A sonogram obtained early in the pregnancy yields the most accurate due date. If there is a discrepancy between the EDD calculated using Naegele rule and the EDD determined by sonogram, the results of the sonogram (if it is done in the first half of the pregnancy) are used to base treatment decisions.

The sonogram done at 20 weeks is the standard prenatal ultrasound. If the health care provider needs further evaluation of the fetus, such as to look for spina bifida or cardiac anomalies, a 3-D or 4-D ultrasound can be performed. A 3-D ultrasound reveals a three-dimensional image, not a flat picture like the standard ultrasound, whereas a 4-D ultrasound looks more like a film and can show images such as the fetus yawning or sucking.

Risk Assessment

The risk assessment takes into account all of the information gathered from the history, physical examination, and laboratory tests. Many factors put a pregnancy at risk. These factors include an unwanted pregnancy, seeking late or no prenatal care, or maternal substance use (alcohol, tobacco, or illicit drugs). A history of complications with previous pregnancies or the presence of maternal disease also put the current pregnancy at risk. Social factors that increase the risk of poor outcomes include inadequate living conditions and domestic violence. If the woman is unaware of the adverse effects of tobacco and alcohol, the benefits of folic acid, or the risk of HIV, the pregnancy is at increased risk for complications and poor outcomes. Age also plays a factor. Young adolescents and women older than 35 years are at higher risk for complicated pregnancies.

TEST YOURSELF

✔ Which obstetric term indicates the number of pregnancies a woman has had?

✔ List four laboratory tests that are routinely ordered during the first prenatal visit.

✔ Using Naegele rule, calculate the estimated due date for a woman whose LMP started on February 1.

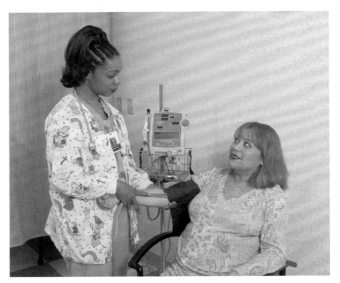

FIGURE 7-2 Measurement of blood pressure at a prenatal visit.

Subsequent Prenatal Visits

Traditionally, the health care provider sees the woman once a month from weeks 1 through 32. Between weeks 32 and 36, prenatal visits are every other week. From week 36 until delivery, the woman is seen weekly. Encourage the woman to keep her appointments and maintain regular prenatal care throughout the pregnancy.

During subsequent visits, weight, blood pressure (Fig. 7-2), urine protein and glucose, and fetal heart rate (FHR) are all data that are routinely collected. At every visit, inquire regarding the danger signals of pregnancy (Box 7-3). Ask the woman about fetal movement, contractions, bleeding, and membrane rupture. Normally the pelvic examination is not repeated until late in the pregnancy closer to the expected time of delivery.

At each office visit, the fundal height is measured (Fig. 7-3). To do this, a tape measure is placed at the base of the uterus, at the symphysis pubis, and then laid against the abdomen. The fundal height is measured in centimeters

BOX 7-3 Danger Signs of Pregnancy

Inquire regarding these warning signals at every visit. Instruct the woman to report any of these signs if she experiences them to her health care provider right away.
- Fever or severe vomiting
- Headache, unrelieved by acetaminophen or other relief measures
- Blurred vision or spots before the eyes
- Pain in the epigastric region
- Sudden weight gain or sudden onset of edema in the hands and face
- Vaginal bleeding
- Painful urination
- Sudden gush or constant, uncontrollable leaking of fluid from the vagina
- Decreased fetal movement
- Signs of preterm labor
  - Uterine contractions (four or more per hour)
  - Lower, dull backache
  - Pelvic pressure
  - Menstrual-like cramps
  - Increase in vaginal discharge
  - A feeling that something is not right

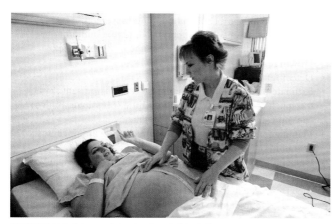

FIGURE 7-3 Measuring the fundal height.

with the reading at the top of the fundus. Between weeks 18 and 32, the fundal height in centimeters should match the gestational age of the pregnancy. For example, if the woman is 18 weeks pregnant, the fundal height should measure 18 cm. If there is a discrepancy between the size and dates, the health care provider needs to determine the cause of the discrepancy; usually this is done by sonogram. A fundal height that is larger than expected could indicate that the original dates were miscalculated, that the woman is carrying twins, polyhydramnios (excessive amniotic fluid, usually more than 2 L), or that there is a molar pregnancy (see Chapter 17). A fundal height that is smaller than expected could indicate that the original dates were miscalculated, oligohydramnios (too little amniotic fluid, usually less than 500 mL), or that the fetus is smaller than expected (see Chapter 20 for discussion of small-for-gestational-age

infants). After 32 weeks, the fundal height does not correlate with gestational age because of variances in fetal growth.

Recommended screenings occur at particular times during the pregnancy. Sometime between 15 and 20 weeks' gestation, a maternal serum alpha-fetoprotein (MSAFP) should be drawn (see the discussion in the section on fetal assessment). Between 24 and 28 weeks, all women should be screened for gestational diabetes. At 28 weeks, a woman who is Rho(D)-negative should be screened for antibodies and given anti-D immune globulin (Rho(D) immune globulin), if indicated (see Chapter 20 for further discussion of hemolytic disease of the newborn). The woman should undergo screening for group B streptococcus. Positive group B streptococcus cultures indicate the need for antibiotic drugs for the woman during labor and close observation of the newborn for 48 hours after birth. To screen for Down syndrome in mothers with a high risk, the health care provider may recommend the woman have a cell-free DNA blood test.

TEST YOURSELF

✔ How many prenatal visits would a woman have if she started prenatal care at the time of her first missed period?

✔ What purpose does measuring the fundal height serve during prenatal visits?

✔ A woman states she was diagnosed with gestational diabetes with her first pregnancy. When would the health care provider want to screen her for gestational diabetes during this pregnancy?

ASSESSMENT OF FETAL WELL-BEING DURING PREGNANCY

Throughout the pregnancy, the health care provider may order tests to observe the well-being of the fetus. Some are screening tests, which means they are not diagnostic. If an abnormal result occurs with a screening test, additional diagnostic testing is recommended. The discussion that follows describes some of the most common tests and procedures. Not every woman will receive every test, although some screening tests are recommended for all pregnant women at certain points during the pregnancy.

Fetal Movement (Kick) Count

A healthy fetus moves and kicks regularly, although the pregnant woman usually cannot perceive the movements until approximately 16 to 20 gestational weeks. The fetus undergoes regular rest/activity cycles that last around 40 to 60 minutes. The woman is instructed to monitor the fetus's movements movements on a daily basis. Instruct the woman to choose a time each day in which she can relax and count the movements. Each kick or position change counts as one movement.

Using a special form provided by the health care provider or a blank sheet of paper, instruct the woman to note the time she starts counting fetal kicks and then keep counting until she counts 10 movements. A healthy fetus will move at least 10 times in 2 hours. If the woman eats or drinks something high in sugar, this may increase the fetal activity during kick counts. If it takes longer than 2 hours for the fetus to move 10 times, or if the woman cannot get her baby to move at all, she should immediately call her health care provider who will order tests to determine the well-being of the fetus.

Ultrasonography

Ultrasound is the gold standard in the United States to determine gestational age, observe the fetus, and diagnose complications of pregnancy (Fig. 7-4). It is a frequently performed procedure that noninvasively monitors fetal well-being and size, placental location, and amniotic fluid. One plus for parents is that with ultrasound, parents can know the gender of the child before it is born if they desire. Many sonographers take a still picture of the fetus and provide this to the parents, also if desired.

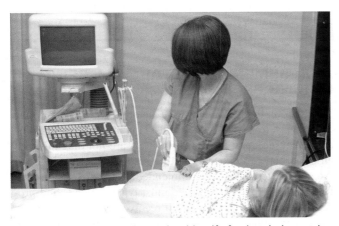

FIGURE 7-4 Ultrasound is used to identify fetal and placental structures during pregnancy.

As stated earlier in the chapter, ultrasound uses sound waves to visualize fetal and maternal structures (Fig. 7-5). The developing embryo can first be visualized at about 6 weeks' gestation. An ultrasound performed at this stage positively diagnoses the pregnancy. Ultrasound captures the fetus's cardiac activity and body movements in real time. Box 7-4 lists ways ultrasound technology is used to monitor the pregnancy and fetal well-being.

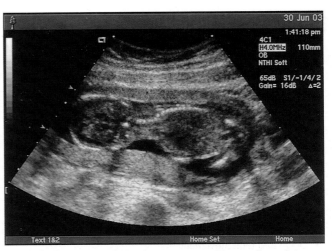

FIGURE 7-5 Fetus viewed via ultrasound. The outline of the fetal head and trunk can be clearly seen in the transverse position.

BOX 7-4 **Uses for Ultrasound Technology During Pregnancy**

- Diagnose pregnancy: intrauterine and ectopic (outside the uterine cavity).
- Diagnose multifetal pregnancies (twins, triplets).
- Monitor fetal heartbeat and breathing movements.
- Take measurements of the fetal head, femur, and other structures to determine gestational age or diagnose fetal growth restriction.
- Detect fetal anomalies.
- Estimate the amount of amniotic fluid that is present. Either too much (polyhydramnios) or too little (oligohydramnios) can indicate problems with the pregnancy.
- Identify fetal and placental structures during amniocentesis or umbilical cord sampling.
- Detect placental problems, such as abnormal placement of the placenta in placenta previa or grade the placenta (determine the age and functioning).
- Diagnose fetal demise (death) by verifying absence of fetal cardiac activity.
- Verify fetal presentation and position.
- Estimate the birth weight, particularly if the fetus is thought to be abnormally large (macrosomic) or small for gestational age.

 Concept Mastery Alert

Ultrasonography is a powerful tool in determining not only maternal dimensions, but also informs the health care provider about the size and well-being of the infant.

Ultrasound can best detect most abnormalities of the fetus, placenta, and surrounding structures between 16 and 20 weeks' gestation. Detailed sonograms can diagnose severe congenital heart, spine, brain, and kidney defects. However, ultrasound cannot pick up all abnormalities. Some anomalies, such as Down syndrome, have subtle characteristics that can be observed on ultrasound, for example, increased nuchal translucency (fetal neck thickness) and shortened long bones (femur or humerus). There are two main ways to perform an ultrasound during pregnancy—the transabdominal or the transvaginal approach.

Transabdominal Ultrasound

For the transabdominal method, the sonographer places a transducer on the abdomen to visualize the pregnancy. In the past, it was recommended that the woman have a full bladder for transabdominal ultrasound. Current recommendations are that the woman does not need to have a full bladder (Shipp, 2020). In fact, a full bladder may actually distort anatomy. If the sonographer cannot see sufficient detail with the transabdominal approach, a transvaginal approach can be used.

If you are assisting during the procedure, place a small wedge (a pillow or folded towel) under one hip to prevent supine hypotension. Explain to the woman that the sonographer will place ultrasonic transducer gel on her abdomen and that the gel will probably be cold. She should not feel any discomfort during the procedure. A darkened room optimizes visualization of fetal structures during the procedure. Although the technician performing the sonogram can see fetal structures and obvious defects during the sonogram, it will take several hours to get the official results because the radiologist, not the sonographer, must review the films and give the diagnosis. After the procedure, clean the excess gel off the woman's abdomen and assist her to the bathroom if necessary.

Here's a Tip!
The woman may be anxious or excited during the ultrasound. Use open-ended questions to determine how she is feeling about the procedure. Do not assume every woman or partner is excited about the ultrasound. Also, some women do not wish to know the gender of the fetus, so inquire about this prior to the procedure.

Transvaginal Ultrasound

For the transvaginal (also referred to as endovaginal) method, the sonographer uses an elongated ultrasound probe that is placed in the woman's vagina. There are several advantages to this method. The transvaginal approach allows for a clearer image because the probe is very close to fetal and uterine structures. This method allows for earlier confirmation of the pregnancy than does the transabdominal method. The transvaginal method is superior for predicting or diagnosing preterm labor because the sonographer can measure and analyze the cervix for changes.

Assist the woman into lithotomy position (as for a pelvic examination) and drape her for privacy. A female attendant must be present in the room at all times during the procedure if the sonographer is male. The examiner covers the probe (which is smaller than a speculum) with a plastic sheath, applies the transducer gel to the covered probe, and inserts the probe into the woman's vagina. Explain to the woman that she will feel the probe moving about in different directions during the test. The probe may cause mild discomfort, but it is generally not painful.

Doppler Flow Studies

Another test that uses ultrasound technology is a Doppler flow study or Doppler velocimetry. A specialized ultrasound machine measures the flow of blood through fetal vessels. The ultrasound transducer on the woman's abdomen allows the sonographer to monitor blood flow through the umbilical vessels and in the fetal aorta, brain, and heart. If the test shows that blood flow through fetal vessels is less than normal, the fetus may not be receiving enough oxygen and nutrients from the placenta, and additional studies will be ordered. Preparation and nursing care for a Doppler flow study are the same as for a transabdominal ultrasound.

Maternal Serum Alpha-Fetoprotein Screening

Alpha-fetoprotein is a protein manufactured by the fetus. The woman's blood contains small amounts of this protein during pregnancy. Measuring maternal serum alpha-fetoprotein (MSAFP) can be done between 15 and 20 weeks' gestation and the optimal time frame is between 16 and 18 weeks' gestation. Abnormal levels (high or low) may indicate a problem and the need for additional testing.

MSAFP levels are elevated in several conditions. Higher than expected levels of MSAFP are seen when the woman is carrying multiple fetuses, or if the fetus has died in utero, or in the presence of neural tube defects. The main reason MSAFP is measured is to check for neural tube defects, such as anencephaly (failure of the brain to develop normally) or spina bifida (failure of the spine to close completely during development). MSAFP levels are usually elevated if the fetus has either of these anomalies. Omphalocele and gastroschisis (both are caused by a failure of the abdominal wall to close) are two other conditions that cause elevated MSAFP levels. Low MSAFP levels may indicate Down syndrome.

Several factors can influence MSAFP results. These include an increased maternal weight, maternal diabetes, and maternal race. It is important that these factors are reported to the laboratory with the MSAFP specimen. Early on in the pregnancy there is higher than normal levels of MSAFP because the neural tube that is developing is still open. This is a normal finding very early in the pregnancy but can be interpreted as a false high if the woman's dates are inaccurate.

It is important for the parents-to-be to understand the reasons for and implications of MSAFP testing. Even when the levels are abnormal, the woman will often deliver a healthy newborn. However, abnormal results increase the likelihood that the fetus has an abnormality, and additional diagnostic testing with ultrasound and amniocentesis will be recommended.

Some women want to have the test done so that they can decide whether to end the pregnancy before the age of viability. Other women feel strongly that abortion is not an option, but they may want to know if an anomaly is present so that they can deliver in a hospital with high-level care and have specialists immediately available to care for the baby. Other women may decide against testing because a false-positive test might be needlessly worrisome and lead to more invasive, riskier tests, such as amniocentesis, even though the fetus might be healthy. Each woman must consider these issues in consult with her partner and the health care provider. No matter what decision the woman makes regarding testing, it is critical to support her decision.

Amniocentesis

An **amniocentesis** is a diagnostic procedure where a needle is inserted into the amniotic sac and a small amount of amniotic fluid is obtained (Fig. 7-6). A variety of biochemical, chromosomal, and genetic studies are possible using the amniotic fluid sample.

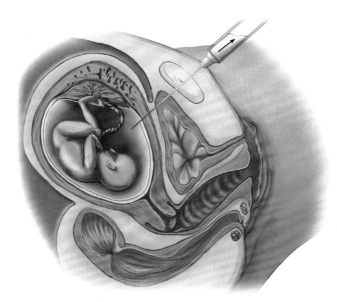

FIGURE 7-6 Amniocentesis. A pocket of amniotic fluid is located by sonogram. A small amount of fluid is removed by aspiration.

The procedure is usually performed between 15 and 20 weeks' gestation, although early amniocentesis (at 12 to 14 weeks' gestation) may be preferable in some cases. Amniocentesis can determine the genetic makeup and gender of the fetus because amniotic fluid contains fetal cells. Box 7-5 lists indications for first- and second-trimester amniocentesis. Third-trimester amniocentesis is usually done to determine fetal lung maturity, which allows for the earliest possible delivery in certain at-risk pregnancies.

Because amniocentesis is an invasive procedure that carries a small risk of spontaneous abortion, injury to the fetus, and chorioamnionitis (infection of the fetal membranes), the woman must give informed consent. The health care provider explains the procedure and risks and answers her questions. If you witness the consent, be certain that the woman has had all her questions answered and that she has not taken any antianxiety medications before she signs. Many women are worried that the procedure will be painful. Although pain is a subjective feeling that varies between individuals, most women find that the procedure is much less painful than they anticipated. Usually women report feeling a slight pinching sensation or vague cramping. Nursing responsibilities during an amniocentesis include observation of the woman and fetus, providing support to the woman, and assisting the health care provider as needed.

Just before the procedure, ultrasound is used to locate a pocket of amniotic fluid. Without ultrasound to guide the needle, there is a high risk that the needle could puncture the placenta or the fetus. After the pocket of fluid is identified (usually on the upper portion of the uterus), the site is prepared with an antiseptic solution and sterile drapes are placed on the abdomen around the site. Sterile drapes also cover the ultrasound transducer. A 20- or 22-gauge spinal needle is inserted into the chosen site and guided into the pocket of fluid. The first 0.5 mL of fluid is discarded to avoid contamination of the specimen with maternal cells. Then, 20 mL (less for early amniocentesis) of amniotic fluid is withdrawn and the needle removed. The fetal heart rate is monitored by ultrasound to ensure fetal well-being. The fluid sample, which is normally straw colored, is placed into sterile tubes, labeled, and sent to the laboratory for analysis. Results are usually available within 2 to 3 weeks and are highly accurate (approximately 99%).

Continuous electronic fetal monitoring is done to observe the fetal heart rate and also for any contractions. Women who are Rho(D)-negative should receive Rho(D) immune globulin after the procedure as there is risk for leaking of fetal blood into the maternal circulatory system from this invasive procedure. Immediately report to the RN or the attending health care provider any maternal temperature elevation, leaking of amniotic fluid from the puncture site or from the vagina, vaginal bleeding, cramps, or contractions. After several hours of monitoring, the woman may go home. Instruct her to remain on bed rest for the rest of the day. The following day she may do light housework chores, and the third day she may resume regular activities. Warning signs she should immediately report to the health care provider include fever, amniotic fluid leakage, decreased fetal movement, vaginal bleeding, and cramping.

As with any medical procedure that carries risk, amniocentesis has advantages and disadvantages that each woman must consider carefully. The most common reason for undergoing amniocentesis is to determine if there is a fetal chromosomal abnormality. If the fetus does have a chromosomal abnormality, knowing in advance allows the medical team and the parents to prepare for the birth. It also allows the health care provider to make better decisions about managing the pregnancy. Every woman who is contemplating amniocentesis should have genetic counseling. At that point, no matter what decision the woman makes, it is critical that the healthcare team supports her decision.

Chorionic Villus Sampling

Chorionic villus sampling is a procedure similar to amniocentesis that can provide chromosomal studies of fetal cells. Indications for chorionic villus sampling are the same as for amniocentesis (Box 7-5). One advantage of chorionic villus sampling testing is that it is done earlier in the pregnancy than amniocentesis. Chorionic villus sampling is typically performed at 8 to 12 weeks' gestation. Because chorionic villus sampling is an invasive procedure, informed consent is required.

Just before the procedure, an ultrasound confirms fetal well-being, the location of the placenta, and gestational age. For the transcervical approach, assist the woman into the lithotomy position in stirrups. The health care provider then performs the procedure. First, cleaning the vagina and cervix with povidone-iodine or other antiseptic fluid is done. Using ultrasound guidance, a small catheter is inserted into the woman's vagina and through the cervix. Placental tissue is then extracted into a syringe to obtain fetal cells for chromosomal analysis. Sometimes a transabdominal approach is used with a needle, similar to the procedure for amniocentesis. The woman usually experiences minimal discomfort and may resume normal activities after the test. Rho(D) immune globulin should be administered after the procedure to Rho(D)-negative women.

One advantage of chorionic villus sampling testing is that the results are available in 7 to 10 days, much faster than with amniocentesis. Another advantage is that testing can occur earlier in the pregnancy. However, there are disadvantages to this technique such as a risk for miscarriage. A second potential disadvantage is that there is no amniotic fluid in a chorionic villus sampling sample; therefore, the fetal alpha-fetoprotein cannot be evaluated as it can with amniocentesis. This means the woman would need to have MSAFP levels drawn at 16 to 18 weeks' gestation to test for neural tube defects. A woman who has amniocentesis performed does not need the MSAFP test because amniocentesis results report the fetal alpha-fetoprotein level, which is a more accurate predictor of neural tube defects than maternal serum levels. The third disadvantage of chorionic villus sampling is that there is a small risk that the cells taken from the placenta will be different from fetal cells. Finally, chorionic villus sampling performed before 9 weeks' gestation can cause fetal limb and digit deformations. Instruct the woman to report postprocedure warning signs that can occur including fever, amniotic fluid leakage, vaginal bleeding, and cramping.

Percutaneous Umbilical Blood Sampling

Percutaneous umbilical blood sampling (PUBS), also known as **cordocentesis**, is a procedure similar to amniocentesis, except that fetal blood is withdrawn from the umbilical cord. The procedure is done in a similar manner as an amniocentesis and also requires informed consent. Ultrasound locates the placenta and fetal structures and confirms gestational age and viability. A thin needle is inserted transabdominally under ultrasound guidance and blood is withdrawn from the umbilical cord close to its insertion with the placenta. The blood is then sent for testing.

Sometimes, PUBS is done specifically to diagnose and treat certain diseases of the blood, such as von Willebrand disease, thrombocytopenia, and hemolytic disease. It can also diagnose cases of fetal infection such as toxoplasmosis, rubella, cytomegalovirus, varicella zoster, human parvovirus, and HIV. Through the technology of cordocentesis, the fetus with thrombocytopenia can receive weekly infusions of platelets until delivery. The fetus with hemolytic disease can receive exchange transfusions (part of the fetus's blood is withdrawn and the same amount replaced with healthy blood). The fetus with an infection can be treated with antibiotic drugs or receive other therapies, depending upon the type of infection. The blood obtained from cordocentesis can also be sent for rapid chromosomal studies. Results are back within 48 to 72 hours. The risks associated with PUBS are approximately the same as those of amniocentesis. As with amniocentesis and chorionic villus sampling, instruct the woman to report any warning signs including fever, amniotic fluid leakage, vaginal bleeding, and cramping.

Nonstress Test

The nonstress test (NST) is a noninvasive way to monitor fetal well-being. After 28 weeks, the fetal nervous system is developed enough so that the autonomic nervous system works to periodically accelerate the heart rate. Therefore, fetal heart rate (FHR) can be observed for accelerations using electronic fetal monitoring (EFM).

The woman requires no special preparation for the NST (see Chapter 10 for in-depth discussion of fetal monitoring). EFM is used to monitor the FHR and the woman may or may not have an event marker to hold. If she uses an event marker, she pushes a button every time she feels the fetus move. In the past, FHR was always monitored in conjunction with fetal movement. Now, it is generally felt that spontaneous accelerations with or without fetal movement are indicative of fetal well-being, so it is not necessary to have the woman track fetal movements, although some health care providers prefer this.

The fetal monitor tracing is evaluated after 20 minutes. Generally, if there are at least two accelerations of the FHR, at least 15 beats above the baseline for at least 15 seconds, the NST is said to be "reactive" provided that the baseline and variability are normal and that there are no decelerations of the FHR. In the presence of a reactive NST, fetal well-being is assumed for at least the next week.

If, however, there are no accelerations or less than two occur within 20 minutes, the strip is said to be "nonreactive." In this case, the monitoring would continue for another 20 minutes in the hopes of obtaining a reactive NST. This is because fetal sleep cycles last for approximately 20 minutes. During fetal sleep, accelerations do not usually occur, so it is prudent to observe for an additional 20 minutes. Sometimes attempts are made to stimulate the fetus. The provider may clap loudly close to the woman's abdomen or may manipulate the fetus through the abdomen, or the woman may be given something cold to drink. Any of these activities might stimulate a sleeping fetus to wake up and result in a reactive tracing. If the tracing remains nonreactive or equivocal (meaning the results cannot be interpreted), additional testing is warranted. In these instances, the health care provider frequently recommends a contraction stress test.

Contraction Stress Test

Uterine contractions cause a momentary reduction of uteroplacental blood flow, which stresses the fetus. A contraction stress test (CST) monitors the fetus's response to contractions to determine fetal well-being. The woman is placed on EFM, as for the NST. There are three ways to obtain uterine contractions for a CST. The easiest way is if the woman is having spontaneous Braxton Hicks contractions because there is no need to induce contractions. Another way is to induce uterine contractions through nipple stimulation. Nipple stimulation causes release of oxytocin from the posterior pituitary gland. The oxytocin then stimulates the uterus to contract. The third way is to start an intravenous drip of oxytocin to induce contractions.

The goal is to have three contractions of at least 40 seconds duration within a 10-minutes period. The fetal monitor strip is then evaluated to determine the reaction of the fetus to the stress of the contractions. If there are no late decelerations

(see Chapter 10) after any of the contractions, the CST is considered negative. A negative CST is a reassuring sign and indicates that the fetus is not suffering from hypoxia and does not need immediate delivery. An equivocal CST occurs when there are late decelerations after some, but not all, of the uterine contractions. This result is suspicious of fetal hypoxia and may cause the physician to decide to perform a cesarean delivery of the fetus. A positive CST is when there are late decelerations after every contraction and is indicative of fetal hypoxia requiring delivery of the fetus. An unsatisfactory CST occurs when there are insufficient contractions. For an unsatisfactory CST, orders may be for the test to be repeated within 24 hours or for a biophysical profile to be performed.

Biophysical Profile

A **biophysical profile** uses a combination of factors to determine fetal well-being based upon five fetal biophysical variables. First, an NST is done to measure FHR acceleration. Then an ultrasound is done to measure fetal breathing, body movements, tone, and amniotic fluid volume. Each variable receives a score of 0 (abnormal, absent, or insufficient) or 2 (normal or present) for a maximum score of 10. A score of 8 to 10 indicates fetal well-being. A score of 6 correlates with possible fetal asphyxia, whereas a score of 4 indicates probable fetal asphyxia. Scores of 0 to 2 indicate poor fetal well-being and require immediate delivery of the fetus.

TEST YOURSELF

✔ How many times should the fetus move in a 2-hours period of time?

✔ What is the difference between a positive CST and a negative CST?

✔ What tissue is extracted for study when chorionic villus sampling is used?

Remember **Stefani Mueller** from the start of the chapter. How would you document her gravida and parity in the chart? Since she had a previous miscarriage, the health care provider would want to monitor this pregnancy closely. What laboratory or diagnostic tests would most likely be ordered for Stefani?

COMMON DISCOMFORTS OF PREGNANCY

Pregnant women tend to experience similar discomforts because of the significant bodily changes they undergo. Some discomforts tend to occur in early pregnancy, some toward the end, and others continue throughout. Table 7-2 lists selected discomforts along with suggestions for helping the woman cope.

TABLE 7-2 Common Discomforts of Pregnancy

DISCOMFORT	CONTRIBUTING FACTOR OR CAUSE	SUGGESTIONS FOR RELIEVING THE DISCOMFORT
Bleeding gums	Stimulating effects of estrogen on the gums.	• Visit the dentist. • Use rinses and gargles to freshen the oral cavity. • Use a soft-bristled toothbrush.
Nasal stuffiness	Effects of estrogen on the nasal mucosa cause vasocongestion and stuffiness.	• Use a cool-air vaporizer. • Try normal saline nasal sprays. • Avoid over-the-counter medicated nasal sprays because initial relief may be followed by rebound stuffiness.
Nosebleeds	The tiny veins of the nasal lining are prone to breaking and causing nosebleeds. Dry nasal passages increase the risk.	• Avoid vigorous nose blowing. • Use a humidifier. • Drink plenty of fluids.
Breast tenderness	Progesterone and estrogen are thought to contribute to the tingling or heavy sensations in the breasts that come and go throughout pregnancy.	• Wear a well-fitted support bra. • Wearing a bra at night might be helpful if breast discomfort is interfering with restful sleep.
Nausea and nausea with vomiting	Rising levels of hCG probably contribute to nausea along with other factors.	• Begin the day with a high-carbohydrate food, such as dry toast, saltines, or other bland crackers. • Change positions slowly, especially when getting up in the morning. • Eat small high-protein meals frequently throughout the day. • If protein is not well tolerated, try high-carbohydrate, low-fat snacks to avoid hypoglycemia. • Wait at least 1 hour after eating to brush the teeth. • Drink small amounts frequently. • Include electrolyte-replenishing liquids for emesis. • Avoid noxious odors. • Take a walk outside in the fresh air. • Delay iron supplementation until the second trimester.
Feeling faint	Postural hypotension can easily develop with the hemodynamic changes that occur in a normal pregnancy as the blood vessels in the periphery relax and dilate.	• Change positions slowly. • Avoid abrupt position changes. • Eat small, frequent, high-carbohydrate meals.
Fatigue	Cause is unknown. Progesterone may contribute.	• Plan for daily naps. • Take frequent rest breaks throughout the day. • Go to bed early.
Shortness of breath	In early pregnancy, the effects of progesterone can create a sense of shortness of breath. In later pregnancy, the uterus pushes on the diaphragm.	• Sit up straight to increase diameter of the chest. • If shortness of breath is interfering with sleep, prop up with pillows.
Heartburn	Relaxation of the lower esophageal sphincter under the influence of progesterone and increased intra-abdominal pressure because of the growing uterus cause acid reflux into the lower esophagus.	• Eat small, frequent meals. • Avoid substances that increase acid production, in particular cigarette smoking. • Avoid substances that cause relaxation of the lower esophageal sphincter, such as coffee, chocolate, alcohol, and heavy spices. • Avoid lying down after a meal. • Avoid lying flat.
Low back pain	Changes in the center of gravity and loosened ligaments.	• Avoid gaining too much weight. • Avoid high-heeled shoes. • Always bend at the knees, not the waist. • Avoid standing for too long at one time. • Keep one foot on a stool when standing. Frequently change the foot that is resting on the stool.

TABLE 7-2 Common Discomforts of Pregnancy (Continued)

DISCOMFORT	CONTRIBUTING FACTOR OR CAUSE	SUGGESTIONS FOR RELIEVING THE DISCOMFORT
Round ligament pain	Sharp, severe pain, usually on the right side brought on by stretching of the round ligaments that support the uterus.	• Avoid sudden changes in positions or sudden movements. • Apply heat. • Lie on the side opposite the pain.
Leg cramps	Not known.	• Avoid plantar flexion. • Rest frequently with the feet elevated. • When cramps occur, extend the affected leg and dorsiflex the foot.
Varicose veins	Increased pelvic pressure, vasodilation in the lower extremities and vagina, along with pooling of blood in the lower extremities can contribute to varicosities of the legs and vagina.	• Exercise daily. • Rest with the legs elevated several times daily. • Wear compression stockings. Put them on before getting out of bed in the morning. • Avoid prolonged periods of standing or sitting. Move around frequently. Stretch and take small walks. • When standing for a long time, frequently exercise the leg muscles and change positions frequently. • Keep within the recommended weight range during pregnancy.
Ankle edema	Progesterone effects, increased pressure in the lower extremities, increased capillary permeability.	• Avoid prolonged periods of standing. • Rest frequently with the feet elevated. • Soak in a warm pool or bath. • Avoid constrictive garments on the lower extremities. • Wear compression stockings.
Flatulence	Relaxation of the gastrointestinal tract under the influence of progesterone, pressure of the uterus on the intestines, air swallowing.	• Avoid gas-producing foods. • Chew foods thoroughly. • Get plenty of exercise. • Maintain regular bowel habits. • Avoid chewing gum.
Constipation and hemorrhoids	Slowing of the gastrointestinal tract under the influence of progesterone and increased blood flow and pressure in the pelvic area.	• Drink at least eight glasses of noncaffeinated beverages per day. • Eat plenty of fiber. • Get adequate exercise. • Use a stool softener if prescribed by the primary health care provider. • Use topical anesthetic agents to treat the pain of hemorrhoids.
Trouble sleeping	Many discomforts of pregnancy, as well as the increase in size of the abdomen, can all contribute to sleepless nights in the third trimester.	• Get adequate exercise. • Try different positions and use pillows to support and wedge. • Try sleeping in a sitting position. • Drink a glass of warm milk before bed. • Have a late-night, high-carbohydrate snack. • Try progressive muscle relaxation or guided imagery.

Nasal Stuffiness and Epistaxis

A pregnant woman is prone to nasal stuffiness and epistaxis (nosebleeds). Estrogen is the hormone most likely responsible for this discomfort because it contributes to vasocongestion and increases the fragility of the nasal mucosa. Sometimes the woman may have symptoms resembling the common cold that persist throughout pregnancy. Menthol applied just below the nostrils before bedtime might help relieve some discomfort from congestion. The woman should generally not use nasal decongestants, other than normal saline nasal sprays, and should consult her health care provider before taking any medications, including over-the-counter or home remedies.

Avoiding vigorous nose blowing may prevent nosebleeds. It is also helpful to keep the nasal passages moist. Using a humidifier in the house and staying well hydrated can accomplish this. If a nosebleed occurs despite precautions, instruct the woman to pinch the nostrils and hold pressure for at least 4 minutes until the bleeding stops. Ice may help stop the bleeding. If the bleeding is heavy or does not stop with pressure, instruct the woman to consult her health care provider.

Nausea

Morning sickness, or nausea, is a common complaint of early pregnancy for many women. Rising levels of hCG are thought to be part of the cause, although it is likely many factors that contribute. Although "morning sickness" is the lay term for the nausea of pregnancy, many women experience nausea at other times during the day, or even throughout the day. Fortunately, nausea generally subsides by the end of the first trimester.

Caloric intake during the first trimester is not as crucial as it is in the second and third trimesters, so nausea is usually not harmful to the pregnancy. However, severe nausea and vomiting can lead to nutritional deficiencies, dehydration, and electrolyte deficiencies, so preventive measures are important. Some helpful suggestions include advising the woman to place a high-carbohydrate, low-fat snack, such as dry toast or saltine crackers, at the bedside before going to sleep. When she wakes, before getting out of bed, she should eat the snack. This can help prevent early morning nausea. Other helpful hints are to encourage the woman to eat small amounts frequently throughout the day, instead of consuming three heavy meals hours apart, and never to let the stomach become completely empty. It also helps to avoid strong odors and spicy and fatty foods. Sometimes it is easier for the woman to eat when someone else prepares the meal. Brushing the teeth causes salivation, which can intensify nausea. In addition, the smell of the toothpaste may cause nausea, so the woman should wait for 1 hour after eating before brushing her teeth. Candies or tea containing peppermint or ginger may help the woman. Taking prenatal vitamins prior to bedtime instead of in the morning helps some women with nausea that is related to the iron in the vitamins. Ginger-containing foods, such as a lollipop or tea, is helpful for nausea without emesis.

When the nonpharmacologic interventions described above do not sufficiently treat the nausea, the health care provider may suggest the woman take pyridoxine (vitamin B_6). Pyridoxine is helpful for nausea but not emesis. Another suggestion the provider might make is for the woman to take an antihistamine drug. Some H1 antagonist drugs (such as doxylamine, meclizine, and diphenhydramine) have been shown to be effective against both the nausea and vomiting associated with pregnancy (Smith, Fox, & Clark, 2020). Remind the woman that she should not take any medications without first discussing them with the health care provider as she may have some medical reason that the medication is contraindicated.

Persistent vomiting may be a sign of hyperemesis gravidarum, a complication of pregnancy that can lead to dehydration and electrolyte imbalances (see Chapter 17). If the vomiting is severe or prolonged (e.g., unable retain any food or fluids for 24 hours), advise the woman to consult her health care provider.

Feeling Faint

Sometimes women feel faint during the first few weeks of pregnancy. Postural hypotension could be the cause. Low blood sugar levels aggravate the situation. Advise the woman to change positions slowly and to avoid abrupt position changes. Eating frequent high-carbohydrate meals helps keep blood sugar levels up. If she feels faint, a walk outside might help. Alternatively, she might need to lie down with her feet elevated or sit with her head lower than her knees until the feeling passes.

Frequent Urination

Frequent urination can be bothersome and interfere with sleep. One cause of frequent urination in the first trimester is the increasing blood volume and increased glomerular filtration rate. Frequency usually diminishes during the second trimester, only to reappear in the third trimester because of pressure of the enlarging uterus on the bladder.

Increased Vaginal Discharge

Leukorrhea, or increased vaginal discharge, is common during pregnancy. Increased production of cervical glands and vasocongestion of the pelvic area contribute to the discharge. If the discharge causes itching or irritation, or if there is a foul smell noted, the woman should contact her health care provider because these are signs of infection. She should avoid douching because douching can upset the normal balance of vaginal flora, increasing the risk of contracting an infection. Sanitary pads may help absorb the discharge.

Shortness of Breath

Shortness of breath may occur during the first trimester because of the effects of progesterone. During the latter half of pregnancy, this symptom results from the pressure of the uterus pushing upward on the diaphragm. Advise the woman to take her time and rest frequently. If shortness of breath occurs during exercise, she may need to decrease the level of intensity. During late pregnancy, shortness of breath may interfere with sleep. Propping up with pillows can help expand the chest and decrease the sensation of being unable to catch her breath. Shortness of breath accompanied by fever, chest pain, coughing up blood, or a smothering sensation is a danger sign that indicates the need for medical intervention.

Heartburn

Heartburn, or pyrosis, is a common complaint. Several factors contribute to this discomfort. Progesterone causes a generalized slowing of the gastrointestinal tract and can cause relaxation of the lower esophageal sphincter. When this sphincter is relaxed, acid content from the stomach can back up into the lower part of the esophagus and cause a burning sensation known as heartburn. The increased pressure in the abdomen from the enlarging uterus contributes to the problem.

Prevention is generally the best way to treat heartburn. Several factors aggravate the condition. Smoking increases the acid content of the stomach. Certain foods and beverages, such as coffee, chocolate, peppermint, fatty or fried foods, alcohol, and heavy spices, can contribute to relaxation of the lower esophageal sphincter and exacerbate heartburn. Explain that the woman should avoid the particular substances that cause her discomfort. The pregnant woman should not smoke or drink alcohol because of the harmful effects on the fetus.

Advise the woman regarding interventions to help prevent heartburn or lessen its severity. The woman should eat smaller meals more frequently and avoid drinking fluids with meals. Filling the stomach with a heavy meal or with food and fluid increases the pressure and contributes to gastric reflux. It is best if the woman avoids lying down after meals. If she must lie down, suggest that she lie on her left side with her head higher than her abdomen. Placing 6-inch blocks under the head of the bed or propping pillows at night to keep her chest higher than the abdomen may help. Chewing gum can help neutralize acid.

If nonpharmacologic interventions are not successful in preventing heartburn, medication may help. However, the woman should not take any over-the-counter medications or remedies without first consulting her health care provider because several commonly used heartburn remedies, such as sodium bicarbonate, are not for use during pregnancy. Antacids may be prescribed. Instruct the woman not to take her vitamins within 1 hour of taking antacids.

Backaches

Most pregnant women experience low back pain at some point during pregnancy. Obesity and previous history of back pain are risk factors. Softening and loosening of the ligaments supporting the joints of the spine and pelvis can contribute to low back pain, as can the increasing lordosis of pregnancy and the changing center of gravity.

The woman can help prevent low back pain by using good posture, proper body mechanics, such as bending the knees to reach something on the floor, rather than stooping over from the waist. She should also avoid high-heeled shoes. Good pelvic support with a girdle might be helpful for some women. Strengthening and conditioning exercises may be beneficial.

Treatment of mild backache includes heat, ice, acetaminophen, and massage. If the woman must stand for prolonged periods, she can put one foot on a stool. She should periodically switch the foot that is on the stool. Severe back pain is usually associated with some type of pathology. The woman should consult her health care provider for severe back pain.

Round Ligament Pain

The round ligaments support the uterus in the abdomen. As the uterus expands during pregnancy, it applies pressure to the round ligaments, which respond by stretching and thinning. Because ligaments are pain-sensitive structures, some women experience round ligament pain. The pain most frequently occurs on the right side and can be severe. The pain can occur at night and awaken the woman from sleep, or exercise can bring it on.

Helpful hints to treat round ligament pain include the application of heat. A heating pad or warm bath might be soothing. Sometimes lying on the opposite side can relieve some of the pressure on the ligament and reduce the pain. Avoiding sudden movements may help prevent round ligament pain. If fever, chills, painful urination, and vaginal bleeding accompany the pain, the woman should seek emergency care because the pain is likely the result of a medical condition.

Leg Cramps

Leg cramps are a common occurrence during pregnancy, but researchers do not know the cause. Preventive measures include getting enough rest, resting several times per day with the feet elevated, walking, wearing low-heeled shoes, and avoiding constrictive clothing. Another preventive measure is for the woman to avoid plantar flexion (pointing the toes forward). Calcium traditionally was recommended as a supplement to prevent leg cramps; however, some studies have shown that magnesium lactate or citrate may be helpful (Bermas, 2020). Other recommendations for helping prevent leg cramps include maintain adequate hydration and consuming adequate potassium, such as in oranges or bananas, through a balanced diet. When cramps occur, the woman's partner can help by assisting her to extend her leg, then dorsiflex the foot so that the toes point toward the woman's head. If she is alone, she can extend her leg and dorsiflex the foot, or stand and rise up on her toes until the cramp resolves.

Constipation and Hemorrhoids

The natural slowing of the gastrointestinal tract under the influence of hormones can lead to constipation during pregnancy, and constipation can lead to hemorrhoids. The best way to treat constipation is to prevent it. The same common sense approaches to preventing constipation that are advisable under normal situations are also helpful during pregnancy. These include drinking at least eight glasses of noncaffeinated beverages each day. Advise the woman to get adequate exercise. Adding fiber to the diet or a bulk-forming supplement, such as psyllium, to the daily routine are also helpful hints.

Hemorrhoids can become a problem during pregnancy because of the increased blood flow in the rectal veins and pressure of the uterus that prevents good venous return. Elevating the legs and hips intermittently throughout the day can help counteract this problem. Hemorrhoids can cause pain, itching, a burning sensation, and occasionally bleeding. Applying topical hemorrhoidal anesthetic agents, or compresses such as witch hazel pads, can relieve the pain and swelling.

Trouble Sleeping

Many of the discomforts discussed previously, such as heartburn and shortness of breath, can contribute to restlessness at night and trouble sleeping. As the pregnancy progresses, it may become increasingly difficult to find a position of comfort in bed. Suggest that the woman try lying on her side with plenty of pillows to support her back and legs. If that position does not help, she may find it easier to sleep in the sitting position in an armchair.

Urinary frequency returns during the third trimester and can contribute to sleeplessness because of frequent trips to the restroom. Drinking the majority of fluids early in the day and limiting fluids in the evening hours can reduce this problem. Heartburn can contribute to reduction in sleep, as can the movements of an active fetus. Some degree of sleeplessness and restlessness at night is an expected occurrence in the third trimester.

SELF-CARE DURING PREGNANCY

During pregnancy, it is important for the woman to maintain self-care. Most women are willing to make lifestyle changes during this time period to benefit the health of herself and the fetus. The woman is usually very aware of her diet but other topics of self-care should be covered. Self-care activities often help to alleviate some of the discomforts of pregnancy as well.

Maintaining a Balanced Nutritional Intake

During the first trimester, the fetus's demands on maternal nutritional stores are less than at other times during the pregnancy. This is helpful because sometimes it is difficult for the woman to eat a well-balanced diet when she is coping with nausea. During the first visit, focus on determining the adequacy of her diet and answering her questions. Emphasize the importance of taking the prenatal vitamins prescribed for her. On subsequent visits review with the woman her diet and examine for adequacy or for any review of information needed. See Chapter 6 for nutritional requirements of pregnancy.

Monitor weight gain throughout pregnancy. There should be a steady increase in weight throughout pregnancy, for a total increase of 25 to 35 lb (11.5 to 16 kg). A sudden weight gain is often associated with fluid retention and may be a sign of developing preeclampsia. Monitor the hemoglobin and hematocrit at the 28-week checkup for any decreases and potential need for iron supplementation.

Dental Hygiene

A pregnant woman needs to continue regular dental checkups and practice daily dental hygiene. This includes at least twice-daily brushing, once-daily flossing, and a nutritious diet. Some women find their gums bleed easily during pregnancy and that a soft bristled toothbrush is less irritating to their gums. If pregnancy gingivitis is a problem, then regular dental checkups are necessary. Untreated gingivitis can damage the gums and result in bone and tooth loss.

Vomiting in association with morning sickness can weaken tooth enamel. Stomach acids in the vomitus can make the teeth more susceptible to injury from the toothbrush. To reduce the impact of this problem, instruct the woman to rinse with water after vomiting, followed by a fluoride rinse or sugarless chewing gum to help neutralize the stomach acid. She should avoid brushing her teeth for at least 1 hour after vomiting to decrease the risk of enamel loss.

Exercise

Exercise is healthy during pregnancy. A woman may generally maintain her normal exercise routine during pregnancy, as long as she does not become overheated or excessively fatigued. Some research indicates that women who exercise during pregnancy experience shorter labors, have fewer cesarean deliveries, and have fetuses that experience fewer episodes of fetal distress. Women who exercise demonstrate positive effects on self-esteem and a return to prepregnancy weight faster than sedentary women. Exercise is also recommended for women who report depressive symptoms. Box 7-6 outlines precautions to increase the safety of exercise for the pregnant woman.

It is recommended that a well-conditioned woman continue her normal pattern of exercise during pregnancy. If the woman is sedentary before pregnancy, she should not start a vigorous aerobic routine. In this situation, walking is the preferred exercise. There are some high-risk conditions, such as premature rupture of membranes, preeclampsia, vaginal bleeding, or incompetent cervix, in which exercise is contraindicated.

BOX 7-6 | **Precautions to Ensure a Safe Exercise Program for the Pregnant Woman**

The pregnant woman should avoid the following activities:
- Contact sports and any activities that can cause falls and even mild trauma to the abdomen, such as ice hockey, kickboxing, soccer, and basketball, gymnastics, horseback riding, downhill skiing, and vigorous racquet sports.
- Scuba diving, which puts the baby at increased risk for decompression sickness and may contribute to miscarriage, birth defects, poor fetal growth, and preterm labor.
- Exercising on the back after the first trimester. Also, avoid prolonged periods of motionless standing. Both can reduce blood flow to the uterus.
- Jerky, bouncing, or high-impact movements that may strain joints and cause injuries.
- High-intensity exercising at high altitudes (more than 6,000 ft) because it can lead to reduced amounts of oxygen reaching the baby.
- Overheating, especially in the first trimester. Drink plenty of fluids before, during, and after exercise. Wear layers of "breathable" clothing and do not exercise on hot, humid days.
- Bathing in hot tubs, saunas, and Jacuzzis.

General common sense guidelines include advising the woman to listen to her body. The woman can use the "talk test" to gauge exertion level; that is, she should not be too short of breath to carry on a conversation while exercising. If she is feeling fatigued, she should slow down or stop. She should not allow her heart rate to exceed 140 beats per minute. In the last trimester as the center of gravity changes, she should take extra care to avoid injury during exercise.

Hygiene

Perspiration and vaginal discharge increase during pregnancy, making personal hygiene a concern for some pregnant women. In general, tub baths or showers can continue throughout pregnancy. Inform the woman that she should bathe in warm, not hot, water. Extreme temperature elevations associated with hot showers, baths, saunas, hot tubs, and fever are dangerous to the developing fetus.

She should take care, particularly in the third trimester, when getting in and out of the tub or shower. Fainting can occur, particularly if the water is too hot. Balancing can become problematic because the center of gravity changes. Handrails in the shower or tub are ideal. Rubber bath mats are also helpful.

Let the woman know that she should avoid douching during pregnancy. This practice increases the risk for bacterial infection. Gentle cleansing of the genital area with warm water and soap is sufficient to control discomfort from increased vaginal secretions.

Breast Care

A pregnant woman should wear a bra that fits well and supports the breasts. She should use only clean water to wash the nipples. Soap dries the nipples and can lead to cracking and potential infection.

Some women wish to condition their nipples for breast-feeding. Exposing the nipples to air and sunlight for a portion of each day is helpful. Manually stimulating the nipples by rolling them between the fingers or oral stimulation of the nipple by the woman's partner, as a part of sexual expression, are additional ways to toughen the nipples. These practices are acceptable as long as there is no history of preterm labor because nipple stimulation can stimulate labor.

Clothing

Clothing should be loose and comfortable. The woman should not wear garments that constrict the waist or legs. If finances are of concern, the woman might try borrowing clothes from a friend or relative rather than investing in expensive maternity clothes. She might also buy used maternity clothes. High heels exacerbate backache and can be a safety hazard for the pregnant woman who has problems with balance. Shoes should fit comfortably.

Sexual Activity

Many couples are fearful that sexual activity during pregnancy might hurt the fetus. Unless there is a history of preterm labor, vaginal bleeding, ruptured membranes, or other medical contraindication, the woman and her partner can safely continue intercourse and other sexual activities throughout pregnancy. Many factors influence the woman's desire for sexual activity. During the first trimester, she may feel nauseous and tired, so her interest in sex might be low. During the second trimester, she often feels better and may have a heightened interest in sex. The increased blood flow to the pelvic area can intensify the sexual experience for the pregnant woman. Some women experience orgasm for the first time during pregnancy. During the third trimester, fatigue may reduce her desire or she might fear hurting the fetus.

The partner's sexual desire is also dependent on several interrelated factors. Some find their partner's pregnant body sexually appealing and desirable. Others may have trouble adjusting to their partner's changing body shape. Some are afraid of hurting their partner or the unborn child during intercourse. It may be helpful to have a tactful discussion regarding sexual concerns with the woman and the partner. During the third trimester a side-lying or woman-superior position might be easier. Vaginal penetration is less deep with the partner facing the woman's back. This position might be more comfortable for the woman.

Sometimes the woman might be content with kissing, cuddling, and caressing as forms of sexual expression. The essential ingredient is ongoing respectful communication between the partners regarding their sexual needs and desires.

A Word of Caution!

If the couple practices anal intercourse, they should not proceed to vaginal intercourse after engaging in anal intercourse. Doing so could introduce the bacteria into the vagina that could cause an ascending infection.

Employment

How long a woman can remain safely employed during pregnancy depends on several factors. In general, a woman with a low-risk pregnancy can continue working until she goes into labor unless there are specific hazards associated with her job. Research demonstrates that women in physically demanding jobs, such as working in the fields (day laborers), experience a higher incidence of low–birth-weight infants, preterm delivery, and hypertension during pregnancy. A woman who is required to stand for long periods as part of her job also is at increased risk for preterm delivery.

When a woman chooses to work during pregnancy, it is most helpful if she can take frequent rest periods. If she must stand for prolonged periods, suggest that she shift her weight back and forth, and that she take frequent breaks to walk around and to sit with her feet elevated. She should avoid excessive fatigue.

Exposure to teratogens, substances capable of causing birth defects, is always a concern when a woman works during pregnancy. Environmental hazards that might put the pregnant woman at risk in the workplace include exposure to chemicals, metals, solvents, pharmaceutical agents, radiation, extreme heat, second-hand smoke, and infection. The woman should investigate the type of chemicals or other substances to which she is exposed during the course of her work and then work with her employer to limit exposure to harmful substances.

Travel

Travel is generally not limited during the first trimester. The woman can travel safely in the second and third trimesters with careful planning. One concern when traveling long distances is the chance that labor will occur while the woman is away. It is advisable for the woman to carry copies of her prenatal records with her when she travels. This practice will increase the odds that she will receive appropriate care if she must seek healthcare away from home.

When traveling by car, encourage the woman to make frequent stops at least every 2 hours so that she can empty her bladder and walk about. Sitting for prolonged periods in one position can predispose the woman to blood clot formation. She should not decrease fluid intake to avoid having to stop to void. Insufficient fluids can lead to dehydration and increase the risk for clot formation, constipation, and hemorrhoids. There is no increased risk with air travel, other than the risk of developing complications in an area remote from the help needed.

The greatest risk to the fetus during an automobile crash is death of the mother. Therefore, all pregnant women should use three-point seat belt restraints when traveling in the car (Fig. 7-7). Instruct the woman to apply the lap belt snugly and comfortably. When driving, she should move the seat as far back as possible from the steering wheel. The airbag should be engaged with the steering wheel tilted so that the airbag releases toward the breastbone versus the abdomen or the head.

Medications and Herbal Remedies

The general principle regarding medication use during pregnancy is that almost all medications cross the placenta and can potentially affect the fetus. The woman should not take any medication, including over-the-counter medications and herbal remedies, during pregnancy without the express approval of the health care provider. Before she takes any medication, the health care provider will make a careful appraisal of risk versus

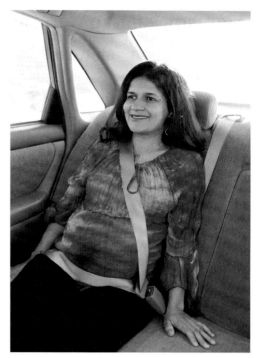

FIGURE 7-7 Proper application of a seat belt during pregnancy.

benefit. Treatment, including medications, for certain diseases and conditions must continue during pregnancy, including epilepsy, asthma, diabetes, and depression (see Chapter 16).

The problem with most medications is that they cross the placenta, but their potential effects on the fetus or pregnancy are not always known. Because of ethical concerns, controlled trials of medication use during human pregnancy are usually not possible. The little that is known about medication effects during pregnancy comes from animal trials and from experience over the years in treating chronic maternal conditions. The problem with animal studies is that there is no guarantee that human pregnancies or fetuses will respond in the same way as the animal that is being studied responds. Box 7-7 describes the Food and Drug Administration's five pregnancy categories for medications.

Many women use herbal remedies. Some remedies are culturally determined, passed from mother to daughter from generation to generation. Some women believe that herbs and alternative therapies are safer than medications. Some studies are verifying the health benefits of certain herbs. However, there are certain herbs that are contraindicated in pregnancy, so it is important for the pregnant woman to report all herbal and over-the-counter remedies she uses. Enhance communication by asking about herbal use in a nonthreatening way.

TIPS FOR REINFORCING FAMILY TEACHING

Major Components of Prenatal Self-Care

- Avoid alcohol. Alcohol harms the fetus; no amount of alcohol is safe during pregnancy.
- Avoid smoking. Smoking harms the fetus. It can lead to lower birth weight and increase the incidence of preterm labor.
- Eat a healthy, well-balanced diet. If you consume a variety of nutritious foods daily, you will likely get the nutrients you need.
- Consume approximately 300 calories more per day than before pregnancy, for example, a peanut butter sandwich that is two slices of bread and two tablespoons of peanut butter is approximately 300 calories.
- Take an extra 400 μg of folic acid per day. If the doctor ordered prenatal vitamins, the recommended dose will be met.
- Avoid dieting during pregnancy. A woman with a normal body mass index should gain 25 to 35 lb (11.5 to 16 kg) during the pregnancy.

- Continue to exercise during pregnancy. However, do not exercise to the point of exhaustion or start a grueling new workout that you were not doing before pregnancy.
- Avoid handling raw meat and cat litter. Wear gloves when gardening to prevent contracting toxoplasmosis from animal droppings, an infection that is very harmful to the baby.
- Handle cold cuts carefully. Heat thin slices of meat in the microwave until steaming hot. Wash hands with hot soapy water after handling deli meats to avoid listeriosis, a bacterial infection that is harmful to the baby.
- Avoid douching. Douching during pregnancy increases the risk for bacterial infection.
- Avoid taking any medication (other than acetaminophen) or over-the-counter herbal remedy unless your health care provider has approved it.

TEST YOURSELF

✔ List three suggestions for reducing nausea in early pregnancy.

✔ Name three actions the pregnant woman can take to reduce constipation.

✔ Why should the pregnant woman avoid hot showers or baths?

SUBSTANCE USE AND ABUSE DURING PREGNANCY

The woman is often more receptive to making lifestyle changes during pregnancy than at other times in her life. She may view this as "wanting what is best for the baby" or may see it as a protective reaction "I don't want the baby to be harmed by my substance use." It is important for the nurse to be nonjudgmental when reinforcing teaching related to substance use and abuse. Some women may feel guilty for their substance abuse. The nurse should use therapeutic communication and listening to the woman when she expresses her feelings.

Substance use is a term that simply refers to use of a substance, whereas the term substance abuse specifically indicates that a person has a problem with the use of the substance. Although many substances have the potential for abuse, this section covers caffeine, tobacco, alcohol, and recreational drug use. Chapter 20 provides more in-depth coverage of the fetal/neonatal effects of alcohol and recreational drug use during pregnancy.

Caffeine

There is controversy and uncertainty regarding the role of caffeine use during pregnancy. Current recommendations are that the pregnant woman may safely consume coffee and caffeine in moderation. The March of Dimes

---

BOX 7-7 **FDA Pregnancy Categories of Medications**

The Food and Drug Administration (FDA) has delineated five categories for medication use during pregnancy. In any case, the woman should not take any medication during pregnancy unless there is a clear benefit for its use.

Category A: Adequate studies in pregnant women have not demonstrated a risk to the fetus in the first trimester of pregnancy, and there is no evidence of risk in later trimesters.

Category B: Animal studies have not demonstrated a risk to the fetus, but there are no adequate studies in pregnant women. Animal studies have shown an adverse effect, but adequate studies in pregnant women have not demonstrated a risk to the fetus during the first trimester of pregnancy, and there is no evidence of risk in later trimesters.

Category C: Animal studies have shown an adverse effect on the fetus, but there are no adequate studies in humans; the benefits from the use of the drug in pregnant women may be acceptable, despite its potential risks. There are no animal reproduction studies and no adequate studies in humans.

Category D: There is evidence of human fetal risk, but the potential benefits from the use of the drug in pregnant women may be acceptable despite its potential risk.

Category X: Studies in animals or humans demonstrate fetal abnormalities or adverse reaction; reports indicate evidence of fetal risk. The risk of use in a pregnant woman clearly outweighs any possible benefit.

(2020a) recommends a pregnant woman limit her caffeine to 200 mg per day which is about the amount found in 12 oz of coffee.

Tobacco

Smoking is contraindicated during pregnancy. Smoking increases the risk for low birth weight; preterm delivery; early pregnancy loss; stillbirths; sudden infant death syndrome; birth defects, such as cleft lip and palate; and neonatal respiratory disorders, including asthma. Smoking exposes the fetus to carbon monoxide and nicotine while decreasing the amount of available oxygen, leading to fetal hypoxia. It also affects the placenta, causing it to age sooner than normal, resulting in reduced blood flow to the fetus that then results in hypoxia and stunted fetal growth. Although aids to stop smoking, such as nicotine gum and the new drug varenicline, are pregnancy Category C drugs and the transdermal patch is in pregnancy Category D (Box 7-7), the health care provider will weigh the risk of injury caused by smoking against the risk of harm from these drugs.

Alcohol

There is no safe amount of alcohol consumption during pregnancy. The rate of women who reported drinking during pregnancy, including amounts from occasional to binge drinking, increased from the 2015 to 2017 study as compared to the studies done prior to that time period (Chang, 2020a). A woman should not drink any alcoholic beverages during pregnancy because alcohol is a known teratogen. For years, the risk of fetal alcohol spectrum disorder has been linked to the use of large amounts of alcohol during pregnancy. Characteristics of fetal alcohol spectrum disorder include **microcephaly** (a very small cranium), facial deformities, growth restriction, and cognitive deficits. Although smaller amounts of alcohol may not lead to a severe case of fetal alcohol spectrum disorder, subtle features of the syndrome might present to include milder forms of cognitive deficits and learning disabilities. See the section Newborn of a Mother with Substance Abuse in Chapter 20.

Marijuana

There are conflicting data about the effects of marijuana on pregnancy. Some studies suggest that marijuana use in pregnancy may slow fetal growth and possibly increase the risk for premature delivery and stillbirth. Infants born to women who smoke marijuana during pregnancy tend to have high-pitched cries, tremors, and low birth weight (March of Dimes, 2020b). Researchers continue to study the long-term effects of marijuana use in pregnancy on the child.

Cocaine

Cocaine is not reported as frequently as cigarettes or alcohol during pregnancy, but it has many negative effects on pregnancy. Pregnancy increases the cardiovascular dysfunction associated with cocaine use. Cocaine causes vasoconstriction and hypertension which can cause placental damage (Chang, 2020b). Cocaine use is associated with a higher rate of early pregnancy loss and premature labor. Infants born to women who use cocaine during pregnancy tend to be small and have a higher incidence of low birth weight and preterm birth. Cocaine use during pregnancy can cause the placenta to pull away from the uterine wall prematurely (placental abruption), leading to fetal and maternal hemorrhage. Infants exposed to cocaine in utero exhibit withdrawal behaviors after birth and must receive special treatment for the withdrawal (see Chapter 20).

HELPING THE WOMAN PREPARE FOR LABOR, BIRTH, AND PARENTHOOD

Being prepared for labor, birth, and parenting boosts the woman's confidence and increases her use of positive coping measures. Many women search the internet and read books that address the birth and parenting experience. Lists of resources available in the local community should be provided to the woman. Available resources may include classes on a variety of topics offered by private practices, not-for-profit educational organizations, or by hospitals.

Packing for the Hospital or Birth Center

As the woman prepares for the birth of her baby, she may begin to gather items she will need at the hospital or birth center. She should pack articles she will want while she is in labor, items for her postpartum stay, and for the infant to wear at discharge (Box 7-8). Many childbirth classes cover this information as well.

Labor and Birth Preparation

It is important for the woman to feel comfortable communicating her desires regarding labor and birth. Some women feel very strongly about having natural childbirth or breast-feeding. Others want an epidural as soon as possible after they go into labor. These are only a few examples

---

BOX 7-8 **What to Pack for the Hospital or Birth Center**

Labor Items
- Lotion for massage or effleurage
- Sour lollipops (counteracts nausea, moistens mouth, gives energy)
- Lip balm
- Socks
- Tennis ball, ice pack, back massager
- Picture or object for focal point
- Phone and charging cord
- Camera (check with hospital regarding policies on videoing during delivery)
- Relaxation music
- Contact lens case and solutions (if used)
- Hair brush and hair band to get hair off neck
- Hand fan

Postpartum Items
- Nursing gowns
- Robe and slippers/nonskid socks
- Nursing bras
- Toiletry articles (e.g., toothpaste, toothbrush, hairbrush, deodorant)
- Cosmetics
- Pen and paper to write down questions on
- Loose-fitting clothes for the trip home
- Clothes for newborn to wear home
- Baby blankets appropriate for weather
- Car seat

of expectations a woman may have. Encourage the client to write down her questions and expectations and to communicate these to the health care provider. Some women develop written birth plans (Box 7-9) to communicate their desires. These can be helpful to the woman and the provider. If the woman communicates her expectations early in the pregnancy, there is time for her to find another health care provider if her current provider cannot or is unwilling to meet her labor and birth expectations.

Choosing the Support Person

The expectant mother may have choices involving her labor support team if she delivers in the hospital or birth center. Some hospitals limit her to one or two persons for labor support. Other women may have the option of having more support persons for labor. The woman may choose the father of the baby as her main support person. In other situations, the primary support person might be her mother, sister, other family member, or friend. The woman's culture plays a large role in who will support her during labor and who will be in attendance during the actual birth.

The woman may choose to have a **doula** with her as a nonmedical support person. The woman may contract with a doula during her pregnancy to provide support for labor and birth and help with establishing breast-feeding. The doula's role may include assisting the woman and her partner in preparing for and carrying out their plans for the birth; providing emotional support and physical comfort measures; and advocate for the woman get the information she needs to make good decisions. A doula can also provide support for the postpartum period.

Childbirth Education Classes

Since the 1970s, many parents have begun to prepare for labor and childbirth by attending prenatal classes. Today, childbirth educators offer classes in private practices, not-for-profit organizations, and hospitals. Some classes adhere to the philosophy of one method of childbirth (Box 7-10), whereas others combine philosophies of two or more methods of childbirth. Still, others tend to focus on the medical procedures and routines that she can expect upon admission to the hospital. Some programs combine information about birth, baby care, and breast-feeding in one series of classes. Others offer separate classes for which the woman and her partner can register. Box 7-11 lists common topics included in childbirth education classes.

BOX 7-9 | **Topics for Birth Plan**

The following are items that are often covered in birth plans. Some birth plans contain all of this information, or more, while others may be more simplified. Birth plans often are phrased as "I would prefer to avoid…" or "I would like to have…."

Identifying Information
- Client's name and due date
- Name of obstetrician/midwife and newborn's pediatrician/health care provider
- Name of hospital/birth center

Labor Support
- Person(s) to be present during labor and delivery including name and relationship

Laboring
- Treatments such as enemas, shaving of pubic hair
- Movement and positions during labor, specialty items such as birthing ball
- Environment during labor such as music and lighting
- Hydrotherapy (bath, Jacuzzi, shower)

Use of Fetal Monitors

Stimulation of Labor
- Artificial rupture of membranes
- Position

Medication and Anesthesia (Preferred or to Avoid)

C-Section
- Who to be present
- Type of anesthesia preferred (unless emergency)

Episiotomy

Pushing
- Position
- Pushing technique (see the section Effective Pushing Techniques in Chapter 10)

After Delivery
- Who to cut cord
- When mother to hold newborn
- Where newborn to be evaluated
- Skin to skin contact
- Delay of newborn medications (eye ointment and vitamin K) for a few hours after birth
- Disposal of placenta and umbilical cord blood

Newborn Feeding/Care
- Type of feeding (breast or bottle) and desired time of first breast-feeding
- Supplements
- Pacifier
- First newborn bath

Photo/Video

BOX 7-10 Methods of Prepared Childbirth

Dick-Read Method

In *Childbirth without Fear* (1942), Dr. Grantly Dick-Read described a fear-tension-pain cycle with the laboring woman tensing in fear at the beginning of each contraction resulting in an increase of pain which reinforces the belief that labor is painful causing the woman to tense prior to the next contraction, continuing the cycle. He believed that relaxation and knowledge about the birth process were important to pain reduction during labor.

Lamaze Method

In 1951 Dr. Fernand Lamaze introduced a childbirth method where the woman practices a variety of relaxation techniques, including breathing and attention focusing, during pregnancy. These help her to relax during the birth process and reduce her pain level by blocking the pain stimulus. Additionally, the woman's partner is taught to support the laboring woman by offering encouragement, assisting with attention focusing and comfort measures including position changes and massage.

Bradley Method

In 1947 Dr. Robert Bradley described a childbirth method with six important components: quiet, darkness and solitude, comfort measures, abdominal breathing, relaxation, and closed eyes with the appearance of sleep. He also felt that having the father present during labor and able to support the woman was important. His work was instrumental in having the father present in the labor room.

Leboyer Method

In *Birth without Violence* (1974), Dr. Frederick Leboyer recommended decreased stimulation for the newborn during the birthing process and immediately thereafter. This includes turning down the lights, limiting noise and loud talking, warmth, gentleness, and not separating the woman and her newborn.

Water Birth Method

Soaking in a warm bath enhances relaxation and reduces weight bearing and sensory stimulation. This results in a reduction of stress-related hormones and an increase in endorphin secretion. Within 10 to 15 minutes of entering the water there is a decrease in maternal blood pressure. Soaking in water increases the elasticity of the perineum, which reduces the frequency and severity of perineal tearing during birth.

Hypnobirthing

Hypnobirthing incorporates the beliefs that the woman who is prepared physically, mentally, and spiritually can experience the joy of birth. Forms of hypnosis, relaxation, visualizations, and affirmations are integral parts of the method.

BOX 7-11 Common Topics Included in Childbirth Education Classes

- Psychological and emotional aspects of pregnancy
- Anatomic and physiologic changes involved in pregnancy and childbirth
- Fetal development
- Communication with obstetrician/pediatrician/health care provider
- The normal, natural process of labor and birth
- Stages/phases of labor: physical and emotional changes of each
- Partner's role in providing support for each stage/phase of labor
- Comfort measures for labor
- Medication and anesthesia options for labor and birth
- Possible complications of labor
- Possible medical procedures including indications for vaginal examinations, routine laboratory work, fetal monitoring, artificial rupture of membranes, IVs, and assisted birth techniques (see Chapter 11).
- Cesarean birth
- What to pack for the hospital
- Breast-feeding
- Physical and emotional aspects of the postpartum period
- Sibling preparation and possible reactions

of pregnancy, are included, as well as exercises that allow the woman to be able to utilize beneficial labor positions comfortably.

Baby Care Classes

These classes are offered to the parents-to-be. Basics such as infant bathing, diapering, and feeding are covered. Information on newborn sleeping and waking patterns and infant comforting and rousing techniques are also provided. Safety information such as handling of the baby, car seat safety, and safety proofing the home is included. Routine well-baby check and immunization schedules are covered. Signs of illness and guidelines for when to call the health care provider are also an important part of this class.

Breast-feeding Classes

An international board-certified lactation consultant often teaches breast-feeding classes; however, certified breast-feeding educators or specially trained nurses may also conduct these classes. Usually offered in the last trimester of pregnancy, this class educates the woman on the benefits of breast-feeding, signs of good latch and position, and establishing a good milk supply. Selection of and using a breast pump and milk storage are topics of interest in this class, as many women plan to return to work and continue to nurse their infants. Attendance of this class by the woman's partner increases their support and ability to provide assistance, thus contributing to the success of breast-feeding. The instructor usually provides contact information for lactation support resources in the community.

Pregnancy Exercise Classes

The purpose of these classes is to enhance endurance as well as to strengthen the arms, legs, pelvic floor, back, and abdomen. A certified childbirth educator or a nurse usually offers these classes. Some fitness centers also offer pre- and postnatal exercise classes. Basic pregnancy exercises, such as the pelvic tilt, Kegel, tailor sit, tailor stretch, and stretches as comfort measures to combat some of the discomforts

Siblings Classes

Many hospitals provide siblings classes for children who are soon-to-be big brothers and big sisters. Class goals include preparing children for the time of separation from the mother while she is in the hospital and helping the children accept the changes resulting from the arrival of the new baby in the family. The instructor demonstrates basic infant safety, with emphasis on how the child can be included or help with the tasks related to baby care. The class usually includes tours of the maternal–child areas of the hospital. The instructor shares suggestions with parents on ways to help the older siblings accept changes in the household after the baby arrives.

In hospitals that allow siblings to attend births, siblings' classes may include information on how to help prepare the older child for being present at delivery. Most hospitals require an adult to be responsible for children at birth, in addition to the partner who is caring for the laboring woman.

TEST YOURSELF

✔ Identify at least five ways smoking adversely affects the fetus.

✔ A pregnant woman asks you "How much alcohol is it OK for a pregnant woman to drink?" How would you respond to her question?

✔ Describe the role of a doula.

Nursing Process and Care Plan
for the Woman Seeking Prenatal Care

Don't Make Unfounded Assumptions!

Do not assume that just because this is not the woman's first baby, or because she is educated, or even that she is a nurse, that she has the information she needs to maintain a healthy pregnancy. Evaluate her knowledge level by asking her direct questions and answering any questions she may have.

Nurses are in a unique position to influence behaviors of the pregnant woman and to increase the probability she and her baby will stay healthy. Through consistent use of the nursing process, most problems can be identified in order to intervene or assist the health care provider in intervening, and supporting the woman. Providing the pregnant woman with information and the safety of the woman and the fetus remains the primary nursing care focus throughout the pregnancy.

Assessment (Data Collection)

Ongoing data collection is an essential component of prenatal visits. During the first prenatal visit, pay close attention to cues the woman may give regarding her feelings toward the pregnancy. Ambivalence is normal. The woman may express feelings of doubt about the pregnancy or her ability to be a good parent. These are normal reactions when a woman first finds out she is pregnant. Reassure her that her responses are normal. Withdrawal or consistently negative remarks are warning signs. Report these observations to the RN or health care provider.

If you administer the initial questionnaire, show the woman all the pages and assist her in completing it if necessary. Review the document carefully when she is done to ensure completeness. Look for answers that indicate the need for further evaluation. Alert the RN or the health care provider of possible risk factors identified in the history.

Observe for signs of nervousness and anxiety. The woman may express her nervousness by being restless or tense or by being quiet and withdrawn. Be attuned to signals she is giving regarding her comfort level. At every visit, inquire carefully regarding current medications, food supplements, and over-the-counter remedies she is using.

Note if the woman has been experiencing nausea and vomiting. Pay close attention to signs that might indicate poor nutritional status. Weight is an obvious clue. If the woman is overweight or underweight, she will need special assistance with nutritional concerns throughout the pregnancy. Other warning signs of poor nutritional status include dull, brittle hair; poor skin turgor; poor condition of skin and nails; obesity; emaciation; or a low hemoglobin level. Ask the woman to write down a typical day's food consumption pattern, and then determine if her diet is adequate for her nutritional needs.

Determine her education level and knowledge of pregnancy and prenatal care. If she is highly knowledgeable, she may ask high-level questions that indicate an understanding of basic issues. Conversely, she may ask basic questions, or no questions at all, which could indicate a knowledge deficit.

Cultural Snapshot

Just because the woman does not ask questions may not mean that she does not have questions. In some cultures, it may be improper to ask questions to the health care provider, as it may seem that the client is questioning the provider's authority. Also, if the woman's first language is not English, you may want an interpreter present to assure that the woman is getting the information in her native language to avoid gaps in the information she is given and to answer her questions completely.

During subsequent visits, you may assist with observing for signs of fetal well-being. These observations include obtaining fetal heart tones with an ultrasonic Doppler device (Fig. 7-8) beginning in week 10, and asking questions about fetal movements after quickening occurs (weeks 16 to 20). Pay close attention to the blood pressure and urine protein levels. Monitor for danger signs of pregnancy (Box 7-3).

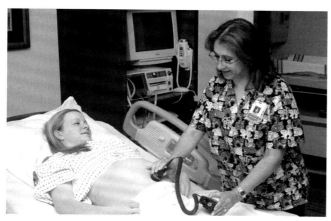

FIGURE 7-8 The nurse listens to fetal heart tones with a Doppler device.

Nursing Care Focus

When determining the focus of nursing care for the pregnant woman seeking prenatal care, consideration should be given to the woman's knowledge related to pregnancy and any previous experience she has had with pregnancy. It is also important to remember that the woman may be anxious about the pregnancy, even if this is not her first pregnancy. Regardless of her prior experiences, prenatal fetal and maternal assessments will still be performed. Many women experience similar discomforts during pregnancy and the woman often seeks information on the changes occurring to her body during this time.

Outcome Identification and Planning

Maintaining the health of mother and fetus is the primary goal of nursing care during the prenatal period. Other important goals during this time frame are to relieve anxiety and also to ensure that the woman has the information she needs to adequately care for herself during pregnancy and the information needed to prepare for delivery.

Nursing Care Focus

- Injury risk related to complications of pregnancy

Goal

- The woman and fetus will remain free from injury.

Implementations for Injury Risk Related to Complications of Pregnancy

Monitor the pregnant woman at every visit for warning signs that might indicate problems with the pregnancy (Box 7-3). If she reports experiencing any of the warning signs, notify the RN or health care provider immediately. If at any time during the pregnancy an elevated blood pressure is noted, report this finding immediately to the RN or health care provider, particularly if it is accompanied by elevated urine protein levels, headache, epigastric pain, or blurred vision.

Inquire about fetal movement. Reinforce teaching related to self-care and injury prevention related to fall prevention, seat belt use, avoidance of substances that can cause harm to the fetus, and not taking medications or herbal supplements prescribed or approved by the health care provider.

Evaluation of Goal/Desired Outcome

- The woman does not experience injury from falls.
- The woman avoids substances that can harm the fetus.
- The woman immediately reports any symptoms that suggest a pregnancy complication might be occurring.

Nursing Care Focus

- Acute anxiety related to prenatal procedures

Goal

- The woman will display decreased signs and symptoms of anxiety.
- The woman will verbalize her concerns related to the pregnancy.

Implementations for Acute Anxiety Related to Prenatal Procedures

Monitor for signs and symptoms of anxiety the woman may be exhibiting and the level of her anxiety. Note if her anxiety level increases. Encourage the woman to verbalize her concerns and fears. It is important to develop a trusting relationship with the woman. The more confidence she has in the nurse, the more likely she will be willing to describe her feelings. Use active listening and encourage positive coping behaviors.

Escort the woman to the examination room. Explain normal procedure and describe what she can expect during the visit. When the woman knows what to expect, she will be much less anxious. Maintain a calm, confident demeanor while giving care.

Be mindful of the woman's perspective. Routine procedures and tests are not "normal" for the woman and can increase anxiety. Reassure her that these feelings are normal. Protect the woman's privacy during all procedures, especially invasive examinations. Anticipate concern when fetal testing is required. Solicit questions and correct misconceptions the woman may have. Provide information concerning the treatment plan.

Evaluation of Goal/Desired Outcome

- The woman reports a decrease in her anxiety and exhibits a decrease in symptoms of anxiety.
- The woman discusses her pregnancy concerns to the nurse or health care provider.

Nursing Care Focus

- Impaired comfort related to physiologic changes of pregnancy

Goal

- The woman will describe measures to increase her comfort during pregnancy.

Implementations for Impaired Comfort Related to Physiologic Changes of Pregnancy

Help the woman to anticipate the pregnancy changes that may cause her discomfort by providing literature that she can review at her own pace. Provide her with a list of trusted websites that supplement this information. Let her know that there can be misinformation from well-meaning individuals and that she should contact the health care provider's office before doing any self-treatment. Reinforce teaching that has been provided. Offer nursing interventions to help relieve the discomforts she verbalizes.

Evaluation of Goal/Desired Outcome

- The woman identifies common discomforts of pregnancy.
- The woman describes measures to deal with the common discomforts of pregnancy.

Nursing Care Focus

- Knowledge deficiency related to self-care activities during pregnancy

Goal

- The woman feels confident in her ability to care for herself throughout pregnancy.

Implementations for Knowledge Deficiency Related to Self-Care Activities During Pregnancy

The woman is usually too distracted during the first visit to absorb and retain much information. Keep information sessions brief and give her printed materials to read at home. A handout with a list of resources, such as books and websites, is helpful to give to the woman at the end of the visit. Tailor information topics to the individual needs of the woman during subsequent visits. Tips for Reinforcing Family Teaching: Major Components of Prenatal Self-Care highlights key topics to discuss with the pregnant woman during the course of prenatal care.

Reinforce information related to self-care during pregnancy at each prenatal visit. Information that should be reviewed includes the woman's diet, exercise, and medications or herbal remedies that the woman is taking.

Evaluation of Goal/Desired Outcome

- The woman verbalizes an understanding of how to modify her lifestyle to accommodate the changing needs of pregnancy.
- The woman describes self-care measures to perform during pregnancy.

Recall **Stefani Mueller** from the start of the chapter. She was worried about this pregnancy after a previous miscarriage. Since she is worried about the pregnancy, what signs would you instruct her to report? What would be appropriate nursing interventions for Stefani?

KEY POINTS

- The goal of early prenatal care is to increase the chances that the fetus and the mother will remain healthy throughout pregnancy and delivery.
- The main goals of the first prenatal visit are to confirm a diagnosis of pregnancy, identify risk factors, determine the due date, and provide education regarding self-care and danger signs of pregnancy.
- The history at the first prenatal visit includes chief complaint, reproductive history, medical–surgical history, family history, and social history. The reproductive history includes the obstetric history, which looks at previous pregnancies and their outcomes. Determining the gravida and parity of the woman is an important part of the obstetric history. The parity is usually further subdivided into the number of term deliveries, preterm deliveries, abortions (spontaneous or induced), and living children.
- A complete physical examination will be done during the first visit to include a breast examination, a speculum examination with a Pap test, and a bimanual examination of the uterus.
- Laboratory assessments done in conjunction with the first prenatal visit include a complete blood count, blood type and screen, hepatitis B, HIV, syphilis, gonorrhea, chlamydia, rubella titer, and a urine culture.
- To calculate the estimated due date by Naegele rule, add 7 days from the first day of the last menstrual period, then subtract 3 months to obtain the due date.
- Other methods for estimating the due date use uterus size, landmarks in the pregnancy, and ultrasonographic measurement of fetal structures.
- Any abnormal part of the history, physical examination, or laboratory work can put the pregnancy at risk. A history of difficult pregnancy or pregnancy complication puts subsequent pregnancies at risk.

- Subsequent prenatal visits are shorter and focus on the weight, blood pressure, urine protein and glucose measurements, fetal heart rate, and fundal height. Inquiry is made regarding the danger signals of pregnancy at each prenatal visit.

- Fetal movement (kick) count is done by the woman at the same time each day. It should not take longer than 2 hours to get to 10 counts. If it does, the woman should call her health care provider.

- Ultrasonography uses sound waves to visualize fetal and maternal structures. Ultrasound is done to determine or confirm gestational age, observe the fetus, and diagnose fetal and placental abnormalities.

- Maternal serum alpha-fetoprotein testing is recommended for every pregnant woman between 16 and 18 weeks. Elevated levels are associated with various defects, in particular fetal spinal defects.

- Triple-marker screening involves a blood test to determine levels of three hormones—maternal serum alpha-fetoprotein, hCG, and unconjugated estriol. This test screens for chromosomal abnormalities, but an abnormal result does not mean that something is definitely wrong with the fetus. Further tests are needed.

- Amniocentesis involves aspiration of amniotic fluid through the abdominal wall to obtain fetal cells for chromosomal analysis. Amniocentesis is usually done between 15 and 20 weeks' gestation.

- Chorionic villus sampling is similar to amniocentesis, but it can be performed earlier, usually at 10 to 12 weeks. Placental tissue is aspirated through a catheter that is introduced through the cervix or it can be done transabdominally.

- Percutaneous umbilical blood sampling (PUBS) is similar to an amniocentesis; however, fetal blood is withdrawn from the umbilical cord for testing, rather than amniotic fluid.

- The nonstress test (NST) measures fetal heart rate acceleration patterns. A reactive NST is reassuring.

- The contraction stress test (CST) is done to determine how well the fetus can handle the stress of contractions. Three contractions are needed within a 20-minutes period. These can occur spontaneously or they may be induced by nipple stimulation or oxytocin infusion. A "negative" (desired) result occurs when there are no decelerations during the test. A negative CST is reassuring. If decelerations occur with one half or more of the contractions, this is a "positive" (undesirable) result. A positive CST indicates probable hypoxia or fetal asphyxia.

- The biophysical profile combines the NST and several ultrasound measures, breathing, movements, tone, and amniotic fluid volume to predict fetal well-being.

- Symptoms that indicate a potential threat to the mother or fetus must be reported immediately and include an elevated blood pressure, sudden weight gain, epigastric pain, vaginal bleeding, decreased fetal movement, or signs of preterm labor.

- Providing the pregnant woman with information on relieving common discomforts of pregnancy, self-care during pregnancy, and preparation for labor and delivery is a major nursing intervention during the prenatal period.

INTERNET RESOURCES

Pregnancy
www.marchofdimes.com
http://www.childbirthconnection.org/healthy-pregnancy/your-body-throughout-pregnancy.html

Prenatal Care
https://medlineplus.gov/prenatalcare.html

Childbirth Education
www.icea.org

Childbirth
www.lamaze.org

Doulas
http://dona.org

NCLEX-STYLE REVIEW QUESTIONS

1. A woman reports that her LMP occurred on January 10, 2018. Using Naegele rule, what is her due date?
   a. October 17, 2018
   b. October 17, 2019
   c. September 7, 2018
   d. September 7, 2019

2. A woman presents to the clinic in the first trimester of pregnancy. She has three children living at home. One of them was born prematurely at 34 weeks. The other two were full term at birth. She has a history of one miscarriage. How do you record her obstetric history on the chart using GTPAL format?
   a. G3 T2 P1 A1 L3
   b. G4 T3 P0 A1 L3
   c. G4 T2 P1 A1 L3
   d. G5 T2 P1 A1 L3

3. A woman who is 28 weeks' pregnant presents to the clinic for her scheduled prenatal visit. The nurse-midwife measures her fundal height at 32 cm. What action does the nurse expect the midwife to take regarding this finding?
   a. The midwife will order a multiple-marker screening test.
   b. The midwife will order a sonogram to confirm dates.
   c. The midwife will schedule more frequent prenatal visits to monitor the pregnancy closely.
   d. The midwife will take no action. This is a normal finding for a pregnancy at 28 weeks' gestation.

4. A G1 at 20 weeks' gestation is at the clinic for a prenatal visit. She tells the nurse that she has been reading about "group B strep disease" on the internet. She asks when she can expect to be checked for the bacteria. How does the nurse best reply?
   a. "I'm glad that you asked. You will be getting the culture done today."
   b. "The obstetrician normally cultures for group B strep after 35 weeks and before delivery."
   c. "You are only checked for group B strep if you have risk factors for the infection."
   d. "You were checked during your first prenatal visit. Let me get those results for you."

5. Results of an early chorionic villus sampling test show that a woman's baby has severe chromosomal abnormalities. When the obstetrician explains the findings to her, she becomes tearful. She shares with the nurse that it is against her religious beliefs to have an abortion. How would the nurse best respond to her?
   a. "Abortion is really the best thing for the baby. He has no chance of a normal life."
   b. "I agree with you. It is against my religious beliefs, too."
   c. "It is dangerous to carry a fetus with chromosomal abnormalities to term. You really should consider an abortion to protect your health."
   d. "You don't have to decide what to do today. Take some time to talk this over with your family. I will support whatever decision you make."

6. Which of the following increase the probability of the woman having a small infant at birth? Select all that apply.
   a. Twin pregnancy
   b. Maternal smoking during pregnancy
   c. Maternal gestational diabetes during pregnancy
   d. Postterm birth
   e. Maternal cocaine use during pregnancy

STUDY ACTIVITIES

1. Do an internet search on "genetic counseling." Identify three genetic counselors in your area to which a pregnant woman could be referred.

2. Using the following table, fill in key points for each topic regarding self-care during pregnancy. Note any special precautions for that topic that would be important to emphasize to the pregnant woman.

Topic	Key Points	Special Precautions
Nutrition		
Dental hygiene		
Exercise		
Hygiene		
Breast care		
Clothing		
Sexual activity		
Employment		
Travel		
Medication use		

3. Develop a list of tips that can be used for pregnant women who are at 20 weeks' gestation or further related to common discomforts of pregnancy that they are likely to encounter during the last half of pregnancy.

CRITICAL THINKING: WHAT WOULD YOU DO?

Apply your knowledge of the nurse's role during pregnancy to the following situations.

1. Theresa Martinez presents to the clinic because she thinks she might be pregnant.
   a. What nursing assessments should be completed?
   b. During the history, Theresa reports that there is a history of type 2 diabetes in her family, and that her mother delivered large babies (10 and 11 lb/4,500 and 5,000 g). What should you do with this information?

2. Amanda Jones calls the clinic. She is a G2 P1 at 28 weeks' gestation. She is worried because she thinks the baby is moving less than usual.

   a. What should you tell Amanda to do first?

   b. Amanda comes to the office to be checked because she is still worried about the baby. What is the priority nursing assessment that should be completed at this time? Why?

   c. Because Amanda has decreased fetal movement, a biophysical profile has been ordered. How would you explain this test to Amanda? Which part of this test would you normally expect to be a nursing function?

3. Rebecca Richards is pregnant for the first time. She is 40 years old. The obstetrician has suggested chromosomal studies.

   a. Explain the advantages and disadvantages of chorionic villus sampling versus amniocentesis.

   b. Rebecca tells you that she is opposed to abortion for any reason. She asks why she should go through chorionic villus sampling because she will not accept an abortion. How would you respond to Rebecca?

   c. What is the rationale for the chromosomal studies being ordered?

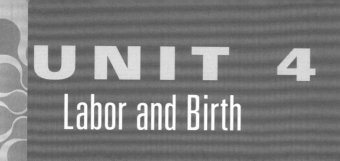

UNIT 4
Labor and Birth

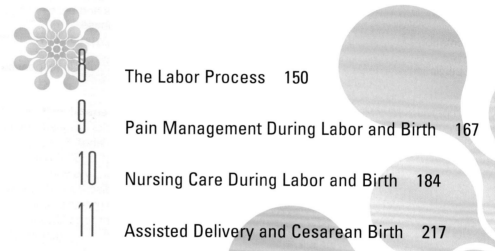

The Labor Process

Key Terms

android pelvis
anthropoid pelvis
caput succedaneum
cardinal movements
cephalohematoma
duration
effacement
engaged
false pelvis
fetal attitude
fetal lie
fetal presentation
frequency
gynecoid pelvis
intensity
molding
platypelloid pelvis
station
true pelvis

Learning Objectives

At the conclusion of this chapter, you will:

1. Explain the four essential components of the labor process and how they work together to accomplish birth.
2. Discuss current theories regarding causes of labor onset.
3. List anticipatory signs of labor.
4. Differentiate between false labor and true labor.
5. Describe the seven mechanisms or cardinal movements of a spontaneous vaginal delivery.
6. Identify the stages and phases of labor and events that occur in each stage or phase.
7. Discuss ways the woman physiologically and psychologically adapts to labor.
8. Describe fetal physiologic responses to labor.

During a routine prenatal visit, your client, Brenda Hines, a G1P0 who is 36 weeks pregnant, mentions that she is anxious about going through labor. She states, "I just don't think a baby can come out of me," and "I'm afraid I won't know when I'm about to go into labor." As you read the chapter, think about topics that you can discuss with her about her body and the labor process that might help reduce Brenda's anxiety. What signs would you want to tell Brenda to look for that might indicate that she is about to go into labor?

As a nurse, it is essential for you to understand the components of labor, how these components work together in the process of labor, and how the woman and fetus adapt to labor in normal situations. This knowledge allows you to support the laboring woman appropriately and assist her through a safe labor and delivery. This chapter explores each component of labor and birth separately and then discusses the combined components during the process of labor. Normal maternal and fetal adaptations to labor are examined.

Your knowledge and understanding of the principles of labor are important when caring for the pregnant woman either in the clinic or in the hospital. A woman may come to the health care provider's office for a checkup and may be in labor. Clients in labor are cared for by registered nurses. Your role in caring for the laboring client includes following guidelines set by the healthcare institution as well as the guidelines related to your scope of practice.

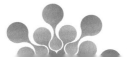

FOUR ESSENTIAL COMPONENTS OF LABOR

There are four essential components of labor. These are known as the "four Ps" of labor: passageway, passenger, powers, and psyche. A problem in any of these four areas will negatively influence the labor process.

Passageway

The passageway consists of the woman's bony pelvis and the soft tissues of the cervix and vagina.

Bony Pelvis

The bony pelvis forms the rigid passageway through which the fetus must navigate to deliver vaginally. The flared upper portion of the bony pelvis is the **false pelvis** (in lay terms this is the "hips"). The false pelvis is not part of the bony passageway. The portion of the pelvis below the linea terminalis is the true pelvis. The **true pelvis** is the bony passageway through which the fetus must pass during delivery. Important landmarks of the true pelvis include the pelvic inlet (entrance to the true pelvis) and the pelvic outlet (exit point). Figure 8-1 illustrates important landmarks of the pelvis.

The basic shape and dimensions of the true pelvis may either favor a vaginal birth or may interfere with the ability of the fetus to descend.

Pelvic Shape

The shape of the pelvic inlet determines the pelvic type. There are four basic pelvic shapes: gynecoid, anthropoid, android, and platypelloid (Fig. 8-2). Most women have pelvises that are various combinations of the four types.

The **gynecoid pelvis** is most favorable for a vaginal birth. The rounded shape of the gynecoid inlet allows the fetus room to pass through the dimensions of the bony passageway. The **anthropoid pelvis** is elongated in its dimensions. The anterior–posterior diameter is roomy, but the transverse diameter is narrow compared with that of the gynecoid pelvis. This type of pelvis can prevent a vaginal delivery in some women. The **android pelvis** is heart shaped. Large babies often become stuck in the birth canal and must be delivered by cesarean, whereas a smaller baby may be able to navigate the narrow diameters of the android pelvis. The least common type is the **platypelloid pelvis**. This pelvis is flat in its dimensions with a very narrow anterior–posterior diameter and a wide transverse diameter. This shape makes it extremely difficult for the fetus to pass through the bony pelvis. Therefore, women with platypelloid pelvises must usually deliver the fetus by cesarean section.

Pelvic Dimensions

Early in the pregnancy, particularly if a woman has never delivered a baby vaginally, the health care provider may take pelvic measurements to estimate the size of the true pelvis. This helps determine if the size is adequate for vaginal delivery. However, these measurements do not consistently predict which women will have difficulty delivering vaginally, so most health care providers allow the woman to labor and attempt a vaginal birth.

> **Take Note of This Detail**
> You cannot determine the shape and dimensions of the pelvic inlet by the size of the woman. A woman might be small in stature but have a roomy gynecoid pelvis. A larger woman may have a small, contracted platypelloid or android pelvis.

Soft Tissues

The cervix and vagina are soft tissues that form the part of the passageway known as the birth canal. In early pregnancy, the cervix is firm, long, and closed and measures approximately 2 cm in length. As the time for delivery approaches, the cervix usually begins to soften. Then, when labor begins, uterine contractions change the cervix in two ways. First, the cervix begins to get shorter and thinner, a process called **effacement**. Cervical effacement is recorded as a percentage. At a length of 1 cm, the cervix is 50% effaced. When the cervix is completely effaced, it is paper thin and is called 100% effaced.

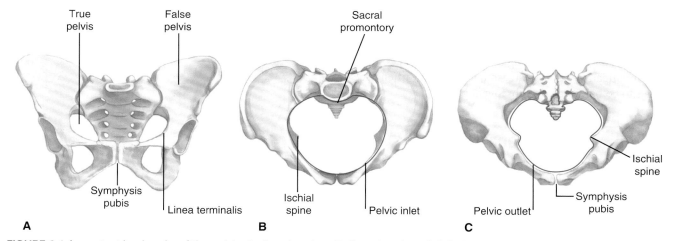

FIGURE 8-1 Important landmarks of the pelvis. **A.** Anterior view. **B.** Superior view. **C.** Inferior view.

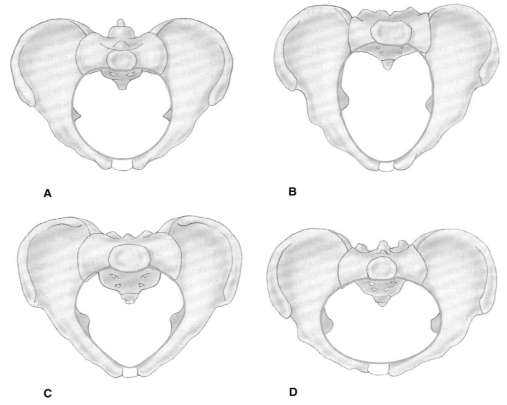

FIGURE 8-2 Pelvic shapes. **(A)** Gynecoid, **(B)** anthropoid, **(C)** android, and **(D)** platypelloid.

The second cervical change that occurs during normal labor is dilation. The cervix must dilate (open) to allow the fetus to be born. Dilation is measured in centimeters. When the cervix is dilated completely, it measures 10 cm. Normally, a primiparous woman experiences effacement before dilation. For a multiparous woman, both processes usually occur at the same time. Often, the multipara's cervix dilates 1 to 2 cm several weeks before labor begins. Figure 8-3 illustrates the processes of cervical effacement and dilation as they normally occur for the primipara.

The vaginal canal participates in childbirth via passive distention. During birth, the rugae of the vaginal walls stretch and smooth out, allowing for considerable expansion. The muscles and soft tissues of the primipara provide greater resistance to stretching and distending than do those of the multipara. This is one reason the first baby often takes longer to be born than do subsequent babies.

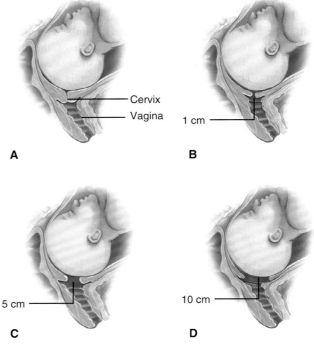

FIGURE 8-3 Cervical effacement and dilation. **A.** Before labor: Cervix is not effaced or dilated. **B.** Early effacement, early dilation to 1 cm. **C.** Complete effacement, mid-dilation to 5 cm. **D.** Full dilation to 10 cm.

TEST YOURSELF

✔ Why is the false pelvis not considered part of the passageway?

✔ How is cervical effacement recorded?

✔ How many centimeters wide is the cervix when it is fully dilated?

Passenger

The "passenger" refers to the fetus. The size of the fetal skull and the way the fetus is situated (which includes fetal lie, presentation, attitude, position, and station) can significantly affect labor progress. Each concept will be defined and discussed in relation to its influence on the progression of labor.

Fetal Skull

The skull is the most important fetal structure in relation to labor and birth because it is the largest and least compressible structure (Fig. 8-4). The diameters of the fetal skull must be small enough to allow the head to travel through the bony pelvis. Fortunately, the fetal skull is not entirely rigid. The cartilage between the bones allows the bones to overlap during labor, a process called **molding** which elongates the fetal skull, thereby reducing the diameter of the head. The newborn of a primipara often has significant molding.

Fetal Lie

Fetal lie describes the position of the long axis of the fetus in relation to the long axis of the pregnant woman. There are three basic ways that the fetus can lie in the uterus: in a longitudinal, transverse, or oblique position (Fig. 8-5). A longitudinal lie, in which the long axis (spine) of the fetus is parallel to the long axis (spine) of the mother, is the most common. When the fetus is in a transverse lie, the long axis

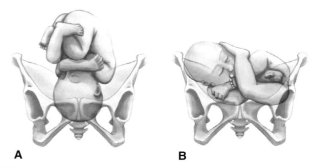

FIGURE 8-5 Longitudinal versus transverse lie. **A.** Longitudinal lie (the fetus lies parallel to the maternal spine). **B.** Transverse lie (the fetus lies crosswise to the maternal spine).

of the fetus is perpendicular to the long axis of the woman. The fetus appears to be lying "sideways" in the uterus instead of up-and-down. An oblique lie is in between a longitudinal and a transverse lie.

Fetal Presentation

Fetal presentation refers to the foremost part of the fetus that enters the pelvic inlet. There are three main ways that the fetus can present to the pelvis: head (cephalic presentation), feet or buttocks (breech presentation), or shoulder (shoulder presentation). A cephalic presentation is the most common presentation.

Breech presentations occur in approximately 3% to 4% of term pregnancies. This percentage increases with preterm deliveries (Gray and Shanahan, 2020). Figure 8-6 illustrates different types of breech presentations. Shoulder presentations are the least common, occurring in less than 0.3% of all term pregnancies. Shoulder presentation is associated with a transverse lie.

Fetal Attitude

Fetal attitude refers to the relationship of the fetal parts to one another. In a cephalic presentation, there are several different ways the head can present to the maternal true pelvis. The most common attitude, and the one that is most favorable for a vaginal birth, is an attitude of flexion, also called a vertex presentation. When the fetus curls up into an ovoid shape, they present the smallest diameters of the skull to the true pelvis. When the fetus is neither flexed nor hyperextended, they are in a military presentation and a larger head diameter is presented to the true pelvis. If the fetus' neck is partially extended, the brow (called the frontum) becomes the presenting part. If the fetus' neck is fully extended, the face presents first to the true pelvis. Figure 8-7 shows variations of cephalic presentation in association with fetal attitude.

Fetal Position

The health care provider will determine fetal position by first establishing the presenting part (occiput, brow, etc.). Table 8-1 lists the position name for the different presenting parts. The provider then determines if the part is facing the maternal right or left side and also which direction it is facing in relation to the maternal pelvis.

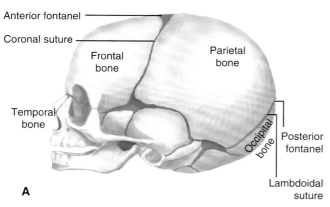

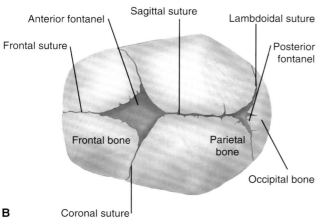

FIGURE 8-4 Sutures and fontanels of the fetal skull. **(A)** Lateral view and **(B)** anterior view.

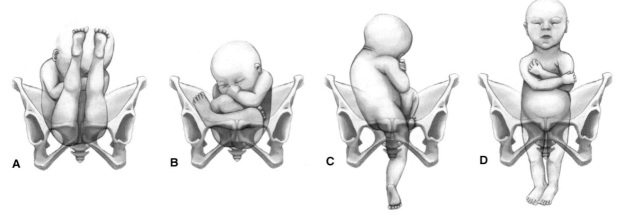

FIGURE 8-6 Breech presentations. **A.** Frank breech. **B.** Complete breech. **C.** Single footling breech. **D.** Double footling breech.

Fetal position is documented in the clinical record using abbreviations (Box 8-1). The first letter describes the side of the maternal pelvis toward which the presenting part is facing ("R" for right and "L" for left). The second letter of the abbreviation indicates the fetal presenting part ("O" for occiput, "Fr" for frontum, etc.). The last letter of the abbreviation specifies whether the presenting part is facing the anterior (A) or the posterior (P) portion of the maternal pelvis or whether it is in a transverse (T) position.

For example: the occipital bone, or occiput, is the presenting part in a vertex presentation. If the occiput is facing the right anterior quadrant of the pelvis, the position is recorded as right occiput anterior (ROA). If the occiput was instead facing the left anterior quadrant of the pelvis, the position would be recorded as left occiput anterior (LOA). Figure 8-8 illustrates examples of different positions in a vertex presentation and how the positions would be documented. The most favorable positions for vaginal birth are occiput anterior, either ROA or LOA.

Fetal Station

Station refers to the relationship of the presenting part of the fetus to the ischial spines of the pelvis (Fig. 8-9). When the widest diameter of the presenting part is at the level of the ischial spines, the station is zero (0). If the presenting part is above the level of the ischial spines, the station is recorded as a negative number and is read "minus." If the presenting part is below the level of the ischial spines, the station is recorded as a positive number and is read "plus." For example, in a cephalic presentation, if the widest part of the fetal head is 1 cm above the level of the ischial spines, the station is reported as a minus one and recorded as −1. If, on the other hand, the presenting part is 1 cm below the level of the ischial spines, the station is reported as a plus one and recorded as +1.

> **Be Careful!**
> A transverse position is not the same as a transverse lie. Transverse lie refers to the way the fetus' body is aligned in the uterus, whereas transverse position refers to the way the presenting part is aligned to the maternal pelvis.

> **Think About This**
> When the fetus is floating, they are high in the pelvis. A high station is recorded as a negative (minus) number. On the other hand, if the fetus has moved deep into the pelvis, the station is low and is recorded as a positive (plus) number. As the fetus is being born, the station is recorded as a plus four (+4).

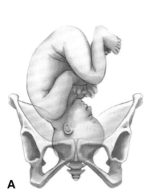
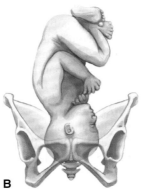
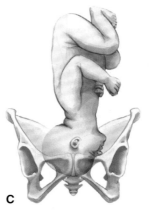
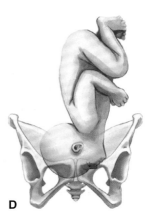

FIGURE 8-7 Fetal attitude affects the type of presentation in cephalic (head-first) presentations. The degree of fetal flexion affects whether the presentation is classified as **(A)** vertex, **(B)** military, **(C)** brow, or **(D)** face.

TABLE 8-1 Fetal Position and Corresponding Presenting Parts

POSITION	FETAL PRESENTING PART
Vertex	Occiput
Brow	Frontum (brow)
Face	Mentum (chin)
Breech	Sacrum
Shoulder	Scapula (acromial process)

When the station is a minus four (−4) or higher, the fetus is said to be floating and unengaged. When the fetus is floating, the presenting part has not yet entered the true pelvis. When the presenting part has settled into the true pelvis at the level of the ischial spines, the fetus is said to be **engaged** and is reported to be at a station of zero (0).

TEST YOURSELF

✔ What term is used to describe the fetal part that enters the true pelvis first?

✔ How is the fetal skull designed to decrease its diameter during birth? Would an infant delivered by cesarean section have significant molding? Describe why or why not.

✔ How is fetal lie described if the fetus is lying perpendicular to the maternal spine?

Powers

The primary force of labor comes from involuntary muscular contractions of the uterus. These labor contractions cause effacement and dilation of the cervix during the first stage of labor. Secondary powers are voluntary muscle contractions of the maternal abdomen during the second stage of labor that help expel the fetus (i.e., when the woman is pushing).

Each involuntary uterine contraction is composed of three phases—increment, acme, and decrement—followed by a relaxation period (Fig. 8-10). The increment, or building up of the contraction, is the longest phase. During the increment, the contraction gains strength until it reaches the acme, or peak, of the contraction. The decrement is the letting-up phase, as the uterus relaxes gradually to baseline.

Contractions are documented using three descriptors: frequency, duration, and intensity. **Frequency** refers to how often

This is an Important Point

Because each contraction interrupts blood flow to the placenta temporarily, there is decreased oxygen available to the fetus. It is as if the fetus must hold their breath during each contraction. Therefore, the fetus cannot tolerate contractions that last too long, that are too strong, or that have no rest period between them for prolonged periods.

The health care provider documents fetal position as an abbreviation using the following criteria:

First Designation
Refers to the side of the maternal pelvis in which the presenting part is found[1]
• Right (R)
• Left (L)

Second (Middle) Designation
Reference point on the presenting part
• Occiput (O)—vertex and military presentations
• Frontum or brow (Fr)—brow presentation
• Mentum or chin (M)—face presentation
• Sacrum (S)—breech presentation
• Scapula (Sc)—shoulder presentation

Third (Last) Designation
Refers to the front, back, or side of the maternal pelvis in which the reference point is found
• Anterior (A)—front of the pelvis
• Posterior (P)—back of the pelvis
• Transverse (T)—side of the pelvis

[1]This designation is not included in the notation if the reference point is exactly in the middle and is turned neither to the left nor to the right.

the contractions are occurring and is measured by counting the time interval from the beginning of one contraction to the beginning of the following contraction. **Duration** is the interval from the beginning of a contraction to its end. **Intensity** refers to the strength of the contraction. Intensity is recorded as mild, moderate, or strong and can be estimated by palpating the fundus at the peak of the contraction. Intensity can also be measured directly with an intrauterine pressure transducer.

It is extremely important to the well-being of the mother and the fetus that there is a period of relaxation between contractions. Each contraction constricts the blood vessels that supply the placenta, thereby decreasing the amount of oxygen that flows to the fetus. The relaxation period allows the vessels to fill with oxygenated blood to supply the uterus and placenta. Relaxation is also necessary so that maternal muscles do not become overly fatigued and allows the laboring woman momentary relief from the discomfort of labor.

Psyche

Many factors affect the psychological state or psyche of the laboring woman (Box 8-2). When the woman feels confident in her ability to cope and finds ways to work with the contractions, the labor process is enhanced. However, if the laboring woman becomes fearful or has intense pain, she may become tense and fight the contractions. This situation often becomes a cycle of fear, tension, and pain that interferes with the progress of labor.

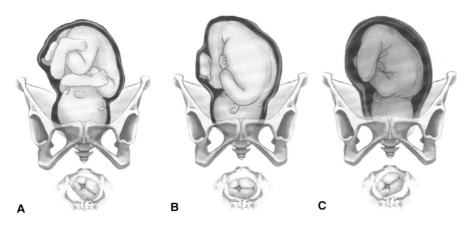

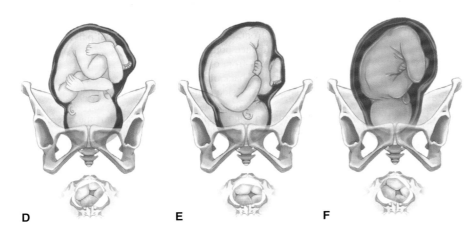

A B C

D E F

FIGURE 8-8 Examples of fetal position in a vertex presentation. **A.** Left occiput posterior (LOP). **B.** Left occiput transverse (LOT). **C.** Left occiput anterior (LOA). **D.** Right occiput posterior (ROP). **E.** Right occiput transverse (ROT). **F.** Right occiput anterior (ROA). In each illustration, the lie is longitudinal, and the attitude is one of flexion. Notice that the smaller illustrations show the anterior view of the fetal skull that would be presented with the woman in a dorsal recumbent position. The LOA and ROA positions are emphasized as they are the most favorable positions for a vaginal delivery.

TEST YOURSELF

✔ What is another name for the peak of the contraction?

✔ How is the frequency of uterine contractions measured?

✔ What is the purpose of the relaxation period between uterine contractions?

Think back to Brenda Hines. She was anxious about how she could deliver a baby. What can you tell her about her body and how it is designed to deliver the baby? What might be some other concerns she might have regarding the delivery process?

THE PROCESS OF LABOR

Labor is a process in which the four components (passageway, passenger, powers, and psyche) work simultaneously to accomplish birth. It is important to remember that during the labor process, a problem in any of the components can negatively affect the duration or outcome of the labor.

Onset of Labor

A question that is frequently asked is, "What is the trigger that causes labor to begin?" As pregnancy nears term, the pregnant woman is more concerned with when labor will begin than with what causes labor to begin. She often asks the health care provider, "When will I go into labor?" This section will explore both questions.

Theories Regarding Causes of Labor Onset

There are several hypotheses regarding what causes labor to begin. A single causative factor of labor has not yet been determined. Studies indicate labor onset results from a combination of several maternal and fetal hormones working together. Some of these hormones include progesterone, oxytocin, prostaglandins, and fetal cortisol (Norwitz, 2019).

Anticipatory Signs of Labor

There are some signs that indicate that labor might be nearing. Approximately 2 weeks before labor, engagement may occur, causing the pregnant woman to sense that the baby has "dropped." This subjective feeling is called "lightening." The woman is able to breathe more easily, and she may need to urinate more frequently because of the pressure of the fetus on the urinary bladder. Not all women experience lightening before the onset of labor. Multiparous women often do not experience lightening until labor begins or the fetus may engage prior to 2 weeks in advance of labor.

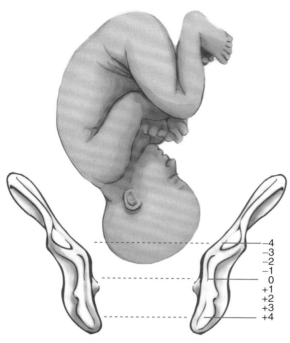

-4
-3
-2
-1
0
+1
+2
+3
+4

FIGURE 8-9 Fetal station.

Braxton Hicks contractions occur more frequently and are more noticeable as pregnancy approaches term. These irregular contractions usually decrease in intensity with walking and position changes. These contractions are not part of labor and do not cause effacement or dilation to occur. The woman may experience gastrointestinal disturbances, such as diarrhea, heartburn, or nausea and vomiting, as labor approaches. Sometimes the mucus plug is expelled a week or two before labor begins. When the mucus plug passes, the woman will notice a one-time clear or pink-tinged discharge that is the consistency of jelly.

Frequently, the woman experiences a burst of energy 24 to 48 hours before the onset of labor. She may have the energy and desire to do thorough cleaning or some other big project in anticipation of the baby's arrival, a phenomenon known as the nesting urge. Caution the woman regarding the nesting urge, and advise her to conserve her energy for the work of labor.

Clinical signs that labor is approaching include ripening (softening) and effacement (thinning) of the cervix. Dilation of the cervix may accompany ripening and effacement, particularly in multiparous women. The health care provider informs the woman of these changes if a pelvic examination is done during a scheduled office visit.

Differences Between False and True Labor

False labor (prodromal labor) refers to the increase in Braxton Hicks contractions that occur toward the end of pregnancy. These practice contractions can be quite uncomfortable, making it difficult to distinguish true labor from "false" labor. See Table 8-2 for differences between true and false labor. Sometimes the woman presents to the labor facility because she thinks she is in labor. After the initial assessment by the health care provider, the woman may be instructed to walk for an hour or two. Then, a vaginal examination is repeated to determine any cervical changes. If there are changes, the laboring woman is admitted to the facility. If there are no changes, the woman may go home with instructions to return if the contractions become stronger, more regular, or if other signs of true labor occur, such as rupture of membranes ("bag of waters breaks") or presence of bloody show (mucous vaginal discharge that is pink or brown tinged which occurs as the blood vessels in the cervix start to rupture as effacement and dilation are beginning).

> **True Labor Changes the Woman**
>
> By definition, true labor results in progressive dilation and effacement of the cervix. If the woman is having contractions but the cervix is not getting thinner (effacing) or opening (dilating), she is not in true labor.

Mechanisms of a Spontaneous Vaginal Delivery

For a vaginal birth to occur, the fetus (passenger) must pass through the birth canal (passageway). The turns and

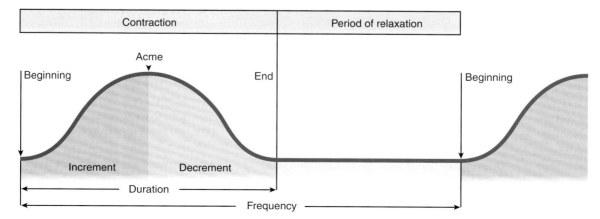

FIGURE 8-10 The three phases of a uterine contraction are the increment (building up in intensity), acme (peak intensity), and decrement (decreasing intensity). A period of relaxation normally follows the contraction.

Factors that may affect the woman's psyche during labor include the woman's:

- Current pregnancy experience
  - Unplanned versus planned pregnancy
  - Amount of difficulty conceiving
  - Presence of risk factors or complications of pregnancy
- Previous birth experiences
  - Positive or negative feelings regarding previous delivery experience
  - Complications encountered during previous delivery
  - Mode of delivery (cesarean vs. vaginal)
  - Birth outcomes (e.g., fetal demise, birth defects)
- Expectations for current birth experience
  - View of labor as a meaningful or a stressful event
  - Realistic and attainable goals versus idealistic views that conflict with reality (a situation that can lead to disappointment)
- Preparation for birth
  - Type of childbirth preparation
  - Familiarity with institution and its policies and procedures
  - Type of relaxation techniques learned and practiced
- Presence and support of a birth companion
- A woman's culture influences and defines:
  - The childbirth experience
    - Shameful versus joyful
    - Superstitions and beliefs about pregnancy and birth
    - Prescribed behaviors and taboos during the intrapartum period
  - Relationships
    - Interpersonal interactions
    - Parent–infant interactions
    - Role expectations of family members
    - Support person involvement
  - Pain
    - Meaning and context of pain during labor
    - Acceptable responses to pain during labor
  - The significance of touch
    - Soothing versus intruding
    - May be a symbol of intimacy

movements made during birth are referred to as the **cardinal movements** (or cardinal mechanisms) of delivery. These seven movements are engagement, descent, flexion, internal rotation, extension, external rotation, and expulsion (Fig. 8-11). Although the movements are discussed separately, it is important to understand that they may overlap or occur simultaneously.

- *Engagement.* Initial descent of the fetal head results in engagement when the presenting part descends to the level of the ischial spines. Engagement may occur as early as 2 weeks before labor or not until after the onset of labor. Engagement is more likely to occur earlier in the primigravida and later in the multigravida.
- *Descent.* Descent may begin before labor when the fetus "drops." Descent is measured by station, which is the relationship of the fetal-presenting part to the maternal ischial spines. Descent continues throughout labor until the fetus reaches a fetal station of plus four (+4).
- *Flexion.* As the head descends during labor, the fetus encounters resistance from the soft tissues and muscles of the pelvic floor. This resistance normally coaxes the fetus to assume an attitude of flexion. Flexion is the attitude that presents the smallest diameters of the fetal head to the dimensions of the pelvis.
- *Internal rotation.* Frequently, in early labor, the fetal head presents to the pelvis in a transverse position because the inlet of the pelvis is widest from side to side. During active labor, the fetal head typically rotates 45 degrees from a transverse position to an anterior position so that the head can accommodate the pelvic outlet, which is wider from front to back. This movement is called internal rotation. If the fetus does not rotate, the widest diameters of the fetal head present to the outlet of the pelvis, resulting in a less than optimal fit between the head and the bony passageway. This can prolong labor.
- *Extension.* Typically, the fetal head is well flexed with the chin on the chest as the fetus travels through the birth canal.

TABLE 8-2 Characteristics of False (Prodromal) Versus True Labor

	TRUE LABOR	FALSE (PRODROMAL) LABOR
Cervical changes	Progressive dilation and effacement	No change
Membranes	May bulge or rupture spontaneously	Remain intact
Bloody show	Present	Absent; may have pinkish mucus or may expel mucus plug
Contraction pattern	Regular (may be irregular at first) pattern develops in which contractions become increasingly intense and more frequent	Pattern tends to be irregular, although the contractions may seem to have a regular pattern for a time
Pain characteristics	Often starts in the small of the back and radiates to the lower abdomen; may begin with a cramping sensation	May be described as a tightening sensation; usually the discomfort is confined to the abdomen
Effects of walking	Contractions continue and become stronger	May decrease the frequency or eliminate the contractions altogether

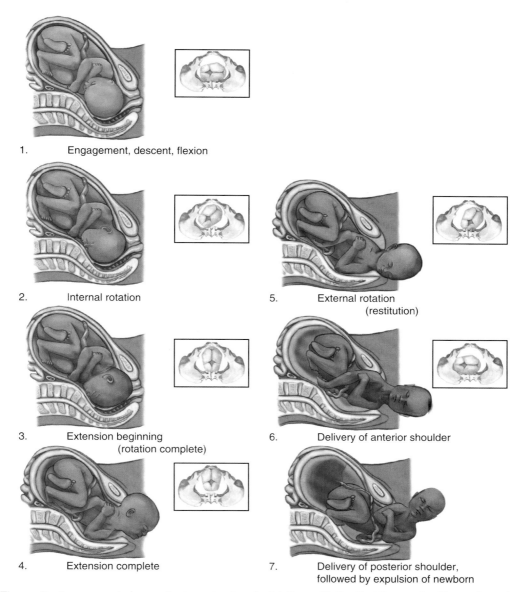

1. Engagement, descent, flexion

2. Internal rotation

3. Extension beginning
(rotation complete)

4. Extension complete

5. External rotation
(restitution)

6. Delivery of anterior shoulder

7. Delivery of posterior shoulder,
followed by expulsion of newborn

FIGURE 8-11 The cardinal movements (or cardinal mechanisms) of delivery. Notice that the smaller illustrations show the anterior view of the fetal skull that would be presented with the woman in a dorsal recumbent position.

When the fetus reaches the pubic arch, it must extend under the symphysis pubis.

- *External rotation.* As the head is born, external rotation lines the head up with the shoulders.
- *Expulsion.* Expulsion (birth) occurs after delivery of the anterior and posterior shoulders.

Think This Through

If the fetus is in an occiput posterior position, the fetal head must rotate 90 degrees versus 45 degrees. The typical result is a prolonged and painful "back" labor.

TEST YOURSELF

✔ List three anticipatory signs of labor.

✔ A woman calls the labor and delivery unit stating she is in labor. What questions would you want to ask her to determine if she is in true labor?

✔ List the cardinal movements of delivery in order.

Stages and Duration of Labor

Labor is categorized into four stages, and the first stage is further divided into three phases. Each stage and phase of labor has unique characteristics that help the nurse and physician, or midwife, determine if labor is progressing as expected. It is important to note that individual labors vary greatly with regard to length. Many factors affect the progress of labor such as parity, the use of agents to soften the cervix, labor induction techniques, and type of anesthesia (if any) used. These factors are discussed in other chapters.

This Can Be Confusing

Although technically a woman who has never delivered a viable child is a nullipara, when she goes into labor, she is usually referred to as a primipara.

Each stage of labor is discussed in regard to important landmarks, physical findings, and approximate length of time for each stage. Because parity influences labor progress, typical differences between a primiparous woman and a multiparous woman are noted. Time frames can be shorter than listed and a woman can have a much shorter (quicker) labor than "typical." Table 8-3 summarizes the stages of labor.

First Stage: Dilation

The first stage of labor begins with the onset of true labor and ends with full dilation of the cervix at 10 cm. This stage is subdivided into three phases: latent, active, and transition.

Early Labor (Latent Phase)

Early labor begins when the contractions of true labor start and ends when the cervix is dilated at 4 cm. Contractions during this phase are of mild intensity and typically occur at a frequency of 5 to 10 minutes (although they may occur as infrequently as every 30 minutes), with a duration of 30 to 45 seconds. In a normal labor, the pattern of contractions during the latent phase becomes increasingly regular with shorter intervals between contractions.

The latent phase lasts on average approximately 8 to 9 hours for a primiparous woman but generally does not exceed 20 hours in length. Multiparous women usually experience shorter labors (an average length of approximately 5 hours, with an upper limit of 14 hours).

Here's a Tip for Encouraging the Woman

The nulliparous woman may become discouraged during the early phase of labor if many hours have passed and the cervix is still dilated less than 3 cm. Explain to the woman that her cervix is making progress because it is effacing. Reassure her that the cervix will begin to dilate more rapidly with the contractions of active labor.

Active Labor (Active Phase)

The active phase begins at 4 cm cervical dilation and ends when the cervix is dilated at 8 cm. Contractions typically occur every 2 to 5 minutes, last 45 to 60 seconds, and are of moderate to strong intensity. Progressive cervical dilation and fetal descent normally occur in this phase.

For primiparas, dilation should occur at approximately 1.2 cm/hr. Multiparas progress at a slightly faster pace of 1.5 cm/hr. These designations are only approximations and may vary a great deal if the woman receives medication, anesthesia, or other medical intervention during labor. Fetal descent is often slow in the first stage of labor, regardless of parity. Occasionally, the fetus does not descend during active labor.

Transition (Transition Phase)

Transition is the most difficult part of labor. This phase of the first stage of labor starts when the cervix is dilated at 8 cm and ends with full cervical dilation. The contractions are of strong intensity, occur every 2 to 3 minutes, and are of 60 to 90 seconds in duration. The woman often feels "out of control" as the contractions are frequent, longer, and more intense than during the latent and active phases. It is important for the nurse to help the woman with relaxing between contractions and comfort measures during contractions. This is usually the shortest phase of the first stage of labor.

Frequently, the woman experiences a strong urge to push as the fetus descends. It is important for the woman to resist the urge to push until the cervix is dilated completely. Pushing against a partially dilated cervix can cause swelling, which slows labor, or the cervix can develop lacerations, leading to hemorrhage.

Second Stage: Birth

The second stage begins when the cervix is dilated fully to 10 cm and ends with the birth of the infant. Contractions usually continue at a frequency of every 2 to 3 minutes, last 60 to 90 seconds, and are of strong intensity. The average length of the second stage is 1 hour for primiparas and 20 minutes for multiparas, although it is normal for a primipara to be in this stage for 2 hour or longer.

During the second stage, the woman is encouraged to use her abdominal muscles to bear down during contractions while the fetus continues to descend and rotate to the anterior position. Fetal descent is usually slow but steady for the primipara, from the active phase of the first stage through the second stage. Frequently, the fetus of a multipara may not descend significantly during active labor but may rapidly descend during the second stage. In this scenario, the baby may be born with one or two pushes. When the fetus is at a station of +4, they proceed to move through the cardinal movements of extension and external rotation, followed by delivery of the shoulders and expulsion of the rest of the body.

Third Stage: Delivery of Placenta

The third stage of labor begins with the birth of the baby and ends with delivery of the placenta. This stage normally lasts from 5 to 20 minutes for both primiparas and multiparas. Signs that indicate the placenta is separating from the uterine wall include a gush of blood, lengthening of the umbilical cord, and a globular shape to the fundus.

The placenta usually delivers spontaneously by one of two ways. If the fetal or shiny side of the placenta presents first, it is referred to as Schultze placental delivery. If the maternal or rough side of the placenta presents first, it is

TABLE 8-3 Stages of Labor

	DEFINITION	CONTRACTIONS	CHARACTERISTICS	MATERNAL RESPONSE
First stage: dilation	Onset of true labor through full dilation of cervix at 10 cm			
Latent phase	Contractions of true labor through dilation of cervix to 4 cm	*Frequency:* every 5–10 minutes *Duration:* 30–45 seconds *Intensity:* mild	Contractions may be irregular at first followed by increasing regularity Cervical effacement (thinning) generally occurs before dilation for the primipara	Excited, very talkative, some women are apprehensive
Active phase	Cervical dilation of 4 cm to cervical dilation of 8 cm	*Frequency:* every 3–5 minutes *Duration:* 40–60 seconds *Intensity:* moderate to strong	Contractions are regular and progressively increase in frequency, duration, and intensity Progressive cervical dilation Fetal descent	Conversations more limited, woman is focused on contractions, rests with eyes closed between contractions, diaphoresis
Transition phase	Cervical dilation of 8 cm to cervical dilation of 10 cm (complete dilation)	*Frequency:* every 2–3 minutes *Duration:* 60–90 seconds *Intensity:* strong	Most difficult phase Woman must resist if she has a strong urge to push	Nausea and vomiting, irritability, diaphoresis, inability to relax between contraction, feelings of loss of control
Second stage: birth	Complete cervical dilation (10 cm) through birth	*Frequency:* every 2–5 minutes *Duration:* 60–90 seconds *Intensity:* strong	Fetal descent is most pronounced during second stage Woman should push when she feels the urge	Feelings of being more in control, rests between contractions, less irritable
Third stage: delivery of placenta	From birth through delivery of the placenta	Variable	Signs of placental separation: gush of blood, lengthening of umbilical cord, fundus becomes globular	Asks about infant, may close eyes and briefly rest
Fourth stage: recovery	From delivery of the placenta through 2–4 hours post delivery	Afterpains: variable	In general, afterpains are more noticeable for the multipara and for the breast-feeding woman	Awake, talkative, excited, wanting to touch and see infant, shaking of extremities, may shiver and be cold, may have periods of crying even though she is happy

referred to as Duncan placental delivery. Regardless of which side presents first, the delivery attendant will examine the placenta for intactness to make sure no parts of the placenta broke off and were retained inside the uterus.

Fourth Stage: Recovery

Because of the tremendous changes that the new mother's body goes through during the process of labor and delivery, the period of recovery

This Advice May Be Helpful on a Test!

It is easy to confuse phases of the first stage of labor (latent, active, and transition) with stages of labor (first, second, third, and fourth). Be sure you are able to clearly define each stage and phase so that you do not confuse phases with stages during an examination.

after delivery of the placenta is considered to be a fourth stage of labor. This recovery stage may last from 1 to 4 hours. During this fourth stage, observe the woman frequently for signs of hemorrhage or other complications. Vital signs, uterine tone, and vaginal bleeding are assessed every 15 minutes initially until stable.

MATERNAL AND FETAL ADAPTATION TO LABOR

Maternal Physiologic Adaptation

Labor has an effect on the woman as if she were engaged in moderate to vigorous aerobic exercise. There is an increased demand for oxygen during the first stage of labor, most of this due to the energy used for uterine contractions. To meet the demand, there is a moderate increase in cardiac output throughout the first stage of labor. During pushing (second stage), cardiac output may be increased as much as 40% to 50% above the prelabor level. Immediately after birth, it may peak at 80% above the prelabor level.

The pulse is often at the high end of normal during active labor. Dehydration and maternal exhaustion can increase the woman's heart rate and temperature. Blood pressure, however, does not change much during normal labor, although the stress of contractions may cause a 15 mm Hg increase in the systolic pressure. The increased demand for oxygen and the discomfort of uterine contractions cause the respiratory rate to increase, which puts the laboring woman at risk for hyperventilation. If the woman shows signs of hyperventilation or notices a tingling sensation in her fingers, she should be encouraged to breathe into her cupped hands or a paper bag. Mouth breathing and dehydration contribute to dry lips and mouth.

Labor prolongs the normal gastric emptying time. This change often leads to nausea and vomiting during active labor and increases the woman's risk for aspiration, particularly if general anesthesia is required. Traditionally, the laboring woman received intravenous fluids while solid food and fluids were withheld. However, research shows that the risk for aspiration remains high, even if the woman maintains a nothing-by-mouth status, because gastric secretions become more acidic during periods of fasting. Women tend to desire fluids and food during early labor, but the desire declines as labor progresses. Current recommendations are to allow the laboring woman to have clear liquids, unless there is a high likelihood that she will deliver by cesarean.

Pressure on the urethra from the presenting part may cause overfilling of the bladder, a decreased sensation to void, and edema. A full bladder is uncomfortable and slows the progress of labor. As the bladder fills, it rises upward in the pelvic cavity, which puts pressure on the lower uterine segment and prevents the head from descending. Sometimes the use of an in-and-out (straight) urinary catheter becomes necessary to empty the woman's bladder.

Labor affects some laboratory values. The stress of vigorous labor may cause an increase in the white blood cell count to as high as 30,000 cells/microliter (mL). This increase is the body's normal response to inflammation, pain, and stress. Frequently the urine specific gravity is high, indicating concentrated urine, and there may be a trace amount of urinary protein because of increased metabolic activity. Gross proteinuria is never normal during labor and is a sign of complication.

Maternal Psychological Adaptation

Labor is hard work that puts a demand on the woman's coping resources. The woman's response changes as labor progresses. During early labor, the woman is often excited and talkative, although anxiety and apprehension are common responses. As labor becomes active, the woman becomes more introverted and focuses her energies on coping with the stress of contractions. Women who are unprepared psychologically for labor lose control easily during the active phase and may resort to crying, screaming, or thrashing about during contractions. This response may impede the labor process by causing muscular tension. Tense muscles work against cervical dilation and fetal descent.

Transition is the most intense phase of the first stage of labor, and many women, even ones who have had natural childbirth classes, have a difficult time maintaining positive coping strategies during this phase of labor. Many women describe feeling out of control during this phase of labor. A woman in transition needs support, encouragement, and positive reinforcement. Once pushing efforts begin, the woman usually feels more in control and is better able to cope.

Maternal responses to the actual birth vary widely. Many mothers are excited and eager to see and hold the baby. Others are exhausted and may doze intermittently. Most new mothers are anxious about the baby's health. When the woman holds the baby for the first time, it is normal for her to use fingertip touching and for her to explore the infant and count their fingers and toes.

Fetal Adaptation to Labor

Normal labor stresses the fetus in several ways. Intracranial pressure increases as the fetal head meets resistance from the birth canal. Sometimes this increased pressure results in a slowing of the fetal heart rate at the peak of a contraction—a normal phenomenon described in Chapter 10. Placental blood flow, the source of oxygen for the fetus, is temporarily interrupted at the peak of each contraction. Pushing efforts interrupt placental blood flow for even longer periods. For these reasons, relaxation in-between contractions is important for fetal oxygenation. Because of these changes, even the healthy fetus experiences a slowly decreasing pH throughout labor. Some health care providers will take a sample of cord blood to test the pH of the fetus. Box 8-3 describes normal and abnormal fetal pH levels. Although labor stresses the fetal cardiovascular system, a healthy fetus is able to compensate and maintain the heart rate within normal limits (see Chapter 10). This ability to compensate demonstrates the presence of a well-oxygenated fetus with a healthy neurologic system.

BOX 8-3   Implications of Fetal Scalp pH

Fetal pH
- >7.25
  - Reassuring
  - Associated with normal acid–base balance
- Between 7.20 and 7.25
  - Worrisome
  - May be associated with metabolic acidosis
- <7.20
  - Critical
  - Represents metabolic acidosis
- <7
  - Damaging
  - Frequently associated with fetal neurologic damage

C u l t u r a l   S n a p s h o t

The woman's culture influences her outward response to labor. In some cultures, the woman is expected to accept pain stoically. In other cultures, loud expressions of pain are accepted. It is important to perform a careful assessment of a woman's discomfort and to determine measures the laboring woman thinks would be helpful to relieve the pain. Just because the woman is quiet during labor does not mean that she is not experiencing pain. (Refer to Chapter 9 for an in-depth discussion of management of discomfort during labor.)

The act of passing through the birth canal is beneficial to the fetus in two ways. The process of labor increases surfactant secretion in the fetal lungs to promote respiratory adaptation at birth. Also, as the fetus descends, maternal tissues compress the fetus' body, a process that helps clear the respiratory passageways of fetal lung fluid. Infants who are born by cesarean section usually require more frequent suctioning because they have not had the benefit of this compression.

Pressure on the fetus caused by progress through the birth canal may result in areas of ecchymosis or edema, particularly on the presenting part. In the vertex presentation, pressure may cause formation of a **caput succedaneum**, swelling of the soft tissue of the head, or development of a **cephalohematoma**, collection of blood under the scalp (see Chapter 13 for a discussion of these two findings). In a breech presentation ecchymosis may be seen on the buttocks of the infant. In a facial presentation, facial ecchymosis may be present and can be confused for cyanosis.

TEST YOURSELF

✔ How many centimeters must the cervix dilate before a woman is in active labor?

✔ Which stage of labor requires the woman to help by pushing?

✔ In which stage of labor does delivery of the placenta occur?

Recall Brenda Hines, your client from the beginning of the chapter. She was wondering how she would know if she was going into labor. What would be some signs that she might go into labor in the next few weeks? How would she know if she was in true labor?

KEY POINTS

- Four essential components of the labor process are the passageway (maternal pelvis and soft tissues), passenger (fetus), powers (involuntary and voluntary muscle contractions), and psyche (psychological state of the woman).

- The bony pelvis is the rigid passageway through which the fetus must pass. There are four basic pelvic shapes: gynecoid, anthropoid, android, and platypelloid. The gynecoid type is the most favorable type for vaginal birth.

- The cervix, part of the soft tissue of the passageway, must completely efface (thin) and dilate (open) for the fetus to be born. Full dilation is equal to 10 cm.

- The fetal skull is the most important fetal structure because it is the largest and least compressible. The bones in the fetal skull can overlap some to decrease the diameter of the fetal head during delivery.

- The majority of fetuses enter the pelvis head first, a condition referred to as a cephalic presentation. When the feet or buttocks present first, the fetus is in a breech presentation. Shoulder presentation is uncommon.

- The part of the fetus that is closest to the cervix is the presenting part. Presentation and fetal attitude (vertex, military, brow, or face) together determine the presenting part.

- To determine fetal position, the presenting part and location to the reference point (occiput, frontum, mentum, sacrum, etc.) are described and then described in relation to maternal pelvic quadrants. ROA and LOA are the most favorable fetal positions for vaginal birth.

- Station is a determination of the relationship of the presenting part to the ischial spines. Zero station occurs when the presenting part is at the level of the ischial spines. When the fetus is high in the pelvis (above the ischial spines), the station is recorded as a negative number. A low station (below the ischial spines) is recorded as a positive number.

- The primary power of labor comes from involuntary uterine contractions, which serve to efface and dilate the cervix. Maternal pushing efforts supply secondary powers during the second stage of labor.

- The contraction pattern (frequency, duration, and intensity) and the resting interval are important to assess because the fetus can become hypoxic if contractions are too close together, too strong, or if there is not an adequate rest period between contractions.

- Maternal psyche is an important influence on the labor process. Nursing interventions can help break the cycle of fear, tension, and pain that can interfere with labor.

- There are both maternal and fetal factors that stimulate the onset of labor, and research is ongoing as to the exact cause of labor onset. Both the maternal and the fetal factors prepare the cervix to dilate, stimulate labor to begin, and allow for delivery of the fetus.

- Anticipatory signs of labor include gastrointestinal disturbances, expelling the mucus plug, engagement (lightening), Braxton Hicks contractions, and a burst of energy (the "nesting urge").

- True labor results in progressive effacement and dilation of the cervix. In true labor, contractions become progressively stronger and occur more frequently and are not stopped with walking.

- There are seven cardinal movements a fetus goes through during birth. These seven movements are engagement, descent, flexion, internal rotation, extension, external rotation, and expulsion.

- Labor occurs in four stages: the first stage is from 0 to 10 cm dilation; the second stage is from full (10 cm) dilation to birth; the third stage is from birth of the infant to expulsion of placenta; and fourth stage is the recovery period.

- The first stage of labor is composed of three phases: latent, active, and transition. Each phase has unique characteristics that differentiate it from other phases.

- Labor affects the mother in much the same way as vigorous exercise does. The heart rate, cardiac output, and respiratory rate increase to meet the body's increased oxygen need. Other systems, notably the gastrointestinal and urinary systems, are also affected.

- The healthy fetus is able to withstand the stress that labor places on the cardiovascular system. A vaginal birth helps mature the respiratory system and clears fetal lung fluid from the respiratory tract.

INTERNET RESOURCES

Labor Signs and Symptoms
www.emedicinehealth.com/labor_signs/article_em.htm

Labor and Delivery
https://www.mayoclinic.org/healthy-lifestyle/labor-and-delivery/
 in-depth/stages-of-labor/art-20046545
https://www.healthline.com/health/pregnancy/labor-and-delivery
https://americanpregnancy.org/labor-and-birth/first-stage-of-labor-893

Workbook

NCLEX-STYLE REVIEW QUESTIONS

1. A 32-year-old woman is dilated 4 cm. The health care provider states that she has a roomy pelvis and the baby is in a right occiput anterior (ROA) position at +1 station. Her contractions are occurring every 10 minutes, lasting 30 to 40 seconds, and palpate mild in intensity. She is calm and relaxed. Given these data, which essential component of labor is unexpected and likely to slow the progress of labor at this time?
   a. Passageway
   b. Passenger
   c. Powers
   d. Psyche

2. A woman near the end of pregnancy comments to the nurse, "I'm curious. What causes labor to begin?" Which reply by the nurse is the most accurate?
   a. "It is a mystery. No one knows."
   b. "It is believed that several factors work together to stimulate labor to begin."
   c. "The pituitary gland in the brain releases a special hormone that signals labor to begin."
   d. "You don't need to worry about that. The baby will come when he is ready."

3. The fetus is in a cephalic presentation. The occiput is facing toward the front and slightly to the right of the mother's pelvis, and the fetus is exhibiting a flexed attitude. How is the position of the fetus documented for this situation?
   a. LOA
   b. LOP
   c. ROA
   d. ROP

4. A woman has just delivered a healthy baby, but the placenta has not yet delivered. What stage of labor does this scenario represent?
   a. First
   b. Second
   c. Third
   d. Fourth

5. Place the following events in correct order:
   a. Extension
   b. Expulsion
   c. Flexion
   d. Engagement
   e. Internal rotation
   f. External rotation
   g. Descent

6. Which of the following statements made by the woman indicate false labor? Select all that apply.
   a. "My bag of waters just broke."
   b. "The contractions are irregular."
   c. "The contraction feels tight and located in my abdomen."
   d. "Walking has made the contractions stop."
   e. "I am having a lot of bloody, mucus-type vaginal discharge."

STUDY ACTIVITIES

1. Using the table below, write a brief definition or explanation of each of the "four Ps" of labor. List critical nursing observations/assessments for each area, and briefly describe what should be documented.

Four Ps of Labor	Definition or Explanation	Observations (What to Look for)	Documentation
Passageway			
Passenger			
Powers			
Psyche			

2. Develop a teaching aid or poster explaining the stages of labor to a first-time pregnant woman.

3. Conduct an internet search using the terms "culture" and "labor and delivery." Choose three different cultures, and research the typical responses during labor and delivery, support persons present at the birth, and food preferences. Have a discussion with your clinical group about the way culture affects behaviors and choices regarding labor and birth.

CRITICAL THINKING: WHAT WOULD YOU DO?

Apply your knowledge of the components of labor to the following situation.

1. Anna, a 25-year-old gravida 2, has been in labor for several hours, but her cervix is not dilating. The health care provider says that Anna's pelvis is roomy and adequate for a vaginal delivery.
   a. In what way do you anticipate the journey of the fetus through the passageway will be affected because Anna's cervix is not dilating?
   b. Discuss two possible causes of the failure of Anna's cervix to dilate.

2. Anna's midwife performs a vaginal examination and states the fetus is "occiput posterior."
   a. Anna asks you, "What does it mean that the baby is occiput posterior?" How would you explain this position to Anna?
   b. What will you tell Anna's partner regarding the probable progress of labor because the fetus is in a posterior position?

3. Anna has been in active labor for 7 hours. She has been quietly coping with contractions with the help of her partner. Now she begins to cry, "I can't stand it anymore!" She screams at her partner, "This is all your fault. You're not helping me at all!"

   a. How far do you expect Anna to be dilated? What stage and phase of labor is most likely represented in this scenario?

   b. How will you advise Anna's partner to be helpful and understanding during this difficult part of labor?

4. Anna progresses to the second stage of labor. The fetus has not rotated to an anterior position, so the baby is delivered face up.

   a. What does the health care provider document in the delivery note regarding the position of the baby at birth?

   b. How would you expect the baby's head to look after his long journey through the birth canal?

   c. How do you expect Anna will react to the birth of her baby?

9

Pain Management During Labor and Birth

Key Terms
analgesia
anesthesia
effleurage
epidural
intrathecal
opioids

Learning Objectives

At the conclusion of this chapter, you will:

1. Explain how the pain of labor and birth differs from other types of pain.
2. Describe sources of labor pain.
3. List factors influencing the woman's experience of labor pain.
4. Discuss principles of labor pain management.
5. Compare nonpharmacologic interventions to manage labor pain.
6. Explain various relaxation techniques that help a woman cope with labor.
7. Differentiate analgesia from anesthesia.
8. Describe advantages and disadvantages of opioid administration during labor.
9. Compare methods of regional anesthesia.
10. Explain major complications associated with epidural and spinal anesthesia.
11. Discuss reasons why general anesthesia is risky for a pregnant woman and her fetus.

Kayleigh Webber comes to the labor and delivery unit stating she is in labor. While you are helping her to the labor room, she begins to experience a contraction. She closes her eyes, bends over, clenches her teeth, and is squeezing her partner's hand. After you observe her react to several contractions this way, she starts to cry and says, "This hurts so bad! I can't do this!" As you read this chapter, think about what interventions could help Kayleigh's discomfort during her labor and birth.

Pain is an individual, subjective, sensory experience. A complex interplay of physiologic, psychological, emotional, environmental, and sociocultural factors influences the way a person perceives and responds to pain. A woman's response to labor pain is influenced by all of these factors, including her expectations about labor and her confidence in her ability to cope with labor. Additionally, her previous experience with pain, birth, and any coping strategies she has utilized in the past will also influence her response to labor pain with this birth. As a licensed practical/vocational nurse, you assist the registered nurse (RN) to manage the pain associated with labor and birth.

THE PAIN OF LABOR AND CHILDBIRTH

Uniqueness of Labor and Birth Pain

The pain of labor and birth is different from other types of pain in several ways. In most instances, pain is a warning sign of injury, but labor pain is associated with a normal physiologic process. In other types of pain, greater intensity is often associated with greater injury. During labor, intensity increases as the woman approaches birth, which is the desirable and positive outcome. Although the pain of labor often begins without warning, once labor is established, it occurs in a predictable pattern with respite from pain between contractions. This characteristic is different from most other types of pain. Because it is predictable, the woman can prepare for and better cope with the pain.

Physiology and Characteristics of Labor Pain

Pain sensations associated with labor originate from different places, depending on the stage of labor. During the first stage of labor, the stretching required to efface and dilate the cervix stimulates pain receptors in the cervix and lower uterine segment. During the second stage of labor, the main source of pain is from pressure on the perineum and birth canal as the fetus descends.

Labor pain in the first stage of labor has characteristics similar to other types of abdominal pain. It is often diffuse in nature, occurs in the lower abdomen, and may be referred to the lower back, buttocks, and thighs. Women often describe contractions as wavelike, with some "waves" more powerful than others. The contraction begins as a sensation of cramping in the lower abdomen or lower back and gradually increases in strength to the peak of the contraction, and then it slowly subsides.

Women sometimes describe the pain of birth as the most extreme sensation of pain. Most women experience an intense sensation of burning in the perineum as the tissues stretch in response to the fetus pressing against them during descent. Often the sensation is so powerful that the health care provider can perform an episiotomy (cut into the perineum) without anesthesia and the woman does not feel it.

Factors Influencing Labor Pain

There are two general concepts related to pain that are helpful to understand: threshold and tolerance. The pain threshold is the level of pain necessary for an individual to perceive pain. Pain tolerance refers to the ability of an individual to withstand pain once it is recognized. Each woman has her own pain threshold and tolerance of pain. Each woman responds to labor in a unique way, and women report the experience of labor differently. In addition, with each subsequent birth, a woman experiences labor uniquely.

Many factors influence the pain of labor and birth, making it a multidimensional experience. These include both psychosocial and physiologic factors. Psychosocial influences include the level of the woman's fear and anxiety, her previous labor experiences or her knowledge about the birth process, her culture, and the circumstances surrounding the birth experience, such as whether the pregnancy is planned or unplanned, the child is wanted or unwanted, the birth is preterm or term, and if the fetus is living or dead.

Psychosocial factors can also influence the woman's perception of her pain. For example, the younger the woman, the more likely she is to report severe pain. Women bearing children for the first time also report more intense levels of pain. High levels of anxiety and fear correlate with high levels of perceived pain. A woman who is physically conditioned or a trained athlete usually reports lower levels of pain during labor and birth.

Physiologic factors directly related to the birthing process also affect the perception of pain. In general, the longer the labor, the more likely the woman is to report extreme pain. The woman also usually reports more pain when she is experiencing abnormal labor. Obstructed labor can result from fetopelvic disproportion and abnormal fetal positions, causing an increase in reported labor pain. When labor contractions are induced with oxytocin, women report them as extremely strong, intense, and lacking the gradual ebb and flow of naturally occurring contractions. Back labor is when intense discomfort, during and even between contractions, is felt in the woman's lower back instead of mostly in the abdomen. Back labor is usually perceived as being intensely painful, even excruciating. Some women report that back labor feels as if the back is literally breaking in two. When a woman experiences back labor, her pain may not completely resolve between contractions.

Caution!

Don't assume that the woman who reports severe pain has low pain tolerance. Always do a thorough assessment because pain that is not controlled with normal interventions may be a signal that the woman is experiencing a complication of labor or a medical emergency.

PAIN MANAGEMENT PRINCIPLES AND TECHNIQUES

There is no one "perfect way" to control labor pain. Each woman responds to the experience uniquely. Pain management during labor should be planned and implemented, keeping several principles in mind. These principles include interventions, safety, and involvement of the woman in her pain relief. The specific techniques used to manage pain can be divided into two major categories: nonpharmacologic interventions and pharmacologic interventions. Most commonly, a woman uses a combination of techniques to cope with labor. She may need assistance coping before medication is used or in conjunction with medication. Safety considerations for the woman and her fetus are an important part of the nursing care for both categories.

Principles of Pain Relief During Labor

Women identify being involved in their pain management and adequate control of their pain as important factors in their overall labor experience. Inform the woman of pain management options, and be supportive of the choices that she makes. Remember that the woman has the right to change her mind about the acceptability of any particular pain management technique at any time before or during labor.

Rarely is there a completely pain-free labor. Even when a woman plans for an **epidural**, pain medication given through a small catheter placed in the epidural space of the spinal column by an anesthesiologist or anesthetist, she frequently reports pain before the epidural is administered. Caregivers may underrate the severity of pain when compared with the woman's ratings. It is important to accept the woman's description of the severity of the pain, even when she may not appear to be in pain. Women often report that it is not the amount of pain they have during labor that contributes to a satisfactory birth experience but rather how their pain is managed.

Sensitivity and Understanding Go a Long Way

It is important to be nonjudgmental when assisting a woman coping with pain. Some nurses feel strongly that a woman should have a "natural" childbirth without medication. Other nurses don't understand why any woman would want to "suffer" through labor without an epidural. In both situations, the nurse is in danger of not providing the support that the laboring woman needs and deserves if the nurse influences the woman with personal opinions.

Cultural Snapshot

A woman's culture influences the way that she responds to pain. Some women are very vocal. They may cry or moan with pain. Some women display a stoic response to pain. They may be quiet or appear to be resting. Caregivers frequently underestimate the pain of both types of women. The woman who is vocal may be labeled a "difficult" client who does not handle pain well. The stoic woman may be labeled a "good" client. However, neither woman is likely to get the pain control that she needs unless the nurse does a careful pain assessment.

Ideally, the woman discusses labor pain management with her primary care provider during the pregnancy and attends prenatal classes. The woman who enters labor with realistic expectations usually copes well and reports a more satisfying labor experience than does a woman who is not as well prepared. Regardless of whether the woman is prepared or not, update the woman on what to expect during each stage and phase of labor, assist her in coping, offer pain management techniques as appropriate, and provide information and emotional support to her labor partner.

Nonpharmacologic Interventions

Almost every woman uses some type of nonpharmacologic pain intervention during labor, even when pharmacologic methods are used. There are numerous methods of nonpharmacologic pain relief. Some interventions are evidence based. Other interventions need more research to demonstrate efficacy. In general, the intervention that works for the woman is frequently the best one to use. Typically, a woman needs a variety of interventions throughout labor. As labor becomes more intense, the woman may need to switch to a different method of coping. For example, effleurage and distraction are often helpful in early labor, but not as effective in active labor and transition. Table 9-1 compares selected nonpharmacologic interventions.

Continuous Labor Support

Continuous labor support with a trained nurse or doula (a trained layperson, who supports and coaches a woman during labor) has been shown to be effective in increasing the coping ability of the laboring woman. Additional benefits include fewer requests for pain medication, fewer obstetric interventions, and a lower rate of cesarean delivery. Women do not experience the same benefit when nurses provide intermittent labor support, as is typical for busy labor and delivery settings. Prenatally, the woman can be given information on local doula services, particularly if the woman desires childbirth with minimal medical intervention.

Comfort Measures

The need for comfort measures during labor should not be underestimated. Mouth breathing during labor can lead to a dry mouth. Lip balm can help keep the lips hydrated during labor, whereas ice chips, lollipops, and clear liquids (if allowed) can be helpful to moisten the mouth.

Change linens soiled with perspiration or body fluids. Most facilities have pads to place under the buttocks to catch bloody show and amniotic fluid during labor. Explain to the woman that it will be impossible to keep her completely dry, but reassure her that you will change the pads frequently. Give perineal care with warm water after she uses the restroom and before changing the linens.

Relaxation Techniques

Relaxation is the objective of almost every nonpharmacologic intervention. When the woman becomes anxious or apprehensive, she tenses her muscles. This action can slow the labor process and decrease the amount of oxygen reaching the uterus and the fetus. When the woman maintains a state of relaxation during, and between contractions, she is actually working with her body to facilitate the labor process. Some of these relaxation techniques require training and practice before labor to be most effective; however, you can inform the woman and her partner about some of the basic techniques when she presents to the delivery suite, which will benefit her even without practice.

Patterned Breathing

In the past, childbirth educators encouraged the use of very structured breathing techniques for labor. Now the trend is to

TABLE 9-1 Comparison of Selected Nonpharmacologic Interventions for Relief of Labor Pain

INTERVENTION	EFFECTIVENESS TO RELIEVE LABOR PAIN	ADVANTAGES	DISADVANTAGES
Continuous labor support	• Highly effective throughout labor. May increase the woman's perception of personal control, a factor that correlates with higher satisfaction with the labor experience	• Low-technologic/high-touch intervention • Addresses the emotional and spiritual aspects of labor and birth	• Most busy labor and delivery hospital settings cannot provide this level of support for the laboring woman, so the woman must usually hire a doula if she desires continuous labor support
Patterned breathing	• Can be very effective when the woman has practiced before labor and has an attentive labor coach	• Does not require any special tools • Promotes relaxation • Basic patterns can be taught by the nurse when the woman presents in labor	• Requires training and practice before labor to be most effective
Imagery	• Can be very effective for some women	• Is noninvasive • Requires no special tools • Incorporates spirituality with the birthing process	• Requires discipline and practice to achieve maximum benefit • May not be appropriate for individuals with mental illness or history of emotional trauma
Effleurage	• Can be helpful during early labor to decrease the sensation of pain	• Is easy to learn and simple to perform • Does not require any special tools	• Is less effective during active labor as the contractions become more intense • Fetal monitor straps on the abdomen may interfere with the woman's ability to use this technique
Hydrotherapy	• Highly effective in promoting relaxation and decreasing the sensation of pain, especially during the first hour or two of use	• Many women find water very comforting during labor • Promotes relaxation	• Requires availability of a tub—equipment that is not always available in the hospital setting • May slow labor if used too early • The woman may notice decreased effectiveness over time
Hypnosis	• Carefully selected women can benefit from hypnosis during labor	• Requires no special tools • Promotes the woman's sense of control over her pain • Involves a holistic approach to labor	• Special training by a therapist is required • Can be expensive and may not be covered by insurance • Does not work for all women • History of psychosis is a contraindication
Water injections	• Very effective in relieving back pain during labor	• Can be administered by the nurse	• Invasive (requires an injection) • Not effective for abdominal discomfort associated with contractions
Acupressure and acupuncture	• Anecdotal reports suggest that these therapies may be helpful in reducing the pain of labor	• Addresses the holistic nature of labor and incorporates spiritual and emotional aspects • Acupressure is noninvasive	• Requires a trained practitioner to perform • Acupuncture is invasive and requires special needles

demonstrate basic principles of patterned breathing without emphasizing strict patterns. Frequently, the woman begins with a slow-paced breathing pattern. She maintains the slow-paced pattern until it is no longer working to enhance relaxation, and then she switches to a higher level. Table 9-2 describes the basic breathing patterns often taught in childbirth preparation classes.

All breathing patterns should begin and end with the woman taking a cleansing breath. A cleansing breath is a deep, relaxed breath that signals the woman to relax and provides deep ventilation. Encourage the woman to breathe through the nose or through the mouth, whichever is most comfortable and natural for her. If she uses mouth breathing, pay particular attention to measures to keep the mouth moist.

Breathing should be comfortable and should not cause the woman to hyperventilate. If she feels short of breath, she may need to take deeper breaths. If she notices a tingling sensation in her hands and around her mouth, she is probably hyperventilating. She should slow her breathing and breathe into her cupped hands or a paper bag until the tingling stops.

Attention Focusing

Many childbirth classes discuss methods of attention focusing, or concentration. Women attending Lamaze-oriented classes are encouraged to focus internally or externally, whichever is more effective. Bradley classes advocate an internal focus based on the belief that external focus distracts the woman from the job of "listening to her body" while laboring.

TABLE 9-2 Patterned Breathing Techniques for Labor

BREATHING PATTERN	DESCRIPTION
Slow-paced breathing	The woman takes slow, deliberate breaths while she focuses on maintaining a relaxed stance. She may use effleurage, music, or any technique that encourages relaxation while using slow-paced breathing. The rate is approximately 6–10 breaths per minute
Modified-paced breathing	The woman begins taking slow, deep breaths at the beginning of the contraction. She then increases the rate while decreasing the depth of respirations as she reaches the contraction peak, after which she slows the rate and increases the depth
Patterned-paced breathing or the "pant-blow" technique	This technique is similar to modified-paced breathing with the addition of a rhythmic pattern. The woman takes four light breaths and then blows out through her lips, as if she is blowing out a candle. The woman repeats this pattern through the peak of the contraction

Attention focusing, or concentration, helps the woman to work with her body, instead of panicking.

Another name for internal focus is imagery. Imagery is a technique used to help the woman associate positive thoughts with the birth process. The method engages the senses and promotes relaxation. The woman is encouraged to visualize a positive, healing situation during contractions. For example, some childbirth educators encourage the woman to visualize each contraction as a wave. As the contraction strengthens, the tide rises. As the contraction fades away, the tide ebbs. Or the woman may visualize her body opening and allowing the fetus to pass through. Sometimes, the woman visualizes herself at a favorite relaxing place, such as the beach or in a comfortable chair at a vacation cabin. Music used in association with imagery sometimes helps the woman focus and relax.

The woman who focuses externally opens her eyes and focuses on a picture, person, or object that is helpful to her. For example, one woman used a picture of her grandmother as her focus. As she looked into her grandmother's face during her contractions, she drew strength remembering that her grandmother had birthed 11 babies, all at home without medications. Another woman used a picture of a mountain she and her husband had climbed as her focus. As she labored, she remembered her feelings as she overcame the challenges of the ascent of the mountain and likened it to the challenge of her labor. Remembering the feeling of accomplishment when she reached the peak of the mountain, she felt strengthened knowing she would have a strong sense of achievement when she felt her baby slide from her body and held him in her arms. Focusing on sounds, music, voices, relaxation, and breathing may also benefit the laboring woman.

Movement and Positioning

Changing positions frequently can be helpful during labor. A mixture of ambulation, standing, and other positions helps the woman to tolerate early labor. Any position of comfort is acceptable, as long as the fetal heart rate stays within the normal range. If the woman wants to be on her back, be certain to place a pillow or a wedge under one hip to prevent supine hypotension. The woman may find a birthing ball to be helpful. The ball allows her to rock and move to a position of comfort. Women who ambulate and reposition themselves as needed during labor tend to report higher satisfaction levels with the birthing process. Figure 9-1 illustrates several positions the woman can try during labor.

Touch and Massage

Effleurage, a form of touch that involves light circular fingertip movements on the abdomen, is a technique the woman can use in early labor (Fig. 9-2). The theory is that light touch stimulates the nerve pathways to the brain and keeps them busy, thereby blocking the pain sensation. As contractions become stronger during active labor, effleurage becomes less effective. At that point, the woman can use deeper pressure. Pressure is applied with the hands directly over the area of greatest pain intensity, often above the pubic bone or on the upper thighs. Either the woman or a support person may apply the deep pressure.

Massage can be used throughout labor as a way to provide support and comfort and promote relaxation. If the woman is experiencing intense back labor, it is often helpful for the nurse or a support person to give the woman a massage over the lower back or to use a fist, palm of the hand, or a tennis ball to apply counterpressure (Fig. 9-3).

Hydrotherapy

Exposure to warm water during the first stage of labor, either by showering or bathing in a tub or whirlpool, can increase the comfort of the laboring woman, increase her ability to cope with uterine contractions, and reduce labor discomfort. For hydrotherapy, the water temperature should be at or slightly above the woman's body temperature. The woman's temperature should be monitored for hyperthermia, which could be a sign of infection. Recommendations are that the woman should not be in water longer than 2 hours, as this could increase labor pain after that time and possibly prolong labor, and that it is only for women who have uncomplicated pregnancies and are between 37 and 41 weeks' gestation (Caughey, 2019).

Hypnosis

Hypnosis helps some women relax, and it may decrease the pain of labor. The woman attends several sessions with a trained therapist during pregnancy. At each session, she learns how to induce a trancelike state that she can use during labor. The woman who does self-hypnosis during labor often reports it to be an effective form of pain

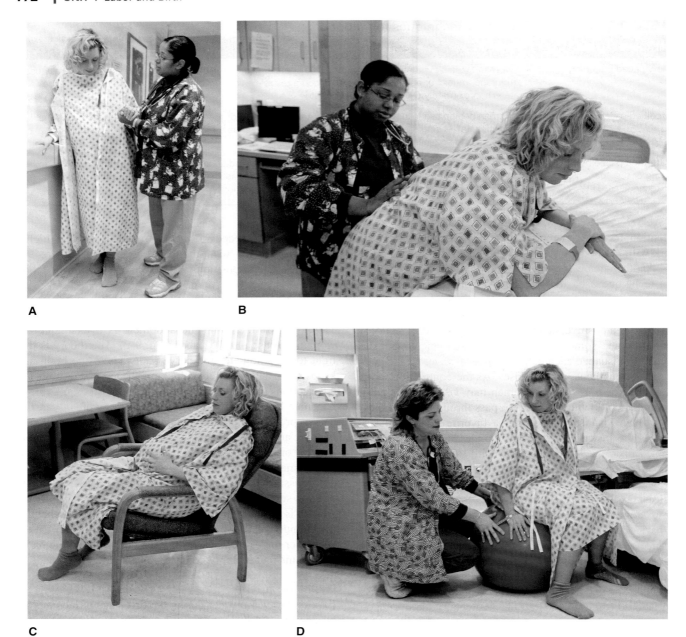

FIGURE 9-1 Various positions for use during labor: **(A)** ambulation, **(B)** leaning forward, **(C)** sitting in a chair, and **(D)** using a birthing ball.

management. Hypnosis is contraindicated for women with a history of psychosis (Caughey, 2019).

Water Injections

Subcutaneous or intracutaneous injections of sterile water can effectively relieve the pain of back labor. The RN administers four injections of 0.05 to 0.1 mL sterile water using a 25-gauge needle into the subcutaneous or intracutaneous tissue in the lower back (Fig. 9-4). Sterile water is used, not normal saline, as normal saline has not been shown to be effective. Important client information to provide before the procedure includes that the injections cause a significant stinging sensation for up to 1 minutes

after being placed and that pain relief generally lasts for 1 to 2 hours (Caughey, 2019). Injections may be repeated as needed.

Acupuncture and Acupressure

Acupuncture involves the use of placing needles at specific acupuncture points to decrease muscle tension, promote relaxation, and decrease the sensation of pain. Acupuncture must be done by a trained health care provider. Acupressure is noninvasive, with pressure applied at specific points using either the practitioner's fingertips or beads. Common acupressure points for controlling labor pain are on the tibia and the back of the hand.

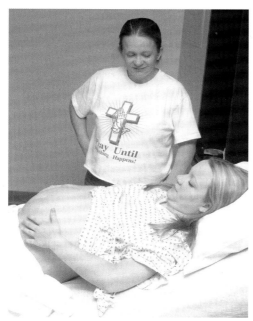

FIGURE 9-2 Effleurage. The woman uses her fingertips to lightly touch her abdomen using circular strokes. This form of light touch often decreases the sensation of pain in early labor.

TEST YOURSELF

✔ Name the two general principles of pain relief during labor.

✔ List three nonpharmacologic methods of labor pain management.

✔ Describe three relaxation techniques that help increase the woman's ability to cope with labor pain.

Remember Kayleigh Webber. What techniques for nonpharmacologic pain relief would you want to suggest if she had never been in labor before and had not prepared for childbirth? How would your approach be different if she had been through labor before? What signs would you observe for that would indicate she might need pharmacologic pain relief instead?

Pharmacologic Interventions

There is currently no perfect method to relieve the pain of labor. The ideal pharmacologic method would provide excellent pain relief and still allow the woman to freely change positions and ambulate and would not impair the woman's cognitive state. Additionally the ideal method would not cross the placenta and would not have potentially severe side effects on the fetus.

One reason women began to choose the hospital as a place to deliver their infant was for the pharmacologic pain relief methods that were available. The pendulum has swung back

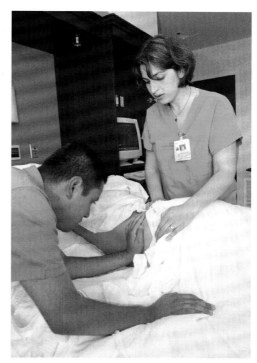

FIGURE 9-3 The woman's partner uses the palm of his hand to apply counterpressure to the woman's lower back.

and forth regarding the favor in which pharmacologic methods are viewed. In the 1950s, women were given strong medications that caused them to forget the pain of labor. Beginning in the 1960s and 1970s, women demanded to have more control and say over the birth process, and natural childbirth came into favor as the "best" way to experience labor and birth. Currently, many women choose to deliver in hospitals so that they can get pain relief with epidural analgesia or anesthesia.

It is important to understand the difference between analgesia and anesthesia, although the terms are sometimes used interchangeably. **Analgesia** is the use of medication to reduce the sensation of pain. **Anesthesia** is the use of medication to partially or totally block all sensation to an area of the body. Anesthesia may or may not involve loss of consciousness. Table 9-3 compares pharmacologic medications used to relieve labor pain.

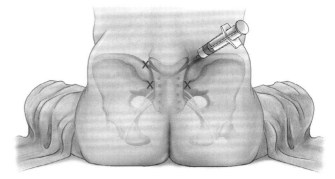

FIGURE 9-4 Location of intradermal water injections. The nurse administers four sterile water injections to relieve the pain of back labor.

TABLE 9-3 Comparison of Selected Pharmacologic Interventions for Relief of Labor Pain

MEDICATION CLASS	ADVANTAGES	DISADVANTAGES	ASSOCIATED SIDE EFFECTS
Sedative drugs	• Promote sleep in the early stage of labor • Decrease anxiety • Promethazine and hydroxyzine may be administered with an opioid to decrease nausea and vomiting • Nurse may administer	• May increase effectiveness of uterine contractions • Do not provide pain relief • Can produce neonatal respiratory depression if given within 12–24 hours of birth	• Excessive sedation and central nervous system depression • Decreased fetal heart rate (FHR) variability
Opioids (narcotic analgesic drugs)	• Increase the woman's ability to cope with uterine contractions • Nurse may administer	• Reduce but do not eliminate pain sensations • Associated with neonatal central nervous system and respiratory depression • May inhibit neonatal sucking and delay effective feeding • May decrease neonatal alertness	• Nausea and vomiting • Pruritus • Delayed gastric emptying • Dysphoria • Drowsiness • Hypoventilation • Decreased FHR variability • Neonatal depression
Paracervical block	• Provides excellent pain relief for the first stage of labor • Does not interfere with maternal mobility • Is an alternative when epidural block is contraindicated	• Requires multiple injections because the duration of pain relief is short • Cannot be used for pain relief in the second stage of labor • Rapidly crosses the placenta, which can lead to fetal central nervous system depression • Can cause constriction of the uterine artery, with resultant decrease in blood flow to the placenta • Is not used frequently because of the association with fetal bradycardia	• Fetal bradycardia
Epidural analgesia/anesthesia	• Provides more effective pain relief than opioid analgesia • Often completely eliminates pain sensation • Anesthesia can be continued for longer periods • If the woman needs a cesarean section, the epidural can be used to provide anesthesia, which saves time in an emergency situation	• Often impairs motor function, which decreases the ability to walk during labor • Women frequently require urinary catheterization • Increases the need for labor augmentation with oxytocin, particularly when administered before 5 cm of dilation (dilatation) • Increases the duration of the second stage of labor • Assisted delivery may be required (see Chapter 11) • Increases the likelihood of maternal fever, which can be confused with infection • Must be administered by an anesthetist or anesthesiologist • Requires complex nursing care	• Hypotension, which often requires administration of medication to raise the blood pressure • Maternal fever • Shivering • Itching (if opioids are used) • Inadvertent injection of anesthetic agent into the bloodstream • Accidental intrathecal puncture with possible postdural puncture (spinal) headache • Inadequate pain relief or failed block • Fetal distress
Intrathecal anesthesia (spinal block)	• Rapid onset of analgesia • Provides excellent pain relief • It is the anesthetic method of choice for planned cesarean birth	• A complete block results in the woman's lower extremities being temporarily paralyzed • Used alone for labor, the dose might wear off before labor is completed • Must be administered by an anesthetist or anesthesiologist • Requires complex nursing care	• Hypotension • Shivering • Postdural puncture (spinal) headache
General anesthesia	• Especially useful in emergency situations because total anesthesia can be accomplished rapidly • Provides total pain relief	• Requires intubation, which is more challenging during pregnancy • All agents used to induce and maintain general anesthesia cross the placenta and can cause severe neonatal depression	• Hypertension during intubation • Hypotension during maintenance • Difficult or failed intubation • Aspiration of stomach acid/contents • Malignant hypothermia • Uterine atony

Analgesia and Sedation

Sedation is a state of reduced anxiety or stress. Sedative drugs promote sedation and relaxation; however, they do not provide direct pain relief (analgesia). Barbiturates, such as secobarbital and pentobarbital, may be given in early labor to promote sleep. These medications can cause respiratory and central nervous system depression in the newborn if given within 12 to 24 hours of birth.

Opioids (also known as narcotic analgesic drugs) are medications with opiumlike properties and are the most frequently administered medications to provide analgesia during labor. Opioids are most commonly given by the intravenous (IV) route because this route provides fast onset and more consistent drug levels than do the subcutaneous or intramuscular routes. Opioids, such as meperidine, fentanyl, and morphine, are frequently ordered to assist the laboring woman to better tolerate labor pain, but each medication has its drawbacks as well. These include short duration of pain relief and the potential for maternal and neonatal sedation. The laboring woman must be observed for any side effects including oversedation, inadequate ventilation, or a rapid onset of delivery.

It is important to note that opioids cross the placenta and remain in the fetal circulatory system, which can cause changes in the fetal heart pattern. This can also cause side effects in the infant right after delivery including neonatal respiratory depression. All newborns born to mothers who received pain medication prior to delivery need careful monitoring during the neonatal transition period.

Be Very Careful!

Always warn the woman and her support person to call you before she tries to get up after receiving IV sedation. Women have fallen when attempting to ambulate after IV sedation and have even delivered their babies unattended in the bathroom because they mistake the urge to push for the need to have a bowel movement.

TEST YOURSELF

✔ What is the difference between analgesia and anesthesia?

✔ What is another name for opioids?

✔ Name two effects opioids have on the mother and newborn.

Anesthesia

There are three basic types of anesthesia: local, regional, and general. Local anesthesia is used to numb the perineum just before birth to allow for episiotomy and repair. Regional anesthesia can provide excellent pain relief during labor and birth and is the preferred type of anesthesia for nonemergent cesarean births. General anesthesia is reserved for emergencies in which the fetus must be delivered immediately to save the life of the fetus, mother, or both.

Regional Anesthesia

Regional anesthesia involves blocking a group of sensory nerves that supply a particular organ or area of the body. Local anesthetic agents and opioids are given to induce regional anesthesia/analgesia. The types of regional anesthetic agents that may be used during labor are pudendal block, epidural anesthesia, combined epidural/spinal anesthesia, and spinal block.

Any time an anesthetic agent is administered using any of the techniques described, there is a chance that the local anesthetic agent will inadvertently enter the bloodstream and cause a toxic reaction in the woman. This situation rarely occurs; however, be prepared to assist with a full resuscitation if one is needed. Every facility in which regional anesthetic agents are administered must have emergency equipment available. This includes oxygen, oral airway, emergency intubation equipment, cardiac monitoring, and emergency medications.

It is the nurse's role to assist the anesthesia provider and to monitor the woman and her fetus during and after administration of anesthesia. Most of these techniques require IV access. Monitor maternal vital signs and fetal heart rate frequently during the procedure. Maternal vital sign assessments should be continued until the woman is completely recovered from the effects of anesthesia.

Pudendal Block. A pudendal block is given just before the fetus is born to provide pain relief for the birth. The health care provider injects a local anesthetic agent bilaterally into the vaginal wall to block pain sensations to the pudendal nerve. A pudendal block can be helpful for instrument-assisted deliveries and for repair of an episiotomy or perineal tear. If an incomplete block occurs, the health care provider may have to inject additional local anesthesia for episiotomy repair. This method is not effective to relieve the pain of labor.

TEST YOURSELF

✔ List three types of regional anesthesia.

✔ Why is it critical for all facilities in which regional anesthesia is provided to have emergency equipment available?

✔ Describe the role of the nurse when a laboring woman receives anesthesia.

Epidural Anesthesia. Epidural anesthesia for the management of labor pain has become increasingly popular in the United States. This method usually provides excellent pain relief, often completely blocking pain sensation. The anesthesiologist or nurse anesthetist places a small catheter into the epidural space and then injects the catheter with local anesthetic agents or opioids to provide pain relief. Sometimes a one-time dose of medication is placed into the spinal fluid (in the subarachnoid space), which is called an **intrathecal** injection, in conjunction with epidural anesthesia. The advantage of the combined epidural/intrathecal technique is that the intrathecal dose is effective almost immediately. It provides pain relief until the epidural begins to work.

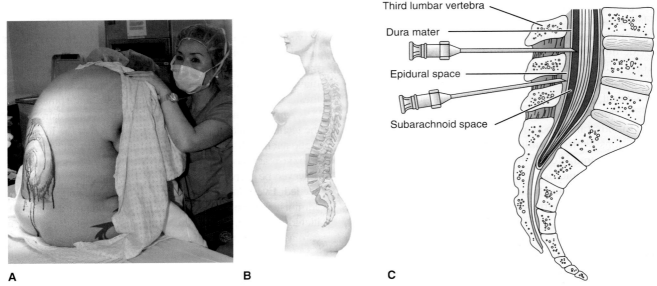

FIGURE 9-5 Epidural or intrathecal anesthesia. **A.** The laboring woman is correctly positioned for epidural anesthesia. **B.** Shaded area shows location of epidural placement. **C.** The different locations for an epidural and an intrathecal needle are shown.

Although its use is popular, epidural anesthesia is not without risk. There is significant risk of maternal hypotension that often requires treatment with vasopressors (medication to raise the blood pressure). Before a woman receives epidural anesthesia, an IV line must be in place. A 500- to 2,000-mL IV fluid bolus is given before the epidural is started to reduce the risk of hypotension. Because it is an invasive procedure, informed consent is required.

The anesthetist must evaluate the woman before placing an epidural. The anesthetist reviews the medical history and laboratory results and interviews the woman. They explain the procedure, answer the woman's questions, and obtain informed consent. Assist the RN, as directed, with vital signs and positioning the woman for epidural placement. The woman can be sitting up on the edge of the bed with her feet dangling or she may be side-lying. In either case, it is important for her to arch her spine because this position opens up the spaces between the vertebrae and allows for easier insertion of the catheter. The nurse holds the woman in position or assists the support person in doing so (Fig. 9-5A). The nurse monitors the woman's pulse and oxygen saturation continuously during the procedure. The blood pressure is also monitored every 3 to 5 minutes because of the potential hypotensive side effect from the epidural.

When the woman is in the proper position, the anesthetist prepares a sterile field with the supplies and medications that will be needed. The woman's back is prepared with alcohol and povidone-iodine. A local anesthetic agent is injected to numb the planned insertion area. The anesthetist inserts a special needle into the epidural space (just outside the dura mater, see Fig. 9-5C) and administers a test dose. The anesthetist questions the woman regarding how she feels and what she is experiencing to detect any adverse reaction. If there is none, the anesthetist proceeds to place the epidural catheter, remove the needle, and tape the catheter securely to the woman's back. At this point, assist the woman to a position

of comfort. If the woman desires to be on her back, place a wedge under the right hip to avoid supine hypotension. Assist the mother in changing positions as needed. The woman's safety is a prime nursing care focus when she has an epidural.

Once the epidural catheter is in place, the anesthetist may intermittently bolus the catheter when the woman begins to feel pain, or a continuous infusion can be set up and connected to the catheter. In either case, it is critical that the epidural catheter be clearly marked so that epidural medications are not administered inadvertently into the IV and vice versa. Management of the epidural is the role of the anesthetist. Monitor for and report any side effects such as hypotension, tinnitus, pruritus, nausea and vomiting, respiratory depression, fever, and fetal bradycardia.

After delivery, the RN stops the continuous infusion, removes the epidural catheter, and applies a sterile pressure dressing to the site. Nursing care during recovery from epidural anesthesia includes assessment of return of sensory and motor function to the lower extremities and monitoring for urinary retention. Instruct the woman not to ambulate without assistance. Allow the woman to dangle her legs for a while before she attempts to ambulate. Be available to provide immediate assistance if needed during initial ambulation attempts.

Intrathecal Anesthesia. Intrathecal anesthesia, also known as a spinal block, is similar to epidural anesthesia. The main difference is the location of the anesthetic agent. Instead of injecting local anesthesia and opioids into the epidural space, these medications are placed in the subarachnoid space into the spinal fluid (see Fig. 9-5C). This type of anesthesia is used most frequently for planned cesarean deliveries. The disadvantage to using a spinal block during labor is that the anesthetic drug might wear off while the woman is still in labor. Nursing care is similar to that provided for epidural anesthesia.

Complications Associated With Epidural and Intrathecal Anesthesia. Hypotension is the most frequent side effect associated with epidural or intrathecal anesthesia. As noted, prehydration with IV fluids helps prevent or decrease the severity of this side effect. Other symptoms associated with hypotension include maternal lightheadedness or nausea and fetal bradycardia from decreased utero-placental perfusion. If the blood pressure falls dramatically, ephedrine may be given intravenously to raise the blood pressure.

Total spinal blockade is a rare, but potentially fatal complication that can occur with epidural or intrathecal anesthesia. The condition results from inadvertent injection of a local anesthetic drug into the intrathecal space instead of the epidural space or from the anesthetic drug traveling too high up the woman's body, causing paralysis of the woman's respiratory muscles. Without immediate supportive care, respiratory and cardiac arrest will occur.

 A Personal Glimpse

I was 37 weeks pregnant with my first baby. I started to have some contractions while I was at work. Nothing big; I wasn't even sure they were contractions because they didn't hurt, but I was able to time them at 10 to 15 minutes apart. I went home at lunchtime and called my husband to tell him that I thought I was in labor. He hurried home to be with me. I stayed home the rest of the day and did some light housework. Around 6 PM, the contractions started to get more intense. I ran some warm water and soaked in the tub. It made me feel better for a while. My husband kept timing the contractions until they were 5 minutes apart. I called the hospital, and the nurse told me to come on in. We arrived at the hospital at about 8 PM. The nurse checked me and said I was at 4 cm and 95% effaced. The nurse suggested that we walk the hallways to speed things along. Sure enough, 45 minutes later, I was a good 5 cm. She asked me if I wanted anything for the pain, and I said no. I was hanging in there just fine. The pain wasn't as bad as I thought it would be. After approximately 45 minutes, the contractions became more intense, and I begged my husband to call the nurse. The nurse checked me, and I was 7 cm. By now, I was begging for an epidural. The anesthesiologist came in and asked me some questions and told me about some risks. I didn't care. I just wanted the epidural. I had to sit very still through several contractions while the doctor put in the epidural, but it was worth it because the pain went away right away. An hour after the epidural was inserted, I was dilated to 8 cm. I was very excited, but then I got stuck at 8 cm for several hours. The doctor thought that the epidural must have slowed down my labor. They were having a hard time monitoring my baby with the external device, so they had to insert an internal monitor. Then the nurse started me on Pitocin to help me progress. Sure enough, after an hour of Pitocin, I was completely dilated and ready to push. For me, pushing was the hardest part. I still felt no pain because of my epidural, so the nurse had to tell me when I was having a contraction so that I could start pushing. I threw up several times from pushing so hard. However, the baby just didn't come down. After 2 hours, I was totally exhausted. The nurse asked if I wanted her to call the doctor and have her

come and use the vacuum to help get the baby out. I was just so tired that I said yes. Elizabeth Michelle was born after just two pushes with the vacuum. She didn't cry at first, so the nurse rushed her to the warming table and gave her some oxygen. Then I heard the most beautiful sound in the world, a cry. My husband and I were thrilled. After the nurse dried the baby, I got to hold her for a while before they took her to the nursery. The baby weighed 7 lb (3,175 g) even, and was 19½ in. long. She was worth everything I went through to have her.

Laura

Learning Opportunity: *What nonpharmacologic measures could the nurse have offered Laura? Do you think these measures would have helped Laura's pain?*

Postdural puncture (spinal) headaches occur rarely because of advanced techniques and smaller needle sizes than those used in the past. A postdural puncture (spinal) headache is suspected when the woman has an intense headache in the upright position that is relieved when she lies down and is still. Without treatment, the postdural puncture (spinal) headache resolves in 7 to 10 days and symptomatic treatment of oral analgesic agents and caffeine can give temporary relief. An epidural blood patch provides lasting relief for severe postdural puncture (spinal) headache. In a procedure similar to that used to provide epidural anesthesia, the anesthesia provider injects 10 to 20 mL of the woman's blood into the epidural space to form a clot over the leakage site.

When narcotic drugs are used in addition to anesthetic agents, pruritus is a common side effect. Most women tolerate the itching, particularly because the pain relief is generally excellent for the first 24 hours after surgery. Nalbuphine, an opioid agonist–antagonist; naloxone, an opioid antagonist; and diphenhydramine, an antihistamine drug, are medications that may be ordered to treat severe pruritus.

Respiratory depression is another possible side effect when narcotic drugs are used for spinal and epidural anesthesia. For this reason, naloxone should be readily available at all times. Sometimes the anesthesiologist may order continuous pulse oximetry for the first 24 hours. In all cases, it is prudent to take vital signs and to check on the woman at least every 15 minutes for the first hour and then every 2 hours during the first 24 hours after spinal or epidural narcotic drugs have been administered.

The woman who has epidural or intrathecal anesthesia should be monitored for urinary retention and may need urinary catheterization if she is unable to void.

General Anesthesia

General anesthesia is not used frequently in obstetrics because of the risks involved. The pregnant woman is at higher risk for aspiration. It requires more skill to intubate a pregnant woman because of physiologic changes in the trachea and thorax. In addition, general anesthetic agents cross the placenta and can result in the birth of a severely depressed neonate who requires full resuscitation. Because of these risks, general anesthesia is only used in emergent cases where delivery of the fetus must be done quickly.

When general anesthesia is to be used, the anesthetist usually orders preoperative medications to reduce the risk of harm should aspiration occur. Sodium citrate 30 mL may be given orally if there is time. IV antacid drugs often are given before surgery.

The anesthetist may use an inhalation agent, an IV agent, or more commonly both to induce anesthesia. The woman is preoxygenated with 100% oxygen and then rapidly anesthetized. The RN gives cricoid pressure (pressure with the thumb and forefinger over the cricoid cartilage in the trachea), which closes off the esophagus and decreases the risk of aspiration. Cricoid pressure is maintained until the woman is intubated and the cuff inflated. The anesthetist then manages the airway and continues to administer anesthetic agents and muscle relaxants as needed throughout surgery. Every attempt is made to deliver the fetus as quickly as possible after the woman is anesthetized to avoid neonatal depression. Be prepared to assist in resuscitating the newborn, if necessary.

When the surgery is completed, the anesthetist removes the endotracheal tube when the woman is awake and has regained her protective reflexes (swallowing and gagging). The woman is transported to the postanesthesia care unit. The RN completes a full assessment; administers oxygen; and monitors oxygen saturation, vital signs, and the continuous electrocardiogram. The RN must be especially vigilant to monitor for hypoventilation after general anesthesia.

Malignant hyperthermia is a rare but potentially life-threatening complication of general anesthesia. It is an inherited condition that causes sustained muscle contractions in the presence of certain anesthetic agents. For this reason, a thorough history is important before general anesthesia is given. Ideally, a pregnant woman with a family history of malignant hyperthermia is identified in the prenatal period so the health care team can be prepared to care for the woman if general anesthesia becomes necessary. In these cases, it is best for the woman to receive epidural anesthesia during labor. This practice allows for safe anesthesia if a cesarean delivery is required. For planned cesarean delivery, the woman usually receives spinal anesthesia.

Be alert to the development of signs and symptoms of malignant hyperthermia. Early signs include severe muscle rigidity, tachycardia, irregular heart rhythm, decreased oxygen saturation, and cyanosis. Body temperature can rapidly increase to lethal levels; however, this may be a late sign. Dantrolene sodium given intravenously is the drug of choice to treat malignant hyperthermia.

Postoperative nursing care of the woman who receives general anesthesia is similar to that of the woman who receives regional anesthesia. However, careful assessment for hypoventilation and uterine atony are indicated.

TEST YOURSELF

✔ Describe the nursing care for the laboring woman who has been given an epidural.

✔ Identify safety measures that need to be taken with a client who has an epidural.

✔ List the side effects to monitor/assess for with a client who has epidural or spinal anesthesia.

✔ What interventions are implemented when hypotension is noted after an epidural is placed?

Nursing Process and Care Plan *for the Woman in Labor*

Nurses are in a unique position to impact the woman's labor experience. Women report a positive labor experience when they are included in their pain management plan and when they receive support during labor. Providing the laboring woman with relaxation techniques, pain management efforts, and safety considerations remain the primary nursing care focus throughout the labor.

Assessment (Data Collection)

Ongoing data collection and pain assessment is an essential component of nursing care for the laboring woman. When collecting data, alert the RN or the health care provider of any data that deviate from the woman's baseline.

Ask if she has any preferred methods of relaxation or pain relief. Use a standardized scale (e.g., 1 to 10 pain scale or a face type scale) to measure her pain. Be alert to nonverbal signs of pain such as facial expressions, tensing of her body, clenching hands or jaw, and holding her breath. Consider the woman's culture before using loud vocalizations or silence as measures of pain. Observe for signs of anxiety.

Determine her education level and knowledge of labor and birth. If she has had previous labors, inquire about the length of the labor, any pain relief measures and medications she used, and if there were any complications. Ask if she has attended birth preparation classes with this pregnancy or in the past. Ask if she has a birth plan written; if she does, make sure a copy of it is placed in her medical record.

Vital signs should be taken when the woman is not having a contraction, as the contraction can elevate all vital signs. Observe her breathing pattern during contractions to make sure she is not hyperventilating. Pay close attention to maternal blood pressure. Monitor for danger signs of pregnancy (see Box 7-3). Vital signs will need to be taken after pain medication is administered. Blood pressure should be monitored before, during, and after and epidural is placed.

Observe the woman's contractions for frequency, duration, and intensity (see Figure 8-10). Observe her contraction pattern (see Chapter 10) and report any nonreassuring patterns to the RN and birth attendant. Observe for signs of fetal well-being. These observations include obtaining fetal heart tones and monitoring fetal movement.

Gather information about her support system. Find out who will be with her during labor and also during the birth. Do not assume her labor support person will also be present during the actual birth. If she is alone during the labor and birth, be sure to provide her support.

Safety of the laboring woman should be continuously assessed. During labor, interventions that help to reduce her pain could also put her at a safety risk. Someone should walk with her as she ambulates so she does not slip; if she needs assistance, they can call out for help. Hydrotherapy increases her risk for slips or changes in blood pressure. Medications can alter her level of consciousness or gait. Utilize side rails as appropriate while she is in bed. Provide assistance when she gets out of bed, ambulates, or uses the toilet. After an epidural or spinal anesthesia, be sure to assess her breathing, blood pressure, feelings of sensation in her legs, and any side effects such as pruritus or urinary retention.

Nursing Care Focus

When determining the focus of nursing care for the woman in labor, safety of both the woman and the fetus should always be primary. Also, consideration should be given to the woman's knowledge related to labor and any previous labor experiences she has had. It is also important to remember that the woman may be anxious about the labor even if this is not her first birth. Regardless of her prior experiences with birth or pain, her labor pain and her coping with that pain are to be assessed frequently. The woman's support person also needs to be included in the reinforcing of information and may also need support to continue to help the woman.

Outcome Identification and Planning

The woman and fetus not being harmed during labor is the primary goal of nursing care. Other important goals during this time include relieving anxiety, ensuring that the woman has the support she needs during labor, and ensuring the woman is provided with pain management options and coaching with techniques used. Nursing implementations should be directed at meeting these goals.

Nursing Care Focus

- Acute pain related to uterine contractions

Goal

- The woman will verbalize or demonstrate relief of pain.

Implementations for Acute Pain

Perform a pain assessment at least every hour during labor to include pain description, location, duration, and intensity. Assess the woman's pain using an appropriate, standardized pain assessment tool. Observe for nonverbal cues of discomfort, such as restlessness, muscle tension, or altered vital signs. A thorough pain assessment will evaluate the woman's response to current pain control methods and reveal the need for more intensive interventions to control the pain of labor. Severe, unrelenting pain may be associated with a complication of labor and be reported immediately to the RN or the health care provider. Inform the client about the phase of labor she is in and how long the pain can be expected to last. Encourage the client to verbalize if she needs a different pain management method.

Assess general comfort at least every hour. Note the condition of the woman's lips and offer lip balm as needed. Offer ice chips and lollipops, if allowed, to relieve complaints of dry mouth. Give perineal care as indicated, and change the under-buttock pad frequently. Change the linen when it becomes moist with perspiration or other body fluids. Mouth breathing during labor increases the drying of the oral mucosa, and comfort measures increase the ability of the woman to cope with labor. It is more difficult for the woman to cope if she has dry, cracked lips, dry mouth, and moist linens and if she feels uncomfortable with amniotic fluid and blood on her perineum. Adjust the environment as necessary. A too hot or too cold room temperature can alter the woman's comfort between contractions.

Assist the woman in changing positions frequently, and encourage her to assume a position of comfort. Position changes can help the woman to cope. If she remains "frozen" in one position, she is more likely to become tense, which increases the perception of pain. Position changes help with increasing blood flow and help decrease the risk of a deep vein thrombosis.

Provide nonpharmacologic comfort measures. Encourage the use of relaxation techniques. Reinforce the use of patterned breathing. Encourage the use of effleurage for as long as it is helpful. Encourage the use of counterpressure when effleurage is no longer helpful. The use of touch, such as effleurage and pressure, can interrupt the sensation of pain. Offer complementary therapies to increase comfort, such as a birthing ball or hydrotherapy, as appropriate. Allow alternative pain treatments that are culturally relevant to the client, if not contraindicated during labor.

Administer medications, as prescribed and with the woman's permission, to reduce pain; monitor for effect. Monitor vital signs and respiratory status frequently after administering pain medications. Remain supportive of the woman's decision to use pharmacologic methods for pain relief including requesting an epidural. The woman has the right to change her mind about pain relief interventions and to choose interventions that will best help her to cope. Reassure her support person that the woman's request for pain medication does not represent a failure on their part as her coach. Support the woman's labor support person. It is a common feeling that the coach may feel that they have somehow "failed" when pharmacologic interventions are requested, especially if the woman did not want medications going into labor.

If the woman has had an epidural placed, perform a pain assessment every 30 minutes after the epidural is placed. Report new complaints of pain to the anesthesiologist. New reports of pain may signal the need for a bolus of medication through the epidural catheter. Observe for a sudden increase in pain that is accompanied by a rigid hard uterus; these could be signs of a complication and need immediate evaluation by the RN or health care provider. Notify the RN or health care provider for any change in the woman's pain.

Evaluation of Goal/Desired Outcome

- The woman expresses that methods used help her to cope with pain from contractions.

Nursing Care Focus

- Injury risk

Goal

- The woman will not be injured during labor.

Implementations for Injury Risk

Assist the woman with mobility (getting out of bed, ambulation) and toileting as appropriate. Instruct her support person on the need to assist the woman and that it is for her safety. The labor support person or the nurse should be with the woman at all times during labor. This is for the woman's emotional comfort as well as physical safety. If the woman is left alone and falls, she and the fetus could be seriously injured. Instruct the woman to rise slowly from lying in bed to a standing position. The woman could have postural hypotension, which could increase her fall risk.

Institute safety measures and review them with the woman and her labor support person. This includes having the call light close to the woman, the bed in the lowest position, foot lighting on if she wants the room lights dim during labor, keeping the floors clear of debris, and side rails up when she is in bed. Socks may become wet with amniotic fluid or blood and could pose a slip hazard. Have her change socks if they are damp. The woman may choose to stand on a towel instead. Safety is a prime concern during hydrotherapy, especially when the woman is getting into or out of the tub/shower. Observe the woman for lightheadedness during hydrotherapy. The woman should never be left alone during hydrotherapy.

Monitor the woman's neurologic status. If the woman is hyperventilating during contractions, she is also at risk for fainting. Medications or hypotension can make her lightheaded and increase her risk for falling. Some medications may make her drowsy and have an unsteady gait. Times that are important for monitoring include after medications are given, after an epidural is placed, after rising from a lying position (especially if she had been lying supine), and when there is a rapid progression in her labor.

Turn the woman who has had epidural or spinal anesthesia at least every 2 hours. This will aid her comfort, promote blood flow, and prevent injury from pressure points. Use pillows between her knees and ankles. Ensure that side rails are up. The side rails are for safety and also help the woman with turning in bed. Be sure that her bed is free from debris that could increase pressure risk, such as medication caps; medical equipment such as a blood pressure cuff; or items that were used for comfort such as lip balm, glasses, and handheld fans.

Evaluation of Goal/Desired Outcome

- The woman does not fall or sustain an injury during labor.

Nursing Care Focus

- Hypotension risk

Goal

- The woman will maintain a blood pressure that does not drop below 90/60 mm Hg.
- The woman will maintain an oxygen saturation above 90%.
- The fetal monitor strip will remain above 120 with reactive patterns noted.

Implementations for Hypotension Risk

Assess vital signs when the woman first arrives to the labor and delivery unit. This will provide baseline data for comparison. Educate the client on the signs and symptoms of low blood pressure, including dizziness, lightheadedness, fainting, blurred vision, nausea, fatigue, or lack of concentration. Have the woman avoid lying supine. Instead have her side-lying or place a wedge under her hip. This will help to avoid supine hypotensive syndrome (see Chapter 6). Monitor intake and output, as ordered, and document accurate totals.

Assess vital signs and monitor the woman receiving IV fluids prior to an epidural placement.

Prehydration with IV fluids helps decrease the risk of hypotension. Monitor the blood pressure, pulse, and oxygen saturation every 3 to 5 minutes during an epidural. Frequent monitoring allows for early detection of changes that may indicate the development of a complication. Once the epidural catheter is taped in place, assist the woman to a side-lying position. The side-lying position enhances blood pressure and placental perfusion.

Monitor oxygen saturation with pulse oximetry. If the woman becomes hypotensive, the fetus is at risk for a decreased oxygen supply. A decrease in oxygen saturation should be immediately reported to the RN or health care provider and will be treated with supplemental oxygen, which will help prevent adverse fetal effects. Monitor fetal heart tones and reactivity. Monitoring is done to detect nonreassuring changes (see Chapter 10), which may indicate inadequate placental perfusion. Immediately report any nonreassuring fetal heart rates or contractions to the RN or health care provider.

Evaluation of Goal/Desired Outcome

- The woman's blood pressure did not drop below 90/60.
- The woman's oxygen saturation remained >90%.
- The fetal heart rate did not drop below 120 bpm and was without nonreassuring contraction patterns.

Remember Kayleigh Webber. She was experiencing pain with her contractions that were overwhelming for her. Kayleigh asks you if an epidural is a safe option for her. How would you respond? What assessments and nursing implementations would you need to make regardless of the type of medication she received?

KEY POINTS

- Labor pain differs from other types of pain because it is associated with a normal physiologic process, increases in intensity as the desired outcome (birth) approaches, and is predictable.

- Sources of pain during the first stage of labor are the thinning and stretching of the cervix in response to uterine contractions. Sources of pain during the second stage of labor are the stretching of tissues in the perineum as the fetus descends.

- Factors that influence the woman's experience of labor pain include her threshold and tolerance to pain, age, parity, anxiety level, culture, physical conditioning, length of labor, size and position of the fetus, induced versus natural labor, and whether the labor is dysfunctional.

- Major principles of labor pain management include the following: Women are more satisfied when they have control over the pain experience; caregivers commonly underrate the severity of pain; and women who are prepared for labor usually report a more satisfying experience than do women who are not prepared.

- Nonpharmacologic interventions to relieve labor pain include continuous labor support, comfort measures, various relaxation techniques, intradermal water injections, and acupressure and acupuncture.

- Relaxation techniques that help a woman cope with labor include patterned breathing, attention focusing, movement and positioning, effleurage, hydrotherapy, and hypnosis.

- Most nonpharmacologic interventions are noninvasive, address emotional and spiritual aspects of birth, and promote the woman's sense of control over her pain. Disadvantages include that many of the interventions require special training and practice before birth, and these methods are not effective for every woman.

- Analgesia reduces the sensation of pain. Anesthesia partially or totally blocks all sensation to an area of the body.

- Advantages of opioid administration during labor include an increased ability for the woman to cope with labor, and that the medications may be nurse administered. Disadvantages include short-term pain relief requiring frequent repeat doses of the medication and frequent occurrence of uncomfortable side effects, such as nausea and vomiting, pruritus, drowsiness, and neonatal depression; pain is also not eliminated completely.

- Types of regional anesthesia include pudendal block, epidural anesthesia, combined epidural/spinal anesthesia, and spinal block. A pudendal block provides pain relief for the birth. Epidurals provide pain relief during labor.

- Complications associated with epidural and spinal anesthesia include hypotension, maternal fever, pruritus, respiratory depression, urinary retention, and postdural puncture (spinal) headache.

- General anesthesia is risky for the pregnant woman because of the increased risk for aspiration. It is risky for the fetus because the medications cross the placenta and may result in severe neonatal depression that requires intensive resuscitation.

- Malignant hyperthermia is a rare, life-threatening complication of general anesthesia. Dantrolene sodium is the treatment of choice for malignant hyperthermia.

INTERNET RESOURCES

Nonpharmacologic Methods of Pain Relief During Labor and Delivery
https://www.mayoclinic.org/healthy-lifestyle/labor-and-delivery/in-depth/labor-pain/art-20044845

Medications for Pain Relief During Labor and Delivery
http://www.acog.org/Patients/FAQs/Medications-for-Pain-Relief-During-Labor-and-Delivery

Epidural Anesthesia
http://americanpregnancy.org/labor-and-birth/epidural/

Workbook

NCLEX-STYLE REVIEW QUESTIONS

1. A 22-year-old gravida 2, para 0 is in the health care provider's office for a checkup at 36 weeks' gestation. Which comment by the woman indicates that she needs additional information about pain relief during labor?
   a. "I have discussed pain relief options with the doctor and my childbirth educator."
   b. "I'm so glad that I won't have any pain because I'm going to have an epidural."
   c. "I've been practicing the relaxation exercises I learned in my childbirth class."
   d. "I want to have medications through the IV if the pain gets so bad that I can't handle it."

2. The labor nurse reports to the nurse on the oncoming shift, "The woman in labor room 2 is handling her pain very well. She smiles whenever I go in to talk to her, and she doesn't complain at all." What assessments by the oncoming labor nurse would best reveal if the offgoing labor nurse's observations were correct?
   a. Asking the woman to describe her pain and rate it on a scale of 0 to 10
   b. Observing for grimacing, moaning, and other nonverbal indicators of pain
   c. Taking the woman's vital signs and observing her interactions with visitors
   d. No additional assessments are indicated until the woman begins to report pain

3. A woman asks the nurse during a prenatal office visit, "What pain relief method is best during labor?" What answer by the nurse best answers the question?
   a. "Epidurals are best because they provide complete pain relief."
   b. "Most women need IV pain medications at some point during labor."
   c. "It is best to learn about the different types of pain relief available, as every woman experiences labor pain differently."
   d. "There is no one best way. However, natural childbirth is best for the baby."

4. A 34-year-old gravida 3, para 2 is experiencing severe back pain with each contraction. She is extremely uncomfortable and upset because she never had this type of pain with her other labors. What interventions are most likely to help in this situation?
   a. Comfort measures, intermittent labor support by the nurse, and reassurance that the pain is temporary
   b. Counterpressure with a fist or tennis ball to the lower back and water injections
   c. Effleurage, ambulation, and frequent position changes
   d. Hypnosis, imagery, and slow chest breathing

5. The nurse is preparing a woman for epidural anesthesia. The woman asks, "Why am I getting more IV fluids?" What reply by the nurse is best?
   a. "Don't worry. This is a routine procedure in preparation for an epidural."
   b. "I'll slow the IV down so you won't feel so cold."
   c. "IV fluids help prevent postdural puncture (spinal) headaches."
   d. "IV fluids help prevent the blood pressure from dropping too low."

6. Which of the following are complications from epidural anesthesia? (Select all that apply.)
   a. Hypotension
   b. Aspiration
   c. Pruritus
   d. Urinary frequency
   e. Respiratory depression
   f. Malignant hyperthermia

STUDY ACTIVITIES

1. Use the following table to compare advantages and disadvantages of pain relief methods for labor.

Method	Advantages	Disadvantages
Natural childbirth		
IV analgesia		
Epidural anesthesia		
General anesthesia		

2. Research the different nonpharmacologic pain relief methods used in labor. Develop a chart on these methods to present to a childbirth education class.

3. Interview the following caregivers in the community regarding their recommendations for pain relief during labor: a doula, a nurse-midwife, a family practice physician, and an obstetrician. What similarities did you find in their answers? In what ways did they disagree? Which argument did you find most convincing? Share your findings with your clinical group.

CRITICAL THINKING: WHAT WOULD YOU DO?

Apply your knowledge of pain management during labor to the following situation.

1. Betty, a 30-year-old gravida 1, reports that she wants to try natural childbirth.
   a. What recommendations will you make to increase the chances that she will be able to experience natural childbirth?
   b. About what will you caution her to decrease the likelihood that she will have unrealistic expectations about pain relief during labor?

2. Betty presents to the labor suite in labor. She is 3 cm dilated, 90% effaced, and at −1 station. Her contractions are every 3 to 5 minutes apart and of moderate intensity.
   a. What nonpharmacologic pain interventions are most helpful at this point in Betty's labor?
   b. Several hours later, Betty is 5 cm dilated, 100% effaced, at 0 station. She is requesting IV analgesia. How will you reply?
   c. When Betty reaches 8 cm, she is screaming at the peak of contractions. She says, "I can't stand the pain anymore. I want an epidural." How will you reply?

Nursing Care During Labor and Birth

10

Key Terms

accelerations
amnioinfusion
early deceleration
electronic fetal monitoring (EFM)
episodic changes
late decelerations
lochia
open-glottis pushing
periodic changes
spontaneous rupture of
   membranes (SROM)
urge-to-push method
uteroplacental insufficiency
variability
variable deceleration
vigorous pushing

Learning Objectives

At the conclusion of this chapter, you will:

1. Discuss assessments and procedures the nurse performs during the woman's admission to the hospital.
2. Describe external and internal methods for monitoring uterine contractions.
3. Compare and contrast advantages and disadvantages of intermittent auscultation of fetal heart rate (FHR) with those of continuous electronic fetal monitoring.
4. Compare and contrast advantages and disadvantages of external fetal monitoring with those of internal fetal monitoring.
5. Explain how to apply the external fetal monitor.
6. Identify the role of the licensed practical/vocational nurse (LPN/LVN) in the interpretation of FHR patterns.
7. Define three major deviations from the normal FHR baseline.
8. Differentiate between early, variable, and late decelerations with regard to appearance, occurrence in relation to uterine contractions, causes, and whether the pattern is reassuring or nonreassuring.
9. Outline appropriate nursing interventions for each major periodic change: early, variable, and late deceleration patterns.
10. Describe common symptoms seen in each stage of labor.
11. Identify nursing interventions for each stage of labor.

Lidia Chu is a 23-year-old primigravida. She arrives at the labor and delivery unit stating she is in labor. For the intake assessment, you need to gather data about her and her pregnancy. What information do you need to gather? What would be your priority questions? Based upon the information you collect, the registered nurse asks you to admit her to a labor, delivery, and recovery room.

The onset of labor begins the transition from pregnancy to motherhood and the transformation of the fetus to a newborn. The woman experiences the process in many dimensions, including physiologic, psychological, social, and spiritual, and no woman's labor experience is identical to another's. When the powers, passageway, passenger, and psyche work together, the miracle of birth progresses in an orderly and predictable sequence.

The role of the licensed practical/vocational nurse (LPN/LVN) in labor and delivery is to provide care and support to the laboring woman under the supervision of a registered nurse (RN). You must have a basic understanding of the processes of labor and birth to provide care

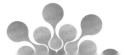

to the woman and her family. It is important for you to be able to recognize deviations from the "normal" or expected sequence of labor and birth and to report deviations immediately. Your understanding will also help you answer the woman's and her support person's questions regarding labor and birth. Although you may not independently perform many of the procedures and assessments described in this chapter, a basic understanding of these procedures and assessments is necessary to effectively assist the RN or health care provider.

The role of the obstetric nurse is central to the care of the laboring woman and her family. You facilitate the labor process and ensure safe passage of the laboring woman and fetus through this critical life event. To be an effective obstetric nurse, you must maintain an attitude of acceptance of the woman's preferences during labor and birth, utilize supportive actions, and develop keen observation skills to detect subtle changes in maternal or fetal status.

Although labor and birth are normal physiologic events, you must be prepared to recognize and report complications that may arise during the process. It is also critical to be prepared to give intensive support to the laboring woman and her birth partner.

Every woman's labor is unique, and if a woman bears more than one child, she experiences each birth differently. This chapter focuses on the nursing care of a woman undergoing normal progression of labor and birth for the first-time who does not experience complications. Common deviations associated with the nursing care of the multiparous woman are noted. For purposes of this chapter, it is assumed that the delivery environment is a labor, delivery, and recovery (LDR) room in a hospital setting. Similar nursing interventions apply to other settings, and the labor process is the same regardless of the environment in which birth occurs.

THE NURSE'S ROLE DURING ADMISSION

The woman may present to the birthing suite at any phase of the first stage of labor. Therefore, it is important to monitor birth imminence, fetal status, risk factors, and maternal status immediately. If birth is not imminent and the fetal and maternal conditions are stable, perform additional data collection including the full labor admission health history, a complete maternal physical assessment, the status of labor, and any labor, birth, and cultural preferences the woman may have.

Immediate Assessments
Birth Imminence
Observing for signs that birth is imminent begins from the moment the woman arrives in the labor and delivery unit. If the woman is inwardly focused and stops to breathe or pant with each contraction, you can infer that she is in an advanced stage of labor. In addition, if the woman makes statements such as

"I feel a lot of pressure," "The baby is coming," or "I want to have a bowel movement," it is likely the woman is in the second stage of labor, and the fetus will be born soon. Other signs that birth is imminent include sitting on one buttock (if the woman presents to the unit in a wheelchair) and bearing down or grunting with contractions. When any of these signs is present, it is prudent to quickly move the woman to a labor bed, assist the RN in performing a vaginal examination if the presenting part is not yet visible, and be prepared to assist with the birth.

Nursing Judgment is in Order!

If the woman presents to the hospital in an advanced stage of labor and it appears that delivery is imminent, the admission history and physical is abbreviated to focus on current status. The history can be completed later, even after delivery, if necessary.

Precipitous Delivery
Rarely, you may be the only person available to assist delivery of the fetus. Figure 10-1 shows the steps to follow for an emergency birth. Call for help. There may not be time to perform all the steps listed. Do the best you can with the time and equipment available. Instruct the woman to remain calm and reassure her that you know what to do to assist with the delivery. Instruct her to blow out through her lips in little puffs (as if she were blowing bubbles) so that she will not forcefully expel the fetus in an uncontrolled manner. Then follow the steps in Figure 10-1 to assist with the birth.

Once the neonate delivers, it is not necessary to cut the cord immediately. However, in most facilities, the protocol is to double clamp the cord soon after birth, and then cut between the clamps. Dry the newborn thoroughly to prevent heat loss. Place the newborn under a radiant warmer for resuscitation, or place in skin-to-skin contact with the woman and cover them both with a blanket.

If signs of placental separation occur (a gush of blood, lengthening of the cord at the introitus), allow the placenta to deliver and then massage the uterus to help it contract. Another way to prevent excessive blood loss immediately after delivery of the placenta is to place the newborn to the woman's breast. The suckling action of the newborn will stimulate the woman's body to release oxytocin, which helps her uterus to contract and control bleeding.

Fetal Status
When the woman arrives at the hospital, determining fetal status is a priority nursing intervention. This can be done by placing the woman on a fetal monitor for continuous monitoring, or to check the fetal heart rate (FHR) by fetoscope or by Doppler ultrasonography for the low-risk woman. The FHR should be strong and regular, with a baseline between 110 and 160 beats per minute (bpm) with no late decelerations and should remain so throughout all phases and stages of labor. See "The Nurse's Role: Ongoing Assessment of Uterine Contractions and FHR" section for in-depth information on assessment of FHR.

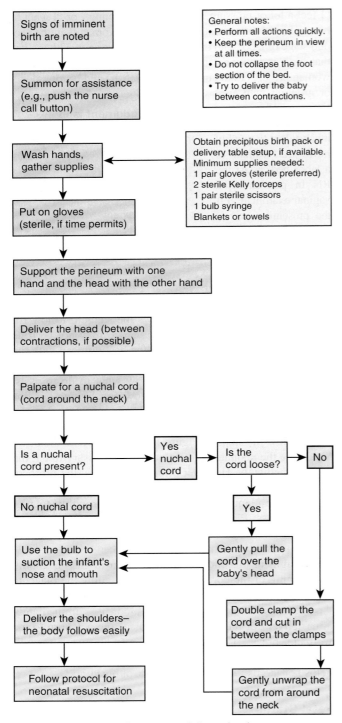

General notes:
- Perform all actions quickly.
- Keep the perineum in view at all times.
- Do not collapse the foot section of the bed.
- Try to deliver the baby between contractions.

Obtain precipitous birth pack or delivery table setup, if available. Minimum supplies needed:
1 pair gloves (sterile preferred)
2 sterile Kelly forceps
1 pair sterile scissors
1 bulb syringe
Blankets or towels

FIGURE 10-1 Emergency delivery by the nurse.

Risk Assessment

Another initial nursing intervention is determining the status of the membranes (some women refer to this as the "bag of waters"). Some women will say, "My waters broke." Signs indicating that the membranes have ruptured include reports by the woman of a gush or continual leaking of warm fluid from the vagina. This is referred to as **spontaneous rupture of membranes (SROM)**. Sometimes the woman will report intermittent leaking of fluid, and it may be unclear if the membranes have ruptured. In this instance, it is important to look for objective signs of rupture. The RN may use a speculum to check for pooling of fluid in the vagina and test the fluid using the Amnisure ROM™ test. If Nitrazine paper is used to check the fluid, amniotic fluid has a pH of 7.0 to 7.7. If the status of the membranes is still in doubt, a fern test may be performed. The RN collects a fluid sample and smears it on a slide, which is then examined under a microscope. If a ferning pattern is seen, the fern test is positive, and membrane rupture is confirmed.

Other important characteristics of the amniotic fluid to observe include the color, odor, amount of fluid, and the time of rupture. The fluid should be clear and without a foul odor. If several hours have passed since the membranes ruptured, assess the woman for signs of infection, such as elevated maternal temperature, cloudy or foul-smelling fluid, and fetal tachycardia. Report the findings to the RN. Green amniotic fluid signals the presence of meconium in the amniotic sac and may indicate that the fetus is distressed. This finding must be reported to the RN and the health care provider immediately. Box 10-1 summarizes the nurse's role in monitoring the status of the membranes.

Observe for vaginal bleeding. The presence of bloody show is an expected finding, but heavy bleeding (heavier than a normal menstrual period) or bright red blood is not normal. Immediately report the bleeding to the RN or the charge nurse along with the FHR. In addition to the amount of bleeding, note other important characteristics, such as color (dark or bright red), amount and type of associated pain (abdominal or back pain, uterine tenderness), and time that the bleeding began.

It is important to ask the woman if she experienced any problems with this pregnancy, such as preterm labor, high blood pressure, or gestational diabetes. Determine if any prenatal fetal assessment tests were done and if any complications were diagnosed. Verify the expected due date and the current fetal gestational age. Ask if there were any complications in previous pregnancies. Establish the approximate number of times the woman saw the health care provider for prenatal care and during what month of pregnancy prenatal care began.

Each of these observations is important to determine if risk factors are present that might require a specialist to be present at the delivery.

Maternal Status

A quick physical assessment of the woman's status upon admission to the hospital is crucial. Document the woman's vital signs, including temperature, pulse, respiration, and BP, and observe for signs of infection, hypertension, or shock.

Some Nurses Find This Approach Helpful!

Bleeding can be scary to the pregnant woman. If the woman presents to the labor unit complaining of bleeding, ask her how many times she has changed sanitary napkins. Her answer will help you determine the approximate amount of bleeding.

BOX 10-1 Monitoring the Status of Membranes

- Observe for spontaneous rupture of the membranes.
- Assist when the birth attendant performs an artificial rupture of the membranes.
- Observe the color of the fluid (should be clear); report green or cloudy fluid.
- Document time and method of rupture, characteristics and amount of the fluid, and FHR pattern.
- Monitor for signs of umbilical cord prolapse (see Chapter 18) immediately after the membranes rupture, when the risk for prolapse is greatest.
  - Continue ongoing fetal assessments because prolapse can occur any time after the membranes have ruptured.

Additional Assessments

Maternal Health History and Physical Assessment

The labor admission health history is part of the initial assessment and includes an obstetric history, determination of current labor status, the woman's medical–surgical and social histories, desired plans for labor and birth, and desires/plans for the newborn. Box 10-2 lists examples of a labor admission health history. Review the prenatal record, if available, to obtain baseline vital signs and weight and to identify other pertinent information.

> **This is Critical to Remember!**
>
> Always perform a quick assessment to determine if the woman has signs of preeclampsia, a serious complication of pregnancy. Immediately report BP greater than 140/90 mm Hg, brisk reflexes or presence of clonus, protein in the urine, edema of the hands or face, sudden weight gain, or if the woman reports headache, visual disturbances, abdominal or epigastric pain, or demonstrates a change in level of consciousness (LOC).

Obtain the woman's current weight and compare it with her most recent weight (Fig. 10-2). Sudden weight gain indicates fluid retention and may signal the onset of preeclampsia (see Chapter 17). Measure vital signs, which should be similar to the woman's baseline. It is normal for the pulse to increase slightly during labor, but the BP, measured during the relaxation phase of a contraction, should not be elevated. Collect a urine specimen to screen for the presence of protein, ketones, glucose, blood cells, or bacteria.

Gather data from a head-to-toe physical assessment. Critical measurements include lung sounds, the presence or absence of right upper quadrant (RUQ) pain or tenderness, brisk deep tendon reflexes (DTRs), clonus, and amount and location of any edema. These observations should be reported to the RN or health care provider right away.

Labor Status

Document the woman's contraction pattern to include frequency, duration, and intensity (see "The Nurse's Role: Ongoing Assessment of Uterine Contractions and FHR" section for in-depth information on monitoring uterine activity).

BOX 10-2 Components of the Labor Admission Health History

Obstetric History
- Number and outcomes of previous pregnancies in GTPAL (gravida, term, preterm, abortions, living) format (see Chapter 7 for a detailed explanation of these terms)
- Estimated delivery date
- History of prenatal care for current pregnancy
- Complications during pregnancy
- Dates and results of fetal surveillance studies, such as ultrasound or nonstress test (NST)
- Complications, if any, with previous labor and delivery

Current Labor Status
- Time of contraction onset
- Contraction pattern including frequency, duration, and intensity
- Status of membranes
- Presence of bloody show or bleeding
- Fetal movement during the past 24 hours

Medical–Surgical History
- Chronic illnesses
- Current medications (including prescribed, over the counter, and herbal remedies)

Social History
- Support system
- Domestic violence screen
- Cultural/religious considerations that affect care
- Amount of smoking during pregnancy
- Drug and alcohol use during pregnancy

Desires/Plans for Labor and Birth
- Presence of a partner, coach, or doula
- Pain management preferences
- Presence of a birth plan
- Plans for feeding—breast or formula

The health care provider or RN will determine fetal lie, presentation, attitude, position, and station when the laboring woman first presents to a birthing facility. This process begins with Leopold maneuvers (Fig. 10-3). Fetal presentation, position, and attitude often can be determined using this technique.

The initial vaginal examination is done by the birth attendant, or in some facilities by the RN, to assess dilation and effacement of the cervix and to determine specific information regarding the fetal (passenger) progress through the birth canal. The examiner can confirm presentation, position, attitude, and fetal station. This information helps the health care provider determine if the woman is in true labor.

> **A Little Sensitivity is in Order!**
>
> If the woman is not in true labor and is discharged home, she may feel embarrassed or upset. Reassure her that it is normal for a woman to present to the hospital before she goes into true labor. Instruct the woman when to return to the hospital, and encourage her to call with concerns or questions.

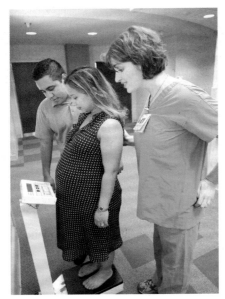

FIGURE 10-2 The nurse measures the woman's weight during the admission process to labor and delivery. (Photo by Joe Mitchell.)

The LPN assists with vaginal examinations but does not perform them. There is no firm rule that establishes how frequently vaginal examinations should be performed during labor; however, the best practice is they should only be done when necessary. Because vaginal examinations are invasive, performing them frequently increases the risk for infection; therefore they should be performed using sterile technique. The RN observes for cues that labor is advancing, so that vaginal examinations are done only as is necessary to evaluate labor progress. A vaginal examination may be done prior to pain medications being administered, when the amniotic sac ruptures, if the woman has an urge to push, or for the sudden onset of deep variable decelerations. Record the results of the vaginal examination in the woman's clinical record.

Be Very Careful!

Vaginal examinations should never be done if the woman presents with bright red painless bleeding until placenta previa (see Chapter 17) is ruled out.

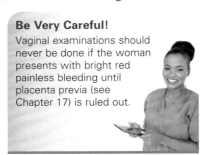

Labor and Birth Preferences

One very important part of the admission intake is to determine if the woman and her partner have special requests for labor and birth. Some women go to great lengths to plan the birth. Ask if the woman has a written birth plan. Ideally, she has reviewed the plan with her birth attendant well ahead of time, and the birth attendant has approved the document. Read the plan and notify the RN of the contents. Birth plans often contain preferences regarding practices related to mobility during labor, intravenous (IV) fluids during labor, episiotomy, presence of friends and family at the birth, fetal monitoring, pain management, and food and fluids during labor.

Many women do not have written birth plans. However, it is important to ask the woman specific questions regarding her preferences and needs. What expectations does she have about the labor process? How does she expect her pain will be managed? Did she attend childbirth class? Does she want to try natural childbirth? What individuals, if any, does she want in the delivery room with her? It is important to reassure her that she can change her mind at any time. If some of her requests are outside the normal protocols and procedures used at the facility, inform the RN or the health care provider.

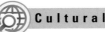

Cultural Snapshot

A woman's culture has a tremendous impact on the type and quantity of support she needs and also on her methods of coping during labor. Some cultures frown on the presence of men during the labor and birth process. In these cases, it would be counterproductive for the nurse to encourage the man to be the support person.

Ask the woman to identify who should provide support. Inquire regarding the relationship of the support person to the woman. Ask the woman to identify any special methods that might help her cope with labor. This information will help you individualize care while taking into account the woman's culture.

Performing Routine Admission Orders

After the admission history and assessment is completed, a full report is given to the health care provider. Sometimes additional observation is ordered to determine if the woman is in true labor or if she should be sent home to wait until active labor ensues. If the woman is to be admitted, admission orders may include some type of IV access be inserted to allow for medication administration or a fluid bolus. Some health care providers and facilities do not routinely insert an IV as part of the admission procedure.

Laboratory studies are often part of the routine labor admission orders, especially if the prenatal record is unavailable or the woman has not had any prenatal care. Compare the results with the prenatal record to determine if changes have occurred during pregnancy. For example, a VDRL or RPR serology test is drawn to determine if the woman has

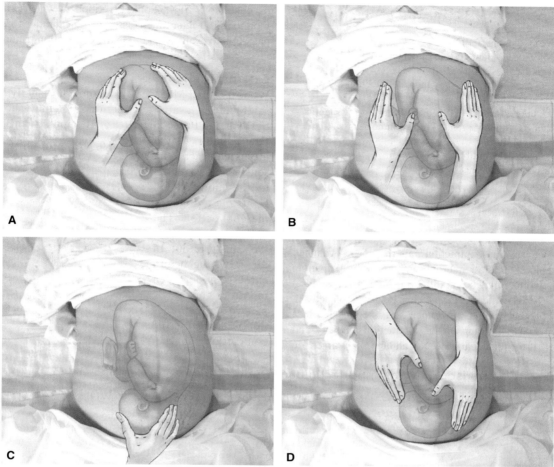

FIGURE 10-3 Leopold maneuvers, a noninvasive method of assessing fetal presentation, position, and attitude. This technique can also be used to locate the fetal back before applying the fetal monitor. **A.** Determining presentation. Stand beside the woman, facing her. Place both hands on the uterine fundus and palpate the fundus. If the buttocks are in the fundus (indicating a vertex presentation), you will feel a soft, irregular object that does not move easily. However, if the head is in the fundus indicating a breech presentation, you will palpate a smooth, hard, round, mobile object. **B.** Determining position. Place both hands on the maternal abdomen, one on each side. Use one hand to support the abdomen while you palpate the opposite side with the other hand. Repeat the procedure so that you palpate both sides of the abdomen. Try to determine the location of the fetal back and extremities in relationship to the maternal pelvis. The back will feel hard and smooth, and the extremities will be irregular and knobby. **C.** Confirming presentation. Place one hand over the symphysis pubis and attempt to grasp the part that is presenting to the pelvis between your thumb and fingers of one hand. In the vast majority of cases, you will feel a hard, round fetal head. If the part moves easily, it is unengaged. If the part is not movable, engagement probably has occurred. If the breech is presenting, you will feel a soft, irregular object just above the symphysis pubis. **D.** Determining attitude. Begin the last step by turning to face the woman's feet. Using the finger pads of the first three fingers of each hand, palpate in a downward motion in the direction of the symphysis pubis. If you feel a hard bony prominence on the side opposite the fetal back, you have located the fetal brow, and the fetus is in an attitude of flexion. If the bony prominence is found on the same side as the fetal back, you are palpating the occiput, and the fetus is in an attitude of extension.

developed a syphilis infection during pregnancy so that woman and newborn can be treated if necessary. Box 10-3 lists routine laboratory work for a woman admitted to the delivery suite.

TEST YOURSELF

✔ Name three signs that indicate that birth is imminent.

✔ List the four characteristics that must be charted regarding ruptured membranes.

✔ What information is important to gather regarding the woman's birth preferences?

THE NURSE'S ROLE: ONGOING ASSESSMENT OF UTERINE CONTRACTIONS AND FHR

It is important to assess uterine activity and fetal heart rate (FHR) frequently during labor. These assessments are necessary to determine adequacy of the labor pattern and to detect signs of fetal well-being or distress. Table 10-1 compares the advantages and disadvantages of each of the methods discussed in the text for monitoring both uterine contractions and fetal status during labor.

Monitoring Uterine Contractions

Evaluate the uterine contraction pattern every time you assess the FHR. See Box 10-4 for monitoring of the uterine

BOX 10-3 | **Admission Laboratory Studies**

- Complete blood count (CBC):
  - White blood cell count (WBC) may increase to 20,000/mm^3 with the stress of labor
  - Levels above 20,000/mm^3 may indicate infection
- Blood type and Rh factor
- Serologic studies, such as VDRL or RPR, to test for syphilis
- Rubella titer (not done if prenatal record indicates the woman is immune)
- ELISA to detect HIV antibodies
- Vaginal or cervical cultures (if indicated):
  - Gonorrhea
  - Chlamydia
  - Group B streptococci
- Urinalysis (clean-catch specimen)

contraction pattern. The contraction pattern can be evaluated using electronic external or internal methods or by palpation. The laboring woman may be monitored using **electronic fetal monitoring (EFM)** where a monitoring device is placed on, and secured to, the woman's abdomen and is connected to a machine that makes a graph of the contraction intensity and length as well as the fetal heart rate. Not all laboring women are

on continuous EFM. Some practitioners will use intermittent monitoring. If intermittent assessment techniques are used, use palpation to evaluate and time the contraction pattern.

External Methods

When using EFM, a tocodynamometer (usually referred to as "toco") measures contraction frequency and duration. See Nursing Procedure 10-1 on the application of external fetal monitor. As the uterus contracts, the sensor sends a signal to the monitor and prints out a graph of the contraction. The FHR is recorded on the same printout. In this way, the health care provider can monitor the FHR pattern in conjunction with the uterine contraction pattern.

Here's a Helpful Hint!

Here is a handy way to determine the intensity of uterine contractions by palpation. If the fundus feels like the tip of your nose at the peak of a contraction, the contraction is mild. If the fundus feels firmer, as when you touch your chin, the contraction is of moderate intensity. A fundus that cannot be indented, one that feels like you are pushing on your forehead, is indicative of a strong contraction.

TABLE 10-1 Comparison of Monitoring Techniques During Labor

TECHNIQUE	DESCRIPTION	ADVANTAGES	DISADVANTAGES
Intermittent fetal heart rate (FHR) auscultation	Fetoscope, Doppler, or fetal monitor used to periodically check FHR	• Noninvasive • Increases maternal comfort and mobility • Focus of health care provider is the laboring woman, rather than the technology	• Requires one-to-one nurse-to-client staffing ratios • Subtle signs of distress may be overlooked
Continuous external electronic fetal monitoring (EFM)	External transducer placed on maternal abdomen with straps to detect the FHR via ultrasound technology	• Noninvasive • Provides a continuous tracing of FHR • Allows for detection of signs of fetal compromise	• An active fetus or maternal movement can interfere with the continuity of the tracing • Generally confines the laboring woman to bed, unless telemetry unit is used
Continuous external monitoring of uterine contractions	External toco placed on maternal abdomen with straps to detect uterine contraction	• Noninvasive • Shows the frequency and duration of uterine contractions • Allows for comparison of FHR pattern with uterine contraction pattern	• Does not accurately depict the intensity of uterine contractions • Tends to be confining and limits maternal movement
Continuous internal electronic fetal monitoring (EFM)	Electrode is placed on the fetal scalp and connected to a reference electrode on the maternal thigh to record electrical activity of the fetal heart	• Allows for continuous monitoring of active fetus • Allows for more accurate recording of the FHR • Allows for continuous monitoring even if laboring woman is restless and changes positions frequently	• Invasive; requires that the membranes be ruptured and the cervix be at least partially dilated • Requires a specially trained health care provider for insertion • Increased risk for complications, such as chorioamnionitis, fetal scalp cellulitis, or osteomyelitis (rare)
Continuous internal monitoring of uterine contractions	Intrauterine pressure catheter inserted into a pocket of amniotic fluid to detect pressure changes within the uterus and record the contraction pattern	• Allows for more accurate determination of contraction intensity than external techniques • Useful for labors in which there is a risk for uterine rupture (e.g., previous uterine incision or induction with oxytocics)	• Invasive; requires that the membranes be ruptured and the cervix be at least partially dilated • Requires a specially trained health care provider for insertion • Increased risk for complications, such as chorioamnionitis

- Document baseline FHR, variability, accelerations, and any decelerations.
- Report fetal bradycardia or tachycardia, or any decelerations.
- Report tetanic contractions (those lasting longer than 90 seconds and of strong intensity) or failure of the uterus to relax between contractions.

Contraction frequency and duration are determined by palpation or by evaluating the EFM tracing. However, unless the woman has an internal uterine pressure catheter, you must palpate the contractions to evaluate intensity. As you will recall from Chapter 8 (see Fig. 8-10), the height of the contraction is an estimate of its intensity. However, many factors affect the height of the contraction on an external tracing. For example, a small woman with minimal adipose tissue may be having mild contractions, but on the monitor strip, the contractions appear tall and pronounced. On the other hand, an obese woman may be having strong contractions that barely register on the tracing. For these reasons, palpation is the most accurate way to estimate intensity when using external monitoring. Nursing Procedure 10-2 describes how to palpate uterine contractions.

Internal Method
Another method of monitoring contractions is the internal method during which an intrauterine pressure catheter is used. The trained birth attendant places the catheter tip above the presenting part in a pocket of amniotic fluid and then connects the catheter to the fetal monitor. In addition

NURSING PROCEDURE 10-1 Application of External Fetal Monitors

EQUIPMENT
Electronic fetal monitor
Tocodynamometer (toco)
Transducer
Two belts
Ultrasonic gel
Monitor paper

PROCEDURE
1. Thoroughly wash your hands.
2. Locate the fetal back through the use of Leopold maneuvers (Fig. 10-3).
3. Assist the woman to a position of comfort. If she wishes to be on her back, a wedge should be placed under one hip to tilt the uterus off the great vessels.
4. Place ultrasonic gel on the transducer and turn on the power to the fetal monitor.
5. Place the transducer on the woman's abdomen over the fetal back.
6. Turn up the volume, and move the transducer over the abdominal wall until the heartbeat is clearly heard.
7. When the monitor is consistently recording the FHR, secure the transducer in place with a belt.
8. Check the maternal pulse either radially or apically to ensure that the transducer is picking up the fetal, not maternal, heart pattern.

9. Next locate the hardest part of the uterine fundus.
10. Place the toco over the fundus, and secure it to the maternal abdomen with a belt (see figure).
11. Check to make sure the paper is recording the FHR and uterine contraction pattern.

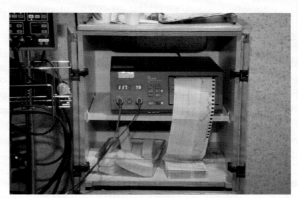

12. Label the EFM strip with the laboring woman's identification data, the date and time the EFM was applied, and maternal vital signs and position.
13. Be sure the call light is within reach before you leave the room.
14. Thoroughly wash your hands.

Note: It is important to position the woman comfortably before attempting to locate the fetal heart. If you wait until after you locate the FHR to reposition, you may lose the FHR and need to relocate the transducer.

NURSING PROCEDURE 10-2 Palpation of Uterine Contractions

EQUIPMENT
Warm, clean hands

PROCEDURE
1. Explain the procedure to the woman and her partner.
2. Wash hands thoroughly.
3. Locate and place one hand on the uterine fundus.
4. Use the tips of your fingers to feel changes in the uterus as it contracts.
5. At the beginning of the contraction, you will feel the muscle begin to tighten.
6. Note the time the contraction begins.
7. Use your fingertips to evaluate how strong the contraction gets before the muscle begins to relax. Intensity is measured at the strongest point (the acme) of the contraction.
8. Note the time the contraction ends to determine duration.
9. Continue with your hand on the fundus through the next three contractions. Note if the uterus completely relaxes by becoming soft between contractions.

10. Note the time from the beginning of one contraction to the beginning of the following contraction to determine frequency. Frequency is documented as a range when appropriate (e.g., every 3 to 5 minutes, or every 2 to 3 minutes), unless they are occurring regularly (e.g., every 2 minutes, every 5 minutes).
11. Wash hands.
12. Chart the contraction pattern (frequency, duration, and intensity) in the labor record. Document whether or not the uterus is fully relaxing between contractions.

Note: It is best to time several contractions consecutively before charting frequency because it is rare for contractions to be exactly "x" minutes apart. It is more common that the contraction pattern occurs every "x" to "y" minutes apart (e.g., every 3 to 5 minutes). Palpation is a method that takes practice. It is best to learn to palpate contractions in conjunction with the use of EFM. In this way, you can see the contraction begin and concentrate on perceiving the tightening of the uterus with your fingertips. You can also see the acme (the strongest/highest part of the contraction), which lets you know when to evaluate intensity.

---

to recording the frequency and duration of contractions, the internal catheter accurately measures the intensity of uterine activity. This information is particularly useful when the woman is undergoing labor after a previous cesarean delivery or when she is receiving an oxytocin infusion to induce labor.

Monitoring FHR

Labor is stressful not only for the woman but also for the fetus. If there is decreased blood flow to the placenta or if the fetus is subjected to chronic hypoxia, the fetus may not be able to withstand the stress of labor. General characteristics of the FHR and changes that occur with uterine contractions give clues as to fetal status. For these reasons, the FHR is monitored in relation to the contraction pattern.

Intermittent Auscultation of FHR

Another method for monitoring FHR in a low-risk pregnancy is to use intermittent auscultation (IA). The most common practice is to place the woman on an external fetal monitor for 20 to 30 minutes to get a baseline evaluation of the FHR. If the pattern is reassuring, then a fetoscope, hand-held Doppler device, or the external fetal monitor is used to monitor the FHR at intermittent intervals. Auscultation of the FHR occurs with the same frequency as is recommended for continuous monitoring methods. See Box 10-5 about when to monitor fetal heart rate. The FHR is auscultated for at least one full minute and throughout at least one uterine contraction. If any abnormalities are noted, or if there is slowing of the FHR with or after contractions, apply the fetal monitor for continuous monitoring.

Continuous EFM

As with monitoring uterine contractions, there are two ways to monitor the FHR using a continuous fetal monitoring device. Continuous EFM can be accomplished using external (indirect) methods or by using an internal (direct) monitoring device.

External EFM

The most common way to assess fetal status during labor is with the use of an external fetal monitor. The external monitor works on the principle of ultrasound. The transducer picks up the fetal heart sounds and transmits them to the monitor. Characteristics of the FHR pattern can then be monitored visually on the video display and with a continuous printout. As stated before, the toco monitors the contraction pattern, which when used in conjunction with a transducer allows for monitoring of the FHR pattern in conjunction with the uterine contraction pattern.

External EFM helps screen for signs of fetal compromise. It is noninvasive and used widely. However, it is sometimes difficult to get a consistent tracing if the fetus is small or extremely active or if the woman is obese. Maternal positioning can adversely affect the quality of the tracing, and many women find external monitoring uncomfortable and confining.

BOX 10-5 **Monitoring Fetal Heart Rate (FHR)**

- Upon admission for 20 to 30 minutes
- For the low-risk laboring woman, every 1 hour during latent phase of labor and every 30 minutes during active phase of labor
- For the at-risk laboring woman, every 30 minutes during latent phase of labor and every 15 minutes during the active phase of labor
- Every 15 minutes during the second stage of labor
- Before and after medication administration during labor and at time of peak medication action
- Before and after any invasive procedure (e.g., vaginal examination, urinary catheterization, amnioinfusion)
- Before and after ambulation
- After any increase in frequency, duration, or intensity of uterine contractions
- The at-risk laboring woman is always on continuous EFM—not intermittent
- Document FHR per facility protocol

Some fetal monitors have telemetry units, which provide wireless transmission of FHR patterns and uterine activity to the monitoring device so that the woman is not attached by cables to the fetal monitor. These units allow for continuous EFM while the woman ambulates, alternates her position, or uses a birthing ball. Some telemetry units can be used in water to allow for monitoring of the FHR during hydrotherapy.

Internal EFM

Internal EFM is an invasive procedure in which a spiral electrode is attached to the fetal scalp just under the skin and extends out the woman's introitus and is taped to the laboring woman's inner thigh (Fig. 10-4). The scalp electrode sends the FHR signal to the monitor, and it is recorded in the same manner as are the results of the external transducer. With internal EFM it is easier to obtain a consistent tracing, regardless of fetal activity, as compared to external monitoring, and maternal position changes usually do not cause interference. When internal techniques are used, the most common combination is that of internal fetal scalp electrode with an external toco to record the contraction pattern. Less frequently, an intrauterine pressure catheter is used with internal EFM. Two criteria for the use of internal EFM are that the fetal membranes must be ruptured and the cervix must be adequately dilated. Internal monitoring procedures increase the risk of maternal and fetal infection and injury.

This is Important!

Because internal monitoring techniques are invasive, both the woman and the fetus are at an increased risk of developing an infection when these are done. Internal methods should be used only when the health care provider determines the benefit clearly outweighs the risk.

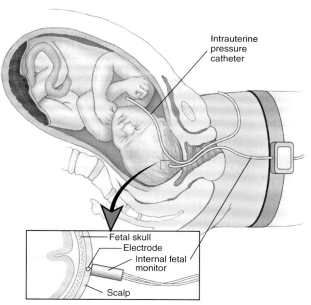

FIGURE 10-4 Continuous internal EFM. The internal fetal scalp electrode is placed on the fetal scalp and connected to the reference electrode which is taped to the maternal thigh and connected to the fetal monitor.

When interpreting a fetal monitor tracing, the first element to evaluate is the baseline FHR. The baseline rate is measured between uterine contractions during a 10-minute period. The normally accepted baseline rate is between 110 and 160 bpm.

Another element to evaluate is the **variability**, fluctuations of the FHR from the baseline rate. Variability is normal if the fluctuations are greater than 6 bpm and less than 25 bpm from baseline (Fig. 10-5). Box 10-6 gives definitions of variability. The presence of moderate variability is a reassuring sign that the fetus is well oxygenated.

There are three major deviations from a normal FHR baseline: tachycardia, bradycardia, and absent or minimal variability. Fetal tachycardia is a rate greater than 160 bpm, and an FHR below 110 bpm is fetal bradycardia. The abnormal rate must continue for at least 2 minutes for identification of tachycardia or bradycardia. The absence of variability is also a nonreassuring sign. Table 10-2 lists examples of conditions that can cause fetal tachycardia, bradycardia, and absent variability.

A Word of Caution is in Order!

Make certain that a nonreassuring pattern is not attributable to medical intervention. For example, fetal bradycardia may result from maternal hypotension secondary to epidural anesthesia, and some medications can cause decreased variability. Often, correcting the maternal condition remedies the nonreassuring pattern.

Periodic Changes

The next step after evaluating the baseline is to check for **periodic changes**, variations in the FHR pattern that occur in conjunction with uterine contractions, and **episodic changes**, variations in the

---

TEST YOURSELF

✔ Name two situations when internal monitoring of labor would be appropriate.

✔ Describe the difference between internal and external EFM of contractions.

✔ How do you evaluate the uterine contraction pattern when external EFM is used?

Evaluating FHR Patterns

Baseline FHR

The obstetric nurse is responsible for monitoring FHR patterns. The RN must not only assess and interpret the pattern accurately, but also know how to intervene and when to notify the birth attendant, either a physician or certified nurse-midwife (CNM). The LPN/LVN is not expected to make a final decision about the FHR pattern; that is the responsibility of the trained RN. However, you must be able to recognize reassuring and nonreassuring signs in order to get help when indicated.

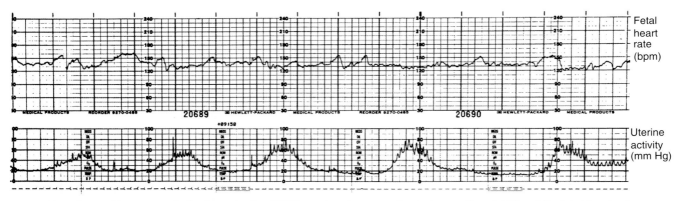

FIGURE 10-5 The electronic fetal monitoring (EFM) tracing shows moderate (normal) variability of the fetal heart rate.

FHR pattern *not* associated with uterine contractions. Because the clinical implications are the same for periodic and episodic changes, the text will refer to periodic changes. Periodic changes can be reassuring, benign, or nonreassuring.

Spontaneous elevations of the FHR, **accelerations**, above the baseline by at least 15 bpm for at least 15 seconds, are considered to be reassuring. Early decelerations are considered benign periodic changes while variable and late decelerations are considered nonreassuring. Figure 10-6 illustrates the appearance and causes of certain periodic changes.

Sometimes, instead of accelerations, there is a slowing of the FHR. If the dip in the FHR tracing occurs in conjunction with and mirrors a uterine contraction, it is an **early deceleration**. This type of deceleration looks like a U on the fetal monitor tracing, like that of an upside down contraction. To be classified as an early deceleration there must be three criteria present: (1) The FHR begins to slow as the contraction starts; (2) the lowest point of the deceleration, the nadir, coincides with the acme (highest point) of the contraction; and (3) the deceleration ends by the end of the contraction.

Early decelerations are caused by pressure on the fetal head as it meets resistance from the structures of the birth canal. The contraction pushes the fetal head downward, causing pressure, which in turn leads to a slowing of the FHR. As long as the baseline remains within normal limits and the variability is good, early decelerations are benign. Therefore, no specific nursing intervention is indicated other than to continue to monitor the tracing and observe closely for the development of nonreassuring patterns.

A **variable deceleration** may occur at any point during a contraction, and it has a jagged, erratic shape on the fetal monitor tracing. The FHR suddenly drops from the baseline and then recovers. A variable deceleration is variable in timing and in shape. It may resemble a U, V, or W.

BOX 10-6 Fetal Heart Rate (FHR) Variability Definitions

- Absent: No fluctuations of FHR
- Minimal: ≤5 bpm from baseline FHR
- Moderate (normal): 6 to 25 bpm from baseline FHR
- Marked: >25 bpm from baseline FHR

The presence of variable decelerations indicates some type of acute umbilical cord compression. When repetitive variables occur on the strip, the cause often becomes apparent at delivery when the umbilical cord is wrapped around a body part, such as the neck (nuchal cord) or foot or it results from an occult (hidden) cord prolapse (see Chapter 18). It is important to note that the cord compression is not continuous when variable decelerations are occurring. The compression occurs when the uterus contracts and squeezes the cord against the fetus. It is relieved when the uterus relaxes between contractions. When compression is continuous, prolonged decelerations or bradycardia occur.

Variable decelerations require careful observation. If the baseline is within normal limits, variability is present, and the variables recover quickly (within the space of a normal contraction), there is no immediate cause for alarm. However, you should be aware that the cord compression stresses the fetus because the umbilical cord is how oxygen reaches the fetus. It is similar to you holding your breath during the length of the contraction. Therefore, nursing interventions are aimed at relieving the compression.

First, assist the woman to change positions. Try to find a position that is comfortable for the woman that relieves the compression. If the variables stop after the position change, you will know that the compression has been relieved. However, if the variables continue, try a variety of position changes, including the left lateral or knee–chest positions.

Pay Attention to the Details!

Here's how to tell if variable decelerations indicate distress. Repetitive variable decelerations with loss of variability that last longer than 1 minute or dip deeper than 60 bpm below the baseline are nonreassuring.

Other interventions for persistent or prolonged variables include stopping any oxytocic infusion, increasing the rate of IV fluids (if they are infusing), starting oxygen via facemask at 10 to 12 L/minute, and notifying the charge nurse and health care provider. The RN or birth attendant may perform a vaginal examination to rule out a prolapsed cord. Sometimes the health care provider will order an

TABLE 10-2 Conditions That Can Influence the Fetal Heart Rate (FHR) Baseline

BASELINE FHR DEVIATION	POSSIBLE CAUSES
Tachycardia (>160 bpm) Mild 161–180 bpm Severe >180 bpm	Maternal conditions • Infection • Dehydration • Fever • Hyperthyroidism Fetal conditions • Infection • Hypoxemia (acute or chronic) • Anemia • Premature Medications given to the woman in labor • Tocolytics (medications used to stop preterm labor) • Any drug that causes maternal tachycardia (e.g., caffeine, epinephrine, or theophylline) • Street drugs
Bradycardia (<110 bpm) Moderate 80–110 bpm Severe <80 bpm	Maternal hypotension Supine hypotensive syndrome Vagal stimulation Fetal hypoxia or decompensation

Decreased or absent variability	• Medications
	  • Narcotics
	  • Magnesium sulfate (to treat preterm labor or preeclampsia)
	  • Tocolytics (medications to stop labor)
	• Fetal sleep (normal fetal sleep cycle is 20 minutes)
	• Prematurity
	• Fetal hypoxemia

amnioinfusion, infusion of normal saline into the uterus, to cushion the umbilical cord and relieve compression.

The most ominous type of nonreassuring periodic change is a pattern of **late decelerations**. These decelerations appear smooth and U shaped on the EFM tracing, like early decelerations, but unlike early decelerations, they begin late in the contraction and recover after the contraction has ended. Figure 10-7 shows how early and late decelerations look on a fetal monitor tracing.

Late decelerations are associated with **uteroplacental insufficiency**, diminished or deficient blood flow to the uterus and placenta. This pattern occurs from chronic interruption of the blood supply to the placenta. This is a grave situation because the placenta is the fetus's sole source of oxygen. Interventions are aimed at improving blood flow to the placenta. Some maternal conditions, such as hypoxemia, decreased cardiac output, or hypotension, can also affect the oxygen supply to the fetus. Notify the RN or the birth attendant of any late decelerations noted.

Don't Forget the Importance of Your Observation Skills!

It is easy to be so concerned about the fetal monitor tracing that you overlook or downplay the skills of inspection and palpation. Always begin your assessment by performing a quick visual inspection of the woman and her environment. If there are no immediate problems, then you may turn your focus to reading the EFM strip.

The following nursing interventions are indicated for a pattern of late decelerations. Position the woman on her right or left side to relieve compression on the maternal abdominal aorta and inferior vena cava, which in turn improves blood flow to the placenta. Discontinue the infusion of oxytocics (if present). Apply oxygen via a facemask at 10 to 12 L/minute. Immediately notify the RN and health care provider. Sometimes tocolytics (medications to relax the uterus) will be ordered in an attempt to improve blood flow to the placenta. Box 10-7 lists signs of an increasingly distressed fetus.

 Concept Mastery Alert

Umbilical cord compression is more likely to result in variable decelerations. Late decelerations are more likely caused by uteroplacental insufficiency.

TEST YOURSELF

✔ Why is a late deceleration of more concern than an early deceleration?

✔ What is the baseline FHR?

✔ How does a late deceleration appear on the fetal monitoring tracing?

✔ What interventions should be implemented when a pattern of late decelerations is detected?

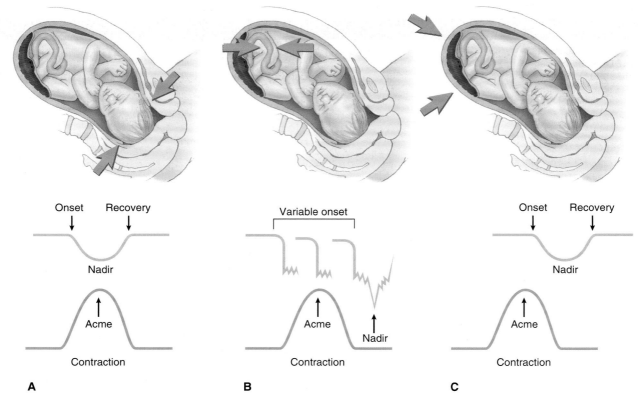

FIGURE 10-6 Appearance and causes of periodic changes. **A.** Early decelerations mirror uterine contractions and are caused by head compression. **B.** Variable decelerations are variable in onset and shape and are caused by cord compression. **C.** Late decelerations are offset from uterine contractions and are caused by uteroplacental insufficiency.

Remember **Lidia Chu** from the start of the chapter. She asks you, "How long will I have to be on the monitor?" How would you respond to her question? What data will guide your response? You notice some early decelerations and her birth partner asks, "What do the dips in the baby's heart rate mean?" What would be your response to their question? What nursing interventions would you implement?

THE NURSE'S ROLE DURING THE FIRST STAGE OF LABOR: DILATION

The first stage begins with the onset of labor and ends when the cervix is 10 cm dilated and 100% effaced. The first stage of labor is divided into three phases: latent, active, and transition. See Table 8-3 for a review of the different stages of labor and their characteristics. The LPN/LVN's role during this stage of labor focuses on maternal and fetal observation, providing physical care to the woman (which in turn provides care for the fetus), providing psychological care to the woman and her birth partner, and keeping both the RN and the health care provider informed about labor progress (see Box 10-8).

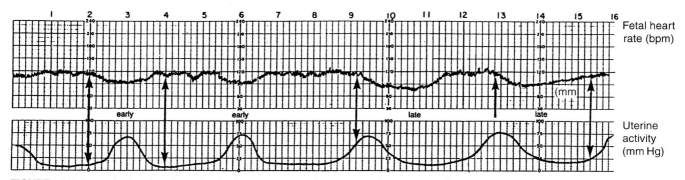

FIGURE 10-7 An early deceleration mirrors the contraction, is caused by head compression, and is benign, requiring no intervention. A late deceleration is offset from the contraction and is caused by uteroplacental insufficiency. Late deceleration interventions are aimed at improving blood flow and oxygenation to the placenta.

As the fetus becomes hypoxic, certain physiologic signs can be noted. These signs are listed in order of least distress to most distress. As you move down the list, the signs are indicative of worsening hypoxia.
1. Absent accelerations
2. Gradual increase in FHR baseline
3. Loss of baseline variability
4. Late deceleration pattern develops
5. Decelerations gradually increase in length and take longer to recover to baseline
6. Persistent bradycardia
7. Death

Latent Phase

The latent phase is sometimes referred to as early labor. This phase starts with the onset of true labor contractions and lasts until the cervix is 4 cm dilated. Contractions during early labor are typically 5 to 10 minutes apart, last 30 to 45 seconds, and are of mild intensity. Initially the contractions may be irregular but become more regular as the phase progresses. The cervix dilates from 1 to 3 cm, and effacement begins. The woman is often easily distracted during contractions and may be talkative or engaged in an activity (such as playing cards or a game on her phone) between contractions. Nursing care is focused on regular assessments, maintaining the safety of the laboring woman and her fetus, and providing comfort to the woman. The laboring woman and her birth partner will also need support and reinforcing of teaching. Support is given even if it is not the woman's first birth as every birth experience is different.

Assessment (Data Collection)

Monitor the woman's vital signs every hour. Temperature may be taken every 4 hours unless the membranes are ruptured, which then requires hourly monitoring of the temperature. Continue to monitor the status of the membranes and the characteristics of any amniotic fluid. Mild tachycardia may be associated with anxiety or the stress of labor contractions. Immediately report elevations in the BP or temperature.

During the latent phase of labor, observe fetal and labor status and record the FHR and uterine contraction pattern at least once every hour. The woman may be on continuous

BOX 10-8 **Nursing Care for the First Stage of Labor**

- **Monitor Maternal Vital Signs**
  - If membranes are intact, monitor temperature every 4 hours.
  - If membranes are ruptured, monitor temperature every 1 hour.
    - An elevated temperature may be associated with dehydration or infection.
  - Measure blood pressure, pulse, and respirations every 60 minutes during the latent phase of labor.
  - Measure blood pressure, pulse, and respirations every 30 minutes during active labor and transition.
    - When certain procedures are done, such as induction of labor or placement of epidural anesthesia, take the vital signs more frequently.
    - Document vital sign per facility protocol.
- **Monitor Maternal Hydration Status**
  - Maintain and document strict intake and output.
  - Observe IV site and IV fluids, if present.
  - Offer ointment for dry lips.
  - Provide frequent mouth care.
  - Offer fluids and ice chips if allowed/desired.
  - Encourage voiding every 2 hours.
  - Check for the presence of glucose or protein in the urine.
- **Provide Maternal Comfort Measures**
  - Regulate environmental temperature; a fan may be helpful if the woman is hot.
  - Soft lighting or darkening the room promotes relaxation.
  - Encourage frequent position changes.
  - Some women find a shower relaxing.
  - Change absorbent pads placed under the hips and buttocks frequently along with providing perineal care.
    - An increase in bloody show may be a sign of advancing labor.
    - Heavy bleeding is a sign that a complication of labor is developing.
- **Monitor Maternal Coping**
  - Assess effectiveness of labor partner or doula in supporting and comforting the woman.
  - Promote positive coping.
    - Demonstrate/reinforce patterned breathing techniques (Chapter 9).
    - Encourage rituals and creative approaches to dealing with contractions.
    - Administer analgesia appropriately if desired by the woman.
    - Assist with the administration of anesthesia as ordered, if desired by the woman.
- **Provide Supportive Care to the Woman and Her Partner/Support Person**
  - Provide privacy.
  - Keep the woman and her partner informed of labor progress and purpose of procedures.
  - Be aware of noise and conversation.
    - Some women need absolute quiet during a contraction.
    - Unnecessary conversations should be kept to a minimum.
    - Some women find music to be soothing.
  - Be a role model for the support person.
    - Actively involve the labor partner if so desired by the laboring woman. Remember some cultures discourage participation by the father in the birthing process.
    - Demonstrate techniques that aid with maternal comfort or coping with contractions.
    - Encourage the support person to take breaks as needed.
- **Monitor Fetal Heart Rate (FHR)**
- **Monitor the Uterine Contraction Pattern Each Time the FHR is Assessed**
- **Monitor Status of Membranes**
- **Assist the RN or Birth Attendant with Vaginal Examinations**

or intermittent fetal monitoring. Report extended periods of reduced variability, FHR decelerations, or other signs of fetal compromise.

It is also important to observe the woman's psychosocial state during the latent phase of labor. She may be talkative and express feelings of confidence and excitement. Conversely, she may be fearful, particularly if she feels unprepared for the event, or she may experience anticipatory anxiety.

Safety During the Latent Phase

Encourage the woman to move around as she is comfortable and as her status allows. She should change positions frequently. Instruct her to avoid lying on her back to avoid supine hypotension. Encourage her birth partner to ambulate with the woman to provide support during contractions. If the woman receives medications during this phase observe the fetal heart rate prior to and after the medication.

Relieving Anxiety

Anxiety causes the release of catecholamines (fight-or-flight hormones), which slow down the labor process. Continuous labor support by a caring nurse or doula can help to decrease a woman's anxiety during labor. As the LPN/LVN, you are in a wonderful position to provide supportive care during labor and influence birth outcomes in a positive way.

Encourage the woman to verbalize her fears and uncertainties. It may be helpful to ask what concerns her most about labor. Often, anxiety decreases when the woman verbalizes her fears. When the source of anxiety is determined, implement measures to decrease the anxiety based on the cause. For example, if the woman is unsure she will be able to withstand the pain of labor, a discussion of pain relief options may be helpful. If she does not know what to expect, she may benefit from a brief explanation of the normal process of labor.

The woman may also fear losing control. In this instance, it may be appropriate to involve the partner in developing a plan to assist her if she starts to lose control. Verbal cues and position changes may be part of the plan. Inquire about coping behaviors that have been helpful to her during other stressful situations. In this way, you can assist the couple to adapt previously successful coping strategies to assist coping efforts during labor.

Promoting Comfort

It is important to support the woman and her partner in their attempts to cope with the discomfort and stress of labor. If the membranes are intact, encourage the woman to ambulate. Even if the membranes are ruptured, she may ambulate with a support person or nurse if the fetus is engaged and well applied to the cervix. Ambulation and upright positions are frequently helpful throughout the labor process. If the woman chooses not to ambulate, assist with comfort measures and position changes.

Provide comfort measures including changing of soiled or wet linens and oral care. Encourage distraction techniques. Engaging in conversation, watching television, and shopping are examples of diversionary activities that may be helpful during the latent phase of labor. Food and beverage intake during labor is a subject of debate (Box 10-9).

BOX 10-9 Food and Fluid Intake During Labor

In the United States for the past several decades, the normal practice has been to withhold food and fluids from the laboring woman. The rationale for this practice was to prevent the woman from aspirating in the event that anesthesia was needed for a cesarean delivery. However, the woman needs fluids during labor to prevent dehydration and ketosis. Practices vary at hospitals across the country. The general consensus is for the woman to avoid solid food but allow clear liquids. Many health care providers prefer to give IV fluids to every woman in active labor and allow only ice chips, whereas others allow clear liquids. The nurse should follow the birth attendant's recommendations and facility policy regarding food and fluid intake during labor (Funai & Norwitz, 2021).

If the woman and her birth partner are well prepared for labor, they may decide to stay at home during the latent phase. This practice is permissible as long as the membranes are intact, and some health care providers encourage it to allow the woman more control over the early labor process.

Reinforcing Prior Teaching

The latent phase of labor is an excellent time to reinforce prior teaching about the process of labor to the woman and her birth partner. An important point to include is what the woman can expect to experience during each phase and stage of labor. Explain pain relief options and discuss appropriate timing of analgesia and anesthesia. Briefly describe the frequency and purpose of nursing assessments and interventions common to each stage of labor.

It is important that the woman and her birth partner understand how to work with the labor process and how to avoid fighting against it. If the woman has not attended childbirth preparation classes, use this time to demonstrate and practice basic relaxation techniques with her. Otherwise, review and reinforce breathing and relaxation techniques that the woman learned in childbirth preparation class (see Chapter 9 for discussion of techniques).

The birth partner needs encouragement regarding the importance of their role during labor. Give information regarding measures the woman may find comforting during each stage of labor, and encourage the partner to take breaks periodically to conserve energy for the duration of labor. Explain the importance of using the nurse as a resource and source of support for the partner and the woman throughout labor. When the woman knows what to expect and receives support during labor, she has less anxiety and fear which enhances the labor process.

TEST YOURSELF

✔ Which criteria define the first stage of labor?

✔ Describe four important nursing interventions during the latent phase of labor.

✔ What observations during the latent phase of labor would need reporting to the RN or birth attendant?

Active Phase

The active phase is sometimes referred to as active labor. This phase starts when the cervix is 4 cm dilated and lasts until the cervix is 8 cm dilated. In the active phase, contractions typically occur every 2 to 5 minutes, last 45 to 60 seconds, and are of moderate to strong intensity. During contractions the woman will not easily be distracted as she was during the latent phase. Between contractions she will want to rest and often will tune out activity in the room and not want to carry on conversation. She will be inwardly focused during contractions. The fetus descends steadily, although descent does not typically progress as rapidly as does cervical dilation. As the fetus descends below the level of the ischial spines, station is described in positive numbers.

Nursing care is focused on regular assessments, assisting the woman with coping with the discomfort of contractions, promoting effective breathing patterns, providing comfort measures for the woman, and preventing infection. Nursing care for the woman's safety, comfort measures, and reinforcing prior teaching are the same as what is done during the latent phase.

Assessment (Data Collection) During the Active Phase

Assessments during the active phase are similar as for the latent phase. There are three main areas the assessments focus on. These are the progress of labor, fetal status, and maternal status. Immediately notify the RN and the birth attendant for any change in the status of the woman or the fetus.

Exercise Caution!

When the membranes rupture, whether spontaneously or artificially, check the FHR for one full minute immediately afterward. If fetal bradycardia or deep variable decelerations occur, assist the woman to the knee–chest position and call the RN immediately to perform a vaginal examination to check for a prolapsed cord.

Assessment (Data Collection) of Labor Progress

Be present for any vaginal examinations and document the findings in the woman's record. Observe the woman's psychosocial state. Note if the woman is becoming more introverted, restless, or anxious; if she is feeling helpless or fears losing control; or if distraction techniques are failing to promote coping. These behaviors signal that the woman is moving into the active phase of labor. Also assess the birth partner's ability to assist the woman during and between contractions. Continue to monitor the status of the membranes and the characteristics of any amniotic fluid. Monitor for signs of infection such as elevated temperature, fetal and maternal tachycardia, and cloudy, foul-smelling amniotic fluid.

During the active phase, monitor the contraction pattern every 30 minutes. It is also critical to observe whether the uterus is relaxing completely between contractions. An adequate relaxation period allows for sufficient blood flow to the placenta and promotes oxygenation of the fetus. Observe the ability of the woman to relax in between contractions.

Assessment (Data Collection) of Fetal Status

Observe and document fetal status at least every 30 minutes. Record the baseline FHR every 30 minutes, and evaluate the fetal monitor tracing for nonreassuring patterns. Variability should be present, except for brief periods of fetal sleep or when the woman receives narcotics or other selected medications. Accelerations of the FHR are reassuring. No late decelerations should be present.

Assessment (Data Collection) of Maternal Status

Observe maternal status every 30 minutes when collecting data on the fetal status. The woman becomes more introverted during active labor because the contractions are closer together, of a stronger intensity, and longer than during early labor.

Measure the temperature every 4 hours if the amniotic sac is intact and hourly after the membranes have ruptured. Box 10-10 lists danger signs to watch for during labor that should be reported immediately.

Vital signs should be taken every hour. The woman's blood pressure (BP) may rise slightly but should be lower than 140/90 mm Hg. It is important to take the BP between contractions because the stress of a uterine contraction can cause the BP to rise briefly, resulting in an inaccurate measurement.

Pulse and respirations may also increase with the work of labor. Monitor for tachycardia. Evaluate breathing patterns frequently. Observe for signs of hyperventilation, which include tachypnea, feelings of lightheadedness or dizziness, complaints of tingling around the mouth or in the fingers, and carpopedal spasms (Fig. 10-8).

A falling BP and a rising pulse could indicate the onset of shock; stay with the woman and immediately report this finding to the RN and birth attendant. Several labor complications can cause shock, including hemorrhage or uterine rupture (see Chapter 18).

Observe the presence and character of pain at least hourly during active labor. Ask the woman to rate her pain on a standardized pain scale. Anxiety and tension often decrease the woman's ability to cope with contractions; therefore, it is important to document how the woman

---

BOX 10-10 Danger Signs During Labor

If any of the following signs occur during labor, immediately notify the RN or the health care provider.

- Elevated maternal blood pressure (BP) (≥140/90 mm Hg)
- Low or suddenly decreased maternal BP (≤90/50 mm Hg)
- Elevated maternal temperature (>100.4°F)
- Amniotic fluid that is green, cloudy, or foul-smelling
- Nonreassuring FHR patterns
- Prolonged uterine contractions (>90 seconds duration)
- Failure of the uterus to relax between contractions
- Heavy or bright red bleeding
- Maternal reports of unrelenting pain, RUQ pain, or visual changes
- Maternal reports of difficulty breathing or shortness of breath

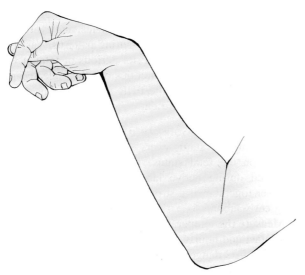

FIGURE 10-8 Carpopedal spasms.

and her partner are coping and to determine if the coping strategies are helpful. For example, if the woman is using patterned breathing techniques to manage contractions, she may hyperventilate and need assistance to regain control of her breathing technique.

Monitor the woman's urinary output. A full bladder can interfere with the progress of labor. Every 2 hours, palpate the area just above the symphysis pubis, feeling for a rounded area of distention, which indicates the bladder is full. Failure of the fetus to descend is another sign that the bladder might be full. Offer the bedpan every 2 hours or assist the woman to the toilet if allowed. If the woman is unable to void, a sterile in-and-out catheterization procedure may be indicated.

Check for dry cracked lips, thick saliva, and a coating on the tongue that may be caused by mouth breathing or restricted oral intake. If the woman is placed on oxygen, it can be drying to the oral membranes. Frequent mouth care stimulates saliva production, which helps keep the oral mucosa moist. Suggest that the woman brush her teeth or gargle with normal saline when her mouth feels dry. Chewing gum also stimulates saliva production and leaves a pleasant taste in the mouth. Providing ice chips, sips of clear liquids, flavored ice, or hard candy (if allowed) can be soothing. Lip balm is comforting if the lips are dry or chapped. If the woman does not have lip balm, water-soluble lubricant effectively moistens the lips. Avoid petroleum based lip products as these are contraindicated if the woman is receiving oxygen.

Immediately report any signs of nonreassuring FHR patterns that do not respond to position changes and other accepted interventions. Report abnormal maternal vital signs, heavy bleeding, or failure of the uterus to relax between contractions.

Check Out This Tip!

A full bladder may interfere with fetal descent. Encourage the woman to void at least every 2 hours during labor.

Providing Pain Management

Continue to observe the woman's ability to cope with the discomfort of contractions. Observe the ability of the birth partner to assist her during contractions. Provide suggestions if needed on different positions or nonpharmacologic relief measures. Let the woman know what pharmacologic options she has ordered if she wants them. The active phase of labor is the time when most women request pain relief measures. If her chosen method of pain relief is not working, remind her that she can change her mind about pain relief options. You may need to repeat earlier instruction and reassure the woman and her birth partner that it does not represent a failure on the woman's part if she chooses an alternate method of pain management. If she starts to lose control, assist the birth partner to use verbal cues and position changes to help the laboring woman regain control. Epidural anesthesia may be initiated or narcotic analgesia may be administered (see Chapter 9); however, it is critical to respect the woman's preferences for pain control. If the woman desires a natural childbirth, she will need intensive support throughout the active phase of labor.

Implementing general comfort measures can help manage the pain and discomfort of labor. Work closely with the birth partner to demonstrate distraction and relaxation techniques, such as effleurage, back rubs, or application of pressure to the lower back during contractions (see Chapter 9). A cool, damp washcloth to the forehead is often comforting.

Perspiration, amniotic fluid, and bloody show frequently soil linen and gowns during active labor. Change linens and her gown as needed to promote comfort and avoid chilling. Place absorbent pads, under her hips and replace as needed. Provide frequent perineal care. At a minimum, perform perineal care after any invasive procedure involving the vagina and after elimination.

Promoting Effective Breathing Patterns

Reinforce breathing techniques appropriate to the active phase of labor (see Chapter 9). Often it helps to make eye contact and perform the breathing patterns with the woman during her contraction to help keep her focused (Fig. 10-9). Vigorous application of breathing techniques can lead to hyperventilation. If hyperventilation occurs, breathing into cupped hands or a paper bag usually relieves the problem.

Some women do not benefit from the use of patterned breathing techniques. Frequently, these women will develop personalized an individualized way of dealing with the discomfort of labor. For example, one woman might find it helpful to close her eyes and attempt to visualize a peaceful scene during contractions. Another woman might involve her partner by squeezing their hands throughout each contraction. Still another woman might assume a particular position during contractions. As long as these individual approaches to coping with the discomfort of labor are helpful, encourage and support their use. When the approach is no longer helping the woman to cope, assist the woman in trying other approaches.

Do You Know the Why of It?

Hyperventilation can cause respiratory alkalosis. Breathing into a paper bag retains CO_2, reverses alkalosis, and relieves the symptoms associated with it such as the tingling of her fingers or mouth.

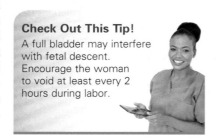

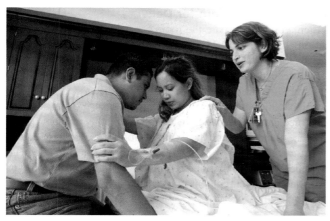

FIGURE 10-9 The nurse instructs the birth partner to maintain eye contact and breathe with the woman during contractions to help keep her focused. (Photo by Joe Mitchell.)

Preventing Infection

Handwashing remains the number one way to prevent the spread of infection. Wash your hands thoroughly before and after providing care. Encourage the woman and her partner to wash their hands before and after any contact with the perineum and after using the toilet.

Frequent vaginal examinations are discouraged, particularly if the membranes are ruptured. Usually, it is best for the woman not to have a cervical check unless there is a clear indication that one is necessary. Assist the examiner to maintain sterile technique when it becomes necessary to perform a vaginal examination.

Invasive procedures increase the risk for infection. Perform urinary catheterization only if there are clear indications for its use. Strict adherence to sterile technique is critical to minimize the risk for infection. Assist the birth attendant with sterile technique when other invasive procedures are done, such as placement of a fetal scalp electrode.

TEST YOURSELF

✔ Why is it important for the laboring woman to void frequently?

✔ What assessment findings are associated with hyperventilation?

✔ List five nursing interventions appropriate for the active phase of labor.

Transition Phase

The transitional phase of labor starts when the cervix is 8 cm dilated and ends when the woman is completely dilated at 10 cm and the cervix is completely effaced (thin). During transition, contractions typically occur every 2 to 3 minutes, last 60 to 90 seconds, and be of strong intensity. The woman feels like she cannot rest between contractions because they happen quickly. This is the shortest phase but

also the most intense phase of the first stage of labor. The woman often reports "feeling out of control" and is very irritable. She may make statements such as, "I can't do this anymore" or "I want to leave the hospital."

Nursing care during transition is focused on fetal and maternal assessments, pain management, assisting with maternal coping, and support of the woman and her birth partner. It also includes the nursing care previously performed during the latent and active phases in regard to safety, comfort, and preventing infection. A new nursing task during the transition phase includes preparing the room for delivery.

Assessment (Data Collection)

Observe for signs that the woman has reached the transition phase of the first stage of labor. Look for an increase in bloody show and a strong urge to push. Observe the woman's psychosocial state. She will often express irritability and restlessness and feel out of control. She may tremble, vomit, or cry. It is also important to observe for hyperventilation during this phase.

> **Do You Know the Why of It?**
> Nausea and vomiting are common occurrences during labor because of decreased gut peristalsis and delayed gastric-emptying time. If vomiting occurs, assist the woman to turn to her side to help prevent aspiration.

Monitor the contraction pattern every 30 minutes. The uterus should relax completely between uterine contractions. This is important for the oxygenation of the fetus. It is essential to continue to evaluate fetal status at least every 30 minutes. The FHR baseline should remain between 110 and 160 bpm and should not significantly increase or decrease. It may be normal to see variable decelerations as the fetal head descends. Variability in the FHR should be present. There should be no late decelerations or prolonged bradycardia.

Promoting Pain Management

Reassure the woman that although this phase of labor is the most intense, it is usually the shortest. Continue to assist the woman's labor partner in providing comfort and support during uterine contractions. Frequent position changes, breathing with the woman during contractions, and providing other comfort measures may help decrease the intensity of the pain stimulus. If she feels the urge to push during this time, explain the importance of resisting the urge to push until full cervical dilation is determined. Panting or blowing during contractions helps to minimize the urge to push.

Narcotics are not given during this phase of labor to prevent delivery of a neonate with respiratory depression. Some women request epidural anesthesia during transition; sometimes by the time the anesthetist has arrived and prepared for the insertion, the woman has rapidly progressed and birth is imminent. The woman should know that an epidural given during transition might delay effective pushing in the second stage of labor.

Assisting the Woman With Coping

Accepting behavioral changes of the laboring woman is an important nursing intervention during this forceful period of labor. You will need to provide intensive psychological support for both the woman and her support person. Remind them this is the shortest phase of labor and these behavioral changes are normal. Most women do not feel like carrying on a conversation between contractions and may become irritated by extraneous conversation while they are resting. Take cues from the woman and provide directions to visitors and the birth partner as needed during this time.

> **This Advice Could Shorten the Day!**
>
> If the woman is feeling a strong urge to push and she is not fully dilated to 10 cm, assist her to pant during the contraction and then blow at the peak of the contraction when the urge is most intense. Pushing efforts before the cervix is fully dilated can result in cervical lacerations or can cause edema of the cervix and slow dilation or delivery of the fetus.

Supporting the Woman Through Fatigue

Relaxing and using coping mechanisms during contractions may be almost impossible for some women. Fatigue is common during this phase of labor. Encourage the woman to relax or even sleep between contractions. Help her find a comfortable position. Support her position with pillows. Placing a cool cloth to her forehead or giving her a back rub may help her relax between contractions (Fig. 10-10). Some women find music to be soothing whereas others may become irritated by it. Some women may not be able to verbalize what support or comfort measures she desires. Continue to utilize different nursing interventions to help her through this phase. When the woman is able to relax between contractions, she conserves energy that she will need during the next stage in order to push effectively. The birth partner is often fatigued as well; encourage them to take breaks as necessary.

Preparing the Room for Delivery

Often, you will prepare the room for delivery during the transition phase (Fig. 10-11). Many delivery units have preference cards so you can prepare the equipment and supplies most often needed by the birth attendant. Prepare the table maintaining surgical asepsis and sterility so that a sterile field is available during delivery. It is important to ensure that supplies and medications needed for the birth are readily available. Turn on the infant warmer. Check the newborn resuscitation equipment to ensure it is working properly, turned on, and adequate supplies are readily available. Replace any missing supplies or malfunctioning equipment immediately.

> **TEST YOURSELF**
> ✔ Discuss signs associated with the transition phase of labor.
> ✔ What responsibilities does the nurse have for supporting the woman's labor partner during the transition phase of labor?
> ✔ Why is it important that the woman refrain from pushing until the cervix is completely dilated?

THE NURSE'S ROLE DURING THE SECOND STAGE OF LABOR: DELIVERY OF THE FETUS

The second stage of labor begins when the cervix is 10 cm dilated and 100% effaced and ends with the birth of the newborn. The fetal station is usually 0 to +2.

Nursing care during this stage of labor focuses on providing physical and psychological support to the woman while she pushes the fetus through the birth canal. Observation of maternal and fetal well-being during this stage is crucial. In addition, the nurse provides assistance to the birth attendant as needed.

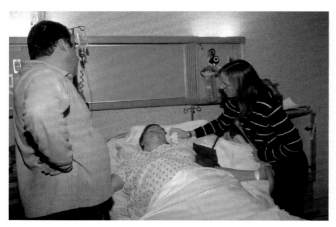

FIGURE 10-10 The birth partner provides comfort measures, such as a cool washcloth to the face and forehead, to help the woman relax as much as possible during the transition phase of labor. (© B. Proud.)

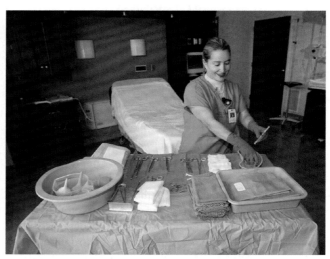

FIGURE 10-11 The nurse prepares the labor room for delivery. (Photo by Joe Mitchell.)

Assessment (Data Collection)

During the second stage of labor, close observation of the laboring woman and her fetus is indicated. Monitor the BP, pulse, and respirations every 15 to 30 minutes. Observe the contraction pattern every 15 minutes. Observe for the woman's report of an uncontrollable urge to push, which is caused by pressure from the descending fetal head.

Observation of the fetus during the second stage is essential. As the fetus descends into the pelvis, the pressure on their head is very intense. There may also be pressure on the umbilical cord during contractions. Frequently, the fetal monitor strip reveals early or variable decelerations. Variables are usually not ominous at this stage as long as the FHR returns quickly to baseline as the contraction relaxes; the baseline remains between 110 and 160 bpm; and variability is present. Check the FHR every 15 minutes for the low-risk woman and every 5 minutes for the woman who is at risk for labor complications.

Evaluate the woman's psyche; the laboring woman may feel more in control and able to cope with the contractions now that she can push. Often, she is less irritable and more cooperative. Observe the woman's level of fatigue. If the second stage is prolonged, she may become extremely fatigued and experience difficulty finding the energy to push. Many women rest deeply and do not want to converse between pushes.

Promoting Effective Pushing Despite Fatigue

All of the comfort measures appropriate to active labor continue to apply during the second stage, particularly while the woman is pushing. Using comfort measures, such as applying a cool cloth to the forehead and offering ice chips and mouth care, can promote relaxation between contractions, which helps conserve energy and prevent exhaustion.

Assist the woman to the chosen position for pushing and provide support throughout each pushing effort. For instance, if the woman is using the sitting position to push, you and the woman's labor partner can assist her to the sitting position when the contraction starts and support her back while she pushes.

If the woman has experienced a prolonged labor and is having a difficult time pushing effectively, it may be appropriate to position her on her side for comfort and allow her to rest for 30 minutes to an hour in order to regain her strength. As long as the fetal monitor tracing remains reassuring, allowing for a break from pushing is acceptable. Often the woman is able to push more effectively after the break.

Effective Pushing Techniques

Once the cervix is fully dilated, the woman can begin pushing efforts. Traditionally, obstetric nurses have taught women to use vigorous pushing techniques. When **vigorous pushing**, also called Valsalva pushing, is used, the woman is told to take a deep breath, hold the breath, and push while counting to 10. She is encouraged to complete three "good" pushes in this manner with each contraction. This form of

pushing, however, may increase the rate of maternal fatigue during the second stage of labor and it has not been shown to be a more effective form of pushing as compared to the open-glottis or urge-to-push methods of pushing.

 A Personal Glimpse

After 2 days of doctors trying to induce labor, I was about ready to request a cesarean section. Although I truly desired a vaginal birth, my husband and I were at our wits' end after having tried every measure available to start labor. During those frustrating days, the nurses I had were so supportive. They encouraged me to think positively and hold onto hope that I would eventually have a vaginal birth. When I was finally able to push, my labor and delivery nurse, Mary Ellen, was so supportive. Somehow, she convinced me that every push was the first one. With her gentle guidance, I believed I could get my baby out, even when it seemed it would never happen. I will never forget how helpful and tender she was. She told me time and again that I was "almost there" while my doctor shook his head in disagreement. Having spent more time with Mary Ellen than with the doctor who would eventually deliver my child, I believed her assessment far more than his! I don't think I even remember his name, but I will always remember Mary Ellen for her reassurance and gentle care.

Sara

Learning Opportunity: *Describe three supportive nursing behaviors that can encourage a woman to not give up when labor seems overwhelming. How can the nurse impact the woman's experience in a positive or negative way?*

The two forms of pushing currently suggested for the woman in labor are open-glottis pushing and the urge-to-push method. **Open-glottis pushing** is characterized by pushing with contractions using an open glottis so that air is released during the pushing effort. You may also encourage the woman to use the **urge-to-push method**, in which the woman bears down only when she feels the urge to do so using any technique that feels right for her. No matter what pushing technique is used, never leave the woman alone during pushing efforts.

Watch Out!

When the woman is pushing effectively, delivery can occur rapidly. Monitor for signs of imminent delivery, which include grunting, bulging of the perineum, crowning of the fetal head, or the woman exclaiming "the baby is coming!"

Positions for Pushing and Delivery

There are many different positions that are acceptable for pushing and for delivering the fetus. However, in the United States, most women deliver in a modified dorsal recumbent position in which the woman's legs are on foot pedals and the head of the bed is elevated approximately 45 degrees. Occasionally, the birth attendant will ask for woman to be in a lithotomy position (sometimes with the woman's legs supported by stirrups). Dorsal recumbent and lithotomy positions allow for greater control by the birth attendant but may not be the most comfortable or effective positions for enhancing delivery.

One major disadvantage of the lithotomy position is that gravity does not assist the birth. Other positions use gravity to aid in the pushing process, which conserves energy during the second stage of labor. Some positions, such as hands and knees, encourage rotation of the fetus, which shortens the second stage of labor. The hands and knees position enhances blood flow to the placenta, resulting in fewer nonreassuring EFM tracings. Table 10-3 illustrates and compares positions used for pushing and delivery of the fetus.

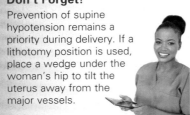

Don't Forget!

Prevention of supine hypotension remains a priority during delivery. If a lithotomy position is used, place a wedge under the woman's hip to tilt the uterus away from the major vessels.

Preparing for Delivery of the Newborn

Nursing judgment is necessary to decide when to prepare the woman for delivery. You may observe bulging of the perineum (Fig. 10-12) or crowning of the fetal head, which indicates imminent delivery. Preparation of the primipara is typically done when the fetus is crowning, whereas preparation of the multipara may be done when the fetus reaches +2 or +3 station. However, the RN may decide to prepare the woman sooner in both cases if the fetus is descending rapidly.

If the woman has been laboring in a birthing bed and she will deliver in the semisitting or lithotomy position, the bed is "broken"—the lower part of the bed is removed to allow room for the birth attendant to control the delivery. Often, you will place the woman's feet on foot pedals. If stirrups are used, take care to position the stirrups properly, then lift both legs together and place them in the stirrups. Position the instrument table close to the birthing bed and uncover it. If the urinary bladder is full, the birth attendant may request that you perform an in-and-out catheterization.

Prepare the equipment necessary to care for the newborn in anticipation of the birth. This preparation involves

TABLE 10-3 Comparison of Positions for Pushing and Delivery

POSITION	ADVANTAGES	DISADVANTAGES
Lithotomy: This was the position used by the majority of health care providers in the 1960s to 1980s. It is still used occasionally. The woman is positioned on a flat delivery bed with her legs in stirrups.	Easy access to the perineum and greater control of delivery by birth attendant	Greater risk of supine hypotensive syndrome and positioning injuries (e.g., clot formation from compression or muscle strain from improper placement in stirrups)

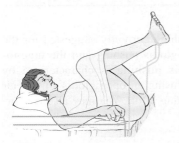

POSITION	ADVANTAGES	DISADVANTAGES
Modified dorsal recumbent or semisitting: This is a common pushing position. When it is time for delivery, the woman's feet are placed on foot pedals and the birthing bed is "broken" in preparation for delivery.	Easy access to the perineum and good control of delivery by birth attendant.	May be uncomfortable for the woman. May not be the best position to facilitate expulsion of the fetus.

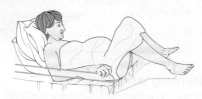

POSITION	ADVANTAGES	DISADVANTAGES
Side-lying 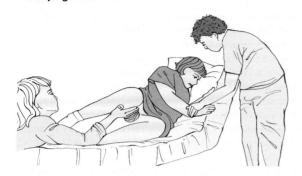	May increase comfort of the woman	Decreases access to the perineum by the birth attendant. Requires high degree of cooperation from the woman and possible assistance of the nurse or support person to hold the upper leg during delivery
Squatting 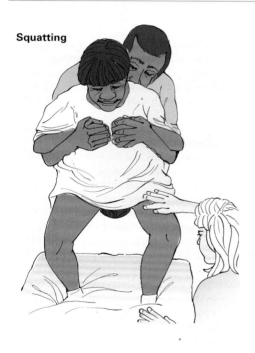	Highly likely to increase the comfort of the woman. Uses gravity to facilitate expulsion of the fetus.	Difficult access to the perineum. Requires a birth attendant who is flexible and willing to use this approach. The woman may lose her balance in this position. A pushing bar can help maintain balance, or a birthing stool may be used.
Hands and knees: The woman is assisted to her hands and knees on the birthing bed to push and deliver the fetus. 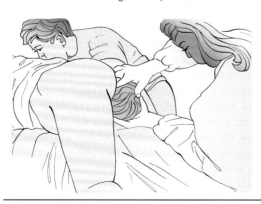	Encourages rotation of the fetal head, which hastens delivery. Enhances placental blood flow, which decreases fetal stress. Allows for the perineum to stretch better than other positions so that an episiotomy is less often required. Allows for greater access to the perineum by the birth attendant than some of the other alternative positions.	May be more tiring for the woman. Does not allow for the use of instruments to assist delivery. Requires a birth attendant who is flexible and willing to use this approach.

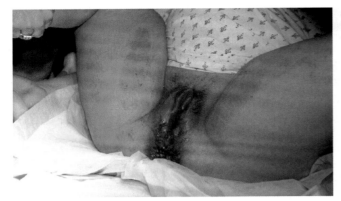

FIGURE 10-12 Bulging of the perineum is an indicator of imminent delivery. (Photo by B. Proud.)

turning on the radiant warmer and placing warm blankets under the warmer. Be sure that the forms to begin the newborn's chart are in the room and check the resuscitation equipment once more before delivery.

The RN is responsible for overseeing events during the birth. Surgical terms describe the role of the RN during delivery; therefore, the RN is the circulator for the delivery. The RN should remain in the delivery room until after the fetus is born, the placenta delivers, and woman and neonate are stable. Box 10-11 lists the major responsibilities of the nurse in the delivery room, including immediate care of the newborn (see Chapters 13 and 14 for comprehensive coverage of newborn care). Figure 10-13 shows a delivery sequence from crowning through birth of the newborn.

This Advice Could Be a Lifesaver!
The risk for splashing of bodily fluids is high during a delivery. Eye shields, gowns, and gloves are necessary for protection from contact with bodily fluids.

TEST YOURSELF

✔ What instructions should be given to the laboring woman regarding pushing?

✔ What are the major responsibilities of the nurse in the delivery room?

THE NURSE'S ROLE DURING THE THIRD STAGE OF LABOR: DELIVERY OF PLACENTA

The third stage of labor begins with the birth of the newborn and ends with delivery of the placenta. During this stage of labor nursing care focuses on monitoring for placental separation, monitoring blood loss, and providing physical and psychological care to the woman.

BOX 10-11 Responsibilities of the Nurse in the Delivery Room

- Closely monitor the laboring woman.
  - Record vital signs and status assessments per facility protocol.
  - Assess for maternal response to anesthesia/analgesia.
- Closely monitor the fetus. Assess FHR:
  - every 15 minutes for low-risk labors.
  - every 5 minutes for at-risk labors.
- Maintain accurate delivery room records.
  - Note and record the time of delivery.
  - Record all nursing procedures performed and maternal/newborn response.
- Provide immediate newborn care (refer to Chapters 13 and 14 for in-depth discussion of newborn adaptation and care).
- Maintain warmth.
  - Immediately dry the newborn on the woman's abdomen or under the radiant warmer.
  - Wrap the newborn snugly, and place a cap on the head when not in skin-to-skin contact with the woman or when not under a warmer.
- Assess adaptation to extrauterine life. Assess and record Apgar scores (see Chapter 14 for a discussion of Apgar scoring).
- Maintain a patent airway.
  - Position the newborn to facilitate drainage.
  - Suction secretions with a bulb suction device or with wall suction.
- Provide for safety and security. Before the newborn and the woman are separated after delivery:
  - obtain the newborn's footprints and the woman's thumb or fingerprint (if part of the facility protocol).
  - place identification bands with matching numbers on the newborn and the woman. Two bands are placed on the newborn and one on the woman. In some facilities, a band is also placed on the woman's partner or support person.
- Promote parental–newborn bonding.
  - Allow and encourage the woman and her partner to hold the newborn.
  - Allow and encourage breast-feeding immediately after delivery.
  - Encourage skin-to-skin contact with the newborn.
  - Point out positive characteristics of the newborn.
- Assist the birth attendant.
  - Perform sponge and instrument counts.
  - Ensure that supplies are available for episiotomy and repair, if needed.
  - Obtain additional supplies as needed, such as forceps or vacuum extractor for difficult deliveries, or extra suturing material.

Assessment (Data Collection)

Observe the woman's psychosocial state after she gives birth. Immediately after birth, the woman often experiences a sense of relief that the birth has been accomplished and contractions have ceased. Monitor for signs of placental separation, which generally occur within 5 to 20 minutes after delivery. These signs begin with a uterine contraction, then the fundus rises in the abdomen, the uterus takes on a globular shape, blood begins to trickle steadily from the vagina, and the umbilical cord lengthens as the placenta separates from the uterine wall.

The placenta may deliver in one of two ways (Fig. 10-14). The most common way is for the smooth, shiny,

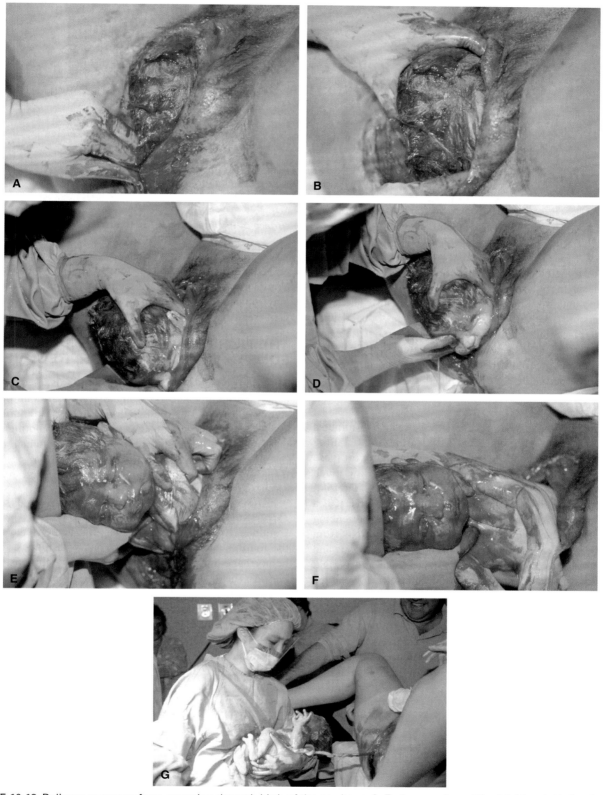

FIGURE 10-13 Delivery sequence from crowning through birth of the newborn. **A.** Early crowning of the fetal head. Notice the bulging of the perineum. **B.** Late crowning. Notice that the fetal head is appearing face down. This is the normal OA position. **C.** As the head extends, you can see that the occiput is to the woman's right side—ROA position. **D.** The cardinal movement of extension. **E.** The shoulders are born. Notice how the head has turned to line up with the shoulders—the cardinal movement of external rotation. **F.** The body easily follows the shoulders. **G.** The newborn is held for the first time! (Photo by B. Proud.)

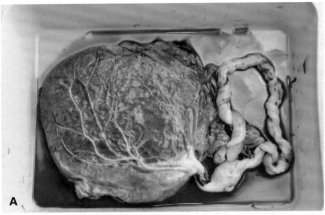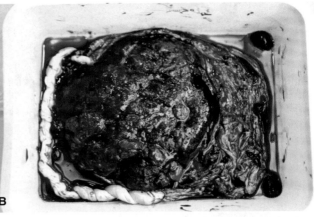

FIGURE 10-14 A healthy placenta after delivery. **A.** Notice the shiny surface of the fetal side. **B.** The maternal side is rough and divided into segments (cotyledons). (Photos by Joe Mitchell.)

fetal side to deliver first (Schultze mechanism). Sometimes, the edge of the placenta appears at the introitus, revealing the rough maternal surface (Duncan mechanism). The latter mechanism of delivery is more frequently associated with retained placental fragments. After the placenta delivers, the birth attendant inspects it for completeness. Palpate the fundus to make certain the uterus is firm and contracted. Monitor the perineum for excess bleeding.

Preventing Fluid Loss

Monitor the woman's vital signs at least every 15 minutes during the third stage of labor. Tachycardia and a falling BP are signs of impending shock; immediately report these signs to the RN and the birth attendant. Note how much time has passed since the birth of the newborn. The placenta normally separates within 20 minutes of delivery. If a longer period has passed, the woman may be experiencing retained placenta, which can lead to acute fluid loss from hemorrhage. If the woman has an IV, monitor the IV site and fluids to ensure patency and document intake and output. Encourage the woman to drink oral fluids to prevent the development of dehydration.

Oxytocin is frequently given in the third stage of labor to prevent hemorrhage. Some health care providers prefer to give oxytocin before the placenta delivers to hasten its delivery, whereas others administer oxytocin as soon as the placenta delivers. When the placenta separates from the uterine wall, it leaves an open wound that is subject to hemorrhage if the uterus does not contract effectively. When oxytocin is given after the placenta delivers, it causes the uterus to contract, which puts pressure on the open blood vessels at the former placenta site. The oxytocin may be added to the IV fluids or it may be given via intramuscular injection.

> **Try Nature's Way!**
>
> Encourage the woman to breast-feed immediately after delivery. Breast-feeding stimulates oxytocin release from the posterior pituitary, which helps the uterus to contract and control bleeding.

Monitor the woman for any sudden change in status. Complaints of shortness of breath, chest pain, or tachypnea may indicate the development of an amniotic fluid embolism (see Chapter 18).

THE NURSE'S ROLE DURING THE FOURTH STAGE OF LABOR: RECOVERY

The fourth stage of labor begins with delivery of the placenta and ends when the woman's physical condition has stabilized (usually within 2 hours). Nursing care during this stage focuses on continued assessments, promoting parental–newborn attachment, and care of the woman including minimizing bleeding, preventing infection, promoting urinary elimination, managing discomfort, and reducing fatigue.

Assessment (Data Collection)

Continue to monitor the woman for hemorrhage during the fourth stage of labor. The woman is at highest risk for hemorrhage during the first 2 to 4 hours of the postpartum period. The woman's vital signs and a fundal check (see Nursing Procedure 12-1) should be done every 15 minutes. To do a fundal check, palpate the fundus for position and firmness. The fundus should be well contracted, at the midline, and approximately one fingerbreadth below the umbilicus immediately after delivery. Observe the **lochia** (vaginal discharge after birth) for color and quantity. The lochia should be dark red and of a small to moderate amount. If the woman saturates more than one perineal pad in an hour, assist the woman to void (if she has not done so recently), palpate and massage the fundus, and notify the RN.

Monitor for signs of infection. The temperature may be elevated slightly right after delivery, as high as 100.4°F, because of mild dehydration and the stress of delivery. Any elevation above that level may indicate infection and should be reported. The lochia should have a fleshy odor but should not be foul-smelling.

The woman should void within 6 hours after delivery. Trauma from the birth may have caused edema in the perineal area or anesthesia may persist, leading to an inability to sense a full bladder. Both conditions can lead to urinary retention. Monitor for suprapubic distention and a high fundus displaced to the right. These signs indicate that the urinary bladder is full. A full bladder can prevent the uterus from contracting and lead to increased bleeding.

Observe the woman's comfort level. There are many sources of pain during the immediate postpartum period. Cramping from uterine contractions (referred to as "after-birth pains") and perineal pain from edema or episiotomy repair are common sources of pain for the woman. Ask the woman to describe the location of the pain and to rate it on a standardized pain scale. Many women have uncontrollable shaking in their lower extremities and postpartum shivering immediately after delivery. Reassure her these are temporary and will subside on their own, usually within a few minutes to an hour. Warmed blankets are often helpful and provide comfort to the woman.

Observe the woman's psychosocial state during the fourth stage. Typically, the woman is fatigued and hungry. It is normal for her to be self-absorbed and demonstrate dependent behaviors. She also has an intense need to talk about the labor and delivery experience. The woman may experience a rapid change in her emotions immediately after birth. She may be elated about the birth and a few moments later cry, even if she is happy. This is usually seen in the first hour after birth.

Observe initial attachment behaviors of the new family. It is normal for parents to want to hold and touch the newborn as soon as it is born. You may notice that the parent begins initial inspection of the newborn with the fingertips; this is normal behavior and indicates positive beginning attachment.

Be careful about documenting inadequate attachment in the immediate time after delivery. Some women are so fatigued or uncomfortable that they may not desire, or be capable of, prolonged interaction with the newborn beyond the initial inspection. Behaviors that indicate a risk for inadequate attachment include turning away from the newborn or making disparaging comments about the newborn.

Provide comfort measures for the woman. After the birth attendant has completed their tasks, inspect and cleanse the perineum. Remove the soiled drapes and linen, and place an absorbent pad under the buttocks with two sterile perineal pads against the perineum. Place a warm blanket (from a blanket warmer, if possible) over the woman. Reassemble the birthing bed. If the woman is in stirrups, remove both legs from the stirrups at the same time. Some health care providers will order an ice pack to be placed against the perineum during the fourth stage.

 Cultural Snapshot

Be aware of the woman's cultural beliefs that she practices. In some cultures, such as the traditional Chinese culture, childbirth makes the body cold, and therefore the woman will avoid cold waters and showers during labor and for a month after delivery. They will also want to consume hot foods such as ginger.

Promoting Parent–Newborn Attachment

While the birth attendant is suturing any lacerations or episiotomy and making a final inspection of maternal tissues, it is important to promote parental attachment with the newborn. Hand the newborn to the woman as soon as it is determined that they does not need resuscitation. If the woman's partner is present at the delivery, encourage holding and interacting with the newborn (Fig. 10-15). This is a good time for the new woman to attempt breast-feeding for the first time. If the woman permits it, place the newborn skin-to-skin against her body and place several blankets over them. This technique (called kangaroo care) keeps the newborn warm and promotes bonding.

If the newborn requires resuscitation, is premature, or has a birth defect, it can impact the attachment process. Pointing out positive aspects of the newborn or resemblances to the woman helps with attachment. If the newborn is taken to the nursery or neonatal intensive care unit (NICU) for support, it is helpful to provide the woman with a photo and emotional support as well as updates on the newborn's status during this time.

Minimizing Bleeding

Continue to monitor the woman for signs of fluid volume deficit or hemorrhage. Take vital signs every 15 minutes during the fourth stage of labor. Falling BP and tachycardia may indicate fluid volume deficit or hemorrhage and should be reported to the RN immediately. Massage the fundus every 15 minutes, and inspect the lochia for amount and color. The fundus should be firm or should quickly become firm when gently massaged. Continue to monitor any IV fluids infusing and offer food and fluids to the woman. Keep accurate records of intake and output.

Preventing Infection

Continue to use an excellent handwashing technique. Wash hands before and after care, between clients, and any time contact with bodily fluids occurs. It is critical to use standard precautions. Wear gloves at all times when you perform procedures anywhere near the perineum or dirty linens. Anything that comes in direct contact with the perineum should be sterile. Handle

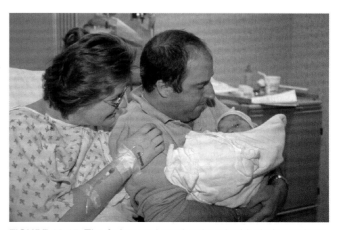

FIGURE 10-15 The father and mother bond with their newborn son soon after birth.

perineal pads from the ends, and do not touch the middle area that will be in contact with the perineum. Instruct the woman to do this as well. Instruct the woman on how to use the peri bottle after she uses the toilet each time or changes her perineal pad.

Promoting Urinary Elimination

If the woman has the urge to void, assist her to the bathroom unless she is still under the effects of anesthesia and does not have complete control of her legs. It is much easier for her to void sitting on a toilet than it is on a bedpan. Have her dangle her feet at the bedside for several minutes before assisting her to a standing position to avoid postural hypotension. Once she is safely in the bathroom, run water or let her soak her hands in warm water if she is having difficulty getting the stream of urine started. An in-and-out catheterization is usually not done unless there is significant suprapubic distention or discomfort from the full bladder, excessive bleeding, or unless 6 hours have passed without voiding.

Managing Discomfort

Nonsteroidal anti-inflammatory drugs (NSAIDs) and oral narcotic analgesics, such as codeine, are often prescribed for discomfort and pain after delivery. NSAIDs are effective at reducing painful uterine cramping (afterbirth pains). These pains can intensify during a breast-feeding session due to the woman's body releasing oxytocin in response to the newborn's sucking. Multiparous women, as compared to primiparous women, often report more intense afterbirth pains. Ibuprofen 600 to 800 mg may be ordered to be given every 6 to 8 hours around the clock. This type of dosing is often more effective at keeping pain under control than is an "as-needed" schedule in which the woman must ask for the medication before it is given.

Combination medications consisting of a mild analgesic, such as acetaminophen, with a narcotic, such as codeine, may be ordered on an as-needed basis for breakthrough pain. Sometimes, codeine is ordered for perineal pain, and NSAIDs are given to control cramping. Assess the woman's pain frequently and administer medications before the pain becomes intolerable.

Warmth to the abdomen may be helpful in reducing the discomfort of uterine cramping. Position changes may also be helpful. If the pain is from an episiotomy or edema of the perineum, it is helpful to apply ice packs. Most labor units have combination perineal pads/ice packs. These are convenient, but a clean glove filled with ice also works as an ice pack. If used, apply the glove between two perineal pads so that a non-sterile object does not come in direct contact with the perineum.

Watch Out!

Extreme perineal pain may indicate the development of a perineal hematoma. Other signs of a hematoma include restlessness, inability to find a comfortable position, and tilting to one side when sitting. A woman who has had an epidural or a local anesthetic may be unaware of a developing hematoma. It is important for you to visually inspect her perineum with each fundal check until she regains full sensation.

Reducing Fatigue

After the initial bonding period, it may be helpful to discourage visitors and promote rest for the woman. Her partner can stay with her to care for the newborn if the newborn is rooming-in or if the hospital provides couplet care. If the newborn is to be stabilized in a newborn nursery, this is a good time for both the woman and her partner to get some much-needed rest and sleep if possible.

TEST YOURSELF

✔ Identify three signs of placental separation.

✔ How often are vital signs checked during the fourth stage of labor?

✔ Name three parameters that should be monitored with each vital sign check during the fourth stage of labor.

✔ What signs should be reported to the RN? What complications might they indicate?

Nursing Process and Care Plan *for the Woman in Labor*

The nursing care plan of the woman in labor is focused on four major areas: assessment of the woman and the fetus including monitoring the contraction pattern and fetal heart rate (FHR), monitoring the progress of the labor, providing comfort to the woman, and providing support to the woman and her birth partner.

Assessment (Data Collection)

The nurse monitors the woman's vital signs each time the FHR and contraction pattern are monitored. If the woman's membranes are ruptured, the woman's temperature is monitored more frequently and the characteristics of the amniotic fluid are also noted. The woman's blood pressure and respiratory pattern are also monitored.

The nurse will collect data on the woman's status regarding the contraction pattern and the woman's physical status. Fetal data collection includes monitoring the FHR, the status of the membranes, and observing the FHR in response to the woman's interventions. The LPN/LVN will need to be ready to assist the RN and the birth attendant if any complications arise during the labor and provide nursing interventions as necessary.

Providing comfort includes not only implementing independent nursing care measures but also assessing the woman's level of discomfort and implementing nonpharmacologic and pharmacologic measures as necessary. The woman will need support in coping with the discomfort associated with the labor and birth processes. The woman's birth partner will need support during the labor and birth as well.

The nurse must be aware of signs that indicate that either the woman or the fetus is not tolerating the stress of labor. The nurse also needs to be aware of signs that the labor is not progressing in an expected manner.

Nursing Care Focus

When selecting a nursing care focus for the woman in labor, safety, including preventing infection, is a prime focus. Being aware of changes in the maternal or fetal baseline status can help the RN and birth attendant to monitor and intervene with the labor as needed. Consideration should also be given to the woman's prior experience with labor and birth and any labor preparation she has done during this pregnancy. Even if this is not her first birth, it will be a different experience for her, so consideration should be given to how she and her birth partner are coping during the labor and the amount of support they require. Additionally, the woman's comfort and pain management are important areas for the nurse to plan care for.

Outcome Identification and Planning

Major goals for the woman in labor include that both she and fetus remain free from harm. This includes harm from an infection; therefore another goal is that she will not exhibit signs of an infection. Other goals that are important for the laboring woman focus on her comfort and management of the discomfort of labor contractions. Remember that every woman experiences labor contractions differently and what may be tolerable for one woman can be described by another woman as excruciating. Planning of nursing activities is based upon these goals. It is important when goal setting to include the woman and her desires for her labor and delivery.

Nursing Care Focus

- Safety

Goal

- The woman will not experience harm during labor.

Implementations for Promoting Safety

The woman in labor is at risk for falls. The woman should have someone with her as she ambulates, gets in and out of the bed, and ambulates to the toilet. Since water increases the risk of slips or falls, someone should be with her at all times when she is in the tub or shower. If she has had epidural, help her to turn and reposition every 2 hours. She should not get up to walk until sensation returns to her legs after the anesthesia.

A decrease in her blood pressure can not only put her at risk for syncope or falling, it also decreases the placental blood flow and thereby the oxygenation of the fetus. To prevent a decrease in her blood pressure, have the woman avoid lying on her back when she is in bed to prevent supine hypotension syndrome. When she gets out of bed, have the woman sit on the edge of the bed and dangle her legs for a few minutes to avoid postural hypotension. If the woman is to receive an epidural follow the health care provider's orders for IV fluid hydration prior to the procedure and monitor the woman's blood pressure before and after the epidural is placed.

Monitor her for danger signs that might indicate complication during labor. These include elevated blood pressure, headache, visual changes, epigastric pain, proteinuria, hyperreflexia with clonus, and in extreme cases, seizures. If she exhibits any of these signs, have her lie on her side in bed, decrease the lights and stimulation in the room and report these findings immediately to the RN and the health care provider.

Monitor the woman's oxygenation status when she receives pain medications as a decrease in her respiratory rate or oxygen level will decrease the fetus' oxygenation. Monitor the woman's breathing pattern and help her to avoid hyperventilation which causes respiratory alkalosis. Signs to monitor for include tachypnea, feelings of light-headedness or dizziness, complaints of tingling around the mouth or in the fingers, and carpopedal spasms. If the woman demonstrates any of these signs have her breathe into her cupped hands or a paper bag.

The fetal heart rate is an indication of the oxygenation status of the fetus. Monitor the fetal heart rate anytime medications are given to the woman, if the woman's membranes rupture, and with any nonreassuring fetal heart rate patterns. If nonreassuring contraction patterns or fetal bradycardia is observed, notify the RN and the birth attendant, have the woman lie on her side, and follow the birth attendant's orders (such as administering oxygen or stopping oxytocin).

Evaluation of Goal/Desired Outcome

The woman:

- does not fall.
- does not experience hypotension or hypertension.
- does not hyperventilate or have a decrease in SaO_2.
- has a FHR between 110 and 160 without decelerations or other signs of fetal distress.

Nursing Care Focus

- Infection risk

Goal

- The woman will remain free from signs of an infection.

Implementations for Preventing and Monitoring for Infection

Frequent and thorough handwashing remains the primary intervention in preventing infection when caring for the laboring woman. The nurse should utilize personal protective equipment (PPE) as appropriate when caring for the woman.

Vaginal examinations, by the RN or birth attendant, should only be done as necessary. Any invasive procedure, including urinary catheterizations, should be done using sterile technique. Assist the birth attendant in maintaining sterile technique when performing vaginal examinations or other procedures such as placing a fetal scalp electrode.

Assess the woman's temperature. Notify the RN and the birth attendant for any elevations in the woman's temperature. If the woman's membranes have ruptured, monitor the amniotic fluid for color and odor. The fetal heart rate increases when there is infection present; therefore monitor the FHR for tachycardia.

Evaluation of Goal/Desired Outcome

The woman:

- remains afebrile.
- has a fetal heart rate that is between 110 and 160 bpm.
- is not tachycardic.
- has clear and odorless amniotic fluid.

Nursing Care Focus

- Coping impairment

Goal

- The woman will exhibit positive coping behaviors during labor.

Implementations for Promoting Coping

Monitor the woman's coping during and in-between contractions. Observe the birth partner's ability to offer support and help the woman cope. Help the woman with, and demonstrate to the partner if necessary, nonpharmacologic interventions including distractions, patterned breathing techniques, back rubs, hydrotherapy, and position changes.

Reinforce prior teaching that was done about the birth process. Offering information helps the woman to know what to expect and to help decrease her fears. Have the woman verbalize her fears/concerns. Address and honor the woman's requests during labor as appropriate (e.g., her birth plan). The woman's coping increases when she feels a sense of being in control and feeling that her voice is being heard. Reinforce that she can change her mind about her prior desires regarding pain interventions.

Evaluation of Goal/Desired Outcome

- The woman copes with contractions during the different stages of labor.

Nursing Care Focus

- Impaired comfort

Goal

- The woman will have her comfort enhanced between contractions.

Implementations for Providing Comfort

The woman's ability to cope during contractions, rest between contractions, and cope with the discomfort of labor are enhanced when her physical comfort needs are met. The nurse independently performs these comfort measures. These include changing any wet or soiled bed linens or the woman's gown. Application of a cool, wet cloth to the forehead and back of the woman's neck can help with feelings of warmth or nausea.

Mouth care is essential during the labor process. The woman does a lot of mouth breathing and vocalization during labor which can dry the lips and oral membrane. In addition, restriction of fluids or oxygen also dries out the mouth as well. Help the woman by providing oral care at regular intervals. Oral care stimulates saliva production which helps with dry mouth. Having the woman suck on sugarless hard candy or chewing gum can help. Ice chips and lip balm are also beneficial.

Encourage the woman to void frequently. It is more comfortable for the woman to void on the toilet than a bedpan. Keep the room free from noxious odors as much as possible. Remove a full emesis basin immediately. Some women feel more comfortable with dim lights and low, or no, conversation or noise (e.g., television or hallway noises) during labor. Adjust the environment, as necessary, and position the woman for comfort.

Educate the woman and her birth partner about addressing comfort issues sooner rather than later, making it easier to cope during and in-between contractions.

Evaluation of Goal/Desired Outcome

- The woman verbalizes satisfaction with her comfort.

Nursing Care Focus

- Acute pain

Goal

- The woman will cope with the discomforts of the contractions and birth processes and utilize pain relief as needed.

Implementations for Managing Pain and Discomfort

Effective coping behaviors can help the woman manage the discomfort of the contractions and in some cases have a medication-free labor and birth. Provide comfort measure which can increase the woman's coping behaviors and thereby minimize her discomfort.

Have the woman identify factors that relieve discomfort and implement those. If those factors become ineffective, help her with alternative measures. Observe for nonverbal cues of discomfort, such as restlessness, muscle tension, or altered vital signs. Offer alternative therapies to increase comfort, such as massage therapy or relaxation therapy, as appropriate. Administer prescribed medications, and monitor for effect.

Evaluation of Goal/Desired Outcome

The woman:

- voices, or exhibits behaviors that demonstrate, her discomfort is manageable.
- uses distraction and relation techniques effectively.
- relaxes between contractions.

Remember **Lidia Chu** from the start of the chapter. From your readings, what information would you need to know about the fetal heart rate and how it responds to contractions? What would be your priority nursing actions during periodic changes? What nursing actions would you perform during each stage of labor?

KEY POINTS

- When a woman arrives at the labor unit, immediate data collection involves observing for signs that birth is imminent, in which case admission procedures are abbreviated until after delivery, as well as determining fetal status, risk factors, and maternal status.
- If the birth is not imminent, the RN will conduct a thorough obstetric, medical–surgical, and social history and a complete physical assessment. Also, determine labor status and the woman's labor and birth preferences. Throughout the labor process, monitor maternal and fetal status and labor progress. Frequent checking of vital signs and fetal heart rate (FHR) are critical nursing functions.
- Uterine contraction patterns are evaluated using external or internal methods. External monitoring always involves palpation when using intermittent auscultation. Palpate to determine intensity of the contraction when the external toco is used during continuous fetal monitoring. Internal monitoring requires the use of an internal pressure catheter. The internal pressure catheter measures intensity as well as frequency and duration.
- Intermittent auscultation of FHR allows for freedom of maternal movement and focuses the nurse's attention on the woman, rather than on the technology. Disadvantages are that intermittent auscultation requires higher staffing levels, and some health care providers fear that subtle signs of fetal compromise may be missed. Continuous electronic monitoring restricts maternal movement and tends to focus the nurse on the monitor versus the woman. Advantages are that the nurse can take care of more clients and can immediately detect changes in fetal status.
- External fetal monitoring is noninvasive and allows for evaluation of FHR patterns. Some external FHR monitoring can be done by telemetry which allows for more mobility by the woman. Internal fetal monitoring requires that the membranes be ruptured and the cervix be at least partially dilated. The woman needs to remain in bed while being internally monitored. Internal FHR monitoring involves a scalp electrode being placed which can increase the risk of infection in the fetus.
- To apply the fetal monitor, first locate the fetal back, and then apply the transducer using ultrasonic transducer gel. Next, locate the fundus, and place the toco on the firmest part of the fundus. Both the toco and transducer are secured to the abdomen with straps.
- LPN/LVNs must be able to detect nonreassuring FHR patterns in order to notify the RN or the health care provider, who then makes a final decision regarding care of the client.
- Three major deviations from a normal FHR baseline are tachycardia (FHR higher than 160 bpm), bradycardia (FHR lower than 110 bpm), and absent or minimal variability (fluctuations at or below 5 bpm from baseline).
- Early decelerations are gradual decreases in the FHR that mirror the contraction. Head compression is the cause, and the pattern is not cause for concern as long as the FHR returns to baseline. Variable decelerations are abrupt decreases in the baseline that are variable in shape and timing (many are shaped like Vs or Ws) and are caused by cord compression. The pattern is nonreassuring when the decelerations are deep and repetitive and when absent variability or changing baseline is present. Late decelerations are gradual decreases in the FHR that start after the peak of the contraction. Late decelerations indicate uteroplacental insufficiency and are nonreassuring.
- No intervention is required for early decelerations, other than continuous monitoring. Nursing interventions for variable decelerations are aimed at relieving cord compression and include maternal position change or assisting the health care provider with amnioinfusion. Late decelerations require aggressive management. The woman is positioned on either side, oxygen is started via facemask, and any oxytocic infusion is discontinued. Sometimes, tocolytics are prescribed to decrease the frequency and duration of uterine contractions, which improves blood flow to the placenta.
- The latent phase of the first stage of labor is marked by maternal feelings of excitement as well as by anticipatory anxiety and fear. Reinforcing prior teaching about the labor process can help reduce anxiety. Distraction techniques are helpful in facilitating coping.
- Contractions become more frequent and stronger during the active phase of labor. Distraction techniques typically do not help during active labor. Support of the woman and her partner include encouragement to continue behaviors that promote coping and assistance in finding alternative approaches when coping is ineffective. Reinforcing breathing techniques and rituals can be helpful.
- The transition phase is the most intense phase of labor. The woman becomes irritable and less cooperative. Assist the woman to rest between contractions and to avoid pushing efforts until the cervix is fully dilated.
- Full dilation of the cervix marks the beginning of the second stage of labor. Because the woman can now participate actively by pushing, she often feels reenergized to deal effectively with the labor.

The open-glottis or natural method of pushing is recommended. Encouragement and reinforcement of pushing techniques are helpful nursing interventions.

- The placenta is delivered in the third stage of labor. Monitor for signs of placental separation and ensure that the fundus remains contracted after the placenta delivers.
- During the fourth stage of labor, or the recovery period, the risk for hemorrhage is high. Close monitoring of the fundus, lochia, and vital signs is a priority intervention. Comfort measures for the woman and observation of attachment are also important nursing interventions.

INTERNET RESOURCES

Labor and Birth
http://americanpregnancy.org/labor-and-birth/

Normal Labor and Delivery Process
https://www.webmd.com/baby/guide/normal-labor-and-delivery-process#1

Stages of Labor
http://www.marchofdimes.org/pregnancy/stages-of-labor.aspx

Workbook

NCLEX-STYLE REVIEW QUESTIONS

1. A woman presents to the labor suite and states, "I have water leaking down my legs." What is the priority data that need to be collected?
   a. Fetal heart rate
   b. Fern test
   c. Blood pressure check
   d. Urine test for protein

2. A primipara is dilated 8 cm and is completely effaced at +1 station. She tells the nurse, "I can't keep myself from pushing when I have a contraction." What intervention is most appropriate in this situation?
   a. Offer comfort measures.
   b. Reapply the fetal monitor.
   c. Assist the woman to blow at the peak of contractions.
   d. Tell the birth partner that it is not good for the baby if she pushes right now.

3. A G1P0 is in the active phase of labor. She is a low-risk client. The nurse evaluates the fetal monitor strip at 10 AM. Moderate variability is present. The FHR is in the 130s with occasional accelerations, no decelerations. At what time does the nurse need to reevaluate the FHR?
   a. 10:05 AM
   b. 10:15 AM
   c. 10:30 AM
   d. 11:00 AM

4. A G3P2 has just delivered a healthy newborn 30 minutes ago. Which of the following nursing interventions will the nurse perform? Select all that apply.
   a. Have her dangle her legs before assisting her to the toilet to void.
   b. Palpate the fundus to make sure it is firm and midline.
   c. Perform an in-and-out catheterization.
   d. Encourage her to send the newborn to the nursery so she can rest.
   e. Take maternal vital signs every 15 minutes.

5. It is most likely that the health care provider would consider performing an amnioinfusion if the EFM tracing shows which contraction pattern?
   a. Consistent early decelerations, variability present, and occasional accelerations
   b. FHR 130 without variability and no decelerations
   c. Occasional mild variable decelerations and moderate variability present
   d. Deep variable decelerations with every contraction

STUDY ACTIVITIES

1. Choose what you think are the three most important nursing assessments and interventions during labor. Using the table below, compare your top three picks for the laboring woman during the active phase, transition phase, and the second stage of labor. Include the frequency of the interventions. What similarities do you see? What differences are apparent?

	Active Phase	Transition Phase	Second Stage
Major nursing assessments			
Major nursing interventions			

2. Do an internet search using the key words "birth plans." How many sites returned? After exploring some of the sites, what are the main issues covered in a birth plan? Does a birth plan seem realistic to use if the woman intends to deliver in the hospital? Why or why not?

3. Interview a labor and delivery nurse. Ask her how her facility handles birth plans. Does she recall a time when parts of the birth plan could not be honored? How was the situation handled? What was the outcome?

CRITICAL THINKING: WHAT WOULD YOU DO?

Apply your knowledge of the labor process and the nurse's role during labor and birth to the following situation.

1. Priscilla, a 26-year-old G1P0, presents to the birthing center because her "labor pains" have begun. She talks excitedly with her husband, who is to be her coach. She says that she is pleased that the happy day is finally here, but she is afraid that she will "lose it" when the contractions get stronger. She and her husband have attended childbirth preparation classes.
   a. What nursing assessments should be completed?
   b. What phase/stage of labor do you suspect Priscilla is in?
   c. What do you expect the vaginal examination will reveal?
   d. What nursing interventions will you implement for Priscilla and her husband?
   e. How would your care be different if the couple had not attended childbirth classes?

2. Several hours after admission to the birthing center, Priscilla is dilated 5 cm, and the cervix is completely effaced. When a contraction begins, Priscilla kneels on the bed, rests her upper body against her husband, closes her eyes, and sways slowly while humming softly. At the end of the contraction, her husband gently places her on her side and she rests with her eyes closed until the next contraction begins.
   a. What phase/stage of labor is Priscilla in?
   b. What nursing assessments need to be completed at this time?
   c. What is your assessment of Priscilla's coping technique?
   d. What nursing actions are appropriate for Priscilla and her partner at this point in her labor?

3. Three hours later, Priscilla becomes agitated and snaps at her husband and the nurse. She exclaims, "I can't stand this anymore! I want to go *home*!"

   a. What nursing assessments should be completed at this time? Why?

   b. What nursing interventions are appropriate for Priscilla and her husband now?

   c. How would you decide whether or not your interventions had been effective?

4. It is the beginning of your shift. The charge nurse gives you a report on Martha Brown, a 29-year-old G2P1. The fetus is in a vertex presentation, and the membranes are intact. A vaginal examination was done 1 hour previously. At that time, her cervix was 4 cm dilated and 80% effaced. The station was +1, and the position was LOT. Continuous EFM is ordered, and IV fluids are infused into her left arm.

   a. What assessments do you make, in what order, when you enter Martha's room?

   b. What behaviors do you expect Martha to exhibit at this time?

5. A few hours later, you go to check on Martha. You notice that she is much more restless than she has been. The fetal monitor tracing shows the FHR baseline in the 140s. Moderate variability is present. During each contraction, the FHR dips into the 120s. The dip is smooth with a gentle slope on both sides, like a contraction, only upside down. The FHR is back to 140 by the end of the contraction. You do perineal care because Martha has a lot of bloody show.

   a. How do you interpret the FHR pattern? Is the pattern reassuring or nonreassuring? Defend your answer.

   b. What should your next action be? Why?

Assisted Delivery and Cesarean Birth

Key Terms

amniotomy
artificial rupture of membranes (AROM)
cephalopelvic disproportion (CPD)
cesarean birth
elective induction
episiotomy
forceps
laminaria
perioperative period
time-out
vacuum extraction
vaginal birth after cesarean (VBAC)

Learning Objectives

At the conclusion of this chapter, you will:

1. Identify medical indications for induction of labor.
2. Explain methods health care providers use to determine labor readiness.
3. Contrast mechanical methods for hastening cervical readiness with pharmacologic methods.
4. Describe the reasons for and nursing care after the procedure for artificial rupture of membranes.
5. Outline essential equipment needed for and possible complications associated with oxytocin induction.
6. Describe indications and risks for an episiotomy, and also describe the difference between mediolateral and midline episiotomies.
7. Describe indications, risks, and nursing considerations for vacuum extraction and forceps-assisted delivery.
8. Name the more common and less common indications for cesarean birth.
9. Explain maternal and fetal complications of cesarean delivery.
10. Differentiate among vertical and transverse skin and uterine incisions.
11. List the responsibilities of the licensed practical/vocational nurse throughout the perioperative period for a cesarean delivery.
12. Compare nursing interventions needed to prepare a family for a planned cesarean birth with those for a family who is to undergo emergency cesarean delivery.
13. Identify criteria for a woman to be a candidate for an attempted vaginal birth after cesarean (VBAC) and criteria that would prevent a woman from attempting a VBAC.

Deidre Jordan has been in the labor unit for 12 hours. This is her second delivery, and she is 39 weeks gestation. Her amniotic sac is intact, and she is dilated 2 cm and 50% effaced. Her first child was born vaginally 3 years ago without any problems during labor. The birth attendant has decided that Deidre's labor is not progressing. As you read the chapter, think about what methods the birth attendant might use to attempt to assist Deidre's labor to help her deliver vaginally.

There are several techniques and tools available to the birth attendant to decrease the risk of labor and birth to the woman and her fetus. Induction techniques are used to initiate labor if delivery is indicated and has not yet started on its own. The birth attendant also has tools to assist the delivery if conditions arise that threaten the safety of the woman or her fetus. Many of these options help avoid cesarean delivery, which subjects the woman and her fetus to all the hazards of major surgery.

Before the advent of surgical asepsis and antibiotics, if a laboring woman could not deliver a child vaginally, there were few options available to the physician or midwife. Sometimes, the woman died. Other times, extreme measures became necessary and the unborn child's life was sacrificed to save the life of the mother. Today, cesarean birth is available if assisted delivery methods do not work or the risk of vaginal delivery outweighs the risk of surgical intervention.

All of the procedures discussed in this chapter carry risk. Many of these procedures are done to correct problems discussed in Chapter 18. Although many of these techniques are frequently used, they should never be considered routine.

INDUCTION OF LABOR

When a condition exists that could endanger the life of the woman or the fetus, the health care provider, usually an obstetrician, may elect to induce, or start, labor rather than wait for the woman to go into labor spontaneously. The rate of induced labors has risen dramatically over the past few years. There are many reasons for this rise, although one contributing factor seems to be an increase in the number of elective inductions. An **elective induction** is one in which the health care provider and woman decide to induce labor in the absence of a medical reason to do so.

Indications

Induction of labor is medically indicated when there is a condition that threatens the well-being of the woman or the fetus, if the pregnancy were to continue. Postdate pregnancy, a pregnancy that persists beyond the expected due date, is probably the most common reason that labor is induced. Other indications for induction of labor include prelabor rupture of membranes (PROM; spontaneous rupture of membranes without the onset of spontaneous labor), chorioamnionitis (infection of the fetal membranes), gestational hypertension, preeclampsia, severe intrauterine fetal growth restriction, fetal demise, or maternal medical conditions such as diabetes or gestational diabetes. In any case, the health care provider weighs the risks of allowing the pregnancy to continue against the risks of labor induction.

Contraindications

Conditions in which spontaneous labor is contraindicated are also contraindications for the induction of labor. Maternal contraindications include complete placenta previa, history of a classical (vertical) uterine incision, structural abnormalities of the pelvis, and invasive cervical cancer. Fetal contraindications include certain anomalies such as hydrocephalus, certain fetal malpresentations (e.g., transverse lie), and fetal compromise or distress. There are certain maternal medical conditions (e.g., active genital herpes lesions) that necessitate a cesarean delivery and therefore would not require induction of labor.

Labor Readiness

Cervical readiness is generally a prerequisite for successful labor induction. One way the health care provider determines cervical readiness is by using the Bishop score (Table 11-1). Five factors are evaluated in the Bishop score: cervical consistency, position, dilation, effacement, and fetal station. The higher the score, the greater the chance that induction will be successful. A cervix that is favorable for induction is called a "ripe" cervix. A Bishop score of 6 or less indicates an "unripe," or unfavorable cervix, and labor induction is less likely to be successful.

Other methods that have been used to predict labor readiness include measuring the cervical length by endovaginal ultrasound (see Chapter 7) and also measuring fetal fibronectin levels in cervical secretions. However, these studies are costly and take time, and are not yet completely predictive. Currently, the Bishop score remains a reliable predictor of cervical readiness that is both cost and time effective.

In addition to cervical readiness, the fetus should be mature before labor induction, unless a condition exists in which the risks of continued pregnancy outweigh the risks of delivering the fetus prematurely. If the pregnancy has completed at least 38 weeks' gestation (as determined by reliable dating methods), the fetus is considered to be mature. The date that fetal heart tones were first audible and other pregnancy milestones can help validate gestational age when determining fetal maturity. Fetal lung maturity is a major point the health care provider will consider when determining if the fetus is mature enough for delivery. See Chapter 17 for a description of determining fetal lung maturity.

TABLE 11-1 Bishop Scoring System

SCORE	DILATION (CM)	EFFACEMENT (%)	STATION	CERVIX	CERVICAL POSITION
0	Closed	0–30	−3	Firm	Posterior
1	1–2	40–50	−2	Medium	Middle
2	3–4	60–70	−1	Soft	Anterior
3	≥5	≥80	≥+1		

Bishop E. H. (1964). Pelvic scoring for elective induction *Obstetrics & Gynecology, 24,* 266.

Cervical Ripening

Frequently a medical reason exists for labor induction, but the cervix is not ready. In this situation, the health care provider may perform a procedure to ripen the cervix before labor induction is started with oxytocin. There are two methods to ripen the cervix: mechanical and pharmacologic.

Mechanical Methods

One of the most common mechanical methods used to hasten cervical readiness is a procedure called "membrane stripping." The health care provider inserts a gloved finger through the internal cervical os and sweeps the finger 360 degrees to separate the membranes from the lower uterine segment. Plasma levels of prostaglandins (one substance associated with the onset of labor) are measurably higher after membrane stripping. Another mechanical method includes dilation of the cervix by the health care provider using a catheter. The tip of the catheter is inserted through the cervix, and the balloon of the catheter is filled with 30 to 80 mL of sterile saline. The inflated balloon rests between the internal cervical os and the amniotic sac.

Laminaria, or cervical dilators, are used to soften and dilate the cervix, usually to induce abortion either therapeutic or elective, or to induce labor when the fetus has died in utero. Laminaria is made from the root of seaweed; the provider can also use a synthetic product. The health care provider places the material in the cervix, where the material slowly expands as it absorbs moisture, a process that dilates the cervix gradually. Synthetic dilators are removed in 6 to 8 hours, whereas laminaria stay in place for 12 to 24 hours.

Pharmacologic Methods

Pharmacologic agents can be used to effectively prepare an unripe cervix for labor. The agents used are called prostaglandins, and they are applied locally to the cervix. The only substance approved by the U.S. Food and Drug Administration (FDA) for this purpose is prostaglandin E_2 gel or vaginal inserts (dinoprostone). Prostaglandin E_1 (misoprostol) is used frequently for cervical ripening, although it is not approved for this use by the FDA. Both prostaglandin E_2 and prostaglandin E_1 are contraindicated in women who have had a previous cesarean birth or who have had a uterine surgery, such as a fibroid (leiomyoma) removal, because of the increased risk of uterine rupture (see Chapter 18 for a description of uterine rupture). Also, these agents can cause fetal heart rate changes. Nursing care of the woman receiving a pharmacologic method of labor induction includes fetal heart rate and contraction monitoring.

Prostaglandin E_2 (Dinoprostone)

Prostaglandin E_2, dinoprostone, is available as a gel or as a vaginal insert. The health care provider inserts the gel into the cervix, whereas the vaginal insert is time-released and is placed into the posterior fornix of the vagina during a vaginal examination. The insert stays in place until spontaneous labor ensues, or for at least 12 hours. One advantage of the insert is that, if uterine hyperstimulation occurs, the insert can be removed by pulling on the string that is attached to it, like a tampon.

The woman receiving prostaglandins should be in a facility that has continuous fetal monitoring capabilities. Assist the RN in placing the fetal monitor on the woman prior to the procedure. At least 20 minutes of fetal heart rate and uterine activity should be documented before the prostaglandins are administered. Assist the health care provider as requested for the vaginal examination, and instruct the woman about the importance of lying in a recumbent position, with a wedge under one hip, for at least 30 minutes after the procedure. Continue the fetal monitor tracing as ordered. The RN will monitor the woman for signs of uterine hyperstimulation and monitor the fetal heart rate for signs of fetal distress.

Prostaglandin E_2 is usually administered in the evening. Many health care providers prefer to keep the woman in the delivery suite overnight to allow for fetal and maternal observation and then begin oxytocin induction of labor in the morning, approximately 6 to 12 hours after dinoprostone is applied.

Names Can Be Misleading
Even though prostaglandin E_2 has the numeral "2" in it, this is the first choice of medications the provider will usually choose for induction of labor by a pharmacologic method.

Prostaglandin E_1 (Misoprostol)

Use of the synthetic prostaglandin E_1, misoprostol, is considered off-label, as misoprostol is approved by the FDA to treat gastric ulcers that are caused by nonsteroidal anti-inflammatory drug (NSAID) use. However, the effects of misoprostol as a cervical ripening agent have been successfully documented. It is administered either orally or vaginally to ripen the cervix. When given via the oral route, misoprostol causes less uterine hyperstimulation than via the vaginal route. Some studies indicate that there is lower chance of cesarean birth with a low oral dose of misoprostol as compared to other routes and also as compared to dinoprostone. Nursing care for the woman receiving misoprostol is similar to that described for dinoprostone.

Artificial Rupture of Membranes

Artificial rupture of membranes (**AROM**), also known as an **amniotomy**, can be done to induce labor or to augment labor that has already begun. The health care provider introduces a hard plastic instrument with a hook on the end, called an amniohook, into the vagina during a digital examination. The health care provider then guides the instrument through the cervix and uses the hook to create a hole in the membranes (Fig. 11-1). At this point, amniotic fluid is usually expelled. This process causes the body to release prostaglandins, which enhances labor.

Oxytocin Induction

Intravenous (IV) oxytocin, a synthetic form of the posterior pituitary hormone that causes the uterus to contract, is the

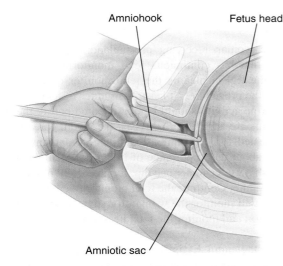

FIGURE 11-1 An amniohook is guided through the cervix by the health care provider to "nick" the fetal membranes, causing them to rupture artificially. (Reprinted with permission from O'Meara, A. M. (2019). *Maternity, newborn, and women's health nursing: a case-based approach.* Wolters Kluwer.)

most common agent used for labor induction. The woman is admitted to a labor and delivery suite and the external fetal monitor is attached. Fetal monitoring is done for at least 20 minutes to obtain a baseline fetal heart assessment, a mainline IV line is started, and the RN connects the oxytocin medication as a secondary IV line. An infusion pump is required for oxytocin administration to ensure precise control of the dose. The RN closely manages the woman receiving oxytocin induction.

Several potential complications are associated with the use of oxytocin for inducing labor. When labor is induced, as compared to the woman going into spontaneous labor, the risk for a cesarean birth increases. There is also a risk that the uterus will be hyperstimulated. Hyperstimulation leads to contractions that occur one after the other without a sufficient rest period in between. This can lead to fetal distress and even uterine rupture. The fetal distress is due to a decrease in blood flow through the placenta causing a decrease in the amount of oxygen the fetus receives. Another potential complication is water retention. Symptoms of water retention include hyponatremia, confusion, convulsions, or coma. Congestive heart failure and death also can occur.

Nursing Care

The role of the licensed practical/vocational nurse (LPN/LVN) during induction depends upon the procedure. Comfort care, including changing lines and supporting the laboring woman, is an important intervention performed by the LPN/LVN. The RN maintains responsibility for monitoring the woman and her fetus during pharmacologic cervical ripening procedures and oxytocin induction and augmentation. However, as the LPN/LVN, you may be asked to assist the health care provider during a pelvic examination in which mechanical methods of cervical ripening are used (i.e., membrane stripping and laminaria insertion) or during an amniotomy.

When assisting with amniotomy, document the fetal heart rate before and after the procedure. Continue to observe the fetal heart rate after the procedure. Notify the RN or health care provider if the fetal heart rate drops from the baseline that was obtained prior to the procedure. One risk associated with AROM is a prolapsed umbilical cord, especially if the fetus is not engaged. See Chapter 18 for a description of umbilical cord prolapse. Nursing care after an amniotomy also includes noting and documenting the color and amount of the amniotic fluid. Monitor for an increase in contraction frequency and strength after the amniotomy as this is an expected response to the procedure.

> ## TEST YOURSELF
> ✔ Name two medical indications for the induction of labor.
> ✔ What nursing interventions are included in the care of the woman whose labor is being induced?
> ✔ List two major complications associated with labor induction.

ASSISTED DELIVERY

Sometimes a problem develops in one of the essential components (passenger, powers, psyche; see Chapter 8) toward the end of labor. For example, the fetus may descend to the pelvic floor without rotating to the anterior position, or the mother may become tired and stop pushing effectively. In cases such as these, the birth attendant may elect to use an operative technique or device to hasten the delivery. Types of assisted delivery include episiotomy, vacuum-assisted delivery, and forceps delivery. Another name for instrument-assisted vaginal delivery (vacuum or forceps) is operative vaginal birth. The surgeon may employ either instrument during cesarean birth as well, although the following discussion focuses on operative vaginal birth.

Episiotomy

An **episiotomy** is a surgical incision made into the perineum to enlarge the posterior part of the vaginal opening just before the baby is born. Rates of episiotomies vary from state to state and hospitals. Some hospitals report a rate of 20% and others as high as 40%. The American College of Obstetricians and Gynecologists (ACOG), World Health Organization (WHO) and other groups have position statements that an episiotomy should not be done routinely during a spontaneous vaginal delivery because of complications associated with its use and should only be done if medically indicated.

A midline episiotomy increases the risk that the perineum will tear into the anal sphincter, a condition that increases maternal discomfort as well as the risk of infection and long-term consequences, such as anal incontinence. Complications from an episiotomy include bleeding, hematoma, infection, and an extension of the episiotomy into

BOX 11-1 Methods to Minimize the Need for Episiotomy

- Prenatal perineal massage
- Using natural pushing techniques, particularly in the side-lying position
- Birth attendant's patience with the delivery process
- Warm compresses to the perineum during second stage of labor
- Delivering the fetal head between contractions

the anal sphincter. Box 11-1 lists several measures that can reduce the need for an episiotomy.

However, an episiotomy is appropriate in certain situations. These include the following:

- The baby's shoulders are stuck in the birth canal after the head is born (shoulder dystocia).
- The head will not rotate from an occiput posterior position (persistent occiput posterior).
- The fetus is in a breech presentation.
- Instruments (forceps or vacuum) are being used to shorten the second stage of labor.

There are two basic types of episiotomies (Fig. 11-2). A median or midline episiotomy extends from the fourchette (the point where the labia minora join at the perineum) straight down into the true perineum. This type of episiotomy increases the risk for extension into the anal sphincter but is easier for the health care provider to repair than a mediolateral episiotomy, which angles to the right or left of the perineum.

The perineum requires repair after an episiotomy. The birth attendant uses local anesthesia to numb the perineum for repair. If the woman had epidural anesthesia, she may not need additional anesthesia for repair. The nurse should have sutures and other supplies readily available according to the birth attendant's preference. Reassure the woman that the sutures are absorbable and do not need to be removed. A sterile ice pack applied to the perineum after repair can help decrease swelling and pain.

A Personal Glimpse

When I was pregnant with my second child, I reread everything about the experience: the pregnancy, the delivery, the recovery, and nursing. Having had one healthy baby before this one, I felt like I was prepared for what was going to happen in the whole process of delivering a baby.

When my water broke at 4 AM on a Saturday, my husband and I rushed to the hospital. The vaginal delivery went well and quickly. However, after our little girl was born, I was told that I had been given an "episiotomy." Of course during the delivery, I was numb from the epidural, and I really had no idea what had gone on other than being told to push numerous times. The nurse left me some cotton pads and told me to keep myself clean until the stitches "melted."

The area of the episiotomy caused me a lot of pain. Every time I sat on the toilet to urinate, my vaginal area would hurt. I would avoid having bowel movements, as those were very painful as well. When I told the nurses about how much it hurt, they would tell me to clean myself better after urinating and got a doctor to prescribe me a stool softener to take home.

It wasn't until I was discharged and my mother was staying at home with me to help out that we figured out what the problem was. I asked my mother to look at my vaginal area, and she saw that one of the stitches had a knot that had irritated the skin around it and caused a sore.

It would have been better if one of the nurses had looked for me (with my giant belly after the delivery, I couldn't see a thing) and figured out what the problem was before I had left the hospital.

Shelly

Learning Opportunity: *Discuss two actions the nurse could take to better prepare this new mother to understand how to take care of her episiotomy. What assessments do you think the nurse should make for a client with an episiotomy?*

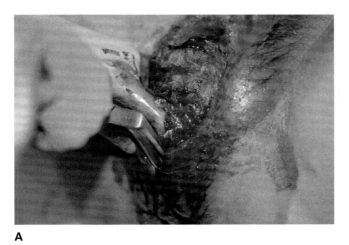

A

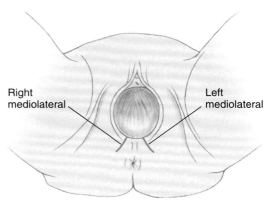

Right mediolateral

Left mediolateral

B

FIGURE 11-2 Two basic types of episiotomy. **A.** Midline episiotomy extends straight down into the true perineum. **B.** Mediolateral episiotomy angles to the right or the left of the perineum.

Vacuum-Assisted Delivery

Another procedure sometimes used to assist the delivery is the **vacuum extraction**, in which the birth attendant places a suction cup, made of plastic or soft silicone, on the fetal head and connects it to a handheld suction device. The RN pumps the device, which applies the suction, to the level directed by the birth attendant. The birth attendant then uses the device to gently guide the delivery of the fetal head (Fig. 11-3). The RN is responsible for providing the necessary equipment, connecting and regulating the suction as instructed by the birth attendant, monitoring fetal status, and supporting the laboring woman during the procedure by keeping her informed of the procedure and progress.

Vacuum-assisted delivery is not without risk. Serious neonatal complications, such as scalp bruising or lacerations, cephalohematoma, subgaleal and intracranial hemorrhage, can occur (Wegner & Bernstein, 2020). The risk increases with the amount of pressure used; the number of times the suction cup suddenly loses suction, commonly called a "pop-off"; and the total amount of time the suction is used.

Forceps-Assisted Delivery

Forceps are metal instruments with curved, blunted blades (somewhat like large flattened spoons) that are placed around the head of the fetus by the birth attendant to facilitate delivery (Fig. 11-4). Low and outlet forceps are more common than midforceps. Outlet forceps are applied when the fetal head can be seen at the introitus. Low forceps are used when the station is equal to or greater than +2, but the head is not yet showing on the perineum. Midforceps are used when the fetal head is well engaged but still relatively high in the pelvis (higher than +2) and are most often used to assist the fetus in rotating to an anterior position.

Operative Vaginal Delivery Indications

Prior to the birth attendant using either forceps or vacuum extraction, there are several requirements that must have already occurred. These include that the cervix must be completely dilated, the membranes must already be ruptured, the fetal head must be engaged, satisfactory maternal anesthesia should be in effect, the woman's bladder is empty, and the woman has consented to the procedure. Any problem that causes the second stage of delivery to be prolonged, or any situation of concern that is likely to be relieved by delivery of the infant, may be an indication for assisted delivery. Maternal indications include fatigue (the woman is too physically exhausted to push); certain chronic medical conditions, such as heart or lung disease; and prolonged second stage of labor. If the fetal strip is nonreassuring and the woman is a candidate for forceps delivery, then the birth attendant may use an episiotomy or forceps to deliver the infant rapidly.

Complications of Operative Vaginal Delivery

Because operative vaginal delivery is invasive, there are associated risks. Neonatal cephalohematoma, retinal, subdural, and subgaleal hemorrhage occur more frequently with vacuum extraction than with forceps. Facial bruising, facial nerve injury, skull fractures, and seizures are more common with forceps. The woman is at higher risk to have episiotomy and for extension of episiotomy into the anal sphincter with operative vaginal delivery. Other maternal complications include uterine rupture, perineal pain, lacerations, hematomas, urinary retention, anemia, and rehospitalization (Wegner & Bernstein, 2020).

Nursing Care

Nursing responsibilities for the LPN/LVN during an assisted delivery include obtaining needed equipment and supplies; monitoring maternal and fetal status before, during, and

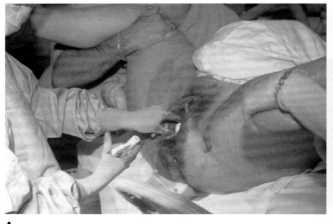
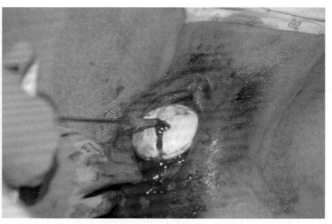

A   B

FIGURE 11-3 Delivery assisted by vacuum extraction. **A.** The birth attendant has just placed the suction cup on the fetal head and is using the hand pump to increase the pressure. **B.** Gentle traction is placed on the fetal head to assist it through the last maneuvers of delivery.

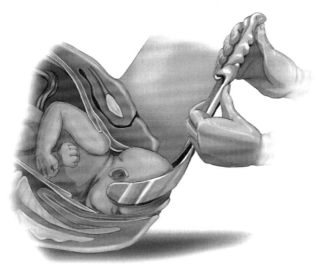

FIGURE 11-4 Forceps-assisted delivery.

Remember **Deidre Jordan**. What interventions might the birth attendant take at this point to assist the progress of the labor? What would you need to include in your nursing care for Deidre? How can you best support her at this point in her labor (2 cm and 50% effaced)? What information would you want to provide her with?

after the procedure; assisting the birth attendant and the RN caring for the woman; providing support for the woman and her labor partner; and documenting the type of procedure, as well as maternal and fetal response. Be aware that use of a technique to assist vaginal delivery may not work, and anticipate the possibility of cesarean delivery. Episiotomy care after delivery is discussed in Chapter 12.

After either a vacuum-assisted or forceps-assisted delivery, the infant should be examined carefully for signs of trauma. This could include cephalohematoma, bruising, edema, caput from the suction cup (often referred to as chignon, as it resembles a bun hairstyle), forceps mark, and facial or shoulder paralysis. Reassure the parents that forceps marks and exaggerated caput from vacuum-assisted deliveries will subside in a few days. Observe the infant who has facial bruising for an elevated bilirubin level (as the blood cells from the bruise as it heals will increase the circulating bilirubin levels) and instruct parents to observe for, and report, any jaundice noted in the newborn the first few days after discharge.

Maternal soft tissue trauma may also result from an operative vaginal delivery. Inspect the perineum for bruising and edema. Monitor closely for excessive bleeding or development of a hematoma. (See Chapter 19 for nursing care of the woman with postpartum hemorrhage.) Monitor for urinary retention by measuring each void the woman has. In addition, provide pain relief, and apply ice to the perineum to promote comfort and decrease perineal swelling. If the swelling is severe, the woman may need an in-and-out or indwelling catheter.

Tell the Whole Story!

It is critical to inform the postpartum and nursery nurses that the birth was instrument-assisted. Complications, although rare, may not appear until several hours after birth. Your report alerts caregivers to monitor for complications.

CESAREAN BIRTH

A **cesarean birth** is the delivery of a fetus through incisions made into both the abdomen and the uterus. Sometimes, the term "cesarean section" is used. This discussion uses the terms "cesarean birth" and "cesarean delivery" because the focus for the nurse and the woman is the birth experience.

Indications

There are many indications for cesarean birth. Some of the more common reasons for a cesarean birth include history of previous cesarean (or other uterine incision), labor dystocia (failure to progress in labor), nonreassuring fetal status, and fetal malpresentation (i.e., breech presentation).

Other less common obstetric indications include placenta previa (placenta covers the cervix), placental abruption (abruptio placentae; placenta separates from the uterus before birth), **cephalopelvic disproportion** (**CPD**; this is when the fetal head is too large to fit through the pelvis), active vaginal herpes lesions, prolapse of the umbilical cord, and ruptured uterus. Sometimes medical and obstetric conditions necessitate premature delivery of the fetus and require cesarean delivery. Examples include maternal diabetes, preeclampsia, erythroblastosis fetalis, and for some fetal malformations (such as spina bifida).

Incidence

Birth by cesarean was rare before the development of antibiotics and antiseptic surgical techniques because of high maternal mortality rates from infection. The cesarean birth rate in the United States in 2018 was 31.9%. The lowest rate of cesarean births in the United States was in 1996 at 20.7% of all deliveries (CDC, 2019). There are many factors that contribute to the increase in cesarean deliveries. Box 11-2 lists some of these factors.

Risks

Cesarean birth is a major surgery and carries with it all the risks associated with surgery combined with the risks of birth itself. A woman who delivers by cesarean is at risk

BOX 11-2 Factors Contributing to the Rise in Cesarean Deliveries

- Change in perception of risk by health care providers and pregnant women regarding cesarean birth
- Rise in the number of older pregnant women
- More labor inductions for nonmedical reasons (e.g., mother wants the infant born on a certain date for a specific reason, to start maternity leave at that time, significance of birth date)
- Almost universal use of continuous electronic fetal monitoring, which carries with it high false-positive indications of fetal compromise (i.e., the tracing indicates compromise when none exists)
- Trend toward delivering breech presentation via cesarean birth
- Return to the adage "once a cesarean, always a cesarean"
- A decrease in VBAC attempts
- Increasing concerns regarding malpractice litigation
- Increased prevalence of multiple gestations
- Increased prevalence of maternal obesity
- New phenomenon of cesarean by demand (women asking for planned cesarean without medical indications)

for anesthesia-related complications, thromboembolic and wound complications, and infection. The normal physiologic changes of pregnancy increase some surgical risk factors. For example, thrombophlebitis is a complication of both surgery and pregnancy, so the risk is higher with cesarean delivery than vaginal delivery.

There are risks to the fetus as well. Inadvertent delivery of a premature fetus is one cesarean risk factor. In addition, a cesarean birth increases the incidence of transient tachypnea of the newborn, a type of respiratory distress, due to the fetal lung fluid not being expressed from vaginal compression during delivery. For these reasons, cesarean delivery should be performed only when the risks of vaginal delivery clearly outweigh the risks of surgery. Because of the higher morbidity and mortality rates associated with cesarean delivery versus vaginal delivery, it is a national goal to decrease the cesarean delivery rate.

Maternal Complications

Maternal complications that can occur during the operation include laceration of the uterine artery, bladder, ureter, or bowel; hemorrhage requiring blood transfusion; and hysterectomy. The most common postoperative complication associated with cesarean birth is infection. Two common infection sites are the uterus and the surgical wound, although sepsis, urinary tract infection, and other infections can also occur. Pneumonia, postpartum hemorrhage, thrombophlebitis, and other surgical-related complications (such as wound dehiscence) can occur during the postoperative period.

Fetal Complications

The two most common fetal complications are unintended delivery of an immature fetus because of miscalculation of dates and respiratory distress because of retained lung fluid. Because the fetus delivered by scheduled cesarean birth does not go through the birth canal, they does not have the chance to get most of the amniotic fluid squeezed out of their lungs, as does a baby born vaginally. Therefore, respiratory distress happens more frequently in these newborns. In addition, general anesthesia given to the woman can depress the fetus's respiratory drive, making it difficult for the newborn to take their first breath. Less commonly, fetal injury can occur. For example, the scalpel cutting through the uterine wall can nick the baby causing a small laceration. Usually, these wounds are superficial and require minimal intervention. The fetus can become wedged in the pelvis after a prolonged second stage with the woman pushing, which can make for a difficult extraction leading to bruising and possibly other injuries.

Incision Types

There are two major incisions made during cesarean birth: one through the abdominal wall and the other into the uterus.

Abdominal Incisions

An incision made into the abdomen is termed a laparotomy and for a cesarean birth it can be either vertical or low transverse (Fig. 11-5). Vertical abdominal incisions are located in the midline of the lower abdomen. A low transverse incision is commonly known as a "bikini cut" (Fig. 11-5B). Although a low transverse incision slightly increases the risk for bleeding, this is usually the preferred method for cosmetic reasons.

Uterine Incisions

An incision made into the uterus is termed a hysterotomy and can be either vertical or low transverse (Fig. 11-6). There are two types of vertical uterine incisions: classical and low cervical. The classical incision (Fig. 11-6A) extends through the body of the uterus to the fundus. This incision is used only in severe emergencies, when it is critical to deliver the fetus immediately or when the fetus is unusually large. Bleeding during surgery is more likely with a classical uterine incision. It carries a higher risk for abdominal infection and the highest risk for uterine rupture in subsequent pregnancies. The low cervical vertical incision (Fig. 11-6B) is smaller and carries a lower risk for uterine rupture than does the classical approach, but it is used infrequently because it is more complicated to perform, carries higher risk of maternal injury, and is associated with a higher risk of uterine rupture than is the low cervical transverse incision. It does have the advantage of allowing for extension of the incision into the body of the uterus, if the surgeon has difficulty extracting the fetus. The low cervical transverse incision (Fig. 11-6C) is the preferred method. This incision is associated with the least risk of uterine rupture, is easier to repair, and is associated with less blood loss (Berghella, 2020a).

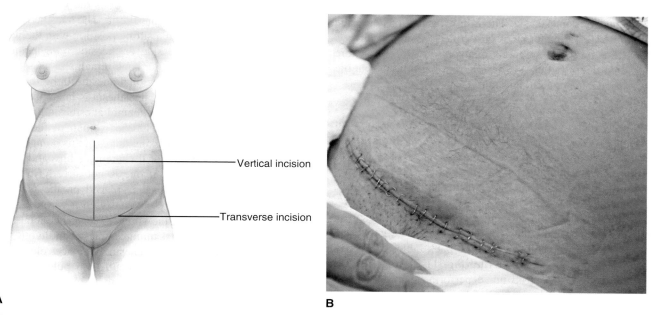

FIGURE 11-5 **A.** Types of abdominal incisions used for cesarean delivery: vertical or low transverse. **B.** Example of a low transverse abdominal incision.

TEST YOURSELF

✔ Name four common indications for a cesarean birth.

✔ Name three possible complications of cesarean birth for both the mother and the fetus.

✔ Cesarean delivery involves incisions into what two structures?

Steps of a Cesarean Delivery

Because cesarean birth involves major surgery, the period encompassing the surgery is the **perioperative period**, which has three phases: preoperative, intraoperative, and postoperative. Care of the woman during the preoperative and intraoperative phases requires a team approach, sometimes referred to as collaborative management. You may be involved in some of the preoperative care to prepare the woman for surgery. You may also be a part of the intraoperative care by functioning in the scrub nurse role. The RN

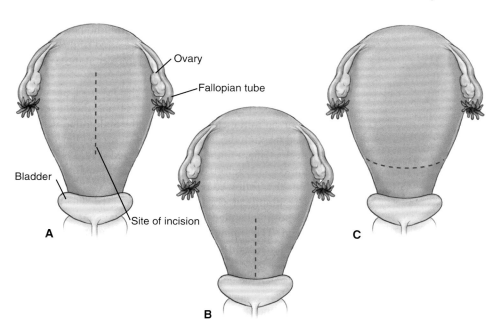

FIGURE 11-6 Types of uterine incisions used for cesarean delivery. **A.** Classical (vertical) approach. **B.** Low (cervical) vertical approach. **C.** Low (cervical) transverse approach.

carries out the immediate postoperative care in the postanesthesia care unit (PACU). You may assume care of the woman during the postoperative phase, after she has sufficiently recovered from anesthesia. The following sections describe and illustrate the major steps of a typical cesarean delivery. Some facilities and surgeons may perform the procedure slightly differently than the description that follows, but the basic principles remain the same.

Preoperative Phase

Preparing the woman for the cesarean birth is the focus of preoperative care. The anesthetist interviews the woman, explains the planned anesthesia to include risks, obtains verbal consent, reviews laboratory results, and orders preoperative medications, such as antacids and, less frequently, a sedative.

The scrub technician or nurse opens the sterile cesarean delivery pack and instruments, puts on a sterile gown and gloves, and proceeds to prepare the back table and instruments keeping everything sterile (Fig. 11-7). Together the circulating RN and scrub nurse perform an initial instrument, sponge, and sharp count. The initial and subsequent counts are extremely important to client safety to help prevent any equipment from being left in the woman. The scrub nurse holds accountability with the circulating RN for accuracy of counts during and after the surgery.

The woman's labor support person changes into operating room (OR) attire, usually a scrub suit or disposable coverall suit, a surgical cap, mask, and shoe covers. The labor support person is often anxious if the surgery is unplanned and will need information on what to expect, how the laboring woman is doing, and an update on the fetus. The RN reviews the preoperative checklist and chart for completeness. An IV is started if the woman does not already have one infusing. A surgical cap is placed on the woman's head to cover her hair, and she is transported to the OR suite by wheelchair or stretcher or she may ambulate with assistance.

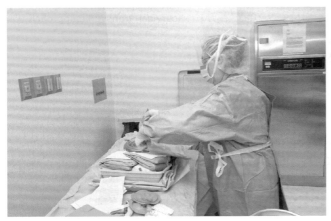

FIGURE 11-7 Cesarean birth: preoperative phase. The scrub nurse sets up the back table in preparation for cesarean delivery.

Intraoperative Phase

The intraoperative phase begins once the woman enters the OR. The circulating nurse positions the woman on the operating table for regional anesthesia. The anesthetist may request the woman to be in a sitting position with the woman's legs dangling to one side or the side-lying position. Support the woman so that her back remains in a C-shaped curve during placement of regional anesthesia by the anesthetist (Fig. 11-8A). (General anesthesia is uncommon; see Chapter 9 for nursing care for general anesthesia.)

The circulating RN assists the woman to the supine position on the OR table. Nursing duties at this point include placing a wedge under one of the woman's hips and inserting an indwelling catheter, if one is not already in place. Additionally, a grounding pad is placed on the woman's thigh, the woman's legs are covered with a warm blanket, and a safety strap secures the woman's legs. The fetal heart rate is checked for at least 1 minutes unless continuous fetal monitoring is in progress. The anesthetist places electrocardiogram leads, a blood pressure cuff, and pulse oximeter device on the woman and connects them to the monitoring equipment. The woman's arms are positioned on arm boards and her wrists are gently immobilized with soft restraints.

The circulating nurse performs a sterile abdominal preparation with alcohol, povidone–iodine, chlorhexidine, or other antiseptic, as per facility policy (Fig. 11-8B). The surgical team performs a time-out. A **time-out** is a procedure that is part of the Universal Protocol developed to reduce the incidence of wrong site, wrong procedure, and wrong person surgery. The Universal Protocol emphasizes accurate client and procedure identification and informed consent. During the time-out, each member of the surgical team, which includes the client, must agree and actively communicate their agreement that the right procedure is being performed on the right client with documented informed consent before the procedure can begin. Then, the health care provider and assistant place sterile drapes on the woman. Individuals who will be attending the newborn and the woman's labor support person are called to the surgical suite. The woman's labor support person sits at the woman's head behind the surgical drapes.

The health care provider tests the level of anesthesia before proceeding (Fig. 11-8C). If the anesthesia level is sufficient, an initial cut is made into the abdominal wall and extended through the layers of skin, fascia, and muscle until the lower segment of the uterus is exposed (Fig. 11-8D). The incision is made into the uterus. The fetal head is delivered (Fig. 11-8E), followed by the body.

The umbilical cord is double clamped and cut; then the newborn is handed over to the medical staff assigned to the infant. The infant may be briefly shown to the mother and support person (Fig. 11-8F) before being taken to the warmer for assessment, drying off, and resuscitation if needed. When the newborn is breathing well and stable, they are double wrapped in prewarmed blankets with a cap on their head and then taken to the woman and support person for initial bonding (Fig. 11-8G).

After the infant is delivered, the health care provider then physically removes the placenta. Then the health care provider brings the fundus and body of the uterus through the incision (Fig. 11-8H) and cleans the inside thoroughly; then the uterine incision is closed and sutured. The circulating nurse and scrub technician perform another instrument count. If the woman desires a tubal ligation, the procedure is performed at this time. The tubes are tied and ligated (Fig. 11-8I) and the specimens handed to the circulating RN, who labels them to be sent to the laboratory. The health care provider then replaces the uterus in the pelvic cavity.

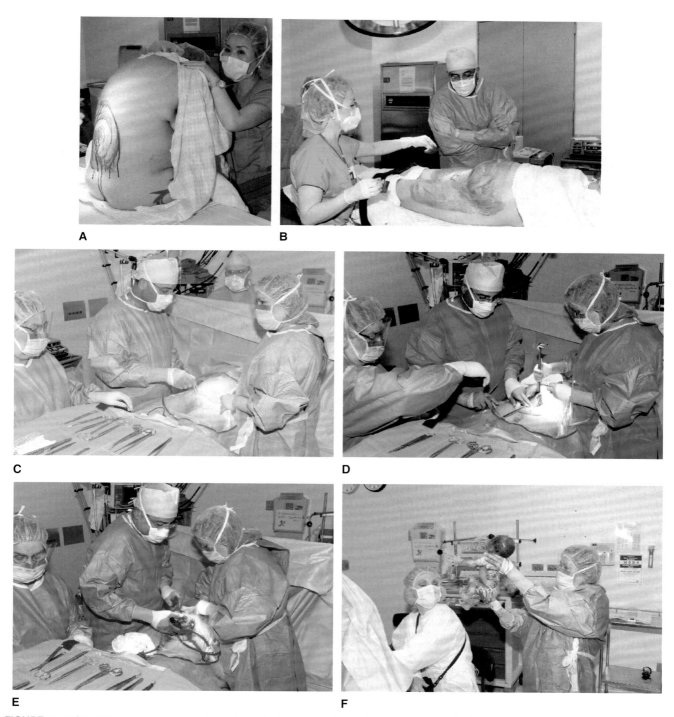

FIGURE 11-8 Cesarean birth: intraoperative phase. **A.** Preparing for regional anesthesia. **B.** Abdominal skin preparation. **C.** Testing anesthesia level before initial incision. **D.** Abdominal incision is complete and now preparing for the uterine incision. **E.** Delivery of fetal head. **F.** The newborn is quickly shown to the client.

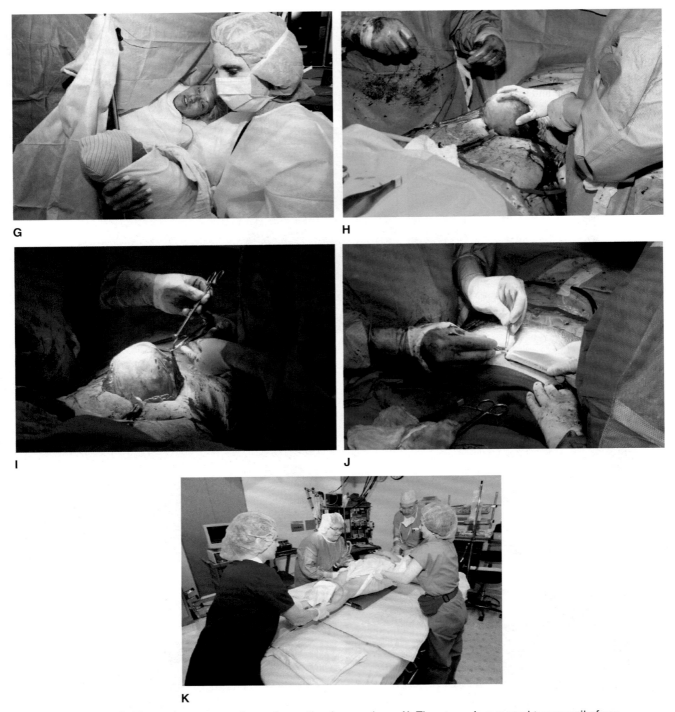

FIGURE 11-8 Cont'd **G.** The support person shows the mother her newborn. **H.** The uterus is removed temporarily from abdominal cavity to make suturing easier. **I.** A fallopian tube is ligated (the mother requested surgical sterilization). **J.** Stapling the skin incision. **K.** The surgical team moves the client to a stretcher.

Repair of muscle and fascia layers is done with absorbable suture while another instrument count is done. An x-ray should be done while the woman is still on the OR table if the counts were not done for any reason or if there is a discrepancy between the initial and subsequent counts. The abdominal incision is closed by the surgical team using staples (Fig. 11-8J) or sutures and a sterile dressing is applied. The circulating nurse removes the drapes, massages the uterine fundus, and places a sterile perineal pad on the woman. The woman is moved from the OR table to a stretcher (Fig. 11-8K) and transported to the PACU for initial recovery from anesthesia.

Your Voice Is Critical!
Never be afraid to speak up if the surgical counts are incorrect. Many client injuries can be prevented by the scrub nurse voicing their concerns.

Postoperative Phase

The circulating RN gives report to the PACU RN. In labor and delivery units, the PACU RN and circulating RN may be the same individual. The woman is placed on a cardiac monitor, an automatic blood pressure device, and a pulse oximeter (Fig. 11-9). The PACU RN performs a thorough assessment to include level of consciousness, cardiac and respiratory status, condition of the dressing, fundal and lochia status, urinary output, condition and patency of IV site, pain status, and a full set of vital signs. The RN completes this assessment at least every 15 minutes for hour or until the woman meets PACU discharge criteria, which vary by facility and anesthetist. The anesthetist writes orders for pain control in the PACU and usually for the first 24 hours after surgery.

Nursing Care

Reinforcing Family Teaching for a Planned Cesarean Birth

The focus of nursing intervention for a planned cesarean is family education (see Tips for Reinforcing Family Teaching: Preparing for a Planned Cesarean Birth). Each time you encounter the client before surgery is an opportunity to explore with the woman and her partner what they know about cesarean delivery. Reinforce the procedural steps to take, such as where to preregister, when and where to have laboratory work drawn, and when and where to present for surgery. Review what they can expect during the surgical experience. Review with the woman and her support person how to help avoid complications in the postoperative period, such as the how and why of taking deep breaths and turning frequently while in bed and why it is important to ambulate as soon as possible after surgery. Reinforce the principles of postoperative pain control and the options that are available to her for pain relief. Reinforcement of teaching is more effective when it occurs over time in multiple sessions, involves repetition of major concepts, and focuses on topics in which the family is interested.

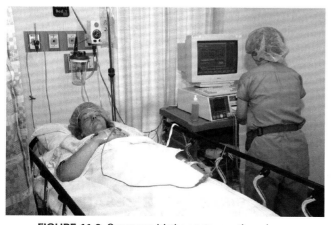

FIGURE 11-9 Cesarean birth: postoperative phase.

TIPS FOR REINFORCING FAMILY TEACHING

Preparing for a Planned Cesarean Birth

- Be sure to preregister and have blood work drawn.[1]
- You will meet the anesthesia provider for preoperative evaluation. Ask for these details when you preregister.
- Be sure to note the date, time, and location to which to present before the surgery.
- Do not eat or drink anything before surgery. Your health care provider will tell you how long you need to be fasting.
- An IV will be placed in the preoperative holding area and will remain in place for approximately 24 hours after the procedure, until you are tolerating liquids by mouth.
- Regional anesthesia (epidural or spinal) is usually performed to decrease the risk to mother and baby associated with general anesthesia.
- An indwelling catheter will be inserted into your urinary bladder and will remain in place for approximately 24 hours after surgery.
- After the surgery, you will spend some time in the recovery area. You will be transferred to your postpartum room as soon as you have sufficiently recovered from anesthesia.
- After delivery, and for the remainder of your hospital stay, the nurse will check your uterus to make sure it is contracted. This is done by pressing on your abdomen near your incision.
- You will need to turn, cough, and deep breathe every 1 to 2 hours after surgery. This is important to help prevent respiratory complications. You will be shown these techniques after delivery.
- Early and frequent ambulation is important to decrease the pain and distention of intestinal gas and to decrease risks associated with major surgery, such as respiratory complications, infection, and thrombophlebitis.
- The anesthesia provider will discuss postoperative pain management strategies with you. After the surgery, be sure to request pain medications before pain becomes severe.
- You may have different sources of pain that respond to different types of treatment (e.g., gas buildup responds best to ambulation and simethicone, incisional pain is usually best treated with opioids, and uterine cramping often responds well to nonsteroidal anti-inflammatory drugs).
- After cesarean, using the football hold when breast-feeding your baby will help decrease pressure on your incision.

---

[1]Some of these procedures will be done on the morning of surgery, depending upon the protocols of the facility at which the woman has chosen to deliver.

Providing Preoperative Care

Nursing interventions to help the woman and her partner prepare for cesarean birth depend on many factors, including whether it is a planned procedure and whether the woman has experienced cesarean delivery in the past. Ideally, the woman and her partner will have attended childbirth classes. Part of childbirth class discussion centers on the possibility of cesarean birth. When a woman is psychologically prepared for the experience, coping is enhanced.

Whether the cesarean is a planned or emergent procedure, several preparations are critical. Always check to see if the woman has given informed consent and that a signed consent form documents it (Fig. 11-10). Ask the woman when she last had anything to eat or drink. Follow facility and anesthetist orders regarding fasting times before surgery. Often, liquids are permissible closer to surgery time than are solids (ACOG, 2018). Frequently, the anesthetist orders an antacid, such as sodium citrate, before surgery to reduce the pH of the gastric contents in order to reduce risk of aspiration while the woman is under the effects of anesthesia. An IV must be in place with a large-bore (generally 18-gauge or larger) catheter. Lactated Ringer solution is a commonly ordered IV fluid. Sometimes clippers are used to remove hair from the abdomen and perineal area. Clippers do not create skin nicks like razors can (skin nicks increase the risk for infection), so clippers are the preferred tool to use. An indwelling catheter must be in place before the surgery begins to decrease the risk that the health care provider might inadvertently cut a full bladder during surgery. Sometimes the catheter is inserted in the preoperative area. Alternatively, the circulating nurse may place it after anesthesia has been administered, which is more comfortable for the woman.

Ensure that required laboratory studies are completed. The routine complete blood count, hemoglobin, and blood type and screen are important presurgical labs to obtain. When a type and screen is done, the laboratory holds at least two units of blood that matches the woman's blood type. The health care provider may also order other laboratory studies, such as electrolytes. When the woman is ready for surgery, assist the RN in transferring the client to the operating suite and then to the operating table.

Remember!

A client can withdraw consent at any time. If she states she has changed her mind, she is not sure, or she needs more information, alert the charge nurse or health care provider immediately so that her concerns can be addressed.

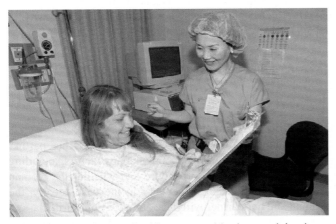

FIGURE 11-10 After the health care provider has explained the procedure, the nurse witnesses signing of the informed consent form.

Providing Support During an Unplanned or Emergency Cesarean Birth

When a cesarean birth becomes necessary because of an unplanned or emergency situation, it is important to quickly prepare the woman for surgery. The woman and her labor support are often anxious and worried about the baby. She may be fearful of the surgery or anesthesia, particularly if she has never had surgery before. There is usually not much time for education; therefore, support of the woman and her family becomes paramount. See Nursing Process and Care Plan *for the Woman Undergoing Assisted Delivery* for in-depth description of support measures.

Providing Care in the Immediate Recovery Phase

Many factors influence nursing care in the postoperative period. Some of these factors are the type of anesthesia that was given, the outcome and condition of the newborn, the stability of the woman, and complications, if any, that occurred during surgery. The type of anesthesia, in large part, influences the timing and process of recovery. Chapter 9 discusses the different types of anesthesia, including recovery considerations.

Assist the RN in transferring the woman from the operative suite to the PACU. The woman will be connected to continuous monitoring devices that record the electrocardiogram, blood pressure, pulse, and oxygen saturation of the blood. The RN is responsible for the assessment of this information. The RN will also take vital signs and pulse oximetry readings every 5 minutes until the readings are stable, and then every 15 to 30 minutes until the client has met predetermined criteria. The RN assesses the client's urinary output to make certain it is at least 30 mL/hr.

In addition to normal PACU activities, the RN must also perform postpartum assessments. The RN evaluates the condition of the fundus and records the findings along with vital signs. The RN uses a hand or a pillow to support the incision while gently massaging the fundus to determine if it is firm. A firmly contracted uterus minimizes bleeding. In conjunction with the fundal check, the RN performs an assessment of the amount and type of lochia (discharge from the uterus after birth). The RN performs and records these assessments at the same time interval as the vital signs. (See Chapter 12 for a full discussion of postpartum assessment and nursing care.)

A Word of Caution Is in Order!

During cesarean birth, the health care provider thoroughly cleans inside the uterus. Therefore, there is less lochia flow than after a vaginal delivery. Check for postpartum hemorrhage if lochia flow is moderate or heavy, or if the woman saturates more than one perineal pad in an hour.

VAGINAL BIRTH AFTER CESAREAN

In the past, the adage "once a cesarean, always a cesarean" guided the practice of obstetrics in the United States, and women with a prior cesarean birth were scheduled for repeat cesareans. During the 1980s, efforts began to decrease the number of cesarean births in the United States by reducing the number of repeat cesarean births, opting instead for **vaginal birth after cesarean** (VBAC). VBAC rates were at the highest in the late 1990s and have steadily declined since then. In 2018, 13.3% of women who had a prior cesarean delivery had a VBAC delivery (CDC, 2019). This is due to several factors including restrictions placed on the procedure by hospitals and insurance companies, client request, and many obstetricians no longer offering this procedure for their clients because of safety and legal liability concerns. ACOG developed guidelines identifying factors for the health care provider to consider before attempting a trial of labor after cesarean (TOLAC). Because of the risks associated with a VBAC delivery, there is continued debate in the medical community regarding the safety and advisability of VBAC.

Prerequisites

The woman attempting a VBAC should not have had a prior cesarean for cephalopelvic disproportion (CPD). The guidelines set by ACOG require the presence of a surgeon, anesthesia provider, and OR personnel in the hospital throughout active labor who are able to perform an immediate cesarean delivery if needed. Prior to attempting a TOLAC, the woman needs to have adequate counseling from her health care provider regarding the benefits and risks as well as the benefits and risks for a repeat cesarean delivery. She needs to give consent to the attempt for TOLAC. The health care provider or RN should be at the bedside to read and interpret electronic fetal monitor tracings because they can recognize the signs and symptoms of uterine rupture.

Contraindications

The risk for uterine rupture during VBAC is much higher when a woman has a classical uterine incision from a previous cesarean delivery; therefore, VBAC is contraindicated when this type of scar is present. Other contraindications include any complication that disqualifies the woman for a vaginal delivery such as placenta previa, history of previous uterine rupture, and lack of facilities or equipment to perform an immediate emergency cesarean.

Risks and Benefits

The greatest concern during TOLAC is uterine rupture. Although the overall risk remains very low, a woman who has a uterine scar, either from a previous cesarean section or from a uterine surgery such as a myomectomy, is more likely to suffer uterine rupture during labor. Uterine rupture becomes an emergency situation that puts both the woman and the fetus's life in danger. There are conflicting opinions over which mode of delivery is safer after a previous cesarean delivery. The risk of uterine rupture depends on several variables including the number of previous cesarean sections the woman has had, the amount of time between pregnancies, type of uterine scar, and if the current labor needs to be induced. Uterine rupture was seen less often in women who had a repeat cesarean section than a VBAC delivery (Landon & Frey, 2020).

Women who experience successful VBAC, as compared to women who have scheduled repeat cesareans, have less incidence of infection, hemorrhage, and blood transfusions. Also, women who have a VBAC have a shortened postpartum recovery time than a woman who has a repeat cesarean.

Several factors impact the likelihood of VBAC success. Factors that increase the likelihood of success include a history of a prior vaginal delivery or successful VBAC and onset of spontaneous labor with a ripe cervix. Factors that decrease a successful VBAC attempt include obesity, short stature, increased maternal age, fetal macrosomia, and induction of labor.

Induction of labor is another source of controversy regarding the woman attempting a VBAC delivery. Most authorities recommend either prostaglandins or oxytocin, but not both, for labor induction in VBAC. The health care provider needs to counsel the woman regarding the increased risk of uterine rupture with labor induction.

Nursing Care

It is outside the scope of practice for the LPN/LVN to care for a laboring woman who has a history of a previous cesarean delivery. An experienced RN will manage the labor. Many facilities require written informed consent that outlines the risks and benefits of VBAC. You may help ensure that the woman understands the plan of care and may witness the woman's signature on the consent form. The woman may verbally withdraw her consent at any time during the course of labor. At the time she withdraws her consent, the trial of labor is discontinued, and the woman is prepared for a cesarean delivery.

During the labor, the RN continuously monitors the electronic fetal monitoring tracing. The RN immediately reports any nonreassuring patterns to the health care provider because a nonreassuring pattern is the most significant sign of a ruptured uterus. Box 11-3 lists signs associated with uterine rupture.

BOX 11-3 *Signs of Uterine Rupture*

- Dramatic onset of fetal bradycardia or deep variable decelerations
- Reports by the woman of a "popping" sensation in her abdomen
- Excessive maternal pain (can be referred pain, such as to the chest)
- Unrelenting uterine contraction followed by a disorganized uterine pattern
- Increased fetal station felt upon vaginal examination (e.g., station is now −3 when it has been −1)
- Vaginal bleeding or increased bloody show
- Easily palpable fetal parts through the abdominal wall
- Signs of maternal shock

Nursing Process and Care Plan for the Woman Undergoing Assisted Delivery

While nurses who work in the labor and delivery department of a hospital are used to seeing these assisted delivery procedures, this is not a routine or expected event for the woman. For this reason, the nurse needs to be aware of the woman's experience and feelings. The nurse should not assume the woman understands what is happening or why the assisted delivery technique is being suggested/done. Fear for her infant and her own safety is a common feeling. Attitudes of the nursing staff can contribute to a positive, or negative, birth experience for the mother. The nurse should intercede to help the woman cope during this time and not wait for the woman to voice concerns. The woman may be too afraid to ask questions or verbalize understanding of information provided. She may be too overwhelmed to express her feelings.

Assessment (Data Collection)

While the woman is having an assisted delivery, regardless of the intervention the birth attendant uses, the woman will require ongoing data collection and support. She will need to be provided with information or have reinforcement of prior teaching done by the RN. Data collection will include overall assessment, vital signs, and fetal observations.

Overall data collection of the woman's status includes her level of consciousness, anxiety level, urinary elimination status, and any changes in amount of vaginal bleeding or changes in amniotic fluid color. The nurse will need to perform ongoing pain assessment and encourage the woman to use appropriate pain management techniques. During assisted delivery, the woman will not be able to utilize techniques such as position of comfort or a birthing ball so she will need to return to techniques such as effleurage and patterned breathing. The nurse needs to be aware of the labor support person's ability to provide support. The person with the mother may also need support during this time. Do not forget to include them in any explanations.

Vital signs need to be done more frequently during assisted delivery to help monitor the woman's status. Vital signs should be done prior to, during, and after any intervention by the birth attendant. Notify the RN or the birth attendant of any deviation from the woman's baseline or of any vital sign value that is at a critical level.

Fetal observations will include fetal movement, fetal heart rate monitoring, and observing fetal heart rate patterns. Contraction monitoring includes observing the contractions for intensity, frequency, and nonreassuring patterns. The LPN/LVN should notify the RN or health care provider of any nonreassuring fetal heart rates or any nonreassuring contraction patterns.

Support is shown in many ways. The nurse can show support of the woman through therapeutic communication, providing information, and a reassuring touch. Avoid platitudes such as "Everything will be ok," or "I know how you feel." Include the woman in conversations instead of talking to other staff as though the woman is not present. Encourage the woman to rest in-between contractions. During these rest periods, avoid conversations that are not related to the delivery (e.g., do not talk about a unit holiday party or a current TV show). A quiet room in-between contractions can help the woman rest and therefore better cope during the intervention or contractions.

Explain procedures as you are doing them. Use short, nontechnical sentences. The woman's anxiety may be elevated and she may not be able to process lengthy or detailed explanations. Repeat information as needed. If the RN or health care provider says the fetal monitor tracing is reassuring, reinforce this important fact to the woman and her labor support person. Explain what sensations she can expect to experience and what procedure to expect next. Be empathic. Acknowledge her feelings and let her know that these feelings are normal considering the situation with which she must cope.

Nursing Care Focus

When determining the focus of nursing care for the woman undergoing an assisted delivery, it is important to remember that this is an unfamiliar and possibly frightening experience for her. The woman may never have heard of, or experienced, the medical intervention before. Her lack of knowledge combined with the unfamiliar aspect can increase her anxiety.

Outcome Identification and Planning

Addressing and reducing the woman's anxiety and providing her with information are main goals to address. Anxiety can increase her pain, which can affect her oxygen levels and blood pressure, which can in turn decrease the amount of oxygen the fetus is receiving. Knowledge about what to expect and how her fetus is doing can help to decrease her anxiety.

Nursing Care Focus

- Acute anxiety related to fetal status and unexpected medical procedure

Goal

- The woman will demonstrate a decrease in her anxiety.

Implementations for Acute Anxiety

Observe the woman for nonverbal signs of anxiety such as jaw or hand clenching, rapid breathing, tics, an inability to focus, or an increase in vital signs. Note the level of the woman's anxiety. If the woman's anxiety is high or critical, the birth attendant may want to administer supplemental oxygen or medications to help decrease her anxiety and to aid fetal oxygenation and perfusion.

Remain with the woman while preparing her for the procedure. Provide therapeutic touch as appropriate to let the woman know you are supporting her and that you are with her. Display a calm and confident manner while providing nursing care and assisting the birth attendant. The presence of the nurse can be reassuring in a stressful situation. The confidence of the nurse helps promote trust. Trust can help decrease anxiety. In urgent situations continue to talk to the woman about what is happening and use a calm, lowered voice, and avoid yelling. This helps the woman to know that the situation is being handled professionally and that she is still the focus of care.

Encourage the woman to express her concerns. If she is unable to state her concerns or states "I don't know," validate that this is normal and that a nurse will remain with her during this time. Do not make promises you cannot keep (e.g., "I won't leave your side until you deliver," or "Everything will be ok").

In-between contractions and during pauses in the procedure, avoid excess conversations and decrease stimulation in the labor room as possible. Shut the door to the labor room, if possible, to decrease noise from the hallway or nurses' desk. Attend to alarms on monitors and IV pumps quickly. Mute phones and intercoms if possible. Handle instruments and open packages softly. Unexpected and extraneous noises can increase stimulation and decrease the woman's coping, which can increase her anxiety.

Explain procedures as you perform them and also what the client and her support person will experience throughout the procedure. Use short sentences with clear, simple language. Give the woman brief instructions on what to do at that moment. Do not tell her what she needs to do during future steps of the procedure. Understanding what is being done and why it is being done will decrease her anxiety. The woman who is already anxious will not be able to comprehend lengthy explanations, detailed medical terminology, or follow multiple instructions.

Encourage the woman's support person to be present and support her (e.g., holding her hand, remaining with her whenever possible) throughout the procedure. Encourage her labor support person to continue to assist her with pain management techniques (e.g., effleurage or patterned breathing). Involve her support person in the plan of care; do not talk only to the woman. Give helpful suggestions on how they can support the woman. Do not yell commands at the support person, rather give them examples of how they can help and demonstrate how you would like them to help. Do not assume they understand your verbal instructions. The presence and touch of a support person can be comforting and help decrease anxiety. If the support person also feels supported and is given information on how to help the woman, they can be more involved in assisting the woman and decreasing her anxiety.

Evaluation of Goal/Desired Outcome

- The woman rests between contractions or medical procedures and does not show signs of anxiety or elevated vital signs.

Nursing Care Focus

- Knowledge deficiency

Goal

- The woman will demonstrate understanding of medical intervention being performed to assist her delivery

Implementations for Knowledge Deficiency

Provide information in simple and clear language. Reinforce information that the birth attendant or RN has given by repeating and restating the information. The woman may need the same information given over and over to understand what is happening. Anxiety can also impede her processing of the information requiring the same information being said several times. Technical language and complex sentences may interfere with the woman understanding the information during a stressful time.

Provide information right before and during all interventions you are doing and what the woman can expect to experience. When telling the woman statements such as "I am going to touch you," wait a moment before actually touching her. Do not say what you are doing at the same moment you are doing the action—this does not help the woman to prepare or to know what is happening and can be startling or increase discomfort.

If needed and appropriate, use diagrams or pictures. Not everyone understands information given verbally. Some clients learn better through visual means. If the woman wears corrective lenses make sure she has those in place while information is given or while looking at visual aids. Visual cues the nurse gives while providing information can help the woman understand what is being said.

When determining if the woman understands the information given, do not use close-ended questions such as "Do you understand?" or "Is that clear?" Have the woman or her support person state back the information you gave. Close-ended questions do not adequately gauge understanding of information. Be mindful of the woman's culture. Some cultures consider questioning the healthcare staff as a sign of disrespect and may not ask questions. Anxiety can impair the woman's understanding of information.

Make certain that client and her support person have had any questions or concerns they have about the procedure addressed. If there are additional questions, notify the RN or birth attendant immediately.

Evaluation of Goal/Desired Outcome

- The woman acknowledges understanding of her procedure.

Remember **Deidre Jordan** from the beginning of the chapter. She has progressed to full dilation, her membranes spontaneously ruptured, and she has been pushing for 2 hours. From your readings, what methods do you think the birth attendant might choose at this point to assist her delivery? Are there any methods discussed that Deidre is not a candidate for? Why would those methods not be appropriate for her? If the methods chosen are unsuccessful, what do you think will happen to Deidre's labor and delivery?

KEY POINTS

- Medical indications for the induction of labor include postdate pregnancy, prelabor rupture of membranes, chorioamnionitis, gestational hypertension, intrauterine fetal growth restriction, fetal demise, or certain medical conditions, such as maternal diabetes.

- The Bishop score helps determine cervical readiness for labor. Five factors are evaluated: cervical consistency, position, dilation, effacement, and fetal station. Newer methods to evaluate cervical readiness include measuring cervical length and fetal fibronectin.

- Mechanical methods to enhance ripening of the cervix include membrane stripping and mechanical dilation (dilation) of the cervix with either a catheter or laminaria.

- Pharmacologic methods to ripen the cervix include local application of prostaglandin gel or vaginal inserts, or insertion of a prostaglandin tablet. Pharmacologic methods require closer monitoring of the woman.

- AROM, also called an amniotomy, is done by the birth attendant to induce or augment labor. The amniotic sac is ruptured by a plastic hook. Nursing care after an amniotomy includes noting the color and amount of the amniotic fluid and fetal heart rate.

- Oxytocin induction requires continuous fetal monitoring, a mainline IV, and a secondary IV line that contains the oxytocin on an IV pump. Complications associated with the use of oxytocin include higher risk for cesarean delivery, hyperstimulation of the uterus with possible uterine rupture, water retention, and fetal distress.

- An episiotomy is a surgical incision made in the perineum to enlarge the vaginal opening just before delivery. Some instances when an episiotomy is used include cases of shoulder dystocia, when the infant must be delivered quickly, or when forceps are used. A midline episiotomy extends straight downward into the true perineum. A mediolateral episiotomy angles to the right or the left of the perineum. Complications of an episiotomy include extension of a midline episiotomy into the anal sphincter or increased risk of blood loss and infection.

- Vacuum extraction involves a suction cup placed on the fetal head, which allows the birth attendant to provide gentle traction to assist delivery. Nursing considerations for the nurse during the procedure include assisting with creating the suction, monitoring the fetal heart rate pattern, and supporting the woman. After delivery, the neonate must be evaluated for complications from the vacuum extraction and the postpartum/nursery report must include the use of vacuum during delivery. The woman must be monitored for pain, excess blood loss, hematoma, urinary retention caused by edema, and infection.

- In a forceps-assisted delivery, hard metal tools shaped like large hollowed-out spoons are applied to the fetal head. Midforceps can help rotate the fetus to an anterior position. Low and outlet forceps can assist delivery when the fetus is at a low station and the woman is too fatigued to push effectively, pushing is contraindicated (e.g., maternal heart disease), the second stage of labor is prolonged, or the fetal monitor tracing is nonreassuring. Nursing considerations are similar to those for a vacuum extraction delivery.

- The most common indications for cesarean delivery are history of previous cesarean, labor dystocia, nonreassuring fetal status, and fetal malpresentation. Other less common indications include placenta previa, placental abruption (abruptio placentae), cephalopelvic disproportion (CPD), active vaginal herpes lesions, prolapse of the umbilical cord, fetal malformation (such as spina bifida), and ruptured uterus.

- Cesarean delivery is a major surgical procedure. For the woman it carries with it all the risks and complications associated with abdominal surgery including excess blood loss, infection, and prolonged recovery time. In addition, the woman who has a cesarean delivery also has the same risks that are associated with normal birth. Fetal complications include respiratory distress and accidental laceration from the scalpel.

- Both skin and uterine incisions can be vertical or transverse. The uterine incision is the important of the two. The classical (vertical) uterine incision is associated with the highest risk for uterine rupture in subsequent pregnancies. The low cervical transverse uterine incision is the preferred method.

- During the preoperative phase of a cesarean delivery, the LPN/LVN may assist the RN in preparing the client for surgery including obtaining vital signs, urinary catheter insertion, and assisting with positioning of the woman for anesthesia and on the operating table. After the woman has fully recovered in the PACU, the LPN/LVN may provide postoperative care for the woman and the newborn after a cesarean delivery.

- Nursing interventions for a planned cesarean birth focus on education to prepare the family for the birth. Interventions for an emergency cesarean include mostly supportive behaviors, such as explaining procedures as they are done and providing appropriate reassurance.

- Much controversy surrounds VBAC deliveries. The greatest concern in a VBAC delivery is the increased risk for uterine rupture during labor. The woman most likely to have a successful VBAC has only had one previous cesarean, has previously delivered a child vaginally, and whose labor has spontaneous onset and does not require augmentation. History of a classical uterine incision or a previous uterine rupture is a contraindication for VBAC.

INTERNET RESOURCES

Labor Induction

https://www.acog.org/patient-resources/faqs/
  labor-delivery-and-postpartum-care/labor-induction

Cesarean Birth

https://www.emedicinehealth.com/cesarean_childbirth/article_em.htm
https://medlineplus.gov/cesareansection.html
https://www.verywellfamily.com/
  cesarean-section-photos-step-by-step-2758512

VBAC

https://www.acog.org/patient-resources/
  faqs/labor-delivery-and-postpartum-care/
  vaginal-birth-after-cesarean-delivery

Workbook

NCLEX-STYLE REVIEW QUESTIONS

1. Which statement is true about episiotomies?
   a. An episiotomy is a routine procedure during a vaginal delivery.
   b. An episiotomy is always done to protect the woman's perineum from hard-to-repair tears.
   c. An episiotomy is an invasive procedure that has associated risks and benefits.
   d. An episiotomy is only indicated for certain extreme emergencies, such as shoulder dystocia.

2. A primigravida is tired of being pregnant. She asks the nurse, "Why can't my doctor just schedule a cesarean delivery? My friend had a cesarean, and everything went very well." What is the best reply by the nurse?
   a. "A cesarean birth involves major surgery, which puts you and your baby at higher risk for complications. Your health care provider will discuss the options with you."
   b. "I will ask your health care provider. Sometimes a first-time mother will be allowed to have a cesarean birth if she wants to do so."
   c. "Oh no. This would not be good for the baby. Try not to think too much about it. It is always better to have a vaginal delivery."
   d. "It is always your choice to have a cesarean delivery if that is what you want to do. Would you like me to help you schedule a date for the surgery?"

3. Which of the following are true regarding cesarean section? Select all that apply.
   a. After a woman has cesarean she will need to have a cesarean for all future deliveries.
   b. One of the most common complications after a cesarean is urinary retention.
   c. A common reason for a woman having a cesarean is failure for the labor to progress.
   d. Respiratory distress is a potential neonatal complication after a cesarean delivery.
   e. A vertical uterine incision places the woman at risk for uterine rupture in future pregnancies.

4. The LPN/LVN is the scrub nurse for a cesarean delivery. The surgeon asks for the scalpel to make the initial incision before a time-out has been called. What response by the scrub nurse is most appropriate?
   a. The nurse does not give the surgeon the scalpel and whispers to the circulating nurse to call the time-out.
   b. The nurse hands the surgeon the scalpel and calls the time-out.
   c. The nurse hands the surgeon the scalpel, but says not to start until the time-out is done.
   d. The nurse states that they will hand the surgeon the scalpel as soon as the time-out is completed.

5. A woman with history of previous cesarean is in labor. She has signed the consent form for a VBAC. She is dilated 7 cm and is making satisfactory progress in labor. She tells her nurse that she has changed her mind and she wants a cesarean. What response by the nurse is best?
   a. "Don't you want to do what's best for the baby? Your baby has a higher chance of having problems if you have a cesarean."
   b. "OK. Since you no longer consent to a VBAC, I will let the health care provider know, and we'll begin preparing you for a cesarean delivery."
   c. "There is no reason to do a cesarean right now. Let me ask your health care provider for an epidural to help relieve your pain."
   d. "You certainly have the right to change your mind. Can you tell me more about your reasons for wanting a cesarean so that we can discuss this further with your health care provider?"

STUDY ACTIVITIES

1. Develop a 15-minutes presentation on cesarean delivery to give to a group of first-time mothers at a prenatal education class.

2. Discuss how care of the newborn during cesarean delivery is different from care of the newborn after vaginal delivery. What additional risk factors does the newborn delivered by cesarean have?

3. Do an internet search on "labor induction." Using the table below, compare methods of labor induction.

Method	Description of the Technique	Prerequisites for Procedure	Contraindications	Nursing Interventions

CRITICAL THINKING: WHAT WOULD YOU DO?

Apply your knowledge of cesarean birth and assisted deliveries to the following situations.

1. Amy Jones is a 21-year-old gravida 1 who is attending a prenatal childbirth education class. She comments that she thinks she will not attend next week's class because cesarean delivery is going to be discussed, and she does not plan to have a cesarean. How would you reply to Amy's comment?

2. A woman who is close to term asks the nurse at a normal obstetric visit, "My doctor says I have a Bishop score of 4. What does that mean?"

a. How would you reply?

b. If the health care provider felt that the woman's labor needed to be induced, what recommendation would they likely make to the woman? Why?

3. You are going to assist the health care provider to perform an amniotomy. What equipment do you need?

4. Ellen Hess, a 30-year-old gravida 2, has chosen to attempt a VBAC. After 4 hours of labor, she reports to you severe pain and a "popping" sensation in her abdomen. What would you do?

UNIT 5
Postpartum and Newborn

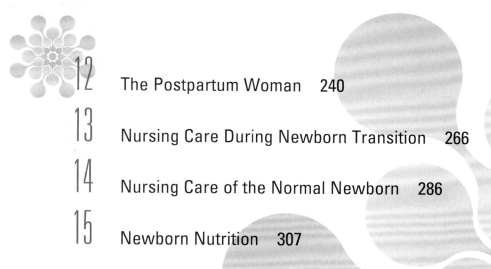

The Postpartum Woman

Key Terms

afterpains
attachment
boggy uterus
bonding
breakthrough pain
colostrum
diastasis recti
en face position
grand multiparity
involution
lochia
postpartum blues
puerperium

Learning Objectives

At the conclusion of this chapter, you will:

1. Describe physiologic adaptations the woman's body goes through during the postpartum period.
2. Discuss psychological adaptation during the postpartum period regarding attachment, bonding, and postpartum blues.
3. Describe the 11 main areas that are covered in a postpartum examination.
4. Describe nursing interventions in the early postpartum period.
5. Compare and contrast the postpartum nursing care of the woman who delivers vaginally with that of the one who delivers by cesarean.
6. Outline the nurse's role in preparing the postpartum woman for discharge.

Mei Chu has just delivered her second child 4 hours ago. Her newborn weighs 9 lb (4,082 g), and she wants to breastfeed. You enter her room to do her postpartum examination. What findings would you expect to see, and what findings would you need to report to the registered nurse (RN)? What might be some of Mei's concerns?

The processes of pregnancy and birth cause the woman to adapt both psychologically and physiologically. During the postpartum period, sometimes referred to as the fourth trimester of pregnancy, the woman must adjust to the reality of her new role as mother while her body recovers from pregnancy and childbirth. The postpartum period, or **puerperium**, encompasses the 6 to 12 (Berens, 2020) weeks after birth. This is sometimes referred to as "the fourth trimester." For ease of discussion, the puerperium is subdivided into three categories: the immediate postpartum period, which covers the first 24 hours; the early postpartum period, or first week; and late postpartum period, which refers to weeks 2 to 12. This chapter discusses the adaptations a low-risk woman makes during the puerperium and the nursing care that promotes healing and wellness.

MATERNAL ADAPTATION DURING THE POSTPARTUM PERIOD

Physiologic Adaptation

The woman's body undergoes tremendous changes during pregnancy. Every body system and organ is affected. During the postpartum period, the body recovers from the changes that occurred and returns to its normal prepregnancy state.

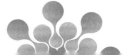

Reproductive System

The organs and hormones of the reproductive system must gradually return to their nonpregnant size and function. **Involution** is the process through which the uterus, cervix, and vagina return to the nonpregnant size and function.

Uterus

Uterine Contraction and Involution. Immediately after the placenta delivers, the uterus contracts inward, a process that seals off the open blood vessels at the former site of the placenta. If the uterus does not contract effectively, the woman will hemorrhage. The clotting cascade is also initiated to help control bleeding. Gradually, the decidua sloughs off, new endometrial tissue forms, and the placental area heals without leaving fibrous scar tissue.

Uterine contraction also leads to uterine involution, which normally occurs at a predictable rate. Uterine involution is monitored by measuring fundal height. Immediately after delivery, the uterus should be contracted firmly with the fundus located midline and at about the level of the umbilicus. The day after delivery, the fundus is found one fingerbreadth (1 cm) below the umbilicus. The normal process of involution thereafter is for the uterus to descend approximately one fingerbreadth per day until it has descended below the level of the pubic bone and can no longer be palpated. This occurs by the 10th to 14th postpartum day (Fig. 12-1).

Several factors promote uterine contraction and involution. Breast-feeding stimulates oxytocin release from the woman's posterior pituitary gland, which stimulates the uterus to contract. Oxytocin given via the IM or IV route can also help the uterus contract. Early ambulation and proper nourishment also foster normal involution.

In addition, there are factors that can inhibit or delay uterine involution. A full bladder impedes uterine contraction by pushing upward on the uterus and displacing it away from the midline. Any condition that overdistends the uterus during pregnancy can lead to ineffective uterine contraction after delivery. Examples include multifetal pregnancy, polyhydramnios, maternal exhaustion, excessive analgesia, and oxytocin use during labor and delivery. Other factors that can hinder effective contraction of the uterus include retained placental fragments, infection, and **grand multi-parity** (five or more pregnancies). When the uterus does not contract effectively, blood and clots collect in the uterus, which makes it even more difficult for the uterus to contract. This leads to a boggy uterus and hemorrhage if the condition is not corrected. A **boggy uterus** is a term used to describe a uterus in the postpartum period that is not contracted and feels soft and spongy, rather than firm and well contracted.

Afterpains. Uterine pain felt after delivery is referred to as **afterpains**. After a multipara delivers, the uterus contracts and relaxes at intervals. This leads to afterpains, which can be quite severe. For the primipara, the uterus normally remains contracted, and afterpains are less severe than that of the multipara. However, breast-feeding, because it causes the release of oxytocin, increases the duration and intensity of afterpains for both the primipara and multipara. For some women, afterpains are severe enough to require medication.

Lochia. The uterus must shed its lining that helped nourish the pregnancy. Blood, mucus, tissue, and white blood cells compose the uterine discharge known as **lochia** during the postpartum period. Lochia progresses through three stages:

- *Lochia rubra:* Occurs during the first 3 to 4 days; is of small to moderate amount; is composed mostly of blood; is dark red in color; has a fleshy odor.
- *Lochia serosa:* Occurs during days 4 to 10; decreases to a small amount; takes on a brownish or pinkish color.
- *Lochia alba:* Occurs after day 10; becomes white or pale yellow because the bleeding has stopped, and the discharge is now composed mostly of white blood cells.

Lochia may persist for the entire 6 weeks after delivery but often subsides by the end of the second or third week. Lochia should never contain large clots. Other abnormal findings include reversal of the pattern (e.g., the lochia has been serosa, then goes back to rubra), lochia that fails to decrease in amount or actually increases versus gradually decreasing, or is malodorous.

> **Warning!**
>
> Normal lochia has a fleshy, but not offensive, odor. If the lochia is malodorous or smells rotten, suspect infection. Report this finding immediately to the RN or health care provider.

Ovaries

Ovulation can occur as soon as 3 weeks after delivery. Menstrual periods usually begin within 6 to 8 weeks for the woman who is not breast-feeding. However, the lactating woman may not resume menses for as long as 18 months after giving birth. Although lactation may suppress

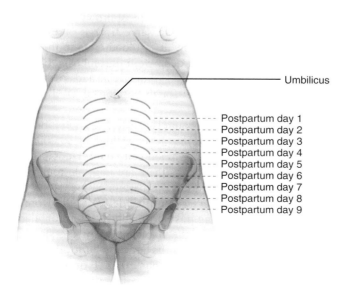

Umbilicus

Postpartum day 1
Postpartum day 2
Postpartum day 3
Postpartum day 4
Postpartum day 5
Postpartum day 6
Postpartum day 7
Postpartum day 8
Postpartum day 9

FIGURE 12-1 Uterine involution.

ovulation, it is not a dependable form of birth control. It is wise for the woman to use some type of birth control to prevent an unplanned pregnancy when she resumes sexual activity.

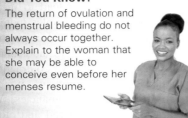

Cervix

During labor, the cervix thins and dilates. This process does not occur without some trauma. Directly after delivery, the cervix is still partially open and contains soft, small tears. It may also appear bruised. The internal os closes after a few days. Gradually, the muscle cells regenerate, and the cervix recovers by the end of the 6-week puerperium. The external os, however, remains slightly open and has a slitlike appearance in comparison with the dimple-like appearance of the cervix of a nulliparous woman (Fig. 12-2).

Vagina and Perineum

The vagina may have small tears that will heal without intervention. Immediately after delivery, the walls of the vagina are smooth. Rugae begin to return to the vaginal walls after approximately 3 weeks. The diameter of the introitus gradually becomes smaller by contraction. Muscle tone in the perineum never fully returns to the pregravid state; however, Kegel exercises may help increase the tone and enhance sexual enjoyment. Because breast-feeding suppresses ovulation, estrogen levels remain lower in the lactating woman, which can lead to vaginal dryness and dyspareunia (painful intercourse).

The labia and perineum may be edematous after delivery and may appear bruised, particularly after a difficult delivery. If an episiotomy was done or perineal tears repaired, absorbable stitches will be in place. The edges of the episiotomy or repair should be approximated (intact). The episiotomy takes several weeks to heal fully. The labia tend to be flaccid after childbirth.

Breasts

Colostrum, the antibody-rich breast secretion that is the precursor to breast milk, is normally excreted by the breasts in the last weeks of pregnancy and continues to be excreted in the first few postpartum days. Prolactin levels rise when estrogen and progesterone levels fall after delivery of the placenta. Suckling at the breast also causes prolactin levels to rise. Prolactin stimulates milk production by the breasts, and the milk normally comes in on the third day. See Chapter 15 for a detailed discussion of breast physiology, milk production, and breast-feeding.

Cardiovascular System

In the early postpartum period, the woman eliminates the additional fluid volume that is present during the pregnancy. This fluid loss occurs via the skin, urinary tract, and through blood loss. The woman who experiences a normal vaginal delivery loses approximately 300 to 500 mL of blood during delivery. If she has a cesarean delivery, normal blood loss is between 500 and 1,000 mL. As the blood volume returns to normal, some hemoconcentration occurs that causes an increase in the hematocrit.

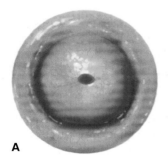

In the postpartum period, plasma fibrinogen levels are elevated, as are other coagulation factors. This helps to protect the woman against hemorrhage, but at the same time it predisposes the woman to the development of blood clots in the deep veins of the legs called deep vein thrombosis (DVT). Dehydration, immobility, and trauma can add to the risk for DVT. (See Chapter 19 for discussion of DVT in the postpartum period.)

The white blood cell count is elevated to approximately 15,000 to 20,000/mL and may reach as high as 30,000/mL. Leukocytosis, a high white blood cell count, helps protect the woman from infection, as there are multiple routes for infection to occur in the early postpartum period.

Immediately or very soon after delivery, the woman may experience shaking postpartum chills. Hormonal and physiologic changes are the likely cause of the shaking and chills. In any event, chills are not harmful, unless accompanied by fever greater than 100.4°F or other signs of infection. Chills normally resolve within minutes, especially if a prewarmed blanket is placed over the woman.

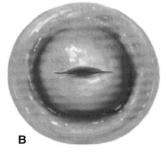

FIGURE 12-2 Appearance of the cervical os. **A.** Before the first pregnancy. **B.** After pregnancy.

Vital Signs

The temperature may be elevated slightly during the first 24 hours because of the exertion and dehydration of labor. After the first 24 hours, a temperature of 100.4°F or greater is abnormal and may indicate infection.

The blood pressure should remain at the woman's baseline level. An elevated blood pressure could be a sign of developing preeclampsia (see Chapter 17) and should be promptly reported. A falling blood pressure, particularly in the presence of a rising pulse, is suggestive of hemorrhage. Monitor the woman carefully for a source of blood loss if her blood pressure drops.

Here's a Clinical Tip!

For accurate blood pressure readings, have the woman sit on the edge of the bed for several minutes before measuring her blood pressure. If you take the blood pressure immediately after she sits up from a lying position, the reading may be falsely low due to orthostatic hypotension.

It is normal for the pulse to be slow in the first week after delivery. The heart rate may be as low as 50 beats per minute. Occasionally, the woman may experience tachycardia. This is more likely to occur after a difficult labor and delivery, dehydration, or it may indicate excessive blood loss.

Musculoskeletal System

The most pronounced changes are evident in the abdominal muscles, although other muscles may be weak because of the exertion of labor. The abdomen is soft and sagging in the immediate postpartum period. Often the woman has to wear loose or maternity clothing for the first few weeks after delivery. The abdomen usually regains its tone with exercise. However, in some women, the abdomen remains slack. In this situation, if another pregnancy occurs, the woman will have more problems with backache. **Diastasis recti** (also referred to as rectus abdominis diastasis) is a condition in which the abdominal muscles separate during the pregnancy, leaving part of the abdominal wall without muscular support. Exercise can improve muscle tone when this condition occurs. A woman is predisposed to poor muscle tone and diastasis if she has weak muscles or is obese before the pregnancy, her abdomen is overdistended during the pregnancy, or if she is a grand multipara.

Gastrointestinal System

Immediately after delivery, the postpartum woman is often very hungry. The energy expended during labor uses up glucose stores, and food has generally been restricted. Restriction of fluids and loss of fluids in labor, in the urine, and via diaphoresis (sweating) often leads to increased thirst.

Constipation may be a problem. Intra-abdominal pressure decreases rapidly after childbirth, and peristalsis is diminished. These factors make it more difficult for feces to travel through the gastrointestinal tract. The woman may be afraid to defecate in the early postpartum period because of hemorrhoidal discomfort and/or perineal pain. Suppressing the urge to defecate complicates the problem of constipation and may actually cause increased pain when defecation finally occurs. Iron supplementation adds to the problem. However, by the end of the first postpartum week, bowel function has usually returned to normal.

Urinary System

The urinary system must handle an increased load in the early postpartum period as the body excretes excess plasma volume. Healthy kidneys are able to adjust to the increased demands. Urinary output exceeds intake. Transient glycosuria, proteinuria, and ketonuria are normal in the immediate postpartum period.

During the process of labor and delivery, trauma can occur to the lower urinary system. Pressure of the descending fetal head on the ureters, bladder, and urethra can lead to transient loss of bladder tone and urethral edema. Trauma, certain medications, and anesthesia given during labor can also lead to a temporary loss of bladder sensation. Prolonged pushing can cause the perineum to become edematous, which can cause pressure around the urethra preventing the woman from being able to adequately void. The result can be urinary retention. Sometimes, the woman voids small amounts but does not completely empty the bladder, or she may not be able to void at all. Voiding may be painful if the urethra was traumatized.

The urinary system is more susceptible to infection during the postpartum period. Hydronephrosis, dilation of the renal pelves of the kidneys and ureters, is a normal change that occurs during pregnancy because of hormonal influences and increased renal blood flow. This condition persists for approximately 4 weeks after delivery. Hydronephrosis and urinary stasis predispose the woman to urinary tract infection.

Check This Out!

If you palpate the fundus and find it above the umbilicus, deviated to the right side, and boggy, the most likely cause is a full bladder. Assist the woman to void, and then reevaluate the fundus. If it does not become firm after she voids, immediately notify the RN or health care provider.

Integumentary System

Diaphoresis occurs in the first few days after childbirth as the body rids itself of excess water and waste via the skin. The woman notices the perspiration particularly at night. She may wake up and be drenched in sweat. This is a normal finding and is not a cause for concern.

The woman will likely have striae (stretch marks) on the abdomen and sometimes on the breasts. Immediately after birth, striae appear red or purplish. Over time, they fade to a light silvery color and remain faintly visible.

The nipples and areolas often darken in color during pregnancy and this color tends to lighten during the postpartum period. In addition, a woman who has linea nigra (see

Chapter 6) may notice it darkening and then lightening in color during the postpartum period.

Weight Loss

Immediately after delivery, approximately 12 to 14 lb (5.5 to 6.4 kg) is lost with the delivery of the fetus, placenta, and amniotic fluid. The woman loses an additional 5 to 15 lb (2.3 to 6.8 kg) in the early postpartum period because of fluid loss from diaphoresis and urinary excretion (Berens, 2020). The average woman will have returned to her prepregnant weight 6 months after childbirth if she was within the recommended weight gain of 25 to 30 lb (11.4 to 13.6 kg) during pregnancy. Some women take longer to lose the additional pounds. In general, the breast-feeding woman tends to lose weight faster than the woman who does not breastfeed because of increased caloric demands.

TEST YOURSELF

✔ A falling blood pressure and rising pulse in the early postpartum period is suggestive of _____.

✔ Name two factors that contribute to constipation in the postpartum period.

✔ Name two conditions to which the postpartum woman's urinary system is susceptible.

Psychological Adaptation

Role change is the most significant psychological adaptation the woman must make. This process occurs with each new addition to the family, but tends to be most pronounced for the first-time mother. Each child is unique with their own temperament and needs, and they must be integrated into the existing family structure. Therefore, the whole family must adapt to the addition of a new member.

As the nurse, you can influence the development of positive family relationships in many ways. Careful monitoring of maternal psychological adaptation and anticipatory guidance regarding postpartum blues and expected psychological adjustments can go a long way toward fostering a positive transition for the woman and the new family.

Becoming a Mother

A woman begins the process of becoming a mother during pregnancy as she anticipates the birth of the baby. She fantasizes about and prepares for her newborn's arrival. After the birth, the woman must take on the role of mother to the newborn. The two critical elements of becoming a mother are development of love and attachment to the child and engagement with the child. Engagement includes all the activities of caregiving as the child grows and changes. This transition is a continuously evolving process throughout the woman's life.

Although each woman takes on the mother role in her own way, influenced by her culture, upbringing, and role models, there are patterns of behavior that are similar for all women. The woman adapts to her new role as mother through a series of four developmental stages:

1. Beginning attachment and preparation for the infant during pregnancy
2. Increasing attachment, learning to care for the infant, and physical restoration during the early postpartum period
3. Moving toward a new normal in the first several months
4. Achieving a maternal identity around 4 months

The stages overlap, and social and environmental variables influence their lengths.

In the early postpartum period, the new mother demonstrates dependent behaviors. She has difficulty making decisions and needs assistance with self-care. She tends to be inwardly focused and concerned about her own physical needs such as food, rest, and elimination. She relives the delivery experience and has a great need to talk about the details. This process is important for her to integrate the experience into her concept of self. She may remain in this dependent, reintegration phase for several hours or days. This is not an optimum time to give the woman detailed newborn care information because the new mother is not readily receptive to instruction. Listen with an attitude of acceptance. No feeling the woman expresses is "wrong." Help her interpret the events of her birth experience.

Most women move quickly from the dependent stage to increasing independence in self- and newborn care. After she has rested and recovered somewhat from the stress of the delivery, the new mother has more energy to concentrate on her infant. At this point, she becomes receptive to infant care instruction. The first-time mother in particular needs reassurance that she is capable of providing care for her newborn. She may feel that the nursing staff is more adept than she is at meeting the newborn's needs. Therefore, it is important to encourage her to perform care for her newborn while providing gentle guidance and support. She responds well to praise for her early attempts at childcare during this phase. This phase lasts anywhere from 2 days to several weeks.

Don't Take Over!

Assist the woman to take care of her newborn rather than do all the care yourself. The new mother needs guidance, practice, and praise to begin to feel confident in her new role.

Development of Positive Family Relationships

Attachment is the enduring emotional bond that develops between the parent and infant. However, this process does not happen automatically. Attachment occurs as parents interact with and respond to their infant. In the early postpartum period, the woman may have a wide range of emotions and responses to her newborn. Humans seem to respond to gains and losses in similar ways. Disbelief and shock are often the initial reactions. The mother may say repeatedly, "I can't believe I just had a baby." Ambivalence is also a normal response. The new parents may communicate uncertainty over their readiness to take on the parent role. Frequently, the new mother may experience negative feelings about the newborn in the first few days after birth. However, she may not express these feelings because of the cultural expectation that "mothers always love their babies." If she does express negativity, such as, "I'm not sure that I like my baby," nurses or family members may reply in a way that denies or dismisses the emotion. "Oh, I'm sure you don't mean that," is one such dismissive response. It is important to remember that negative feelings are part of the process as the mother and newborn adjust to each other and become acquainted. Encourage the woman to express her feelings openly, and then show acceptance and let her know that her feelings are normal.

 Concept Mastery Alert

It is natural for some women to appear to be tentative in handling their newborn. This behavior is not a "difficulty" accepting the role change, but rather a natural response to a dramatic event. The nurse should continue to assess the mother's interactions with the infant before becoming alarmed.

The initial component of healthy attachment is a process called **bonding**. This is the way the new mother and partner become acquainted with their newborn (Fig. 12-3). The bonding process begins with a predictable pattern of parental behavior (Box 12-1). As bonding continues, she begins to spend more time holding the newborn in the **en face position** (the newborn's face is in her direct line of vision and she makes full eye contact with the newborn). The new mother often talks to the newborn using high-pitched tones. She smiles and laughs while she continues the en face posture.

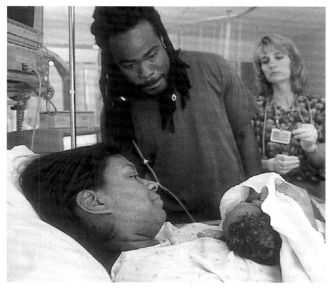

FIGURE 12-3 A mom and dad bond with their newborn immediately after birth.

 BOX 12-1 Progression of Initial Attachment Behaviors

The new mother and her partner both begin their interaction with the newborn in a fairly predictable sequence. Note that this process may take anywhere from minutes to hours to days. The health of the newborn may prevent some of these from happening immediately after birth.

1. Seeing and making eye contact with the infant. This is often accompanied by statements claiming the child (such as "She has my lips.").
2. Exploration begins with light fingertip touching.
3. The new parent explores the newborn's extremities.
4. Fingertip touching progresses to touching with the palmar surface of the parent's hands.
5. Larger body surfaces are touched and caressed.
6. The infant is enfolded with the parent's hands and arms and held closely.
7. Progressively more time is spent in the en face position talking to and smiling at the newborn.

A Personal Glimpse

I delivered my first child after 14 hours of intense labor. I went through my labor naturally without an epidural with the help of my doula. I pushed for 2 hours, so I was pretty exhausted after delivery. The midwife had to cut an episiotomy because she said it was a tight fit. My baby weighed 9 lb (4,082 g)! The next day while the baby was in the room, I remember that everything felt so unreal. I kept telling myself that I should feel happy. But all I really wanted to do was to cry. The nurse came in and told me what a beautiful baby I had and asked me her name. I started to cry and said that I wasn't sure that I could be a good mother. I felt scared and confused and unready to take care of a baby. The nurse told me that the feelings I was having were very normal. She said that this was a huge change for me and that it takes time to get adjusted to the new mother role. She asked me if I had someone to help me at home. I told her that my sister was going to stay with me for several weeks. The nurse gave me a card with the phone number for the hospital. She wrote her name on it and told me that she would be happy to answer any questions I had after I went home. She said that I could talk to any of the nurses, if she wasn't on duty when I called. I felt relieved. The nurse then stayed with me a while and watched while I changed the baby's diaper. She told me that I was a quick learner and that I was very gentle with the baby. I felt so much better. I knew that it was going to be OK.

Holly

Learning Opportunity: *Why do you think this new mother felt better after her interaction with the nurse? In what ways can you in your role as a nurse support the new mother when she expresses negative feelings about her newborn or her abilities as a mother?*

One important component in the development of healthy attachment between the new parents and their newborn is the amount and type of social support available to them. Access to supportive friends and relatives enhances attachment. When a new mother is isolated and without adequate social support, attachment is threatened. In this situation, it is important to assist the woman in finding sources of support. Perhaps there is someone in her neighborhood or community who might be willing to provide support. Discuss the situation with the RN in charge. A referral for home health care visits or social services may be in order.

You Can Do It!

If the new mother makes a negative comment regarding her ability to care for the newborn, make your response accepting and supportive. You might reply, "It is natural to have feelings of uncertainty as you adjust to having a new baby." Be creative, and come up with sincere, supportive phrases.

Cultural Snapshot

In many non-Western cultures, women relatives provide much of the social support and assist the mother at home. It is important to include these relatives in the care of the mother and infant in the hospital. Often this support lasts for 30 to 40 days and may include confining the new mother to her home to protect her and ensure that she rests. This is common in Chinese, Indian, and Middle Eastern cultures.

Healthy bonding behaviors include naming the newborn and calling the newborn by name. Making eye contact and talking to the newborn are other indicators that healthy attachment is occurring. It is important to differentiate between a new parent who is nervous and anxious about her new role and one who is rejecting her parenting role. Warning signals of poor attachment include turning away from the newborn, refusing or neglecting to provide care, and disengagement from the newborn.

Traditional thinking assumed that the mother was the first and most important person to bond with the newborn. We now know that the newborn can make many bonds. The mother's partner benefits from early contact with the newborn immediately after delivery. It is common for the partner to describe strong emotions of pride, joy, and other positive emotions when first holding the newborn and may be engrossed with the newborn. The partner also progresses through a pattern of touching similar to that of the mother.

Cultural Snapshot

Some cultures do not name the newborn until after a naming or presentation ceremony or until the infant is of certain age. The mother and family may refer to the infant as "baby" or "child." This is not a lack of bonding. In addition, some cultures may make limited eye contact or avoid touching the infant's head as a way to protect the infant from unwanted attention from spirits they feel will harm the infant.

Siblings also bond with the newborn (Fig. 12-4). There are special considerations that the parents need to make for older siblings. The birth of a new baby requires a role change for the sibling. Sometimes the newborn does not meet the sibling's expectations. For instance, the baby might be a boy, but the sibling wanted a sister. It is common for the sibling to regress for a few days after the birth or use acting-out behaviors.

Postpartum Blues

Approximately 50% or more of postpartum women experience postpartum blues (Viguera, 2019), sometimes called the "baby blues." **Postpartum blues** is a temporary condition that usually begins about the third day after delivery, lasts for 2 or 3 days, and usually has resolved by 2 weeks postpartum. Women who have had postpartum blues reported having one or more of the following: sadness or tearfulness for no apparent reason, irritability, anxiety, difficulty sleeping or eating, or may have decreased concentration. Women who have a history of premenstrual mood changes, antepartum depressive symptoms, cesarean section, not breast-feeding, family history of depression, or

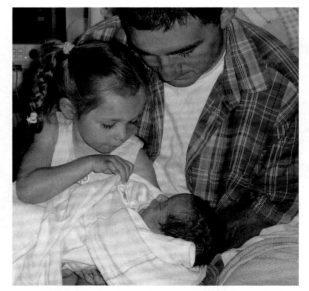

FIGURE 12-4 While the father bonds with his new son, the big sister takes a first peek at her new baby brother.

stress around child care are at risk for the postpartum blues (Viguera, 2019).

Other factors that can contribute to postpartum blues include too much activity, fatigue, disturbed sleep patterns, and discomfort. It is important for the woman and her family to know that this is a normal reaction. Support by the woman's family and friends, help with child care activities, and infant care during the night are beneficial to the woman. The condition resolves in about 2 weeks after delivery.

If the condition lasts for more than 2 weeks, or if the symptoms become severe or interfere with her daily activities (e.g., the woman does not want to feed her infant or refuses to perform activities of daily living), the woman should contact her health care provider or seek medical attention at the emergency department immediately. (See Chapter 19 for a discussion of postpartum depression.)

 Cultural Snapshot

The reported rates of postpartum depression vary among cultures. Reasons for this include the following: terms used to describe depression may not translate across different languages; commonly used postpartum depression screening tools were developed based upon primarily Western populations and may not adequately screen non-Western cultures for the presence of postpartum depression due to terms used; and some cultures consider sadness during the postpartum period as "shameful" and the woman may not be willing to disclose these feelings for fear of discrimination. It is important to screen all women for postpartum depression and provide information on symptoms that require follow-up.

TEST YOURSELF

✔ Describe behaviors that indicate positive attachment.

✔ List the normal progression of interaction that occurs during the initial bonding experience between a new parent and the newborn.

✔ Describe symptoms and risk factors for postpartum blues.

Remember **Mei Chu** from the beginning of the chapter. Since this is her second child and the child was greater than 4,000 g, what findings might indicate a problem with uterine involution? What information would you want to give her about afterpains that might be different than if this was her first delivery?

POSTPARTUM ASSESSMENT AND NURSING CARE

Most women who deliver vaginally go home within 24 to 48 hours after delivery and the woman who has a cesarean birth at about 72 hours after delivery. Therefore, when caring for the woman in the early postpartum period, it is essential to do thorough data collection to detect any complications that might be developing and to use every available opportunity to tell the woman about self- and newborn care.

After the initial recovery period, the woman may be transferred to a postpartum room. If she delivered in a labor, delivery, recovery, and postpartum setting, she will stay in the room in which she delivered. Whatever the setting, it is important to do a thorough initial examination and data collection when you are providing postpartum care.

Much of the data collection is done before the woman delivers and can be found on the initial admission assessment done by the RN upon admission to the labor and delivery unit. It is important to check both the initial assessment and the prenatal record as part of the initial data collection. The labor and delivery nurse gives report to the postpartum nurse upon transfer. The report should include pregnancy history (including significant medical history), labor and birth history, initial postpartum recovery, and general newborn data. If the postpartum nurse will also be caring for the newborn in addition to the mother (i.e., couplet or mother–baby care), then more detailed newborn information will be given to the postpartum nurse.

The medical and pregnancy histories are important because they alert the postpartum nurse to risk factors that might lead to postpartum hemorrhage or other complications and give clues as to bonding potential and nursing interventions. Box 12-2 identifies important information to include in the postpartum report.

At least once per shift, perform a complete head-to-toe examination. A quick visual survey and speaking to the woman reveals her level of consciousness and affect. Assist her in emptying her bladder, if necessary, before beginning the examination. First, take the vital signs. Respirations should be even and unlabored. Be sure to rule out shortness of breath and chest pain. The heart rate should be regular without murmurs and may be as slow as 50 beats per minute. The lungs should be clear in all five lobes (Fig. 12-5).

In addition to the general assessment, there are 11 main areas that must be monitored in the postpartum period: These are breasts, uterus, lochia, bladder, bowel, perineum, lower extremities, pain, laboratory studies, bonding, and maternal emotional status.

Initial Physical Findings in the First Hour Following Delivery

If the woman is going to hemorrhage, she is most likely to do so within the first postpartum hour. For this reason, monitor her closely during this period. Measure her vital signs every 15 minutes during the first hour. With each vital sign check, determine the position and firmness of the uterine

BOX 12-2 **Labor and Delivery Nursing Report to Postpartum Nurse**

Maternal Pregnancy History
- Maternal age
- Gravida and para (should now reflect the current birth)
- Gestational weeks
- Maternal blood type, Rh, and rubella status
- Complications experienced during the pregnancy
- Group B streptococcus culture status
- Any medical problems, including sexually transmitted infections and any preexisting medical conditions

Labor and Birth History
- The length of labor
- Type and time of membrane rupture including color and amount of fluid
- Any events during labor that needed intervention (such as late decelerations)
- Duration of pushing
- Type and time of birth
- Type and timing of analgesia or anesthesia administered
- Type and timing of any medications given (e.g., antibiotics or oxytocin)
- Any assisted birth techniques used (e.g., vacuum extraction, or episiotomy)
- Complications experienced during labor (including lacerations and if they needed repair)

Postpartum Recovery Information
- Status of the fundus, lochia, and perineum
- Last set of vital signs, time and values
- Type of pain, if any, and success of analgesics and comfort measures to control the pain
- Whether the woman ambulated after delivery and how she tolerated it
- Type and amount of IV fluids infusing, if any
- Voiding times and amounts since delivery
- Response of the woman and her partner to the newborn
- Support person(s) for the mother, their names, and relation to the mother
- If woman had a cesarean birth, include type of anesthesia, incisional dressing and incision, pain status, and if foley catheter present or not

Newborn Information
- Gender of infant
- Any significant details related to the infant postdelivery (e.g., low Apgar scores, resuscitation efforts needed after delivery, or congenital anomalies)
- The mother's plans for feeding, times infant fed, and duration of breast-feeding

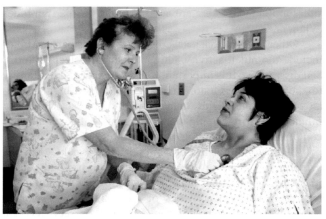

FIGURE 12-5 The nurse auscultates the lungs as part of a complete postpartum examination.

Breasts

Inspect the breasts and nipples for signs of engorgement, redness, or cracks. Palpate the breasts gently to determine if they are soft, filling, or engorged with milk. Note if there are any painful areas. Notice the nipples to determine if they are erect or inverted. The breasts should be soft during the first postpartum day and begin filling on the second and third days. Engorgement may occur on the third day. There should be no reddened areas on the breasts, and the nipples should be intact without cracks or fissures.

Uterus

Assess the uterus of the woman regardless of whether she had a vaginal or cesarean delivery. Make sure the woman has voided prior to checking the fundus. With the woman lying supine, palpate the fundus (Nursing Procedure 12-1). Note the tone (firm vs. boggy), position (midline vs. side-lying), and height of the fundus in relation to the umbilicus. It should be firm, midline, and at the appropriate height in relation to the umbilicus, depending on what hour or day it is after delivery. Some women find this uncomfortable, especially multiparas. It is best to start the palpation gently and then add pressure as needed to palpate the fundus.

If the fundus feels boggy, apply slight pressure as you massage the fundus in a circular motion with the fingertips of your hand that is at the top of the fundus. This should cause it to become firm and the woman may notice a slight gush of lochia. Reassure the woman this is a normal occurrence when the uterus contracts. Avoid vigorous fundal massage as this can overstimulate the uterus and cause it to become flaccid. Notify the RN if the woman required fundal massage and recheck the fundus within 15 to 30 minutes. If she is breast-feeding, encourage her to feed her infant as this will cause her body to release oxytocin, which will stimulate the uterus to contract as well.

For the woman who has had a cesarean birth, remember to check the fundus. It is not necessary to massage the fundus unless it is soft and the woman is bleeding vaginally. Any manipulation of the fundus increases pain. However, it is important to note fundal tone, position, and height. If the

fundus, the amount and character of lochia, and the status of the perineum and monitor for signs of bladder distention. If the woman had a cesarean delivery, also check the incisional dressing for intactness, and determine if there is any incisional bleeding. Some institutions continue monitoring every 30 minutes for the second hour, then every 4 hours during the first 24 hours after delivery.

NURSING PROCEDURE 12-1 Fundal Palpation and Massage

EQUIPMENT
Warm, clean hands
Clean gloves

PROCEDURE
1. Explain the procedure to the woman.
2. Instruct her to empty her bladder if necessary.
3. Wash hands thoroughly.
4. Position her supine with the head of the bed flat.
5. Locate and place one hand on the uterine fundus. It should feel hard and rounded—something like a melon.
6. Place the other hand in a cupped position just above the symphysis pubis, as in the picture. Use this hand to gently support the base of the uterus.
7. Gently palpate the fundus using the hand at the top of the fundus. Note if it is soft or boggy.
8. Notice the height, position and tone of the uterus.
9. If the fundus feels boggy (spongelike) or soft (instead of firm), then use your fingertips at the top of the fundus, apply some pressure, and massage in small circular motions without lifting your hand off the top of the fundus. This should cause the fundus to become firm and you are massaging.
   a. Vigorous fundal massage or overstimulation can cause the uterus to become flaccid rather than helping it contract. Take measures to avoid overmassaging the fundus.
10. Wash hands.
11. Notify the RN of the findings.

12. Document the findings and if fundal massage was needed, and outcome of the massage. The location of the fundus is documented as fingerbreadths above (+) or below (−) the umbilicus or at the level of the umbilicus. Document whether the fundus was midline or deviated to one side.

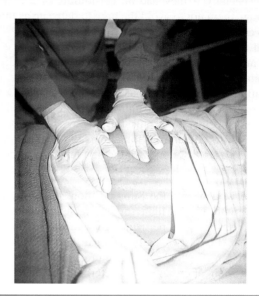

woman has had a cesarean birth, she may find it helpful to place her hand on top of yours as you palpate the fundus. Be mindful of her incision with your supporting hand.

Lochia
Determine the amount and color of the lochia. The amount is documented as scant, small, moderate, or heavy. In the first few days postpartum, the color will be rubra or serosa. Lochia should not have a foul smell. Be sure to check under the woman's buttocks for pooling. Ask her how many times she has changed her peripads (sanitary napkins) since the previous fundal check, and determine if she is saturating pads. The lochia should be rubra of small to moderate amount without large clots and no foul odor. Notify the RN if the postpartum woman is saturating more than one peripad in an hour.

Notice This Difference!
Expect less lochia after a cesarean delivery than after a vaginal delivery. This is because the surgeon cleans out the uterine cavity with surgical sponges before suturing it closed, which removes much of the blood and debris. Report moderate amounts of lochia after a cesarean, as this may signal postpartum hemorrhage.

Bladder
The woman should be voiding adequate amounts (more than 100 mL per each voiding) regularly. Voiding frequently in amounts smaller than 100 mL with associated suprapubic

distention (a rounded area just above the symphysis pubis) is indicative of urinary retention. A full bladder prevents the uterus from contracting and can lead to extra bleeding. Also, the full bladder will cause the uterus to deviate to the side, away from the midline of the umbilicus.

If the woman pushed for a long time or had a large infant, she may have some edema around the urethra, which can prevent her from completely emptying her bladder, leading to some urinary retention. Regardless of her pushing or infant size, all women should be assessed for urinary retention.

The best way to assist the woman with emptying her bladder is to help her up to the restroom to void. However, sometimes this is not possible because of incomplete recovery from regional anesthesia. In this instance, assist the woman to sit up on the bedpan, a position that may promote emptying of the bladder. Be certain that the woman has privacy. If she is having difficulty voiding, running water in the sink or using the peribottle to run warm water over the perineum may help. It also helps to give her plenty of time in which to void. If she feels rushed, this may contribute to urinary retention. If the woman cannot void on her first trip to the bathroom after delivery, it may be appropriate to allow her to wait for a while longer. If she is still unable to void and it has been longer than 6 hours or there are signs of bladder distention, you may need to perform an in-and-out urinary catheterization to empty her bladder. Likewise, catheterization may be necessary if she is voiding small amounts (less than 100 mL) in frequent intervals. Notify the RN if signs of urinary retention are noted.

Bowel

Next, visually inspect the abdomen and auscultate for bowel sounds. Bowel sounds should be present in all four quadrants. Ask the woman if she has had a bowel movement since delivery. Many women are very concerned about if they will have a lot of pain with their first bowel movement, especially if they had an episiotomy or lacerations. Encourage them not to avoid the urge to defecate as this can lead to constipation.

All of the normal measures that help prevent constipation are also helpful in the postpartum period. Adequate fluid intake keeps the feces soft, facilitating passage. Early ambulation stimulates normal bowel peristalsis. Adding plenty of fruits, vegetables, and fiber to the diet also helps to prevent constipation. A bulk-forming agent, such as psyllium, may also be helpful. Sometimes the health care provider orders a stool softener for the first few days after birth.

Perineum

Assist the woman into the Sims position. Lift the top buttock, and with a good light source (such as a penlight or flashlight) inspect the perineum for redness, edema, and ecchymosis (Fig. 12-6). If the woman had an episiotomy or a laceration (tear), check the sutures, and be certain the edges are well approximated. Determine if there is any drainage from the stitches. Palpate gently with a gloved hand to determine if there are any hematomas forming in the area. Note any hemorrhoids. The perineum should be intact with only minimal swelling and no hematomas.

Lower Extremities

Inspect the extremities for edema (Fig. 12-7), equality of pulses, and capillary refill. Check for potential DVT by inspecting the woman's calves. There should be no pain in the calves when the woman is walking. Feel along the calf area for any warmth or redness. The calves should be of equal size and warmth bilaterally. There should be no reddened, painful areas, and there should be no pain in the calves when she walks. Pain and/or one calf with

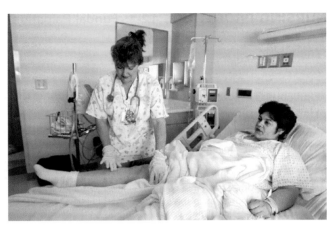

FIGURE 12-7 Monitoring of the lower extremities. The nurse checks the calf for edema, redness, and excess warmth and compares the diameter of both calves.

redness, warmth, and greater size than the other could indicate DVT (see Chapter 19) and must be reported to the RN.

Assist the woman in ambulating as soon as possible after delivery. Early ambulation decreases the chance of thrombus formation by promoting venous return. Encourage liberal fluid intake as dehydration contributes to the risk of thrombus formation. After a cesarean delivery, some health care providers will order compression devices until the woman is ambulating.

Preventing Injury From Falls

The first time the woman gets up, she is at risk for fainting and falling because of postural hypotension. When the woman is going to get out of bed for the first time after delivery, assist her in dangling her legs at the side of the bed for 5 minutes. If she is not feeling dizzy, assist her to the bathroom. Remain with her until she returns to bed. If she begins to feel dizzy at any time, help her sit down with her head forward for a few minutes. If she begins to black out, gently support her to the floor until she comes to. Another time she is at increased risk for fainting is the first time she is in the shower. The warm water may cause peripheral dilation of blood vessels, which leads to hypotension and fainting. Stay in the woman's room while she is showering for the first time. Have a shower chair available for her to sit on if she begins to feel faint.

Pain

Determine if the woman is experiencing any pain. If so, investigate the source (e.g., afterpains, episiotomy, painful urination, pain in the calves). Determine the characteristics, quality, and timing of the pain. Provide comfort and pharmacologic pain measures as appropriate. Note status of pain after pain relief measures are implemented. Some nursing care can cause pain. Fundal palpation can cause afterpains. Exhaustion can exacerbate pain; therefore make sure to cluster care, encourage the woman to rest, and limit visitors as appropriate.

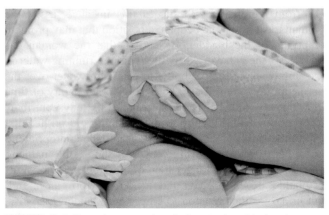

FIGURE 12-6 Postpartum perineal observation. Notice that the woman is in the Sims position. The nurse lifts the upper buttock and inspects the perineum.

NURSING PROCEDURE 12-2 Application of Perineal Ice Packs

EQUIPMENT

A commercial ice pack or a clean glove and ice
  Clean gloves

PROCEDURE

1. Explain procedure to the woman.
2. Wash hands thoroughly.
3. Position her in dorsal recumbent position.
4. Activate the commercial pack as instructed in the directions for use, or fill a clean glove with crushed ice, and tie a knot at the opening at the top of the glove.

5. Cover the pack or the glove with a thin covering, such as a towel.
6. Place the pack on the perineum.
7. Assist her to a position of comfort.
8. Wash hands.
9. Leave in place for 10 to 20 minutes then remove for 10 to 20 minutes. Repeat as necessary for comfort during the first 24 hours postpartum.
   a. If the ice pack is allowed to stay next to the perineum continuously for prolonged periods, tissue damage could result.

Breast Pain

Investigate breast pain to determine if it is unilateral and associated with increased warmth and redness. This could be a sign of mastitis, a postpartum complication discussed in Chapter 19. If the breasts are painful bilaterally because of engorgement, interventions will be chosen based on whether or not the woman is breast-feeding.

If she is breast-feeding, warmth seems to help the most. Have her run warm water over her breasts in the shower, or place a warm washcloth as a compress on the breasts. If the engorgement is preventing the newborn from latching on, advise the woman to express some milk before attempting to breastfeed. Caution her to only express enough to soften the breast to enable the infant to latch. Overexpressing the breast can cause further engorgement.

If the breasts are engorged and the woman is bottle-feeding her newborn, instruct her to keep a close-fitting support bra on 24 hours per day. This will provide comfort by supporting the extra weight in the breasts from the engorgement. It will also help to prevent leaking of milk from the breasts. Cool compresses or an ice pack wrapped in a towel will usually be soothing and help suppress milk production. She should refrain from any type of milk expression including allowing warm water to run over the breasts in the shower. The breasts will replenish any milk that is expressed or released.

If the nipples are painful during breast-feeding attempts, examine the nipples for cracks or fissures. Observe the woman when she puts her newborn to the breast, and ensure that she is positioning the newborn properly to prevent sore, cracked nipples. Encourage the use of a lanolin-based cream to keep the nipples soft and promote healing. A mild analgesic may be helpful. (See Chapter 15 for additional breast-feeding interventions.)

Afterpains

Ibuprofen or other nonsteroidal anti-inflammatory drugs (NSAIDs) are usually helpful if the source of pain is afterpains. The health care provider often will order 600 to 800 mg of ibuprofen every 6 to 8 hours as needed (PRN) for pain. For multiparas, it may be appropriate to schedule the medication around the clock, rather than waiting for the woman to ask for it. Timing administration of the drug so that the woman takes it 30 to 45 minutes before breast-feeding is also helpful because breast-feeding intensifies uterine cramping and associated afterpains. Nonpharmacologic methods that might be helpful include warm compresses to the abdomen, positioning for comfort, adequate rest and nutrition, and early ambulation.

Perineal Pain

If the pain is arising from the perineum, visually inspect the perineum before taking measures to control the pain. Check that the episiotomy is well approximated and that there are no signs of a hematoma. Early intervention within the first 24 hours include ice packs to the perineum (Nursing Procedure 12-2). Ice helps reduce swelling and ease painful sensations. Most institutions use special perineal ice packs that incorporate the cold source into the perineal pad. The ice pack should be on for 10 to 20 minutes, then off for 10 to 20 minutes to be most effective. Be careful not to apply an ice pack without a cloth cover next to the perineum. The cloth cover will help to protect the perineal tissues from trauma caused by the ice pack adhering to the tissue.

 C u l t u r a l   S n a p s h o t

In many cultures of Asian Americans, African Americans, and Americans of Hispanic or Latinx ethnicities, maintaining a hot–cold balance is important, especially in the postpartum and newborn period. Hot–cold balance impacts postpartum bathing/hygiene, room temperature, and dietary practices. The woman's culture may avoid bathing during the postpartum time. The nurse suggesting that the woman take a shower may cause her internal conflict. On one hand she may not want to take the shower but on the other hand may want to respect the authority of the nurse. If the woman believes that she should be as warm as possible, she may be reluctant to use the perineal ice pack and she may want to keep the room very warm and avoid air conditioning. The woman may avoid drinking the ice water that the nurse provides. Inquire about the woman's cultural customs and desires and use her answers to provide individualized, culturally appropriate care.

NURSING PROCEDURE 12-3 Assisting the Postpartum Woman With a Sitz Bath

EQUIPMENT

New sitz bath in manufacturer's packaging with directions
   Clean gloves

PROCEDURE

1. Explain the procedure to the woman.
2. Instruct her to empty her bladder, if necessary.
3. Wash hands thoroughly.
4. Place the sitz bath in the toilet as per the manufacturer's instructions.
5. Place the tubing in the allotted slot, and clamp the tubing.
6. Fill the bag with warm (102°F to 105°F) water and hang it at a level of a few feet above the toilet.
   a. Some women may prefer cooler water temperatures, which is an acceptable practice.
7. Unclamp the tubing, and allow the warm water to fill the basin.

8. Reclamp the tubing, and refill the bag with warm water. Seal the bag with the locking mechanism provided.
9. Assist the woman to sit on the basin so that her perineum is submerged in the water.
10. Ensure that she can reach the emergency call bell.
11. Instruct her to unclamp the tubing periodically to allow water to run over the perineum and into the toilet.
12. Encourage the woman to stay on the sitz bath for at least 20 minutes.
    a. Encourage the woman to use the sitz bath three times per day, or as needed for comfort.
13. Provide a clean towel with which to pat dry and clean sanitary napkins to apply when she is finished.
14. With clean-gloved hands, assist her to rinse out the basin, dry it, and store it for the next use.
15. Wash hands.

After the first 24 hours, warm sitz baths can be especially comforting for a woman with a sore perineum (Nursing Procedure 12-3). Throughout the first few postpartum days, mild analgesics combined with a narcotic are usually most helpful for perineal pain. Examples of combination products include acetaminophen with codeine or hydrocodone. Local anesthetics, such as witch hazel pads or benzocaine sprays, may be helpful in relieving perineal pain. Sitz baths, witch hazel pads, and/or products that contain hydrocortisone can also help reduce the pain associated with hemorrhoids.

> **Be Careful!**
> When administering combination products for pain, be certain you know the dose of each product in the combination. Be particularly watchful that you do not exceed the maximum daily recommended dosage of acetaminophen when giving products that contain this medication.

Pain After Cesarean Birth

Pain management for the woman after cesarean birth is a priority when providing postpartum care. During the first 24 hours, the anesthesiologist usually manages the pain. Generally, if the woman had a spinal narcotic administered, she will have orders for a PRN medication for breakthrough pain. **Breakthrough pain** occurs when the basal dose of analgesia does not control the pain adequately.

Another form of pain control that may be ordered is patient-controlled analgesia (PCA). This type of analgesia allows the woman to control how often she receives pain medication. The PCA pump delivers an opioid (usually morphine) into the IV line. The pump locks to prevent tampering. The health care provider's orders describe how much narcotic the woman receives when she pushes the button. The orders include a lockout interval so that the woman cannot accidentally overdose herself. Many women require reassurance that they cannot self-administer too much medication when using PCA.

Infrequently, the anesthetist orders narcotics only at PRN intervals after cesarean birth. In this instance, consult with the RN about administering the narcotic around the clock for the first 24 hours. It is easier to control pain before it becomes severe, and adequate pain control in the first 24 hours after surgery reduces the total amount of pain medication required. It is important to always assess the woman's pain prior to administering any pain medication and to reassess after the medication has been given.

> **A Word of Caution!**
> Do not push the PCA button yourself, even if the woman does not push the button. Pushing the PCA button for the woman is called analgesia by proxy. This practice is dangerous because you or a family member could inadvertently cause respiratory arrest.

The woman who is breast-feeding may be reluctant to take pain medication out of concern that the newborn may receive the medication. Inform her that adequate pain control is necessary so that she can ambulate well and provide self- and newborn care. Pain medications administered just prior to breast-feeding minimize the amount that the newborn will receive at that feeding.

Pruritus is a common side effect of narcotics given by the spinal or epidural routes. This side effect can become quite uncomfortable and can lead to scratching and excoriation. An antipruritic, usually diphenhydramine, may help control this side effect even though the cause of the pruritus is not from histamine release. Small doses of naloxone, nalbuphine, or naltrexone have been shown to help with the pruritus (Grant, 2020). If nothing is ordered, notify the anesthetist. Other comfort measures include applying lotion, administering a back rub, and using cool compresses or diversion to help control the itching.

Another common source of pain for the woman who delivers by cesarean is gas pain. The woman is at increased risk for gas formation after a cesarean because of decreased peristalsis, the lingering effects of anesthesia and analgesia, and manipulation of the intestines during surgery.

Gas pain is usually not relieved by analgesics. Many surgeons order simethicone around the clock or PRN. Frequent and early ambulation stimulates peristalsis and passing of flatus. Instruct the woman to avoid very hot or very cold beverages, carbonated beverages, chewing gum, and drinking through straws. All of these things can increase the formation and discomfort of gas. Other medical interventions may become necessary, such as rectal suppositories or enemas. Encourage the woman to lie on her left side. This position facilitates the release of gas. Having the woman rock in a rocking chair may also provide comfort from gas pains.

Laboratory Studies

Monitor the hemoglobin and hematocrit (H&H). Note the H&H before delivery. Most health care providers order a postpartum H&H on the morning after delivery. If the values drop significantly, the woman may have experienced postpartum hemorrhage. Note the blood type and Rh. If the woman is Rh-negative, she will need laboratory studies to determine if she is a candidate for a Rho(D) immune globulin injection before discharge. Determine the woman's rubella status. If she is nonimmune, she will need a rubella immunization before she is discharged home. If the woman needs both the Rho(D) immune globulin and rubella vaccine, notify the health care provider. The woman may need to have serum titers 6 to 8 weeks after the vaccination to see if she developed immunity to rubella as the Rho(D) immune globulin may prevent her body from making adequate antibodies. A revaccination may be necessary if she remains nonimmune.

Bonding

Any time the newborn is in the room, note maternal–newborn interactions. Observe the interaction during the infant's feedings. Be aware of the woman's culture and how that impacts her interactions with the newborn. Notice the quantity and quality of social support available to the woman. Inquire about preparations she made for the infant while pregnant and her plans for caring for the newborn after discharge. Box 12-3 lists warning signs of poor attachment.

BOX 12-3 | **Warning Signs of Poor Attachment**

- Making negative statements about the newborn
- Turning away from the newborn
- Refusing to care for the newborn
- Withdrawing
- Verbalizing disappointment with the sex of the newborn
- Failing to touch the newborn
- Limited handling of the newborn

Maternal Emotional Status

Monitor her mood and affect. Reinforce information given to her about postpartum blues. Reassure her that this is a common occurrence. Inquire about help she will have after discharge and how she feels about that help. Reinforce information given to her about postpartum depression. Emphasize that if she notices these symptoms that she should seek help immediately and that having these symptoms does not mean she is not a good mother. Many women are afraid to report symptoms of postpartum depression for fear of stigma.

 Cultural Snapshot

In Asian cultures, in-law conflict between the woman and her mother-in-law can be a significant cause of stress and depression in the postpartum woman. The woman may regard the conflict as a family secret and therefore be unwilling to share this information with the medical staff. However, if the woman and her mother-in-law have a positive relationship and the mother-in-law provides strong postpartum support, this may help protect the woman against postpartum depression.

Promoting Restful Sleep

Sleep and fatigue are contributing factors to the woman's emotional status. To help the woman emotionally during the postpartum period, the nurse should encourage rest for the woman. Monitor the woman's sleep–wake cycle. Encourage her to continue presleep routines that she normally uses at home. Promote a relaxing, low-stress environment before sleep. Dim the lights and monitor noise and traffic near the woman's room during sleep time. Medicate for pain if needed at bedtime. Plan care activities (i.e., cluster care) so that she can sleep undisturbed for several hours at a time. For instance, if the postpartum recovery is going well and vital signs have been stable, consult with the RN about waiting until the morning laboratory draw to obtain vital signs, rather than awaking the client at 2 AM. Or instruct the woman to call you if she awakens in the night to use the restroom; you can perform the vital signs at this time.

Of course, it is challenging for a new mother to get enough sleep because newborns feed every 2 to 3 hours. Encourage the woman to rest when the newborn is sleeping. She may also wish to get in the habit of maintaining a quiet atmosphere and

This is Illuminating!
The woman should always have adequate lighting when feeding the newborn during the night. This is so she can observe the infant's facial color for any signs of cyanosis and also observe the newborn for any signs of choking or respiratory distress while they are feeding.

keeping the lights low when feeding the newborn during the night. This practice helps develop their sleep–wake pattern so that it coincides with light and dark periods of the day. If the lights are on and the parents talk loudly and play with the infant in the middle of the night, they will think it is playtime and stay awake longer.

TEST YOURSELF

✔ List five major components of the woman's history that are important to know when assuming care of the woman after delivery.

✔ Describe the appropriate way to examine an episiotomy after delivery.

✔ Name three important laboratory studies the nurse needs to know the results of after delivery.

Nursing Process and Care Plan *for the Postpartum Woman*

Nursing care in the postpartum period focuses on the woman's safety, comfort, assisting her with caring for herself and the newborn, and providing information. While childbirth is a common experience, it is unique for each woman, regardless if this is her first birth or if she has had more than one child. No labor and delivery experience is identical.

Because of this, it is important to monitor the woman for any potential postpartum complication and to assess her level of knowledge. For example, a woman who has delivered her second child and had an episiotomy with this birth but not her first will need information on caring for the incision—information she did not have with her first birth experience. Additionally, emotions and discomforts experienced by the woman are unique to her. Be attentive to her needs. Nothing she is experiencing is routine for her, even though the nurse may have seen the symptoms many times before.

Since complications can arise during the postpartum period, the woman needs frequent monitoring. As postpartum stays are typically short, it is also important to give the woman information on signs to watch for at home that indicate a need for her to call her health care provider.

The nurse is in an important position to help promote bonding between the woman and her newborn. The nurse is also one of the first individuals to notice if the woman is having difficulty with the bonding process.

Assessment (Data Collection)

Assessment of the postpartum woman should focus on both the general assessment and the postpartum assessment. The postpartum assessment focuses on the 11 areas: breasts, uterus, lochia, bladder, bowel, perineum, lower extremities, pain, laboratory studies, bonding, and maternal emotional status.

Nursing Care Focus

When selecting nursing care focuses for the postpartum woman, consideration should be given to risks to the woman's safety. For the woman, safety includes not only protecting her from falls and monitoring for potential DVT but also monitoring for hemorrhage and infection. The postpartum woman is at risk for infection in the immediate postpartum and also during the 6 weeks after delivery. The nursing care plan should reflect these safety risks. The focus of nursing care should also reflect that the woman has a newborn and that bonding is an important event to monitor.

Outcome Identification and Planning

Major goals for the postpartum woman include remaining free from potential injury and infection as well as exhibiting positive bonding behaviors that indicate the beginning of a healthy attachment with the newborn. Other goals and interventions are planned according to the individual needs of the woman and her partner.

Nursing Care Focus

● Bleeding risk related to uterine atony, undetected lacerations, or hematoma formation

Goal

● The client will not exhibit signs or symptoms of unexpected bleeding.

Implementations for Bleeding Risk

The postpartum woman is at risk for hemorrhage from several different sources. Uterine atony is the most common cause of postpartum hemorrhage. If the uterus feels boggy or soft to palpation, massage it until it firms up beneath your fingers. Notify the RN of the condition. Oxytocin may be ordered to correct uterine atony. Instruct the woman to perform periodic self-fundal massage. Breast-feeding releases oxytocin naturally into the woman's bloodstream and can help prevent uterine atony.

Be Prepared!

When the woman gets up for the first time after delivery, it is normal for the lochia to seem heavy and to flow down her legs. Prepare her before she gets up that this is a normal occurrence caused by lochia pooling in the vagina while reclining and does not signify that she is hemorrhaging.

Monitor the blood loss and source of bleeding. If bright red bleeding occurs in a steady stream in the presence of a firm fundus, the most likely cause is a vaginal or cervical laceration that was not repaired. Report this finding to the RN or the health care provider immediately. Report bleeding from, or separation of the edges of, the episiotomy or laceration. Monitor for and report any painful, soft, and possibly pulsing masses palpable in the perineal area. These are signs of hematoma formation. Monitor vital signs and be alert to subtle changes in the woman's vital signs that might indicate bleeding such as a decreasing blood pressure and increasing heart rate.

Lack of Pain is Not Always Good

It is important to inspect the perineum and not just ask the woman if her perineum is sore or not. If the woman had an epidural, she may have a hematoma and be unaware of it. Perineal hematomas can be a source of postpartum hemorrhage.

The incision site from a cesarean birth can also be a site for bleeding. Monitor the dressing for drainage. Mark any areas of drainage so that you can tell if the area is increasing during subsequent checks. If the dressing becomes saturated, reinforce it, and apply pressure to the site. Notify the RN or health care provider for further orders.

Evaluation of Goal/Desired Outcome

- The fundus is firm and in the midline.
- The lochia flow is rubra (dark red in color) and small to moderate in amount.
- Incisions are approximated and without bleeding.
- Vital signs remain stable.

Nursing Care Focus

- Acute pain related to sore nipples, afterpains, or episiotomy discomfort

Goal

- The woman will verbalize or demonstrate relief of pain.

Implementations for Acute Pain

Assess the woman's pain (characteristics, severity, location, onset, type, precipitating factors, and duration). When monitoring the woman's pain, use an appropriate, standardized pain assessment tool. Interventions for postpartum pain are based upon the pain source. Inform the woman on what causes the pain and how long the pain can be expected to last. Encourage the woman to take medication early on, to prevent instances of severe pain. Administer medications to reduce pain, as prescribed, and monitor for effect. Monitor vital signs and respiratory status frequently for clients receiving sedative or narcotic pain medications.

If the woman reports breast pain, check her breasts for any reddened areas or excess heat. Report any signs of infection to the health care provider. Palpate the breasts to see if they are filling with milk. Instruct the woman to wear a well-fitting bra. If the woman is breast-feeding, observe the infant's latch to make sure it is properly positioned. If the woman is breast-feeding and engorged, encourage to only express a minimal amount of milk as the breasts will replenish any milk that is removed. If the woman

chooses not to breastfeed at all, reinforce teaching about not expressing any milk from the breasts and to wear a tight bra and that acetaminophen or ibuprofen will help the discomfort.

Inform the woman about causes of afterpains, including multiparity and breast-feeding. Instruct the woman about prescribed medications. Taking medications 30 minutes prior to breast-feeding can help lessen the severity of afterpains associated with breast-feeding. Nonpharmacologic relief measures such as warm heat to the abdomen may help provide relief. Assist the woman into a comfortable position.

If the woman reports perineal pain, check her perineum. Observe for hematomas. Inspect episiotomy or laceration repairs for signs of separation or bleeding. Provide medications as ordered. Nonpharmacologic relief includes ice packs in the first 24 hours after delivery and sitz baths as ordered. Instruct the woman on using the peribottle with warm water after every use of the toilet. Assist the woman into a comfortable position. The woman may find comfort from an inflatable ring to sit on or by placing a slight wedge under one hip while sitting to relive perineal pressure.

Evaluation of Goal/Desired Outcome

- The woman reports pain before it becomes severe.
- The woman verbalizes a tolerable pain level and a decrease in pain after interventions.

Nursing Care Focus

- Infection risk related to multiple portals of entry for pathogens, including the former site of the placenta, episiotomy, bladder, breasts, intravenous access sites, and bladder catheterization

Goal

- The woman remains free from infection.

Implementations for Infection risk

There are multiple portals of entry for infection for the postpartum woman. The number one way of preventing infection continues to be handwashing. Wash your hands before and after caring for the client, even if you will be wearing gloves. It is also important to tell the woman to wash her hands before touching her breasts or feeding the newborn, before and after using the restroom or performing perineal care, and before eating. Early ambulation, adequate fluid intake, and good nutrition strengthen the immune system and help prevent infection.

The best way to prevent mastitis (infection in the breast), in addition to frequent handwashing, is to avoid cracked nipples. Assist the woman to position the infant properly at the breast to prevent this complication. Other measures that help prevent cracked nipples are to rub the nipples with a few drops of expressed milk after breast-feeding and allow the nipples to air dry. Lanolin cream may also be a helpful measure. The woman should breastfeed at regular, frequent intervals. Milk stasis can lead to obstruction of a duct, which can lead to inflammation and then infection. If the woman is using breast pads in her bra, she should change them when they become damp to help prevent maceration of the nipples.

Endometritis, or infection of the uterine lining, is another type of infection that can occur in the postpartum period. Inform the woman that the best way to prevent this type of infection is to wash her hands before and after using the bathroom and/or performing perineal care. In addition, the woman should use a peribottle to perform perineal care and change her sanitary napkins/pads at least every 4 hours. Instruct her to fill the peribottle with warm water (she may add a gentle soap, if desired). After using the restroom, she should squeeze the bottle while aiming at the perineum so that the water flows from front to back. She can then use a washcloth or tissue to gently pat and dry the perineum from front to back. Instruct the woman to avoid touching the center part of the peripads (sanitary napkins); she should handle the pads only by the ends. The part of the peripad that touches her perineum should be sterile. These measures can also help prevent infections of the episiotomy.

The postpartum woman is prone to bladder infections because of urethral trauma and perhaps from stasis related to incomplete bladder emptying. Urinary catheterization may be necessary to treat urinary retention; however, this invasive procedure increases the risk for urinary tract infection. Taking steps to avoid urinary catheterization, when possible, is helpful in decreasing the risk for urinary tract infection. Adequate fluid intake and measures to prevent urinary retention are also helpful.

Evaluation of Goal/Desired Outcome

- The woman remains afebrile (temperature less than 100.4°F).
- There is no redness or heat in localized areas of the breast.
- Lochia is without a foul odor.
- Episiotomy remains well approximated without purulent discharge.
- The woman does not report severe pain when voiding.

Nursing Care Focus

- Risk for impaired bonding

Goal

- The woman and her partner demonstrate signs of healthy bonding with the newborn.

Implementations for Impaired Bonding

It is important to allow as much parent–newborn contact as possible during the early postpartum period. Encourage the parents to cuddle the newborn closely. Encourage role model attachment behavior by talking to the newborn and calling the them by name, if appropriate. Point out positive features of the newborn. Encourage the parents to participate in the care of the newborn. Provide privacy for the family to interact with the newborn. Assist the parents with learning the newborn's cues that they are ready for interaction, over-stimulated, hungry, or ready for sleep. Show the parents that a good time to interact with the newborn is during the alert state. Meet the woman's needs for pain relief, rest, and self-care so that she will have the energy to care for and interact with her newborn.

Evaluation of Goal/Desired Outcome

- The woman and her partner interact with the newborn in the en face position.
- The woman and her partner make positive comments about and/or interact positively with the newborn.
- The woman and her partner participate in the newborn's feedings and care.

TEST YOURSELF

✔ Name two ways to promote hemostasis for the postpartum woman.

✔ List three nursing actions that can help a new mother avoid endometritis.

✔ What are the three things you can do to help promote rest and sleep for a new mother?

Nursing Process and Care Plan for Postpartum Care After Cesarean Birth

The woman who has a cesarean birth faces the major postpartum challenges; however, she has also undergone major surgery. This section discusses how postpartum nursing care differs for the woman who has had a cesarean birth. Remember that most of the nursing considerations discussed above for the postpartum woman also apply to the woman who delivers by cesarean section.

Assessment (Data Collection)

The woman who has a cesarean birth has a significantly increased risk for complications than does the woman who delivers vaginally. These include complications of anesthesia, postpartum infection, hemorrhage, and thromboembolism. In addition to the normal postpartum data collection, the woman who has experienced a cesarean delivery requires close monitoring. Auscultate lung sounds at least every 4 hours in the first 24 hours and at least every 8 hours thereafter. The lungs should be clear without adventitious sounds and not be diminished in any lobe.

Monitor the woman closely for signs of respiratory depression if a narcotic, such as morphine sulfate, was used in conjunction with the spinal or epidural anesthesia. Many anesthesiologists have preprinted orders that include how often the nurse should monitor respirations after this type of anesthesia. The orders may be to count the respiratory rate every 1 to 2 hours for the first 24 hours. Report respiratory rates of 12 breaths per minute or less to the RN. Pulse oximetry, either continuous or intermittent, is often ordered. The oxygen saturation should remain above 95%.

Monitor the IV for rate of flow and correct solution. Check the IV site at least every 2 hours for redness, swelling, and pain. The IV usually remains in place for the first 24 hours after delivery. At that time, the health care provider usually gives an order to remove the device or to convert the IV to a saline lock.

The sources of pain and discomfort for the woman who delivers by cesarean are similar to those of a woman who has delivered vaginally. Some women who have had a cesarean birth pushed for several hours prior to the decision being made for the cesarean and therefore may have perineal pain and edema. The abdominal incision is an additional source of pain. The buildup of intestinal gas and referred shoulder pain are other sources of pain. Pruritus (itching) is a common side effect of narcotic administration during regional anesthesia. This can be a source of discomfort for the woman who had a cesarean birth.

The abdominal incision is a site for possible hemorrhage and infection. Monitor for drainage on the dressing in the first 24 hours. Check the incision at least once every 8 hours after removing the dressing. The incision should remain well approximated with sutures or staples. A small amount of redness is normal. Drainage from the incisional site, an increase in the amount of redness, or edema is an abnormal finding and should be reported to the RN.

Monitor bowel sounds at least every 4 hours. Check closely for abdominal distention and pain associated with gas formation. It may be difficult for the woman to pass flatus after cesarean delivery because of decreased peristalsis. Ask the woman if she is passing gas. Instruct her to report bowel movements.

Observe the indwelling catheter for urinary output. The catheter usually remains in place for the first 24 hours after cesarean birth. Output should be at least 30 mL/hr. The urine should be clear yellow or a light straw color. Cloudy urine is associated with infection. After removing the urinary catheter, observe the woman for the first few voids to make certain she is voiding adequately without retention.

Monitor for signs of thrombus formation. The calves should be of equal size without redness, warmth, or pain. Remember, the woman who delivers by cesarean is at even higher risk for thrombus formation than is the woman who delivers vaginally.

Nursing Care Focus

When selecting nursing care focuses for the woman who has just had a cesarean birth, consideration should be given to risks to the woman's safety including her respiratory status, infection, and potential thrombus formation. In addition, the woman has undergone major abdominal surgery and she will have pain from the incision and may have pruritus and gas pains as well. The nursing care plan should reflect these safety risks and discomforts.

Outcome Identification and Planning

After a cesarean birth, major goals for the postpartum woman are the same as after a vaginal birth; however, safety goals focused on the risks associated with the surgical event are also included. Safety goals are focused on the woman maintaining an adequate respiratory rate and oxygen saturation level, and remaining free from injury from either hemorrhage, infection, or thrombus formation.

Nursing Care Focus

- Ineffective airway clearance risk related to respiratory depression from narcotics

Goal

- The woman will maintain effective airway clearance.

Implementations for Ineffective Airway Clearance Risk

If the woman has had narcotics administered via the spinal or epidural routes, monitor her closely for respiratory depression. Monitor her lung sounds frequently during the first 24 hours after she delivers and at least once per shift thereafter. Monitor the respirations at least every 2 hours for the first 24 hours following spinal narcotic administration. Have naloxone readily available. The anesthesiologist will order when the naloxone should be administered, usually if the respiratory rate falls below 10 to 12 per minute. Monitor oxygen saturation as ordered. Report continuous oxygen saturation levels below 95%.

Encourage the use of incentive spirometry as ordered. Encourage the woman to cough and deep breathe. Assist her with turning every 2 hours. Assist her with ambulation as soon as ordered. Encourage her to use nonnarcotic pain relief methods as soon as her pain tolerates.

Evaluation of Goal/Desired Outcome

- The woman maintains an adequate respiratory pattern (16 to 20 breaths per minute).
- Oxygen saturation remains above 95%.
- Lung sounds remain free from adventitious sounds.

Nursing Care Focus

- Acute pain related to incision, discomfort from pruritus, or inability to pass flatus

Goal

- The woman will verbalize or demonstrate relief of pain.

Implementations for Acute Pain

Assess the woman's pain (characteristics, severity, location, onset, type, precipitating factors, and duration). When monitoring the woman's pain, use an appropriate, standardized pain assessment tool. Inform the woman on what causes the pain and how long the pain can be expected to last. Encourage the woman to take medication early on, to prevent instances of severe pain. If the woman has PCA, encourage her to use it as needed. Administer PRN medications, as prescribed, to reduce pain and monitor for effect. Monitor vital signs and respiratory status frequently for clients receiving sedative or narcotic pain medications.

Assist the woman with ambulation as soon as ordered. Walking and sitting up in a chair will help her recovery. Provide pain medication prior to these events. Laying or sitting in bed for prolonged periods will increase her pain when she moves and increases her risk for a DVT. Walking will help relieve gas pains if she has them.

Monitor the woman for pruritus. Provide medication as ordered. Inform the woman the cause of the discomfort and how long she can expect it to last. Provide nonpharmacologic relief measures such as a back rub and applying lotion to the site.

Evaluation of Goal/Desired Outcome

- The woman reports pain before it becomes severe.
- The woman uses PCA as ordered.
- The woman verbalizes a tolerable pain level and a decrease in pain after interventions.
- The woman states pruritus is at a tolerable level.
- The woman reports a relief from gas pain.

Nursing Care Focus

- Infection risk related to stasis of secretions in the lungs, abdominal incision, and presence of the indwelling urinary catheter

Goal

- The woman remains free from infection.

Implementations for Infection risk

One major difference between care of the woman who has delivered vaginally and one who has had a cesarean is that of lung status. Auscultate the lungs of a woman who has experienced cesarean birth carefully at least every 4 hours during the first 24 hours. Also assist the woman to turn, cough, and deep breathe at least every 2 hours. It will not be easy for her to take deep breaths or to cough. Assist her in splinting her incision with a pillow while she coughs. This stabilizes the area and reduces pain. The health care provider usually orders an incentive spirometer. Assist the woman to use it hourly for the first 24 hours when she is awake.

The cesarean birth incision site is another possible site for infection. During the first 24 hours, the original dressing usually covers the incision. After the health care provider removes the dressing, monitor the incision for increasing redness, edema, or drainage. Proper incision care includes washing the hands thoroughly before touching the incision for any reason. Instruct the woman to wash the incision with soap and water, and then thoroughly pat it dry. Nothing wet should remain against the incision.

The indwelling urinary catheter that is in place during the first 24 hours after a cesarean birth is another potential source of infection. Provide frequent perineal and urinary catheter care. Monitor IV fluids to ensure adequate infusion of fluids. As long as the woman remains well hydrated and has a stable blood pressure, her kidneys will produce enough urine to keep a steady flow. The flow helps wash out bacteria. When you discontinue the catheter, assist the woman to void within 6 hours of removal. Continue to monitor the intake and output of the woman.

Evaluation of Goal/Desired Outcome

- The woman's temperature remains below 100.4°F.
- The woman's lungs remain clear to auscultation.
- The woman's incision is clean, dry, and well approximated without redness or drainage.
- The woman's urine remains clear.

Nursing Care Focus

- Venous thromboembolism (VTE) risk related to postpartum status and decreased activity levels

Goal

- The woman will remain free from VTE.

Implementations for VTE Risk

Many women come back from surgery with compression stockings already in place. If not, check for an order to apply them. Pneumatic compression devices also may be ordered during the first 24 hours. These devices stimulate venous return to the heart, an action that helps prevent pooling and thrombus formation. Once the woman can get out of bed and ambulate, advise frequent ambulation. This is the best way to prevent a thrombus from forming. Encourage the client to move her legs while in bed to increase blood flow. Another important nursing action is to ensure adequate fluid intake.

Assess the woman's calves for color, warmth, symmetry, and edema. Assess her for calf pain as she ambulates or moves her legs in bed. Report any of these signs to the RN or the health care provider.

Evaluation of Goal/Desired Outcome

- The woman is without unilateral swelling, redness, or warmth in the lower extremities.
- The woman is without calf pain.
- The woman does not experience shortness of breath or chest pain.

PREPARING THE POSTPARTUM WOMAN FOR DISCHARGE

Discharge planning for the new mother begins upon admission and continues until she leaves the facility. Most interventions related to discharge focus on informing the woman how to care for herself and the newborn when she goes home. Observe how the woman and her partner are adapting to their new roles as parents and support healthy adaptation behaviors.

Bearing a child is a life-changing event. Observe how the parents interact with each other and with the newborn. Watch for interactions between other members of the family, such as grandparents and siblings of the newborn. Determine what behaviors are helping the new family adjust, and note if any actions are getting in the way of positive adjustment.

Because providing information is the focus of most nursing interventions when planning for discharge, it is important to determine the woman's knowledge base. Do not assume that a woman knows how to take care of herself and the newborn based on her educational level, or if she is a nurse, or if she has other children, etc. The only way to know what a woman knows about self-care and newborn care is to ask questions and to observe her behaviors. This section focuses on maternal self-care at home. Newborn care is discussed in Chapter 14.

SUPPORTING HEALTH-SEEKING BEHAVIORS

Reinforce positive family behaviors. Take particular care to acknowledge positive parenting skills exhibited by either the mother and/or her partner. When the parents require assistance as they learn new skills, provide positive verbal support. It is not supportive to tell the mother, "No. That's not the way to do it. Do it like this instead of that way." Remember that there are different ways to swaddle, hold, and bathe a newborn, and while her way may be different than the nurse's, it is not necessarily incorrect. Safety is most important when caring for the newborn. The nurse should instead, focus on the things the mother is doing well, and use positive language to guide her when she is having difficulty with the task. Use words that avoid criticism. Instead say, "Some women find it helpful to do it this way." Or, "the baby might find this to be soothing."

Anticipatory guidance is helpful when siblings are involved. Explain to the parents that it is normal for a young sibling to regress in the first few days after the birth of the newborn. Tell them it helps if they do not focus undue attention on regressive behaviors, such as a return to bedwetting, sucking the thumb, or clinging to a favorite toy or blanket. It is particularly important for the parents not to criticize or belittle the child for regressive behaviors. Explain that the regression is temporary and will pass as the child adjusts to his new role in the family. Suggest that the parents set aside time every day that is just "big brother or sister" time. The sibling will find it easier to adjust if they feel that their

parents still care for and value them. Another helpful suggestion is to provide the older child with a doll, and allow the child to take care of the doll as the parent is caring for the newborn. This activity helps the older child feel included and can help develop nurturing skills. Parents can also read books that are age-specific to the child about becoming a "big brother or sister."

Cultural Snapshot

The woman's culture impacts her postpartum period, including the types of food she will want to consume, her hygiene and physical activities, who will assist her, and her interaction with her partner and the newborn. Some cultures will request foods based upon the hot and cold theory. Some cultures dictate the woman stay inside for 30 to 40 days after birth and may restrict the woman's physical activity. Some cultures discourage the woman from bathing during the immediate postpartum period. It is important to learn what cultural practices the woman will be following and be supportive of her cultural practices.

Preventing Injury From Rh-Negative Blood Type or Nonimmunity to Rubella

Before the woman leaves the hospital, it is important to check to see if the woman who is Rh-negative is a candidate for Rho(D) immune globulin. If the woman is Rh-negative and the newborn is Rh-positive, the woman will need an injection of Rho(D) immune globulin to prevent the development of antibodies to Rh-positive blood. The woman must receive the Rho(D) immune globulin within 72 hours of delivery to be most effective. If the newborn is Rh-negative, the woman does not need Rho(D) immune globulin. Box 12-4 outlines nursing considerations for administering Rho(D) immune globulin.

You must also identify the woman's rubella status. If she is nonimmune to rubella or the rubella titer is less than 1:8, she will need to receive the rubella vaccine before she is discharged. It is important for her to know that she should not get pregnant for at least 3 months after receiving the vaccine. Box 12-5 outlines nursing considerations for giving the rubella vaccine.

One Can Block the Other!

Rho(D) immune globulin can prevent the woman's body from making antibodies to the rubella vaccine. If a mother is both Rh-negative and rubella nonimmune, it is important to inform the health care provider before administering both Rho(D) immune globulin and the rubella vaccine.

PROVIDING CLIENT INFORMATION

Because the postpartum stay is very short, it is important to utilize every available opportunity for providing the woman with information. It is better to give her small sections of

BOX 12-4 Prevention of Antibody Development

Medication: Rho(D) immune globulin

Method of action: Prevents development of antibodies to Rho(D)-positive blood if given to the Rho(D)-negative woman within 72 hours of abortion, invasive procedure such as amniocentesis, or delivery of a Rho(D)-positive infant.

Usual dosage and administration: 1,500 Units given via the intramuscular route, can be given intravenous

Antidote: None

Nursing interventions:

1. Ensure that the woman is a candidate for Rho(D) immune globulin. She is a candidate if she meets all of the following criteria. She:
   a. Is Rho(D)-negative
   b. Has never been sensitized to Rho(D)-positive blood
   c. Has had an abortion, ectopic pregnancy, invasive procedure, or delivered a Rho(D)-positive infant within the past 72 hours
2. Explain that the woman is receiving Rho(D) immune globulin to prevent her from becoming sensitized to Rho(D)-positive blood. This will prevent hemolytic disease of the newborn in subsequent pregnancies.
3. Inform the woman that Rho(D) immune globulin is a blood product. Although it is screened, tested, and treated to reduce the risk of disease transmission, there is still a slight possibility that she could get an infection from the product.
4. Obtain informed consent before administering the Rho(D) immune globulin.
5. Explain that there may be soreness at the site.
6. Ask the woman which site she prefers for the intramuscular injection. The deltoid and gluteal muscles are both acceptable sites.
7. Instruct the woman to call her health care provider immediately if she has fever, chills, shaking, back pain, a change in the color or amount of her urine, sudden weight gain, or swelling in her extremities.
8. She should not take any vaccines for 3 months after treatment with Rho(D) immune globulin because Rho(D) immune globulin may prevent the woman from developing immunity from the vaccine. If the woman receives a vaccine during the 3 months after Rho(D) immune globulin, she should have blood titers drawn at 6 to 8 weeks after the vaccine to see if she developed immunity. If not, a revaccination is necessary.
9. Give the woman a card indicating her Rh status and the date of Rho(D) immune globulin administration. Instruct her to carry the card with her at all times.

BOX 12-5 Development of Immunity to Rubella

Medication: Rubella virus vaccine

Method of action: Causes the body to produce antibodies against the rubella virus, thereby stimulating the development of immunity to rubella.

Usual dosage and administration: 0.5 mL given subcutaneously in the upper, outer aspect of the arm.

Antidote: None

Nursing interventions:

1. Determine whether there are any contraindications for administering the vaccine. Contraindications include that the woman:
   a. Is sensitive to neomycin
   b. Is immunosuppressed
   c. Has received a blood product (including Rho(D) immune globulin) within the past 3 months. If the woman receives the rubella vaccine during the 3 months after Rho(D) immune globulin, she should have blood titers drawn at 6 to 8 weeks after the rubella vaccine to see if she developed immunity. If not, a revaccination is necessary.
2. Explain possible adverse reactions:
   a. Discomfort at the injection site.
   b. Development of rash, sore throat, headache, and general malaise within 2 to 4 weeks of the injection.
3. Obtain informed consent before administering the vaccine.
4. As a precaution, the woman should not get pregnant for 28 days after MMR vaccination. Because the rubella vaccine is a live virus, it could be teratogenic to the fetus.
5. Inform the breast-feeding woman that the rubella vaccine crosses over into the breast milk. The newborn benefits from short-term immunity but may become flushed, fussy, or develop a slight rash. Suggest that the woman speak to the infant's health care provider if she has concerns.

BOX 12-6 Postpartum Danger Signs

- Fever of 100.4°F or higher
- Shaking chills
- Localized reddened, painful area on one breast
- Frequency, urgency, and painful urination
- Sudden onset of shortness of breath and/or chest pain
- Severe unremitting abdominal or back pain that is unrelieved by normal pain measures
- Foul-smelling lochia
- Increased or heavy lochia flow or passage of clots
- Return to lochia rubra after it has been serosa or alba
- Severe pain, redness, or swelling in the episiotomy or cesarean incision
- Swollen, reddened, painful area on the calf
- Prolonged or severe symptoms of depression (extreme sadness, lethargy, loss of interest in activities, feelings of worthlessness, difficulty concentrating)
- Thoughts of harming the infant or self (suicidal thoughts)

information throughout her stay instead of one very lengthy session just prior to discharge. It is best to ask her questions regarding how she plans to care for her breasts, perineum, pain, etc. to determine how much information she has retained and to reinforce areas she may not remember or fully understand. Instruct the woman that she needs to make an appointment with her health care provider for a 6-week postpartum checkup. It is important for the woman to know danger signs that she should report to the health care provider. Box 12-6 lists these danger signs.

Breast Care

Inform the woman about breast care as you are assisting her with breast-feeding or when she is preparing to take a shower. Explain that plain water is sufficient to clean the nipples because soap is drying and can contribute to sore, cracked nipples. Encourage the use of lanolin cream on the nipples. After a feeding, have the woman express a drop of breast milk, rub it into each nipple, and allow the nipples to air dry. She should wear a good support bra at all times.

The woman who chooses to exclusively formula-feed her infant will need information on how to care for her breasts as well. Inform her that her breasts will produce milk even without the infant nursing. The breasts produce milk in the postpartum period based upon a supply-and-demand system. The amount of milk that is removed will be produced again. As long as the milk is not expressed, the woman's body will make less and less each day until it eventually stops producing milk. After the woman's body stops making milk, it will not restart again until after she delivers another child. The lay term for this is that the breasts "dry up." To help this process, the woman should wear a well-fitting slightly tight bra that provides support, avoid letting shower water directly touch the breasts, and not pump her breasts even if they are painful. Cold compresses and an analgesic such as acetaminophen or ibuprofen can help alleviate some discomfort.

Fundal Massage

Show the woman how to do self-fundal massage when you are checking the fundus. Assist her with touching the top of the uterus and massaging it gently as she makes certain it stays firmly contracted. Explain to her that the uterus should no longer be palpable by the 10th day.

Perineum and Vaginal Care

Instruct the woman on proper perineal care the first time she gets up to use the bathroom. As described earlier, advise her on how to clean the perineum using a peribottle and to handle peripads (sanitary napkins) to avoid contaminating the center of the pad. Explain the importance of these instructions to help prevent bladder and episiotomy infections. Explain that she will need to continue to use peripads until the lochia stops. She should not use tampons or douche because these can contribute to uterine infection until the placental site has completely healed. Reinforce that she should continue perineal care after every voiding and defecation until the lochia stops. Encourage handwashing before and after performing perineal care.

Remind the woman that lochia flow should become progressively lighter. Lochia rubra generally lasts for approximately 2 to 3 days. This is followed by lochia serosa for the remainder of the first week after delivery. After the first week, the flow should be lochia alba. She should not saturate peripads, and there should not be any large clots.

To prevent additional trauma and infection, inform the woman to avoid sexual intercourse, tampons, or putting any substance into the vagina until the placental site and episiotomy (or tear) have healed. Healing is indicated when the lochia flow stops and there is no discomfort when two fingers are placed inside the vaginal opening. Hormonal changes associated with breast-feeding sometimes contribute to vaginal dryness and associated dyspareunia. For this reason, breast-feeding mothers may find it helpful to use a water-soluble jelly for lubrication during sexual intercourse.

Advise the woman to use birth control even if she is breast-feeding or if her menses have not yet returned. Women can ovulate without a menses in the postpartum period. Women who are breast-feeding should be encouraged to use a nonhormonal method of birth control to avoid a decrease (or in some cases a complete cease) in their milk supply. If the woman desires a hormonal birth control method, the health care provider may suggest a progestin-only method as it does not seem to interfere with lactation.

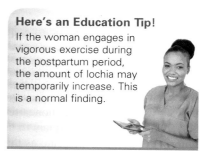

Here's an Education Tip!

If the woman engages in vigorous exercise during the postpartum period, the amount of lochia may temporarily increase. This is a normal finding.

Pain Management

Inform the woman about pain management. Explain that it is more effective to control pain before it becomes severe. Many women are afraid to take pain medication when they are breast-feeding. Reassure her that the analgesics the health care provider has ordered will not harm the newborn. Clarify that it is easier to breastfeed when she is comfortable and pain-free. Tell her the name of the medication that you are giving her, and briefly describe its benefit. For instance, when the woman complains of afterpains, administer the ordered ibuprofen, and explain that ibuprofen is usually effective in controlling the pain of cramping. If she complains that her stitches hurt, administer the ordered analgesic–narcotic combination, and make clear that this medication is most effective at controlling episiotomy or incisional pain. Tell her how frequently she can have each medication and why it is important not to take pain medication more frequently or at higher dosages than what is ordered.

Explain the benefits of using nonmedicinal ways of easing pain, such as applying warmth to the abdomen to help soothe afterpains. When you assist her with the sitz bath, encourage her to continue using it at home until the episiotomy has healed. Some women worry that the stitches will have to be removed and anticipate that this will be painful. Reassure her that the body absorbs the stitches, and they do not need to be removed.

Nutrition

Nutrition is an important aspect of self-care. Meal times are a good time to discuss nutrition with the woman. Determine what her prepregnancy dietary intake was. Give her brochures that explain the recommended amounts of food group intake each person should get. Instruct the woman who is not breast-feeding to resume her prepregnancy calorie intake levels. The lactating woman will need approximately 500 kcal above her prepregnancy calorie requirements to meet the demands of lactation. Instruct the lactating woman to consume a minimum of 8 glasses of water a day and to avoid caffeinated beverages. Dehydration can decrease the lactating woman's milk supply.

Constipation

As you are caring for the woman, explain how different activities contribute to or prevent constipation. Describe how activity helps the bowel regain its tone, which helps prevent constipation. When you fill her water pitcher, explain that she needs to liberally drink noncaffeinated fluids to help keep the stool soft. Explain that caffeine is a diuretic, so it is best to limit or avoid caffeinated fluids. Encourage her to drink fluids that she enjoys. If she does not like water, or uses hot–cold dietary practices, explore alternatives with her, such as noncaffeinated herbal tea, juice, and sugar-free gelatin. Explain to her the importance of not ignoring the urge to defecate as this can contribute to constipation. Inform her about high-fiber foods when you serve her a meal or bring her a snack. If the health care provider has prescribed a stool softener, tell her the name of the medication and its intended effect when you administer it. Offer her a large glass of water when she takes the stool softener, and emphasize the importance of adequate hydration when taking a stool softener.

Some women develop hemorrhoids during pregnancy. If the woman has hemorrhoids, inform her about the importance of adequate fluids, ambulation, preventing and avoiding constipation, and high-fiber foods. These measures will help the woman avoid straining during defecation, which can aggravate hemorrhoids. Sitz baths and topical hemorrhoid creams may help with any itching or discomfort she may have with hemorrhoids.

Proper Rest

It is important for the woman to know that it is easy to overdo it in the first few days after giving birth. Explore the possibility of asking a friend or relative to help out for the first few days. Reassure her that her health and that of her newborn are the most important concerns while she is recovering from childbirth. Give her information such as, "When you are tired, rest. If you are exhausted, you will not have the energy to care for your baby." It might be helpful to suggest that she rest with her feet up when the newborn is napping during the day. Reassure her that house-cleaning chores can wait if she is too tired to do them. The woman should not do heavy lifting. A good rule of thumb is the woman should not lift anything heavier than the infant for the first 6 weeks after delivery. If the woman overtires herself and does not consume enough food or fluids, it may affect her breast milk volume.

When the partner is present, explain how much energy it takes for the woman's body to repair itself after childbirth. This concept is probably easier for the partner to understand if they were present at the birth. If appropriate, encourage the partner to help with household chores and older sibling care while the woman recuperates.

> ### TEST YOURSELF
> ✔ Describe four major ways that the examination of the woman after cesarean delivery differs from that for a woman who delivers vaginally.
> ✔ Explain the proper way to perform perineal care.
> ✔ List four signs of infection that the new mother should report.

Remember **Mei Chu**. What information would you want to cover in her discharge instructions? How would this information be different if this was her first delivery and not her second? What signs would you want her to report to the health care provider immediately?

KEY POINTS

- The reproductive system organs gradually return to the nonpregnant size and function during the process of involution.
- Fundal height decreases at a rate of one fingerbreadth (1 cm) per day until the uterus is no longer palpable on the 10th to 14th postpartum day.
- Multiparas more frequently experience afterpains than do primiparas.
- Lochia progresses from rubra, to serosa, to alba as the uterine lining and other cells are cast away from the uterus.
- Kegel exercises can help the postpartum woman regain tone in the perineal area, although the size and tone of the introitus never fully return to the prepregnant state.
- The extra fluid volume that builds up during pregnancy is eliminated in the early postpartum period, leading to increased urinary output and diaphoresis.
- The woman's temperature may be slightly elevated during the first 24 hours after delivery because of dehydration and exhaustion. After the first 24 hours, temperature should be under 100.4°F. Blood pressure should remain at the level it was during labor. Mild bradycardia (50 to 60 bpm) in the early postpartum period is normal.
- The woman is at risk for a DVT, and her legs should be monitored for edema and excess heat or redness.
- The woman is often very hungry and thirsty after giving birth. Allow her to eat and drink unless medically contraindicated.
- Trauma to the lower urinary tract can lead to urinary retention in the postpartum period.
- The most significant psychological adaptation a woman must make is role change as she becomes a mother. She

usually does this in four overlapping stages: beginning attachment and preparation for the baby; increasing attachment, learning to care for the newborn, and physical restoration; moving toward a new normal; and achieving maternal identity.

- Bonding is the initial component of healthy attachment between a parent and the newborn. It generally occurs in a predictable sequence.

- Postpartum blues is a temporary mood disorder that manifests itself through tearfulness and other signs of mild depression. Postpartum blues is different than postpartum depression (see Chapter 19 for information on postpartum depression).

- The postpartum examination focuses on 11 areas: breasts, uterus, lochia, bladder, bowel, perineum, lower extremities, pain, laboratory studies, maternal–newborn bonding, and maternal emotional status.

- Nursing interventions in the early postpartum period focus on preventing and detecting hemorrhage, treating pain, preventing infection, preventing falls, detecting and treating urinary retention, preventing constipation, preventing and detecting thrombus formation, promoting sleep, and promoting healthy parental–newborn attachment.

- The woman who has a cesarean birth requires additional nursing considerations because she has undergone surgery. Possible complications include respiratory compromise and pain, infection, and separation of the abdominal incision.

- Helping the woman turn, cough, and deep breath and encouraging early and frequent ambulation after cesarean delivery are necessary measures to help prevent respiratory compromise and thrombus formation.

- Prepare the woman for discharge by giving her information on performing self- and infant care and on danger signs that she should report to her health care provider. Self-care includes breast care, fundal massage, monitoring of lochia, perineal care, pain management, prevention of constipation, and prevention of fatigue. Danger signs she should report include fever, pain, dysuria, foul-smelling lochia, increased lochia, calf pain, or feelings of persisting sadness.

INTERNET RESOURCES

Postpartum Resources
https://www.babycenter.com/baby/postpartum-health
https://www.mayoclinic.org/healthy-lifestyle/labor-and-delivery/in-depth/postpartum-care/art-20047233

Resources for New Fathers
https://dadsadventure.com/

Cultural Differences
https://www.mikvah.org/article/jewish_perspectives_on_the_birthing_experience
https://womenshealthtoday.blog/2017/07/30/how-cultures-protect-the-new-mother/

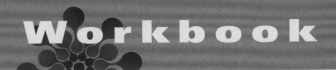
NCLEX-STYLE REVIEW QUESTIONS

1. An 18-year-old primipara is getting ready to go home. She had a third-degree episiotomy with repair. She confides in the nurse that she is afraid to go to her postpartum checkup because she is afraid to have the stitches removed. Which reply by the nurse is best?
   a. "It doesn't hurt when the midwife takes out the stitches. You will only feel a little tugging and pulling sensation."
   b. "It is very important for you to go to your checkup visit. Besides, the stitches do not have to be removed."
   c. "Many women have that fear after having an episiotomy. The stitches do not need to be removed because the suture will be gradually absorbed."
   d. "You cannot miss your follow-up appointment. Don't worry. Your midwife will be very gentle."

2. A woman has just delivered her third child 15 minutes ago. Everything has progressed normally up to this point. When the nurse tries to take the woman's blood pressure, she notices that the woman is shaking and that her teeth are chattering. Which action should the nurse take first?
   a. Finish taking the vital signs, and then decide what to do
   b. Notify the RN immediately
   c. Place two prewarmed blankets on the woman
   d. Put on the call bell to summon for help

3. The night shift LPN is checking on a woman who had a cesarean delivery with spinal anesthesia several hours earlier. The nurse counts a respiratory rate of 8 breaths in one minute. What should the nurse do first?
   a. Administer naloxone, per the preprinted orders.
   b. Awaken the woman and instruct her to breathe more rapidly.
   c. Call the anesthesiologist from the room for orders.
   d. Perform bag-to-mouth rescue breathing at a rate of 12 per minute.

4. Which of the following signs should be reported to the RN immediately? Select all that apply.
   a. Chills and shaking 15 minutes after delivery
   b. A void of 200 mL 3 hours after delivery
   c. Diaphoresis during the first day after delivery
   d. A boggy uterus that does not firm up with massage
   e. Complaints of uterine cramps during breast-feeding
   f. One calf that measures larger than the other
   g. A firm and painful lump on the perineum

5. A woman who has chosen to bottle-feed says that her breasts are painful and engorged. Which nursing intervention is appropriate?
   a. Assist the woman into the shower, and have her run warm water over her breasts.
   b. Assist the woman to place ice packs on her breasts.
   c. Encourage the woman to breastfeed because she is producing so much milk.
   d. Provide a breast pump, and assist the woman in emptying her breasts.

STUDY ACTIVITIES

1. With your clinical group, develop a one-page postpartum instruction sheet to send home with the new mother that covers all of the essential information she needs for self-care at home.

2. Explain how nursing care of a woman after cesarean birth differs from that of a woman who delivers vaginally. What additional risk factors does the woman have after cesarean?

3. Do an internet search on cultural differences of postpartum care. Discuss with your classmates how different cultures view the postpartum period.

4. Using the table below, compare the different sources of postpartum pain.

Pain Source	Possible Causes	Nursing Care to Prevent and Treat
Breast		
Afterpains		
Perineal pain		
Gas pain and distention after cesarean		
Cesarean incision		

CRITICAL THINKING: WHAT WOULD YOU DO?

1. You enter the room of Heather, a 22-year-old primipara, and find her on the floor looking a little dazed. When you ask her what happened, she tells you that she remembers trying to get up to go to the restroom and that she started feeling a bit dizzy and faint. The next thing she knew she was on the floor.
   a. What is the likely cause of Heather's fall? What nursing actions could have prevented this occurrence?
   b. Later that day, Heather reports that she feels like she just "dribbles" when she tries to urinate, and she feels like she is bleeding too much. What data collection should you do first? What do you expect to find?
   c. What measures can the nurse take to help relieve Heather's urinary retention?
   d. On the third postpartum day, Heather says that she is experiencing chills and thinks she is coming down with a fever. In addition to taking the temperature, what other data collection should you make? Why?

2. Marla delivered her fifth child yesterday after a difficult labor that lasted almost 24 hours. The newborn weighed 7 lb 6 oz (3,345 g), and she is breast-feeding.

   a. What factors put Marla at risk for postpartum hemorrhage?
   b. While you are checking Marla's lochia, you notice that her lochia has saturated through two sanitary napkins/pads since you last checked on her an hour ago. What do you think is causing the bleeding? What is your first action and why? What would you do next? Justify your answer.

3. Mindy had a cesarean delivery. This is her second post-operative day. She is in her bed when you come in to take vital signs. She looks miserable, and she says that she just cannot get comfortable.

   a. What data collection should you do first?
   b. You determine that Mindy is suffering from incisional pain and gas pain. What remedies should you offer for these two sources of pain?
   c. You perform a complete postpartum examination and discover that Mindy has a painful right calf that is warm to the touch. What action should you take?

Nursing Care During Newborn Transition

Key Terms

acrocyanosis
Apgar
brown fat
caput succedaneum
cephalohematoma
cold stress
epispadias
Epstein pearls
frontal–occipital circumference (FOC)
Harlequin sign
hyperbilirubinemia
hypospadias
jaundice
lanugo
meconium
milia
molding
mottling
phimosis
physiologic jaundice
pseudomenstruation
simian crease
smegma
surfactant
thermoregulation
thrush
vernix caseosa

Learning Objectives

At the conclusion of this chapter, you will:

1. Identify respiratory adaptations the newborn makes during the transition to extrauterine life.
2. Outline cardiovascular changes that occur in the newborn immediately after birth.
3. Explain the four main methods of heat loss in the newborn.
4. Discuss the role of the liver in adaptation to extrauterine life.
5. Describe expected behavioral characteristics of the newborn.
6. Describe how an Apgar score is assigned.
7. Define newborn hypoglycemia.
8. Explain the major steps of the initial nursing examination of the newborn.
9. Define expected weights and measures of the newborn.
10. Compare and contrast expected versus unexpected findings during the newborn examination.
11. Identify each newborn reflex and explain how to elicit each one.

Keesha Williams is a term infant born to a gravida 1 para 1 mother. She is brought to the nursery for her initial nursing examination. As you assist the RN with Keesha's admission, what signs would indicate the newborn is having difficulty with her transition? How can you help keep her safe during this time period? The nurse performs several routine nursing interventions during this time in addition to the examination. As you read, think about what parts of the data collection differ from the routine data collection of an adult.

The newborn is a unique individual, different from the fetus, older infant, child, or adult. The newborn's anatomy and physiology change immediately at birth and continue to mature as they grow. As the nurse, it is essential for you to be aware of extrauterine adjustments the newborn must make during transition to life outside the womb. It is important to know the characteristics of a normal newborn in order to make accurate observations. This knowledge also enables you to appropriately answer parents' questions and concerns about their newborn. This chapter explores the immediate and ongoing adaptation of the normal newborn to extrauterine life and describes initial nursing care.

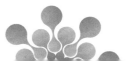

TABLE 13-1   Anatomic and Physiologic Comparison of the Fetus and Newborn

COMPARISON	FETUS	NEWBORN
Respiratory system	Fluid-filled, high-pressure system causes blood to be shunted from the lungs through the ductus arteriosus to the rest of body	Air-filled, low-pressure system encourages blood flow through the lungs for gas exchange; increased oxygen content of blood in the lungs contributes to the closing of the ductus arteriosus (becomes a ligament)
Site of gas exchange	Placenta	Lungs
Circulation through the heart	Pressures in the right atrium greater than in the left; encourages blood flow through the foreman ovale	Pressures in the left atrium greater than in the right; causes the foreman ovale to close
Hepatic portal circulation	Ductus venosus bypasses the majority of the liver; maternal liver performs filtering functions	Ductus venosus closes (becomes a ligament); hepatic portal circulation begins
Thermoregulation	Body temperature maintained by maternal body temperature and warmth of the intrauterine environment	Body temperature maintained through a flexed posture, muscle activity, and metabolism

PHYSIOLOGIC ADAPTATION

The fetus is fully dependent upon the mother for all vital needs, including temperature maintenance, oxygen and nutrition delivery, and waste removal. At birth, the body systems must immediately undergo tremendous changes so that the newborn can exist outside the womb. Table 13-1 compares the anatomy and physiology of the fetus and newborn.

Respiratory Adaptation

Fetal lungs are uninflated and full of fetal lung fluid because they are not needed for oxygen exchange. Immediately after birth, the newborn's lungs must inflate, the remaining fluid must be absorbed, and oxygen exchange must begin.

One factor that helps the newborn clear fluid from the lungs and take the first breath begins during labor. Much of the fetal lung fluid is squeezed out as the fetus moves down the birth canal. This is the important step in helping to clear the airway in preparation for the first breath. It also plays a role in stimulating lung expansion. The pressure of the birth canal on the fetal chest releases immediately when the infant is born. The lowered pressure from chest expansion draws air into the lungs.

Chemical changes stimulate respiratory centers in the brain. When the umbilical cord is clamped oxygen levels fall and carbon dioxide levels rise, causing the newborn's pH to fall. The resulting acidosis and falling oxygen level stimulates the respiratory centers of the brain to begin their lifelong function of regulating respiration.

It is critical for the newborn to make strong respiratory efforts during the first few moments of life. This effort is best demonstrated and stimulated by a vigorous cry because crying helps open the small air sacs (alveoli) in the lungs.

Think About This

A newborn delivered by cesarean does not always have the benefit of the pressure squeezing the chest from the birth canal. This newborn often has more fluid in their lungs, making respiratory adaptation more challenging. Closely monitor this newborn's respiratory rate, lung sounds, and oxygen saturation levels.

Immediately after birth, sensory and thermal changes stimulate the newborn to cry. Inside the uterus, it is warm and dark, sounds are muffled, and the fetus is cradled by the confines of the womb. The environment changes drastically at the moment of birth. It is colder, brighter, louder, the boundaries of the uterus are gone, and the newborn is directly touched for the first time.

Another important factor in the newborn's respiratory adaptation is surfactant. **Surfactant**, a substance found in the alveoli of mature fetuses that decreases the surface tension, keeps the alveoli from collapsing after they first expand after birth. The work of breathing increases (i.e., it is more difficult for the newborn to breathe) when the lungs lack surfactant, such as in a premature newborn. The newborn without enough surfactant expends large amounts of energy to breathe and quickly becomes exhausted without medical intervention. By the end of 35 weeks of gestation, the fetus usually has enough surfactant.

Many things can cause respiratory distress in a newborn. These include infection, stressful labor and delivery, cesarean birth, hypoglycemia, and prematurity. Box 13-1 lists signs of respiratory distress in the newborn. These signs must be reported to the RN or health care provider immediately.

 Concept Mastery Alert

Higher oxygen content of the circulating blood causes the ductus arteriosus to close.

BOX 13-1   **Signs of Respiratory Distress in the Newborn**

- Tachypnea (sustained respiratory rate greater than 60 breaths per minute)
- Nasal flaring
- Grunting (noted by stethoscope or audible to the ear)
- Intercostal or xiphoid retractions
- Unequal movements of the chest and abdomen during breathing efforts
- Central cyanosis

Cardiovascular Adaptation

The cardiovascular system must also make rapid adjustments immediately after birth. Fetal circulation differs from newborn circulation in several important ways. As you will recall from Chapter 5, only a small amount of blood flows to the fetal lungs. The rest flows away from the lungs through fetal shunts. The placenta oxygenates fetal blood, so only blood needed to supply oxygen to the lung tissue goes to the lungs. Because the fetal lungs are small and not inflated, they are resistant to blood flow and characterized by high pressures. The high pressures in the lungs cause the pressures in the right atrium of the heart to be higher than those in the left atrium. These pressure differences help route blood through the foramen ovale and ductus arteriosus, away from the nonfunctioning lungs, back into the general circulation. The ductus venosus shunts fetal blood away from the liver because the woman's liver performs most of the filtering and metabolic functions necessary for fetal life.

Newborn circulation is similar to adult circulation. After birth, deoxygenated blood that enters the heart must go to the lungs for gas exchange; therefore, the fetal shunts must close. Several factors contribute to their closing. The lungs fill with air, causing the pressure to drop in the chest as soon as the newborn takes their first breath. This change results in a reversal of pressures in the right and left atria, causing the foramen ovale to close, which redirects blood to the lungs. The first few breaths greatly increase the oxygen content of circulating blood. This chemical change (i.e., higher oxygen content of the blood) contributes to the closing of the ductus arteriosus, which eventually becomes a ligament. The ductus venosus also closes, allowing nutrient-rich blood from the abdomen to circulate through the newborn's liver.

Thermoregulatory Adaptation

Thermoregulation is the process by which the body balances heat production with heat loss to maintain adequate body temperature. The newborn has difficulty with thermoregulation because of two key factors. First, the newborn is prone to heat loss. The newborn has a large surface area to body mass ratio. This means that they have a large area of their body that can lose heat but not a large mass to produce heat. In other words, the amount of heat-producing tissue, such as muscle and adipose tissue, is small in relation to the amount of skin exposed to the environment. Second, the newborn is not able to produce heat by muscle movement and shivering. These factors make the newborn vulnerable to cold stress. **Cold stress** is a serious, potentially life-threatening condition, where exposure to temperatures cooler than normal body temperature results in the newborn using energy to maintain heat. If left untreated, cold stress can lead to hypoglycemia, respiratory distress, acidosis, and even death.

There are four main ways that a newborn loses heat—conduction, convection, evaporation, and radiation (Fig. 13-1). Conductive heat loss occurs when the newborn's skin

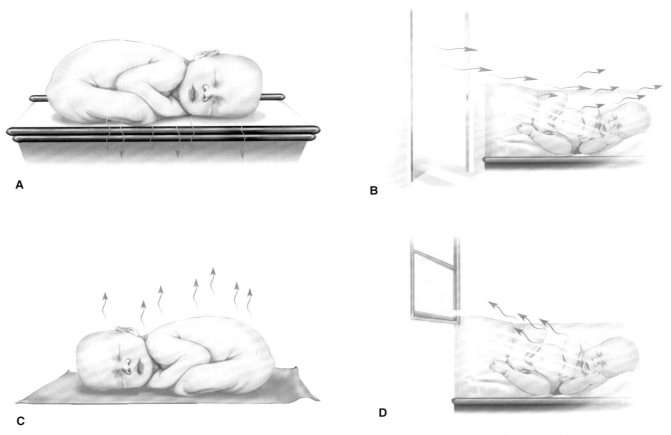

A

B

C

D

FIGURE 13-1 Mechanisms of heat loss. **A.** Conduction. **B.** Convection. **C.** Evaporation. **D.** Radiation.

touches a cold surface, causing body heat to transfer to the colder object. An example of this is when the newborn is placed on a cold scale. Heat loss by convection happens when air currents blow over the newborn's body. An example of this is when the newborn is left in a draft of cool air. Evaporative heat loss happens when the newborn's skin is wet. As the moisture evaporates from the body surface, the newborn loses body heat along with the moisture. This is why it is important to dry the newborn thoroughly after birth and to bathe the newborn under a radiant warmer. It is also important to change the newborn's linens if they become soiled with emesis or urine. Heat loss also occurs by radiation to a cold object that is close to but not touching the newborn. An example of this type of heat loss is when the newborn is close to a cold windowpane, causing body heat to radiate toward the window and be lost.

The normal newborn is not entirely without protection from heat loss. The newborn naturally assumes a flexed, fetal position that conserves body heat by reducing the amount of skin exposed to the surface and conserving core heat. The newborn can also produce heat by burning **brown fat**, a specialized form of heat-producing tissue found only in fetuses and newborns. Deposits of brown fat are located at the nape of the neck, in the armpits, between the shoulder blades, along the abdominal aorta, and around the kidneys and sternum. Unfortunately, brown fat is not renewable; once depleted, the newborn can no longer use this form of heat production. Brown fat is also important in the maintenance of blood glucose levels in the first few days of life.

A Word of Caution Is in Order

It takes oxygen to produce heat. If the newborn becomes cold stressed, they will eventually develop respiratory distress. This is one important reason to protect the newborn from heat loss.

TEST YOURSELF

✔ Name two ways a vaginal birth assists the newborn's respiratory adaptation.

✔ What causes the three fetal shunts to close after birth?

✔ Describe two ways a newborn can lose heat and how the nurse can prevent it in each case.

Metabolic Adaptation

Throughout life, a steady supply of blood glucose is necessary to carry out metabolic processes and produce energy. Glucose is also an essential nutrient for brain tissue. Neonatal hypoglycemia occurs when blood glucose levels drop below 50 mg/dL (Rozance, 2020 and Karlsen, 2013). It is important to be familiar with risk factors for hypoglycemia (Box 13-2). Any condition that adversely affects blood flow to the placenta during pregnancy puts the

---

BOX 13-2 Risk Factors for Hypoglycemia

History of any of the following during the pregnancy increases the risk that the newborn will develop hypoglycemia.
- Gestational hypertension
- Maternal diabetes (preexisting or gestational)
- Prolonged labor
- Fetal distress during labor
- Ritodrine or terbutaline administered to mother

Newborn characteristics that increase the risk for hypoglycemia. Note that many of these conditions result from an at-risk pregnancy.
- Intrauterine growth restriction
- Macrosomia (a very large newborn, >4,000 grams)
- Large for gestational age (LGA)
- Small for gestational age (SGA)
- Prematurity
- Postmaturity
- Hypothermia (cold stress)
- Respiratory or cardiovascular depression requiring resuscitation
- Infection

---

newborn at risk. If the mother's blood sugar was elevated during the latter part of the pregnancy, such as in maternal diabetes, or if she received medications that elevate her blood sugar, the newborn is also at risk for hypoglycemia. Any condition that puts physiologic stress on the fetus, such as prolonged or stressful labor or maternal infection, may deplete fetal glycogen stores, putting the newborn at risk for low blood sugar. Respiratory distress and cold stress are also two stressors that often lead to neonatal hypoglycemia.

Early signs of hypoglycemia in the newborn include jitteriness, poor feeding, listlessness, irritability, low temperature, weak or high-pitched cry, and hypotonia. Respiratory distress, apnea, seizures, and coma are late signs of hypoglycemia.

Hepatic Adaptation

Although immature, the newborn's liver must handle a heavy task. The fetus has a high percentage of circulating red blood cells to make use of all available oxygen in a low-oxygen environment. Because of this, the newborn has a hematocrit about 45% to 65%. After birth, the newborn's lungs begin to function, and more oxygen is available immediately. Therefore, the "extra" red blood cells gradually die and circulate to the liver to be broken down.

Bilirubin (a yellow-colored pigment) is released as the red blood cells are broken down. Normally the liver conjugates bilirubin (i.e., makes it water soluble), and then bilirubin is excreted in the feces. However, the newborn's liver is immature and easily overwhelmed by the large volume of red blood cells. When this happens, the unconjugated bilirubin, which is fat soluble, builds up in the bloodstream, crosses into the cells, and stains them yellow. **Hyperbilirubinemia**, high levels of unconjugated bilirubin in the bloodstream (serum levels of 4 to 6 mg/dL and greater), can lead to **jaundice**, a yellow staining of the skin. Jaundice appears first on the head and face; then as bilirubin levels rise, jaundice progresses to the trunk and then to the extremities in a cephalocaudal manner.

In approximately one half of all term newborns, a condition known as physiologic jaundice occurs. **Physiologic jaundice** is characterized by jaundice that occurs after the first 24 hours of life (usually on days 2 or 3 after birth); bilirubin levels that peak between days 3 and 5; and bilirubin levels that do not rise rapidly (no greater than 5 mg/dL/day). Jaundice that occurs within the first 24 hours is considered pathologic. However, anytime jaundice is present, document and report it. See Chapter 20 for more in-depth discussion of jaundice and its treatment.

The liver manufactures clotting factors necessary for normal blood coagulation. Several of the factors require vitamin K in their production. Bacteria that produce vitamin K are normally present in the gastrointestinal tract. However, the newborn's intestinal tract is sterile because normal flora have not yet been introduced and colonized there yet. Therefore, the newborn cannot produce vitamin K, which in turn causes the liver to be unable to produce some clotting factors. This situation could lead to bleeding problems, so newborns receive vitamin K intramuscularly (IM) shortly after birth to prevent hemorrhage (see Chapter 14 for discussion of the vitamin K administration procedure).

Behavioral and Social Adaptation

Each newborn has a unique temperament and personality that becomes readily apparent. Some newborns are quiet, rarely cry, and are consoled easily. Other newborns are frequently fussy or fretful and are more difficult to console. There are as many variations and characteristics as there are newborns.

In 1973, Dr. T. Berry Brazelton developed the Neonatal Behavioral Assessment Scale based on research he had done on the newborn's personality, individuality, and ability to communicate. Dr. Brazelton's key assumptions include that the newborn is a social organism capable of communicating through behavior and controlling their responses to the environment (The Brazelton Institute, 2020). Dr. Brazelton identified six sleep and activity patterns that are characteristic of newborns. It is important to remember that individual infants display uniqueness in their sleep–wake cycles. The six patterns identified in the newborn are (American Academy of Pediatrics, 2020):

1. *Deep sleep:* The newborn is quiet, not restless, and hard to awaken.
2. *Light sleep:* The newborn appears asleep with eyes closed, some activity is noted, may show sucking behavior.
3. *Drowsy:* The newborn's eyes open and close, the newborn looks sleepy but has intermittent periods of light activity or fussiness.
4. *Quiet alert:* The newborn's eyes are open and is attentive to people and things that are in close proximity. This is a good time for the parents to interact with their newborn.

5. *Active alert:* The newborn's eyes are open and responds to stimuli with activity.
6. *Crying:* The newborn's eyes are tightly closed and thrashing movements are made in conjunction with active crying.

TEST YOURSELF
✔ Identify four risk factors for neonatal hypoglycemia.
✔ What causes physiologic jaundice?
✔ Describe the difference between the active alert and quiet alert states of the newborn.

NURSING EXAMINATION OF THE NORMAL NEWBORN

Initial Assessments at Birth

Immediate observation of the newborn is concerned with the success of cardiopulmonary adaptation. A strong, healthy cry is usually the newborn's first response to external stimuli. A vigorous or lusty cry, heart rate greater than 100 beats per minute (bpm), and natural color without central cyanosis are associated with effective cardiopulmonary adaptation. The registered nurse (RN) makes these assessments rapidly during the first minutes after birth.

A traditional immediate evaluation of newborn adaptation is the Apgar score developed by Dr. Virginia Apgar. The **Apgar** score is a means of quickly assessing the newborn's transition to extrauterine life based upon evaluation of five newborn parameters: heart rate, respiratory effort, muscle tone, reflex irritability, and color. The score is not used to guide newborn resuscitation; however, it is useful to evaluate the effectiveness of resuscitation efforts.

Each of the five parameters in the Apgar score is given a score of 0 to 2 points for a maximum total score of 10 (Table 13-2). The RN attending the birth assigns the Apgar score at 1 and 5 minutes after birth. If the newborn receives a score of less than 7 at 5 minutes, the RN continues to assign a score every 5 minutes until the score is 7 or above or until the newborn is transferred to the nursery.

Apgar scores of 7 to 10 at 5 minutes of life are indicative of a newborn who is adapting well to the extrauterine environment. These newborns typically do well in the regular newborn nursery or rooming-in with their mothers. Scores between 4 to 6 at 5 minutes after birth indicate that the newborn is having some difficulty in adjusting to life outside the womb and need interventions and close observation. These newborns usually go to a special care nursery or neonatal intensive care unit (NICU) where they may receive oxygen and other special monitoring until their condition improves. Newborns who receive a score of 0 to 3 at 5 minutes are experiencing severe difficulty in making the transition to extrauterine life. These infants require resuscitation efforts and care in a NICU.

TABLE 13-2 Apgar Scoring

Apgar scoring is done at 1 and 5 minutes after birth. The newborn is considered to be "vigorous" if the initial scores are 7 and above. If the 5-minute score is less than 7, scoring is done every 5 minutes thereafter until the score reaches 7. The numbers in the left-hand column represent the number of points that are assigned to each parameter when the criteria in the corresponding column are met.

	HEART RATE	RESPIRATORY EFFORT	MUSCLE TONE	REFLEX IRRITABILITY	COLOR
2	Heart rate >100 beats per minute (bpm)	Strong, vigorous cry	Maintains a position of flexion with brisk movements	Cries or sneezes when stimulated[a]	Body and extremities pink
1	Heart rate present, but <100 bpm	Weak cry, slow or difficult respirations	Minimal flexion of extremities	Grimaces when stimulated	Body pink, extremities blue
0	No heart rate	No respiratory effort	Limp and flaccid	No response to stimulation	Body and extremities blue (cyanosis) or completely pale (pallor)

[a]Stimulation is provided by suctioning the infant or by gently flicking the sole of the foot.

Continuing Data Collection During Newborn Transition

During the transition period, continue to observe the newborn for signs of respiratory distress (see Box 13-1) or cardiovascular compromise. Observe for excess mucus, which could obstruct the airway. Measure the heart and respiratory rates at least every 30 minutes during the first 2 hours of transition.

Observe the newborn closely for cold stress. Use a thermal skin probe for continuous temperature monitoring while the newborn is under the radiant warmer. Measure the axillary temperature at least every 30 minutes until the temperature stabilizes above 97.6°F (36.5°C).

Hypoglycemia is a potential problem that can, if prolonged, have devastating effects on the newborn. Therefore, it is critical for you to be able to recognize signs and symptoms of hypoglycemia in the newborn. These signs include the following:

- Jitteriness or tremors
- Exaggerated Moro reflex
- Irritability
- Lethargy
- Poor feeding
- Listlessness
- Apnea or respiratory distress including tachypnea
- High-pitched cry

The main sign of hypoglycemia is jitteriness, which the newborn often exhibits as rapid shaking of the hands, arms, and legs. Conversely, the hypoglycemic newborn may have no symptoms. If hypoglycemia is prolonged without treatment, the newborn may have seizures or lapse into a coma. Permanent brain damage can result, leading to lifelong disability.

This is a Critical Point
Never mistake jitteriness in the newborn for "shivering." If the newborn has shaky movements or an exaggerated startle reflex, immediately check the blood sugar. Remember, newborns can develop hypoglycemia even when there are no recognizable risk factors for its development.

If a newborn is exhibiting signs of or is at risk for hypoglycemia (see Box 13-2), check the glucose level using a heel stick to obtain a blood sample for testing (see Chapter 14 for heel stick procedure). Blood levels between 50 and 60 mg/dL during the first 24 hours of life are considered normal. Levels less than 50 mg/dL are indicative of hypoglycemia in the newborn.

Remember **Keesha Williams**. What assessment data would you expect to see in her if she was experiencing cold stress? What nursing care would you expect to initiate? How could cold stress have been prevented from occurring?

Initial Admitting Examination

The initial newborn nursing examination (sometimes called the admission assessment) is completed within the first 2 hours after birth. The RN, nurse practitioner, or health care provider is responsible for the full assessment, but the LPN/LVN may assist with portions of the examination. Therefore, you should be familiar with the procedure and expected findings.

Review of the woman's history is an important part of a complete newborn nursing examination. The maternal family, medical–surgical, prenatal, and obstetric histories reveal clues to neonatal conditions.

The examination is conducted in a warm area that is free from drafts to protect the newborn from chilling. There should be plenty of light available to facilitate visual inspection. Indirect lighting works best. All equipment (neonatal stethoscope and ophthalmoscope) should be functioning properly and should be readily available. An experienced practitioner can complete a thorough examination in a short time, which is ideal because newborns become easily fatigued when overstimulated.

The general order of progression is from general observations to specific measurements. Least disturbing aspects of the examination, such as observation and auscultation, are completed before more intrusive techniques, such as palpation and examination of the hips. It is generally advisable to proceed using a head-to-toe approach. The overall physical appearance of the newborn is evaluated first, followed by measurement of vital signs, weight, and length. Then a thorough head-to-toe examination follows, ending with checking neurologic reflexes and the gestational age determination. Observation of behavior is integrated throughout the examination as the health care provider notes how the newborn responds to sensory stimulation.

General Appearance, Body Proportions, and Posture

A healthy term newborn's appearance is symmetrical and well-nourished without central cyanosis. Typically, the newborn has a head that is large in proportion to the body. The newborn's neck is short, and the chin rests on the chest. The newborn maintains a flexed position with tightly clenched fists. The abdomen is protuberant (bulging or prominent), and the chest is rounded. Note the newborn's sloping shoulders and rounded hips. The newborn's body appears long with short extremities.

Vital Signs

Vital signs are important because they yield clues as to how well the newborn is adapting to life outside the uterus. The respiratory effort and character should be checked at the beginning of the examination while the newborn is quiet. Respirations are activity dependent and should not be counted during episodes of feeding or crying. The respiratory rhythm is often irregular, a characteristic known as episodic breathing. Momentary cessation of breathing interspersed with rapid breathing movements is typical of an episodic breathing pattern. Extended periods of apnea are not normal. The abdomen and chest rise and fall together with breathing movements. The normal respiratory rate is 30 to 60 breaths per minute and should be counted for a full minute when the infant is quiet. The breath sounds are then auscultated.

Auscultate the heart rate apically for a full minute. The normal heart rate is the same for the newborn as it is for the

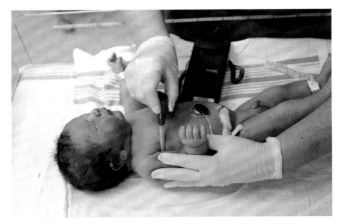

FIGURE 13-2 Measuring the newborn's axillary temperature.

fetus, ranging between 110 and 160 beats per minute (bpm), depending on activity level. When the newborn is sleeping, the heart tends to beat in the lower range of normal and is not considered problematic as long as it stays above 100 bpm. The newborn's heart rate increases with activity and may increase to the 180s for short periods during vigorous activity and crying. The rhythm should be regular. Listen for any abnormal sounds or murmurs. Although most newborn murmurs are benign, always report a murmur to the health care provider for further evaluation.

It's Not So Confusing!
To remember normal newborn heart rate and blood pressure values, think about this. A newborn has a low blood pressure (60/40 mm Hg) and a high pulse (120 to 160 bpm). In the adult, the opposite is true; the blood pressure is high (120/80 mm Hg) and the pulse is low (60 to 80 bpm).

The axilla is the preferred site for newborn temperature measurement (Fig. 13-2). Normal temperature range is between 97.7°F (36.5°C) and 99.5°F (37.5°C). Measure blood pressures on an arm or leg. For blood pressures to be accurate, the cuff must be of an appropriate size and placed correctly on the arm or leg. Table 13-3 outlines the expected vital signs of the term newborn.

TABLE 13-3 Expected Vital Signs of the Term Newborn

VITAL SIGN	EXPECTED RANGE	CHARACTERISTICS
Heart rate	110–160 beats per minute (bpm); during sleep as low as 100 bpm and as high as 180 bpm when crying	Rhythm regular; murmurs may be normal, but all murmurs require medical evaluation
Respiratory rate	30–60 breaths per minute	Episodic breathing is normal; chest and abdomen should move synchronously
Axillary temperature	97.7°F–98.6°F (36.5°C–37°C)	Temperature stabilizes within 8–10 hours after delivery
Blood pressure	60–80/40–45 mm Hg	Some facilities record the mean arterial pressure (MAP) in addition to the systolic and diastolic readings

Physical Measurements

Weight and length of a newborn are dependent on several factors, including country of origin, gender, genetics, and maternal nutrition and smoking behaviors. The normal weight range for a full-term newborn is between 5 lb 8 oz and 8 lb 13 oz (2,500 and 4,000 grams). The average length is 20 inches (50.5 cm) with the range between 19 and 21 inches (48 and 53 cm). Length can be difficult to measure accurately because of the newborn's flexed posture and resistance to stretching. Nursing Procedure 13-1 lists the steps for obtaining the newborn's weight and length.

It is normal for the newborn to lose 5% to 10% of their birth weight in the first few days. For the average newborn, this physiologic weight loss amounts to a total loss of 6 to 10 oz (170 to 285 grams) and the cause is a loss of fluid combined with a low fluid intake during the first few days of life. The newborn should regain the weight within 7 to 10 days, after which they begin to gain approximately 2 lb (900 grams) every month until 6 months of age.

Head and chest circumferences are two additional important newborn measurements. The **frontal–occipital circumference (FOC)** is the widest circumference of the head and is measured by placing a paper tape measure from the occipital prominence around the head to just above the eyebrows (Fig. 13-3A). To measure the chest circumference, place the infant on their back with the tape measure under the lower edge of the scapulae posteriorly, and then bring the tape forward over the nipple line (Fig. 13-3B). The average FOC is between 13 and 14 inches (33 and 35.5 cm), approximately 1 to 2 inches (2.5 to 5 cm) larger than that of the chest.

NURSING PROCEDURE 13-1 Obtaining Initial Weight and Measuring Length

EQUIPMENT
Calibrated scale
Paper to place on the scale
Tape measure
Marker or pen
Clean gloves

PROCEDURE
Weighing the Newborn

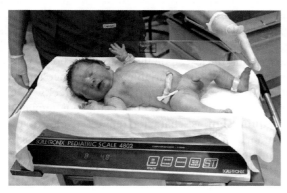

1. Thoroughly wash your hands.
2. Put on a pair of clean gloves.
   a. Gloves are necessary when handling the newborn before the first bath because of traces of blood, mucus, vernix, and other secretions on the body. Use universal precautions to protect yourself from bloodborne pathogens.
3. Place a paper or other designated covering on the scale to prevent direct contact of the newborn's skin with the scale.
4. Set the scale to zero.
5. Remove the newborn's clothes, including diapers and blankets, and place the newborn on the scale.
   a. To avoid inaccurate results, do not leave clothes, including diaper, on the newborn while weighing.

6. Hold one hand just above the newborn's body. Avoid actually touching the newborn. Never turn your back away from the newborn while they are on the scale.
7. Note the weight in pounds and ounces and in grams.

Measuring the Newborn

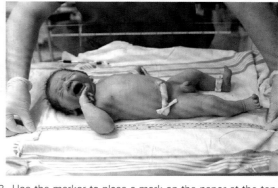

8. Use the marker to place a mark on the paper at the top of the newborn's head.
9. Use one hand to firmly hold the newborn's heels together and straighten the legs.
10. Place a second mark on the paper at the newborn's heel.
11. Measure the area between the two marks with a tape measure. This is the newborn's length.
12. Return the newborn to the crib and redress and recover to prevent cold stress.
13. Remove your gloves, and thoroughly wash your hands.
14. Record the newborn's weight and length in the designated area of the chart.
15. Report your findings to the mother, her partner, and other family members, as appropriate.

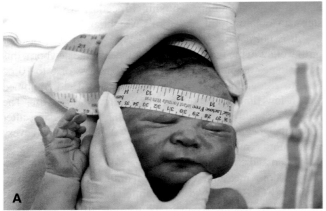

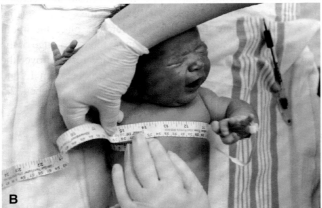

FIGURE 13-3 A. Measuring the head circumference. **B.** Measuring the chest circumference.

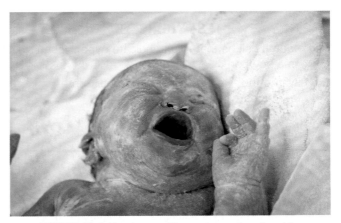

FIGURE 13-4 Newborn with vernix coating the skin.

TABLE 13-4 Average Physical Measurement Ranges of the Term Newborn

MEASUREMENT	AVERAGE RANGE METRIC SYSTEM	AVERAGE RANGE US CUSTOMARY SYSTEM
Weight	2,500–4,000 grams	5 lb 8 oz–8 lb 13 oz
Length (head-to-heel)	48–53 cm	19–21 inches
Head circumference	33–35.5 cm	13–14 inches
Chest circumference	30.5–33 cm	12–13 inches

Table 13-4 summarizes normal ranges for physical measurements of the term newborn.

Head-to-Toe Data Collection
Skin, Hair, and Nails

The normal newborn's skin is supple with good turgor, reddish at birth (returning to the natural color within a few hours), and flaky and dry. **Vernix caseosa** (or vernix), a white cheeselike substance that covers the body of the fetus during the second trimester, is normally found only in creases of the term newborn (Fig. 13-4). Vernix protects fetal skin from the drying effects of amniotic fluid. **Lanugo** is fine downy hair that is present in abundance on the preterm infant but is found in thinning patches on the shoulders, arms, and back of the term newborn. The scalp hair should be silky and soft. Fingernails are present and extend to the end of the fingertips or slightly beyond.

Common newborn skin manifestations are described in Box 13-3. **Milia** are tiny white papules found on the face. Reassure parents that these are very common, harmless, not pimples, will subside spontaneously, and should not be picked at. **Acrocyanosis**, blue hands or feet with a natural color trunk, results from poor peripheral circulation and is not a good indicator of oxygenation status. Acrocyanosis usually resolves itself within 24 to 48 hours after birth. The mucous membranes should be pink, and there should be no central cyanosis. Birthmarks and skin tags may be present. **Mottling** is a red and white lacy pattern sometimes seen on the skin of newborns who have fair complexions. It is variable in occurrence and length, lasting from several hours to several weeks. Mottling sometimes occurs with exposure to cool temperatures. **Harlequin sign** is characterized by a clown-suit–like appearance of the newborn. The newborn's skin is dark red on one side of the body, whereas the other side of the body is pale. Dilation of blood vessels causes the dark red color, whereas constriction of blood vessels causes the pallor. This harmless condition occurs most frequently with vigorous crying or with the infant side lying.

It is important to evaluate the newborn's skin for signs of jaundice. Natural sunlight is the best environment in which to observe for jaundice. If sunlight is not available inside the nursery, use indirect lighting. Press the newborn's skin over the forehead or nose with your finger and note if the blanched area appears yellow. It is also helpful to evaluate the sclera of the eyes, particularly in dark-skinned newborns. A yellow tinge to the sclera indicates the presence of jaundice.

BOX 13-3 Common Skin Manifestations of the Normal Newborn

Milia

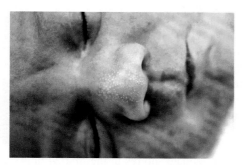

Small white spots on the newborn's face, nose, and chin that resemble pimples are an expected observation. Do not attempt to pick or squeeze them. They will subside spontaneously in a few days.

Erythema Toxicum or Newborn Rash

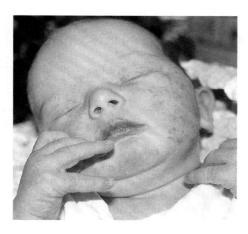

This rash appears commonly on the chest, abdomen, back, and buttocks of the newborn. The rash is harmless and will disappear without treatment.

Congenital Dermal Melanocytosis

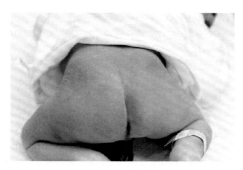

These bluish black areas of discoloration commonly appear on the back, buttocks, or extremities of dark-skinned newborns. These spots should not be mistaken for bruises or mistreatment. They gradually fade during the first year or two of life.

Telangiectatic Nevi or "Stork Bites"

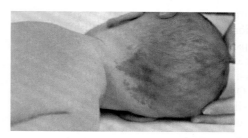

These pale pink or red marks sometimes occur at the nape of the neck, eyelids, or nose of fair-skinned newborns. Stork bites blanch when pressed and generally fade as the child grows.

Nevus Flammeus or Port-Wine Stain

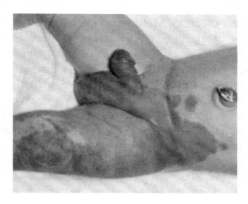

This dark reddish purple birthmark most commonly appears on the face. A group of dilated blood vessels causes the mark. It does not blanch with pressure or fade with time. Cosmetics are available to help cover the stain if it is disfiguring. Physicians have had success fading port-wine stains with laser therapy.

Some skin characteristics are attributable to birth trauma or operative intervention. Bruising may occur over the presenting part or on the face if the labor or delivery was unusually short or prolonged. Swelling may form on the newborn's head from vacuum extraction. Look for a forceps mark on the face or cheek after a forceps-assisted delivery. Occasionally, there will be a nick or cut on the infant born by cesarean, particularly if the surgery was done rapidly under emergency conditions.

> **Be Careful!**
>
> Visual inspection plays an important role in detecting early (i.e., pathologic) jaundice. If you notice jaundice, report it immediately. However, measuring jaundice using the naked eye is not a reliable way to screen for hyperbilirubinemia. Most facilities use transcutaneous bilirubinometers or blood samples to screen for this purpose.

Head and Face

The head may be misshapen because of molding or caput succedaneum (caput). **Molding** is an elongated head shape caused by overlapping of the cranial bones as the fetus moves through the birth canal (Fig. 13-5). **Caput succedaneum** is swelling of the soft tissue of the scalp caused by pressure of the presenting part on a partially dilated cervix or trauma from a vacuum-assisted delivery. These conditions are often of concern to new parents. Reassure them that the molding or caput will decrease in a few days without treatment.

A **cephalohematoma** is swelling that occurs from bleeding under the periosteum of the skull, usually over one of the parietal bones. A cephalohematoma is caused by birth trauma, usually requires no treatment, and will spontaneously resolve. However, the health care provider should evaluate the newborn for signs of anemia or shock from acute blood loss. Infants with a cephalohematoma need to be observed for jaundice as bilirubin will be produced when the infant's body breaks down the blood cells from the site. It is also important to make certain the cephalohematoma does not cross over suture lines. If it does, it suggests a skull fracture. Sometimes it is difficult for the inexperienced examiner

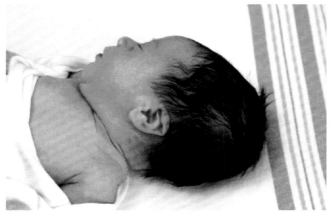

FIGURE 13-5 Molding in the newborn's head.

to tell the difference between a cephalohematoma and caput. Figure 13-6 compares features of these two conditions.

Cranial sutures occur where two cranial bones meet. The normal newborn's sutures are palpable with a small space between them. It may be difficult to palpate sutures in the first 24 hours if significant molding is present. However, it is important to determine that the sutures are present. In rare cases the sutures will fuse prematurely (craniosynostosis). It is important to detect this condition because it will require surgery to allow the brain to grow.

> **You May Notice This Relationship**
>
> Molding and caput are more common or more pronounced in a first-born newborn than in the newborn of a multipara. In addition, many newborns delivered by cesarean do not experience molding or caput unless the fetus is in the birth canal for a prolonged period of time before delivery.

♡ A Personal Glimpse

The doctor was just about to use the vacuum extractor because I had been pushing for 3 hours. I gave one additional strong push and felt the absolute relief of my baby sliding out of my body. The doctor said, "It's a girl." My husband was crying, and I couldn't wait to see our little girl. I wanted to examine her, touch her, feel her, and look into her eyes. They laid our tiny baby girl on my chest, and the first thing I noticed was her very long, pointy head. "Oh, my poor little girl," I thought, "that looks so painful and awful." I had heard and read about molding but had no idea it would be so pronounced. I must have had a look of serious concern on my face because the nurse touched my arm and said, "Don't worry, her head will be back to a normal size and shape in just a day or two." The nurse then covered my sweet baby's pointy head with a soft pink cap, and my baby and I began to get to know each other.

Isabel

Learning Opportunity: *How can nurses' knowledge of normal newborn examination findings provide assurance to new parents? Describe how a nurse's reaction to a common newborn finding could encourage or discourage parents.*

Fontanels occur at the junction where two or more cranial bones meet. The anterior and posterior fontanels are both palpable after birth. The anterior fontanel is diamond-shaped and larger than the posterior fontanel, which has a triangular shape (Fig 13-7). The posterior fontanel closes within the first 3 months of life, whereas the anterior fontanel does not close until 12 to 18 months of life. The fontanels should be flat, neither depressed nor bulging. It is normal to feel pulsations that correlate with the newborn's heart rate over the anterior fontanel. Bulging fontanels may

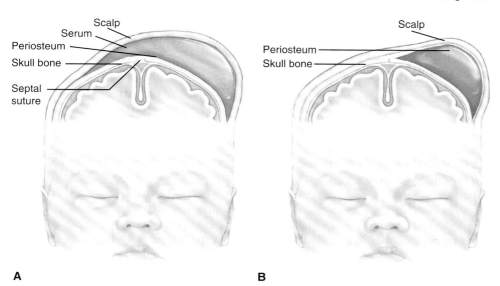

Scalp
Serum
Periosteum
Skull bone
Septal suture

Scalp
Periosteum
Skull bone

A   **B**

FIGURE 13-6 Comparison of caput succedaneum and cephalohematoma. **A.** Caput is a collection of serous fluid (edema) between the periosteum and the scalp caused by pressure of the fetal head against a partially dilated cervix. Caput often crosses suture lines. **B.** Cephalohematoma is a collection of blood between the periosteum and the skull. It does not cross suture lines, unless there is a skull fracture, which is a rare occurrence.

indicate hydrocephalus or increased intracranial pressure. Increased intracranial pressure can occur from crying or can be from a pathologic condition. Sunken fontanels are a sign of severe dehydration.

Facial movements should be symmetrical. Facial paralysis can occur from a forceps delivery or from pressure on the facial nerve as the fetus travels down the birth canal. It is easiest to look for facial paralysis when the newborn is crying. The affected side will not move, and the space between the eyelids will widen. Facial paralysis is usually temporary, but occasionally the deficit is permanent.

Eyes

The eye color of a newborn with light-skinned parents is usually blue-gray, whereas a darker skinned infant usually has a dark eye color. It is normal for the eyelids to be swollen from pressure during birth. See Chapter 14 for discussion of newborn eye prophylaxis done after birth.

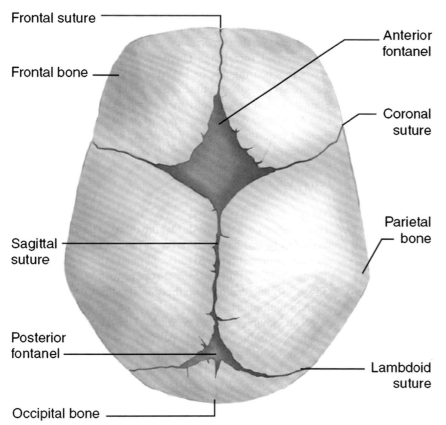

Frontal suture
Frontal bone
Sagittal suture
Posterior fontanel
Occipital bone
Anterior fontanel
Coronal suture
Parietal bone
Lambdoid suture

FIGURE 13-7 Anterior and posterior fontanels. Note the anterior is much larger than the posterior fontanel. To easily locate the posterior fontanel, start the anterior fontanel and lightly feel along the sagittal suture until the posterior fontanel is felt. (From Stephen, T. C., & Skillen, L. D. (2021). *Canadian nursing health assessment: A best practice approach* (2nd ed.). Wolters Kluwer.)

The sclera should be clear and white, not blue. The pupils should be equal and reactive to light. A red reflex should be present. The health care provider elicits the red reflex by shining an ophthalmoscope onto the retina of the eye. The normal response is a red reflection from the retina. Absence of the red reflex is associated with congenital cataracts. Small subconjunctival hemorrhages may be present. These usually disappear within a week or two and are not harmful.

Eye movements are usually uncoordinated, and some strabismus (crossed eyes) is expected. A "doll's eye" reflex is normal for the first few days; that is, when the newborn's head is turned, the eyes travel to the opposite side. Persistence of this reflex after the second week requires evaluation.

The newborn is able to perceive light and can track objects held close to the face. The newborn's vision is sharp at about 8 to 15 inches (20 to 38 cm) from the face. Newborns prefer shapes, the black and white color contrast, and a definite preference for the human face. Crying is usually tearless because the lacrimal apparatus is underdeveloped.

TEST YOURSELF

✔ Name the major nursing actions to take while weighing and measuring a newborn.

✔ Identify five common skin manifestations in the newborn.

✔ Name two differences between caput succedaneum and cephalohematoma.

Nose

The newborn's nose is flat, and the bridge may appear to be absent. The nostrils should be bilaterally patent because the newborn is an obligate nose breather. The newborn clears obstructions from the nose by sneezing. There should be no nasal flaring, which is a sign of respiratory distress. The sense of smell is present, as evidenced by the newborn's turning toward milk and by turning away from, or blinking, in the presence of strong odors.

Both Sides Should Be Equal

To check for nostril patency, use your finger to occlude one naris. The naris on the opposite side is patent if the newborn can breathe easily. Repeat the test on the other side.

Mouth

The mucous membranes should be moist and pink. Sucking calluses may appear on the central part of the lips shortly after birth. The uvula should be midline. Place a gloved finger in the newborn's mouth to evaluate the suck and gag reflexes and to check the palate for intactness. The suck reflex should be strong, the gag reflex should be present, and both the hard and soft palates should be intact. Well-developed fat pads are bilaterally present on the cheeks.

Epstein pearls are small white cysts found on the midline portion of the hard palate of some newborns. They feel hard to the touch and are harmless. Precocious teeth may be present on the lower central portion of the gum. If the teeth are loose, removal is recommended to prevent the infant from aspirating them.

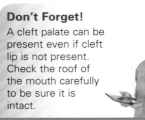

Don't Forget!
A cleft palate can be present even if cleft lip is not present. Check the roof of the mouth carefully to be sure it is intact.

A fungal infection (caused by *Candida albicans*) in the oral cavity, called **thrush**, may be present. The newborn can contract the infection while passing through the birth canal. The fungus causes white patches that resemble milk curds on the oral mucosa, particularly the tongue. It is important not to remove the patches because doing so will cause bleeding in the underlying tissue. An oral solution of nystatin is the treatment of choice for thrush.

Ears

The pinna should be flexible with quick recoil, indicating the presence of cartilage. The top of the pinna should be even with or above an imaginary horizontal line drawn from the inner to the outer canthus of the eye and continuing past the ear (Fig. 13-8). Low-set ears are associated with congenital defects, including those that cause cognitive impairment and internal organ defects.

In recent years, most hospitals have developed newborn hearing screening programs in accordance with recommendations of the American Academy of Pediatrics (AAP) for universal screening. There are two main ways that a newborn's hearing can be tested satisfactorily using current technology: evoked otoacoustic emissions and auditory brainstem response. Both methodologies are noninvasive, take less than 5 minutes, and are easy to perform. Each method monitors hearing differently, and each has unique advantages and disadvantages. It is important for the nurse to make certain that a newborn receives a hearing screen before discharge.

Neck

The newborn's neck is short and thick. The head should move freely and have full range of motion. There should be no masses or webbing. Significant head lag is present when the newborn is pulled from a supine to a sitting position (Fig. 13-9) and can hold up their heads slightly when placed on their abdomens.

The clavicles should be intact. Occasionally, a clavicle fractures during a difficult delivery. Signs of a fractured clavicle include a lump along one clavicle accompanied by crepitus (a popping sensation) at the site. An asymmetrical Moro reflex (discussed later in the chapter) is another indication.

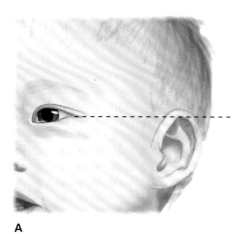

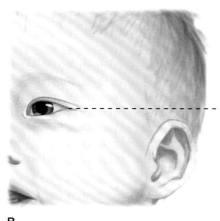

FIGURE 13-8 A. In normal ear alignment, the top of the pinna should be even with or above an imaginary horizontal line drawn from the inner to the outer canthus of the eye and continuing past the ear. **B.** Low-set ears may be seen in children with chromosomal abnormalities.

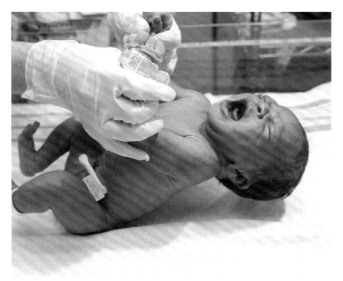

FIGURE 13-9 The newborn exhibits significant head lag when pulled to a sitting position from lying on their back.

Chest

The anteroposterior and lateral diameters of the chest are equal, making the chest appear barrel-shaped. The xiphoid process is prominent. Chest movements should be equal bilaterally and synchronous with the abdomen.

Breast enlargement and breast engorgement is normal for both sexes. This is temporary and caused by maternal hormones. Inspect for supernumerary (accessory) nipples below and medial to the true nipples.

Abdomen

The newborn's abdomen is dome-shaped and protuberant. Respirations are typically diaphragmatic, which make them appear abdominal in nature. Peristaltic waves should not be visible. Bowel sounds should be audible within 2 hours of birth. The abdomen should be soft to palpation without palpable masses. A normal umbilical cord is well formed and has three vessels. The base of the cord should be without redness, drainage, or swelling. The umbilical clamp should be fastened securely. Many facilities utilize a security device attached to the cord clamp to help protect the infant from abduction.

Genitourinary

The newborn should void within the first 24 hours of life. Vigorous newborns may urinate for the first time in the delivery room minutes after birth. The stream of a male newborn should be strong enough to cause a steady arch during voiding, and the female should be able to produce a steady stream. The kidneys are not able to concentrate urine well during the first few days, so the color is light, and there is no odor. It is normal to occasionally find a small amount of pink or light orange color in the diaper when the newborn voids. Excess uric acid in the urine causes this temporary condition.

Both male and female genitalia may be swollen. **Smegma**, a cheesy white sebaceous gland secretion, is often found within the folds of the labia of the female and under the foreskin of the male. It is best to allow the secretion to gradually wear away because attempts at removal can irritate the tender mucosa and cause skin abrasion. Immediately report the presence of ambiguous genitalia (i.e., it is difficult to tell if the newborn is male or female) to the health care provider.

In the female newborn, the labia and clitoris may be edematous. In the term newborn, the labia majora cover the labia minora. A hymenal tag may be present. An imperforate hymen (a hymen that completely covers the vaginal opening) should be reported. A blood-tinged mucous discharge from the vagina, **pseudomenstruation**, results from the sudden withdrawal of maternal hormones. Reassure the parents that this condition is not cause for alarm and will resolve on its own within a few days.

In the male newborn, the urinary meatus should be positioned at the tip of the penis. If the opening is located abnormally on the dorsal (upper) surface of the glans penis, the condition is called **epispadias**. If the opening to the urethra is on the ventral (under) surface of the glans, the condition is termed **hypospadias.** If either of these is noted, circumcision is contraindicated as the foreskin is used during the reconstruction process (see Chapter 21 for a discussion on urinary tract defects). **Phimosis,** tightly adherent foreskin, is a normal condition in the term newborn. The nurse or the parents should not attempt to retract the foreskin over the glans penis in the newborn period. Inform the parents that the newborn's health care provider will instruct them on how and when to do this. Monitor the urinary stream for adequacy. If phimosis interferes with urination, intervention will be needed. Spontaneous erections are a common finding.

The male scrotum is pendulous, edematous, and covered with rugae (deep creases). Dark-skinned newborns have deeply pigmented scrotum. Both testes should be descended. Using a thumb and forefinger, the scrotal sac is gently palpated while pressing down on the inguinal canal with the opposite hand. The procedure is repeated on the opposite side. Cryptorchidism results when the testes do not descend into the scrotal sac during fetal life. This condition requires medical evaluation. A hydrocele, fluid within the scrotal sac, may be present and should be noted.

Extremities

The term newborn maintains a posture of flexion with good muscle tone. The term newborn's extremities return quickly to an attitude of flexion after they are extended. The extremities are short in relation to the body and without deformities. Full range of motion is present in all joints, and movements are bilateral and equal.

Light Easily Identifies a Hydrocele

Take a penlight and hold it against the scrotal sac. If fluid is present (hydrocele), the light will transilluminate the scrotum. If there is no hydrocele, the light will not shine through solid structures.

Ten fingers and 10 toes should be present without webbing between the digits and without extra digits. Syndactyly refers to fusion or webbing of the toes or fingers, whereas polydactyly is the medical term for extra digits. The palms of the hands should have creases. A single straight palmar crease, a **simian crease**, is a finding that is associated with Down syndrome. Brachial pulses should be present and equal.

The legs are bowed and the feet flat because of fatty pads in the arch of each foot. Creases should cover at least two thirds of the bottom of the feet. The femoral pulses should be equal and strong

Practice Makes Perfect

Practice taking the femoral pulse on newborns that are resting quietly. Be patient, and take your time. You will gain confidence as you are consistently able to find the pulse.

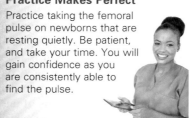

bilaterally. A strong brachial pulse with a weak femoral pulse is abnormal and should be reported (Fig. 13-10).

You may be asked to assist the RN while they attempt to elicit Ortolani and Barlow maneuvers (Fig 13-11) to evaluate the hip for signs of dislocation or subluxation (partial dislocation). A positive sign is associated with subluxation. Other signs of a dislocated hip included uneven gluteal folds or one knee that is lower than the other when the newborn is supine with both knees flexed.

The feet may appear to turn inward because of the way the fetus was positioned in the womb or birth canal. If the feet are easily reducible, that is, they can be easily moved to a normal position, this is positional and will resolve spontaneously. If the feet do not move to a normal position, true clubfoot may be present. A specialist should evaluate this condition.

Back and Rectum

The newborn's spine is straight and flat. The lumbar and sacral curves do not appear until the infant begins to use his back to sit and stand upright. Feel along the length of the spine. There should be no masses, openings, dimples, or tufts of hair. Any of these findings may be associated with spina bifida (an opening in the spinal column) and should be reported to the health care provider.

The anus should be patent. **Meconium,** the first stool of the newborn, is a thick black tarry substance composed of dead cells, mucus, and bile that collects in the rectum of the fetus in utero. Passage of meconium should occur within the first 24 to 48 hours and confirms the presence of a patent anus.

A Word of Caution!

Do not take a rectal temperature in an attempt to make the infant pass the first meconium. A delay in passing the first meconium may indicate Hirschsprung disease (see Chapter 38) or cystic fibrosis (see Chapter 36). It is important to know if there is a delay and not a reaction to rectal stimulation.

TEST YOURSELF

✔ Describe the difference between hypospadias and epispadias.

✔ When should the infant have the first void and first meconium?

✔ Define subluxation of the hip.

Neurologic Examination

General Appearance and Behavior

The first part of the neurologic examination involves quiet observation of the general appearance and behavior of the newborn. The newborn should maintain an attitude of flexion. Hypotonus (decreased tone) is an abnormal finding, as

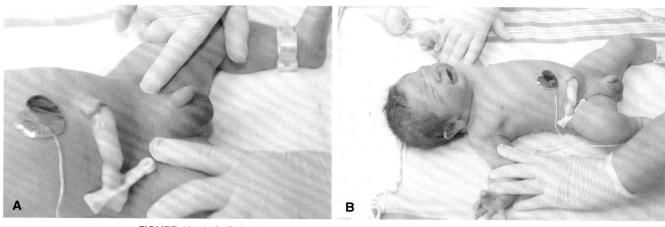

FIGURE 13-10 **A.** Palpating the femoral pulse. **B.** Palpating the brachial pulse.

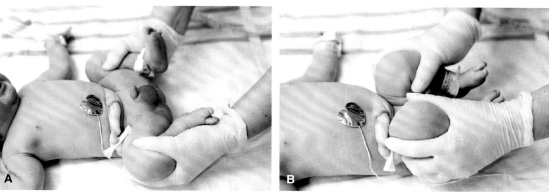

FIGURE 13-11 **A.** The RN checking for Ortolani sign. Sign is positive if a clicking or clunking sound is felt or heard. A positive sign indicates possible dislocation of the hip. **B.** The RN checking for Barlow sign. Sign is positive if the head of the femur is felt to slip out of the acetabulum indicating an unstable joint.

is hypertonus (increased tone), distinct tremors, jitteriness, or seizure activity. Any of these states may be associated with neurologic dysfunction, hypoglycemia, hypocalcemia, or neonatal drug withdrawal. The cry should be vigorous and of medium pitch. A high-pitched, shrill cry is associated with neurologic dysfunction and can also be caused by drug withdrawal.

Reflexes

Normal newborn reflexes (Fig. 13-12) are tested at the end of the examination. Although the list is not exhaustive, the reflexes discussed here are the most commonly assessed reflexes. In addition, the newborn should demonstrate the protective reflexes of sneezing, coughing, blinking, and withdrawing from painful stimuli.

Rooting, sucking, and swallowing reflexes are important to the newborn's nutritional intake. Gently stroking the newborn's cheek brings out the rooting reflex. The newborn demonstrates this reflex by turning toward the touch with an open mouth. Show the new mother how to use this reflex to help the newborn begin breast-feeding (see Chapter 15). Place a gloved finger in the newborn's mouth to test the sucking reflex. The suck should be strong. Swallowing is

evaluated when the infant eats. Listen and watch for coordinated swallowing efforts.

Evaluate the palmar and plantar grasp reflexes by placing a finger in the palm or parallel to the toes. The digits will wrap around the finger and hold on. The grasp should be bilaterally equal and strong. Check the stepping reflex by supporting the newborn in a standing position on a hard surface. The newborn will lift the legs up and down in a stepping motion. Babinski sign is positive (normal) if the newborn's toes fan out and hyperextend and the foot dorsiflexes when a firm object (such as the blunt end of a writing pen) is traced from the heel along the lateral aspect of the foot up and across the ball of the foot. After the infant starts walking, this reflex should disappear and the toes should curl inward (negative Babinski), rather than fanning outward.

The Moro reflex is also known as the startle reflex. When the newborn is startled, they extend the arms and legs away from the body and to the side. Then the arms come back toward each other with the fingers spread in a "C" shape. The arms look as if the newborn is trying to embrace something. The Moro reflex should be symmetrical. This reflex disappears at approximately 6 months of age.

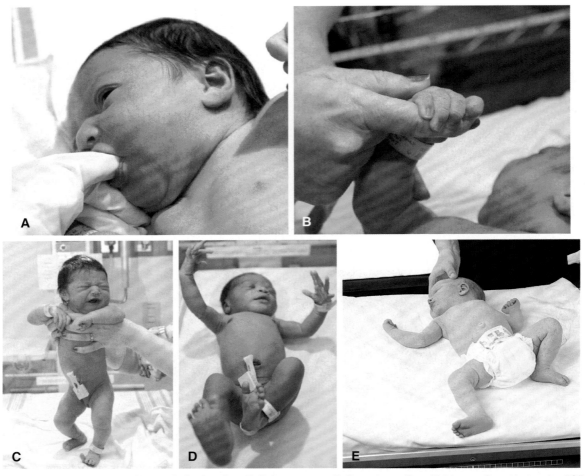

FIGURE 13-12 Normal newborn reflexes. **A.** Suck reflex. **B.** Palmar grasp. **C.** Stepping reflex. **D.** Moro reflex. Notice the "C" shape of the arms. **E.** Tonic neck reflex (fencer's position). Notice how the extremities on the side the newborn is facing are extended, whereas the opposite extremities are flexed.

The tonic neck reflex is another total body reflex. With the newborn lying quietly on their back, turn the head to one side without moving the rest of the body. The newborn responds by extending the arm and leg on the side they are facing and flexing the opposite arm and leg. This position has been called the "fencer's position" because it looks as if the newborn is poised to begin fencing.

Behavioral Examination

It is important to note how the parents react to the newborn's behavior states and how they talk about the newborn. Newborns who demonstrate self-quieting behaviors may be considered "good" babies. Parents usually respond positively to cuddly and sociable newborns. When a newborn resists cuddling or is difficult to console, they may feel rejected, and bonding can be adversely affected.

Instruct the parents to watch for cues as to when the newborn wants to interact. The quiet alert state is a good time for focused interaction with the newborn. When the newborn is in the active alert stage, they like to play. The drowsy state lets the parents know the newborn needs rest. Crying signals that the newborn has a need. Inform the parents to check for physical problems first such as a wet diaper, hunger, or need to burp. If the newborn is still crying, the parents can try soothing actions, such as walking, rocking, or riding in the car. Reassure the parents that, contrary to popular opinion, you cannot spoil a newborn by picking them up when they are crying. Holding reassures and comforts the newborn.

> **This is Vital!**
> Tell the parents *never* to shake an infant. Shaking can cause permanent brain damage. If the parent is frustrated because a crying infant is inconsolable, encourage the parent to lay the infant in the crib and take a minute to stop and count to 10 or ask a friend for help.

Gestational Age Evaluation

The gestational age evaluation is a critical part of the newborn examination. The RN is ultimately responsible for performing the evaluation; however, as the licensed practical nurse, you should be familiar with the instruments used and be able to differentiate characteristics of the full-term newborn from those of the premature newborn. Chapter 20 details the gestational age evaluation and compares the preterm with the full-term newborn.

Remember newborn **Keesha** from the start of the chapter. As you assist the RN with their assessment, what nursing interventions would be performed during this transition period? While doing the data collection, what findings would you see that are considered normal? What findings would be different if Keesha was male instead of female?

KEY POINTS

- The newborn must rapidly adapt to life outside the womb. Respiratory adaptation occurs when the newborn fills their lungs with air, absorbs remaining fluid in the lungs, and begins oxygen exchange.

- All the fetal shunts (foramen ovale, ductus arteriosus, and ductus venosus) must close so that blood will travel to the lungs for gas exchange and to route blood through the liver.

- The newborn has poor thermoregulation because they are prone to heat loss through the skin and cannot produce heat through muscle movement and shivering. Heat is lost through the processes of convection, conduction, evaporation, and radiation. The newborn conserves heat by maintaining a flexed position and produces heat by metabolizing brown fat.

- The newborn's immature liver may not be able to handle the heavy load from the breakdown of red blood cells, and physiologic jaundice appears. This condition is harmless if bilirubin levels do not rise dramatically and if jaundice is not present before the newborn is 24 hours old.

- Not all of the necessary blood coagulation factors are manufactured directly after birth, and the gut is sterile, so vitamin K is given intramuscularly to stimulate appropriate clotting.

- Each infant is unique, but all infants have similar sleep and activity patterns. These include deep sleep, light sleep, drowsiness, quiet alert state, active alert state, and crying.

- The RN performs immediate assessments in the delivery room, including assigning the Apgar score. The Apgar score is a way of determining how well the newborn is transitioning to life outside the womb. Five parameters (respiratory effort, heart rate, muscle tone, reflex irritability, and color) are used to assign a score at 1 and 5 minutes of life. A healthy, vigorous newborn has a 5-minute score of 7 or greater.

- Newborn hypoglycemia is a blood glucose level less than 50 mg/dL. Newborns can be without symptoms or may demonstrate multiple signs. The most common sign is jitteriness.

- The newborn examination is an important way to determine how well the newborn is adapting to life outside the womb. The least disturbing aspects of the examination are completed first. Respiratory rate and heart rate are taken first, while the newborn is quiet. Then examination proceeds in a head-to-toe manner and includes physical measurements and inspection of each body part.

- The expected weight range is 5 lb 8 oz to 8 lb 13 oz (2,500 to 4,000 grams). Length is 19 to 21 inches (48 to 53 cm). Head circumference is 13 to 14 inches (33 to 33.5 cm), and chest circumference is 12 to 13 inches (30.5 to 33 cm).

- The skin should be supple with good turgor and have natural color to it. Many variations are normally present on newborn skin. Acrocyanosis may be present.

- Head and face: Molding may be present. The infant's head should be observed and palpated for the presence of caput or cephalohematoma. The newborn is an obligate nose breather. The hard and soft palates should be intact.

- Neck and chest: The neck is short and thick. Webbing should not be present. Periodic breathing episodes are normal. The infant should be examined for a fractured clavicle. Swollen breast tissue in the newborn is common in both sexes and is temporary.

- Abdomen: The abdomen is protuberant. The cord should be clamped and drying with three vessels present. Bowel sounds should be present and the newborn should pass meconium, the first stool, within the first 24 hours

- Genitourinary: The newborn should void within the first 24 hours Genitalia of both sexes may be swollen.

- The back should be straight and free of hairy tufts, dimples, or tumors. There should be equal and full range of motion of all extremities.

- The main reflexes tested to determine neurologic status are rooting, sucking, swallowing, grasping, Moro, Babinski, and tonic neck.

INTERNET RESOURCES

The American Academy of Pediatrics
https://healthychildren.org/english/ages-stages/baby/Pages/default.aspx

Parent Resources About Newborns
http://kidshealth.org/parent/pregnancy_center/childbirth/newborn_variations.html#

Resources for Professionals: Newborn Assessment Photos
http://med.stanford.edu/newborns/professional-education/photo-gallery.html

Workbook

NCLEX-STYLE REVIEW QUESTIONS

1. An infant is born by cesarean delivery. In what way is respiratory adaptation more difficult for this infant than the one who is born by vaginal delivery?

   a. More fluid is present in the lungs at birth.
   b. Surfactant is missing from the lungs.
   c. The respiratory centers in the brain are not stimulated.
   d. There is less sensory stimulation to breathe.

2. A new mother says, "I think something is wrong with my baby. She looks like she is having a menstrual period!" What is the nurse's best response?

   a. "I don't know. Let me have the charge nurse check her."
   b. "It's nothing to worry about. That's a normal finding."
   c. "This is a normal occurrence. You may clean her with a damp washcloth, and it will go away in a few days."
   d. "This means she was exposed to an infection during birth. I'll notify the doctor at once!"

3. Baby boy Alvarez is 5 minutes old. The nurse gathers the following data: the newborn has a heart rate of 110 bpm, a weak cry, and acrocyanosis. His extremities are held in partial flexion, and he grimaces when a catheter is placed in his nose. What Apgar score does the registered nurse record and what does the score mean?

   a. 5—The newborn is having extreme difficulty transitioning.
   b. 5—The newborn is having moderate difficulty transitioning.
   c. 6—The newborn is having moderate difficulty transitioning.
   d. 6—The newborn is vigorous and transitioning with minimal effort.

4. The nurse is examining a 1-day-old newborn and notices a small amount of white drainage and redness at the base of the umbilical cord. Which of the following is the best response by the nurse?

   a. Call the doctor immediately to ask for intravenous antibiotics.
   b. Carefully clean the area with a damp washcloth, and cover it with an absorbent dressing.
   c. Notify the charge nurse because this finding represents a possible complication.
   d. Show the mother how to clean the area with soap and water.

5. A newborn's axillary temperature is 97.4°F (36.3°C). His T-shirt is damp with spit-up milk. His blanket is loosely applied, and several children are in the room running around his crib. The room is comfortably warm, and the bassinet is beside the mother's bed away from the window and doors. What are the most likely mechanisms of heat loss for this newborn?

   a. Conduction and evaporation
   b. Conduction and radiation
   c. Convection and radiation
   d. Convection and evaporation

6. The nurse is performing a newborn examination on a 12-hour-old term female infant. Which of the following findings should be reported to the RN? (select all that apply)

   a. Bluish colored feet
   b. Swollen labia
   c. Bluish color around mouth
   d. Positive Babinski reflex
   e. Passage of meconium
   f. Cephalohematoma
   g. Respiratory rate of 68 during rest
   h. Presence of milia

STUDY ACTIVITIES

1. Do an internet search using the key words "newborn crying." How many internet sites returned? List three to four that would be good references for new parents. Compare your list to that of your clinical group.

2. Use the table below to describe important newborn criteria for each body system.

Body System	Critical Parameters for Data Collection	Expected Findings	Possible Deviations From Normal
Respiratory			
Cardiovascular			
Gastrointestinal			
Metabolic			
Hepatic			
Skin			

3. Research resources in your community designed to help first-time parents in their new role. How many sources did you find? Were you surprised? Share your findings with your clinical group. Discuss ways the community might be more supportive of new parents.

CRITICAL THINKING: WHAT WOULD YOU DO?

Apply your knowledge of normal newborn adaptation to the following situation.

1. Mary, a 28-year-old woman, delivered her first newborn several hours ago. She and the father of the baby had joyful interaction with the newborn immediately after delivery. The newborn breastfed well with assistance from the delivery room nurse. You are coming on duty for the evening shift and have just entered the room to examine the newborn.

   a. You find the newborn sleeping with only a diaper on in an open bassinet. The bassinet is located against the wall under a window. The baby's skin is mottled, and the newborn's extremities feel cool to the touch. What is your initial determination of the situation? What actions should you take?

   b. What instructions should you give to the parents?

2. On day 3 of life, you notice that the newborn's skin is a light yellow color.

   a. What is the likely cause of the yellow color?

   b. Mary asks you if the yellow color indicates illness. How do you reply?

3. Mary says she is frustrated. She has been trying to "play" with her newborn, but the newborn keeps looking away and yawning. She is worried that her baby does not "like" her.

   a. How should you reply to Mary?

   b. Mary expresses concern about a blue-black spot she found on the baby's back. She is worried that he received a bruise in the nursery. How do you explain this finding to Mary?

14

Nursing Care of the Normal Newborn

Learning Objectives

At the conclusion of this chapter, you will:

1. Explain how to support immediate cardiovascular and respiratory transitions in the newborn.
2. Identify two methods to promote thermoregulation for the newborn.
3. Discuss appropriate interventions for the newborn with hypoglycemia.
4. Describe immediate care of the newborn regarding eye prophylaxis and administration of vitamin K.
5. Explain the nurse's role in protecting the newborn from misidentification in the hospital.
6. Identify effective infection control procedures in the nursery.
7. Describe when and how the newborn receives the first bath.
8. Describe strategies hospitals can take to protect the newborn from abduction.
9. Identify signs of pain in the newborn, and list nursing measures to help decrease or avoid pain in the newborn.
10. Compare the care of the uncircumcised newborn male with that of the circumcised newborn male.
11. List immunizations and newborn screening tests that should be done before the newborn is discharged home.
12. Develop an education plan for the parents regarding normal newborn care.

Matthew Colluci is a 30-minute-old newborn male born to a gravida 4 para 3 mother via spontaneous vaginal delivery that lasted 14 hours. As you assist the RN in the delivery room, you will be asked to perform data collection and assist with procedures. What do you think will be some data collected and procedures performed? Prior to his discharge home, Matthew will need several more routine tests, and his mother will need discharge instructions on his newborn care. What routine tests do you think Matthew will need? When you provide discharge instructions with his mother, what topics will you cover?

As you learned in Chapter 13, the newborn must make rapid adjustments to successfully adapt to life outside of the womb. Your role is to support the newborn as they adapt to these changes, quickly recognize the development of complications, and report changes in condition to the RN to facilitate rapid intervention. Giving parents information on the skills needed to care for

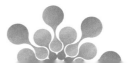

their newborn is another critical role you will play. This chapter discusses the basic nursing care required for newborns and their families.

NEWBORN STABILIZATION AND TRANSITION AFTER BIRTH

The current standard of care for resuscitation of the newborn immediately after birth is outlined in the Neonatal Resuscitation Program (NRP), which is developed and maintained by the American Heart Association (AHA) and the American Academy of Pediatrics (AAP). The basic principles of newborn resuscitation are reviewed in this chapter. Refer to an NRP textbook for detailed guidelines on newborn resuscitation. The Registered Nurse (RN) is responsible for the resuscitation; however, the licensed practical/vocational nurse (LPN/LVN) must be able to initiate resuscitation if necessary and assist throughout the process.

The first 6 to 12 hours after birth is a critical transition period for the newborn. The healthy newborn may stay with the mother immediately after delivery and be cared for by the same nurse who is overseeing the mother's recovery. In some facilities, the newborn is taken to a transition nursery after a short initial bonding period with the parents. In either case, when caring for the newborn during the transition period, you must be alert to early signs of distress and be ready to intervene quickly to prevent complications and poor outcomes.

Immediately after birth, the newborn undergoes rapid transition from fetal to adult circulation and oxygenation. The newborn requires close observation during the first 6 to 12 hours of life, the transition period. Monitoring the newborn's cardiac and respiratory function during this time is essential as is reporting any difficulties noted in the newborn's ability to oxygenate, ventilate, or perfuse. Measure the heart and respiratory rates at least every 30 minutes during the first 2 hours of transition. Monitor the axillary temperature every 30 minutes until it stabilizes in the expected range of 97.7°F to 99.5°F (36.5°C to 37.5°C). Be alert for signs of hypoglycemia.

A nursing examination of the newborn (see Chapter 13), including the gestational age exam (detailed in Chapter 20), is completed within the first few hours of life. During this time, the newborn will also start to breast- or bottle-feed and receive their first medications (eye prophylaxis and vitamin K). Monitoring the newborn's vital signs, first void and bowel movements, feeding ability and tolerance of feedings, and for signs of potential problems (e.g., jaundice and sepsis) are important to report and record. Parental bonding, involvement in and knowledge about the newborn's care are also important observations for the nurse to make.

Maintaining the safety of the newborn during transition from intrauterine to extrauterine life is the primary goal of nursing care immediately after delivery and in the first 6 to 12 hours of life. Nursing care is focused on observing and assisting the newborn to experience adequate cardiovascular, respiratory, thermoregulatory, and metabolic transitions to extrauterine life. An important safety goal is that the newborn will be adequately identified before separation from, and when returning to, the parents.

SUPPORTING CARDIOVASCULAR AND RESPIRATORY TRANSITION

Nursing interventions to support newborn vital functions begin before the birth occurs. If you will be assisting in the immediate care of the newborn, ensure that adequate supplies are present for a full resuscitation in the delivery room and that all equipment is functioning properly and turned on prior to the delivery. Most delivery settings have a newborn resuscitation area that contains needed supplies. Check that oxygen is readily available and that there is a functioning suction source. Ensure that a warmer is in the delivery area, and turn it on several minutes before the delivery is expected. Resuscitation equipment is to always be ready as it cannot be predicted which newborns will need resuscitation after birth. A "normal" labor and delivery may have a neonate who requires assistance with breathing or stabilization immediately after birth.

Observe the newborn carefully at birth. The delivery attendant will usually suction the mouth and nose with a bulb syringe and clamp and cut the umbilical cord. Prior to birth, drape a blanket onto the mother's abdomen and support the newborn there when the birth attendant places the newborn there. Dry the newborn quickly to prevent heat loss from evaporation and to provide stimulation to encourage the newborn's breathing efforts. Remove the wet linens and apply warm dry ones. Quickly palpate the base of the umbilical cord and count the pulse for 6 seconds. Multiply that number by 10 to calculate the heart rate. A pulse above 100 beats per minute and a vigorous cry are reassuring signs that indicate the newborn is making a successful transition.

If the newborn does not cry immediately, quickly place them under the preheated radiant warmer for immediate resuscitation. Continue stimulation of the newborn by rubbing with dry linens. If the newborn still does not make adequate breathing efforts, a bag and mask connected to 100% oxygen are used to provide respiratory support until spontaneous breathing occurs.

Most newborns do not require resuscitation, and the ones who do generally respond well to a short period of positive pressure ventilation with a bag and mask. However, a small number of newborns also require chest compressions, intubation, or medications. The RN will follow the NRP guidelines for complete resuscitation protocols.

Give constant attention to the airway. Newborns often have abundant secretions. The initial airway intervention is to position the newborn on the side to help prevent aspiration of secretions. A bulb syringe is used to suction the mouth first

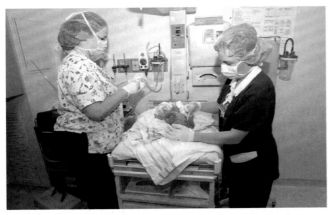

FIGURE 14-1 The nurse uses a bulb syringe to suction the mouth of the newborn before suctioning the nares.

and then the nose (Fig. 14-1). Keep the bulb syringe with the newborn and inform the parents how and when to suction the newborn. If copious secretions are present that do not resolve with a bulb syringe, a small suction catheter connected to a suction source may be used. Be careful not to apply suction for longer than 5 seconds at a time and to minimize suction pressures to avoid damaging the delicate respiratory structures.

M Before N

It is important to suction the mouth of a newborn before the nose. If the nose is suctioned first, the newborn may gasp or cry and aspirate secretions in the mouth.

MAINTAINING THERMOREGULATION

It is critical to protect the newborn from chilling. Cold stress increases the amount of oxygen and glucose needed by the newborn, which can quickly deplete glucose stores and cause hypoglycemia. The newborn can also develop respiratory distress and metabolic acidosis if exposed to prolonged chilling. If the newborn cries vigorously and has an adequate heart rate, they may stay with their mother. Quickly dry the newborn on the mother's abdomen, swaddle them snugly, and apply a cap to prevent heat loss. Another way to maintain the newborn's temperature and promote early bonding is by **skin-to-skin (kangaroo) care**, where the newborn is skin-to-skin with the family caregivers and both are covered with blankets (Fig. 14-2). Skin-to-skin (kangaroo) care is an excellent way to meet the needs of the newborn and provide family-centered care.

It is important to support thermoregulation in the newborn, particularly in the first 24 hours of life. The environmental temperature necessary to maintain a **thermoneutral environment**, an environment in which heat is neither lost nor gained, is slightly higher for the newborn than that required for an older child or adult. Take care to prevent unnecessary heat loss in the nursery. For example, drafts of air can cause convective heat loss, and placing a newborn on a cold surface, such as a

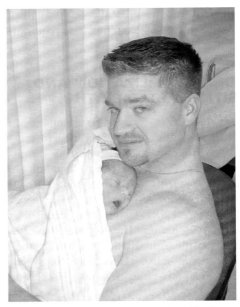

FIGURE 14-2 A new father practices skin-to-skin (kangaroo) care, keeping his newborn warm using skin-to-skin contact. Skin-to-skin (kangaroo) care is also an excellent way for parents to bond with their newborn.

scale, can lead to conductive heat loss (see Chapter 13 for discussion of these terms). Conversely, do not allow the newborn to become overheated. Hyperthermia can be just as harmful as hypothermia. Hyperthermia causes the neonate to increase their metabolic rate, and this causes an increase in oxygen consumption. Hyperthermia can lead to vasodilatation, which can cause hypotension. Another consequence can be dehydration. A skin temperature probe should be in place on the skin anytime the newborn is under the radiant warmer, and alarms should be set to signal if the skin temperature becomes too hot or too cold. Avoid placing the sensor over a bony prominence or areas of brown fat to prevent false temperature readings as these areas tend to be warmer than the rest of the newborn's body.

PREVENTING INJURY FROM HYPOGLYCEMIA

The best way to prevent injury from hypoglycemia is to prevent the condition altogether. If the mother is breast-feeding, encourage early and frequent feedings. If she is experiencing difficulty, it may be necessary to have a lactation consultant assist the mother. See Chapter 15 for detailed information on breast-feeding and nutrition. If the newborn is to be bottle-fed, initiate early feedings.

When a newborn displays signs of, or is at risk for, hypoglycemia (see Chapter 13), perform a heel stick (Nursing Procedure 14-1) and use a bedside glucometer to check the blood sugar level. The bedside glucometer must be calibrated specifically for newborns to accurately detect glucose levels in the presence of higher hematocrit concentrations. If a heel stick specimen reveals a glucose level of less than 50 mg/dL, report the finding to the RN and follow the health care provider's

NURSING PROCEDURE 14-1 Performing a Heel Stick

EQUIPMENT
Alcohol wipe (or other antiseptic, per institution policy)
2 × 2 square gauze pad
Tape
Adhesive bandage
Lancet or other puncturing device
Device to read the glucose level and all supplies needed for its use or laboratory supplies for specimen collection
Clean gloves

PROCEDURE
1. Thoroughly wash your hands.
2. Put on a pair of clean gloves.
3. Hold the foot so that it is well supported with your thumb or finger covering the flat surfaces of the foot to avoid puncturing this area and causing damage to nerves or blood vessels. The highlighted areas on the lateral aspects of the foot in the illustration are appropriate areas from which to perform a heel stick. Do not puncture anywhere over the calcaneus bone.

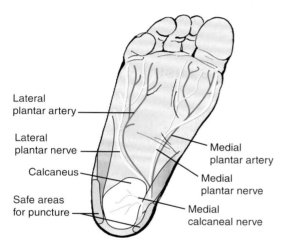

Lateral plantar artery
Lateral plantar nerve
Calcaneus
Safe areas for puncture
Medial plantar artery
Medial plantar nerve
Medial calcaneal nerve

4. Locate a fat pad on either side of the foot. Palpate the chosen site to ensure there is enough padding to avoid puncturing the bone, which could lead to infection.
5. Clean the site with alcohol (or other antiseptic, per institution policy) and allow to air dry.
6. Using the lancet, puncture the site to a depth of no greater than 2 mm. If using a commercial puncturing device, follow

the manufacturer's guidelines for use. Place the lancet in a sharps container.

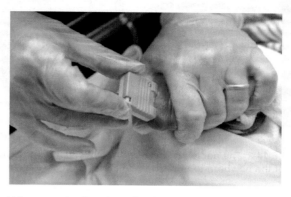

7. Wipe away the first drop of blood. Do not squeeze the tissue close to the puncture site or the reading may not be accurate.
8. Collect the specimen from the second drop of blood. Follow the manufacturer's instructions regarding processing the specimen.

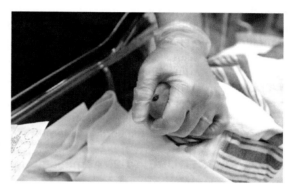

9. Make a pressure dressing from the gauze and tape it over the puncture site. An alternative is to hold pressure for a few moments and then apply an adhesive bandage when the bleeding stops.
10. Remove the gloves and thoroughly wash your hands.
11. Record the glucose level/specimen draw in the designated area of the chart.

---

orders. These may include drawing a venous blood sample and sending it to the laboratory for confirmation as well as feeding the newborn. It is critical, however, that you immediately notify the RN as in some instances the newborn may need intravenous (IV) fluids in addition to the feeding or may need further laboratory testing. Follow institutional policy for frequency of testing newborns at risk for hypoglycemia.

Newborns Are Not Little Adults!
For the newborn capillary blood glucose, you will need to use a glucometer that is calibrated specifically for newborns. Noncalibrated glucometers can give inaccurate readings because of the higher hematocrit levels in newborns.

Most facilities have protocols to guide nursing care in the treatment of hypoglycemia. Many health care providers have preauthorized orders that can be initiated if the glucose level falls below a predetermined level (usually 50 mg/dL). In the past, glucose water was used to treat low blood glucose levels, but current best practice recommends a feeding of breast milk or formula to the alert newborn. If the symptoms are severe enough to interfere with regular feeding (e.g., sleepiness, inability to suck, or tachypnea), intravenous dextrose solutions or gavage feedings are administered.

PREVENTING INFECTION

Within the first hour after birth, an antibiotic agent must be placed in the newborn's eyes (Fig. 14-3) to prevent **ophthalmia neonatorum**, a severe eye infection contracted from the

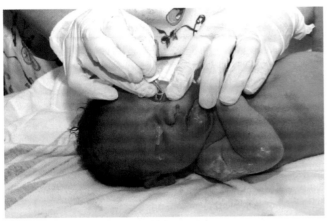

FIGURE 14-3 The nurse administers antibiotic ointment to the eyes of the newborn to prevent ophthalmia neonatorum.

birth canal of a woman with gonorrhea or chlamydia. There are three ophthalmic agents approved for eye prophylaxis: 1% silver nitrate, 0.5% erythromycin, and 1% tetracycline. Silver nitrate is used infrequently because it is irritating to the eyes. In some facilities, it is the practice to instill the eye prophylaxis in the delivery area immediately after birth, but it is recommended that the instillation be delayed up to 1 hour to allow the newborn and parents to bond while the newborn is in a quiet alert state.

Another possible infection site is the umbilical cord stump. Practice careful handwashing, and use strict aseptic technique when caring for the cord. Often an antiseptic solution such as triple dye, bacitracin ointment, or povidone-iodine is used initially to coat the cord to help prevent the development of infection. Follow facility policy for daily care of the stump.

POTENTIAL FOR HEMORRHAGE

One possible cause of hemorrhage and fluid volume loss is an immature clotting mechanism. Vitamin K is necessary in the formation of certain clotting factors. In the adult, normal flora in the intestines manufacture vitamin K, but the intestines of the newborn are sterile as symbiotic bacteria have not yet colonized it. Therefore, it is necessary to supply the newborn with vitamin K to prevent possible bleeding episodes. Within the first hour after birth, 0.5 to 1 mg of vitamin K (phytonadione) is given intramuscularly (Nursing Procedure 14-2).

One potential source of hemorrhage is an unclamped umbilical cord. An unusually large cord may have large amounts of Wharton jelly, which may disintegrate faster than the cord vessels and cause the clamp to become loose. This situation could lead to blood loss from the cord. Another cause could be an improperly applied or defective cord clamp. Inspect the umbilical cord for signs of bleeding.

PREVENTING MISIDENTIFICATION OF A NEWBORN

Fortunately, it is a rare occurrence for newborns to be switched in the hospital and go home with the wrong parents, but it has happened. When the mistake is uncovered, the situation often results in heartache and heart-wrenching choices for all parties involved. Because of the serious consequences of mistaken identity, the delivery

---

NURSING PROCEDURE 14-2 Administering an Intramuscular Injection to the Newborn

EQUIPMENT
Warm, clean hands
Clean (nonsterile) examination gloves
Syringe
0.5-in 23- to 25-gauge safety needle
Alcohol pad
Flat surface

PROCEDURE
1. Wash hands thoroughly.
2. Check health care provider's order for medication and dose.
3. Follow normal nursing procedure for drawing medications from a vial or ampule. Do not draw more than 0.5 mL for intramuscular (IM) injection to a newborn.
4. Identify the newborn by identity band. Place the newborn on a flat surface with good lighting.
5. Select an injection site on the vastus lateralis (anterior lateral aspect of the thigh) or rectus femoris (midanterior aspect of the thigh) muscle.
6. Apply clean gloves.
7. Clean the site with an alcohol pad. Use a circular motion from the center of the chosen site outward in increasingly widening circles. Hold the alcohol pad between two of your fingers.
8. With your nondominant hand, hold the leg in place.
9. Using your dominant hand, insert the needle at a 90-degree angle with a quick darting motion.

10. Stabilize the needle with your nondominant hand, and slowly inject the medication.

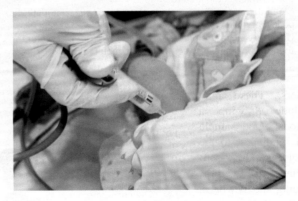

11. Use the alcohol pad to stabilize the skin as you withdraw the needle.
12. Discard the syringe and needle in a sharps container. Discard the gloves in a trash receptacle.
13. Wash hands thoroughly.
14. Document on the medication administration record.

room nurse must take the utmost care to positively identify the newborn before separation from the parents.

Many facilities footprint the newborn and some may fingerprint the mother, but footprints are usually for a memento of the birth and not for identification purposes. Most hospitals use some form of bracelet system. Three to four bracelets with identical numbers on the bands are prepared immediately after delivery and placed on both the newborn and mother. Information included on the bands is the mother's name, hospital number, health care provider, and the newborn's date and time of birth and sex. Two bands are placed on the newborn, one on the arm and one on the leg. A matching band is placed on the mother and another band may be placed on another designated adult. Instruct the mother to always check the bands when the newborn is brought to her to ensure it is her newborn. At some facilities, a clamp with a number matching the bracelet number is placed on the umbilical stump.

TEST YOURSELF

✔ Identify nursing measures the nurse takes in the delivery room prior to the delivery that will support the newborn's transition.

✔ Identify four measures the nurse can take to prevent infection in the newborn.

✔ What is the purpose of eye prophylaxis?

✔ Identify the steps in the identification of the newborn.

GENERAL NORMAL NEWBORN CARE

Nursing care of the normal, stabilized newborn is directed toward controlling risk and early detection of developing complications through vigilant observation and data collection. When caring for newborns, it is important to be familiar with signs that indicate the newborn is successfully transitioning to life outside the womb or if they need special care.

Areas to monitor include continuing observation of cardiac and respiratory status, adequate intake of nutrition, voiding and passing meconium, preventing infection, and skin care. An important safety consideration includes preventing abduction. Observing the newborn's behavior and for pain are also important. The nurse should reinforce information given to the mother and other caregivers during all interactions with them.

ONGOING CARDIAC AND RESPIRATORY MONITORING

Obtain vital signs prior to each feeding or per facility protocol. Note the cardiac rate and rhythm as well of presence of any murmurs. Observe respirations for rate, regularity (keep in mind that newborn respirations are often irregular but should not have periods of apnea greater than 20 seconds), and symmetry, and report any signs of respiratory distress (e.g., grunting noise heard during exhalation, flaring of nostrils, substernal or intercostal retractions, or tachypnea).

The newborn is at risk for aspiration from secretions and mucus that are present in their airway during the first few days of life. Monitor the newborn closely for excessive secretions. Gagging and frequent regurgitation are normal in the first few hours of birth. Signs of respiratory distress or central cyanosis should not be present.

Keep the bulb syringe in the bassinet with the newborn at all times. Turn the newborn on the side and suction frequently as secretions and mucus accumulate. Inform both parents how to use the bulb syringe. Position the newborn on their back for sleep, as recommended by the American Academy of Pediatrics Task Force on Sudden Infant Death Syndrome (2016) to decrease the risk for sudden infant death syndrome (see Chapter 20).

NUTRITIONAL INTAKE

The breast-fed newborn should be nursed every 2 to 4 hours and the bottle-fed newborn every 3 to 4 hours. Observe the mother's technique during the feeding session. Reinforce teaching regarding positing of the newborn, time to nurse or amount to feed, burping, and watching the newborn for any facial cyanosis. Monitor the newborn for signs of feeding intolerance (i.e., spitting up) or difficulty arousing or maintain latch or sucking. The goal of maintaining adequate nutrition and hydration is covered in detail in Chapter 15.

Continue to observe the newborn for number of voids and bowel movements per day. Notify the RN if the neonate has not voided in greater than 6 hours since the previous void or has not had a spontaneous meconium within 24 hours of birth. Remember to never attempt to rectally stimulate the newborn to induce a bowel movement.

PREVENTING TRANSMISSION OF INFECTION

A newborn may contract infection from the mother, visitors, nursery personnel, or the environment. Infection can be particularly devastating for a newborn because the immune system is immature, and the newborn has not yet developed effective defenses against invading pathogens. Therefore, it is essential to practice good infection control techniques when caring for newborns. Handwashing remains the mainstay of infection control, even in newborn nurseries. Many nurseries require a 3-minute surgical-type scrub at the beginning of the shift. Follow the protocol of the facility in which you are working. The hands should be washed thoroughly before and after caring for a newborn. In no instance should you care for a newborn and then proceed to handle or give care to another newborn without physically washing your hands or utilizing hand sanitizer in between newborns. Hand sanitizer is acceptable to use between newborns when visible soiling of the hands has not occurred. Artificial nails have been shown to increase the risk of infection transmission to clients and should not be worn.

Infection can start in the newborn while they are still in the womb, so review both the maternal history and labor and delivery records especially for maternal fever at time of delivery, prolonged rupture of membranes, maternal presence of group B streptococci, or known maternal infection. A mother who had limited or no prenatal care may not have cultures or blood work done to detect potential infections. An infected umbilical cord will show signs of redness and edema at the base and may have purulent discharge. Early signs of sepsis in the newborn include poor feeding, hypoglycemia, irritability, lethargy, apnea, and temperature instability.

Other methods for reducing the transmission of infection include keeping all of the newborn's belongings together in the bassinet and not sharing items between newborns. This practice reduces the possibility of cross-contamination. Wipe reusable equipment, such as a stethoscope, with facility-approved wipes between uses. Rooming-in also reduces the likelihood of cross-contamination. The nurse should drape a clean blanket over their shoulder or front of their body before holding a newborn up against them. This prevents cross contamination between newborns from the nurse's uniform.

It is necessary to use universal precautions for your protection. Do not handle a newborn without gloves until after the bath. After the bath, you may provide care for the newborn without gloves unless contact with bodily fluids is likely, such as during diaper changes and when drawing blood for testing.

NEWBORN SKIN CARE

Perform a thorough skin observation. The skin should be intact and elastic with normal turgor. Inspect the diaper area for signs of rash or breakdown. Observe for jaundice. As you will recall from Chapter 13, jaundice that occurs within the first 24 hours of life is associated with abnormal lysis of red blood cells and is pathologic in nature.

The first bath (Nursing Procedure 14-3) is delayed until the newborn's temperature is stable. Warm water is usually sufficient for bathing; however, a mild soap is permissible. The sponge bath is given under a radiant warmer to minimize heat loss. If a radiant warmer is not used, it is important to bathe the newborn in a warm room, away from drafts and windows, and keep them wrapped; exposing only the body part being washed to avoid causing cold stress. The newborn is not given a tub bath until the cord has dried up and fallen off.

Be Careful

Do not use harsh soaps when bathing newborns because they can irritate the skin. Hexachlorophene in particular should not be used because it can be absorbed through the skin and cause central nervous system damage.

Be careful to wash off all traces of blood off the newborn to minimize transmission of infection. Combing the hair helps remove dried blood. Vernix serves as a lubricant and is protective against infections; therefore, it is best to allow it to wear off naturally.

Encourage the parents to participate in the bath (Fig. 14-4). This is an excellent time to allow them to interact with their newborn and help them gain confidence in parenting skills. When the bath is finished, check the axillary temperature. If it is within the expected range, dress the newborn in a shirt, diaper, and cap. Swaddle the newborn in a blanket, and place them in an open crib. If the temperature is below 97.5°F (36.4°C), return the newborn to the radiant warmer and notify the RN.

Use warm water to clean the newborn's perineal area and buttocks at diaper changes. Frequent diaper changes will help prevent diaper rash and skin breakdown. No special oils or ointments are necessary on clean, intact skin. Do not use talcum powders because they can cause respiratory irritation when particles are inhaled. Fold the diaper down in the front so that the cord is open to air (Fig. 14-5). This action protects the cord area from irritation when the diaper is wet and promotes drying of the cord.

PROVIDING SAFETY FROM ABDUCTION

Keeping the newborn safe from abduction is an important nursing goal. Although infant abduction is a rare event, it has devastating effects on hospital personnel and family members of the victim. Some abductions are from the home setting and not the hospital. The National Center for Missing and Exploited Children has compiled a typical abductor profile (Box 14-1). When taking care of newborns, be especially alert to any suspicious activity by visitors or persons unknown to you. Inform the mother to let only dedicated nursing staff remove the newborn from the mother's presence. Match identification bands prior to leaving the mother's room and upon the newborn's return to her room.

Education and watchful vigilance are the keys to preventing abduction. Each facility that cares for newborns should have specific policies and procedures in place that address this problem. Review these policies, and know the protocols for the facility in which you will be working.

Most nurseries and mother–baby units are in a part of the hospital that has some security features to discourage abductions. Most nurseries are locked and a security code is necessary to gain entrance. Security cameras are usually placed strategically near entrances and exits. Some facilities use security bracelets that set off an alarm if someone attempts to remove it, or it may trip an alarm when a person exits the unit, or gets close to an exit, with a newborn.

The matching identification bands for newborns and parents are also part of the security plan. In many facilities, identification photos are taken of each newborn. Cooperation of the parents is essential to the effectiveness of any security plan, especially because most newborns who are abducted are taken from the mother's room. Tips for Reinforcing Family Teaching: Keeping the Newborn Safe lists key points to discuss with parents regarding the safety of their newborn while in the hospital.

ENHANCING ORGANIZED NEWBORN BEHAVIORAL RESPONSES

Newborns respond to the environment in more predictable and organized ways when caregivers anticipate their needs. The psychosocial task of infants is developing a sense of trust. Newborns begin to develop trust when the adults around them consistently meet their needs. Feeding the newborn, keeping them dry and comfortable, and holding them are all actions that promote trust. Feeding the newborn before they become too upset and will not latch helps them to organize their feedings. Skin-to-skin (kangaroo) care with family caregivers provides comfort and encourages attachment. Swaddling a newborn is comforting and promotes sleep. Nonnutritive sucking on a gloved finger or pacifier can also be comforting.

NURSING PROCEDURE 14-3 Giving the First Bath

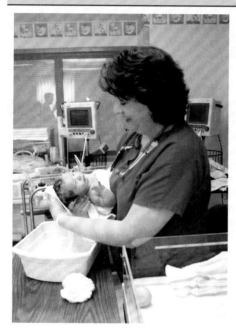

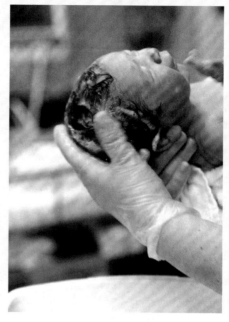

EQUIPMENT
Clean examination gloves
Basin of warm water (98°F to 100°F)
Mild soap and shampoo
Washcloth
Towel
Comb
Cap
Clean diaper
Shirt
Two receiving blankets

PROCEDURE
1. The room should be warm, approximately 75°F (24°C) to prevent chilling. In many facilities, the first bath is given under the radiant warmer.
2. Assemble equipment.
3. Wash hands, and put on clean examination gloves.
4. Use only clear water (no soap) on the eyes first (proceeding from inner canthus to outer canthus), then the rest of the face. Each body area should be washed, rinsed, and then dried before proceeding to the next area to prevent heat loss from evaporation.
5. Hold the newborn with your nondominant arm using the football hold. Use the washcloth with the other hand to wipe off visible blood.
6. Lather the hair with shampoo, and rinse thoroughly.

7. Comb through the hair to remove dried blood and to facilitate drying.
8. Place the newborn back in the crib or under the radiant warmer (per the facility policy).
9. Bathe and rinse the neck and chest. Be sure to remove blood from the creases of the neck and armpits. If vernix is present, do not scrub it off, or you may cause skin abrasions; instead, wipe it gently to remove visible traces of blood.

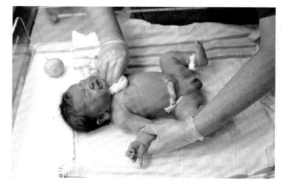

10. Proceed to the abdomen. Take care not to soak the cord in water (a wet cord increases the risk for infection).
11. Wash the extremities, then the back.

NURSINGPROCEDURE 14-3 Giving the First Bath (continued)

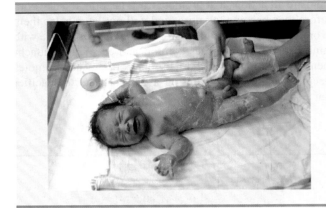

12. Next, bathe the genital region. For boys, do not force the foreskin over the glans. For girls, wash from front to back, avoiding contamination of the urethral and vaginal areas with bacteria from the rectum.
13. Last, bathe the anal region.
14. Apply a clean cap, t-shirt, and diaper.
15. Double wrap the newborn with two receiving blankets.
16. Rinse and dry the basin. Store unused soap, shampoo containers, and comb in the basin in the storage area of the bassinet.
17. Place the towel and washcloth in the dirty linen hamper.
18. Remove gloves.
19. Wash hands.
20. Document the procedure and how the newborn tolerated the bath in the nursing notes.

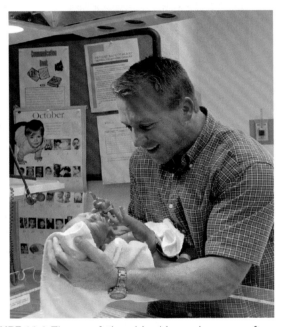

FIGURE 14-4 The new father dries his newborn son after giving him his first bath.

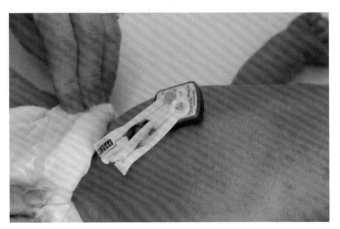

FIGURE 14-5 The diaper is folded down so that it does not cover the drying umbilical cord.

BOX 14-1 Profile of a Typical Infant Abductor

- Usually a female of childbearing age who appears pregnant.
- Compulsive and uses manipulation, lying, and deception to gain access into the newborn care area.
- Often married or cohabiting with a companion.
- Motivated often because the companion has a desire to have a child, or the abductor has a desire to provide her companion with "their" child.
- Familiar with, or lives in, the community in which the abduction takes place.
- A visitor to the nursery or maternity ward prior to the abduction and asks detailed questions about procedures and the maternity floor layout.
- Additionally, the abductor often will:
  - Frequently use a fire exit stairwell for escape.
  - Plan the abduction ahead of time but not necessarily target a specific infant, seizing any available infant when she has the opportunity.
  - Impersonate a nurse or other allied health care personnel.
  - Provide "good" care to the baby after the abduction.

Adapted from http://missingkids.org/theissues/ infantabductions

PAIN IN THE NEWBORN

Watch for signs of pain in the newborn, particularly if they are scheduled for a painful procedure. Until recently, little thought was given as to how newborns perceive pain and what, if any, long-term effects there might be if pain is prolonged or untreated. Many research studies now support the evidence of real physiologic pain responses experienced by the newborn. It appears that untreated pain in the newborn can lead to increased sensitivity to painful experiences later on in life or result in more immediate consequences, such as illness during the neonatal period.

The newborn may experience pain and discomfort from any number of routine procedures. Injections, heel sticks, and circumcision are sources of painful stimuli. Because the newborn cannot express pain verbally, other measures must be used to evaluate pain. Pain can be evaluated in the newborn

TIPS FOR REINFORCING FAMILY TEACHING

Keeping the Newborn Safe

- Never leave the newborn unattended.
- Do not remove the identification bands on the newborn until they are discharged from the hospital; alert the nurses if an identification band falls off or becomes illegible for any reason.
- Do not release the newborn to anyone who does not have a hospital photograph ID that matches the specific security feature (e.g., uniform color, code word, or badge) that identifies personnel authorized to transport and handle newborns.

- Know the nurses caring for you and your newborn.
- Question anyone who does not have the proper identification, or whose picture does not match the identification tag they are wearing, even if they are dressed in hospital attire.
- Alert the nurses immediately if you are suspicious of any person or activity.
- Know when the newborn will be taken for tests, what health care provider authorized the test, and how long the procedure is expected to last.

by paying attention to behavior, such as crying, sleeplessness, facial expression, and body movements. Changes in heart and respiratory rates, blood pressure, and oxygen saturation can also be used to determine physiologic responses to pain.

It is the ethical responsibility of the nurse to prevent and treat pain. Enough research exists to document the adverse effects of unnecessary and untreated pain in the neonate. The best treatment is prevention. When possible, avoid situations that may be painful or distressing to the newborn. If there is a choice between an invasive versus noninvasive procedure, choose the noninvasive procedure whenever practical. Use common sense, and make suggestions to the RN or health care provider as appropriate. For instance, it may be less painful to insert an intravenous device than to give multiple intramuscular injections, or it might be more tolerable for the newborn to have laboratory specimens drawn by venipuncture than to undergo numerous heel sticks.

Provide for a quiet, soothing environment as often as possible. Simple comfort measures can be initiated that decrease the amount of pain perceived by the newborn. Swaddling and holding the neonate securely are soothing measures. Nonnutritive sucking on a pacifier can be comforting. Placing sucrose on the pacifier prior to the procedure, if allowed by hospital policy, adds the benefit of analgesia suitable for minor pain stimulus.

TEST YOURSELF

✔ Identify the steps in the newborn bath.

✔ List four things the nurse can do to decrease the spread of infection to newborns.

✔ Describe three steps parents can take to reduce the risk of infant abduction while in the hospital.

Remember Matthew Colluci? What nursing care would you have performed in the first 12 hours of his life? What information would be important to review with his mother? As this is her third newborn, how would you determine the level of her understanding of newborn care?

PREPARING THE NEWBORN FOR DISCHARGE

Monitoring and promoting healthy adaptation to newborn life, observing for complications, and reinforcing information with family caregivers guide nursing care when planning for discharge of a healthy newborn. Continue to monitor the newborn's respiratory, cardiovascular, thermoregulatory, nutritional, and hydration statuses. Monitor for signs of infection. Check for developing jaundice.

It is also important to monitor the adaptation of the mother and significant other to the parenting roles. Experienced parents may feel comfortable in their roles and carry out newborn care without difficulty, or they may still feel unsure of themselves. New parents may ask many questions or may appear afraid to handle the newborn. Observe for signs of positive bonding with the newborn. Refer to Chapter 12 for an in-depth discussion of bonding.

Prevention of, and relief from, pain are applicable goals throughout the newborn's stay in the hospital; however, these goals become particularly important when the newborn is scheduled for an invasive procedure, such as circumcision. Protection from infection and injury from preventable diseases by immunizing against hepatitis B and screening for phenylketonuria and other metabolic disorders is a critical goal during this time. It is also important to evaluate parental knowledge and ability to care for the newborn throughout the hospital stay, but as the time draws near for discharge, this task becomes particularly important.

Not All Babies Are the Same

Remember, just because the parents have had a previous child, this is a different child and therefore a new parenting situation. Do not assume the family caregivers are without questions because they have more than one child.

Circumcision

Circumcision is the surgical removal of the foreskin of the penis. There has been much debate concerning whether or not circumcision should be routinely performed. The current position of the American Academy of Pediatrics (AAP, 2012) is that "Evaluation of current evidence indicates that the health benefits of newborn male circumcision outweigh the risks; furthermore, the benefits of newborn male circumcision justify access to this procedure for families who choose it." The procedure is contraindicated in newborns who:

- Are still in the transition period.
- Are preterm or sick.
- Have a family history of bleeding disorder until the disorder is ruled out in the newborn.
- Have received a diagnosis of a bleeding disorder.
- Have a congenital genitourinary disorder, such as epispadias or hypospadias.

The AAP advises that parents should be given enough information to make an informed choice and that pain relief measures should be provided if the procedure is done. Box 14-2 compares the advantages and disadvantages of male circumcision. The religious and cultural values of the family caregivers may play a large role in the decision on whether or not to circumcise. These values must be respected. Whatever the parents decide, you must be supportive of their decision and not try to influence their decision based on your beliefs regarding circumcision.

If the parents decide to have their male newborn circumcised, informed consent is necessary. It is the health care provider's responsibility to obtain informed consent, although you may be responsible for witnessing the mother's signature to a written documentation of that consent.

If the parents have unanswered questions, notify the health care provider before the procedure is done. Because of the overwhelming evidence regarding the adverse effects of pain on the newborn, many health care providers will use some type of pain management protocol.

After the mother signs the written consent, prepare for the procedure by gathering all necessary supplies and equipment. Check the health care provider's preference card to determine what procedure they use and what special materials are required. Immobilization is usually provided with a padded circumcision board (Fig. 14-6). If the board is not padded, add blankets or other soft material to the board. Secure the newborn's legs to the board using soft Velcro straps. Swaddle his upper body during the circumcision. Keeping his hands and arms near his face helps him remain calmer than if they are strapped down on the board.

Check the health care provider's orders for preprocedure pain relief methods. Acetaminophen may be given within 1 hour before the procedure and then every 4 to 6 hours afterward during the first 24 hours per health care provider's orders or facility protocol. If an anesthetic cream is to be used for the procedure, it must be applied approximately 1 hour before the procedure to adequately numb the area. The type of anesthesia that provides the best pain relief appears to be a dorsal penile nerve block. The provider performs the nerve block with buffered lidocaine at least 5 minutes before the circumcision to allow for complete anesthesia in the area. Other methods that can decrease the pain sensation include dimming the lights during circumcision, playing soft music or prerecorded intrauterine sounds for the newborn, and offering a sucrose-dipped pacifier to the newborn before and throughout the procedure.

BOX 14-2 Advantages and Disadvantages of Male Circumcision

Advantages
- Lower rates of urinary tract infections. (Note that the overall rate of urinary tract infections in male infants is very small.)
- Risk of penile cancer, a rare disease, is reduced if circumcision is performed in infancy.
- Significant reduction in sexually transmitted infections. (This is an important medical benefit of circumcision; however, practicing safe sexual behaviors remains the best way to prevent these infections.)
- Circumcision for the newborn has fewer complications than when the procedure is performed in adulthood, although medical necessity for adult circumcision is rare.
- Easier hygiene. (Good hygiene of the uncircumcised penis may be as protective as circumcision; however, most uncircumcised boys do not perform adequate hygiene under the foreskin.)

Disadvantages
- Neonates experience pain during circumcision.
- All anesthetic methods to block or reduce the pain of circumcision have side effects and possible complications.
- Circumcision can lead to the complications of hemorrhage and infection (infrequent occurrences, but potentially life-threatening).
- The outcome may not be exactly as the parents expected/ desired it to look.

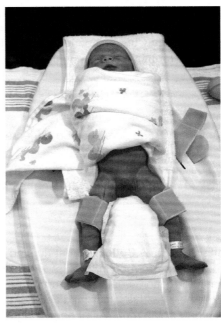

FIGURE 14-6 Medical immobilization in preparation for circumcision.

A Personal Glimpse

The nurse walked into my room and found me crying and holding my newborn son. She asked me if I was in pain or if something was wrong with the baby. I said, "No." She asked if I needed to talk, and I nodded my head. I blurted out, "I just don't know if I should circumcise my son or not. My husband thinks we should, but I don't want my baby to be in pain. I just don't know that it is a necessary procedure."

She sat down on the side of my bed and calmly explained that there was no right or wrong decision. She assured me that she and the other nurses and doctors would support us in any decision we made for our son. Then she gave me several pamphlets to read explaining the pros and cons of circumcision, the pros and cons of choosing not to circumcise, and the latest recommendations from the American Academy of Pediatrics. I felt much better after our talk, and my husband and I were able to make an informed decision about whether or not our son would have this procedure.

Heather

Learning Opportunity: *What things can the nurse tell parents about pain control for painful procedures? In what ways can the nurse act as an advocate for parents when they are trying to decide whether or not to allow procedures on their newborn?*

The health care provider will administer an anesthetic and then cleanse the penis and surrounding tissues with an antiseptic. The three main types of circumcision techniques are the Gomco clamp, Plastibell device, and the Mogen clamp (Fig. 14-7). Immediately after the procedure, place a petroleum gauze dressing as ordered by the provider for a Gomco or Mogen type of circumcision but not for the Plastibell device. The plastic ring of the Plastibell protects the glans of the penis until the site has healed and the ring falls off. Hold and comfort the newborn after the procedure. If the parents are not readily available or cannot perform this action, the nurse soothes the newborn. Administer analgesic medications as ordered for pain. Allow the newborn to do nonnutritive sucking. Monitor the newborn for signs of unrelieved pain.

Examine the newborn every hour for the first 12 hours after circumcision for evidence of bleeding. If bleeding occurs, apply gentle pressure as needed. Carefully observe for return of voiding, and observe the urine stream. Failure to void indicates a complication of circumcision. Report this situation to the RN and the health care provider. Refer to Tips for Reinforcing Family Teaching: Uncircumcised and Circumcised Penis Care for important education points to discuss with parents after circumcision or, if circumcision is not done, how to care for the uncircumcised penis.

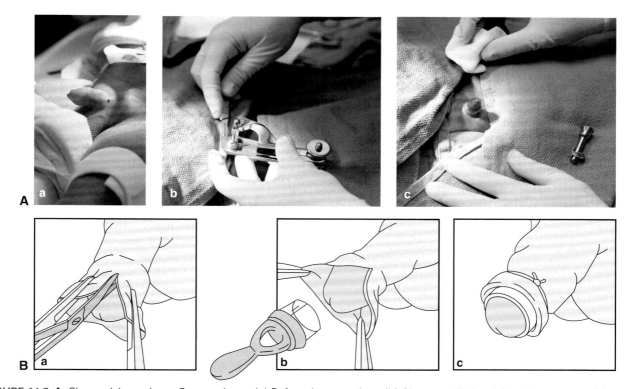

FIGURE 14-7 A. Circumcision using a Gomco clamp. (a) Before the procedure. (b) Clamp applied and foreskin removed. (c) Appearance after procedure. **B.** Circumcision using a Plastibell. (a) Incision made in the top of the foreskin. (b) Plastibell placed over head of penis; foreskin pulled over the Plastibell. (c) Suture tied around foreskin over the tying groove in the Plastibell. In 5 to 8 days, the Plastibell falls off.

TIPS FOR REINFORCING FAMILY TEACHING

Uncircumcised and Circumcised Penis Care

Care for the Uncircumcised Newborn

- Wash the exterior of the penis with each diaper change.
- Avoid forcing the foreskin to retract because bleeding, infection, and scarring can result.
- Educate the child, when he is old enough, to wash under the foreskin daily by gently retracting the foreskin as far as it will go (without using forcible retraction).

Care for the Circumcised Newborn

- Inspect the circumcision site each time the diaper is changed. Call the health care provider if more than a few drops of blood are present in the diaper.
- Wash the penis with warm water squeezed gently from a washcloth at each diaper change. Avoid soap and water washing of the penis until the site has healed.
- Reapply petroleum jelly at each diaper change for the first 24 to 48 hours unless a Plastibell was used.

- Fasten the diaper loosely to prevent unnecessary friction and irritation.
- Do not use any talcum powder in the diaper area.
- Remember that yellow crusting over the area indicates normal healing. The crust should not be removed.
- Hold and comfort your newborn frequently while the site is healing. Nonnutritive sucking with a pacifier may be soothing.
- Call the health care provider if a Plastibell does not fall off within 5 to 8 days.
- Report the following warning signs after circumcision.
  - Bleeding spot larger than a quarter in the diaper.
  - No wet diapers within 12 hours after circumcision.
  - Fever, low-grade temperature.
  - Bad smell to the drainage, pus at the site.
  - Plastibell falls off before 5 days or is displaced.
  - Scarring after the area has healed.

Neonatal Immunization

Hepatitis B virus (HBV) vaccination is recommended by the Centers for Disease Control and Prevention for all newborns before they leave the hospital, regardless of the mother's hepatitis B surface antigen (HBsAg) status. The HBV vaccine requires parental consent. Be sure to obtain the mother's written consent before administering the vaccine. Instruct the family caregivers to follow up with the recommended vaccination schedule for all immunizations, starting at 2 months and continuing throughout infancy.

The HBV vaccination is especially important in newborns of mothers who are infected with hepatitis B or in whom infection is suspected. Many newborns who contract HBV from their mothers become chronic carriers of the disease. In some cases, the newborn develops an acute case of HBV and dies of the infection. In other cases, the newborn has no symptoms but has an increased risk for developing cirrhosis or hepatocellular carcinoma later in life. If the woman is HBsAg-positive, bathe the newborn thoroughly after birth (to remove traces of blood and decrease the risk of transmission from the mother's blood on their skin when receiving the vaccination). In addition, the newborn is given the HBV vaccination and one dose of hepatitis B immunoglobulin within 12 hours of birth. This dosing schedule is 98% to 99% effective in preventing transmission of HBV from an infected mother to her newborn. If the mother's HBsAg status is unknown, the HBV vaccine is given, and the hepatitis B immunoglobulin dose can be postponed as long as 1 week while awaiting the mother's results.

Neonatal Screening

It is crucial to screen newborns for several metabolic and genetic disorders that have the potential to cause lifelong disability if diagnosis and treatment are delayed. Some of these disorders are listed in Box 14-3. The laws in

---

BOX 14-3 Newborn Screening

Disorders for which newborn screening is commonly done:
- Phenylketonuria (PKU)
- Congenital hypothyroidism
- Galactosemia
- Maple syrup urine disease
- Homocystinuria
- Biotinidase
- Sickle cell disease
- Congenital adrenal hypoplasia
- Cystic fibrosis

All 50 states have newborn screening programs with a participation rate of 99.9% according to the National Institute of Health https://www.nichd.nih.gov/health/topics/newborn/conditioninfo/infants-screened#:~:text=Today%2C%20all%2050%20states%2C%20the,Rico%20have%20newborn%20screening%20programs

---

most states require this initial screening to be done within 72 hours of birth. The ideal time to collect the specimen is after the newborn is 36 hours old and 24 hours after the first protein feeding. Using a heel stick, draw blood, and collect a specimen on a special collection card. The card has five rings, and each ring must be completely filled with the newborn's blood (Fig. 14-8). The specimen is then labeled and sent to a special laboratory for testing. A second test is performed at 1 to 2 weeks of age. The parents must be instructed on where and when to take the newborn for the follow-up screening test.

A hearing screen is done on all newborns before they are discharged home. There are two tests that are used to screen a newborn's hearing—the auditory brainstem response and otoacoustic emissions. Both tests use clicks or tones played into the newborn's ear. The auditory

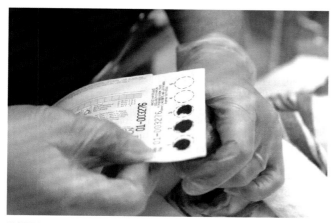

FIGURE 14-8 The nurse collects a blood specimen on a special card to screen the newborn for treatable disorders that otherwise might cause cognitive impairment, disability, or even death.

brainstem response measures how the brain responds to sound through electrodes placed on the newborn's head. Otoacoustic emissions measure sound waves produced in the inner ear. A probe is placed inside the newborn's ear canal, and the response or echo is measured. Both tests are effective screening devices. An abnormal screening result is followed up with more extensive testing. If the newborn is treated with an ototoxic antibiotic, such as gentamicin, the hearing screen must be performed after the antibiotic therapy is completed. Early diagnosis and treatment results in better outcomes, including better chances for improved speech, for newborns who have hearing disorders.

Reinforcing Information

Providing information to parents is an essential part of normal newborn care. The parents need to know many things to effectively meet the needs of their newborn. Because hospital stays are short, it is difficult to educate parents on everything they need to know and to give them time to absorb the information and ask questions. At the very least, instructions should be written so that the parents can refer to them as needed. Tips for Reinforcing Family Teaching: General Tips for Newborn Care at Home provides helpful information for new parents.

Some hospitals have newborn care videos that the parents can take home. Newborn care classes often are available that can be started before discharge and continued for several weeks or months afterward. Some hospitals have home visitation programs in which a nurse, lactation consultant, or clinical nurse specialist follows up with the new family at home. All of these are ways to extend the information session and allow family caregivers to absorb the material and formulate questions. Return demonstrations and home visits allow for direct observation of the parents' ability to care for the child.

Pay Close Attention

If the parents are inexperienced, they need to feel confident in their ability to care for their child. Tactfully role model newborn care; then let them develop their skills while you are available to assist. Sincerely complement them when they do well.

HANDLING THE NEWBORN

New parents are often anxious about picking up the newborn for the first time. Assist them to slide one hand under the neck and shoulders and place the other hand under the buttocks or between the legs before gently lifting the newborn. Because newborns cannot support their heads for the first few months, it is necessary for parents to provide this support when holding the newborn.

Demonstrate different ways to hold the newborn (Fig. 14-9). The football hold is one position that allows the parent to support the head and body with one hand because the body is tucked under the arm. This leaves one hand free for other tasks. Instruct the parents to use the football hold judiciously while walking because the head is largely unprotected with this hold (see Fig. 30-4). Cradling the newborn is familiar to most parents, as is the shoulder hold, which is sometimes comforting for a colicky infant. Newborns should always be placed on their backs to sleep to reduce the risk for sudden infant death syndrome.

Swaddling gives the newborn a sense of security and is comforting. Demonstrate to the parents how to swaddle the newborn. Then let the parents give a return demonstration. Place the blanket in such a way that the newborn is positioned diagonally on the blanket. Fold down the top corner of the blanket behind the newborn's neck. Pull the left corner around the front of the body and tuck it under the right arm. Pull up the bottom corner, and tuck it in the front. Pull the right corner around the front of the newborn and tuck it under the left arm (Fig. 14-10).

Not Too Tight!

Do not swaddle the newborn too tightly as this can impair their breathing and cause respiratory difficulty. Inform the newborn's family caregivers of this important tip.

Handwashing before and after handling the newborn is the best way family caregivers can protect their newborn from infection. They should also encourage visitors to wash their hands before touching the newborn. Anyone with obvious illness should not visit until they are well again.

CLEARING THE AIRWAY

Show the parents how to use the bulb syringe. Depress the bulb first, away from the newborn's face, and then place the tip in the mouth between the gum and cheek, never toward the back of the tongue. Release the bulb to aspirate the secretions. Remove the bulb syringe and depress the bulb onto a cloth to discard secretions. Repeat as needed to clear the mouth. Suction the nose after the mouth using the bulb syringe. Again, depress the bulb away from the face before placing the tip securely against one nare and then release the bulb. Do not force the tip of the bulb syringe into the nare; place only against the opening firm enough to make a seal. Repeat the steps for the opposite nare. Instruct the parents not to overuse the bulb suction on the nares as it can be drying and also cause swelling of the delicate nasal membranes. Clean the bulb with warm water and a mild soap. Sneezing is a normal response

TIPS FOR REINFORCING FAMILY TEACHING

General Tips for Newborn Care at Home

Feeding

- Most newborns eat every 2 to 4 hours. Feeding patterns become fairly regular in approximately 2 weeks.
- Occasional regurgitation (spitting up) is expected. Vomiting should be reported to the health care provider. Frequent vomiting can quickly lead to dehydration. Projectile vomiting may indicate an obstruction and needs to be reported immediately.

Sleeping

- Newborns sleep approximately 16 to 20 hours per day.
- Newborns should be placed on their backs for sleep.
- If you are caring for the newborn, it is a good idea to rest frequently throughout the day and sleep when the baby sleeps.
- For the first 3 to 4 months, it is difficult for infants to fall asleep by themselves. It is helpful to rock, walk, cuddle, or otherwise comfort the infant as they try to fall asleep. After 4 months of age, you can help the baby learn to fall asleep at predictable times.
- There are wide variations of "normal" as to when babies sleep through the night. Some are able to do so by 6 to 7 weeks of age. Others may not until they are 3 or 4 months old.
- It does not help a baby sleep through the night to introduce solid foods too soon. A newborn's digestive system is immature and not ready to handle large protein molecules until approximately 4 months of age. Exclusive breast-feeding is recommended for the first 6 months of life if possible.

Crying

- It is normal for a newborn to cry approximately 2 hours per day for the first 6 to 7 weeks of life. These are often referred to as "crying jags."
- A "fussy period" during the day is to be expected.
- Crying is the way a baby communicates. First, check the baby for physical causes of discomfort, such as a wet or dirty diaper or hunger. Then, try all or some of the following suggestions to help quiet the baby:
  - Rock the baby.
  - Carry the baby, and walk.
  - Take the baby for a stroll in the stroller.
  - Put the baby in a baby swing or a rocking cradle.

- Gently pat or stroke the baby's back.
- Swaddle the baby.
- Take the baby for a ride in the car.
- Turn on some white noise—washing machine, vacuum cleaner, air conditioner, radio not tuned to a station, etc.
- **NEVER** shake a baby for any reason. If you have tried everything and the baby continues to cry, put the baby down in a safe place (such as the crib) and take a time-out. It won't hurt the baby to cry for a short time alone. Also, you could ask someone else to take over for a while.

Sensory Input

- Babies' brains need stimulation to develop. Use the five senses to communicate with the baby.
- Visual stimulation can be as simple as making faces with your baby during periods of alertness. Mobiles are another means of visual enrichment.
- Talking, singing, and reading give the baby auditory stimulation.
- Holding and cuddling the baby and letting them touch different textures and shapes develops the touch sense.
- Pay attention to your baby's cues. They will let you know when they have had enough stimulation and needs rest.

Health Maintenance

- Be sure to make an appointment with the newborn's health care provider within the time frame given to you at discharge, usually at 2 weeks of age.
- Be sure to take the baby for follow-up screenings and immunizations at the appropriate times.
- Recognize signs of illness, and follow up with the health care provider if these signs are present:
  - Fever
  - Vomiting
  - Unusually fussy
  - Diarrhea (frequent, watery stools)
  - Yellow or blue color to the skin
  - Breathing that appears stressed
  - Refuses to eat or has a poor suck
  - Appears listless, hard to wake up

---

to particles in the air and is not indicative of a cold. Yellow or green nasal drainage are signs of illness that the parents should report to the health care provider. If the newborn turns blue or stops breathing for longer than 20 seconds, the parents should seek immediate emergency care by calling 911, and initiate infant CPR if necessary.

MAINTAINING ADEQUATE TEMPERATURE

Inform the parents to protect their newborn from drafts and to adequately dress the newborn. However, sometimes the temptation is to overdress the newborn. The best advice is

to instruct the parents to dress the newborn in the amount and quality of clothes that would keep the parents comfortable in the environment, plus one light blanket. Check the newborn's temperature if they seem ill. Axillary temperatures less than 97.7°F (36.5°C) or greater than 99.5°F (37.5°C) should be reported to the health care provider.

MONITORING STOOL AND URINE PATTERNS

It is normal for the newborn to have 6 to 10 wet diapers per day after the first day of life. Instruct the parents to report if the newborn does not void at all within a 12-hour period.

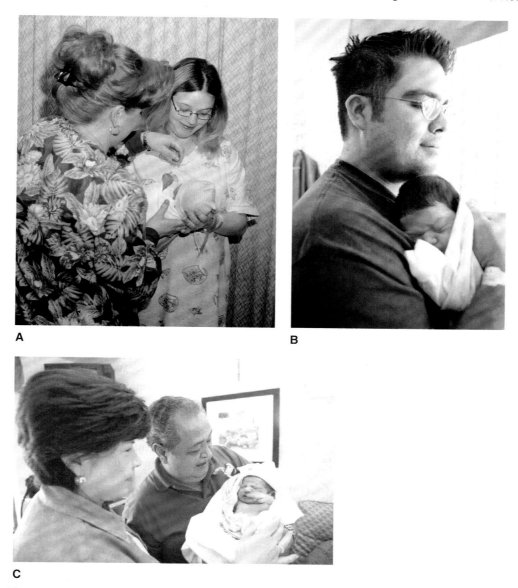

FIGURE 14-9 A. The nurse shows the new mother how to support the newborn using the football hold. **B.** The new father demonstrates the shoulder hold. **C.** The grandfather is using the familiar cradle hold.

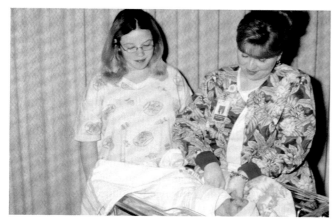

FIGURE 14-10 The nurse shows the new mother how to swaddle her newborn.

Frequent, regular voiding indicates the newborn is getting enough milk.

Newborn stools are initially dark greenish black and tarry. The name for these stools is meconium. Transitional stools are lighter green or light green-yellow and are looser in character. Most newborns are having transitional stools by the time they are discharged home. In general, breast-fed infants have softer, less-formed stools that have a sweetish odor to them. They are often referred to as "seedy" in consistency. Formula-fed infants tend to have more well-formed stools that are a little darker in color with a more unpleasant odor.

Signs of constipation are infrequent hard, dry stools. Babies normally turn red in the face and strain when passing stools. These signs do not indicate constipation. Diarrhea is defined as frequent stools with high water content. Because newborns dehydrate quickly, it is important for parents to notify the health care provider if the newborn has more than two episodes of diarrhea in 1 day.

PROVIDING SKIN CARE

Inform new parents about normal, expected skin changes, such as Mongolian spots and newborn rash (see Chapter 13). Until the cord falls off (approximately 10 to 12 days after birth), the parents should give the newborn sponge baths. Newborns need protection from chilling when they are bathed, from either cool bath water or evaporation. It is also important for parents to monitor the water temperature to prevent scalding the newborn's tender skin. Daily tub baths are not necessary and may dry the skin. The cord site should be cleansed once a day with plain water and a cotton tip applicator.

MAINTAINING SAFETY

Newborns quickly learn to roll over and can move around, even intentionally, on surfaces. For this reason, newborns and infants should never be left unattended on high surfaces, such as on dressing tables or beds. They also should not be left unattended around any amount of water to avoid the possibility of drowning. To protect from suffocation, plastic should not be used to cover crib mattresses or on any object to which the newborn has contact. Pillows are not needed and are considered dangerous for the infant.

Parents need to be able to differentiate normal from abnormal newborn observations and behaviors. A yellow tint to the skin is indicative of jaundice and should be reported to the health care provider promptly. Untreated jaundice can lead to permanent brain damage. Listlessness and poor feeding behaviors are signs of illness that should be reported. Inform the parents about normal behavior states of newborns, and help them learn to read the special cues their newborn gives regarding when and how much interaction the newborn can tolerate (see Chapter 13).

Proper use of car seats is a critical skill for new parents to learn. Car seats save lives. Newborns, and infants, should never be transported in a car without one. Most states have laws regarding their use, and family caregivers must be familiar with these laws. The parents should choose a car seat that is designed for the newborn's weight. Newborns, and infants, are safest in rear-facing seats placed in the middle of the back seat of the car. Parents should never place car seats in the front seat of cars equipped with air bags because death and injury have occurred when air bags deploy. If it is absolutely necessary to place the car seat in the front seat, there must be no air bag or the air bag must be professionally disabled. Parents should be thoroughly familiar with the operation of the car seat they choose.

Nursing Process and Care Plan *for the Normal Newborn*

The nursing care of the normal newborn is focused on three major areas: assessment of the newborn, providing the family caregivers with information about newborn care, and providing safety for the newborn. The newborn needs frequent assessments to monitor adaptation outside the womb. The nurse needs to be alert for subtle signs that the newborn might have an infection or other complication. As hospital stays for term, uncomplicated newborns are typically short, every interaction the nurse has with the family caregivers should involve some aspect of reinforcing the teaching that has been done. Reinforcing teaching should be done for all parents, even if this is not their first child or if they insist they "know what they are doing."

Assessment (Data Collection)

It is important to monitor the newborn's adaptation outside the womb. Immediately after birth, it is vital to observe and collect data on the newborn's cardiovascular, respiratory, temperature regulation, and metabolic status. Immediately report to the RN any abnormal observations.

Observe the newborn's ability to feed and coordinate their sucking and swallowing. Monitor the duration or amount of the feeding and the newborn's tolerance of the feeding. Report any instances of vomiting or cyanosis during feedings immediately to the RN. Monitoring the newborn's voids and bowel movements is also important, especially the timing of the very first one. Assessment of bonding between the mother and newborn should occur during every interaction the nurse is present for.

Check for signs of infection at the umbilical stump site, the circumcision site (if the newborn has had this procedure), and for signs of infection including poor feeding, inability to maintain thermoregulation, or inability to maintain blood glucose levels. Report these findings immediately to the RN. Review the birth record for any potential predisposing factor for infection including prolonged rupture of membranes, maternal fever during labor, or maternal infection such as positive group B streptococci.

Nursing Care Focus

When selecting nursing care focuses for the normal newborn, consideration should be given to the family caregiver's knowledge regarding newborn care and any special events that occurred during delivery or transition. If the newborn has an uncomplicated delivery and transition, the nursing care focus is directed at preventing infection, safety of the newborn, and providing interventions for the newborn's discharge.

Outcome Identification and Planning

Major goals for the newborn include being free from infection, remain free from injury, and being prepared for discharge. Planning of nursing activities is based upon these goals.

Immediately after birth, a full newborn assessment is done including vital signs and monitoring of the newborn's cardiovascular, respiratory, temperature regulation, and metabolic status. During the transition phase after birth, the vital signs are done frequently, as often as every 15 minutes until the newborn is stable. After the transition phase, vital signs and newborn assessments will continue on a regular basis for the duration of the hospital stay. Monitor the newborn's respiratory status for rate and abnormal findings (including grunting, flaring, and retracting). Monitor the newborn's temperature, especially for hypothermia. If low temperatures are noted, notify the RN and the health care provider and initiate warming procedures. Glucose monitoring is done when the newborn exhibits signs of hypoglycemia or if conditions such as maternal gestational diabetes was present or if the infant is macrosomic (>4,000 g).

Once the newborn is stable, the nurse will help the mother initiate the first newborn feeding and monitor the newborn during the entire feeding. During subsequent feedings, the nurse will help the mother start the feeding and monitor the newborn's ability to latch, suck, and swallow. Documentation of the amount or length of the feeding, frequency fed, and the newborn's tolerance of the feedings is done. The nurse should assist the caregivers with feeding, burping, and holding the infant as needed while reinforcing teaching and encouraging the new parents at the same time. Documentation of the newborn's voids and bowel movements is important, especially the very first one. During feedings and when reinforcing teaching, the nurse should assess bonding while keeping in mind the mother's culture and pain status.

Preventing infection is a key nursing intervention. This is seen by the nurse doing meticulous handwashing, cleaning reusable medical equipment (such as scales and stethoscopes) according to manufacturer's directions, avoiding sharing of infant items, using a clean blanket as a barrier between the nurse and newborn, and not wearing artificial nails. Newborns are given eye prophylaxis to prevent ophthalmia neonatorum. Instructing the caregivers on cord care and infant skin care is important for protecting the newborn from infection. Heel sticks or venipunctures should be done with an aseptic technique. Monitor circumcision sites for signs of infection.

Providing for the newborn's safety, and instructing caregivers on newborn safety, is another major focus of nursing care for the newborn. Safety starts at delivery with identification bands being placed on the infant and mother, which are checked at each interaction with the couplet. Vitamin K injections are given to prevent hemorrhage. The nurse should demonstrate and instruct on safe handling of the newborn including never leaving infant unattended, never shaking the infant, avoiding choking hazards, bath safety, and checking formula temperature.

Safety information that should also be covered includes use of car seats, newborn hearing screen, newborn screenings (formally called a PKU test), hepatitis B vaccination (HBV), when to call the provider, and follow up provider visits. Monitoring for jaundice and instructing caregivers on home observation for jaundice, and calling the provider, should also be done.

Nursing Care Focus

- Infection risk

Goal

- The newborn will remain free from infection.

Implementations for Infection Risk

Review the birth history for any predisposing factors that could cause an infection in the newborn such as maternal fever during labor. Observe the newborn for signs of infection. Newborns will not run a high fever so monitor for hypothermia instead. Hypothermia along with hypoglycemia or respiratory difficulty (grunting, flaring, retracting, tachypnea, or apnea) might indicate an infection and should be reported to the RN or health care provider immediately.

The nurse should perform meticulous handwashing before and after handling the newborn. All procedures should be performed with aseptic technique. Administer eye prophylaxis after birth as ordered. Administer hepatitis B vaccination (HBV) as ordered. Monitor potential infection sites, such as the umbilical and circumcision site, for signs of infection.

Evaluation of Goal/Desired Outcome

The newborn:

- receives prophylactic medications.
- maintains an axillary temperature between 97.5°F (36.4°C) and 99.5°F (37.5°C).
- has a drying umbilical cord without purulent drainage or foul odor.
- exhibits regular respiratory pattern without signs of respiratory distress.
- has stable blood sugars.

Nursing Care Focus

- Safety of the newborn

Goal

- The newborn's parents will verbalize actions they can take to help keep the newborn safe.

Implementations for Safety

Newborn safety begins with the nurse doing effective and consistent handwashing. The nurse should also use personal protective equipment (PPE) as appropriate. The nurse should always use a barrier (such as a clean blanket) between the nurse's uniform and the newborn to prevent cross contamination. At every interaction, the nurse should check the identification bands on the newborn and match with the mother's identification bands.

Demonstrate how to position the infant to help prevent aspiration and how to use the bulb syringe, and instruct to have a light on during feedings to monitor the newborn's breathing during feedings. Reinforce to the parents how to warm formula or breast milk by heating the bottle in warm water, not a microwave, which can cause hot spots in the milk that can burn the newborn's mouth. Reinforce signs of poor feeding, which can lead quickly to dehydration and malnutrition, and that formula must be prepared according to the directions or it can cause malnutrition. Demonstrate to the parents how to prevent the infant from falling and to always keep a hand on the newborn. Reinforce that only axillary temperatures, never rectal, should be done. If the newborn had a circumcision, monitor for excessive bleeding. Ensure that the first newborn metabolic screening is done prior to the newborn's discharge. Reinforce to the parents car seat safety.

Evaluation of Goal/Desired Outcome

The newborn's parents will:

- verbalize and demonstrate how to position the newborn and use the bulb syringe.
- verbalize safety measures to take during feedings.
- demonstrate how to take an axillary temperature.
- provide a car seat for the newborn to leave the hospital in.

Nursing Care Focus

- Discharge planning for the uncomplicated newborn

Goal

- The newborn's parents will verbalize understanding of newborn care and follow up visits.

Implementations for Discharge Planning

Discharge planning for the uncomplicated newborn starts at birth. The LPN/LVN should reinforce teaching with every encounter they have with the newborn's parents. Information that needs reinforcing includes newborn care and feeding, newborn safety, routine screening that will occur prior to the newborn's discharge (such as hearing screening and newborn metabolic screening), when to call the health care provider, and when to make routine follow-up visits for the newborn. Some facilities provide videos for parents to watch in addition to the information provided by the nurse.

Evaluation of Goal/Desired Outcome

The newborn's parents will:

- demonstrate the skills needed to care for their newborn.
- describe when to call the newborn's health care provider.
- make arrangements for a follow-up visit with the newborn's health care provider.
- state when to take the newborn for the follow up newborn screening.

Remember **Matthew Colluci** from the start of the chapter. His mother chose to have him circumcised. After the procedure, for what would you observe for, and how would you tell his mother to care for the circumcision? Before Matthew is discharged home, the RN asks you if his routine tests have been completed. What tests is the RN referring to? Matthew's mother asks you what she should expect him to do at home. What information would you tell her?

KEY POINTS

- The delivery room should be prepared for resuscitation of the newborn before birth. Resuscitation supplies should be checked and the warmer turned on in anticipation of the birth. If resuscitation is needed, Neonatal Resuscitation Program guidelines should be followed.
- Steps should be taken to prevent the newborn from becoming overly cold or overly hot. A thermoneutral environment is ideal in which the temperature is maintained at a level so that heat is neither gained nor lost.
- The nurse monitors the newborn for signs of hypoglycemia. Hypoglycemia is best prevented and treated with early and regular feedings. If the newborn cannot or will not eat, gavage feedings or intravenous glucose may be necessary.
- Eye prophylaxis to prevent eye infection from gonorrhea and chlamydia should be instituted within the first hour after birth. Vitamin K is given intramuscularly to prevent bleeding problems.
- Identification bands are immediately placed in the delivery room before newborn and parents are separated. The identification bands should be checked before removing the newborn from the mother's presence and when returning the newborn to their mother.

- Maintaining the newborn's own crib and supplies, using excellent handwashing technique, and minimizing exposure to sick people are all measures nurses take to decrease the risk for cross-contamination and infection in the newborn.

- The newborn receives their first bath when their temperature is stable. A sponge bath is given. The bath should be given under a radiant warmer if possible to avoid cold stress.

- Nurses must be constantly on guard for suspicious activity in and around the labor and delivery, postpartum, and nursery units. The risk for abduction is a real threat. Inform the parents to ask to see identification before releasing their newborn to anyone.

- Newborns show behavioral and physiologic responses to painful procedures. These responses include crying, grimacing, and increased heart and respiratory rates.

- Circumcision remains a controversial procedure. The AAP strongly recommends the use of analgesia and anesthesia for the procedure. If the parents choose not to circumcise, they must be taught proper hygiene for the uncircumcised penis.

- The care for the circumcised penis depends upon the technique used. Gomco and Mogen circumcisions are covered with a petroleum gauze for the first 3 to 5 days after the procedure. Plastibell circumcisions do not have any ointment applied.

- All newborns should receive an HBV vaccination, screening for genetic diseases (e.g., phenylketonuria and congenital hypothyroidism), and hearing screen prior to discharge.

- Parents need to learn how to hold and position their newborn, how to clear the airway, maintain adequate body temperature, monitor stool and urine patterns, provide skin care, maintain safety of the newborn, and make follow-up visits for the newborn to be seen by a health care provider.

INTERNET RESOURCES

Newborn Care
www.nlm.nih.gov/medlineplus/infantandnewborncare.html

Cord Care
www.nlm.nih.gov/medlineplus/ency/article/001926.htm

Vitamin K
https://www.cdc.gov/ncbddd/vitamink/faqs.html

Preventing Newborn Abductions
https://www.missingkids.org/theissues/infantabductions

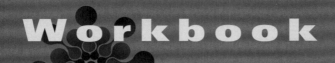

NCLEX-STYLE REVIEW QUESTIONS

1. The delivery room nurse has just brought a 10-lb (4536 grams) newborn to the nursery. The nurse monitoring the newborn during the transition period recognizes that which of the following parameters will most likely inhibit this newborn's transition?

   a. Apgar score
   b. Blood sugar
   c. Heart rate
   d. Temperature

2. The newborn has just been delivered and is placed in skin-to-skin contact with the mother. A blanket covers all of the newborn's body except the head. The newborn's hair is still wet with amniotic fluid, etc. What is the most likely type of heat loss this newborn may experience?

   a. Conductive
   b. Convective
   c. Evaporative
   d. Radiating

3. A woman dressed in hospital scrub attire without a name badge presents to the nursery and says that Mrs. Smith is ready for her newborn. She then offers to take the newborn back to Mrs. Smith. What response by the nurse is best in this situation?

   a. "I don't know you. Are you trying to take a baby?"
   b. "Leave immediately! I'm calling security."
   c. "May I see your identification, please?"
   d. "You must be Mrs. Smith's sister. She said her sister is a nurse."

4. A new mother is not sure if she wants her newborn to be circumcised. Which response by the nurse is best?

   a. "Circumcision is best in order to protect him from diseases like cancer."
   b. "If you do not circumcise your baby, he will always have difficulty maintaining adequate hygiene."
   c. "It is best not to circumcise him because the procedure is very painful."
   d. "There are pros and cons to circumcision. Let me ask the health care provider to come and talk to you about the procedure."

5. Which of the following should the nurse include in the discharge instructions to the parents of a term newborn male? (select all that apply)

   a. "Sponge bathe the newborn every other day until the cord falls off."
   b. "Your son will need to be circumcised before being sent home."
   c. "It is important to bring your son back in a week for his follow-up newborn screening lab test."
   d. "A yellow color to the skin is normal in the first week and ears off."
   e. "Only if he turns blue with crying do you need to call 911."
   f. "Your son will have a hearing test before he is discharged."

STUDY ACTIVITIES

1. Develop a poster that shows nurses ways to prevent transmitting infections in the nursery.

2. Develop a handout for nurses with helpful tips on preventing infant abductions. Use an internet search to help find material for the handout.

3. Make a discharge handout for parents of a newborn.

CRITICAL THINKING: WHAT WOULD YOU DO?

Apply your knowledge of the nurse's role in newborn care to the following situations.

1. A neighbor calls to tell you that their partner just delivered her newborn in the living room. The ambulance is on the way but is not yet there. You run to the house and find the newborn loosely wrapped in a blanket. The neighbor says, "The baby was born approximately 2 minutes before you arrived".

   a. What actions do you take first and why?
   b. The newborn becomes jittery and irritable. What do you suspect may be the problem?
   c. What two interventions will need to be carried out as soon as the newborn and mother can be safely transported to a healthcare facility?

2. Mrs. Mathias just delivered a newborn who cries immediately and is pink. The newborn's cry sounds "wet" and "gurgly."

   a. What action should the nurse take first?
   b. If the respirations continue to sound wet, what step would the nurse take next?

3. Newborn boy Hinojosa is crying and thrashing about after a circumcision.

   a. What is the likely cause of his crying?
   b. What should the nurse do in this situation?

4. A new mother calls the nursery from home. She and her newborn were discharged 2 days ago. She is worried about a small amount of yellow crust she notes at the circumcision site. She is also worried because he has been crying and fussy for the last hour.

   a. How would you advise the mother regarding the yellow crusting?
   b. What suggestions could you give her for the crying?

15

Newborn Nutrition

Key Terms

artificial nutrition
colostrum
engorgement
foremilk
hindmilk
lactation
lactation consultant
mastitis

Learning Objectives

At the conclusion of this chapter, you will:

1. Describe factors that influence the woman's choice of feeding method.
2. Identify advantages of breast feeding for both the woman and the newborn.
3. Discuss situations for which breast-feeding would not be recommended.
4. Discuss the physical and hormonal control of the breast during lactation.
5. Describe the role of the nurse when assisting a woman with breast-feeding.
6. Outline appropriate educational topics for the woman who breastfeeds.
7. Outline appropriate nursing interventions for common problems the woman who breastfeeds might encounter.
8. List signs that a newborn is not breast-feeding well.
9. Differentiate between breast milk and formula.
10. Name situations in which formula-feeding would be beneficial.
11. Compare the various types of formulas available to feed newborns and infants.
12. Outline appropriate educational topics for the woman who formula-feed.
13. List several questions the nurse should ask the parents of a newborn who is not tolerating formula.

Frances Barnes is an 18-year-old gravida 1 para 1. She delivered her son, John, at term via vaginal birth. During the report, you are given the information that Frances would like to breastfeed. When you do your data collection, she states, "I'm worried he won't get enough to eat." How would you respond to her concerns? What information would Frances need about breast-feeding? While you are caring for Frances, her husband states, "I really wanted to feed John." How would you respond to his statement?

In utero, the fetus obtains all of its nutrition in a passive manner. The nutrients cross from the maternal circulation, across the placenta, and enter the fetus's circulation. The nutrients then circulate to the tissues for use at the cellular level. At birth, the passive intake of nutrition ends, and the newborn must actively consume and digest food.

The newborn has unique nutritional needs. The healthy term newborn requires 80 to 100 mL/kg/day to maintain fluid balance and 110 to 120 kcal/kg/day to meet energy needs for growth and development. Breast milk, or an iron-fortified infant formula, provides the newborn with all the calories and fluids necessary. Infants less than 6 months of age who are given water are at risk for hyponatremia. In addition, breast milk and infant formulas are balanced to meet the carbohydrate, protein, and fat needs of the newborn.

SELECTION OF A FEEDING METHOD

There are two main types of nourishment suitable for the healthy term newborn—breast milk and commercially prepared formula. There are also two delivery methods: breast and bottle. The woman can choose to exclusively breastfeed; breastfeed and supplement with expressed breast milk in a bottle; breastfeed and supplement with formula; or she may choose to exclusively formula-feed.

Factors That Influence Choice of Method

Many factors influence the woman's decision about whether to breastfeed or bottle-feed. Some of these factors are culture, sociodemographic factors, prior experience with or exposure to breast-feeding, and intent or need to return to work or school.

Culture

A woman's culture often strongly influences newborn feeding choice. One culturally influenced issue is the acceptability of breast-feeding in public. Bottle-feeding rates are higher in women from cultures that frown upon breast-feeding in public or where there is a taboo against breast-feeding when men are present. The amount and quality of family and community support for breast-feeding is a strong culturally influenced predictor of the type of feeding the woman is more likely to choose.

The question is not only whether to breastfeed or bottle-feed. If breast-feeding is chosen, then culture influences when the woman initiates breast-feeding (e.g., immediately vs. after the "milk comes in"), how many times per day the woman breastfeeds, whether she supplements, and when to stop breast-feeding (i.e., wean the infant). In every culture, there are circumstances in which a woman cannot breastfeed or chooses not to breastfeed for many reasons.

In the United States, women receive mixed messages regarding infant feeding methods. In the media, subtle messages such as picturing infants bottle-feeding versus breast-feeding may give the message that bottle-feeding is preferred. Discussing bottle-feeding may be more comfortable than discussing breast-feeding for some people. Advertising by formula companies suggests that formula is of equal composition to breast milk. Healthcare professionals often contradict one another when giving advice to new mothers. Healthcare workers may promote breast-feeding verbally, but their actions may discourage breast-feeding initiation (e.g., separating the woman and newborn immediately after birth, supplementing with formula in the nursery, or by providing gift bags with bottles and formula).

Breast-feeding rates vary by country of origin. Immigrant women are more likely to follow the practice of their country of origin if they have not completely acculturated. It is important for the nurse to avoid stereotyping whether a woman will or will not breastfeed based upon her origin.

Sociodemographic Factors

Breast-feeding rates differ by age, amount of education, and socioeconomic status. Women older than 30 years have higher breast-feeding initiation rates than do younger women. Slightly less than half of mothers younger than 20 years choose to bottle-feed their newborns. Higher levels of education correlate with higher breast-feeding initiation rates. Fewer women who live in poverty choose to breast-feed compared to women with higher income levels.

Past Experiences of the Woman and Her Support System

A woman's past experience with or exposure to breast-feeding greatly affects her decision whether to breastfeed or bottle-feed. The feeding experiences and attitudes of the individuals who compose the woman's support system strongly influence the woman's choice of feeding method. The woman's mother, her partner, or her friends frequently have previous experiences and strong feelings about which method is best for the newborn. These attitudes may cause these individuals to advise the new mother or put pressure on her to choose a particular feeding method.

Intent to Return to Work or School

The need to return to work or school soon after the newborn's birth plays an important role in the woman's feeding choice. A woman who chooses to breastfeed in the hospital can continue to breastfeed and pump while at work or school, breastfeed when the infant is present and offer formula while she is away, or she can elect to stop breast-feeding. Some women prefer not to begin breast-feeding because of their other obligations and choose to feed formula from the newborn's birth.

Nursing Considerations

As the nurse, your role in assisting the new mother to choose a feeding method is to provide education so that the woman can make an informed choice and to support the woman to provide nutrition to her newborn according to the method she chooses. Although it sounds simple, performing this role can be challenging. On one hand, providing a supportive environment is crucial to the success of the woman who chooses to breastfeed. However, the challenge is to provide this support without making the woman feel guilty if she chooses to bottle-feed her newborn or avoid making suggestions about feeding formula if she is having difficulty with breast-feeding. Exclusive breast-feeding requires a commitment from the woman. Often, women without adequate breast-feeding support (from home, work, school, or other caregivers) have difficulty maintaining the commitment.

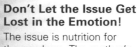

Don't Let the Issue Get Lost in the Emotion!
The issue is nutrition for the newborn. The mother's choice of method is not a reflection of her ability to be a good parent.

BREAST-FEEDING

Breast-feeding is the recommended method for feeding newborns because breast milk is nutritionally superior to commercial formulas. Many organizations, including the American Academy of Pediatrics; the World Health Organization; and the Association of Women's Health, Obstetric, and Neonatal Nurses actively encourage breast-feeding. Each of these organizations has a policy statement that defines their position on breast-feeding and their recommendations for infant feeding.

The American Academy of Pediatrics recommends exclusive breast-feeding until 6 months of age and continuation of breast-feeding until at least 12 months of age and then leaves it up to the woman to decide how long to continue breast-feeding after 12 months. One of the *Healthy People 2030* goals is to increase the proportion of infants who are breastfed exclusively through 6 months of age.

Advantages and Disadvantages of Breast-Feeding

Breast-feeding confers short- and long-term benefits for the woman, her newborn, and the society at large with few (if any) disadvantages.

Advantages

Immediate advantages of breast-feeding for the woman include more rapid uterine involution and less bleeding in the postpartum period. The woman who breastfeeds loses weight faster on average than does the woman who formula feeds her child. Long-term advantages for the woman include decreased incidence of ovarian and premenopausal breast cancers. Women who breastfeed, especially for greater than 3 months, have a lower risk for coronary artery disease, breast and ovarian cancers, and hypertension than women who have formula-fed (Perez-Escamilla and Segura-Perez, 2019).

The advantages of breast-feeding for the newborn are numerous. Breast milk contains substances that facilitate the critical growth and development of vital organs and systems, including the brain, immune system, eyes, and gastrointestinal tract. Breast milk provides immunologic properties that help protect the newborn from infections and strengthen the immune system. Breastfed infants tend to have lower incidences of otitis media, diarrhea, and lower respiratory tract infections. Breast-feeding also provides a possible protective effect against certain conditions or diseases such as sudden infant death syndrome, insulin-dependent diabetes, and allergic diseases.

There are also benefits for the family and society. Breast-feeding is economical. The woman who breastfeeds does not need to purchase formula, bottles, or nipples. Breast milk is always available, needs no preparation or storage, and does not require cleanup of utensils or dishes after the feeding. When away from home, the woman does not need to carry extra equipment or supplies to feed her newborn if her infant is with her. If the newborn is not with the woman, compact, easy-to-use breast pumps can be used to pump the breast and store and save the breast milk for the infant.

Breast-feeding reduces health care costs because breastfed infants are ill less frequently than are formula-fed infants.

Disadvantages

There are no physiologic disadvantages to either the woman or the newborn during breast-feeding, although there may be perceived cultural barriers for some women. There are certain maternal conditions or situations in which breast-feeding is contraindicated. Examples of these conditions include the following:

- Illegal drug use
- Active untreated tuberculosis
- Human immunodeficiency virus infection
- Chemotherapy treatment
- Herpetic lesions on the breast

In addition, certain newborn conditions are contraindications for breast-feeding. Galactosemia, an inborn error of metabolism, requires a specialty formula because the newborn lacks one of the necessary enzymes to break down the sugar in breast milk. With phenylketonuria, another inborn error of metabolism, the newborn requires a special diet that can include breast milk in limited amounts.

Other medical conditions may necessitate that the newborn receive formula. Some women who deliver a preterm infant may have a hard time producing an adequate milk supply by only pumping (if the infant is too premature to breastfeed). In some situations, the woman may produce little to no breast milk. In both instances, a health care provider or lactation specialist should complete a thorough assessment before advising the woman to supplement or switch over completely to formula. Having the mother pump at the preterm infant's crib side during or after skin-to-skin (kangaroo) care may help the woman produce more milk.

There may be misperceptions or perceived barriers to breast-feeding. Some women feel that breast-feeding excludes others from caring for or feeding the newborn. Some fathers express an interest in wanting to feed the newborn and feel that breast-feeding might take away this opportunity. In this circumstance, you can suggest that for some feedings, the woman can pump her breast milk and the father or other caregiver could then feed the newborn the breast milk with a bottle. This way the newborn still receives the superior nutrition of breast milk while allowing the father or other caregiver feeding time with the newborn. This also gives the woman a respite from feeding.

There are other perceived cultural or psychological barriers to breast-feeding. Some women feel that they will be unable to return to work or school if they breastfeed. Others feel that breast-feeding is too difficult or uncomfortable. Some women are uncomfortable touching their breasts or with the idea of the infant sucking at the breast.

The woman or partner may perceive that breast-feeding is sexual in nature or that it detracts from the woman's sexuality. Some women feel restrained by breast-feeding in that it ties them to the infant or they think it will make them "too clingy."

Physiology of Breast-Feeding

Newborn Features That Facilitate Breast-Feeding

The newborn possesses several unique characteristics that make breast-feeding physiologically possible. Specifically, the newborn is born with a uniquely shaped nose and mouth, the rooting reflex, and the innate ability to suck. These characteristics disappear as the infant gets older.

Newborn Facial Anatomy

The newborn is uniquely designed for breast-feeding. The design of the nose, which looks flattened after birth, creates air pockets when up against the breast. This allows the newborn to eat without obscuring the nasal opening. Because newborns are nose breathers, they can breathe while their mouth is full. They do not have to release the breast to take a breath. The newborn's mouth is designed to compress the milk ducts located behind the nipple under the areola. The tongue, pharynx, and lower jaw are unique in shape when compared to those of the older child or adult. The newborn also has fat pads on each cheek that aid in the sucking process.

Rooting and Sucking Reflexes

The newborn's reflexes also assist in breast-feeding. The newborn demonstrates the rooting reflex by turning their head toward the stimulation when the cheek is brushed lightly. Rooting is a feeding cue that lets the woman know her newborn is ready to nurse. When the newborn's lips are lightly touched, the newborn will respond by opening their mouth.

The sucking reflex occurs when the nipple is placed into the newborn's mouth and the newborn begins to suck. The term newborn has the ability to coordinate sucking, swallowing, and breathing in a manner that facilitates nursing and prevents choking. The newborn sucks in a burst pattern, sucking several times and then pausing to rest. The length of the pause should be equal to the time the newborn sucks. The type of sucking also changes during the feeding. At the beginning of the feeding, the newborn nurses with rapid, short sucks. These sucks stimulate the breast to release the milk. When the milk is flowing freely, the newborn nurses with longer, slower sucks.

The Breast and Lactation

The female breast is a unique organ designed to provide the newborn with nourishment through **lactation**, the production and secretion of milk. The breast is very vascular, with a rich lymphatic and nervous supply. Each breast consists of 15 to 20 lobes containing the milk-producing alveoli. The alveoli are clustered together and empty into ducts. Smooth muscle cells surround the alveoli, which help to eject the milk into the ducts. The ducts lead to the nipple, where the milk is released. Figure 15-1 illustrates the anatomy of the female breast.

The breast makes milk in response to several different stimuli. These include the physical emptying of the breast, hormonal stimulation, and sensory stimulation.

Physical Control of Lactation

When breast milk is released (by the newborn sucking, by use of a breast pump, or by other stimulation such as water spray from a shower massaging the breast), the breast responds by replenishing the milk supply. If the breast is emptied incompletely, it will not make as much milk the next time. This is why it is important for the newborn to nurse long enough and often enough to establish a good milk supply. If the woman is pumping, she should allow sufficient time for the pump to drain both breasts. She should not stop pumping until the flow of milk has stopped. If the

FIGURE 15-1 Anatomy of the female breast.

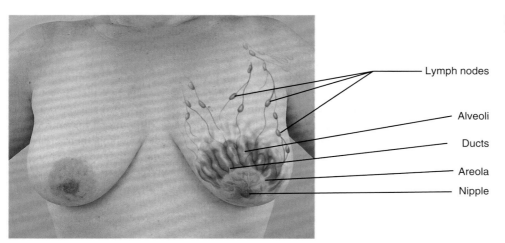

Lymph nodes

Alveoli

Ducts

Areola

Nipple

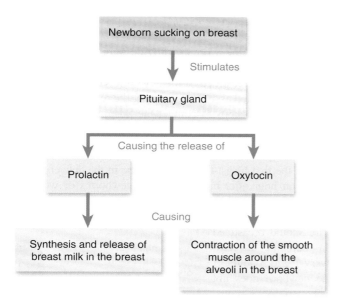

FIGURE 15-2 Diagram of the hormonal effect on lactation.

newborn completely empties the breast and then nurses again shortly after the feeding, the breast is stimulated to increase the amount of milk produced.

Hormonal Control of Lactation

The breast is also under hormonal control. When the newborn sucks on the breast, the woman's pituitary gland releases prolactin and oxytocin. Prolactin stimulates the alveoli to produce milk and then to release it. Oxytocin causes contractions of the muscle cells that surround the alveoli in the breast, which push milk downward toward the nipple (Fig. 15-2).

During the first few days, frequent nursing activates receptor sites in the breasts that respond to lactogen, which aids milk production. If the breast is not stimulated by the newborn's sucking or by a breast pump, the number of receptor sites is reduced. This change can reduce the quantity of the woman's milk supply. Encourage the woman to feed her newborn every 1½ to 3 hours until her milk supply is established. If she is unable to nurse her newborn, as in the case of a premature newborn, she should pump at least every 3 hours around the clock, even during the night.

Did You Know?

The most common reason for insufficient milk supply is infrequent nursing. Help your clients avoid this common pitfall.

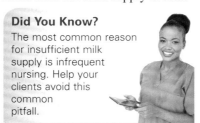

Sensory Stimulation

In addition to the physical emptying of the breast and hormones, the woman's body responds to sensory information from her newborn. As the woman holds her newborn and the newborn touches her breast or grasps her finger with his hand, the woman's skin is stimulated. As the woman looks at her infant, the infant's feeding cues produce visual stimulation. When the infant cries or makes sucking noises, auditory stimulation occurs. Finally, the infant's scent stimulates the woman's sense of smell. The woman's brain processes all of these sensations and then sends messages to the breasts to produce the letdown reflex, which allows milk to flow to the newborn during breast-feeding. This is why a woman may have a letdown reflex when she hears a stranger's baby cry.

Here's a Quick Tip

Maternal alcohol consumption can inhibit the letdown reflex, so the woman who breastfeeds should avoid drinking alcoholic beverages.

Composition of Breast Milk

Breast milk is a unique substance that commercial formulas have been unable to duplicate, especially with regard to the immunologic factors in breast milk. The woman's breast does not produce milk until approximately 3 to 5 days after birth. Until this time, the breast produces a substance called colostrum. **Colostrum** is a thick, yellowish gold substance that is higher in antibodies, lower in fat, and higher in protein content than is breast milk. There are between 2 and 20 mL of colostrum available for each feeding until the woman's milk comes in. The woman's breasts may start to produce colostrum during the second trimester.

Breast milk supplies 20 cal/oz on average. There are two different compositions of breast milk: foremilk and hindmilk. **Foremilk** is the first milk the infant receives during the nursing session and is watery, thin and may have a bluish tint. As the session progresses, the foremilk is replaced by hindmilk. **Hindmilk** is thicker, whiter, and contains a higher quantity of fat than foremilk and therefore has a higher caloric content. The hindmilk satiates the infant between feedings. If the infant is thirsty or not very hungry, they will not nurse long and will receive only the foremilk. The hungry infant nurses longer to get the hindmilk.

It's OK to Reassure the Woman

Until her milk comes in, the woman may feel that her newborn is not getting enough to eat. Assure the woman that her newborn is getting enough calories and that the frequent nursing will aid in establishing an ample milk supply.

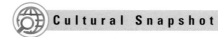

Cultural Snapshot

Some cultures feel that the colostrum is "old" or "dirty" milk; women from such cultures may not want to breast-feed until her milk comes in.

Nutritional Needs of the Woman Who Breastfeeds

The woman who breastfeeds does not need to radically increase the amount of food she eats to produce milk for her infant. In order to meet the energy requirements of lactation, she does need to consume approximately 300 to 500 kcal/day above her prepregnant needs depending upon her age, prepregnant health status, and activity level. The lactating woman needs plenty of fluids. If the woman does not consume enough fluids to satisfy her thirst or does not rest and eat a balanced diet, she may notice that she stops producing breast milk or that the quantity of her breast milk diminishes. A daily multivitamin will not make her breast milk more nutritious but will help ensure she obtains sufficient vitamins and minerals for her own body.

Nursing Care of the Woman Who Breastfeeds

As the nurse, you have several roles when assisting a woman who is breast-feeding. These roles include determining breast-feeding readiness, assisting with and observing the breast-feeding technique, monitoring newborn fluid intake, and providing information about special breast-feeding topics.

Determining Breast-Feeding Readiness

Certain situations or conditions require extra planning and nursing support. Observe the woman's breasts for flat or inverted nipples and inquire about any history of breast surgery, her attitudes toward breast-feeding, and attitudes and amount of support for breast-feeding. A **lactation consultant** is a nurse or layperson who has received special training to assist and support the woman who breastfeeds. Be sure to ask one of these specialists to consult with the woman who breastfeeds who has special needs or unusual difficulty nursing her infant.

Although she will need extra support in the beginning until she and the newborn become comfortable with nursing, the woman with flat or inverted nipples can still breastfeed. She may need to use a breast pump for a few minutes before nursing to help pull out and harden the nipples so the newborn can make a good latch. If the infant is unable to latch, notify the RN and the lactation consultant.

The woman who has had breast augmentation or reduction surgery may still be able to breastfeed, depending on the type of surgery. She needs to be emotionally prepared for the possibility that she may not be able to exclusively breastfeed or that she may not be able to breastfeed at all depending on the involvement of the breast surgery. This woman may need the services of a lactation consultant.

Some women are opposed to or repulsed by the thought of the newborn sucking on the breast. The woman with this concern may choose to pump and feed her newborn expressed breast milk from a bottle once she understands the benefits of breast milk for herself and her newborn.

Inquire about the woman's support systems. If the woman has family members or friends who have breast-fed before or are supportive of her decision to breastfeed, the woman is more likely to continue to breastfeed. On the other hand, if the woman's support system is opposed to breast-feeding, she may become discouraged and stop breast-feeding or not even begin because of the negative influences and comments.

Assisting With and Observing the Breast-Feeding Technique

While assisting the woman, provide support and encouragement because many breast-feeding women are unsure of their ability to breastfeed. If the newborn will not nurse after you have provided assistance, contact the registered nurse in charge and take steps to contact the hospital lactation consultant for additional help.

Beginning the Breast-Feeding Session

Ideally, the first breast-feeding should be in the delivery room within an hour after birth unless the newborn's or woman's condition prevents this. Thereafter, the newborn should breastfeed on demand at least every 1½ to 3 hours. If the newborn does not wake up by 3 hours, the woman should wake the newborn and encourage them to feed.

Be Careful!
It is not helpful to give supplemental water or glucose solutions. Supplements give the newborn a feeling of fullness causing them to not nurse as frequently, which may in turn decrease the woman's milk supply.

🤍 A Personal Glimpse

Todd is my second baby. My husband and I hadn't been planning for another child when I found out that I was pregnant. The pregnancy was completely normal with a few more aches and pains than I remembered with my first child, Richard. Right after the delivery, I felt completely exhausted and ravenous. The nurse was insisting that I breastfeed and kept giving me a lot of information. I just couldn't deal with it. It seems like such a blur. I feel guilty that I didn't listen more. They whisked the baby away an hour after he was born. I was kind of relieved because I was so tired. But then when they brought him back to my room the nurse said, "They told me that you breastfed in the delivery room. And since this is your second child, I'm sure you remember how to do it. He should feed for 5 to 10 minutes on each breast." I just looked at her. She handed me the baby and told me to call if I needed anything. Todd was fussy. I kept trying to get him to latch on but couldn't seem to figure out how to do it. I was sitting up in bed and having trouble getting comfortable. My stitches were hurting. But I didn't want to ask the nurse for help because I was afraid she would think I was dumb for not remembering how to get started with breast-feeding. The truth is I was very sick with my first child, so I only breastfed for a couple of weeks, and it seemed so long ago. I finally gave up and called the nursery for a bottle. Todd immediately gulped down an ounce and a half. After that, he didn't seem interested in breast-feeding. Now that he is a year old, I sometimes wish I had tried a little harder to breastfeed. I feel that somehow I missed out on a very special experience.

Rowena

Learning Opportunity: What assumptions did the nurse make that discouraged the mother from asking for help? How could the nurse have approached this situation to give the new mother the help that she needed?

Some women may become discouraged if their newborn is sleepy, will not latch immediately, or is crying vigorously and will not latch. Reassure the woman that the newborn will nurse. Take steps to rouse a sleepy newborn: change the diaper, gently rub the back or head, and wash the newborn's face with a wet washcloth. If the newborn is crying and not exhibiting signs of hunger, check for other causes of crying, such as a wet or dirty diaper or constricting clothing. Try to calm the newborn before attempting to put the newborn to the breast.

In the hospital when you bring the newborn to the woman for feedings, first check the identification bands of both the newborn and the mother and make sure they match. After confirming identity, provide privacy by pulling a curtain around the bed or closing the door. Then, assist the woman into a comfortable position. The woman should sit up in bed or in a chair or lie on her side in bed. Use pillows as needed to support the woman's back and arms. Make sure there is nothing constricting or obstructing the breast, such as a too-tight bra or a cumbersome hospital gown that is in the woman's line of sight or falls between her and the newborn.

 Concept Mastery Alert

The infant should be awake and alert for best breast-feeding. Just positioning the infant near the breast is not sufficient and stroking the infant's cheek can cause confusion for the infant about where to turn their head.

 Cultural Snapshot

Some cultures place a high importance on privacy and modesty. The woman who breastfeeds may not want to expose herself completely to breastfeed or she may not want to breastfeed in your presence, especially if the nurse is a male.

Positioning the Newborn

There are three basic positions for a woman to hold her newborn while nursing. These are the cradle hold, football hold, and side-lying position (Fig. 15-3). Women who have breastfed before may already know these three basic holds. However, a woman who does not have experience breast-feeding or who has just had surgery needs more help with positioning the newborn correctly, even if this is not her first child. Correct positioning and latching on of the newborn will help avoid nipple tissue trauma and sore nipples.

Cradle Hold. In the cradle hold, the newborn's abdomen is facing and touching the woman's abdomen. Make sure the newborn is not lying on their back and turning the head over the shoulder to reach the breast. The newborn should be on their side and "tummy-to-tummy" with the woman. Assist the woman to tuck the newborn's lower arm between her arm and breast. In this position, the woman should use her free hand to support the breast that she is offering to the newborn (Fig. 15-3A).

Football Hold. For the football hold, the woman is in a sitting position, and the newborn lies on their back on a pillow beside her. The woman tilts the newborn slightly to the side and supports the infant's back with her arm. She supports the head with the palm of her hand. This is a good position for the woman who has undergone surgery, the woman with large breasts, or the mother with twins. It also facilitates an unobstructed view between the newborn and woman (Fig. 15-3B).

Side-lying Position. For the side-lying position, both the woman and the newborn lie on their sides facing each other. A blanket roll behind the newborn's back provides support to prevent rolling backward during the feeding. As with the cradle hold, the woman's and the newborn's abdomens should be touching. The newborn should not be flat on their back with the head turned to the side (i.e., having to reach over their shoulder to latch on the breast) during the nursing session (Fig. 15-3C). The side-lying position facilitates maternal rest and is also good for a woman who has undergone surgery.

Latching On

After correctly positioning the newborn, the next step is for the infant to latch onto the breast. The newborn's mouth needs to be wide open with the tongue down at the floor of the mouth, as during a yawn. When the newborn latches onto the breast, they must take the entire nipple and part of the areola into the mouth (Fig. 15-4). If only the nipple is in the mouth, the newborn will not sufficiently compress the milk ducts in order to empty the breast. It will also cause the woman's nipple to become sore and cracked and bleeding.

Have the woman make a "C" shape with her free hand and grasp the breast with four fingers underneath and the thumb on top. Make sure that the woman's hand does not bump into the newborn's jaw or prevent the jaw from making a good latch. The woman may need to reposition her hand so that it is closer to the chest wall and farther from the newborn's jaw.

When the newborn is latched onto the breast, make sure the woman does not dimple the breast near the newborn's mouth and nose. Many women do this because they think they are providing breathing space for the newborn. However, this action can interfere with breast-feeding in several ways. It can cause the nipple to be pulled out of the mouth completely or can cause the nipple to be pulled to the front of the mouth and lead to sore nipples. The pressure from the mother's finger can put pressure on the milk ducts, thereby reducing the flow of milk to the newborn and preventing the breast from emptying completely.

Monitoring the Breast-Feeding Session

Once the newborn is nursing, evaluate the effectiveness of the latch and sucking. A newborn that is correctly latched onto the breast will resist being pulled off the breast. Audible swallowing and rhythmic jaw gliding are positive signs that the newborn is sucking effectively.

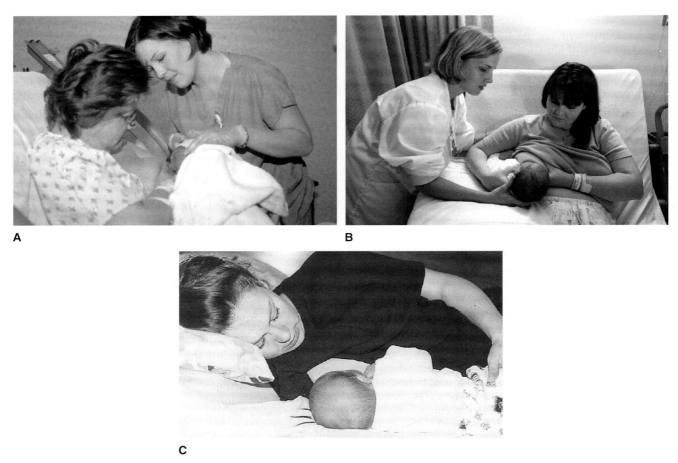

A

B

C

FIGURE 15-3 **A.** The nurse is assisting the woman using the cradle hold to breastfeed her newborn (photo © B. Proud). **B.** The nurse is assisting the woman using the football hold to breastfeed her newborn. **C.** In the side-lying position, the woman can rest while feeding her newborn.

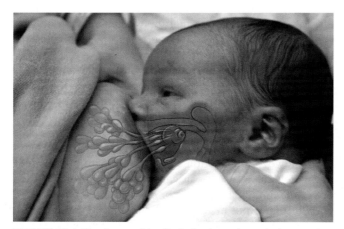

FIGURE 15-4 Newborn with all of nipple and areola in mouth, correctly compressing milk ducts.

After the newborn has been nursing for a few minutes, many women report an increase in the flow of lochia or uterine cramping. This is a good indication that the newborn is nursing well because effective sucking causes the release of oxytocin from the posterior pituitary, which in turn causes uterine contractions. After her milk has come in, the woman may report leaking from the opposite breast or a letdown reflex. This is another good indication that the newborn is latched on and sucking well at the breast.

Ending the Breast-Feeding Session

The nursing session should last approximately 10 to 20 minutes per breast. When the newborn stops sucking vigorously and moves to nonnutritive sucking, the woman should remove the newborn from the breast by placing her finger in the mouth, between the gums and cheek, to break the suction, and then gently pull the newborn away from the breast. The woman should leave the flaps of her nursing bra open to allow her nipples to air dry.

After the feeding session, the woman may wish to burp her newborn. A breastfed infant may not always burp after eating because they swallow less air at the breast than when drinking from a bottle. There are three ways for the woman to hold the

This Tip May Help Prevent Sore Nipples

Tell the woman that it is important for her to break the suction before pulling the newborn from the breast. If she does not, tissue damage can occur, resulting in sore, cracked nipples.

newborn while burping: by placing them over her shoulder, sitting them upright, or laying the newborn across her lap with the head elevated slightly above the level of the stomach.

Monitoring Newborn Fluid Intake

There are several ways to monitor the newborn's fluid intake. A small bit of milk left in the mouth after the feeding is a good indication the newborn is sucking well. The newborn should be satiated between feedings and after nursing appear to be drowsy or asleep. By the end of the third day of life, the newborn should have at least six wet diapers and about three bowel movements per day. Newborns that are breast-fed exclusively will have a yellow or mustard-colored seedy type of bowel movement that is very loose and not formed. Explain to the woman that this is normal for the breastfed newborn and is not diarrhea. Many breastfed newborns will have a bowel movement during the nursing session.

Monitor the newborn's weight daily during the hospital stay. The breast-feeding newborn should lose no more than 10% of his birth weight and should return to birth weight by 7 to 14 days of age. Evaluate the newborn's weight and feeding status, and notify the registered nurse and the health care provider if problems exist.

Remember **Frances Barnes.** She was concerned that her son wouldn't get enough to eat. How would you respond to her concern? What data would you want to collect that would indicate that he is getting enough to eat during breast-feeding? How is this information different in the first few days after birth as compared to after her milk comes in?

Relieving Common Maternal Breast-Feeding Problems

The woman who breastfeeds needs information regarding problems she may encounter at home. Some of the most commonly reported problems include sore nipples, engorgement, a plugged milk duct, or mastitis. For some women, these common problems may become frustrating and cause her to stop breast-feeding sooner than expected.

Sore Nipples

Some nipple sensitivity is normal during the first few days of breast-feeding. It is normal for the nipples to feel sensitive during the first minute after the newborn begins sucking. Incorrect latch is the most common cause of tissue trauma leading to sore nipples. If the woman reports sore nipples or cracked and bleeding nipples, observe how the newborn latches on. The newborn's mouth must open wide, and they must take all of the nipple and part of the areola into the mouth. Other reasons for sore nipples are that the newborn may be a vigorous breastfeeder or the woman may have sensitive or tender skin.

Some women find rubbing a few drops of expressed breast milk onto their nipples after the nursing session

helpful. A purified lanolin ointment may help some women. Contact the lactation consultant if the woman continues to have sore nipples despite correct positioning and latch.

Engorgement

Engorgement refers to swelling in the breast that first occurs when the breast starts producing milk. The breasts may become hard and warm to the touch and can be quite painful. Frequent breast-feeding is the best way to prevent and treat engorgement, as long as the newborn is emptying the breast with each feeding. First, check to see that the newborn is able to obtain a good latch. A poor latch does not allow for complete emptying of the breast and can exacerbate engorgement. If the breast is so firm that the nipple is flat and unable to become erect, the infant will be unable to make a good latch. The woman may need to express a small amount of milk to soften the nipple before putting the newborn to the breast. Treatments to alleviate discomfort include cold packs to the breast and taking a mild analgesic such as ibuprofen or acetaminophen. It may help the woman to stand in a warm shower several times per day and let the water flow over her breasts. This may stimulate milk release and relieve some of the pressure. Reassure the woman that engorgement is temporary and will go away within a few days. Tell the woman not to empty her breasts by pumping between feedings, as this will increase her milk supply beyond the newborn's needs.

> **This is Helpful Advice**
>
> Milk may leak from the breasts during engorgement. If the woman uses bra pads to help absorb the leaking milk, advise her to change the pads as they become damp to avoid maceration or possible infection of the nipple and areola.

Plugged Milk Ducts

A plugged milk duct is a common problem. This happens when one of the milk ducts becomes obstructed, causing a backup of the milk. The woman usually notices a sore, reddened, hard lump in one area of her breast. The woman should continue nursing. Sometimes it helps to position the infant with the chin close to the lump to facilitate drainage. She should avoid constricting clothing or bras, including underwire bras. Instruct the woman to place a warm wet washcloth to the area and then massaging it before nursing. It is helpful to change positions the infant nurses in instead of always holding the infant in the same position. Some women find relief by laying the infant on its back and letting the breast hang down toward the infant. This position uses gravity to help drain the breast and can aid in unplugging the duct. Interventions to treat discomfort are the same as those to treat the discomfort of engorgement. If the site does not improve within a few days, develops red streaks, the reddened area enlarges or becomes wedge shaped (like a triangle), or she develops a fever, then she should contact her health care provider.

Mastitis

Another common problem associated with breast-feeding is **mastitis,** an infection of the breast tissue. Women with mastitis usually describe having a run-down feeling or flu-like symptoms with a low-grade fever. Tell the woman not to ignore these signs and symptoms but to report them immediately to her health care provider. Treatment consists of antibiotics, analgesics, bed rest, and fluids. The woman needs to know that she can continue to breastfeed during this time. Mastitis will not affect her milk quality, and the antibiotics prescribed usually do not affect the newborn or infant. If the health care provider prescribes medication that is contraindicated for breast-feeding and there is no alternative medication, the woman can pump her breasts and dump the expressed breast milk until she is able to resume breast-feeding when the medication course is complete.

Informing the Woman About Breast-Feeding Special Concerns

Nurses play a crucial role in informing the woman who breastfeeds. Items to be covered include signs that the newborn is not feeding well; normal increases in the newborn's feeding schedule to accommodate for growth spurts; available resources for the woman who breast-feeds; using supplements; breast-feeding amenorrhea; contraception while breast-feeding; and pumping and storing breast milk.

Signs the Newborn Is Not Feeding Well

The woman also needs to know how to evaluate how well her newborn is nursing and when to call for help. Dry mouth, not enough wet diapers per day, difficulty rousing the newborn for a feeding, not enough feedings per day, and difficulty with latching on or sucking are signs that the newborn is not receiving enough breast milk. Explain to the woman that if she notices any of these signs, she should immediately contact the newborn's health care provider and a lactation consultant. Newborns can become dehydrated and suffer from a lack of nutrition very quickly and may need hospitalization.

Growth Spurts

Another important information topic for the woman who breastfeeds is about how the newborn increases the milk supply. Newborns have growth spurts in which they will nurse longer and more frequently for a few days and then space out their feedings after those few days. This causes the woman's breasts to increase their milk volume to match the growing newborn's needs. A woman who does not understand that the newborn increases the frequency and duration of feedings over a period of days to increase the milk supply may misinterpret the situation and think that she does not have enough milk to feed her newborn. This may cause the woman to stop breast-feeding unnecessarily.

Available Resources for the Woman Who Breastfeeds

The woman who breastfeeds needs to be aware of the many resources available to assist her and her newborn with breast-feeding. Lactation consultants, the La Leche League, and breast-feeding support groups in the community can give both practical and emotional support to the woman who breastfeeds.

Lactation consultants work in the hospital, in the community, and sometimes in the health care provider's office. In the hospital, lactation consultants can help the woman with positioning and getting the newborn latched on and sucking. After discharge, the hospital may provide follow-up visits or telephone calls to the woman to help ensure that the newborn is breast-feeding as expected. The newborn's health care provider may have an agreement with a lactation consultant who can provide assistance to the woman who breastfeeds.

The La Leche League is a national organization that provides support, education, and literature to the woman who breastfeeds. The woman can find the group listed online or the hospital may provide the woman with the telephone number of the local chapter. In addition, the hospital may have a list of breast-feeding support groups the woman can join. These groups can provide both breast-feeding support and socialization.

Using Supplements

Many women have questions about supplements for their nursing newborn. The newborn who is breastfed does not need supplemental bottles of water. Exclusive breast-feeding provides the newborn with all fluid needs. In the hospital, newborns are not started on any vitamin or iron supplements. The follow-up health care provider will instruct the woman on when and what types of supplements the newborn may need. By the time the infant is 4 months of age, breast milk typically does not provide adequate amounts of iron. For this reason, until the infant is consuming solids that can meet the infant's iron needs, most providers will recommend the infant receive a daily dose of supplemental oral liquid iron.

The woman needs to know that her breast milk is nutritionally superior to any other newborn food and that she should not introduce any solids, including rice cereal, until the infant is at least 6 months of age. If there is a family history of allergies, solids should be delayed even longer.

Breast-Feeding Amenorrhea

An important topic for the lactating woman is breast-feeding amenorrhea. The return of the woman's menstrual cycle occurs between 6 and 10 weeks after delivery. Approximately 75% of women do not ovulate during the first postpartum menstrual cycle. The woman who is breast-feeding exclusively (i.e., without providing any supplemental bottles or solids) may experience breast-feeding amenorrhea. Some women who exclusively breastfeed may not have a return of their menstrual cycle for several months. The woman needs to know that ovulation can happen in the absence of a menstrual period, and she can become pregnant. It is important for her to use contraception during this time.

TABLE 15-1 Contraceptive Choices for Women Who Breastfeed

NONHORMONAL		HORMONAL
PERMANENT	TEMPORARY	NONESTROGEN
Tubal ligation Vasectomy	Abstinence Condom Diaphragm Spermicide	Progestin only

Contraception While Breast-Feeding

Women who breastfeed need information about their choices in contraception. Contraception that contains hormones, especially estrogen, can lead to a decrease in the milk supply in women who breastfeed. The woman should be informed of this and make alternative contraceptive choices if breast-feeding is to continue. The first choice of contraception for women who breastfeed should be nonhormonal. If she chooses a hormonal type of contraception, a progestin-only pill is preferred over one that contains estrogen. Table 15-1 summarizes different contraceptive choices for women who breastfeed.

Pumping and Storing Breast Milk

The woman should wash her hands before pumping her breasts and use clean equipment. Before beginning pumping, it may be necessary for the woman to use techniques to aid the letdown reflex, which include bilateral breast massage and applying warm packs. The woman may also find that looking at a picture of her infant and mentally thinking about her infant's smell, texture, and sounds helps induce a letdown reflex. At home, the woman may want to pump one breast while having the infant nurse on the opposite breast. The breast-feeding will stimulate the letdown reflex and allow her to collect more breast milk.

It is recommended that the woman use a hospital-grade, dual-sided electric breast pump (i.e., pumps both breasts at the same time) (Fig. 15-5). Pumping of both breasts at the same time increases the quantity of milk expressed at one sitting. The woman should be encouraged to pump until the flow of milk has stopped, usually about 15 to 20 minutes. She should avoid a "bicycle horn" style of hand breast pump. This type of hand pump creates suction when the bulb is squeezed, but the suction cannot be controlled and can cause trauma to the breast tissue.

When she is finished pumping, the expressed breast milk can be refrigerated, frozen, or fed to her infant. She also needs to clean the equipment right after pumping. Tap water and a small amount of dish soap are usually sufficient to clean the equipment.

After pumping, she may want to rub a small amount of breast milk onto her nipples and allow them to air dry before covering them with a bra. If the woman experiences soreness with the breast pump, check to make sure she is using it properly and starting the pumping session at the lowest suction necessary.

Breast milk should be stored in hard plastic bottles or breast milk bags, not in glass containers or plastic bottle liners. The leukocytes in breast milk adhere to the glass, and this decreases the bacteriostatic properties of the milk. The proper way to reheat breast milk is to place the bottle/bag into a pan of hot water. Heating in the microwave kills the antibodies in breast milk. In addition, milk reheated in the microwave may have hot spots that could burn the newborn's mouth and esophagus. Breast milk that has been frozen and thawed should never be refrozen. Table 15-2 provides guidelines for breast milk storage.

Returning to Work or School

The woman who returns to work or school after giving birth does not need to give up breast-feeding. The woman should breastfeed exclusively for at least 6 weeks before introducing the bottle. After 6 weeks, if she has established a good milk supply and the newborn is nursing well, she should introduce one feeding per day of expressed breast milk. She should pump her breasts during this bottle-feeding so she will not reduce her milk supply. Mothers who continue to breastfeed during this time express satisfaction with continuing to breastfeed and often state it helps them during the time away from the infant to pump and be able to continue to provide milk for them.

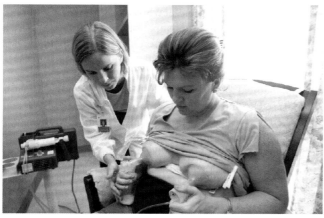

FIGURE 15-5 The nurse is assisting the woman to use a hospital pump to pump milk from both breasts at the same time.

TABLE 15-2 Freshly Expressed Breast Milk Storage

LOCATION OF STORAGE	DURATION OF STORAGE
Room temperature 77°F (25°C)	4 hours
Refrigerator 40°F (4°C)	Up to 4 days
Freezer 0°F (−18°C)	6 mo
Thawed after being frozen	24 hours

Adapted from Centers for Disease Control and Prevention. (2021). *Proper storage and preparation of breast milk.* https://www.cdc.gov/breastfeeding/recommendations/handling_breastmilk.htm

FORMULA-FEEDING

Artificial Nutrition, that is, infant formula or another type of animal milk, has been given to infants since ancient times. In the United States, commercially prepared infant formula has been available since the early 1900s. Today there are several brands available to women who choose not to breastfeed or who need a supplemental formula. There are also alternative formulas to meet specific infant nutritional needs.

It's Not the Same!

Infants younger than 12 months should not be given cow's milk. Cow's milk has higher concentrations of proteins and minerals and less iron than human breast milk or commercial infant formula. The infant's kidneys cannot adequately tolerate the extra proteins and minerals and the low iron can lead to anemia if given to the infant.

Advantages and Disadvantages of Formula-Feeding

Infant formulas are helpful in certain circumstances. Many women choose to forgo breast-feeding and feed their infant only formula. No one should attempt to make the woman who chooses to do so feel guilty regarding her decision. However, make sure that the woman has made an informed decision and has heard the advantages of breast-feeding before feeding her infant formula.

Advantages

There are specific circumstances in which formula-feeding is necessary. These include adoption or cases in which breast-feeding would be harmful to the infant, as discussed earlier in the chapter. In some cases, the woman may need to temporarily stop breast-feeding, such as for surgery or while taking a medication that can pass to the infant through the breast milk. Sometimes the woman's breast milk supply dries up sooner than expected or she does not produce enough milk to meet her infant's needs.

For some women, being able to quantify how much the infant has consumed with formula-feeding reduces their worries about the infant getting enough to eat. Some women feel it is easier to formula-feed than to breastfeed the infant. Formula-feeding also allows others to be involved in the infant's care by feeding the infant and preparing the formula and bottles for feeding.

Disadvantages

Formula-feeding has several disadvantages. It is inferior nutrition and has none of the immunologic properties provided by breast milk. Formula is harder for the newborn to digest than breast milk. There is a higher correlation between infants who are formula-fed and some illnesses, such as otitis media and allergies.

Infant formula is expensive. If the family is on a limited budget, formula-feeding creates additional financial needs. In addition to buying the formula, the family will need to purchase bottles, nipples, and the equipment needed to clean these items.

Make Sure the Woman Is Informed!

If the woman is on the Women, Infants, and Children program, the woman will need to purchase some formula because the program is only supplemental.

There are more steps involved in formula-feeding the newborn than in breast-feeding. With formula-feeding, the woman or caregiver must mix the right amount of powder or formula concentrate to water, store the mixed preparation, warm it when the newborn is ready to eat, and then wash all of the utensils afterward. Formula is available for purchase in three forms: ready to feed, concentrate, and powder. Because of the differences in formulation, there can be errors with the proper dilution of the formula. Errors in preparation can lead to under- or overnutrition of the newborn. These errors can result in serious illness and even death.

Composition of Formula

There are three main types of formula: milk-based, soy-based, and hypoallergenic formulas. Most term newborn formulas are derived from cow's milk, and the main carbohydrate source is lactose or corn syrup solids. The protein used is a whey–casein blend to simulate that found in breast milk. The iron composition in infant formula is either high or low. Iron-fortified formulas contain 1.2 mg of iron per 100 mL. Iron-fortified or high-iron formula is the preferred formula to give to the healthy term newborn. Some women are reluctant to feed their newborn iron-fortified formula, thinking it will cause constipation. Studies have shown that there is no significant difference in constipation rates between infants fed iron-fortified and low-iron formulas.

Alternative formulas are available for newborns with special medical needs. Soy-based infant formulas are for newborns who have galactosemia or whose parents do not want the child to have a formula made from an animal protein. Hypoallergenic formulas are for newborns with allergy or malabsorption problems. The proteins are partially or completely broken down in these formulas. There are also a variety of formulas specially designed for specific medical conditions, including carbohydrate or lactose intolerance, impaired fat absorption, cystic fibrosis, congestive heart failure, and intestinal resection or short gut problems. The newborn should not receive these formulas unless specifically

TABLE 15-3 Comparison of Common Infant Formulas

CATEGORY	FORMULA NAME (MANUFACTURER'S NAME)	FORMULA DESIGNED FOR WHICH NEWBORN POPULATION/MEDICAL CONDITION
Milk-based term formulas	Enfamil (Mead Johnson) Gerber Good Start (Nestle) Similac (Abbott)	For full-term healthy newborns
Soy-based formulas	Isomil (Abbott) ProSobee (Mead Johnson)	Newborns whose parents desire to feed a nonanimal protein formula or newborns with galactosemia
Lactose issue	Lactofree (Mead Johnson) Lactose Sensitivity (Abbott)	Lactase deficiency, galactosemia
Specific medical conditions	Alimentum (Abbott) Nutramigen (Mead Johnson) Pregestimil (Mead Johnson)	Milk protein allergy Fat absorption difficulty
	Enfamil AR (Mead Johnson) Similac Lactose Sensitivity (Abbott)	Gastroesophageal reflux/spit-up
	Phenyl-free (Mead Johnson) Phenex-1 (Abbott)	Phenylketonuria
	Enfamil Premature 24/Enfacare (Mead Johnson) Similac/Neosure (Abbott)	Premature infants

Note: This is not an exhaustive list of all of the manufacturers, types of formulas, or conditions for which formulas may be used.

ordered by the infant's health care provider. Some providers treat esophageal reflux with a formula thickened with some rice cereal or a specialized formula that already has rice cereal added to it.

There are many different compositions of formulas in the hospital. Formulas vary based on the needs of the newborn. Preterm formulas differ from term formulas in the amounts of vitamins and minerals and caloric and iron content. Preterm formulas have higher levels of sodium, potassium, calcium, and iron than do term infant formulas. Term formula, like breast milk, has 20 cal/oz, whereas preterm formulas have 22 or 24 cal/oz. See Table 15-3 for a comparison of different brands of formulas.

Nursing Care of the Woman Who Formula-Feed

As the nurse, you have three major roles when assisting the woman who bottle-feed in the hospital. These are assisting with formula-feeding technique, observing the woman who formula-feed and newborn, and informing her about special concerns related to formula-feeding.

Assisting With Formula-Feeding Technique

In the hospital, standard infant formula comes ready to feed. This means that you do not need to mix or add any additives to the formula before feeding the newborn. The first step in feeding the formula-fed newborn is to check the health care provider's order. Many providers have a preference regarding which formula the woman should feed her newborn. Check the label on the formula bottle before taking it to the woman to feed her newborn. Make sure the brand, caloric content, and iron composition match those of the health care provider's order.

Compare the newborn's and woman's identification bands to ensure a match. Use pillows as needed to ensure the woman is in a comfortable position and can hold and see her newborn easily. Make sure the woman is in a comfortable position sitting upright. The woman who formula-feed should not feed her newborn in a lying down position. The newborn should be in a semireclined position in the woman's or other caregiver's arms. An angle of at least 45 degrees is preferred (Fig. 15-6).

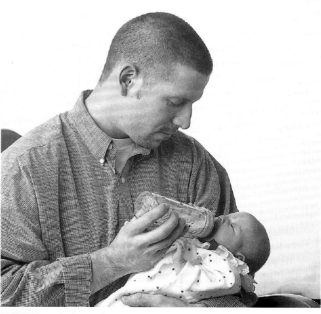

FIGURE 15-6 A newborn receives a formula-feeding from her father. Notice the correct positioning.

Show the woman how to observe her newborn for hunger cues and inform her about the newborn's ability to suck, swallow, and breathe during the feeding. The woman should also observe her newborn's color while eating. Instruct the woman on what to do if the newborn starts to choke during the feeding. Make sure the nasal aspirator and a burp cloth are within the woman's reach.

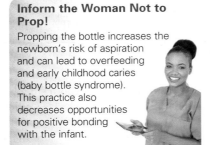

This Tip Could Save a Life!

It is easier for the newborn to aspirate while sucking from a bottle. Instruct the woman to keep the light on in the room so that she can observe her newborn during the whole feeding.

Gently shake the bottle of formula because some settling of contents may occur. Attach a sterile nipple and ring unit to the bottle. The woman should feed 1 to 2 oz per feeding in the immediate newborn period. She should burp her newborn after every 0.5 oz. As the newborn grows, she should advance the feeding amount slowly, no more than 0.5 to 1 oz at a time. Instruct the woman regarding cues that the newborn is satiated and finished eating. If the newborn consumes too much formula at one time, emesis or diarrhea may result.

Inform the Woman Not to Prop!

Propping the bottle increases the newborn's risk of aspiration and can lead to overfeeding and early childhood caries (baby bottle syndrome). This practice also decreases opportunities for positive bonding with the infant.

You may assist the woman who bottle-feed by feeding the newborn if the woman is unable to (e.g., she is having surgery) or if she is sleeping and requests her newborn to be fed in the nursery during the night.

Monitoring the woman who formula-feed and Newborn

Observe the newborn's feeding ability, amount of formula consumed at each feeding, tolerance of the infant formula, and the woman's comfort level with formula-feeding. Also, monitor the newborn's bowel movements. Explain to the woman that her newborn's stool should progress from meconium to transitional and then to a pasty yellow solid consistency (Chapter 14).

Report signs of difficulty to the RN immediately. These signs include that the newborn is not sucking well, has difficulty swallowing and breathing, or is not tolerating the formula. Emesis and diarrhea may indicate that the newborn is not tolerating the formula.

Informing About Formula-Feeding Special Concerns

Topics to discuss with the woman who formula-feed include how to prepare bottles of formula, adding supplements to the bottle, maternal breast care, and managing common problems in the formula-fed newborn. Formula-fed infants do not require additional bottles of water as the formula provides all the infant's fluid requirements.

Preparing Bottles of Formula

Inform the woman about the different forms of formula and how to mix each type. Powder formula is the least expensive and requires the addition of water. Concentrate also requires the addition of water but is more costly than the powder form. Ready-to-feed formula is the most expensive but does not require the addition of any water to the formula before feeding.

Warn the woman that the newborn could be injured if formula is not mixed according to the package directions. Some women may be unable to afford formula and try to make the formula last longer by adding more water than the directions specify. This will cause malnutrition in the newborn. If too much powder is added to the water, the newborn will receive more calories per ounce. This can lead to an overweight infant or formula intolerance with resulting diarrhea or emesis.

The woman will need to know what type of water to add to the powder or concentrate type of formula. This depends on what type of water she has available (e.g., city tap, well, or purified bottled water). She should mix only as much formula as the newborn needs in 24 hours. After mixing, the formula needs to be refrigerated. After 24 hours, she should discard unused formula.

Show the woman how to warm cold formula. She should place the bottle containing the formula in a pan of hot water until the formula is warm, then she should shake the bottle before feeding the newborn. Warn the woman never to use the microwave to warm the formula because it can create hot spots that could burn the newborn. When the newborn has finished eating, tell the woman to discard any remaining formula. This is because as the newborn sucks saliva mixes with the formula and remains in the bottle and then digestive enzymes in the saliva begin to break down the remaining formula. The woman should wash the feeding utensils in hot soapy water or in the dishwasher after every feeding. Sterilizing the bottles and nipples is not necessary after each feeding.

Adding Supplements

The newborn's health care provider will determine if and when the newborn needs any type of supplementation, such as multivitamins. Formula-fed infants who receive an iron-fortified formula do not need iron supplementation. Inform the woman that the newborn does not need any other type of nutrition (e.g., cows' milk or juices). Instruct her not to add anything to the formula. Some providers tell parents to offer infant cereal mixed with formula, but not juice, at around 4 to 6 months. The woman should not begin to feed solid foods until the infant's health care provider has recommended it, usually around 6 to 8 months of age. Around 12 months of age, the infant's provider will discuss with the parents about weaning the infant from the formula.

Maternal Breast Care

Women who choose to formula-feed exclusively need to know how to care for their breasts in the immediate postpartum period. Explain to the woman that she will produce milk, even though she is not nursing, and that this is a normal physiologic process in response to giving birth. The woman will experience engorgement when her milk comes in. She should not express any milk because this will stimulate milk production. She should wear a tight bra; the constriction will help prevent leaking and aid in the drying up of the milk supply. In addition, a tight bra will help lessen discomfort from the full breasts. Some women benefit from having their breasts bound tightly with an elastic-type bandage. In the past, some health care providers prescribed medication that would aid in the drying up of the woman's milk supply. However, it was determined that the benefits of their use did not outweigh the associated risks and are no longer prescribed.

Contradict a Common Myth

Some women add rice cereal to the formula because they have heard that doing so will make the newborn sleep longer. This should only be done if it is prescribed by a health care provider for a specific medical reason, such as reflux.

Common Problems in the Formula-Fed Newborn

The woman needs to monitor for problems in the formula-fed newborn. These include the newborn not wanting to eat, not tolerating the formula, and dental caries.

The woman who is formula-feeding is able to accurately determine how many ounces per feeding and per day the newborn is receiving. Table 15-4 lists the amount of formula and other foods the newborn and infant should be receiving at different ages. If the newborn or infant is not taking in enough formula for his age and weight, dehydration may result, and the infant may not gain sufficient weight to develop appropriately and be healthy. If a newborn or infant is refusing to eat, the woman should contact the health care provider because there may be an underlying medical condition.

Some newborns take in the recommended amount of formula and then have large amounts of emesis after or during feedings. The woman should report this situation to the newborn's health care provider because this is not an acceptable situation for growth and nutrition. This may be a symptom of overfeeding, gastroesophageal reflux, formula intolerance, or an underlying medical condition. Ask the woman the following questions: How much formula is the newborn taking per feeding and per day? When does emesis occur (during or after the feeding, with burps, or with repositioning)? How much emesis does the newborn have per episode? What is the consistency of the emesis? Which formula is the infant eating, and how is it prepared? What other foods are included in the infant's diet? The answers to these questions will assist the registered nurse and the health care provider with determining the probable cause of the emesis.

Diarrhea also requires investigation. Again, ask specific questions: How much and what type of formula is the newborn eating, and how is it prepared? How many episodes of diarrhea has the newborn had in the past 24 hours? What is the consistency of the bowel movement, and is there blood present in the stool? It is important to monitor and document the newborn's intake and output to check for dehydration and to perform a physical examination. Possible causes are overfeeding, illness, formula intolerance, or an underlying medical condition.

Inform the parents that newborns and infants can dehydrate much more quickly than adults can. For this reason, the parents must quickly report any cases of emesis or diarrhea.

Infants can develop dental caries from frequent sucking on a milk- or juice-filled bottle. This situation is known as "early childhood caries" (baby bottle syndrome). Often this happens when parents give the infant a bottle at bedtime and the infant sucks on the bottle throughout the night. The frequent exposure of the immature teeth to high levels of sugars found in the milk or juice leads to dental caries. The parents should not give the infant a bottle in the crib. They also should not allow the toddler to carry a bottle around; this practice of continual drinking of formula increases the risk of damage to the infant's teeth and is associated with a higher incidence of aspiration and otitis media.

TABLE 15-4 Amount of Formula and Other Foods the Newborn and Infant Should Receive

AGE	AMOUNT OF FORMULA	OTHER FOODS
Birth to 4 months	2–6 oz/feeding 18–32 oz/day	None
4–6 months	4–6 oz/feeding 27–45 oz/day	Infant cereal mixed with breastmilk or formula can start being added if advised by the health care provider
6–8 months	6–8 oz/feeding 24–32 oz/day	Baby cereal, soft mashed fruits and vegetables, no more than 3–4 oz of fruit juice
8–10 months	7–8 oz/feeding 21–32 oz/day	Same as 6–8 mo and may begin to add pureed meats
10–12 months	16–32 oz/day	Same as 8–10 mo but consistency may be firmer and portions may be slightly bigger

Note: The American Academy of Pediatrics (AAP) and the World Health Organization (WHO) recommend exclusive breast-feeding until 6 months of age and continuation of breast-feeding until at least 12 months of age.

Remember **Frances Barnes** from the start of the chapter. She wanted to breastfeed her newborn John. From your readings, how would you respond to her concern about painful breast-feeding? What information will you give to Frances as compared to a mother who wanted to formula-feed? Her husband had expressed a desire to feed their son. What information would you give to these new parents to address their concerns and desires?

KEY POINTS

- Several factors influence the woman's decision to breastfeed. These include culture, age, education, past experience with breast-feeding, and the woman's intent to return to work or school.

- Maternal advantages of breast-feeding include more rapid uterine involution, less bleeding in the postpartum period, and less ovarian and premenopausal breast cancers. Newborn advantages to breast-feeding include a strengthened immune system, less risk of becoming overweight, and lower incidences of certain infections such as otitis media, diarrhea, and lower respiratory tract infections.

- Maternal contraindications to breast-feeding include a woman actively using illegal drugs, one who has untreated tuberculosis, one with human immunodeficiency virus, or a woman receiving chemotherapy medications. A newborn condition that would contraindicate breast-feeding includes galactosemia.

- The breast is under both physical and hormonal control to stimulate lactation. The hormones prolactin and oxytocin stimulate milk production and release from the breast. The newborn sucking on and emptying the breast also leads to milk production.

- When assisting a woman with breast-feeding, provide for privacy, help the woman into a comfortable position, help the woman hold her newborn correctly, and monitor the newborn for correct latching on and positioning on the breast. Observe the woman's breasts and nipples, her comfort level with breast-feeding, her support system, and the newborn's feeding ability.

- Give women who breastfeed information about common problems including signs the newborn is not feeding well, growth spurts, available resources, supplements, contraception, and pumping and storing breast milk.

- When caring for a woman with sore nipples, observe the latching on and the positioning of the newborn during nursing. A few drops of expressed breast milk or a purified lanolin treatment applied to the nipples after breast-feeding may help with soreness.

- When caring for a woman with engorgement, observe the infant for a good latch and advise the woman to breastfeed frequently. Cold packs to the breast and taking a mild analgesic help alleviate discomfort. Letting warm water flow over her breasts several times per day may stimulate milk release and relieve some of the pressure.

- When caring for a woman with a plugged milk duct, advise her to apply warm packs to the site, take a warm shower, take acetaminophen, nurse in different positions, avoid constrictive clothing or bras, and massage the site.

- When caring for a woman with mastitis, advise a woman who breastfeeds to contact her health care provider, take the antibiotics as prescribed, and continue to breastfeed even on the affected side. If breast-feeding is too uncomfortable on the affected side, she should pump the milk at each feeding so her milk supply does not diminish.

- Signs that a newborn is not breast-feeding well include dry mouth, fewer than expected wet or dirty diapers, difficulty rousing the newborn for feedings, increased weight loss, and not enough feedings per day.

- Breast milk is superior to formula because it is easier to digest and has immunologic and bacteriocidal properties that cannot be duplicated in artificial nutrition. Breast milk is economical and ready to feed and requires no special preparation or storage.

- Formula-feeding is beneficial in cases in which the woman is unavailable to breastfeed, such as adoption, surgery, or if she is taking a medication that passes through the breast milk and would be harmful to the newborn. Formula-feeding is also beneficial when the newborn has certain medical conditions, such as galactosemia.

- There are many types of formulas available. The ingredients vary by protein source, caloric content, and mineral and electrolyte concentration. The health care provider considers the newborn's gestational age and medical needs before recommending a specific formula.

- Show the woman who formula-feed how to feed her newborn and how much and when to increase feedings, how to prepare and store the formula and care for the equipment, how to care for her breasts after delivery, and when to notify the RN and health care provider.

- For the formula-fed newborn who is having emesis or diarrhea, ask the parent: What type of formula is the newborn on and how is it prepared? How much is the newborn eating per session and per day? What does the emesis/bowel movement look like? What other foods is the newborn eating? How much emesis is there per episode? How many episodes has the newborn had in the last 24 hours?

INTERNET RESOURCES

Baby Friendly Hospital Initiative
http://www.babyfriendlyusa.org/

International Lactation Consultant Association
http://ilca.org/

La Leche League International
www.llli.org

Government Sources
www.cdc.gov/breastfeeding

Women, Infants, and Children
www.fns.usda.gov/wic

Formula Information
http://www.nlm.nih.gov/medlineplus/ency/article/002447.htm

World Health Organization
http://www.who.int/maternal_child_adolescent/topics/child/nutrition/
   breastfeeding/en/

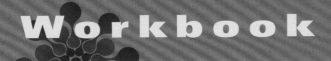

NCLEX-STYLE REVIEW QUESTIONS

1. A woman tells the nurse, "I don't need to use any contraception because I plan on breast-feeding exclusively." On which fact should the nurse base her response?
   a. Women who exclusively breastfeed do not ovulate.
   b. Ovulation can occur even in the absence of menstruation.
   c. The birth control pill is the best form of contraception for breast-feeding women.
   d. Breast-feeding women should not use contraception because it will decrease their milk supply.

2. During a prenatal visit, an 18-year-old gravida 1 para 0 in her 36th week says to the nurse, "I don't know if I should breastfeed or not. Isn't formula just as good for the baby?" On what information should the nurse base her response?
   a. The benefits of breast-feeding are equal to those of formula-feeding.
   b. It is ultimately the woman's choice whether she wants to breastfeed or not.
   c. The immunologic properties in breast milk cannot be duplicated in formula.
   d. The economic status of the woman is an important breast-feeding consideration.

3. The nurse is assisting a woman who breastfeeds during a feeding session. Which data collection has priority during the feeding session?
   a. Observe the position, latching on, and sucking of the newborn.
   b. Observe the woman's visitors and their opinions regarding breast-feeding.
   c. Check the woman's perineal pad for increased lochia flow.
   d. Determine if the woman needs a visit from the lactation consultant.

4. Which statements are true regarding breast-feeding? (Select all that apply.)
   a. Breastfed infants are ill less frequently than formula-fed infants.
   b. Previous breast-feeding experiences do not affect how the mother will breastfeed this infant.
   c. The woman with mastitis is unable to breastfeed.
   d. Medications the woman takes can pass to the infant via the breast milk.
   e. The woman cannot breastfeed until her milk comes in.
   f. The woman will not ovulate while breast-feeding.

STUDY ACTIVITIES

1. Use the following table to compare information contained in your nursing pharmacology reference with information the hospital lactation specialist has on medications and their use during breast-feeding. If the two references disagree, from where did the lactation specialist get her information? Which information do you think is more accurate? Why?

Medication	Pharmacology Reference	Lactation Specialist
Magnesium sulfate		
Phenobarbital		
Depo-Provera		
Vicodin		
Coumadin		

2. Call your local Women, Infants, and Children (WIC) clinic. Interview the nurse to determine what she does to encourage the woman to breastfeed the newborn.

3. Interview the lactation consultant at the local hospital. What foods does she tell the woman to avoid when she is breast-feeding, and why? How many calories should the woman consume? How much liquid should she drink? Share your findings with your clinical group.

4. Do an online search of home remedies to treat sore nipples and engorgement. What would you recommend to a mother who wanted to use these remedies?

CRITICAL THINKING: WHAT WOULD YOU DO?

Apply your knowledge of newborn nutrition to the following situations.

1. You are working in the prenatal clinic. Here is a list of several of the clients you encounter and the questions they ask you.

   a. Sally is a 20-year-old gravida 1 para 0. She tells you she is unsure about feeding her newborn and asks you if she should breastfeed or bottle-feed. How would you respond?

   b. Betsy, a gravida 3 para 1, states she needs to return to work 6 weeks after the baby is born. "I don't know if it's even worth it to begin to breastfeed when I know I'll just have to stop in 6 weeks. It seems like a lot of work." How would you respond?

   c. Elizabeth is a 15-year-old gravida 1 para 0. She asks you, "I don't want to breastfeed, but I heard you still make milk after the baby is born. How do you stop it from happening?" How would you respond to Elizabeth's question?

2. You are working in the mother–baby unit at the hospital. Here are some of your clients for the day and the questions they ask you.

   a. Susan is a 24-year-old gravida 3 para 1. She delivered a day ago and wants to breastfeed. When you examine her newborn, she tells you that she thinks she does not have enough milk to feed her baby and asks you to give her baby a bottle so he does not starve. How would you respond?

   b. It has been 3 days since Alicia's cesarean delivery, and she is formula-feeding her newborn a milk-based formula. She tells you her baby spits up with every feeding. What questions would you ask her and why?

   c. Lanya is a 30-year-old gravida 2 para 2 who had a postpartum tubal ligation earlier today. It is time to breastfeed her baby, but her abdomen is sore. How would you suggest Lanya feed her newborn and why?

   d. Tricia is a 28-year-old gravida 1 para 1 who is formula-feeding. She asks you how to mix formula and how she should care for the bottles and nipples. What information would you give her and why?

   e. Maria is a 24-year-old gravida 1 para 1. She has some questions for you about how long her breast milk is good for after she pumps it. How would you respond?

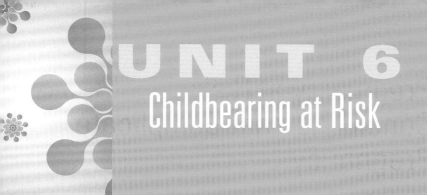

UNIT 6
Childbearing at Risk

16

Pregnancy at Risk: Conditions That Complicate Pregnancy

Key Terms

dermatome
euglycemia
gestational diabetes
hyperglycemia
hyperinsulinemia
hypoglycemia
macrosomia
polyhydramnios
pregestational diabetes
status asthmaticus
status epilepticus
TORCH

Learning Objectives

At the conclusion of this chapter, you will:

1. Compare and contrast the three major classifications of diabetes in the pregnant woman.
2. Differentiate between the care of the pregnant woman with pregestational diabetes and one with gestational diabetes.
3. Explain treatment goals for the pregnant woman with diabetes.
4. Describe nursing interventions for the pregnant woman with diabetes.
5. Explain the goals of treatment and nursing care for the pregnant woman with heart disease.
6. Differentiate between pregnancy concerns for the woman with iron-deficiency anemia and one with sickle cell anemia.
7. List treatment considerations for the pregnant woman with asthma.
8. Detail the risk to pregnancy from epilepsy and its treatment.
9. Describe the impact on pregnancy from the TORCH infections.
10. Differentiate among common sexually transmitted infections (STIs) according to cause, treatment, and impact on pregnancy.
11. Describe nursing considerations for the pregnant woman with an STI.
12. Describe nursing interventions for the pregnant woman who is the victim of intimate partner violence.
13. Identify special concerns associated with adolescent pregnancy.
14. Describe the impact of childbearing for women over 35 years old.

Melissa Hightower is an 18-year-old woman who presents to the clinic. She appears to be in the second trimester of pregnancy. When asked her chief reason for being at the clinic today, she states, "I think I might be sick and need medicine so the baby doesn't get sick." Upon further questioning she says this is her first pregnancy, she has not been to a health care provider yet for prenatal care, she has symptoms of a yeast infection, and she does not smoke or use illicit drugs. As you read this chapter, think about what complications of pregnancy Melissa might be having. What would be the effect of the disorders on both her and her unborn fetus? What follow-up care will most likely be ordered for Melissa?

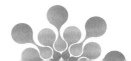

n the very recent past, many women with chronic conditions were unable to become pregnant and give birth. Now that there are effective treatments available for many of these conditions, more women are entering pregnancy with chronic medical conditions. As the licensed practical/vocational nurse (LPN/LVN), you will assist the registered nurse (RN) with providing care for the pregnant woman at risk.

The woman with a condition that complicates pregnancy needs specialized care. A perinatologist is an obstetrician who has received advanced training and specializes in the care of at-risk pregnancies, whether from a preexisting medical condition or from a complication of pregnancy. The perinatologist may consult with the obstetrician or other health care provider who is managing the pregnancy, may comanage the woman's pregnancy, or may be the primary health care provider during the pregnancy.

 Concept Mastery Alert

The specialist who provides care for the patient experiencing a high-risk pregnancy is known as a perinatologist.

PREGNANCY COMPLICATED BY MEDICAL CONDITIONS

Chronic medical conditions and pregnancy complications are both risk factors for the pregnant woman. Pregnancy and medical conditions can be interrelated in the following ways: Pregnancy can affect the underlying disorder; the normal physiologic changes of pregnancy sometimes intensify the symptoms of illness; medical conditions can affect the progress and outcome of pregnancy; or chronic medical conditions of the woman may adversely affect the fetus.

Diabetes Mellitus

Diabetes mellitus (DM) is a disease in which glucose metabolism is impaired by a lack of insulin production by the pancreas or by ineffective insulin utilization in the body. DM, particularly if it is poorly controlled, can adversely affect pregnancy outcomes. At the same time, pregnancy affects glucose metabolism, which makes the disease challenging to manage.

The woman may have diabetes mellitus (type 1 or type 2) prior to becoming pregnant; this is called pregestational diabetes, or she may develop diabetes during her pregnancy, a condition called gestational diabetes mellitus. Type 1 and type 2 DM both affect glucose metabolism, but type 1 is characterized by a lack of insulin in the body, whereas type 2 is most often associated with insulin resistance. Gestational diabetes is similar to type 2 DM. The treatment of the woman does not depend upon the type of diabetes, but rather her symptoms.

To understand the complications of diabetes during pregnancy, it is important to first recognize normal changes in the endocrine system of the pregnant woman related to blood glucose levels and insulin. During pregnancy, maternal tissues become resistant to insulin to provide sufficient levels of glucose for the growing fetus. The woman during pregnancy is in a diabetogenic state due to three normally occurring responses:

1. Blood glucose levels are lower than normal (mild **hypoglycemia**) when fasting.
2. Blood glucose levels are higher than normal (mild **hyperglycemia**) after meals.
3. Insulin levels are increased (**hyperinsulinemia**) after meals.

Pregestational Diabetes Mellitus

Pregestational diabetes describes the condition where a woman enters pregnancy with either type 1 or type 2 diabetes mellitus (DM). Historically, the woman with pregestational type 1 DM had a higher incidence of early pregnancy loss (miscarriage). If the woman was able to carry the pregnancy to term, the fetus was at high risk for congenital anomalies and stillbirth. Maternal and fetal outcomes have improved greatly with strict control of blood glucose levels and fetal surveillance. However, the woman with poorly controlled pregestational DM, particularly in the early weeks of pregnancy, is at risk for complications such as birth defects, stillbirth, hypertensive disorders, **polyhydramnios** (excess levels of amniotic fluid), preterm delivery, and macrosomia.

Gestational Diabetes Mellitus

Gestational diabetes mellitus (GDM) occurs only during pregnancy but is similar to the disease process of type 2 DM. As with type 2 DM, the underlying pathophysiology of GDM is insulin resistance. GDM develops when the woman's body cannot tolerate the physiologic changes seen with the diabetogenic state of pregnancy. Box 16-1 lists selected maternal risk factors for GDM.

Women who develop GDM do not always experience symptoms; therefore, screening for GDM is a standard of obstetric care for all women, not just those at risk. Screening for GDM is done at approximately 24 to 28 weeks of pregnancy, although some health care providers may screen as early as 20 weeks. If the woman has a prior history of GDM, screening often occurs at the first prenatal visit. The traditional diagnosis of GDM depends on the results of the oral glucose tolerance test, also known

| BOX 16-1 | Selected Risk Factors for Gestational Diabetes Mellitus |

- History of a large-for-gestational-age infant
- History of GDM
- Previous unexplained fetal demise
- Advanced maternal age (>35 years)
- Family history of type 2 DM or GDM
- Obesity (>200 lb)
- Non-Caucasian ethnicity
- Fasting blood glucose >140 mg/dL
- Random blood glucose >200 mg/dL

as the glucose challenge test. Box 16-2 outlines values of the oral glucose tolerance test.

The woman who develops GDM is at increased risk for developing type 2 DM after pregnancy. Up to half of women with GDM will go on to develop type 2 DM within 5 to 20 years after delivery.

BOX 16-2 **Diagnostic Values for the Oral Glucose Tolerance Test**

Normal values are the following:
- Fasting: <95 mg/dL
- 1 hour: <180 mg/dL
- 2 hour: <155 mg/dL
- 3 hour: <140 mg/dL

Gestational diabetes mellitus (GDM) is diagnosed if two or more values meet or exceed the levels listed above.

Fetal Complications From Maternal Diabetes

Regardless of the type of diabetes, the fetus born to a mother with diabetes is at increased risk. These risks include placental issues, fetal growth, hypoglycemia after birth, birth trauma, lung maturity issues, and increased health risks later in life (refer to Chapter 20 for a more detailed description of the newborn of the woman with diabetes). The diabetic woman is more likely to experience a cesarean birth than is a woman who does not have DM.

Diabetes mellitus (DM) causes damage to blood vessels, affecting major organs like the eyes and kidneys. In the pregnant woman, this damage also affects the placenta. In a woman with long-standing DM, the placenta tends to be smaller and maternal–fetal circulation is often decreased, which may lead to chronic fetal hypoxemia and growth restriction. The fetus born to a mother with DM can also be large for gestational age because of elevated maternal blood glucose levels.

The greatest risk for the fetus of the woman with GDM is excessive growth, resulting in macrosomia. **Macrosomia** is defined as either birth weight over 8.8 lb (4,000 grams) or as ≥90th percentile for gestational age. As with any disproportionate intake of sugar, the excess calories are stored in the fetus's body in the form of fat, which increases the risk for macrosomia. The macrosomic fetus is at increased risk for birth trauma including shoulder dystocia.

Insulin does not cross the placenta; however, blood sugar does. When the woman's blood sugar levels are elevated, large amounts of glucose cross the placenta. The fetus does not have insulin resistance, like the pregnant woman does, so the fetal pancreas produces increased levels of insulin to handle the high sugar load. After delivery, this increase in insulin levels can lead to hypoglycemia in the newborn of a diabetic mother.

Delayed lung maturity is another complication that the fetus of a woman with DM or GDM is at risk for. Additionally, children born to mothers with DM or GDM have an increased risk later in life for health issues including hypertension, impaired glucose tolerance, and obesity.

Treatment of Diabetes During Pregnancy

Prepregnancy Care

The woman who has pregestational DM should consult with her health care provider before she becomes pregnant. Persistent maternal **hyperglycemia** (elevated blood glucose levels) is harmful to the growing fetus, particularly during the first 8 weeks of pregnancy when organogenesis is occurring. Cardiac defects can occur from hyperglycemia during the period of organogenesis. Since the woman often does not know she is pregnant during the early weeks of organogenesis, it is important for the woman to attain a state of **euglycemia** (normal blood glucose levels) in the months before becoming pregnant to help prevent or minimize birth defects. Several months before becoming pregnant, the woman with diabetes should also start taking a daily multivitamin supplement that contains at least 1 mg of folic acid. Adequate folic acid intake is the best way to prevent neural tube defects, for which the diabetic woman's fetus is at an increased risk.

Glycemic Control

For the woman with pregestational diabetes, the most important goal of treatment is to maintain tight blood sugar control before and throughout pregnancy. An important part of this goal is to check blood sugar levels. This is done by the woman measuring her blood sugar via finger stick testing, or if she has a continuous blood sugar monitor, and by lab values. Lab values can be glucose values or glycosylated hemoglobin (HbA_1C) levels. The HbA_1C determines the average blood sugar levels during the past 4 to 8 weeks by looking at the percentage of red blood cells (RBCs) that have glucose incorporated in the hemoglobin. Sustained periods of hyperglycemia result in higher HbA_1C levels. Pregnancy reduces HbA_1C levels; therefore, HbA_1C expected values are lower for the pregnant women with diabetes than those of nonpregnant women with diabetes.

During pregnancy, the woman often has periods of fluctuating energy needs, which differ from prepregnancy needs. To accommodate for this, the woman with DM must check her blood sugar frequently. Common times include upon awakening, after breakfast, before and after lunch, before and after dinner, and before bedtime. The goal is to maintain fasting blood glucose levels of less than 95 mg/dL, and to not exceed 120 mg/dL 2 hours after meals.

There are three main components to glycemic control for the woman with pregestational DM: insulin, diet, and exercise (Fig. 16-1). For the woman with GDM, glycemic control focuses on diet and exercise. If these two therapies fail to control the diabetes, the woman with GDM begins insulin therapy to maintain blood sugar levels at therapeutic levels.

Insulin Therapy. Blood glucose levels vary throughout pregnancy. In the first trimester, the woman's insulin requirements fluctuate widely, and she is at risk for episodes of hypoglycemia, particularly between meals. This phenomenon occurs because the rapidly growing embryo requires a constant supply of glucose, which may deplete maternal blood sugar levels.

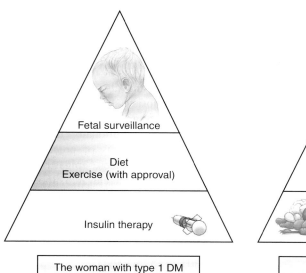

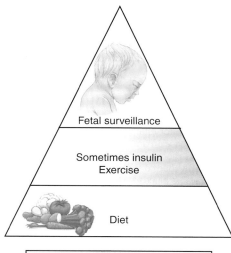

The woman with type 1 DM

The woman with GDM

FIGURE 16-1 Treatment overview for diabetes in pregnancy. For women with pregestational type 1 diabetes mellitus (DM), the foundation of glycemic management is insulin therapy along with dietary management, exercise, and fetal surveillance. For the woman who develops gestational diabetes mellitus (GDM), dietary modification is generally the foundation of treatment. Some women with GDM require insulin therapy, and others do not. Exercise and fetal surveillance are also important facets of care.

At the beginning of the second trimester, insulin requirements stabilize and then begin to increase at approximately 24 weeks' gestation, continuing to increase until term. During labor, insulin needs are variable, and in the first 24 hours after delivery, insulin requirements fall dramatically.

In type 1 DM, the pancreas does not produce insulin, which requires the woman to be on an insulin regimen. The woman may self-administer insulin via several scheduled subcutaneous injections throughout the day or she may use an insulin pump (Fig. 16-2) to administer insulin in low doses throughout the day. The insulin pump mimics that of a healthy pancreas by a continuous basal flow of insulin, which helps keep her blood sugar stable throughout the day. She can also give herself an insulin bolus by pushing a button before eating or if her glucose level is elevated above a predetermined level.

Insulin therapy is recommended for women with GDM when diet and exercise fail to keep fasting blood sugar levels lower than 95 mg/dL or 2-hour postprandial (after meals) levels below 120 mg/dL.

Oral Hypoglycemic Agents. The oral hypoglycemic agents glyburide and metformin have been used in the management of blood glucose levels for the pregnant woman with diabetes. It is recommended that the woman be transitioned to insulin therapy during pregnancy to help keep her blood glucose levels more consistent.

Diet Therapy. Another important part of diabetes management during pregnancy is diet therapy. In fact, the cornerstone of treatment for GDM is diet therapy, although insulin may be required depending upon the severity of glucose intolerance. The goals of dietary intervention for any type of DM during pregnancy are to supply the nutritional needs of the woman and her fetus, maintain blood sugar levels in the normal range, and prevent ketoacidosis. Consultation with a registered dietitian is recommended, preferably one who is also a certified diabetic educator, because diet requirements are individualized.

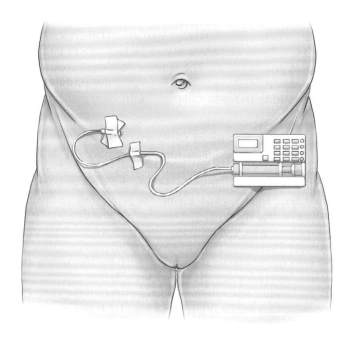

FIGURE 16-2 Using an insulin pump during pregnancy is the best administration method to keep insulin levels constant.

Exercise. Exercise is another way to help control blood sugar for the woman with diabetes. However, the pregnant woman should always consult with her health care provider before exercising. This is important if her diabetes is poorly controlled or if she has diabetes complications such as vascular damage, hypertension, or renal insufficiency.

Fetal Surveillance

Fetal surveillance is critical for the woman with diabetes. An initial sonogram during the first trimester determines gestational age and fetal viability. A more detailed, high-level sonogram is done at 18 to 20 weeks to look closely for structural defects, including heart defects, in the fetus. The sonogram enables careful assessment of fetal anatomy and for measurement of amniotic fluid volume. Maternal serum alpha-fetoprotein levels are measured at 16 to 20 weeks to screen for neural tube defects. If HbA_1C levels were elevated in early pregnancy, a fetal echocardiogram is recommended in the second trimester. Repeat sonograms may be ordered in the third trimester to continue to monitor fetal size.

> **Give Your Client the "Why" of It**
> It is important to monitor fetal growth in the diabetic woman. Macrosomia occurs more commonly in women with GDM due to the high levels of available glucose. Conversely, the woman with long-standing DM or vascular disease may have a fetus that is growth restricted (smaller) due to vascular changes that are complications of the diabetes.

Third trimester fetal surveillance is done to help detect signs of fetal stress. The mother initiates daily fetal activity counts at 28 weeks' gestation. Other tests that may be ordered include a nonstress test (NST) and biophysical profile (BPP). The woman may need contraction stress tests (CSTs) if the NST is nonreactive or the BPP is nonreassuring (refer to Chapter 7 to review prenatal fetal testing).

Determining Timing of Delivery

Determining the optimum time and method of delivery is critical for the woman with diabetes. The challenge is for the health care provider to schedule the delivery to avoid fetal injury while giving the fetus time to mature fully. Elevated maternal glucose levels can delay fetal lung maturation, which predisposes the newborn to respiratory distress. Therefore, third-trimester amniocentesis may be done to document fetal lung maturity by measuring the lecithin-to-sphingomyelin ratio. Some health care providers will induce labor in the diabetic woman if the cervix is favorable and the fetal lungs are mature. If the pregnancy progresses for too long, there is an increased chance for delivery complications, such as shoulder dystocia and fetal demise. Some health care providers attempt to prevent shoulder dystocia by inducing labor in the woman as soon as amniocentesis verifies fetal lung maturity. Alternatively, a cesarean delivery may be performed if macrosomia is suspected.

Multidisciplinary Care

Specialists should be involved in the care of the pregnant woman with DM or GDM. The health care provider, usually an obstetrician, may consult with an endocrinologist or perinatologist who then manages the woman's diabetes throughout her pregnancy. A team approach to the management of diabetes during pregnancy results in the best outcomes. Team members include the primary health care provider, the RN, a certified diabetic educator, and a registered dietitian. Endocrinologists, social workers, and pastoral caregivers may also be team members.

Pregnancy Complications From Diabetes

The woman with diabetes mellitus is at increased risk for pregnancy-related hypertension and also the severe pregnancy complication, preeclampsia (see Chapter 17). At every office visit, blood pressure and urinary protein measurements should be performed. Additionally, the woman should be carefully screened for signs of preeclampsia, including headache, visual disturbances, epigastric pain, generalized edema, urinary protein, and elevated blood pressure. Inform the woman to immediately call her health care provider if she experiences any of these symptoms.

Nursing Process and Care Plan for the Pregnant Woman With Diabetes

The nursing care plan for the pregnant woman with diabetes mellitus (DM) focuses on the measuring and management of her blood sugar levels and the monitoring of the fetus. Glucose levels will be monitored by the woman performing blood glucose checks and by the healthcare team monitoring her lab values. Blood sugar management includes diet, exercise, and for some women, insulin therapy. Fetal surveillance is done by both the woman and the healthcare team.

Assessment (Data Collection)

Diagnosis of type 1 DM usually occurs during childhood or adolescence. Therefore, the woman may be accustomed to monitoring her blood glucose levels and regulating her diet. She may also be used to self-administering insulin. However, she will likely need to increase the number of times she monitors her blood glucose levels during the day. Have the woman demonstrate how she performs self-monitoring of glucose levels and recording of the results. Be sure that she has a log and understands the importance of recording her blood sugar levels.

The woman who has been diagnosed with gestational diabetes mellitus (GDM) will need instructions on how to check her blood sugar levels. Determine the woman's understanding of the plan of care ordered for her. Instruct the woman to bring her blood sugar log to every prenatal visit. Review the log with her and discuss blood sugar patterns noted. Determine her ability to self-manage her condition.

The woman with diabetes should be monitored for signs and symptoms of urinary tract infection (UTI) and vaginal candidiasis (yeast infection). Increased blood sugar levels can increase her risk for these infections. In the third trimester, fetal surveillance should be performed regularly. During labor, frequent monitoring of blood glucose levels is required, sometimes as frequently as every hour. If the woman is unable to maintain normal glucose levels, an intravenous (IV) insulin drip may be initiated, with the insulin dose titrated to maintain glucose levels within a predetermined range.

Nursing Care Focus

When selecting the focus of nursing care for the pregnant women with diabetes, consideration should be given to the woman's understanding of her condition, her comfort level with performing self-monitoring of glucose levels and insulin injections, and her willingness to adhere to the plan of care. Nursing care is also focused on the health of the fetus. Additionally, it is important to determine the amount of support she will have at home with the glucose checks and additional appointments needed for her lab tests and fetal surveillance tests.

Outcome Identification and Planning

Safety is a priority goal for all clients. Appropriate safety goals for the pregnant woman with diabetes include that she will be free from injury from hypoglycemia or hyperglycemia and will remain free from infection. Appropriate safety goals for the fetus include that the fetus will be appropriate size for gestational age at birth and that regular fetal surveillance is done to monitor the health and growth of the fetus.

Nursing Care Focus

- Hypoglycemia and hyperglycemia risk

Goal

- The woman will maintain baseline glucose levels.

Implementations for Preventing Hypoglycemia and Hyperglycemia

The pregnant woman with diabetes is at risk for unstable blood sugar levels and the associated risks. Take particular care to review the signs and symptoms of hypoglycemia (Box 16-3) with the woman and her family. Explain that it is also important to pay attention to the warning signals because she is prone to hypoglycemia during pregnancy.

BOX 16-3   Signs of Hypoglycemia

It is particularly important for the pregnant woman and her family to be familiar with the signs and symptoms of hypoglycemia because she is more vulnerable to the condition during pregnancy. Sometimes it helps to remember that the symptoms of hypoglycemia mimic those of the fight-or-flight response. The woman may experience any of the following symptoms:
- Anxiety
- Shakiness
- Confusion
- Headache
- Tingling sensations around the mouth
- Hunger
- Sudden behavior change
- Pale skin
- Cold, clammy skin
- Increased pulse
- Seizure·
- Unresponsiveness

Review with the woman when to perform her self-monitoring of glucose levels. Have her perform return demonstrations if needed, especially if she is newly diagnosed with diabetes. Information obtained regularly by self-monitoring of glucose levels gives the woman immediate feedback on effect of diet, activity, and medications on glucose levels. At every office visit, carefully review the woman's blood sugar log. If she is having difficulty maintaining her blood glucose levels within the expected parameters, explore with her possible reasons.

Dietary recall for the past 3 days may be helpful for identifying patterns of food intake that interfere with blood sugar control. Refer the woman for a consult with a registered dietitian if she is having difficulty following the prescribed dietary regimen. Review with the woman her exercise patterns to determine if improved blood sugar control might result from implementation of an exercise regimen.

Carefully explore the woman's compliance with insulin administration. If she is having difficulty controlling her blood glucose levels, ask her to do a return demonstration by having her check her blood sugar levels. If possible, request that she do a return demonstration of insulin preparation and administration. Assist her to correct her technique, if necessary.

The cause of frequent episodes of hypoglycemia may be too much insulin or too little food; too little insulin or too much food may cause frequent hyperglycemia. Explore the woman's pattern of food intake in conjunction with insulin administration. Be certain she is eating three regular meals and three snacks daily. Food intake should follow insulin administration. A pattern of regular exercise may decrease insulin needs. Notify the health care provider of frequent episodes of hypoglycemia, particularly if the woman began a regular exercise program 3 to 4 weeks previously.

Pay Close Attention!

Hypoglycemia can be deadly. The woman needs a ready source of glucose (e.g., a candy bar or glass of milk) close by. A family member must administer glucagon if the woman loses consciousness.

Although any woman with diabetes is at risk for developing diabetic ketoacidosis (DKA), the woman with type 1 diabetes mellitus during pregnancy is at highest risk. She should know the signs of hyperglycemia and avoid triggers for DKA (Box 16-4).

Evaluation of Goal/Desired Outcome

The woman will:

- recognize and treat hypoglycemia promptly.
- recognize hyperglycemia and take measures to prevent DKA.
- monitor and record blood sugar levels as ordered.
- adjust her diet to recommendations by the health care provider and dietitian.
- exercise at least three times per week using recommended exercises.
- self-administer insulin if prescribed.

BOX 16-4 | **Diabetic Ketoacidosis and Pregnancy**

The onset of diabetic ketoacidosis (DKA) is marked by the classic symptoms of hyperglycemia, which include the following:
- Polydipsia (excessive thirst)
- Polyuria (increased frequency and amount of urine)
- Polyphagia (excessive hunger)

As DKA develops, the following symptoms appear:
- Glucose >300 mg/dL
- Ketonuria
- Kussmaul respirations
- Acetone (like alcohol) breath
- Sleepiness
- Language slurring
- Decreased consciousness

Triggers for DKA include (but are not limited to) the following:
- Too little insulin or too much food
- Infection
- Tocolytic therapy (to prevent preterm labor)
- Corticosteroid use
- Insulin pump failure

Nursing Care Focus

- Infection risk

Goal

- The woman will be free from infection.

Implementations for Infection Risk

The woman with diabetes is at increased risk for infections because of elevated blood sugar levels. Review with the woman the signs of a UTI, which include increased frequency, voiding small amounts, pain with urination (dysuria), and cloudy urine. Instruct her to drink 8 to 10 glasses of noncaffeinated beverages every day to help prevent UTI and to wipe from front to back after using the restroom. Frequent handwashing continues to be the best way to prevent infection. Remind the woman that if a UTI occurs, prompt treatment is essential because a UTI can cause premature labor.

Vaginal candidiasis is another problem the woman with diabetes is more likely to develop. Signs include white, cheesy-type vaginal discharge, severe itching, and discomfort. The discharge does not have a foul odor but is highly irritating to tender vaginal tissue. Fluconazole is an oral tablet sometimes prescribed for the woman with vaginal candidiasis. However, fluconazole is not regularly prescribed during pregnancy for the treatment of candidiasis, only when the benefits of treatment with this medication outweigh the possible risks to the fetus. The health care

provider will discuss these risks with the woman. Most frequently, treatment is done with over-the-counter vaginal creams and suppositories to control the symptoms during pregnancy. Verify that the woman understands treatment recommendations.

Evaluation of Goal/Desired Outcome

The woman:

- will remain afebrile.
- will have no signs of vaginal discharge.
- will be free from dysuria, cloudy urine, or other signs of a urinary tract infection.

Nursing Care Focus

- Injury risk to the fetus

Goal

- The fetus will remain free from injury and concerns.

Implementations for Injury Risk

It is important for the pregnant woman with diabetes to understand the risk for fetal injury, which can include fetal demise. The risk for fetal concerns increases if blood sugar levels are difficult to control and the woman requires insulin to manage her diabetes. The third trimester is generally the time of greatest danger. Instruct the woman to follow the diet and exercise plan. Review with the woman any prescribed insulin therapy. Have the woman demonstrate how she performs self-monitoring of blood glucose levels and insulin injections (if prescribed). Review with her times during the day she should perform self-monitoring of glucose levels.

Fetal surveillance is done per the health care provider's orders. It is always appropriate to tell the woman to monitor fetal activity and movement (kick) counts, starting at approximately 26 to 28 weeks' gestation. Twice-weekly nonstress tests (NSTs) may be ordered. Give the fetal monitor tracing to the RN to assess and report results to the health care provider. If the NST is nonreactive, anticipate follow-up with a contraction stress test (CST) and a biophysical profile (BPP).

The fetus of the woman with diabetes is at risk for disproportionate growth resulting in fetal growth restriction or macrosomia. The fundal height should be measured at each prenatal visit. Report findings that do not correlate with gestational age (refer to Chapter 7 to review fundal height measurement). Larger-than-expected size may be related to a large fetus or polyhydramnios; both are complications of diabetes.

Ultrasounds may be done to monitor the growth of the fetus. Instruct the woman on the importance of serial sonograms to estimate the fetal weight. The macrosomic infant is much more likely to experience shoulder dystocia (difficulty delivering fetal shoulders after delivery of the head) during birth, leading to birth trauma.

Evaluation of Goal/Desired Outcome

- The fetus will be active each day.
- The woman will monitor her blood glucose levels and take insulin as needed.
- The woman will comply with scheduled fetal surveillance tests as ordered.
- NST is reactive.
- BPP score is greater than 7.
- CST is negative.

TEST YOURSELF

✔ What test is used to monitor long-term glucose control during pregnancy for the woman with diabetes?

✔ What term is used to describe the fetus whose weight exceeds 4,000 grams?

✔ What are the three cornerstones of therapy for the pregnant woman with diabetes?

Cardiovascular Disease

Cardiovascular conditions were the leading cause of maternal deaths from 2014 to 2017 (CDC, 2019). Common heart disease conditions include coronary heart disease, pulmonary hypertension, and congenital heart disease but do not include cardiomyopathy or preeclampsia.

Significant cardiovascular changes occur in a normal pregnancy. During pregnancy, there is an increase in blood volume, heart rate, and cardiac output with a drop in systemic vascular resistance. The normal healthy woman is able to tolerate these cardiovascular changes. However, for the woman with heart or vessel disease, the normal physiologic increases that occur in pregnancy can cause discomfort or lead to cardiac failure. A woman with undiagnosed heart disease might be newly diagnosed based upon symptoms she reports; in the woman with preexisting disease, the symptoms can worsen. The periods of greatest risk for the pregnant woman with cardiac disease are at the end of the second trimester (when blood volume peaks), during labor, and in the early postpartum period due to fluid shifts (Waksmonski & Foley, 2020).

The World Health Organization (WHO) has classified the risk for the pregnant woman with cardiovascular conditions (Table 16-1). Generally, women with class I or II heart disease have a good prognosis for pregnancy. However, women with class III or IV are at much higher risk for poor pregnancy outcomes and require more extensive monitoring and treatment throughout the pregnancy. In addition, the risk of maternal and fetal complications increases if the woman has any of the following conditions: cyanosis, pulmonary hypertension, history of arrhythmia, or if she is currently taking anticoagulants (Waksmonski & Foley, 2020). Measurement of maternal oxygen saturation levels is one of the most important predictors of maternal and fetal outcomes. Oxygen saturation levels below 85% are associated with poor fetal outcomes.

Clinical Manifestations and Diagnosis

Preconception counseling is imperative for the woman with known cardiac disease. Tests to evaluate the woman's heart include a 12-lead electrocardiogram, echocardiogram, and Doppler study.

TABLE 16-1 World Health Organization Classification of Cardiovascular Disease Risk During Pregnancy

CLASS	CONDITIONS	RISK OF MATERNAL MORBIDITY/MORTALITY	PREGNANCY PROGNOSIS
I	• Small patent ductus arteriosus (PDA) • Mild pulmonic stenosis • Mitral valve prolapse • Successfully repaired atrial or ventricular septal defect or PDA • Isolated atrial or ventricular ectopic beats	No identifiable elevated risk	Good
II	• Unrepaired atrial or ventricular septal defect • Repaired tetralogy of Fallot or coarctation of the aorta • Marfan syndrome without aortic dilation	Mild elevated maternal mortality risk Moderately elevated morbidity risk	Good
III	• Mechanical heart • Unrepaired cyanotic heart disease • Some cases of Marfan syndrome	Substantially elevated maternal mortality risk Severely elevated morbidity risk	Moderate; woman needs regular cardiac monitoring throughout and after pregnancy
IV	• Severe mitral or aortic stenosis • Marfan syndrome with dilated aorta • Pulmonary hypertension • Preexisting cardiomyopathy	Extremely elevated maternal mortality risk Severely elevated morbidity risk	Poor; pregnancy contraindicated Monitoring done closely, as in Classification III

Adapted from Iftikhar, S. F., & Biswa, M. (2020). *Cardiac disease in pregnancy.* https://www.ncbi.nlm.nih.gov/books/NBK537261

Signs and symptoms (Box 16-5) vary depending on the underlying cause of heart disease. Tachycardia that lasts for more than several minutes accompanied by dizziness or lightheadedness requires further investigation. Pregnancy is particularly dangerous for the woman with severe pulmonary hypertension.

BOX 16-5 Signs and Symptoms of Heart Disease

The woman may complain of the following:
- Dyspnea
- Orthopnea
- Nocturnal cough
- Dizziness
- Fainting
- Chest pain

Physical examination may reveal the following:
- Cyanosis
- Clubbing of the fingers
- Neck vein distention
- Tachycardia
- Heart murmurs
- Edema

The earliest warning sign of cardiac decompensation is persistent rales in the bases of the lungs. The woman will probably notice a nocturnal cough. A sudden decrease in the ability to perform normal duties, dyspnea upon exertion, or attacks of coughing with a smothering feeling are serious signs of heart failure. Other symptoms such as tachycardia, edema, and hemoptysis may be noted.

Treatment

A team approach to management of the pregnancy complicated by heart disease is ideal. The obstetrician, cardiologist, and perinatologist often collaborate in the care of the pregnant woman with heart disease. Treatment varies depending on the etiology of the heart condition; however, there are general principles for management. These principles involve activity, stress management, diet, and medication. No matter the underlying cause of the condition, the main goal is prevention, early detection, and early treatment of cardiac decompensation.

Management During Pregnancy

Activity is allowed as tolerated. The woman is cautioned to rest frequently and not allow herself to become overly fatigued. Because pregnancy greatly increases the workload of the heart, bed rest is sometimes necessary, particularly for the woman who is severely compromised.

Any unusual stress that increases demands upon the cardiovascular system can precipitate heart failure. Examples include infection, anemia, dehydration, underlying medical disorders, and excessive emotional or physical stress. Pneumococcal and influenza vaccines are recommended because infection is particularly harmful for the pregnant woman with heart disease. Antibiotic prophylaxis to prevent endocarditis may be ordered before invasive procedures.

Diet is individualized. In some cases, sodium restriction is helpful. The woman can usually continue to take her cardiac medications during pregnancy. The three main medications or classifications of medications that are contraindicated in pregnancy are warfarin, angiotensin-converting enzyme (ACE) inhibitors, and angiotensin II receptor blockers (ARBs). Warfarin crosses the placenta and increases the risk of congenital anomalies. An alternative is treatment with heparin. The large molecules of heparin do not cross the placental barrier. ACE inhibitors and ARBs can lead to fetal renal failure and increase the risk of newborn mortality (DeCara, Lang, & Foley, 2018).

Management During Labor and the Postpartum Period

During labor, cardiac output increases, placing the woman with cardiac disease at risk for decompensation. Although no pregnant woman should be flat on her back during labor, it is particularly important for the woman with heart disease to avoid a supine position. Lying supine can cause supine hypotensive syndrome, which can lead to decreased placental perfusion, which can compromise the fetus. The condition can also increase maternal cardiac output and quickly lead to maternal complications.

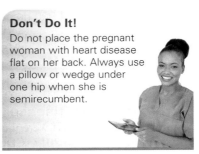

Don't Do It!
Do not place the pregnant woman with heart disease flat on her back. Always use a pillow or wedge under one hip when she is semirecumbent.

The health care provider may perform amniocentesis to determine fetal lung maturity in anticipation of early delivery if the woman's cardiac status begins to deteriorate in the third trimester. The woman who is at risk for endocarditis needs antibiotic prophylaxis. The antibiotic therapy begins when labor begins. Administration continues through the first postpartum day.

Spontaneous onset of labor is ideal instead of having labor induced. Vaginal birth is preferred if possible. Benefits of vaginal versus cesarean birth include decreased oxygen demands, minimal blood loss, and less chance of postoperative complications, such as infection and pulmonary issues like pneumonia. Cesarean delivery may be recommended in some situations, including cephalopelvic disproportion or the presence of an aneurysm, where the risk to the fetus or mother is greater than the risk of surgery.

The stress and pain of labor greatly increases demand on the heart, making pain relief a crucial part of labor management for the woman with heart disease. Epidural analgesia is acceptable for managing the woman's discomfort. During the second stage of labor, vigorous pushing using Valsalva maneuver can lead to cardiac decompensation; therefore, the fetus should be allowed to descend without maternal pushing. The woman remains at risk for heart failure in the postpartum period. Postpartum hemorrhage, anemia, infection, and thromboembolism are complications that greatly place the woman with heart disease at risk.

The woman should have frequent vital signs and cardiac monitoring during labor. Due to the woman's oxygenation status, the fetus remains at risk for hypoxia, and therefore her labor should have continuous fetal monitoring (versus intermittent monitoring).

Nursing Care

Thorough nursing observation and reporting of abnormal findings is critical when caring for the pregnant woman with heart disease. Monitor for and report jugular distention, clubbing, and slow capillary refill time. If an irregular pulse is noted, compare it with the apical pulse.

The most important nursing action is to monitor for signs of cardiac decompensation. Listen to breath sounds at each office visit and during labor. Report crackles in the bases of the lungs and complaints of nocturnal coughing to the RN and the health care provider. Ask her how many pillows she usually sleeps on at night and if she has needed to increase the number to help her breathe easier. Elevated blood pressure and tachycardia are other warning signs that require immediate reporting. Increased respiration, shortness of breath, and productive coughing may indicate the development of pulmonary edema or pulmonary emboli; both are life-threatening.

It is especially important for the pregnant woman with heart disease to protect herself from infection. Instruct her to avoid crowds and anyone with signs of respiratory infection, even the common cold. Explain that exposure to second-hand smoke increases the risk of contracting an upper respiratory infection. Advise her of the importance of frequent handwashing. Administer pneumococcal and influenza vaccines as ordered. Remind the woman of the importance of reporting her heart condition to all health care providers, including the dentist.

Encourage the woman to lie on her side when she is in bed or resting. If she must lie on her back, instruct her to put a wedge under one hip to avoid compromising the great vessels. She should minimize the amount of time she spends standing in one position or sitting with her knees flexed and legs dependent. She should avoid dehydration, which can further increase her risks of blood clots. Antiembolic stockings may be recommended.

Advise the woman to get adequate rest and avoid strenuous physical activity. Discuss the importance of avoiding overheating. A cool, dry environment is therapeutic. It is also helpful to give the woman information about what to expect throughout the pregnancy and during labor. This intervention can relieve anxiety and decrease the risk for cardiac decompensation.

Inquire regarding illicit drug use and cigarette smoking in a nonjudgmental way. Explain that illicit drugs and cigarette smoking adversely affect the heart and increase the risk for vasoconstriction and cardiac decompensation. Make clear that IV drug use increases the risk for infective endocarditis, a potentially lethal complication.

Explain to the woman the need for fetal surveillance to monitor the growth and well-being of the fetus. Instruct the woman to do fetal movement (kick) counts in the second and third trimesters. She should immediately report decreased fetal movement.

Monitor the woman closely during labor. Monitor pain levels frequently. Administer analgesia as ordered, and provide nonpharmacologic pain relief measures. Assist with epidural anesthesia administration as needed. Monitor the IV site. IV fluids should not be rapidly infusing. Maintain strict intake and output. Monitor vital signs as recommended. Do not encourage active maternal pushing during the second stage of labor. Anticipate forceps or vacuum-assisted delivery. Continue to observe for signs of cardiac decompensation in the postpartum period. Immediately report fever, increased bleeding, and any signs of decompensation to the RN and the health care provider.

Anemia

Anemia is a condition in which the blood is deficient in RBCs, hemoglobin, or in total volume. Anemia is not itself a disease. Rather, it is a symptom of an underlying disorder. There are three main causes of anemia: blood loss, hemolysis (increased RBC destruction), and decreased production of RBCs. Iron-deficiency anemia is the most common anemia experienced during pregnancy. Other anemias that could complicate pregnancy include megaloblastic anemia from folate deficiency, pernicious anemia from vitamin B_{12} deficiency, sickle cell anemia, and thalassemia. This section focuses on iron deficiency and sickle cell anemia.

Iron-Deficiency Anemia

Reduced production of RBCs characterizes iron-deficiency anemia. This situation occurs because the body does not have enough iron to manufacture the hemoglobin molecule. The RBCs that are produced are often smaller (microcytic) and are pale in color (hypochromic). Because the pregnant woman has increased iron requirements, she is particularly vulnerable to iron-deficiency anemia.

Common signs and symptoms of iron-deficiency anemia in the pregnant woman include tachycardia, tachypnea, dyspnea, pale skin, low blood pressure, heart murmur, headache, fatigue, weakness, and dizziness. Pica (ingestion of nonfood substances, such as clay or laundry starch) and pagophagia (frequent chewing or sucking on ice) are both associated with severe iron-deficiency anemia. If the pregnant woman has a hemoglobin level less than 11 g/dL or a hematocrit level less than 33% she is classified as anemic (Bauer, 2020).

Treatment for iron-deficiency anemia includes a diet rich in iron and folate in addition to iron, folate, and vitamin C supplementation. Folate and vitamin C increase the effectiveness of iron therapy. In some cases, iron injections may be ordered. Rarely does the pregnant woman with anemia require a blood transfusion.

The woman with iron-deficiency anemia needs counseling regarding foods that are high in iron. These include animal protein, dried beans, fortified grains and cereals, dried fruits, and any food cooked in cast iron cookware. Instruct her that vitamin C enhances iron absorption. Therefore, she should try to eat foods high in vitamin C along with iron-rich foods. Drinking orange juice when she takes her iron supplement will increase absorption. Her diet should also contain adequate amounts of folate. Foods high in folic acid include fortified grains, dried beans, and leafy green vegetables. A 3-day food diary is often helpful in identifying any dietary deficiencies.

Iron supplements predispose the woman to constipation. The pregnant woman may be tempted to stop taking iron supplements because of constipation. Instruct her regarding the importance of continuing iron supplementation. All of the normal measures that help prevent constipation, such as maintaining adequate fluid intake, a high fiber diet, getting enough exercise, and establishing regular bowel habits, are helpful for the pregnant woman taking iron supplements. If these measures are not helpful, report this to the RN and the health care provider for further evaluation determining if laxatives or stool softeners are needed. Follow-up hemoglobin and hematocrit lab studies will be ordered.

Sickle Cell Anemia

Sickle cell anemia is a hemolytic anemia that is caused by an abnormal hemoglobin molecule called hemoglobin S (Hgb S). Individuals who have sickle cell anemia inherit two copies of the genetic mutation for Hgb S, one from the father and one from the mother. Some people are carriers of the trait because they inherit only one copy of the mutation. Individuals who are carriers have sickle cell trait. In the United States, sickle cell anemia most commonly occurs in African American, White, and Hispanic individuals (Vichinsky, 2020).

Sickle cell anemia is a chronic condition characterized by acute exacerbations of the disease, called "crises." A crisis is typically caused by stress from infection, hypoxia, trauma, cold, or dehydration. In a crisis, the abnormal hemoglobin causes RBCs to "sickle," which means they change physical shape from round to crescent. The abnormal cells are sticky and clump together in such a way that they cannot flow easily through the capillaries. If enough of the cells clump, the clumping blocks blood flow to the area, causing tissue ischemia and pain at the site of blockage. Unfortunately, the bone marrow cannot produce enough RBCs to replace the damaged ones, so anemia results.

The pregnant woman with sickle cell anemia is at risk for decreased renal function, stroke, heart dysfunction, leg ulcers, and sepsis. Newborns born to the woman with sickle cell anemia are more likely to be born prematurely or to be small for gestational age.

The woman with sickle cell anemia is at risk for a sickle cell crisis at any time during the pregnancy. Depending upon which area of the body is affected, the woman may experience recurrent bouts of pain in the joints, bones, chest, and abdomen. She also may experience nonspecific symptoms of anemia, such as fatigue, tachycardia, and dyspnea. Physical examination may reveal enlarged lymph nodes, enlarged spleen (splenomegaly), hematuria (bloody urine), or jaundice.

Prevention of crises is the focus of treatment for the pregnant woman with sickle cell anemia. Maintaining adequate hydration, avoiding infection, getting adequate rest, and eating a balanced diet are all strategies that decrease the risk of a crisis. Pneumococcal and influenza vaccines are recommended. Medications used in the treatment of a sickle cell crisis are often not recommended for the pregnant woman due to the risks to the infant.

As the woman's pregnancy is considered high risk, she will have more frequent than normal prenatal visits. The recommended schedule for prenatal visits is every 2 weeks in the second trimester and every week throughout the second trimester. Ultrasound examinations may be ordered to measure fetal growth and amniotic fluid in the latter part of pregnancy.

When the woman experiences a painful crisis, a CBC, type and cross match, and sometimes arterial blood gas measurements are ordered. IV fluids will be administered to the woman for hydration and to decrease blood viscosity. Narcotics are generally required to control the pain that occurs during a crisis. Fetal heart rate monitoring is necessary. The woman may require supplemental oxygen by facemask if her oxygen saturation is low. Antibiotics treat infection if it is present. Blood transfusions may be ordered.

The woman with sickle cell anemia needs support throughout her pregnancy. Emphasize the importance of avoiding dehydration and stressful or extreme cold situations to prevent crises. Instruct the woman to wash her hands frequently and to avoid highly crowded areas to decrease her risk of contracting an infection. Pneumococcal and influenza vaccines are recommended. Adequate diet and rest are important for maintaining health in the pregnant woman with sickle cell anemia. Inform her of the importance of keeping prenatal appointments.

> ### TEST YOURSELF
> ✔ What is the earliest sign of cardiac decompensation?
> ✔ How does iron-deficiency anemia differ from sickle cell anemia?
> ✔ Describe two conditions or situations that might trigger a crisis for the woman with sickle cell anemia.

Asthma

Asthma is a chronic, inflammatory disease of the airways characterized by acute exacerbations of reversible airway obstruction; it is also known as reactive airway disease (RAD). The severity of the woman's prepregnant asthma is indicative of how severe her asthma will be during pregnancy. Risk factors for increased severity of asthma include the pregnant woman who is obese or who has had an increased weight gain during the first trimester. About one-third of the women with asthma had attacks during the second trimester. Studies show that the pregnant women with asthma have a slight increased risk for preeclampsia and preterm delivery (Weinberger & Schatz, 2020). If the condition is well controlled throughout pregnancy, maternal and fetal outcomes are similar to those of the general population.

During an acute asthma episode, the respiratory rate increases, and the woman feels short of breath and anxious. An expiratory wheeze is characteristic. Retractions of the respiratory muscles may be noted. Other symptoms frequently include a cough and chest tightness. Pulsus paradoxus, a pulse that weakens during inspiration, is often noted.

The goals of asthma management are prevention of acute episodes, control of symptoms, maintenance of normal pulmonary function, and avoidance of emergency department visits and hospitalizations.

Here's an Opportunity to Correct a Myth

Explain to the woman with asthma that it is much safer for her fetus if she takes her asthma medications. Poorly controlled asthma is not good for the pregnant woman or her fetus.

A thorough history regarding the woman's asthma includes medications, the frequency of acute episodes, the severity of the disease, history of hospitalizations, and any known environmental stimuli that are asthma triggers for the woman.

Maintenance care at home includes self-monitoring of lung function, proper control of the environment to reduce asthma triggers, and medication therapy. In order to control asthma triggers, the woman must first identify her triggers and then take measures to reduce them. Inhaled medications, such as albuterol and corticosteroids, are the frontline treatment agents. Oral asthma control medications are ordered for severe cases.

Management of an acute attack may require hospitalization for the pregnant woman. Treatment may take place on an observation status, or her condition may necessitate a full admission. Pulmonary function tests and arterial blood gases are done to evaluate the woman's respiratory status. Orders may include oxygen by nasal cannula to maintain oxygen saturation greater than 95%. The woman receives IV fluids for hydration, which helps loosen mucus in the airways. Frequent metered dose inhaler (preferred method) or nebulizer treatments with albuterol help bring the attack under control. If those medications do not resolve the attack, other medications including corticosteroids may be ordered. Fetal monitoring is done to observe the infant's response to the asthma attack.

Status asthmaticus is a severe asthma attack that does not respond to treatment (such as bronchodilators) and leads to hypoxemia (low O_2 levels in the blood) and hypercapnia (increased CO_2 levels in the blood) and can lead to respiratory failure. The pregnant woman in status asthmaticus will need aggressive treatment with intravenous medications, early intubation, and mechanical ventilation in the intensive care setting.

There are several important points to remember about managing the woman with asthma during labor. Labor will not exacerbate asthma symptoms, and the woman should continue to receive her regularly scheduled asthma medications throughout labor. Adequate hydration and analgesia minimize the risk of bronchospasm. Fentanyl or butorphanol are the pain relievers of choice during labor because they do not cause histamine release, which could lead to bronchospasm.

A major role when providing nursing care for the pregnant woman with asthma is to reinforce information she has been given. Be sure that the woman does a return demonstration of the use of her inhaler. Do not assume that she knows how to use it. She should also do a return demonstration for use of the peak flow meter. Remind her of the importance of monitoring fetal activity and movement (kick) counts during the second and third trimesters. Instruct the woman to avoid exposure to substances to which she is allergic. She should also avoid dust, tobacco smoke, and other environmental pollutants. Tips for Reinforcing Family Teaching: Managing Asthma During Pregnancy outlines the major points to make when educating the pregnant woman with asthma.

TIPS FOR REINFORCING FAMILY TEACHING

Managing Asthma During Pregnancy

- Do not stop taking your asthma medications. The risk to you and your baby is much higher from uncontrolled asthma than it is from taking your medications.
- Check with your doctor before taking any over-the-counter medications. Some of these medications have been shown to cause harm to your developing baby.
- Protect yourself from your known asthma triggers. Also you should:
  - avoid cigarette smoke, exposure to animals, and dusty, damp environments.
  - stay inside when pollen, pollution, smoke, or mold index is high.
  - wear a mask or scarf over your mouth on excessively cold days to help warm the air.
  - protect yourself from colds and flu because respiratory infections can trigger acute asthma attacks. Do this by avoiding crowds, performing frequent and thorough handwashing, and getting the flu vaccine (it is based on a killed virus, so it is safe to use during pregnancy).
  - avoid foods or chemicals that might have caused a reaction in the past.
- Continue your allergy shots as long as you are not having reactions to the shots. If you are not currently taking allergy shots, it is usually not advised to begin doing so during pregnancy because of the risk of reactions.
- Monitor your peak expiratory flow rate (PEFR) regularly as recommended by your health care provider, as a decrease in the PEFR usually precedes an acute asthma attack hours to days before physical symptoms begin.
- At the first sign of breathing difficulties, measure your PEFR. If it is low or has decreased from your last reading, notify your health care provider immediately. Other warning signs of an impending attack may include a headache, itchy throat, sneezing, coughing, or feeling tired.
- Develop a crisis management plan in consultation with your health care provider. The plan should include how to recognize warning signs and what to do when early signs of worsening status occur. Go immediately to the nearest emergency department if any of the following occur after rescue drugs are taken:
  - Rapid improvement does not result.
  - Improvement is not sustained.
  - Condition worsens.
  - The episode is severe.
  - Fetal movement decreases.

Epilepsy

Epilepsy is a group of neurologic disorders that involve a long-term tendency to have recurrent unprovoked seizures. The vast majority of women with epilepsy have healthy pregnancy outcomes.

Pregnancy presents several difficulties that relate to the condition of epilepsy. Drug metabolism changes during pregnancy, making it more difficult to maintain therapeutic antiepileptic drug levels. The major risk to the pregnancy from epilepsy is from blunt trauma that occurs during a seizure episode. Trauma can lead to miscarriage, premature rupture of membranes, and placental abruption.

Some medications used to treat epilepsy cause fetal defects (i.e., are teratogenic). Cleft lip and palate and neural tube defects comprise the majority of malformations noted in the fetus born to a woman taking antiepileptic medications.

Preconception care is highly recommended for the woman with epilepsy who wishes to become pregnant. The health care provider will be in consultation with a neurologist when following the woman with epilepsy. The goal is to control the seizures with the fewest number of drugs at the lowest possible doses and to use the medications with the lowest incidence of teratogenesis. The woman is advised to wait at least 6 months after seizures are under control before trying to become pregnant (Pennell & McElrath, 2020).

The woman should receive at least 1 mg of folate supplementation daily in the preconception period and continue daily throughout the pregnancy. If the woman is on an antiepileptic drug that has a high incidence of teratogenesis (e.g., valproate), she may be advised to take a high dose (4 to 5 mg daily) of folate supplementation in the 1 to 3 months preceding and throughout pregnancy because antiepileptic drugs increase the risk for neural tube defects. The medication valproate is used as a last resort as it is associated with a high incidence of congenital malformations and autism (Pennell & McElrath, 2020). Screening for neural tube defects will be done using a high-resolution sonogram in addition to maternal serum alpha-fetoprotein levels drawn at 14 to 16 weeks' gestation.

Epilepsy is not usually an indication for cesarean delivery. Most women can expect a normal vaginal delivery with few women experiencing seizures either during labor or after delivery. IV medications are usually sufficient to control a seizure should it occur. The difficulty is for the health care provider to determine if the seizure is due to epilepsy or if it is from the severe pregnancy complication, eclampsia (see Chapter 17).

Status epilepticus is an emergency complication of epilepsy whereby seizure activity continues for 5 to 30 minutes or more or when three or more seizures occur without full recovery between seizures. The healthcare team takes immediate measures to protect the woman from injury while protecting the airway. At least two IV lines are necessary to allow for IV administration of benzodiazepines, such as diazepam or lorazepam. Emergency intubation with mechanical ventilation is sometimes required.

Inform the woman about the importance of carefully following her medical treatment regimen and of maintaining regular prenatal care. Emphasize the importance of eating a diet high in folic acid and of taking folic acid and vitamin K supplementation. Inform the woman about the need for adequate sleep and to avoid stress as much as possible as fatigue and stress can be trigger factors for a seizure. Assist her with scheduling laboratory work at regular intervals. Provide emotional support during prenatal testing for fetal anomalies.

Remember **Melissa Hightower**. What do you think could be the cause of her yeast infection? What further tests do you think the health care provider might order? What fetal effects might be seen if Melissa has a pregnancy complicated by gestational diabetes?

PREGNANCY COMPLICATED BY INFECTIOUS DISEASES

Infectious diseases are a threat to the pregnant woman in several ways. The disease may cause in the woman illness that requires treatment. Unfortunately, the best treatment for the woman is not always good for the developing fetus. The infection itself can be harmful to the fetus, leading to birth defects or active infection of the newborn. Prevention is the best treatment. Table 16-2 defines terminology associated with infectious diseases.

TABLE 16-2 Definitions of Terms Associated With Infectious Diseases During Pregnancy

TERM	DEFINITION
Immunoprophylaxis	Prevention of disease by the production of active or passive immunity. The individual acquires passive immunity when they receive antibodies from the mother across the placenta or when they receive an injection of antibodies to a particular infection, such as hepatitis B. Active immunity occurs when the individual's immune system produces antibodies that fight against a particular disease, such as chickenpox. Active immunity develops when a person becomes ill with the disease, such as chickenpox.
Perinatal or vertical transmission	Transmission of the infectious agent from mother to child during pregnancy, childbirth, or breast-feeding.
Suppressive therapy	Treatment that suppresses the infectious agent but does not cure the individual.
Viral load	The amount of virus in the blood. High viral loads are associated with increased illness symptoms.

TORCH

TORCH is an acronym for a special group of infections that can be acquired during pregnancy and transmitted through the placenta to the fetus (Box 16-6). The "T" stands for toxoplasmosis, the "O" for other infections (hepatitis B, syphilis, varicella, and herpes zoster), the "R" for rubella, the "C" for cytomegalovirus (CMV), and the "H" for herpes simplex virus (HSV).

Each infection is teratogenic, and the effects are different depending upon when the infection occurs during the pregnancy. Cognitive impairment, microcephaly, hydrocephalus, central nervous system lesions, jaundice, hepatosplenomegaly, hearing deficits, and chorioretinitis are examples of conditions that may be seen in the newborn infected with one of the TORCH agents. Fetal infection may also lead to early pregnancy loss, intrauterine growth restriction (IUGR), stillbirth, and premature delivery. Prevention is the focus of interventions because many of the TORCH infections do not have effective treatment regimens.

The TORCH infections that are routinely screened for during pregnancy are hepatitis B, syphilis, and rubella. If the health care provider has reason to believe the woman might have one of the other TORCH infections, they may perform a TORCH screen. In addition to the TORCH screen, antibody titers may be ordered to see if the infection is active or an older infection.

Toxoplasmosis

Toxoplasmosis is an infection caused by the protozoan *Toxoplasma gondii*, also referred to as "*T. gondii.*" Transmission is via undercooked meat, unfiltered water, contaminated soil, and cat feces. Toxoplasmosis is a common infection in humans and usually produces no symptoms. However, when the infection passes from the woman through the placenta to the fetus, a condition called congenital toxoplasmosis can occur. A newborn with congenital toxoplasmosis may present with chorioretinitis and hydrocephalus. The newborn will need ophthalmic and hearing evaluations.

Toxoplasmosis is difficult to diagnose because it rarely produces symptoms in the woman. This infection is particularly harmful if the fetus contracts the parasite between 10 and 24 weeks of pregnancy. The woman can decrease the risk for infection through several common-sense approaches. Advise the pregnant woman to have someone else clean the cat litter box daily. If there is no one else to perform this duty, she should wear gloves and wash her hands thoroughly before and after cleaning the cat's litter box. The woman should wear gloves when working in the garden or when doing yard work. She should wash her hands thoroughly before and after handling raw meat, and she should eat only meats that have been completely cooked to 152°F or higher (i.e., no rare or medium rare meats). Instruct the woman to thoroughly clean in hot, soapy water any surface or item that is touched by raw meat. All fruits and vegetables need to be washed carefully before being served.

Other Infections: Hepatitis B, Syphilis, Varicella, and Herpes Zoster

Hepatitis B

Hepatitis B virus (HBV) is transmitted sexually or through contact with blood or body fluids. Transmission to the fetus can occur across the placenta or by contact with vaginal secretions and blood during delivery. Fortunately, due to routine vaccination of infants, school-age children, and adults at risk, the incidence of HBV infection has decreased in the United States.

Pregnant clients are screened for hepatitis B surface antigen (HBsAg) early in the pregnancy and then again at delivery. If the newborn that is born to a woman who is positive for HBsAg is not treated, the infant is highly likely to develop HBV infection. If the mother is HBsAg-positive, the neonate should receive hepatitis B immunoglobulin (HBIg) and the hepatitis B vaccine within 12 hours of birth. The immunoglobulin provides immediate protection, and the vaccine provides long-term protection from infection. Regardless of the woman's HBV status, all infants need a three-dose immunization series against hepatitis B with the first dose given at birth.

Syphilis

Syphilis is an STI caused by the bacterium (spirochete) *Treponema pallidum* (*T. pallidum*). The bacteria spread via

---

BOX 16-6 TORCH Infections

TORCH (an acronym for the infections)

Toxoplasmosis
Other: hepatitis B, syphilis, varicella, and herpes zoster
Rubella
Cytomegalovirus (CMV)
Herpes simplex virus (HSV)
All cross the placenta and are teratogenic. Fetal effect is determined by gestational age at exposure. TORCH syndrome is characterized by IUGR, microcephaly, hepatosplenomegaly, rash, thrombocytopenia, and CNS findings, such as ventricular calcifications and hydrocephaly.

Maternal Assessment (Data Collection)
1. History: Flu-like symptoms, fatigue, cat exposure, genital lesions, rash, or exposure to sick children
2. Physical examination: Lymphadenopathy, headache, malaise, jaundice, nausea/vomiting, low-grade temperature, rash, and ulcerated and painful lesions of the genitals

Diagnostics
1. Serologic tests
   - TORCH screen
   - CBC
   - HBsAg and HBeAg
   - Liver function tests
2. Cultures
   - CMV
   - HSV
3. Pap test
4. Serial ultrasounds (monitor for IUGR and other defects throughout pregnancy)

sexual contact or through broken skin. The main symptom of primary syphilis is a painless red pustule, which usually appears within 2 to 6 weeks after exposure. The pustule quickly erodes and develops a painless, bloodless ulcer called a chancre. Because it is painless, the newly infected person may not notice the chancre. The chancre, which sheds infectious fluid, usually appears on the body part that served as the portal of entry for the bacteria.

If the pregnant woman acquires a syphilis infection, the bacteria readily cross the placenta, causing infection in the developing fetus. A woman who contracts syphilis early in pregnancy and does not receive treatment is at increased risk for a early pregnancy loss (miscarriage). Other consequences of active syphilis infection include fetal demise, IUGR, nonimmune hydrops fetalis, preterm birth, congenital infection, and neonatal death.

Most infected infants are without symptoms at birth. Hepatomegaly, jaundice, snuffles (rhinitis with a white or bloody discharge), and long bone abnormalities are symptoms that might be seen. The nasal discharge is highly infectious. Symptoms can develop as long as weeks to months or years later (Dobson, 2019).

Every pregnant woman is screened for syphilis by either the RPR or VDRL laboratory test in the early part of pregnancy. A positive screen requires further testing that is more specific to *T. pallidum*. Syphilis is curable if properly treated. The treatment of choice for syphilis is benzathine penicillin G administered intramuscularly either as a single-dose or two-dose series. Penicillin may be given during pregnancy and is safe to use while breastfeeding. Individuals who are sensitive to penicillin receive erythromycin. Penicillin is also the treatment of choice for newborns with congenital syphilis.

Varicella and Herpes Zoster

Varicella zoster is the virus that causes chickenpox. Herpes zoster is the recurrent form of the virus that lies dormant in the dorsal root ganglia of the spinal cord. Reactivation of herpes zoster results in shingles. Varicella zoster and herpes zoster are both members of the herpes virus family.

Varicella zoster is spread by respiratory droplets and is highly contagious. The virus incubates for approximately 2 weeks and is contagious 2 days before onset of the skin lesions until the lesions crust over, generally 5 days after the initial onset. Herpes zoster (shingles) is characterized by a localized rash within a **dermatome**, an area on the body surface supplied by a particular sensory nerve. The rash is very painful. Occasionally pain precedes the rash. Anyone who has had chickenpox is at risk for developing shingles.

With widespread immunizations of the varicella vaccine, currently the incidence of varicella zoster during pregnancy is low, and transmission of varicella zoster by the pregnant woman to her unborn child is very rare. The highest risk occurs if the woman contracts varicella in the second trimester, between 13 and 20 weeks' gestation. However, the severity of fetal varicella syndrome should not be ignored. Fetal varicella syndrome is associated with low birth weight, scar-producing skin lesions, limb hypoplasia, and contractures. The syndrome can also result in damage to the ears, eyes, and central nervous system, leading to cognitive impairment, paralysis, and seizures. If the woman contracts varicella from 5 days before to 2 days after delivery, the newborn is at risk for neonatal varicella, a severe form of chickenpox that can be fatal. Another danger of varicella during pregnancy is the risk to the woman of developing varicella pneumonitis. This form of pneumonia can be severe and even fatal. Even if the woman survives, the severity of pneumonia could result in death of the fetus.

Any pregnant woman who reports a possible exposure to chickenpox or shingles should have a serologic test performed to detect varicella antibodies. Varicella zoster immunoglobulin administered within 10 days of exposure helps prevent the development of chickenpox. The neonate may be treated with the varicella zoster immunoglobulin if the woman develops chickenpox 5 days before or within 48 hours after delivery.

The best treatment is prevention. A woman of childbearing age who has not had chickenpox should be vaccinated. She should avoid pregnancy for at least 1 month after vaccination. Vaccination is not appropriate for pregnant women; however, susceptible individuals in the household of a pregnant woman who is susceptible to chickenpox should receive the vaccine. This is the most effective way to prevent transmission to the pregnant woman. The nonimmune woman should receive one dose of varicella vaccine immediately after delivering her newborn and a second dose at the 6-week postpartum visit.

Rubella

Rubella, also known as German measles, is a virus that caused epidemics in the United States. Rubella is usually a mild illness when it occurs in adults and children. Of rubella infections, 25% to 50% are "silent"; that is, there are no symptoms. When symptoms occur, they are generally mild and include low-grade fever, rash, lymphadenopathy, general malaise, and conjunctivitis. The problem occurs when a woman contracts rubella while she is pregnant. Congenital rubella infection can result with consequences including early pregnancy loss, stillbirth, preterm delivery, and congenital anomalies. Hearing impairment is the single most common defect associated with congenital rubella infection, followed by eye disorders, heart defects, and neurologic abnormalities including cognitive impairment. The greatest risk occurs if the woman develops rubella in the first trimester, which can result in multiple anomalies. Maternal rubella infection contracted after 20 weeks of pregnancy has a low incidence of birth defects.

There is no cure for congenital rubella infection. Treatments are supportive and directed toward control of symptoms and complications. The best treatment for congenital rubella infection is prevention. Ideally, all women of childbearing age should obtain preconception care, which includes testing for immunity to rubella. Nonimmune women should be vaccinated before becoming pregnant and should wait at least 28 days after vaccination before attempting pregnancy. Routine prenatal care includes testing for immunity to rubella in early pregnancy. Authorities do not recommend giving rubella vaccine during pregnancy due to the small risk of congenital rubella syndrome. The nonimmune woman should carefully avoid anyone with flu-like symptoms or rash while she is pregnant. The woman receives the vaccine in the early postpartum period before discharge from the hospital or birth center with instructions to avoid pregnancy for 28 days. Breast-feeding is not a contraindication to rubella vaccination.

Cytomegalovirus

CMV infection is a silent disease because most individuals who contract the virus have no symptoms or only mild flu-like symptoms. About half of the people in the United States will have had a CMV infection. It is caused by a virus in the herpes family. Transmission is by contact with infected bodily fluids, such as saliva, blood, breast milk, urine, and semen. Once a person is infected, they will test positive for the virus for life.

A woman who contracts CMV for the first time during pregnancy can pass the infection to the fetus. CMV infection during the first 20 weeks of pregnancy causes more severe defects. Most infected newborns are without symptoms at birth but may go on to develop progressive hearing loss that is usually unilateral but may affect both ears. About 10% of newborns with congenital CMV have symptoms present at birth which include microcephaly, petechiae, seizures, small size for gestational age, hepatosplenomegaly, jaundice, and rash (Demmler-Harrison, 2020).

Because there is no cure for congenital CMV, prevention is extremely important. Pregnant women who have contact with small children should practice meticulous hygiene. Although CMV is present in breast milk, the woman usually may breast-feed because CMV infection contracted while breast-feeding rarely causes serious problems. Tips for Reinforcing Family Teaching: Preventing CMV Transmission During Pregnancy lists important points to help decrease the woman's chance she will develop CMV infection.

Protect Yourself

A nurse who is pregnant or thinking about becoming pregnant should not take care of a client who has a documented or suspected CMV infection due to the increased risk of transmission to the nurse.

TIPS FOR REINFORCING FAMILY TEACHING

Preventing CMV Transmission During Pregnancy

- Practice good handwashing with soap and water after contact with saliva and urine.
- Carefully dispose of all soiled diapers, tissues, or other potentially infected items.
- Avoid direct contact with the saliva of young children. Suggestions are to not participate in the following behaviors with young children (particularly those in day care):
  - Kissing on the lips
  - Sharing food, drinks, utensils, or straws

- If you develop a flu-like illness (sore throat, low-grade fever, swollen lymph glands, body aches, and fatigue) during pregnancy, call your health care provider to be evaluated for CMV infection. Your health care provider may have lab work done on you to see if you have the infection. There are no medications to treat this infection.
- In most cases, the benefits of breast-feeding outweigh the minimal risk of the infant acquiring CMV from the breast milk.

Herpes Simplex Virus

HSV is a sexually transmitted infection caused by herpes simplex virus 1 (HSV-1) and herpes simplex virus 2 (HSV-2). The virus spreads by direct contact. In general, HSV-1 causes oral herpes, also known as cold sores, and HSV-2 causes genital herpes. However, both types can be transmitted to the mouth or genital region through kissing, oral–genital sex, and other sexual contact, and both types can cause serious illness in a newborn.

Symptoms of genital herpes usually develop within 2 to 14 days after exposure to the virus. Without antiviral treatment, the lesions may last for as long as 20 days. The first attack is generally the most severe, although many individuals with primary HSV infections have no symptoms. Painful lesions develop in the area exposed to the virus, usually the genital or anal regions. The lesions eventually completely heal and do not cause scarring. However, the virus lies dormant in the nervous system and can cause recurrent attacks.

Tenderness, burning, and pain usually occur several hours to several days before a recurring attack.

The majority of cases of neonatal herpes are contracted by contact with active virus in the birth canal, although small percentages of fetuses contract the infection in utero. The highest risk for neonatal herpes occurs in infants of women who develop herpes for the first time during the last trimester of pregnancy and who have active lesions in the birth canal at the time of delivery. A neonate that is infected with HSV manifests the infection in one of three ways: skin, eye, or mouth involvement; central nervous system with encephalitis; or multiple organs involved with symptoms seen throughout the body.

Treatment during pregnancy often includes a 1- to 2-week course of therapy with acyclovir for a first episode of HSV. Suppressive therapy (see Table 16-2) may be ordered beginning at 36 weeks' gestation because this seems to reduce the risk of an active outbreak at the time of delivery (Riley & Wald, 2020).

If the woman has a lesion at delivery, the safest alternative is cesarean delivery to prevent the infant from coming in contact with the virus in the birth canal. Vaginal examinations are withheld if there are active lesions. If there are no lesions present when the woman goes into labor, the American Congress of Obstetricians and Gynecologists recommends a vaginal delivery. Internal monitoring with a fetal scalp electrode is not recommended during labor in the woman with a history of genital herpes as the electrode causes a small break in the fetal scalp and can serve as a portal of entry for the virus. Additionally, forceps and vacuum extraction should also be avoided.

Sexually Transmitted Infections

A sexually transmitted infection (STI) is an infection transmitted primarily by sexual contact or through contact with blood or bodily fluids. STIs previously were referred to as sexually transmitted diseases (STDs). Several of the TORCH infections are STIs, including hepatitis B, syphilis, and herpes simplex. Other STIs that can affect the pregnant woman include chlamydia, gonorrhea, genital warts, trichomoniasis, and human immunodeficiency virus/acquired immunodeficiency syndrome (HIV/AIDS).

Many STIs are reportable diseases tracked by the CDC and include syphilis, chlamydia, gonorrhea, and HIV/AIDS. Some states require additional STIs to be reported. One increasing concern is that many STIs increase the risk for the individual to contract HIV/AIDS. If the symptoms of the STI infection include a break in the integrity of the skin or mucous membranes, these sites can provide a portal of entry for HIV.

Chlamydia

Chlamydia is one of the more common STIs in the United States and is caused by the bacterium *Chlamydia trachomatis*. Most women who have chlamydia have no symptoms, which can delay diagnosis of the infection. Although it is a prevalent STI, it is underreported due to its asymptomatic nature. Symptoms may include vaginal discharge, abnormal vaginal bleeding, and abdominal or pelvic pain. Chlamydia is usually detected by testing the urine or cervical secretions.

The most frequent complication of untreated chlamydia is pelvic inflammatory disease (PID), a serious infection of the reproductive tract that can lead to infertility and chronic pelvic pain. Inflammation of the fallopian tubes that occurs with PID often results in scarring, which increases the risk of ectopic pregnancy and subsequent infertility. A pregnant woman who contracts chlamydia is at increased risk for early pregnancy loss (miscarriage), preterm rupture of membranes, and preterm labor. The postpartum woman is at higher risk for endometritis. The fetus can encounter bacteria in the vagina during the birth process. If this happens, the newborn can develop pneumonia or conjunctivitis that can lead to blindness.

Chlamydia is treated with antibiotics, usually oral erythromycin or amoxicillin. As with other STIs, the sexual partners of the individual also require treatment.

Gonorrhea

Gonorrhea is caused by the bacterium *Neisseria gonorrhoeae* (*N. gonorrhoeae*) and is one of the more common STIs in the United States. Transmission of the bacteria occurs during sexual contact. The primary site of infection for the woman is the cervix, although infection can occur in the rectum and throat depending upon the type of sexual encounters the woman has. A culture taken from the cervix, rectum, or throat is the diagnostic method of choice.

Initial symptoms, which usually develop within 2 to 10 days of exposure to the bacteria, are mild and may go unnoticed. The woman who contracts gonorrhea may have vaginal bleeding during sexual intercourse, pain and burning while urinating, and a yellow or bloody vaginal discharge.

Untreated gonorrhea can lead to PID, which can leave the woman infertile or susceptible to ectopic pregnancy because of scarring in the reproductive tract. The bacteria can also spread through the bloodstream and infect joints, heart valves, or the brain.

The woman with an untreated gonococcal infection is at increased risk for preterm labor. The newborn is at risk for infection of the eyes through contact with vaginal secretions during birth, causing a condition known as ophthalmia neonatorum. Newborn blindness can result from this infection; however, cases are rare because all newborns receive prophylactic ocular treatment within 1 hour after birth (see Chapter 14).

Treatment is usually with a combination of two antibiotics that treat both gonorrhea and chlamydia because these infections often occur together. Treatment includes one intramuscular dose of ceftriaxone along with oral azithromycin. This treatment is appropriate for pregnant women. One emerging problem in the treatment of gonorrhea is that antibiotic resistant strains of *N. gonorrhoeae* exist.

Human Papillomavirus

Human papillomavirus (HPV) is the most common viral STI in the United States. HPV spreads by skin-to-skin contact, usually during sexual activity, whereas other STIs are spread by contact with bodily fluids. This virus can cause condylomata acuminata (genital warts) and cervical cancer. An individual with HPV infection without symptoms can unknowingly pass the virus on to sexual partners.

Condylomata acuminata develop in clusters on the vulva, within the vagina, on the cervix, or around the anus. The lesions may remain small, or they can develop into large clusters of warts that resemble cauliflower. An abnormal Papanicolaou (Pap) smear may be the first indication of HPV infection.

Genital warts have a tendency to increase in size during pregnancy. This may result in heavy bleeding during vaginal delivery. The pregnant woman can pass HPV to her fetus during the birth process. In rare instances, the newborn is at risk for laryngeal papillomas from the HPV infection. Hoarseness in the newborn is a symptom that should be reported to the RN and health care provider.

Genital warts can disappear without treatment. The type of treatment chosen depends on many factors, including age of the client; duration, location, extent, and type of warts; the client's immune status; risk of scarring; and pregnancy status. Several medical treatments are available, most of which consist of topical applications. Many of these treatments involve the use of teratogenic substances that are not for use during pregnancy. Surgical removal of the warts is done through a variety of techniques, including blunt dissection, laser, and cryosurgery.

A vaccine for HPV is available and is administered as a series of two injections over the course of 6 months. The vaccine helps protect against cervical cancer and genital warts. The FDA approved the vaccine for use in males and females 11 to 26 years of age.

Trichomoniasis

Trichomoniasis, or infection with *Trichomonas*, is an STI caused by one-celled protozoa. It can infect the urethra, vagina, cervix, and structures of the vulva. It is possible for the woman to transmit trichomoniasis to the fetus during vaginal delivery, although this is a rare occurrence.

Symptoms of trichomoniasis include large amounts of foamy, yellow-green vaginal discharge, vaginal itching, unusual vaginal odor, painful sex, and dysuria. Many women with trichomoniasis have no symptoms. The most common diagnostic test is the wet mount where a swab of the vaginal secretions is examined under the microscope. A culture is more sensitive than a wet mount, but results are not available for several days. Trichomoniasis can cause premature rupture of membranes, preterm delivery, and low birth weight.

The treatment for trichomoniasis is oral metronidazole given as a single dose. Although metronidazole is available in vaginal suppository and cream formats, oral dosing is recommended because of its increased effectiveness in treating *Trichomonas* infection. Expected side effects of treatment with oral metronidazole are metallic taste and dark urine. Nausea and vomiting can occur with high doses or when the woman drinks alcohol during treatment.

HIV/AIDS

Acquired immunodeficiency syndrome (AIDS) is caused by the human immunodeficiency virus (HIV), which attacks and destroys the protective cells of the immune system (the T-helper lymphocytes/CD4+) that direct the immune response to infections and remove some malignant cells from the body.

Transmission of HIV most often takes place during unprotected sexual activity with an infected partner. This can be through heterosexual or homosexual sex. The virus can enter the body through the mucous membranes of the genitals, rectum, or mouth. Also, exposure to HIV-infected blood by sharing needles for IV drug use, intramuscular injections of anabolic steroids, or tattooing can result in HIV infection. People infected with HIV often do not look or feel sick and may transmit the virus to others before they know they are infected.

A woman who has HIV during pregnancy is at risk for transmitting the infection to the fetus during pregnancy or childbirth and to the newborn while breast-feeding. Receiving appropriate antiretroviral treatment during pregnancy and childbirth and avoiding breast-feeding the newborn substantially reduce the risk of perinatal transmission of HIV to the infant.

The pregnant woman may contract HIV during pregnancy, or she may already have the HIV infection when she gets pregnant. It is important for the health care provider to know the pregnant woman's HIV status. The CDC recommends that confidential HIV testing be offered at the beginning of pregnancy and again during labor. The woman may refuse testing, but the health care provider is encouraged to counsel the woman and explore reasons for refusal.

> **Be Alert!**
>
> The HIV-positive woman may be at higher risk for domestic violence and homelessness. Perform a careful data collection on the woman's emotional status and levels of social support.

The two main goals of treatment for the pregnant woman infected with HIV are to prevent progression of the disease in the woman and to prevent perinatal transmission of the virus to the fetus. The best way to prevent perinatal transmission is to identify HIV infection before pregnancy or as early as possible during pregnancy. Therefore, early prenatal care for all women, regardless of risk, is important.

Nursing Process and Care Plan *for the Pregnant Woman With an STI*

Although different organisms cause STIs, avoiding high-risk behaviors can prevent them all. As the nurse, you can help identify women who are at risk for STIs, provide information, and assist with specimen collection. For women who are negative for an STI, provide education regarding safe behaviors to prevent contracting an STI in the future. For women who are positive, provide nonjudgmental, compassionate care, and assist the woman in coping with the diagnosis and treatment.

Assessment (Data Collection)

Health care providers, including nurses, should perform thorough health histories on their clients, which includes sexual histories. Inquire regarding risk factors for STIs in a way that makes the woman feel safe to answer honestly. Box 16-7 outlines techniques for taking a sexual history.

BOX 16-7 Taking a Sexual History

BOX 16-7 Taking a Sexual History

Create a Conducive Environment
- Be relaxed, and pursue the history as you would for any other medical problem.
- Make certain the client is in a private location, free from distractions.
- The client should be dressed (not in an examination gown).
- In almost all circumstances, it should just be you and the client.

Introducing the Topic of Sexual Activity
- Explain that you take a sexual history on every client (so the individual does not feel singled out), acknowledge the sensitive nature of the questions, and reinforce confidentiality.
  - An example of what to say is: "I take a sexual history on all clients as part as their health history. I know some questions may be sensitive, but the answers are important so we can provide adequate care. Any information you give me is strictly confidential and will stay between us."
- Integrate the sexual history into the lifestyle component of data collection (smoking, alcohol, caffeine intake, etc.) or into the genitourinary system review.

Techniques for Asking Questions
- Begin with open-ended questions such as "Tell me about…" which encourages a more complete history and avoid leading questions.
- Use words appropriate for the level of understanding. Avoid generalities such as "down-there" and if the client uses these terms clarify the meaning.
- Be matter-of-fact and sensitive but avoid appearing bored. The professional tone of the interview will help put the client at ease.
- The nurse's nonverbal communication should convey comfort and responsiveness. Avoid crossing arms or always looking at chart or computer screen.
- Introduce questions by a generalizing statement, such as "people have sex in many different ways." This is less threatening for the client who will not feel like they are the only one engaging in these activities and may feel more comfortable describing the behavior.
- Do not act surprised, shocked, or embarrassed by the answers you get. Do not be judgmental.

- Speak clearly with words that the client can easily understand. For example, use the word "sore" or "scab" versus "lesion" or "breakdown."
- Be careful not to talk down to the client.

Partners
- Ask about gender and number of partners in the past 4 months.
- Inquire about the gender of sexual partners (e.g., *"Do you have sex with men, women, or both?" "Tell me about your sexual partner(s)…"*) before asking any questions that are gender-specific.
- The client should be assured that revealing their sexual orientation will not result in poor care, a negative reaction, or abandonment.

Prevention of Pregnancy and Protection From STIs
- Ask if the client is trying to get pregnant or prevent pregnancy.
- Ask what conception prevention measures the client, or the client's partner, uses.
- Ask about protection from STIs.
- If no protection is used, inquire about the reasons.

Practices
- Ask about specific sexual activities.
  - Example: "Do you engage in oral sex?"

Past History of and Risk for STIs
- Ask about the client and their partner's STI and drug history.
  - Example: "Have you or any of your partners ever injected drugs?" or "Have any of your partners exchanged money or drugs for sex?"

Culture
- Consider if the client would prefer a specific caregiver taking the sexual history.
- For language barriers, consider obtaining the services of an interpreter. Do not assume nodding is a sign of understanding information given.
- Lack of eye contact or minimal responses may be culturally appropriate especially in response to sexual questions.

Adapted from information in the following reference: Workowski, K. A., & Bolan, G. A. (2015). Sexually transmitted diseases treatment guidelines, 2015. *MMWR Recomm Rep*, 64(RR-03), 1–137. https://www.ncbi.nlm.nih.gov/pmc/articles/PMC5885289/

Reassure the woman that you will protect her confidentiality. Provide information on STIs in an open, nonjudgmental manner. Explain the importance, and benefits, of knowing results of the STI

Tact and Understanding Are in Order

It is best not to pressure the woman to reveal risky behaviors. Instead, you can make her aware of behaviors that increase her risk of contracting an STI.

tests so that treatment can be started. Determine the woman's understanding regarding how to protect herself from an STI. Inform her of the need to let her sexual partners know about any positive test results so they can seek treatment as well.

Therapeutic communication is an important nursing intervention to use when talking to the client about STIs. Maintain an open, accepting demeanor when interacting with the woman. Ensure she is in a comfortable, private place before interviewing her. Avoid asking potentially embarrassing questions in the presence of others. Avoid negative criticisms and judgmental questions such as "Why didn't you…?" or "You should have…" Ask questions to determine the woman's understanding of the risk of an STI to herself and to her fetus. Encourage the woman to verbalize her feelings. Use active listening. Ask for clarification when you do not understand.

The history should include questions and a physical exam regarding symptoms of STI including vaginal discharge, painful sex, bleeding during or after sex, swollen lymph nodes, low-grade fevers, rashes or skin lesions, and night sweats or lost weight.

Psychosocial issues to consider that affect the woman's compliance with the treatment plan include the following: substance abuse, psychiatric disorders, inadequate housing, support system, work conditions, and ability to pay for or acquire medications.

Nursing Care Focus

When selecting the nursing care focus for the pregnant woman who may have an STI, it is important to determine the woman's knowledge level regarding STIs, determine her understanding of the treatment plan, and risk to the fetus if the infection is not treated.

Outcome Identification and Planning

Goals for a pregnant woman with an STI include minimizing risk to the woman and fetus from the infection, initiating treatment for the infection, preventing the spread of the infection, and providing the woman with adequate knowledge regarding the cause and prevention of STIs.

Nursing Care Focus

● Infection risk

Goal

● The woman will verbalize how STIs are transmitted.

Implementations for Infection Risk

Provide the woman with information related to the risks of contact with infected bodily fluids and blood. Clarify that women are at higher risk than are men for contracting an STI during heterosexual intercourse. Make clear that the highest risk of STI transmission is engaging in any type of sexual activity without a condom. Emphasize the importance of using a latex condom for every act of sexual intercourse, including anal sex, and a latex barrier for oral sex. Inform the woman to avoid sexual intercourse, including oral or anal sex, when there are open lesions or discharge on the mouth or genitals of her partner or herself.

The woman needs to know that infection with one STI puts her at higher risk for contracting another STI. This is particularly true for STIs that cause lesions or skin breakdown. Explain the importance of having all sexual partners treated for the infection. The pregnant woman with an STI should take her medication as prescribed.

Evaluation of Goal/Desired Outcome

The woman:

● is able to describe actions she can take to protect herself from contracting or transmitting STIs.
● will verbalize how to obtain and use a condom.
● remains free of additional infections.

Nursing Care Focus

● Knowledge deficit related to STI's

Goal

● The woman will state the signs of an STI and how an STI is treated.

Implementations for Reinforcing Teaching

Provide the woman with information on how an STI is transmitted, what the symptoms of infection are, how to avoid spreading the infection to her sexual partners, how to decrease the risk of transmitting the infection to her fetus, and what her treatment plan and goals are.

Verify understanding of the treatment regimen by asking the woman to describe the medications she is taking and when and how she is to take them. Have her explain the expected action of each medication, as well as side effects. Instruct her to immediately report side effects she experiences. Explain the importance of completing the full course of treatment even after symptoms subside to prevent the development of resistant strains of the organism.

Give factual information. Correct any misperceptions or misinformation the woman may have. Use up-to-date facts from reliable sources to avoid false reassurances. Help her understand the disease without causing unnecessary fear, and emphasize the positive. For example, for the woman who has HIV, you can explain that more than 98% of babies born to women with HIV who receive appropriate treatment will be born free of infection and will remain so.

Evaluation of Goal/Desired Outcome

The woman:

● verbalizes the signs of an STI.
● explains how an STI is transmitted.
● describes how to prevent transmission to sexual partners and decrease the risk of transmission to the fetus.
● verbalizes understanding of her treatment regimen.

TEST YOURSELF

✔ Which infection is best prevented by instructing the pregnant woman to avoid changing the cat litter box?

✔ Which STI is most frequently diagnosed with a wet mount?

✔ When should a rubella nonimmune woman receive the rubella vaccine?

PREGNANCY COMPLICATED BY INTIMATE PARTNER VIOLENCE

Intimate partner violence (IPV) is abuse perpetrated by an individual against an intimate partner. The goal of the abusive behavior is to exert and maintain power and control over the partner. Abuse refers to any type of injury committed against a person, including physical, emotional, psychological, and sexual maltreatment (Box 16-8). An intimate partner is any person who is or who has been in an intimate relationship with the victim and includes present and former spouses, boyfriends, girlfriends, and dating partners. IPV occurs in relationships without regard to sexual preference. In other words, IPV occurs between same-sex partners, as well as between heterosexual partners. IPV occurs in all social, cultural, religious, and economic boundaries. Other terms used to describe IPV are domestic violence, spouse abuse, domestic abuse, and battering.

It is difficult to determine the extent of IPV, partly because it is unknown how many cases of IPV go unreported. Varied definitions used to collect and report these data contribute to the confusion. Although men can be the victims of IPV, more women report abuse. Pregnancy is a vulnerable time for a woman. IPV may begin or escalate during pregnancy, particularly if the pregnancy is unplanned. Researchers estimate that 4% to 8% of all pregnant women experience abuse during the pregnancy, and some victims may even die as a result of the abuse. The pregnant woman is at risk for certain complications associated with abuse. A pregnant woman who is a victim of domestic violence is at a risk of antepartum hemorrhage, fetal growth restriction, fetal death, preterm labor, and low birth weight of her infant.

Clinical Manifestations

Abuse may begin slowly and escalate with time, or abusive episodes may begin early in a relationship. The cycle of violence (Fig. 16-3) explains the behaviors and patterns associated with IPV. Abuse usually progress in three identifiable phases:

1. Tension-building phase
2. Explosion phase
3. Absence of tension or the "honeymoon phase"

Although it is not always possible to identify IPV during interactions with the victim, there are signs that might indicate

BOX 16-8 Examples of Abusive Acts

The terms "abuse" or "abused" are often misunderstood to refer only to egregious acts of violence that result in serious physical injury. Therefore, it is important for the health care professional to give specific examples of abuse when screening for intimate partner violence (IPV).

Physical Acts of Abuse
- Punching
- Hitting
- Kicking
- Slapping
- Shoving
- Biting
- Scratching
- Grabbing
- Choking
- Poking
- Shaking
- Hair pulling
- Burning

Emotional Acts of Abuse
- Threats of harm to self, the victim, pets, or others
- Refusing to interact with the victim without explanation ("silent treatment")
- Name calling
- Put-downs or derogatory comments (Example: "You're so ugly," or "You're not smart enough to get a job.")
- Any act of control
  - Financial (controlling all the money)
  - Decision making (without consulting the victim)
  - Isolating victim from family or friends
  - Prohibiting victim access to transportation or telephone
  - Preventing victim from reading text messages or listening to voicemail
- Threatening or completing acts of violence against pets or children
- Destroying property the victim cares about
- Blaming the victim for the abuser's violent outbursts

Sexual Acts of Abuse
- Forcing the partner to watch or perform any sexual act against their will

IPV. The abuser often exhibits an overly protective attitude toward the victim, may accompany the victim to all office visits, and may answer questions for the victim. It is important to remember that the abuser may seem pleasant and congenial. Conversely, they may make degrading remarks about the victim in front of health care providers or others. Be suspicious if the partner refuses to leave the room so that the client cannot be alone. If this happens, look closer for other signs of abuse and immediately notify the RN and the health care provider of your observations. The victim may appear quiet and passive. She may avoid eye contact. She may have an unkempt appearance and may appear depressed. She may exhibit anxiety, nervousness, and suicidal tendencies. She may abuse alcohol or drugs in response to the abuse. Box 16-9 lists signs that should raise the suspicion of abuse.

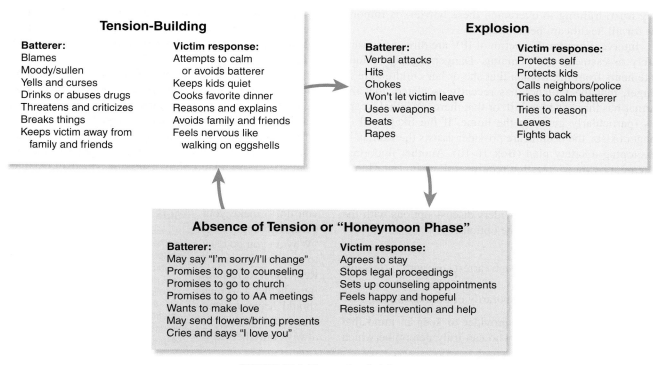

FIGURE 16-3 The cycle of violence.

BOX 16-9 Signs That May Indicate IPV

It is important to remember that a victim who is being abused may not show obvious signs of abuse. Any of the following signs should raise the suspicion of possible intimate partner violence (IPV):
- History of:
  - repeated assaults
  - drug or alcohol abuse
  - depression
  - suicide attempts
- Injury (bruises, scrapes, scratches, or cuts, as well as burns, broken bones, etc.) to the head, face, or neck
- Loose or broken teeth
- Injury to the breasts or abdomen
- Types of injury to include:
  - injury inflicted by a weapon
  - cigarette and rope burns
  - bite marks
  - bruises and welts

- Pattern and distribution of injury to include:
  - injuries on areas normally covered by clothes
  - injuries occurring on both sides of the body (often on extremities)
  - defensive posture injuries (such as to the hands or feet that occur when the victim tries to ward off the attacker)
- Injuries in various stages of healing
- Injuries that do not match the cause of trauma described by the individual or their partner

Signs unique to the pregnant client may include the following:
- Presenting for late prenatal care or having no prenatal care
- Attending prenatal visits sporadically
- High gravidity and parity rates
- Poor weight gain during pregnancy
- History of:
  - early pregnancy loss
  - STIs
  - previous fetal death

Screening and Interventions

Because every woman is at risk for IPV, routine screening of all women is the key to identifying victims and assisting those who are ready to report abuse and receive help. Routine screening and direct questioning about abuse increases the likelihood that the abuse will be detected. In particular, the prenatal period presents an excellent opportunity for screening for IPV. Prenatal visits offer frequent opportunities for the health care provider to develop rapport and trust with the woman. The perinatal period is also a unique time of opportunity because the woman may

be motivated to think about the future and the safety of her unborn child.

Although screening is a powerful tool, common barriers may get in the way. The health care provider may feel that there is not enough time to ask about IPV or may be uncomfortable addressing the issue. The provider may be afraid of embarrassing or offending the woman. Many times, providers avoid screening because of personal feelings or prior encounters with IPV victims. Because screening is a critical intervention for the victim of IPV, and because a victim may confide in a healthcare person they trust, training to overcome these barriers is important for all healthcare personnel.

Interventions for the victim of IPV are directed toward safety assessment and planning. Danger signals include statements from the woman that she or her children are in danger, that the violence has recently escalated, that the partner has threatened to kill, or that there are lethal weapons (particularly guns) in the home. If the likelihood of danger exists, the health care provider assists the woman in developing a safety plan (Box 16-10). Another important statement by the victim that requires follow up is, "Things will be all better now," as victims of IPV are at increased suicide risk.

Trained health care providers discuss options with the woman. The woman has three options:

- Stay with the abuser.
- Remove the abuser through arrest or with protective orders.
- Leave the relationship temporarily or permanently.

It is important for the provider to keep in mind that the woman is the only one who can truly determine which option is best for her.

Nursing Care

There are many reasons that it is difficult to discuss domestic violence with clients. Myths abound, such as IPV happening only in certain socioeconomic or ethnic groups or that the woman could just leave if she were not so weak or codependent. Often a nurse's own discomfort leads to avoidance of the subject. Health care providers may feel powerless to do anything about the situation and therefore do not bring up the subject, or they may lack knowledge about how to screen for abuse. Whatever the barrier, you can learn to screen pregnant women for IPV.

Always screen the woman alone, away from children and the abuser. Provide privacy. Ask simple, direct, open-ended questions in a nonjudgmental way to show the victim that you are a safe person when she is ready to disclose such information. Avoid questions that imply that the woman is responsible for the violence or that it is easy to walk away from a violent relationship. Questions to avoid include, "Why do you not just leave?" or "What did you do to make your partner so angry?" or "Why do you go back to your partner?" Remember, determining whether a woman should leave an abusive relationship is always only her decision to make.

It Is Better to Err on the Side of Caution

If you suspect or are unsure if the woman is a victim of IPV, it is better to report your suspicions of abuse to an RN or the health care provider. However, do not allow your discomfort with the subject to hinder you from learning how to screen for violence.

Always document the woman's responses to questioning about IPV. If the woman denies being in an abusive relationship, document her denial. It is important to quote the woman directly. Do not use terms such as "alleges" when you are documenting the woman's replies. This terminology may cast doubt on the truthfulness of the woman's answers if the medical record becomes evidence in a court of law.

If the woman discloses IPV, be careful to respond with supportive statements. One of the most important things you can communicate to the victim of abuse is the fact that the abuse is not her fault. You can say, "This is not your fault. No one deserves to be treated this way." Examples of other helpful statements include, "I'm sorry that you've been hurt," or "I am concerned for your safety," or "You have options. Help is available."

Document your data collection objectively. If there are physical indications of abuse, draw these on a body map, then use measurable terminology to describe each lesion or observation. Photographs can be invaluable aids in a courtroom. You must get the woman's written consent before photographing her.

Be knowledgeable about local resources that are available for the victim of IPV. Resources include office and hospital personnel with specialized training, IPV advocacy groups, women's shelters, hotlines, child protective services, and law enforcement resources.

By showing compassion and developing the trust of the abused woman, you can help break the cycle of abuse. Recovery from IPV does not happen in only one or two interventions; rather, a consistent atmosphere of encouragement and esteem building may assist the victim in becoming a survivor. For some victims, it may take years to leave the abusive relationship.

BOX 16-10 Components of a Safety Plan

Whether or not the client elects to stay in the abusive relationship, they should have a safety plan. The safety plan includes that the client should:

- Memorize the National Domestic Violence Hotline: 1-800-799-SAFE (7233) or 1-800-787-3224 (for hearing-impaired or deaf victims).
- Pack a bag in advance with cash, credit cards, and clothes for them and any children. The bag should remain at a trusted friend or family member's house.
- Have important personal documents readily accessible. These include the following:
  - Birth certificates
  - Driver's license
  - Bank account information
  - Important telephone numbers
  - Insurance information and cards
  - Court documents or orders
  - Copies of utility bills
- Establish a code word with family and friends to indicate when violence is escalating and help is needed.
- Identify a safe place to go. This may be a shelter or other safe place. Each community has unique resources that should be identified for the client.

PREGNANCY COMPLICATED BY AGE-RELATED CONCERNS

The typical childbearing years include the ages of 15 through 44 years; however, females can and do become pregnant anywhere from ages 9 to 56 years. At either end of the age spectrum, pregnancy carries higher risk for morbidity and mortality for the woman and her fetus. Although age-related concerns warrant special "at-risk" considerations, they are not in the pathophysiologic category, as are the medical conditions discussed earlier in the chapter. Instead, they are a natural part of the reproductive process requiring additional monitoring throughout the perinatal period.

Adolescent Pregnancy

Adolescent, or teen, pregnancy is pregnancy occurring at 19 years of age or younger. The consequences of pregnancy in this age group are well documented. Young mothers tend to have lower education levels and higher levels of poverty, and are more likely to participate in behaviors that increase the risk for poor birth outcomes, such as smoking; late, sporadic, or no prenatal care; and failure to gain sufficient weight. The pregnant adolescent is more likely to experience pregnancy complications, such as preeclampsia. Infants of adolescent mothers are more likely to be below normal birth weight, be premature, and have a higher neonatal mortality rate than do infants of older mothers (Chacko, 2020).

Adolescent pregnancy and birth rates in the United States have steadily declined since 2009. In 2018 the birth rate among women ages 15 to 19 was 17.4 per 1,000 which was a decrease from 2017, which was 18.8 births per 1,000 (Martin, Hamilton, Osterman, & Driscoll, 2019). Racial disparities still exist in adolescent pregnancy and birth rates, with African Americans and Hispanics disproportionately affected (Chacko, 2020). In addition, in the United States there is not consistency in adolescent birth rates between the states.

Clinical Manifestations

Many pregnant adolescents either seek prenatal care later, often in the third trimester, or do not receive prenatal care altogether. Those that do receive care often return sporadically for prenatal visits. In addition to prenatal care, the social situation and maturity level of the pregnant adolescent, rather than age itself, place her at increased pregnancy risk. She is more likely to be unmarried, have less education, be a member of an ethnic minority, and live in poverty (Chacko, 2020).

There are many reasons the pregnant adolescent may receive inadequate prenatal care. She may be fearful of disclosing her pregnancy to her parents or caregivers and therefore may attempt to hide the pregnancy by wearing loose clothing and avoiding prolonged interaction with adults. Some adolescents are unaware of basic body physiology and she may therefore be unaware of the pregnancy. Some adolescents deny that they are, or could be, pregnant. She may lack family support or transportation to attend prenatal visits regularly. Because body image is extremely important

to the adolescent, she may use behaviors associated with eating disorders, such as purging or self-starvation, to avoid weight gain during the pregnancy. She may have inadequate nutrition secondary to poor food choices. There is increasing evidence that pregnant adolescents are at increased risk for domestic violence. Whatever the reason for not receiving adequate prenatal care, the pregnant adolescent is at increased risk for complications, such as inadequate weight gain, anemia, and preeclampsia–eclampsia. All of these conditions can result in fetal complications, such as intrauterine growth restriction (IUGR), low birth weight, and preterm birth.

Diagnosis of adolescent pregnancy is made with the same tests used for other women. However, the diagnosis can be missed if the health care provider does not keep in mind the possibility of pregnancy when performing a history and physical examination on the adolescent. Adolescents often deny the possibility of pregnancy (even to themselves), making diagnosis even more challenging. A pregnancy test should be done if the adolescent reports irregular periods, nausea and vomiting, or fatigue.

Treatment

The best treatment for adolescent pregnancy is prevention. Many health care providers are actively involved in programs designed to prevent adolescent pregnancy. Others are involved in research studies attempting to discover which methods work and which do not. Much of the literature on adolescent pregnancy concentrates on prevention.

It is important to obtain information about any pregnant woman's physical and psychological responses to pregnancy and the social support available to her. This component of the history is vital to collect for the pregnant adolescent. If the adolescent does not have adequate social support, she is more likely to experience adverse outcomes. Areas to discuss include her perception of options available to her, risk factors for STIs, and school plans. Because perinatal and postpartum depression and intimate partner violence (IPV) are associated with adolescent pregnancy, it is particularly important to screen for these as well.

An important role for nurses and health care providers caring for the pregnant adolescent is to be her advocate, which includes giving information in an open, nonjudgmental way and supporting her choices. This treats the adolescent with dignity and respect, provides for and protects her right to privacy and confidentiality, and allows the adolescent to make choices without coercion.

 Cultural Snapshot

Remember that each adolescent is an individual. Her culture influences her beliefs and values. Plan interventions based on her unique needs. Different cultures may have different acceptable ages for pregnancy. Young brides may be acceptable in some cultures.

One crucial part of management includes helping the adolescent develop an adequate support network. Parents, teachers, friends, and the father of the infant are all potential resources for the pregnant adolescent. These individuals may benefit from guidance on ways they can effectively help.

Nursing Care

Caring for Developmental Needs

Keep in mind the developmental needs of the pregnant adolescent. Pregnancy does not change the developmental tasks, although it may complicate the issues. According to Erikson (1963), developing an identity is an essential developmental task during this age. It is important to help the pregnant adolescent work on identity issues while she also begins to adapt to the role of motherhood.

As with others in this age group, the pregnant adolescent's normal priorities include acceptance by her peer group and focusing on appearance. In addition, the adolescent, particularly the very young adolescent, is typically self-centered, a characteristic that can make it difficult for her to consider the needs of others. Take into account these priorities and characteristics as you plan your nursing care.

Caring for Physical Needs

Adequate nutrition is essential to the health of the pregnant adolescent. However, nutritional considerations may not be a high priority for her. Assist in identifying healthy foods that are appealing and easy to prepare. It may help to determine what foods she normally eats and then suggest healthier alternatives. For instance, rather than forbidding desserts, help the adolescent choose desserts that have nutritional value, such as fresh fruit or frozen yogurt. You might suggest that she eat low-salt tortilla chips, baked potato chips, or whole-grain crackers rather than regular potato chips.

Cultural Sensitivity is in Order

Do not forget that culture influences food choices. Be sure that you understand the adolescent's cultural context when you counsel her regarding prenatal nutrition.

Pregnant adolescents are at higher risk for delivering prematurely, particularly if they experience a repeat pregnancy during their teen years. One way to help decrease the risk of a repeat pregnancy is to counsel the adolescent regarding birth control methods. STIs are another potential risk. Encourage the use of barrier methods of birth control, in particular male use of latex condoms, which supply protection from STIs.

Caring for Emotional and Psychological Needs

The emotional and psychological needs of the adolescent are complex. With the added emotional demands of pregnancy, the strain can be tremendous. The pregnant adolescent is at an increased risk for suicide. It is frequently helpful to include significant support people in the care planning. It is

easier for them to provide meaningful support if they know how pregnancy might affect emotional functioning.

Be knowledgeable regarding community resources for the pregnant adolescent. If referrals for other services are made, follow up to make certain the adolescent receives the services for which she was referred. If she does not, determine the barriers to care that exist, if any. Assist her to work through the barriers to obtain needed services.

Remain nonjudgmental and open-minded when dealing with pregnant adolescents. Scolding, scare tactics, and punishment are not helpful interventions. These measures tend to push the adolescent away and do little to resolve the real issues with which she must deal with.

Pregnancy in Later Life

Although adolescent birth rates have declined over time, births for women older than 50 have risen. Assisted reproductive techniques have enabled women to become pregnant at a later age (Fretts, 2019).

There are risk factors that are associated with childbearing for the woman over 35 years of age. For women, fertility naturally declines with age. Although assisted reproductive technology is much more effective than it was in the past, there is a higher incidence of multiple fetal pregnancies (i.e., twins, triplets) when these technologies are used to help a woman get pregnant. A woman older than 35 years is more likely to conceive a child with chromosomal abnormalities, such as Down syndrome. She is also at higher risk for early pregnancy loss (miscarriage), preeclampsia, gestational diabetes, preterm delivery, bleeding and placental abnormalities, and ectopic pregnancy. She has a higher risk than a younger woman of having a fetal demise, cesarean delivery, or a low–birth-weight infant (Fretts, 2019). It is helpful to remember that the majority of pregnancies to women older than 35 years end with healthy babies and healthy mothers.

Clinical Manifestations

In general, the woman who has a child in her late 30s or early 40s has more education than her younger counterparts do. She may have chosen to postpone childbearing or may have been dealing with fertility issues. She is most likely to be married, to have financial resources, and to have planned the pregnancy. She is also more likely to have a chronic condition, such as diabetes or hypertension.

Some women over 35 years of age report more discomforts during pregnancy, whereas others do not. If she is physically fit, it is less likely that the pregnancy will cause excessive tiredness and distress. The hormonal changes of pregnancy are often a cause of facial skin breakouts, even for a woman in this age group.

Treatment

A preconception visit is recommended for any woman who wishes to become pregnant. For the woman over 35 years old, it is especially important that she have a complete physical examination before becoming pregnant, particularly if she has a chronic medical condition. Because it may be more difficult for her to conceive, fertility experts recommend that she seek medical help if she is not pregnant within 6 months of trying.

The woman over the age of 35 years old should be offered genetic testing and counseling. The miscarriage rate is higher as the woman ages, most likely because of chromosomal abnormalities of the conceptus. Trisomy 21 (Down syndrome), trisomy 18 (Edwards syndrome), and trisomy 13 (Patau syndrome) all occur with greater frequency as the woman ages. Genetic testing can be done by chorionic villus sampling or early amniocentesis. In addition, a high-level ultrasound in the second trimester may be done to screen for structural defects in the fetus.

Nursing Care

Approach the woman without bias and in a nonjudgmental manner. Be ready to answer questions and to suggest pregnancy and parenting resources. A woman who is pregnant after 35 years of age usually does not appreciate the label "older" pregnant woman, neither does she want constant reminders of the increased risks associated with late childbearing. If the woman complains of receiving "rude" remarks from strangers about her age, suggest that it is OK to ignore such remarks. If she has a good sense of humor, she may be able to make a joke out of the situation.

 A Personal Glimpse

My husband and I married in our late 20s. We decided to wait until we were both in our 30s to have children because we had lots of school loans to pay off and wanted to be financially secure before raising a family.
I got pregnant with my daughter when I was 33. It was a normal pregnancy; I felt great, and the baby and I were completely healthy throughout. When Libby was 3 years old, we decided to try and have another baby. I conceived easily and eagerly made my first doctor appointment to officially confirm the pregnancy. I assumed that this pregnancy would be as uncomplicated as my first. Imagine my surprise when I sat down with the nurse and she started grilling me about the potential for genetic problems and health problems in my baby because I was over 35 years old. She started talking about the need for me to have special blood tests and an amniocentesis. It was all rather overwhelming and scary. I was shocked. How could 3 years make such a difference in the way that my pregnancies would be managed?

Julia

Learning Opportunity: *How can the nurse present information to the woman at risk without increasing her anxiety level? Does the risk level dramatically increase at the age of 35? Why or why not?*

Provide information tailored to the needs of the woman. Encourage her to discuss her concerns and questions at each visit. It is also helpful to review the sources of her information and help her decide if these sources are credible.

TEST YOURSELF

✔ True or false? IPV occurs only in heterosexual relationships.

✔ List three components of a safety plan for a victim of IPV.

✔ Name two dysfunctional behaviors the pregnant adolescent might use to keep from gaining weight during pregnancy.

Remember **Melissa Hightower** from the start of the chapter. She was 18 years old and in her second trimester of pregnancy but had not started prenatal care and had signs of a yeast infection. What further complications could Melissa and her fetus be at risk for, especially if her current health practices are not changed? What tests/treatments do you think will be ordered for Melissa? Why would those tests/treatments be done?

KEY POINTS

- The three major classifications of diabetes in the pregnant woman are diabetes mellitus (DM), type 1 and type 2 and gestational diabetes mellitus (GDM). The pancreas of the woman with type 1 DM does not produce insulin, so she must receive insulin. The woman who requires insulin can self-inject insulin or use an insulin pump. The cornerstone of therapy for GDM is diet therapy.

- Care for the woman with pregestational diabetes includes glycemic control to prevent or minimize fetal consequences from hyperglycemia. Glucose levels are determined by finger stick measurements and measuring glycosylated hemoglobin (HbA_1C). Care also includes diet therapy and ongoing fetal surveillance.

- Fetal surveillance is critical for the pregnant woman with any classification of diabetes. Monitoring fetal growth is done to observe for macrosomia. Fetal activity counts and nonstress test (NST) are done to determine fetal well-being. Amniocentesis to determine fetal lung maturity in the third trimester may help determine the optimum time for delivery.

- Nursing interventions for the pregnant woman with diabetes include monitoring the therapeutic regimen and screening for maternal and fetal injury risk, the woman's risk for infection, and fetal macrosomia.

- The main goal of treatment for the pregnant woman with heart disease is prevention and early detection of cardiac decompensation. Nursing interventions include monitoring activity levels, managing stress, diet modification, and medication therapy.

- Iron-deficiency anemia requires iron supplementation and a diet high in iron-rich foods. Iron supplements are best absorbed with vitamin C. Because iron supplements may predispose the woman to constipation, inform her about the importance of adequate hydration, exercising regularly, and consuming plenty of fiber in her diet.

- Preventing a crisis is the goal of treatment for the woman with sickle cell anemia. Interventions involve maintaining adequate hydration, avoiding infection and stress, and getting adequate rest.

- Treatment considerations for the pregnant woman with asthma include reinforcing information the woman has had previously. The woman should continue taking her asthma medications during pregnancy. She should protect herself from asthma triggers and infection.

- Preconception care for the woman with epilepsy minimizes the risk to the woman and fetus and allows for stabilization on antiepileptic medications that cause lower risk to the fetus. The woman takes high-dose folic acid supplements before and throughout pregnancy to help prevent neural tube defects. Vitamin K supplementation during the last weeks of pregnancy helps to prevent neonatal hemorrhage.

- TORCH stands for toxoplasmosis, other (hepatitis B, syphilis, varicella, and herpes zoster), rubella, CMV, and herpes simplex virus (HSV). These infections can lead to serious fetal anomalies and other complications. Prevention of infection is the best treatment strategy because many of the TORCH infections do not have effective treatment.

- The bacterium *Chlamydia trachomatis* causes chlamydia infection. Chlamydia spreads through sexual contact. It is frequently asymptomatic but easily treated with antibiotics. Chlamydia can increase the woman's risk for preterm labor.

- The bacterium *Neisseria gonorrhoeae* causes gonorrhea. Antibiotics treat the infection. Gonorrhea increases the risk of PID, early pregnancy loss, and preterm delivery.

- Human papillomavirus (HPV) is a virus that causes genital warts. The warts have a tendency to increase in size during pregnancy and can lead to heavy bleeding during delivery. The fetus can contract HPV through contact with vaginal secretions during birth.

- A protozoan causes trichomoniasis. Metronidazole given orally is the treatment of choice. Trichomoniasis can increase the woman's risk for preterm labor.

- The pregnant woman with HIV/AIDS can pass the infection to her unborn child during pregnancy or childbirth or while breast-feeding. Highly active antiretroviral therapy is prescribed to keep viral loads low throughout pregnancy. Breast-feeding is contraindicated.

- Nursing considerations for the pregnant woman with a sexually transmitted infection (STI) include informing the woman about her risk for additional infections and need for protection, risk for fetal complications from the infection, and her treatment plan. The pregnant woman with an STI is at an increased risk for preterm delivery.

- Nursing care for the woman who is a victim of intimate partner violence (IPV) includes screening of all pregnant women to identify victims of IPV. Interventions are directed toward safety assessment and planning. Development of a safety plan is a key intervention.

- The cycle of violence describes the typical pathophysiology of IPV. Tension building is followed by the explosion phase, which then leads to the honeymoon phase.

- Special concerns for the pregnant adolescent include prenatal care, screening for domestic violence, anemia, preterm delivery, and preeclampsia–eclampsia. Inquire about body image, as it is an important consideration that may lead to attempts to limit weight gain during pregnancy. Nutrition and social support are important areas for data collection with the pregnant adolescent.

- The impact of childbearing for women over 35 years old is an increased risk for complications of pregnancy. However, the woman is frequently mature, has a career, is financially stable, and married. Most pregnancies to older women end successfully with a healthy mother and a healthy child. Preconception care is ideal.

INTERNET RESOURCES

Gestational Diabetes and Pregnancy
http://www.mayoclinic.org/diseases-conditions/gestational-diabetes/basics/definition/con-20014854
http://www.diabetes.org/diabetes-basics/gestational/

Asthma and Pregnancy
https://www.aaaai.org/conditions-and-treatments/library/asthma-library/asthma-allergies-and-pregnancy

TORCH Infections and STIs
https://www.webmd.com/children/what-is-torch-syndrome#1
https://www.cdc.gov/std/pregnancy/stdfact-pregnancy.htm

HPV Vaccine
https://www.cdc.gov/hpv/parents/index.html

Intimate Partner Violence
www.thehotline.org

Workbook

NCLEX-STYLE REVIEW QUESTIONS

1. A woman presents to the prenatal clinic for her 28-week prenatal visit. She has gestational diabetes mellitus (GDM). Which type of diabetes does GDM *most* closely resemble?

a. Type 1
b. Type 2
c. Undetermined
d. Uncontrolled

2. A woman with class III heart disease is in for a prenatal visit. If she is in early heart failure, which sign is the nurse *most* likely to discover?

a. Audible wheezes
b. Persistent rales in the bases of the lungs
c. Elevated blood pressure
d. Low blood pressure

3. A 30-year-old gravida 1 has sickle cell anemia. She is not currently in crisis. Providing education on which topic is the highest nursing priority?

a. Avoidance of infection
b. Constipation prevention
c. Control of pain
d. Iron-rich foods

4. A 25-year-old woman is in for her first prenatal visit at 28 weeks' gestation. Which finding would cause the nurse to further investigate the possibility of intimate partner violence?

a. A calm demeanor
b. Bilateral pedal edema
c. A small bruise on her upper thigh
d. Multiple bruises in varying stages of healing

5. The LPN/LVN is assisting with the admission of a 28-year-old G1P1 at 37 weeks' gestation to the labor and delivery unit. Which of the following statements made by the woman should be reported to the RN? (select all that apply)

a. "I've been having irregular contractions since yesterday."
b. "This is my first pregnancy."
c. "I was treated for a yeast infection last week."
d. "I checked my blood sugar this morning and it was about 250."
e. "The baby has been very sleepy today."

STUDY ACTIVITIES

1. Use the following table to list and compare differences between gestational diabetes and type 1 diabetes during pregnancy.

	Gestational Diabetes	Type I Diabetes
Clinical presentation		
Treatment		
Nursing care		

2. Research the Internet to find at least five reliable websites that give client education information regarding sickle cell anemia.

3. Investigate your community for resources to help adolescents during pregnancy and parenting. Share your findings with your clinical group.

CRITICAL THINKING: WHAT WOULD YOU DO?

Apply your knowledge of medical conditions during pregnancy to the following situation.

1. Elizabeth, a 32-year-old gravida 2, has just received a diagnosis of gestational diabetes mellitus.

a. What test diagnoses the condition? What were the results of the test?
b. What risk factors for GDM may be present in Elizabeth's history?
c. Explain the priorities of care for Elizabeth during her pregnancy.

2. Tanya is 29 years old and has asthma. She is pregnant with her first child.

a. What will pregnancy likely do to Tanya's asthma severity?
b. Outline an information plan for Tanya.

3. Rachel is pregnant with her third child. Her HIV test just came back positive. Rachel says she does not know how she contracted HIV. She thinks it could have been from a blood transfusion she received after her last delivery.

a. What are the most common methods of HIV transmission? Name three risk factors for HIV.
b. What are the priorities of care for Rachel?
c. What medication will most likely be prescribed for her?
d. Rachel wants to know how best to protect her unborn child from the infection. How will you respond?
e. Rachel asks if her other children should be tested. How do you respond? Explain your response.

17

Pregnancy at Risk: Pregnancy-Related Complications

Key Terms

abruptio placentae
cerclage
cervical insufficiency
eclampsia
ectopic pregnancy
gestational hypertension
gestational trophoblastic neoplasia
hydatidiform mole
hyperemesis gravidarum
placenta previa
preeclampsia
proteinuria
salpingectomy
salpingitis
spontaneous abortion
vasospasm

Learning Objectives

At the conclusion of this chapter, you will:

1. Choose appropriate nursing interventions for the woman with hyperemesis gravidarum.
2. Explain the threat to pregnancy posed by ABO and Rh incompatibilities.
3. Describe clinical manifestations of ectopic pregnancy.
4. Compare and contrast the six types of spontaneous abortions.
5. Discuss the treatment for cervical insufficiency.
6. Explain treatment and nursing care for the woman experiencing a hydatidiform mole.
7. Compare and contrast placenta previa and abruptio placentae according to characteristics of bleeding and other clinical manifestations.
8. Apply the nursing process to the care of a pregnant woman with a bleeding disorder.
9. Differentiate four categories of hypertensive disorders in pregnancy.
10. Discuss treatment and nursing interventions for the woman with preeclampsia–eclampsia.
11. Contrast the management of a multiple gestation pregnancy with that of a singleton gestation.

Shakeba Winters is a 20-year-old gravida 1 para 0 who is in for her regular prenatal visit at 30 weeks. When you take her vital signs, you note that her blood pressure is 145/94. Her last visit was 2 weeks ago, and her blood pressure then was 140/90. Her urine specimen shows a protein value of 2+. She denies any pain or vaginal bleeding. As you read this chapter, identify gestational conditions Shakeba is at risk for. What observations would be most important for the nurse to make? If her condition worsens, what symptoms would be seen, and what nursing measures will be implemented?

Chapter 16 examined the effect of preexisting and acquired medical conditions on pregnancy. This chapter focuses on pregnancy-related conditions that place the woman and fetus at risk. The role of the licensed practical/licensed vocational nurse (LPN/LVN) includes identification of risk factors for pregnancy-related complications through both the client interview and data collection. Although the registered nurse (RN) must oversee the care for a woman with a complicated pregnancy, the LPN/LVN must be able to identify signs of complications and know

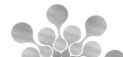

what problems need prompt intervention. An understanding of the basic pathology and clinical manifestations of these conditions will allow the nurse to intervene appropriately, update the woman about her condition and care, and answer questions confidently.

Do not forget or ignore the tremendous psychological and emotional impact of a complicated pregnancy. A complication that results in loss of the fetus can be devastating. The woman and her family will need support and guidance to help them cope with the loss. Sometimes the pregnancy complication puts the woman's life in danger, leaving the family to face difficult treatment choices. Often the risk to the mother of continuing the pregnancy must be weighed against the risk to the fetus if they are delivered early. This chapter highlights information you will need to provide basic physiologic and emotional care for the woman with an obstetric-related complication of pregnancy.

HYPEREMESIS GRAVIDARUM

Hyperemesis gravidarum is a disorder of early pregnancy that is characterized by severe nausea and vomiting that results in weight loss, nutritional deficiencies, and electrolyte and acid–base imbalance. Hyperemesis occurs in less than 2% of pregnancies with a higher incidence among underweight and younger women (Ogunyemi, 2017). The disorder most often appears between 8 and 12 weeks' gestation and usually resolves by week 20. The exact cause is unclear, although there is an association between hyperemesis and high levels of human chorionic gonadotropin (hCG). The risk of hyperemesis is increased with a multiple gestation (pregnancy with more than one fetus), molar pregnancy, or when the woman has a history of hyperemesis gravidarum. Stress and psychological factors can contribute to the condition.

Clinical Manifestations

This disorder is distinguished from "morning sickness" because the nausea and vomiting are severe and result in dehydration, weight loss, and electrolyte imbalances, particularly hypokalemia. Acid–base imbalances may occur. Before the health care provider diagnoses hyperemesis gravidarum, other causes of nausea and vomiting need to be excluded, such as hepatitis, hyperthyroidism, and disorders of the liver, gall bladder, and pancreas. An ultrasound is done to rule out a molar pregnancy.

Clinical features of the disorder include symptoms of dehydration, such as poor skin turgor, postural hypotension, and elevated hematocrit. Although rare, esophageal tears or perforation can occur with ongoing, forceful vomiting. Prolonged starvation from severe or untreated hyperemesis can lead to thiamine deficiency and Wernicke encephalopathy, a severe neurologic disorder marked by inflammation and hemorrhage in the brain.

Treatment

Nonpharmacologic treatment is aimed at avoiding triggers such as odors, heat, and iron preparations and having the woman eat frequent, small meals; consume peppermint teas or candy; and eating cold foods that are not spicy or odorous. Alternative therapies such as hypnosis, acupressure, or acupuncture may help some women. Ginger, found in lollipops or teas, has shown to be beneficial (see the Cultural Snapshot).

 Cultural Snapshot

- Ginger is a herbal remedy commonly used to treat nausea. Some cultures consider ginger to be a "hot" herb that treats "cold" conditions. Although there is no information regarding possible adverse fetal effects during pregnancy, recent research demonstrates that ginger can reduce nausea significantly.
- Acupuncture/acupressure, specifically stimulation of the "P6 Neiguan point," located on the palmar aspect of the forearm above the wrist, has been shown to reduce nausea and vomiting in some women. Some researchers recommend this traditional therapy as a first-line treatment before prescribing antiemetic medications.

If the nausea and vomiting is unrelieved by nonpharmacologic measures and becomes severe, the woman may need to be hospitalized. Treatment at that time is directed toward correcting fluid, electrolyte, and acid–base imbalances. Hospitalization becomes necessary when severe dehydration is present. Normal saline or lactated Ringer solutions are typical intravenous (IV) solutions used to treat the dehydration. Additives may include glucose to give the woman an energy source so that the body does not break down protein and fat for energy. Potassium is added if the woman's potassium is low because untreated hypokalemia can lead to cardiac disturbances. Other electrolytes or multivitamins may be added to the IV fluids as indicated to correct imbalances.

The woman takes nothing by mouth (NPO) for the first 24 hours or until the vomiting stops. Pyridoxine (vitamin B$_6$) has been shown to be helpful in decreasing nausea and vomiting (Smith, Fox, & Clark, 2020). Often the combination of rehydration and pyridoxine is enough to control the vomiting. If pyridoxine does not help the nausea and vomiting, then a combination of pyridoxine and doxylamine may be tried. If those measures do not work, then antiemetics may be added to the regimen.

Antiemetics, if prescribed, are usually more effective when given on a regular, around-the-clock schedule versus as-needed (PRN) dosing. These medications are given by parenteral injection or via rectal suppository until the vomiting is under control. Once the vomiting has subsided, the woman can take antiemetics by mouth. Because many of these medications are in pregnancy category C (see Box 7-7), the health care provider must carefully weigh the benefits of using the drug against the possible harmful effects to the fetus.

In severe cases that do not respond to conventional treatment, the health care provider must consider additional measures. Steroid therapy is sometimes helpful for intractable (hard-to-treat) cases, or the woman may require enteral feeding or parenteral nutrition.

Once the vomiting has stopped, the treatment plan addresses nutrition. A clear liquid diet is given and then advanced, as tolerated, to a bland diet. A dietitian assists in determining caloric requirements. Many health care providers order thiamine supplements to prevent Wernicke encephalopathy.

Nursing Care

Monitor the woman for nausea and administer medications, as ordered. It is also important to observe the amount and character of emesis. Record intake and output, and weigh the woman daily. Monitor for signs of dehydration, such as poor skin turgor and weight loss. Check laboratory values. An elevated hematocrit is associated with dehydration. Observe potassium levels as ordered. Hypokalemia may result from severe vomiting, or hyperkalemia can occur with potassium supplementation. The woman may be placed on a cardiac monitor to observe for any cardiac arrhythmias. Monitor the fetal heart rate (FHR) at least once per shift. Remove or avoid any of the woman's triggers if possible. Immediately remove any emesis basis or bedside commodes.

After the vomiting has stopped, implement measures to promote intake. A relaxed, pleasant atmosphere is conducive to eating. The area for eating should be well ventilated and free of unpleasant odors. In addition, eating with others can promote intake. Instruct the woman to eat before or as soon as she notices that she is hungry, because an empty stomach aggravates nausea. Make every effort to provide foods that the woman enjoys. Carbohydrates, such as breads, cereals, and grains, are sometimes easier to tolerate than other food types. She should avoid foods high in fat because such foods may exacerbate nausea.

Not Too Much!
A small amount of food taken at frequent intervals is easier to tolerate than one large meal, particularly for someone who is experiencing nausea. Large quantities of fluids at one time should also be avoided.

Assist the woman with mouth care before and after meals. This reduces unpleasant tastes in the mouth, thereby encouraging intake and retention of food. In addition, it is a good idea to restrict oral fluids at mealtime to avoid early satisfaction of hunger before she consumes sufficient nutrients.

Observe family dynamics. Because psychological factors can contribute to this disorder, the woman may benefit from a psychiatric or social worker consult. Discuss with the RN regarding this possibility. It may be therapeutic to allow the woman to ventilate her feelings regarding the pregnancy, her condition, and the hospitalization.

BLOOD INCOMPATIBILITIES

Incompatibilities between the woman's blood and the fetus's blood can cause problems for the fetus. Normally the two bloodstreams never meet, but occasionally some type of trauma occurs that allows intermingling of the two bloodstreams. This situation is more likely to occur during invasive procedures, such as amniocentesis. The risk also increases during active labor or an early pregnancy loss (miscarriage), or when the placenta separates at birth. Two types of blood incompatibilities are Rh incompatibility and ABO incompatibility.

Rh Incompatibility

The Rho(D) factor is an antigen (protein) that is found on the surface of blood cells. When this factor is present on the blood cells, the individual is Rh-positive, and when the factor is lacking, the person is Rh-negative. If a woman who is Rh-negative is exposed to Rh-positive blood (e.g., through an incorrectly crossmatched blood transfusion) her immune system produces antibodies to fight the Rho(D) antigen. Once her body has produced antibodies to the Rho(D) factor, she is sensitized to Rh-positive blood, a condition referred to as isoimmunization.

The problem arises when an isoimmunized Rh-negative woman carries a fetus with Rh-positive blood. In this case, the isoimmunized woman's antibodies to the Rho(D) factor readily cross the placenta and attack the fetus's blood cells (that are Rh-positive). The fetus develops hemolytic anemia and often requires exchange transfusions in utero or shortly after birth. In years past, a woman who was Rh-negative often became sensitized while carrying her first child. Sensitization most often occurred during childbirth, when fetal blood can leak into the woman's bloodstream during delivery. Thereafter, with each subsequent pregnancy, the fetus with Rh-positive blood would develop hemolytic anemia, with the disease becoming increasingly severe with each subsequent pregnancy. Now, sensitization rarely occurs because the Rh-negative woman receives anti-D immune globulin within 72 hours of delivering an Rh-positive baby.

Clinical Manifestations

Routine blood and Rh typing during the first prenatal visit identify the woman at risk for Rh incompatibility. Antibody screening determines whether the woman is already sensitized. If sensitization has occurred (i.e., the antibody screen is positive), the woman will have no symptoms at all; however, the fetus may be severely affected. Amniocentesis or cordocentesis is done to diagnose and assess hemolytic disease in the fetus. If sensitization has not occurred (i.e., the antibody screen is negative), the woman will be instructed about treatment and prophylaxis with anti-D immune globulin.

Treatment

Anti-D immune globulin is a product derived from blood that prevents the Rh-negative woman from developing antibodies to the Rho(D) factor. It is critical for a woman who is Rh-negative to receive anti-D immune globulin after any invasive procedure (e.g., amniocentesis or chorionic villus sampling), trauma of any kind (e.g., motor vehicle collision or physical trauma), and delivery, whether it be by an abortion (elective termination of pregnancy), early pregnancy loss (miscarriage), removal of ectopic pregnancy, or vaginal or cesarean birth. It is during these times that fetal blood is most likely to contact maternal blood. Most health care providers also administer a prophylactic dose at 28 weeks of pregnancy.

If the woman is sensitized, she is not a candidate for anti-D immune globulin, and the fetus requires close observation. As the pregnancy progresses, fetal well-being is assessed with amniocentesis, cordocentesis, BPP, NSTs, or contraction stress tests. If hemolytic disease is severe, the fetus may require exchange transfusions or may be delivered to prevent further disease involvement (see Chapter 20 for discussion of hemolytic disease of the newborn).

It is important to note that Rh incompatibility does not occur if the woman is Rh-positive. It does not matter what the fetus's Rh factor is; if the woman is Rh-positive, she is not a candidate for anti-D immune globulin. An Rh-negative woman who delivers an Rh-negative child is not given anti-D immune globulin postpartum. Because the gene for Rh-negative blood is autosomal recessive, if the woman's partner is Rh-negative and she is Rh-negative, the fetus will be Rh-negative, and anti-D immune globulin will be unnecessary. The newborn is never a candidate for anti-D immune globulin.

Think of it This Way

Rh incompatibility can only exist if the woman is Rh-negative. First, determine the woman's blood type. If she is Rh-positive, then no further treatment is needed. If she is Rh-negative, treatment is only needed if the fetus is Rh-positive.

Nursing Care

Before discharging a woman after any invasive procedure, early pregnancy loss, abdominal trauma, abortion (elective termination of pregnancy), ectopic pregnancy, or childbirth, check her blood type. If there is a discrepancy between laboratory reports and the prenatal record, consult with the health care provider before proceeding. If the woman is Rh-negative, determine whether she is a candidate for anti-D immune globulin. The criteria for giving anti-D immune globulin are as follows:

- The woman must be Rho(D)-negative.
- The woman must not have anti-D antibodies (i.e., must not be sensitized).
- The infant must be Rho(D)-positive.
- In cases where the fetus's blood type is unknown (e.g., after an early pregnancy loss or abortion), it is assumed the fetus was Rho(D)-positive.
- Tests on maternal blood or performed on cord blood at delivery must indicate presence of antibodies.

If the woman is a candidate, administer the anti-D immune globulin after the provider has written the order and the woman has given informed, signed consent. Instruct her regarding the purpose and importance of anti-D immune globulin to subsequent pregnancies. Make certain that she understands under what circumstances she is to receive anti-D immune globulin in the future.

ABO Incompatibility

ABO incompatibility is another cause of hemolytic disease of the newborn (see Chapter 20). The problem most frequently arises when the woman's blood type is O and the fetus's blood type is A, B, or AB. Type O blood has naturally occurring antibodies against types A, B, and AB. These antibodies are large and generally do not cross the placenta. However, occasionally during pregnancy, fetal blood may leak into the maternal circulation, causing the woman's immune system to produce antibodies to fetal blood. These antibodies are smaller than the naturally occurring antibodies and readily cross the placenta, where they work to destroy fetal blood. Fortunately, this type of blood incompatibility usually results in a much less severe form of hemolytic disease than does Rh incompatibility. The neonate rarely requires exchange transfusions, although they will likely require treatment for jaundice.

Concept Mastery Alert

The neonate with type A/B/AB blood born to a type O woman is at increased risk for jaundice after birth.

TEST YOURSELF

✔ An elevation in what hormone is associated with hyperemesis gravidarum?

✔ Name two situations that place the fetus at increased risk for blood incompatibilities.

✔ What product is administered to an Rh-negative woman after she has delivered an Rh-positive fetus?

BLEEDING DISORDERS

Bleeding disorders can occur during early, mid, or late pregnancy. Bleeding disorders that occur during early pregnancy include ectopic pregnancy and early pregnancy loss. Although cervical insufficiency is not technically a bleeding disorder, it is discussed in this section because it is a cause of recurrent pregnancy loss in midpregnancy. Diagnosis of a molar pregnancy occurs most commonly in early pregnancy, but occasionally the condition is not identified until midpregnancy. Placenta previa and abruptio placentae are bleeding disorders that become apparent during late pregnancy. Bleeding disorders can lead to hemorrhage during pregnancy and the birth process. You must be alert to signs and symptoms of a bleeding disorder and notify the RN and health care provider if you suspect one. A prompt diagnosis may prevent the woman from experiencing hypovolemic shock from a bleeding episode.

Ectopic Pregnancy

The term "ectopic" refers to an object that is located away from the expected site or position. An **ectopic pregnancy** is a pregnancy that occurs outside of the uterus. The fertilized ovum implants in another location other than the uterus. The common term for this condition is "tubal" pregnancy. The majority of ectopic pregnancies implant in the fallopian tube; however, other sites, such as the abdomen, ovary, or cervix, can serve as implantation sites (Fig. 17-1). The current estimate is that approximately 0.5% to 1% of pregnancies become ectopic pregnancies and is the leading cause of maternal pregnancy-related death in the first trimester accounting for 4% to 10% of pregnancy-related deaths (Tulandi, 2020).

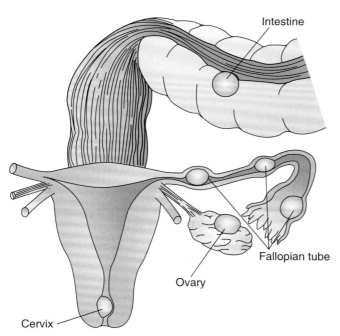

FIGURE 17-1 Possible implantation sites for an ectopic pregnancy.

Ectopic pregnancy occurs because some factor or condition prevents the fertilized egg from traveling down the fallopian tube, so it implants before it reaches the uterus. Adhesions, scarring, and narrowing of the tubal lumen may block the zygote's progress to the uterus. Any condition or surgical procedure that can injure a fallopian tube increases the risk. Examples include **salpingitis** (infection of the fallopian tube), endometriosis, pelvic inflammatory disease, history of prior ectopic pregnancy, any type of tubal surgery (e.g., tubal ligation reversal), congenital malformation of the tube, or multiple abortions (elective termination of pregnancy).

Clinical Manifestations

Symptoms usually appear 6 to 8 weeks after the last menstrual period, although the woman may not seek medical treatment until 8 to 12 weeks. The most commonly reported symptoms are pelvic pain and vaginal spotting. Other symptoms of early pregnancy, such as breast tenderness, nausea, and vomiting, may also be present or they may be less pronounced than an intrauterine pregnancy due to decreased levels of hCG.

Rarely, a woman may present with late signs, such as shoulder pain or hypovolemic shock. These signs are associated with tubal rupture, which occurs when the pregnancy expands beyond the fallopian tube's ability to stretch. The risk of tubal rupture increases with advancing gestation. Therefore, prompt diagnosis is critical to preventing rupture. If the tube ruptures, hemorrhage occurs into the abdominal cavity, which can lead to hypovolemic shock. Manifestations of shock include rapid, thready pulse; rising respiratory rate with shallow, irregular respirations; falling blood pressure; decreased or absent urine output; pale, cold, clammy skin; faintness; and thirst.

The diagnosis is not always immediately apparent because many women present with complaints of diffuse abdominal pain and minimal to no vaginal bleeding. Steps are taken to diagnose the disorder and rule out other causes of abdominal pain. A serum or urine pregnancy test is done to detect the presence of hCG. Transvaginal ultrasound is used to locate the gestational sac and is often diagnostic. Laparoscopy may be required to confirm the diagnosis.

Treatment

Management depends on the condition of the woman. If she presents in shock with abdominal bleeding from a ruptured tube, she requires immediate surgery for exploratory laparotomy, control of hemorrhage, and removal of the damaged tube. The surgeon leaves the ovaries and uterus intact if possible. The woman may need volume expanders and blood transfusions if massive hemorrhage occurs.

In nonemergent diagnosed cases of tubal pregnancy, the health care provider must decide how best to remove the pregnancy. Laparoscopic surgery is the most common method of removing an ectopic pregnancy. If the woman desires to have children in the future, an attempt to save the tube by using microsurgical techniques and minimally invasive surgery is done. A **salpingectomy**, removal of the fallopian tube, is performed when the tube is not salvageable or if the woman has finished childbearing. A newer method of treating a small, unruptured ectopic pregnancy is intramuscular injections of methotrexate, an antineoplastic (anticancer) drug. The medication works by interfering with DNA synthesis, which disrupts cell multiplication. Because the cells of the zygote are rapidly multiplying, methotrexate targets the pregnancy for destruction. Sometimes a single dose is sufficient, or multiple injections may be ordered. The advantage to this approach is avoidance of surgery on the tube. Regardless of the treatment method, the Rh-negative, nonsensitized woman requires anti-D immune globulin.

Think About This

Because surgery on a fallopian tube is a risk factor for ectopic pregnancy, treating an ectopic pregnancy with the anticancer drug methotrexate instead of with surgery can help prevent future ectopic pregnancies.

Nursing Care

Suspect ectopic pregnancy if the woman presents to the emergency department with abdominal pain and absence of menstrual periods for 1 to 2 months. Obtain a urine or blood specimen for hCG levels. Measure and record vital signs every 15 to 30 minutes. Observe for any sudden changes such as a drop in blood pressure or increase in pulse as these may be signs of shock. Monitor the amount and appearance of vaginal bleeding. Frequently monitor pain level, site, and quality. Immediately report heavy bleeding, signs and symptoms of shock, or change in pain level or quality to the health care provider or RN.

If surgery is necessary, assist the RN in preparing the woman. An IV line is started and laboratory testing done. At a minimum, a complete blood count and blood type and crossmatch are ordered. Check to see that the woman signs a written surgical consent and that the surgical preparatory checklist is complete.

Once the woman is in stable condition, emotional issues become the focus of nursing care. Be available for emotional support of the woman and her family. It is important to remember that the woman is grieving a loss, and each individual has her own way of expressing grief. Suggest outside sources of support, such as pastoral care or grief counseling.

Before discharge, instruct the woman regarding danger signs she should report including fever, severe abdominal pain, or a vaginal discharge with bad odor. Explain that weekly follow-up care with her health care provider is necessary to measure hCG levels. Discuss contraceptive options and advise the woman that she should not attempt pregnancy until her hCG levels have returned to nonpregnant levels. If the woman desires more children, explain the possibility of another ectopic pregnancy and review the symptoms of ectopic pregnancy. Encourage her to seek grief counseling or attend a support group after discharge.

Early Pregnancy Loss

Early pregnancy loss (EPL) is the most common complication of pregnancy. A clinical term used to describe early pregnancy loss is **spontaneous abortion**, which is the loss of a pregnancy before 20 weeks of gestation, which in lay terms is often called a miscarriage.

The rate of EPL is difficult to determine because many losses occur before the woman realizes she is pregnant. The rate of EPL when the woman is known to be pregnant is 10% and they mostly occur during the first trimester (Prager, Micks, & Dalton, 2021). Factors that increase the risk for EPL include advancing maternal age, history of previous EPL, smoking, alcohol and substance abuse, increasing gravidity, uterine defects and tumors, active maternal infection, intimate partner violence, and chronic maternal health factors, such as diabetes and renal disease.

It is difficult to determine the exact cause of miscarriage. Frequently, multiple factors contribute, and many times the cause cannot be determined. There are three overall categories of causation: fetal, maternal, and environmental. Fetal factors are usually genetic in nature. In fact, the most common cause of EPL in the first trimester is chromosomal defects in the fetus. Faulty implantation and defects in the sperm or ovum are other fetal-related causes. There are multiple maternal-related causes. Some examples are advanced maternal age, autoimmune diseases, uterine anatomic abnormalities and fibroids (leiomyomas), cervical incompetence, infection, endocrine dysfunction, and coagulation disorders. Environmental factors include poor nutrition; exposure to tobacco, chemicals, or radiation; and use of alcohol, street drugs, or certain prescription drugs.

Some authorities classify EPL according to the timing of the loss. Early spontaneous abortion occurs before 12 weeks, and late spontaneous abortion occurs between 12 and 20 weeks. Fetal factors typically cause early spontaneous abortion, whereas maternal factors tend to cause late spontaneous abortion.

Be Sensitive!

It is best to use the term "miscarriage" or "early pregnancy loss" when talking to clients about spontaneous abortion because the term "abortion" carries negative connotations for some people.

Clinical Manifestations

Typical symptoms of EPL include cramping and spotting or frank bleeding, which can be severe. The woman may expel blood clots or tissue. Abdominal and suprapubic pain are common and may radiate to the lower back, buttocks, and perineum. Fever and chills are associated with sepsis.

TABLE 17-1 Comparison of Spontaneous Abortion Types

ABORTION TYPE	CLINICAL MANIFESTATIONS	TREATMENT
Threatened abortion	Vaginal bleeding or spotting; possibly cramping; no cervical dilatation. Symptoms may resolve and the pregnancy may progress to term, or threatened abortion can lead to one of the other types	Vaginal rest (e.g., no sexual intercourse, tampons, or douches); bed rest or light activity precautions. The woman is to report bleeding heavier than a normal menstrual period, accompanied by cramping or fever. She should save expelled tissue for examination by the health care provider
Inevitable abortion	Cramping and spotting or vaginal bleeding with cervical dilatation; amniotic fluid may leak	There are three treatment options: • Expectant management (wait for the miscarriage to occur on its own) • Misoprostol orally to induce contractions • Surgical removal of the pregnancy; the type of procedure performed depends largely on the gestational age. Dilatation and curettage (D&C) is the procedure of choice for pregnancies under 14 weeks (refer to "Induced Abortion" in Chapter 4)
Incomplete abortion	Some, but not all, of the products of conception are expelled. Most commonly, the fetus delivers, and the placenta and membranes are retained	Treatment is similar to that used for inevitable abortion
Complete abortion	All of the products of conception (fetus, membranes, and placenta) are expelled	Surgical procedures are usually unnecessary. The woman goes home with instructions to monitor for complications such as heavy or increased bleeding or fever
Missed abortion	The fetus dies, but remains in utero. Signs of pregnancy (e.g., nausea, breast tenderness) decrease, and the fundus does not grow as expected in a normal pregnancy and may regress (get smaller). No fetal heart tones are present	Ultrasound confirms the diagnosis. If the woman carries the dead fetus for longer than 4 weeks, the risk of hemorrhage is high; therefore, a coagulation profile is drawn. The uterus is surgically evacuated by D&C or medically by inducing labor with oxytocin or prostaglandin
Habitual (recurrent) abortion	The loss of three or more consecutive pregnancies before the fetus is viable	Attempts are made to determine and treat the cause. For example, cervical insufficiency is often a cause of habitual abortion

Spontaneous abortion occurs along a continuum: threatened, inevitable, incomplete, complete, and missed (Table 17-1). The definition of each category is related to whether or not the uterus is emptied, or for how long the products of conception are retained.

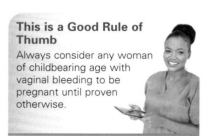

This is a Good Rule of Thumb

Always consider any woman of childbearing age with vaginal bleeding to be pregnant until proven otherwise.

To make the diagnosis, the health care provider often orders laboratory and imaging studies. An hCG level is drawn to confirm that the woman is pregnant. A complete blood count can identify anemia associated with blood loss and can provide evidence of infection. Blood typing is important to determine if the woman is Rho(D)-negative. Blood crossmatching and coagulation studies may be ordered in cases of severe blood loss. Urinalysis rules out a urinary tract infection. Transvaginal ultrasound is done to visualize the uterine cavity and determine if any products of conception are present and whether or not the embryo or fetus is alive.

Treatment

Treatment depends on which type of early pregnancy loss is occurring. Treatment for a threatened pregnancy loss is conservative because currently there is no specific therapy that can reliably prevent a threatened loss from progressing to spontaneous abortion. The health care provider often uses a "wait-and-see" approach. Usually rest and pelvic rest are ordered. Pelvic rest is where the woman does not place anything into the vagina and includes sexual intercourse, douches, or tampons. The woman should report heavy bleeding, cramping, or fever. Most other types of spontaneous abortion require some type of intervention, unless all the products of conception are expelled (complete abortion). The prostaglandin misoprostol may be given by mouth to induce uterine contractions. Vacuum aspiration or dilatation and curettage (D&C) are the most common surgical methods used to clear the uterus of the products of conception (see Chapter 4). After uterine evacuation, the health care provider often orders IV oxytocin or oral methylergonovine maleate to help prevent bleeding. Ibuprofen controls discomfort associated with uterine cramping.

Nursing Care

Record the woman's vital signs, amount and appearance of vaginal bleeding, and pain level. Count the number of perineal pads used or weigh perineal pads to monitor the amount of bleeding. Document whether or not the pad is saturated, and note if clots are present. Report a falling blood pressure and rising pulse, or other symptoms of shock, and an elevated temperature, which is associated with infection. If the pregnancy is greater than 10 to 12 weeks, the FHR should be checked with a Doppler device. Save all expelled tissue for evaluation by the health care provider. The health care provider will order the administration of anti-D immune globulin if the woman is Rho(D)-negative.

After the products of conception deliver, either spontaneously or through surgical intervention, continue to monitor vital signs and bleeding. Administer oxytocin or methylergonovine maleate as ordered to control bleeding. Provide analgesics as ordered and comfort measures to treat pain. Usually the woman may go home a few hours after vacuum aspiration or D&C if she is in stable condition. Tips for Reinforcing Family Teaching: Self-Care After Early Pregnancy Loss explains self-care at home.

Grief reactions are to be expected. Allow the woman and her partner or support person privacy to discuss their feelings with each other. Offer parents the opportunity to view the fetus if they desire. It is important to acknowledge the loss. Avoid nontherapeutic statements such as "You can always have more babies" or "It wasn't his time to be born,"

TIPS FOR REINFORCING FAMILY TEACHING

Self-Care After Early Pregnancy Loss (Miscarriage)

- Return for follow-up care if you experience any of the following danger symptoms:
  - Large amount of vaginal bleeding (soaking more than one pad in 1 hours)
  - Foul-smelling discharge
  - Severe pelvic pain
  - Temperature higher than 100.4°F (38°C)
  - Do not place anything in the vagina for approximately 2 weeks. Do not use tampons or douche and refrain from sexual intercourse
- Return for weekly health care provider visits to monitor hCG levels if ordered.
- Avoid sexual intercourse or use contraception until hCG levels become negative.
- You will likely experience intermittent menstrual-like flow and cramps during the week after miscarriage. Ibuprofen helps to control painful cramping.
- Resume regular activities when you feel well.
- Grief counseling is beneficial.

as these are hurtful to grieving persons. The woman must work through her feelings and come to terms with the current loss before it is helpful or appropriate to focus on future pregnancies.

This is Important!

If a woman is Rho(D)-negative, she should receive Rho(D) immunoglobulin any time a pregnancy is ended for any reason. The length of pregnancy or type of termination does not change this need.

The intensity and range of emotional responses of the woman experiencing an early pregnancy loss vary greatly. The woman may feel overwhelmed by grief. She may feel guilty that she might have done something to cause the pregnancy loss. She may express anger with a divine power for allowing her to lose the baby. Accept and support the woman's emotions. The woman needs ongoing grief support after discharge; be sure to refer the woman for this service.

♥ A Personal Glimpse

I was shocked when I found out I was pregnant with our fourth child. I was almost 40 years old and had an adolescent and two school-aged kids. At first, my husband and I were not eager to return to the days of sleepless nights and changing diapers. However, the idea of a sweet, new baby in our family grew on my husband and me, and our three kids were thrilled and excited. During the 10th week of my pregnancy, I started to have cramping and slight bleeding. I called my OB's office, and the nurse said to come to the office immediately. I called my husband at work and asked him to come home and take me to the doctor. While I was waiting for him to arrive, the cramping grew stronger and the bleeding grew heavier. I started to cry because I knew I was losing my baby. After examining me, my doctor confirmed my fear; I had experienced a miscarriage. I was told that the miscarriage wasn't complete and that they would have to do a procedure to remove what remained in my uterus. No one really explained the procedure to us, and I felt so lonely lying on the table. After the procedure, the nurse gave me some medicine for pain and made sure I was comfortable; she told me that I could probably go home in a few hours. Before leaving the room, the nurse turned to my husband and me and said, "I know this has been difficult for you, but you and your husband are very fortunate to have three children at home." Although she may have meant no harm, this nurse made me feel guilty for grieving the loss of this unexpected, but wanted pregnancy.

Elisabeth

Learning Opportunity: *In what ways can the nurse acknowledge that the loss of a pregnancy is a unique and deeply personal experience for the woman and her family? Describe helpful things the nurse can say when a woman has a miscarriage. Describe unhelpful responses.*

Cultural Snapshot

Culture often influences expressions of grief. Some cultures discourage displays of emotion, whereas others encourage dramatic expression of grief. You cannot determine the degree of grief by the presence or absence of emotional expression.

Cervical Insufficiency

Cervical insufficiency (formerly known as incompetent cervix) presents with painless cervical dilatation with bulging of fetal membranes and sometimes fetal parts through the external os. Cervical insufficiency occurs in the second trimester. Pregnancy loss is frequently inevitable. Cervical insufficiency is a leading cause of recurring midpregnancy loss.

The exact cause of cervical insufficiency is unknown, but there are several risk factors. Congenital defects in the reproductive tract, such as a short cervix or other structural abnormalities, increase the risk. History of trauma to the cervix is another risk factor for cervical insufficiency. Cervical trauma can be related to surgery (e.g., D&C, conization, or cauterization of the cervix) or childbirth, such as cervical lacerations and prolonged second stage of labor.

Standard treatment is cervical **cerclage** (Fig. 17-2), placement of a purse-string type suture in the cervix to keep it from dilating. Generally, cerclage is done between 14 and 26 weeks of gestation following a diagnosis of cervical insufficiency in a previous pregnancy. Sometimes emergent cerclage (procedure performed when the cervix is dilated and effaced) can maintain the pregnancy long enough for corticosteroids to enhance fetal lung maturity or to allow the fetus to mature to viability. The health care provider removes the suture when the pregnancy is at term or the woman goes into labor.

Gestational Trophoblastic Disease

Gestational trophoblastic disease includes two related diseases of trophoblastic tissue (the tissue that develops to form the placenta). These two conditions are **hydatidiform mole** or *molar pregnancy*, characterized by benign growth of placental tissue, and **gestational trophoblastic neoplasia**, malignancy of the uterine lining.

There are two types of molar pregnancies: partial and complete. Both types involve errors in chromosomal

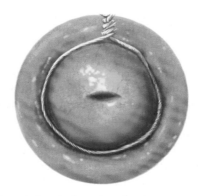

FIGURE 17-2 Cervical cerclage in place around cervix.

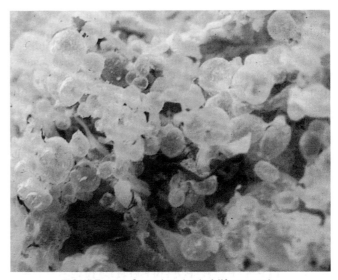

FIGURE 17-3 Complete hydatidiform mole.

duplication during fertilization. The consequence is grape-like (hydatidiform) swelling of the chorionic villi and trophoblastic hyperplasia; there may be no fetus (complete mole) (Fig. 17-3) or fetal tissue with chromosomal abnormalities (incomplete mole). A molar pregnancy has some features of a malignancy in that the trophoblastic tissue proliferates (multiplies) out of control. In fact, approximately 20% of women who experience a complete molar pregnancy develop gestational trophoblastic neoplasia within 6 months to 1 year after molar pregnancy (Burkowitz & Horowitz, 2020).

In the United States, the rate of hydatidiform mole is 1 per 1,200 pregnancies (Moore, 2018). A history of previous gestational trophoblastic disease increases the risk for a complete mole. Risk factors also include extremes of age; young women in their early adolescence and older women who are near the end of their reproductive lives are at highest risk. Women older than 40 years have a 5- to 10-fold increase in risk compared with younger women.

Clinical Manifestations

Before the widespread use of ultrasound, diagnosis of molar pregnancy occurred most frequently in the second trimester. Now the condition is diagnosed most often in the first trimester, before classic symptoms are evident. The most common presenting sign for both partial and complete moles is vaginal bleeding. Typically, the woman presents between 8 and 16 weeks' gestation with complaints of painless (usually) brown to bright red vaginal bleeding. The bleeding may be intermittent or continuous and can be severe. The hCG level is usually higher than expected for gestational age. Hyperemesis gravidarum can be caused by the higher than normal hCG levels. Transvaginal ultrasound reveals an intrauterine mass made up of many small cysts caused by grapelike vesicles that fill the uterus.

If a complete molar pregnancy continues into the second trimester undetected, other signs and symptoms appear. The woman often presents with complaints of dark to bright red vaginal bleeding and pelvic pain. Infrequently, she will report passage of grapelike vesicles. The physical examination may reveal a uterus that measures larger than expected for dates. Fetal heart tones are absent, and the examiner cannot detect fetal parts. Abdominal ultrasound reveals the characteristic tumor, and in 50% of the cases, there are giant ovarian cysts, which are the source of pelvic pain. Other findings include preeclampsia before the 24th week and hyperthyroidism (Moore, 2018).

Treatment

If the woman is hemorrhaging when she presents, the clinical team must move quickly to stabilize her condition. She requires IV volume expanders and blood transfusions. Clotting studies may be ordered to detect coagulation disorders that can develop as a complication of hemorrhage.

Once the woman is in stable condition, preparation for surgery begins. A chest x-ray is obtained as this is the most common site of metastasis. Blood samples are drawn to establish the baseline hCG level and to type and crossmatch the blood if this has not been previously accomplished.

Surgical treatment options include evacuation of the uterus by suction curettage if the woman wishes to have children in the future. Abdominal hysterectomy is the treatment of choice if the woman does not desire continued fertility. Labor induction techniques are not used because of the danger of hemorrhage. After the uterus is evacuated, anti-D immune globulin is given to the woman who is Rho(D)-negative.

Continuous follow-up for 1 year is extremely important. The woman returns to the doctor's office every 1 to 2 weeks to have hCG levels drawn. This monitoring is necessary to detect malignancy, which is highly treatable if caught early. Follow-up is important since one in five women with hydatidiform mole will develop cancer. The woman should avoid pregnancy for at least 6 months to a year after a molar pregnancy by using a highly reliable form of birth control such as oral contraception. The reason for this is that the woman is at increased risk for another molar pregnancy and the symptoms for molar pregnancy and a normal pregnancy are the same.

Nursing Care

The woman is at risk for several complications; therefore, it is important to watch her closely during the postpartum period. Frequently monitor for vaginal bleeding, and check the condition of the uterine fundus. Observe vital signs and the woman's level of consciousness because shock can result from hemorrhage caused by uterine atony or accidental perforation of the uterus during surgery. Oxytocin may be ordered for control of uterine atony. Methylergonovine maleate or carboprost tromethamine are other medications that may be ordered to stimulate the uterine muscle to contract.

Disseminated intravascular coagulation (DIC), a bleeding disorder related to lack of clotting factors, is another possible complication. Molar tissue releases substances that break down clotting factors, increasing the woman's risk for DIC. Review clotting studies for abnormal values, and monitor IV and injection sites for bleeding. Immediately report continual oozing from these sites.

Trophoblastic embolus or pulmonary edema secondary to fluid overload is a possibly fatal condition; therefore, every nursing exam should include a thorough observation of respiratory status and auscultation of the lung fields. Report immediately to the RN or health care provider respiratory distress or crackles in the lungs.

In addition to nursing measures directed at preventing hemorrhage and detecting respiratory distress, emotional support is an important nursing function. The woman has to cope with a complication of pregnancy that can cause severe illness, but a baby will not result from her ordeal. Tips for Reinforcing Family Teaching: Follow-Up Care After Molar Pregnancy lists important aspects of client education for a woman being discharged after treatment for a molar pregnancy.

TEST YOURSELF

✔ What procedure is used to treat cervical insufficiency?

✔ How is hydatidiform mole diagnosed?

✔ Name three important discharge education points for the woman who has experienced a molar pregnancy.

TIPS FOR REINFORCING FAMILY TEACHING

Follow-Up Care After Molar Pregnancy

- You will need to see your health care provider at frequent intervals for 1 year after termination of a molar pregnancy to check for cancer.
- Blood samples will be drawn at every visit to monitor serum hCG levels. Because rising hCG levels are associated with cancer, additional testing is necessary if your levels rise.
- Do not get pregnant for at least 6 months to a year after a molar pregnancy. This is important because hCG levels rise during pregnancy making it difficult to detect cancer if it develops.
- Immediately report unexpected or irregular vaginal bleeding because this could be a sign of developing cancer.
- Report severe persistent headaches, cough, or bloody sputum. These are symptoms of metastasis, which requires immediate, aggressive treatment.
- If you become pregnant in the future, be sure to tell your health care provider about the history of molar pregnancy. Although the overall risk is very small, you are at a higher than average risk to experience another molar pregnancy. A sonogram done early in the pregnancy allows for immediate treatment if needed.

Placenta Previa

Placenta previa is a condition in which the placenta is implanted close to or covers the cervical os. Normally, the placenta implants in the upper uterine segment. In placenta previa, the placenta implants in the lower part of the uterus. As the pregnancy progresses, blood vessels in the part of the placenta that covers the cervix rupture and cause vaginal bleeding.

The exact cause is not known. Any condition that could potentially scar or damage the uterus increases the risk. If scarring is present, the embryo may implant in a site that is more favorable for placental development. Conditions that increase the risk for placenta previa include history of abortions (elective termination of pregnancy), multiparity, advanced maternal age (older than 35 years), previous cesarean birth or uterine incisions, maternal smoking, and prior placenta previa. The condition occurs approximately 3.5 to 4.6 times for every 1,000 deliveries (Lockwood & Russo-Stieglitz, 2019).

Placenta previa is classified according to the degree to which the placenta covers the cervix. Total placenta previa occurs when the placenta completely covers the cervix. Total placenta previa is often associated with breech and transverse lie. It is thought that the abnormally located placenta prevents the fetus from assuming the expected head-down presentation. The term partial placenta previa is used if the placenta covers part of the cervix. Sometimes the placenta does not cover the cervix but is located on the border of the cervix; this condition is called marginal placenta previa. Figure 17-4 shows the three classifications of placenta previa. Sometimes a marginal or partial previa diagnosed early in the pregnancy becomes a normal implantation as the uterus enlarges. However, a complete placenta previa diagnosed in the second trimester rarely resolves to a normal implantation at delivery.

Clinical Manifestations

Painless, bright red bleeding that begins with no warning is a strong indicator of placenta previa. Bleeding may be light to severe and usually stops spontaneously. The bleeding starts before 30 weeks' gestation in about one third of women with placenta previa (Lockwood & Russo-Stieglitz, 2019).

For any pregnant woman who presents with painless bleeding, a digital examination of the cervix should not be done until placenta previa has been excluded by either transvaginal or abdominal ultrasound. This precaution is necessary because digital manipulation of placental tissue through the cervical os can cause uncontrollable bleeding. Usually

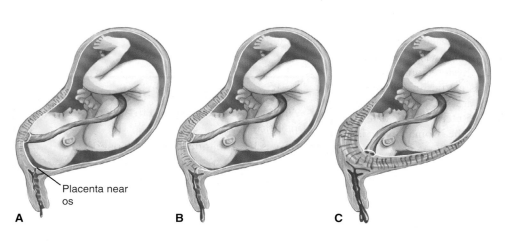

Placenta near os

A   B   C

FIGURE 17-4 Three classifications of placenta previa: **(A)** marginal, **(B)** partial, and **(C)** complete.

the first bleeding episode does not harm the fetus, unless it is unusually severe. The FHR should be within normal limits. In severe bleeding episodes, the fetus can become anemic, hypoxic, or develop hypovolemic shock because of blood loss and decreased oxygen transport across the placenta.

Be Careful!

Never assist with a vaginal examination on a pregnant woman who is bleeding until the health care provider is sure that there is no placenta previa. During the examination, the provider's fingers could penetrate the placenta, causing massive hemorrhage.

Treatment

If the initial bleeding episode does not stop or is massive, an immediate cesarean delivery is a life-saving measure for the woman and her fetus. If the initial bleeding episode stops and the fetus is still immature, hospitalization with bed rest is indicated. IV access is maintained, and at least 2 units of blood are placed on hold for immediate transfusion, if necessary.

If the woman is Rho(D)-negative, a Kleihauer–Betke test is performed to determine if fetal blood cells are in the maternal circulation, which indicates fetal–maternal hemorrhage. Anti-D immune globulin is injected for each bleeding episode to prevent isoimmunization (development of antibodies against Rho(D)-positive blood) in the pregnant woman.

Nonstress tests (NSTs) are ordered to monitor fetal well-being. Continuous electronic fetal monitoring (EFM) is required during acute bleeding episodes. In some instances, the woman is allowed to go home after the bleeding stops, but she must have someone with her at all times who can transport her immediately to the hospital if bleeding begins again.

TIPS FOR REINFORCING FAMILY TEACHING

Home Care for the Woman With Placenta Previa

- Arrange for a dependable person with transportation to be available immediately to transport you to the hospital should a bleeding episode occur.
- Perform fetal movement (kick) count at least daily. If your baby moves less than 10 times in 2 hours, or if your baby is not moving at all, immediately call your health care provider.
- Stay in bed at home. You may get up to use the bathroom. Do no housework or lifting. Moderate to vigorous activity could bring about a bleeding episode.
- Vaginal rest is essential. Do not insert anything into the vagina (e.g., no sexual intercourse, no douching, no tampons). These activities could stimulate bleeding.

A cesarean delivery is necessary in all cases of total placenta previa. If allowed to labor, the woman with total placenta previa would incur massive hemorrhage because placental blood vessels would break open and bleed as the cervix dilates. The delivery is scheduled as soon as it is reasonably certain that the fetal lungs are mature. Maternal and fetal outcomes are better when the delivery is scheduled, as opposed to being done emergently during an acute bleeding episode. Occasionally, a woman with a marginal placenta previa can deliver vaginally, as long as the fetus is stable and heavy bleeding does not occur during labor.

Nursing Care

The woman with placenta previa requires careful nursing observation. Continuous IV access is important. Monitor the IV site. Institute a perineal pad count to quantify bleeding. Monitor the vital signs at regular intervals, and observe for signs of shock. Assist with NSTs as ordered, and check the FHR at least every 4 hours. Instruct the woman to perform and record fetal movement (kick) count (see Chapter 7). If the woman is discharged home before she delivers, give her instructions for self-care (Tips for Reinforcing Family Teaching: Home Care for the Woman With Placenta Previa).

Postpartum care of the woman with placenta previa is the same as for other women. However, it is important to observe her closely for signs and symptoms of infection and postpartum hemorrhage. She is at higher risk for both of these complications because of the proximity of the open, bleeding vessels at the former placenta site to the opening of the uterus. Also, the lower segment of the uterus cannot contract as effectively as can the upper segment; therefore, sometimes not enough pressure is exerted on the blood vessels to stop the bleeding.

Placental Abruption (Abruptio Placentae)

Abruptio placentae, or placental abruption, is the premature separation of a normally implanted placenta. The incidence of abruptio placentae is about 1% (Ananth & Kinzler, 2020). Although the placenta is located in the normal place, it prematurely pulls away from the uterine wall either during pregnancy or before the end of labor. The cause of abruptio placentae is unknown; however, there are associated risk factors. Conditions characterized by elevated blood pressure put the woman at risk for abruption. Preeclampsia and preexisting chronic hypertension fall into this category. Advanced maternal age (older than 35 years) and multiparity increase the risk for placental abruption. Trauma (e.g., motor vehicle collisions or domestic violence), cigarette smoking, alcohol consumption, cocaine use, and preterm premature rupture of the membranes are additional risk factors for abruption.

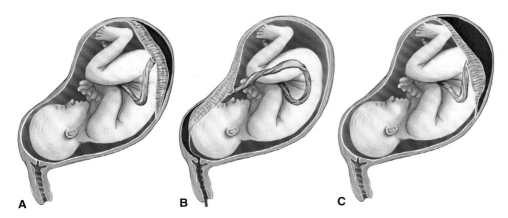

FIGURE 17-5 Types of placental abruption. **A.** partial abruption, concealed hemorrhage; **B.** partial abruption, apparent hemorrhage; **C.** complete abruption, concealed hemorrhage.

A placental abruption is classified in several ways. The bleeding is either concealed (hidden) or apparent, and the degree of abruption is either partial or complete (Fig. 17-5). If the middle portion of the placenta separates but the edges remain attached, massive hemorrhage can occur behind the placenta but the bleeding may remain concealed. Alternatively, a small edge of the placenta may pull away from the uterine wall and the bleeding might be readily apparent.

Maternal complications of abruptio placentae include hemorrhagic shock, disseminated intravascular coagulation (DIC), uterine rupture, renal failure, and death. Severity and type of fetal complications relate to the degree of placental separation and maturity of the fetus. Hypoxia, anemia, growth restriction, and even fetal death may occur. When preterm delivery is indicated, the neonate is at risk because of prematurity.

Clinical Manifestations

The classic signs are pain, dark red vaginal bleeding, a rigid, boardlike abdomen, hypertonic labor, and fetal distress. Pain has a sudden onset and is constant. Bleeding is apparent in most cases. The uterus may not relax well between contractions, the amniotic fluid often is bloody, and signs of maternal shock and fetal distress may be present. The fundal height may increase with severe intrauterine bleeding.

Ultrasound may assist the woman's health care provider with the diagnosis, but a negative sonogram does not rule out the possibility of abruption. A biophysical profile (BPP) gives additional information regarding fetal status. As with other bleeding disorders, disseminated intravascular coagulation (DIC) is a potential complication of placental abruption. The health care provider carefully monitors

> **Know How to Spot the Difference!**
> You can tell the difference between placenta previa and abruptio placentae because the bleeding with previa is bright red and *painless*, whereas the bleeding with an abruption is usually dark red and *painful*.

fibrinogen levels and other clotting studies to detect the development of DIC.

Treatment

For cases of abruptio placentae with severe bleeding, IV fluids are infused via a large-bore IV until cryoprecipitate, fresh frozen plasma, or whole blood is available for transfusion. Four units of crossmatched packed red blood cells should be readily available from the laboratory. Oxygen is administered via facemask. If the condition of either the woman or her fetus becomes unstable, the fetus is delivered by emergency cesarean birth. After delivery of the fetus, if the bleeding is unable to be controlled, a hysterectomy may be required to save the woman's life.

Vaginal delivery is preferred to cesarean birth for small abruptions in which the woman and fetus remain hemodynamically stable or when the fetus has died. Contraindications for a vaginal birth include fetal distress, bleeding severe enough to threaten the life of the mother and fetus, or unsatisfactory progress of labor. The health care provider may rupture the membranes artificially to induce or augment labor, and oxytocin may be used.

Nursing Care

The woman with a suspected or diagnosed placental abruption requires careful monitoring. She must remain NPO until her condition is stable as she may require emergency cesarean birth. Monitor for signs of shock. Watch for bleeding from the gums, nose, and venipuncture sites, which may indicate disseminated intravascular coagulation (DIC). Monitor the IV site as IV fluids and blood products may be ordered. Continuous EFM is necessary. The RN should evaluate the strip frequently. Immediately notify the RN if any signs of fetal distress become evident. Be prepared for an emergency cesarean birth if ordered.

After delivery, the woman requires close monitoring for postpartum hemorrhage because she is at risk for uterine atony. Continue to observe for signs of DIC. This complication may develop after delivery. Monitor strict intake and output. Pay particular attention to the urinary output. Acute renal failure can occur. Notify the RN if the urinary output is less than 30 mL/hour.

The nursing care plan for the woman with a pregnancy bleeding disorder focuses on the safety and health of the mother and the fetus. Tests will be done to assess the status of the pregnancy. If the bleeding causes the pregnancy to end, the woman's feelings regarding the loss of the pregnancy are also a priority.

Assessment (Data Collection)

Obtain thorough data collection on the woman's obstetric history, unless the severity of the bleeding necessitates immediate intervention. It is important to ask about the chief complaint and history of the current condition and to note any risk factors for antepartum hemorrhage (e.g., grand multiparity, advanced maternal age, or previous history of a bleeding disorder).

During an acute bleeding episode, determine the characteristics of bleeding. How much is the woman bleeding? What is the color and consistency? Is pain present? If so, where is the pain located and how severe does the woman rate it? In some conditions, bleeding can be hidden, such as a ruptured ectopic pregnancy and some placental abruptions. Obtain frequent vital signs to determine if shock is present. Initial symptoms of shock include cool, clammy skin, restlessness, apprehension, and confusion. Late signs of shock include tachycardia and when blood loss is severe, hypotension.

Apply the EFM; obtain and record the baseline FHR. Review the monitor strip for indications of fetal distress. Fetal tachycardia that progresses to bradycardia and decreased variability with late decelerations are ominous signs that must be reported to the RN and health care provider at once. Absence of the FHR is associated with fetal death or hydatidiform mole.

Palpate the uterus to determine if the resting tone is soft and to evaluate the characteristics of contractions if present. Measure fundal height and compare it to previous measurements as a sudden size increase may occur when there is concealed hemorrhage.

Evaluate the woman's pain. Pelvic or shoulder pain in early pregnancy is associated with ectopic pregnancy. Pain is generally not associated with placenta previa, unless the woman is also experiencing labor, in which case the pain will subside with each contraction. Cramping and abdominal pain may accompany early pregnancy loss and abruptio placentae.

Nursing Care Focus

When selecting the focus of nursing care for the woman with a bleeding disorder, consideration should be given to the type of disorder she is having, the health of the fetus, and the tests and treatments the woman will have. Her knowledge level of what is happening with the pregnancy and her anxiety level must also be considered.

Outcome Identification and Planning

Maintaining the safety of the pregnant woman and her fetus is the primary goal when planning care. Goals and interventions are planned according to the individual needs and situation of the woman. Appropriate goals may include that the woman's fluid volume will be maintained and that she will not sustain injury. Additional goals for the woman include that she will express the ability to cope with her pain and that her anxiety will be reduced. Planning of nursing activities is based upon these goals.

Nursing Care Focus

- Hypovolemia risk

Goal

- The woman will be free of any signs of hypovolemia.

Implementations for Preventing and Monitoring for Hypovolemia

The priority of care for any woman who is bleeding is to prevent and treat shock. For acute bleeding episodes, or when the potential for hemorrhage exists, the woman should have an IV line with a large-bore catheter present. The RN will infuse IV fluids, as ordered, to maintain circulatory volume. Important interventions include sending blood specimens for type and crossmatching and making certain that 2 to 4 units of blood is available at all times for possible transfusion. If there is severe bleeding, the RN will administer blood or blood products as ordered.

It is important to monitor vital signs closely for signs of shock. Maintain strict intake and output monitoring with special attention to the urine output, which should remain above 30 mL/hour. In addition, maintain the woman in a lateral position to promote placental perfusion. Oxygen by facemask will be ordered if bleeding is heavy or if there are signs of fetal distress.

Bleeding episodes during pregnancy have the risk of surgery, either emergently to control the bleeding or on a planned basis to prevent hemorrhage. In a planned situation, make sure the woman has signed informed consent, carry out preoperative orders, and complete the preoperative checklist. When the woman must be prepared for surgery emergently, move quickly and efficiently to assist the RN in getting the woman ready (see Chapter 11 on emergency cesarean birth).

If active bleeding is not occurring, but the potential for hemorrhage exists (e.g., placenta previa), assist the woman to remain on bed rest with bathroom privileges as ordered. It is important to maintain an ongoing perineal pad count to monitor for increased bleeding.

Evaluation of Goal/Desired Outcome

The woman:

- remains alert, awake, and responsive.
- has a blood pressure that is stable and not decreasing.
- is not tachycardic.
- does not have pale, cold, clammy skin.
- has a urinary output of at least 30 mL/hour.

Nursing Care Focus

- Injury risk

Goal

- The woman will remain free from injury.

Implementations for Preventing Injury

When the pregnancy has reached the point of viability (usually considered 20 weeks or more), monitor the fetus continuously during bleeding episodes until the woman is in stable condition. Watch the fetal monitoring tracing closely for signs of fetal distress such as loss of variability, a gradually increasing or decreasing baseline, or late decelerations. If any of these signs are present, reposition her to a side-lying position and notify the RN or health care provider immediately. The health care provider may order oxygen to be administered to the mother and also increase the rate of IV fluids.

If the woman's condition is stable and there are no signs of fetal distress, the woman may remain hospitalized for observation. Assist her to maintain bed rest, as ordered, and institute preterm labor precautions (see Chapter 18). Betamethasone may be ordered to increase fetal lung maturity in the event delivery must occur before term.

Maternal injury can occur from complications, such as disseminated intravascular coagulation (DIC), which are sometimes the sequelae (consequence) of a bleeding disorder. Obtain specimens for laboratory studies as ordered. Typical blood work includes a complete blood count to detect the presence of anemia and infection. Often, coagulation studies are necessary because some disorders (such as abruptio placentae) are associated with a high risk of clotting dysfunction. Coagulation studies include platelet and fibrinogen levels and prothrombin time/activated partial thromboplastin time.

In addition to close monitoring of laboratory results, observe for and report any bleeding from the nose, gums, and venipuncture sites and observe the skin carefully for petechiae and purpura as these can be signs of DIC. Watch for cough, dyspnea, fever, confusion, and disorientation. Monitor the blood urea nitrogen and creatinine levels as these levels may be elevated secondary to renal failure.

Injury can result from bleeding that allows fetal blood to mix with maternal blood. This is why blood typing is so important with any bleeding disorder of pregnancy. The woman who is Rho(D)-negative may need a Kleihauer–Betke test to determine if any fetal blood has entered her circulation. Every woman who is Rho(D)-negative should receive anti-D immune globulin if there is risk of fetal–maternal hemorrhage. All bleeding episodes, trauma, delivery, or early pregnancy loss increase this risk.

Evaluation of Goal/Desired Outcome

The woman:

- exhibits normal clotting values clotting values.
- does not exhibit abnormal, uncontrolled bleeding.
- receives anti-D immune globulin if she is Rh-negative.

Nursing Care Focus

- Acute pain

Goal

- The woman will verbalize or demonstrate relief of pain.

Implementations for Monitoring and Controlling Pain

Carefully monitor the woman's pain. It is important to ask the following questions regarding pain: Where is it? What is it like? When did it start? How often does it occur? What makes it worse? What makes it better? Evaluate intensity using a pain scale. Ask the woman to rate the pain on a scale of 0 to 10 with 0 representing no pain at all and 10 representing the worst pain imaginable. If a standardized pain scale is used, it can more effectively evaluate the success of nursing interventions.

Give the woman information about what is causing the pain (if you have that information) and how long she can expect it to last. Explain to her the medications the health care provider has ordered to help decrease her pain, and tell her how frequently she can have them. For acute pain, it is often better to schedule the pain medications, rather than waiting for the woman to ask for them. Explain that it is easier to treat pain before it becomes severe. Consider non-pharmacologic methods of pain relief, such as warm or cold applications, massage, or relaxation techniques.

Be sure that the room temperature, lighting, and noise level are at a comfortable level for the woman. It is also helpful to try to eliminate any factors that might be interfering with her ability to cope with the pain (e.g., if the woman is overly fatigued or bored, it will be more difficult for her to deal with the pain sensation). Be sure to inform the RN and the health care provider right away if measures to reduce pain are ineffective.

Evaluation of Goal/Desired Outcome

The woman:

- reports an acceptable pain level on a standardized pain scale.
- states measures help reduce or eliminate her pain.

Nursing Care Focus

- Acute anxiety

Goal

● The woman will display decreased signs and symptoms of anxiety.

Implementations for Relieving Anxiety

Take care to attend to the woman's emotional needs. It can be frightening when there is active bleeding and health care providers are moving quickly to intervene. Use a calm and confident manner. Explain all procedures and treatments as they are being performed, using language the woman and her family can understand. Use therapeutic communication skills to encourage the woman to express her feelings. Encourage the presence of supportive family members and friends, as appropriate. Provide quiet time and decreased environmental stimulation.

Help the patient identify appropriate coping strategies that have worked in the past, and support the use of these strategies. Encourage the woman to rest as appropriate. Fatigue can increase anxiety. Monitor vital signs, as indicated by the patient's condition. Provide supplemental oxygen, as needed.

If the fetus dies because of complications of the bleeding disorder or if the woman requires an unplanned, emergency hysterectomy, she will need additional support to deal with these losses. Consult with social services to provide the patient (and family, as indicated) for spiritual support or counseling, as appropriate, and arrange for visitation.

Evaluation of Goal/Desired Outcome

The woman:

● relaxes between procedures and assessments.
● is able to focus during explanations and repeat back information given.
● identifies a coping strategy she can utilize to decrease her anxiety.

TEST YOURSELF

✔ Name two characteristics that are different between abruptio placentae and placenta previa.
✔ Name three symptoms of shock.
✔ Name one way to evaluate the extent of concealed hemorrhage.

Remember **Shakeba Winters** from the beginning of the chapter. What gestational condition do you think Shakeba is experiencing? What would place her at risk for this condition? For what symptoms would you need to monitor her for?

HYPERTENSIVE DISORDERS IN PREGNANCY

Hypertension during pregnancy is one of the top four leading causes of maternal morbidity and mortality in the United States. These disorders are not only dangerous for the pregnant woman, but they also significantly increase the risk for the fetus. There are four basic categories of elevated blood pressure during pregnancy:

1. Gestational hypertension
2. Preeclampsia/eclampsia
3. Chronic hypertension
4. Preeclampsia superimposed on chronic hypertension

Gestational Hypertension

Gestational hypertension is the current term used to describe elevated blood pressure (systolic ≥140 mm Hg or diastolic ≥90 mm Hg) that develops for the first time during pregnancy after 20 weeks' gestation, without the presence of protein in the urine. Gestational hypertension may resolve spontaneously after the baby is born, in which case the condition is classified transient hypertension. If the blood pressure remains elevated 12 weeks after delivery, the diagnosis becomes chronic hypertension. The concern is that gestational hypertension may develop into the more serious preeclampsia–eclampsia syndrome; therefore, at each obstetrical visit, the urine is checked for protein, and the blood pressure is monitored closely. If the blood pressure increases to a level that might endanger the woman or her fetus, the health care provider may prescribe antihypertensives.

Preeclampsia–Eclampsia

Preeclampsia is a serious condition of pregnancy in which the blood pressure in a woman who has had normal blood pressures rises to ≥140 mm Hg systolic or ≥90 mm Hg diastolic on two separate occasions and is accompanied by **proteinuria**, the presence of protein in the urine. The condition may develop into **eclampsia**, the presence of seizure activity or coma in a woman with preeclampsia. Signs and symptoms of preeclampsia usually appear after the 20th week of gestation and resolve when the pregnancy ends. The syndrome may develop gradually or it may appear suddenly without warning. The underlying cause of this disorder is unknown. Preeclampsia occurs only in pregnancy, but it is not known what causes some pregnant women to develop sensitivity to the tissue, whereas others do not. Box 17-1 lists risk factors for preeclampsia.

Medical researchers want to find ways to prevent and predict preeclampsia–eclampsia because of the severe effects this condition can have on the woman and her fetus (Table 17-2). Various methods have been tried to prevent the condition, including high-protein, low-salt diets and calcium supplementation. However, none of these therapies have been preventive to date. Recent studies have shown aspirin to reduce risk in women who have moderate to high risk factors for preeclampsia but not preventative for women with low risk factors (August & Jayabalan, 2021).

BOX 17-1 **Risk Factors for Preeclampsia**

- Family history of preeclampsia–eclampsia
- Nulliparity
- Preexisting medical conditions such as:
  - Chronic hypertension
  - Systemic lupus erythematosus
  - Renal disease
  - Diabetes
- Obstetric complications including:
  - Multiple gestation
  - Hydatidiform mole (molar pregnancy)
  - Carrying a fetus that develops erythroblastosis fetalis
- Extremes of age
  - Younger than 20 years (increased risk probably due in large part to nulliparity)
  - Older than 35 years (increased risk most likely related to presence of chronic diseases)

Because there are no diagnostic tests available that can predict which woman will develop preeclampsia, early detection through regular prenatal care is the standard of care. Early prenatal care reduces morbidity and mortality associated with preeclampsia–eclampsia.

Preeclampsia occurs in approximately 3% to 5% of pregnancies in the United States. In the United States, it is one of the four most common causes of maternal death (August & Sibai, 2021) and is a leading cause of maternal death in underdeveloped countries. Women who receive no prenatal care are more likely to die of complications of preeclampsia and eclampsia than women who receive any prenatal care.

In a normal pregnancy, a woman's blood pressure does not rise significantly above her baseline. In fact, during the second trimester, the blood pressure decreases. However, in a pregnancy complicated by preeclampsia, the blood pressure rises. The elevated blood pressure occurs because in preeclampsia the woman's blood vessels undergo vasospasm and vasoconstriction, which increases peripheral resistance and blood pressure. The kidneys reinforce this rise in pressure when they respond to decreased blood flow by releasing substances that further raise the blood pressure.

The primary problem underlying the development of preeclampsia is generalized **vasospasm**, spasm of the arteries, which affects every organ in the body. Vasospasm causes generalized vasoconstriction, which leads to hypertension. The elevated blood pressure adversely affects the central nervous system (CNS) and decreases blood flow to the kidneys, liver, and placenta. Vasospasm also leads to endothelial damage, which causes abnormal clotting. Tiny clots (microemboli) cause damage to internal organs, especially the liver and kidneys. Edema of the tissues, body organs, or both may result from this process (Fig. 17-6).

Clinical Manifestations

Preeclampsia is diagnosed when blood pressures of greater than 140 mm Hg systolic or 90 mm Hg diastolic develop after the 20th week of gestation. The hypertension must be documented on at least two different occasions and be accompanied by proteinuria (measured by dipstick of a clean-catch or catheterized urine specimen followed by a 24-hour urine collection). The presence of edema or weight gain is no longer a criterion for diagnosis of this disorder because edema occurs commonly in pregnancy and is not specific to preeclampsia. However, edema is significant if it is nondependent or if it involves the face and hands.

Depending on symptoms, preeclampsia is categorized as mild or severe (Table 17-3). Symptoms of mild preeclampsia are limited to slightly elevated blood pressure and small amounts of protein in the urine. Severe preeclampsia manifests with blood pressure above 160/110 mm Hg, greater than 2+ protein in the urine, and symptoms related to edema of body organs and decreased blood flow to tissues. The CNS, especially the brain, is sensitive to small changes in fluid volume. Nervous system irritability occurs, resulting

TABLE 17-2 Complications of Preeclampsia–Eclampsia That Can Cause Maternal and Fetal Injury or Death

EFFECTS OF PREECLAMPSIA–ECLAMPSIA	POTENTIAL COMPLICATIONS
Maternal Effects of Preeclampsia–Eclampsia	
Seizure activity	Bodily injury (especially the tongue), aspiration, placental abruption, or cerebral hemorrhage
Endothelial damage to pulmonary capillaries	Pulmonary edema
Severely elevated blood pressure and cerebral edema	Cerebral bleeding and complications associated with cerebral vascular accident (CVA or stroke). This complication is rare
Edema and reduced blood flow to the liver	HELLP syndrome and rupture of the liver
Platelet aggregation and consumption of clotting factors	Thrombocytopenia and disseminated intravascular coagulopathy (DIC)
Fetal Effects of Preeclampsia–Eclampsia	
Reduced blood flow to the placenta	IUGR, oligohydramnios, and placental abruption
Preterm delivery to save mother or baby	Respiratory distress syndrome and other complications of prematurity

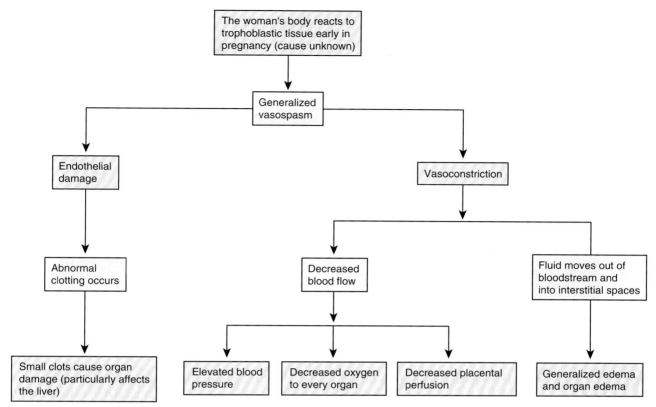

FIGURE 17-6 Pathophysiology of preeclampsia. Every body organ is affected.

TABLE 17-3 Comparison of Mild and Severe Preeclampsia and Eclampsia

	MILD PREECLAMPSIA	SEVERE PREECLAMPSIA	ECLAMPSIA
Blood pressure	140/90 mm Hg or higher; diastolic pressure remains below 100 mm Hg	150/100 mm Hg or higher	Same as for severe preeclampsia
Proteinuria	Trace to 1+ in a random specimen; 300 mg or greater in a 24-hour specimen	Persistent 2+ or more; 500 mg or greater in a 24-hour specimen	Same as for severe preeclampsia
Serum creatinine	Normal	Elevated	Elevated
Platelet count	Normal	Low (thrombocytopenia)	Same as for severe preeclampsia; may develop HELLP syndrome
Liver enzymes	Normal to minimally elevated	Markedly elevated	Same as for severe preeclampsia
Headache, visual disturbances, epigastric (abdominal) pain	Absent	Present	Present; epigastric pain is an important warning of an impending seizure
Fetal growth	Normal (not restricted)	May be restricted, unless there is a sudden onset near term and the baby is delivered promptly	Same as for severe preeclampsia
Edema	Trace to 1+ pedal, if present	May or may not be present; edema of the face or hands is significant	May or may not be present
Pulmonary edema	Absent	May be present	May be present
Seizure activity or coma	Absent	Absent	Present

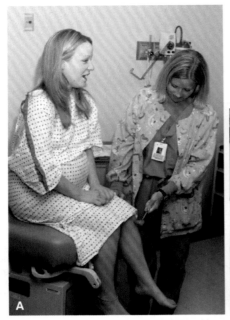

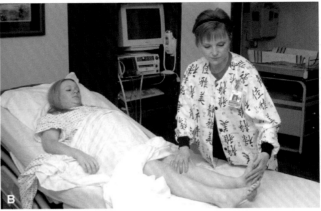

FIGURE 17-7 A. The nurse checks the patellar reflexes. **B.** The nurse checks for clonus.

in hyperactive deep tendon reflexes and clonus (Fig. 17-7). A severe headache may indicate the presence of cerebral edema. If the retina of the eye becomes edematous, the woman will report blurred or double vision and spots before her eyes. Visual changes and a severe headache indicate that a seizure is likely to occur. Liver involvement results in elevation of liver enzymes. Severe edema of the liver causes nausea and pain in the epigastric region. In addition, a low platelet count may result in prolonged bleeding time, and pulmonary edema may occur when the disease process affects the lungs.

If the woman with severe preeclampsia experiences a convulsion or a coma, she has progressed from preeclampsia to eclampsia. Typically, seizures are generalized tonic–clonic in nature and only rarely progress to status epilepticus. Potential complications of eclamptic seizure activity include aspiration, cerebral hemorrhage, stroke, hepatic rupture, abruptio placentae, fetal compromise, and death of the woman or fetus. The woman with preeclampsia remains at risk for seizure activity throughout pregnancy, labor, and in the first few days of the postpartum period. In fact, the signs of preeclampsia–eclampsia may occur suddenly in the postpartum period even if they were not noticeable before delivery.

Be Careful!
Don't let the term "mild" (when applied to preeclampsia) fool you. Mild preeclampsia can progress rapidly to severe preeclampsia or eclampsia with seizures or coma. Closely monitor all pregnant women with elevated blood pressures.

HELLP syndrome is a severe complication of preeclampsia–eclampsia. HELLP is an acronym for *h*emolysis, *e*levated *l*iver enzymes, and *l*ow *p*latelets, which are the laboratory findings in a woman with this syndrome. HELLP syndrome is typically seen in the pregnant woman with severe preeclampsia but may also occur in few cases of pregnant women who do not have proteinuria and elevated blood pressures (Sibai, 2020). HELLP increases the mortality rate during pregnancy.

Symptoms of HELLP, in addition to the change in laboratory values, are similar to preeclampsia, which makes it hard to identify in some cases. Symptoms the client complains of are primarily epigastric pain and tenderness, nausea and vomiting, and less frequently visual disturbances and headache. The symptoms may be mistaken for flu or another viral illness, which can delay diagnosis and treatment.

Treatment

The primary goals of treating preeclampsia are to deliver a healthy baby and restore the woman to a healthy state. The most important decision regarding management of preeclampsia involves the timing of delivery because the only cure for preeclampsia is delivery of the fetus. If the fetus is at term (over 37 weeks), the labor will usually be induced because a vaginal birth is preferred to a cesarean delivery. If the fetus is preterm, management depends on the severity of the disease and determination of fetal lung maturity. The benefits and risks of conservative management (bed rest and observation) are weighed against the benefits and risks of a preterm delivery. If the woman's condition deteriorates rapidly or the fetus becomes unstable, delivery of the fetus is done promptly to save the life of the woman, the baby, or both.

Conservative management may be appropriate for the woman with mild preeclampsia. If she is compliant with the treatment plan and understands the danger signals, she may receive care at home. Otherwise, hospitalization is required with activity restriction that usually involves bed rest in a lateral position with bathroom privileges. The woman should stay in a minimally stimulating environment; therefore, visitors are usually restricted to one or two support persons. In addition, the woman's room should have dim lighting, be away from main doorways, and should not have the television on.

If the health care provider plans conservative management to allow a preterm fetus to mature, closely observe fetal well-being. Instruct the woman to perform fetal movement (kick) count after every meal. Nonstress tests are done at least twice weekly. A biophysical profile (BPP) (see Chapter 7 for a description of fetal surveillance tests) and serial sonograms help monitor fetal status and growth. An amniocentesis may be done to determine lung maturity using the lecithin/sphingomyelin (L/S) ratio. A ratio of 2:1 is indicative of lung maturity. If imminent delivery seems necessary and the baby is preterm, the woman's health care provider may order glucocorticoids (usually betamethasone) in an attempt to hasten maturity of the fetal lungs.

Preventing maternal seizures is another important goal of therapy. If severe preeclampsia ensues, the woman should be placed on bed rest in a darkened, quiet room, and visitors should be restricted. Television, computer, and phone screen activity should be avoided to decrease stimuli. The most effective medication to prevent and treat eclamptic seizures is magnesium sulfate, usually administered intravenously (Box 17-2). The drug works by directly relaxing skeletal muscles and is a CNS depressant which helps to decrease the risk of seizures. IV magnesium sulfate is the drug of choice to treat eclamptic seizures, but other anticonvulsants, such as phenytoin or diazepam, are sometimes ordered.

The pregnant woman on magnesium sulfate must be closely monitored for signs of toxicity. The therapeutic level of magnesium sulfate is 4 to 8 mg/dL. This level is effective to prevent seizures without causing toxicity. Magnesium toxicity begins when serum magnesium levels approach 9 mg/dL. First, the reflexes disappear, then as the levels increase, respiratory depression and cardiac arrest can follow. For this reason, monitor the reflexes and respiratory rate of the woman receiving magnesium sulfate at frequent intervals. Serum magnesium levels are ordered. Calcium gluconate is the antidote to magnesium sulfate. The RN gives this medication by IV push to treat magnesium overdose.

Magnesium sulfate leaves the body via the kidneys. If the kidneys do not function well, blood magnesium levels rise, which can lead to toxicity. Because preeclampsia can damage the kidneys, pay close attention to urinary output by measuring it hourly. Report hourly outputs of less than 30 mL.

BOX 17-2 **Prevention and Treatment of Eclamptic Seizures: Magnesium Sulfate**

Note: The RN administers and regulates this medication. However, the LPN/LVN may assist with monitoring of the woman who is receiving IV magnesium.

Method of Action
Magnesium sulfate prevents seizures by relaxing muscles and through direct action on the CNS.

Usual Dosage and Administration
IV route: Loading dose of 4 to 6 grams diluted in 100 mL fluid infused over 15 to 20 minutes, followed by maintenance dose of 2 grams/hour.
Antidote: Calcium gluconate 1 gram IV push over 2 minutes.

Nursing Interventions
1. Carefully prepare and administer magnesium sulfate exactly as ordered.
2. Use a pump to regulate flow when administering via IV route.
3. Monitor vital signs per facility protocol every 15 to 30 minutes.
4. Perform hourly observations on the following:
    a. Urinary output and protein levels
    b. Deep tendon reflexes
    c. Edema
    d. Respiratory status (including rate and depth)
5. Request serum magnesium levels every 4 to 6 hours as ordered.
6. Discontinue magnesium sulfate and notify the health care provider if deep tendon reflexes are absent, respirations are less than 14 per minute, or urinary output is less than 30 mL/hour.
7. Therapeutic levels of magnesium sulfate are between 4 and 7 mEq/L. Patellar reflexes disappear and respiratory arrest are signs of toxic levels of magnesium sulfate.

Because magnesium sulfate causes muscular relaxation, it inhibits uterine contractions. Therefore, if delivery is indicated, the woman usually requires oxytocin induction of labor. She is also at risk for postpartum hemorrhage because the uterine muscle may be unable to contract effectively. Carefully monitor for this complication after delivery.

The treatment of hypertension is controversial. Generally, antihypertensives are prescribed only in the presence of severely elevated blood pressure (150/100 mm Hg or over) because a rapid drop in the blood pressure can lead to decreased placental perfusion, resulting in fetal distress, and also because the hypertension is from preeclampsia and delivery of the fetus is the correcting factor for the elevated blood pressure. Labetalol or hydralazine is the antihypertensive drug of choice during pregnancy. Nifedipine is another antihypertensive that may be ordered.

Nursing Care
Care of the woman with preeclampsia or eclampsia involves frequent monitoring, informing the woman of the reasons for the treatments ordered, and providing emotional support. The woman and fetus require frequent monitoring for

BOX 17-3 Measuring Blood Pressure in the Preeclampic Woman

- Assist the woman to the same position for each reading.
  - Measuring blood pressure with the arm at heart level is best accomplished with the woman in a sitting position. If she cannot sit up, be sure to take the pressure with the arm at heart level. If the arm is higher than the heart, the pressure reading will likely be lower than the actual pressure. Likewise, a lower than actual reading will likely result if you take the pressure with the woman in the supine position.
- Take care to choose a cuff that fits the woman correctly.
  - If the woman is large and you use a small cuff, the reading may be falsely elevated. Conversely, if the woman is very thin and you use a large cuff, the reading may be lowered falsely.
  - Most facilities use automated blood pressure equipment. These devices tend to underestimate the blood pressure in women with preeclampsia; therefore, manual blood pressures are the standard. If you use an automated device, first verify accuracy of the machine readings by comparing them with manual measurements.
- If the pressure is greater than 140/90 mm Hg, reposition the woman to her left side, wait 5 to 10 minutes (to avoid falsely elevated readings from the pressure of the cuff), and then repeat the reading.
- If the pressure continues to be elevated, determine if the woman is experiencing headache, blurred vision, or epigastric pain.
- Reposition the woman comfortably on her left side, supported by pillows.
- Immediately report blood pressures greater than 140/90 mm Hg and abnormal symptoms to the RN and health care provider.
- Record the blood pressure per facility protocol. Document each reading, noting the time and maternal position for each.

BOX 17-4 Nursing Care During an Eclamptic Seizure

When the Seizure Begins
1. If you are in the room when a seizure begins, summon help with the call bell and note the time the seizure began.
2. Gently attempt to place the woman on her side, if possible. Do not force her to this position if injury will result.
3. Provide oxygen by facemask per orders/standing protocol.

During the Seizure
1. Stay with the woman, even when help arrives.
2. Suction PRN, if it is safe to do so, because aspiration is a real threat.
   a. Do not place the suction catheter into the mouth, particularly if you are using a hard plastic suction tip.
   b. Do not place anything in the woman's mouth.
3. The RN will prepare and administer IV magnesium sulfate or another antiepileptic medication per orders/standing protocol to stop the seizure.
4. If IV access is not in place, assist the RN in establishing access as soon as it is safe to do so.
5. Watch for signs of spontaneous birth of the baby. Sometimes a seizure will precipitate birth.
6. Note the characteristics of the seizure so that you may accurately document the details after the seizure is over.

After the Seizure
1. Continue to suction PRN.
2. Continue administering oxygen to prevent/treat maternal–fetal hypoxia.
3. Begin continuous monitoring of the FHR if a continuous monitor is not already in place.
4. Talk to the woman. Explain to her that she had a seizure and that she is safe and that you will stay with her.
   a. She may appear disoriented, drowsy, or as if she is sleeping, but she can still hear you.
   b. It may be hard for her to speak, answer questions, or follow commands immediately after the seizure during the postictal state.
5. Notify the health care provider of the seizure.
6. Document the following parameters.
   a. Time the seizure began
   b. Characteristics of the seizure including tonic–clonic activity, fecal or urinary incontinence, cyanosis
   c. All nursing actions completed and medications administered
   d. Response of the woman to interventions
   e. Evaluation of the EFM tracing

symptoms of worsening condition. The RN is responsible for assessment and care of the woman with preeclampsia, although you may assist.

In the hospital, monitor blood pressure at least every 4 hours for mild preeclampsia and more frequently for severe disease. See Box 17-3 for nursing considerations when measuring blood pressure in the preeclampic woman. In addition, it is important to auscultate the lungs every 2 hours. Adventitious lung sounds may indicate developing pulmonary edema. Weigh the woman daily on the same scale at the same time of day while she is wearing the same amount of clothing. Report any sudden increase in weight.

Inform the woman to report headache, visual changes, and epigastric pain, which are warning signs of worsening of her condition and may occur prior to seizures. Check deep tendon reflexes and determine if clonus is present at least once per shift. It is important to keep the environment quiet and nonstimulating because bright lights and loud noises could precipitate a seizure. It is important that the woman be told why it is important for her to avoid having the television on (even at low volume) and why she should avoid talking on the phone or playing any handheld games or looking at internet sites. Implement seizure precautions, which include padding the side rails and keeping suction equipment, an oral airway, supplemental oxygen, and medications readily available for use at the bedside. If a seizure does occur, follow proper procedure (Box 17-4).

The woman should remain on bed rest in the left lateral position, although some women with mild preeclampsia may have bathroom privileges. Maintain strict monitoring of intake and output. IV fluids may be ordered. Infusion of

IV fluids will be done carefully with an IV pump to regulate flow rates that will maintain adequate hydration without causing overload. Report urinary output of less than 30 mL/hour. An indwelling catheter may be ordered to accurately document hourly urinary output and also to assist the woman with minimal stimulation.

Adequate nutrition is important to promote fetal growth and maternal well-being. There is no special diet for preeclampsia, but careful attention is needed so that nutrients are consumed in adequate amounts (see Chapter 6). Salt restriction below normal levels is not necessary, but the woman should take care to avoid excessive salt intake.

Remember to care for the psychosocial needs of the woman hospitalized for preeclampsia. Boredom may be an issue because of prolonged bed rest. Encourage the woman with mild preeclampsia to read, keep a journal, or do crafts. The woman may be anxious about the well-being of her fetus or because she had to leave older children at home. Keep the woman informed of the results of NSTs and other tests of fetal well-being. Reassure her that she can monitor fetal well-being by doing fetal movement (kick) count regularly. Allow her to ventilate her feelings of fear or frustration. Short daily visits by older children or telephone calls may also help alleviate anxiety.

Postpartum care of the woman varies depending on whether the woman received magnesium sulfate during the intrapartum period. If so, the woman receives care in the labor and delivery unit or a high-risk antepartum unit for the first 24 to 48 hours after delivery. During that time, magnesium sulfate administration continues with close monitoring of respirations, deep tendon reflexes, clonus, and urinary output as before delivery. The woman will need to be closely observed for postpartum hemorrhage related to uterine atony caused by magnesium sulfate.

The infant born to a woman who received magnesium sulfate will also need careful observation as the medication crosses the placenta. The infant will need to be observed for decreased muscle tone, respiratory depression, and poor feeding until the medication clears from their system.

If magnesium sulfate was not administered, the woman may be transferred to a postpartum unit. In addition to normal postpartum care, closely observe the blood pressure and monitor for other signs of worsening preeclampsia because a seizure can occur several days after delivery. Observe the woman closely because she is at increased risk for postpartum hemorrhage. Monitor the platelet count, as ordered, and watch for development of complications, such as bleeding from the mouth, gums, nose, or injection sites. If the neonate is in the neonatal intensive care unit, assist the woman to visit as soon as she is able. If she cannot visit, provide pictures of the infant and provide a daily update on the baby's condition.

Chronic Hypertension and Preeclampsia Superimposed on Chronic Hypertension

Chronic hypertension is high blood pressure that is present before the woman becomes pregnant. When a woman with

Medical Complications
- Ventricular hypertrophy
- Heart failure
- Cerebrovascular accident (CVA or stroke)
- Chronic renal damage

Complications of Pregnancy
- Superimposed preeclampsia
- Placental abruption
- Fetal growth restriction

preexisting hypertension becomes pregnant, the pregnancy is already at risk. Sustained high blood pressure can be damaging to blood vessels and eventually can decrease placental perfusion, leading to fetal growth restriction. In addition, the woman with chronic hypertension is at a much higher risk of developing superimposed preeclampsia. Box 17-5 lists complications associated with chronic hypertension in the pregnant woman.

Clinical Manifestations

The definition of chronic hypertension is blood pressure that is elevated consistently above 140/90 mm Hg when the woman is not pregnant. If hypertension develops before the 20th week of gestation, chronic hypertension is suspected but is not confirmed until after pregnancy. If the blood pressure remains elevated after the pregnancy, the woman has chronic hypertension. Some women with preexisting hypertension may begin the pregnancy with mild disease but then experience severe disease after the 24th week.

The woman with chronic hypertension has superimposed preeclampsia when she experiences proteinuria. Preeclampsia superimposed on chronic hypertension is a particularly lethal combination. In these cases, the preeclampsia tends to develop earlier in the pregnancy and runs a more severe course. The risk of placental abruption and incidence of fetal growth restriction rises significantly.

Treatment and Nursing Care

Ideally, the woman with chronic hypertension meets with the health care provider before becoming pregnant to modify her treatment regimen. If she is taking antihypertensive medications that may be teratogenic (see Chapter 5 regarding teratogens), the health care provider may change her medication to one more appropriate for pregnancy. The provider often recommends a sodium-restricted diet, explains work and exercise limitations, and recommends weight loss if the woman is overweight. During pregnancy, prenatal visits occur at more frequent intervals, usually every 2 weeks during the first half of pregnancy and weekly thereafter. Fetal surveillance is done more frequently with serial ultrasound tests, frequent NSTs, and BPPs.

Mild, uncomplicated cases of chronic hypertension tend to fare well without significant increases in perinatal mortality. In fact, the woman with mild disease may not require medication. However, in cases of severe hypertension (i.e., if the diastolic blood pressure exceeds 110 mm Hg), the woman will likely need antihypertensive therapy.

Methyldopa is the antihypertensive drug of choice for maintenance therapy. Beta blockers and calcium channel blockers may be added to the regimen if methyldopa alone is insufficient to control the blood pressure. The benefit of treatment with one of these agents generally outweighs the risk of fetal effects when hypertension is severe. Angiotensin-converting enzyme inhibitors and angiotensin II receptor antagonists/blockers are contraindicated, and thiazide diuretics are not recommended for use during pregnancy because of adverse fetal effects.

Nursing Process and Care Plan *for the Woman With Preeclampsia*

The nursing care plan for the woman with preeclampsia focuses on monitoring the woman and the fetus and observing for signs that indicate the condition is worsening. This is done by frequent nursing assessments and by implementing the health care provider's orders for fetal surveillance tests and maternal blood work.

Assessment (Data Collection)

It is important to assess the preelamptic woman frequently. When she comes to the health care provider's office, reinforce the warning signs that indicate that the preeclampsia is worsening and monitor for those signs. Warning signs include blood pressure that is increasing, elevated proteinuria, headache, visual changes, and epigastric pain.

In the hospital, continue to monitor the vital signs and perform the assessments every 4 hours. Additionally, monitor deep tendon reflexes (DTRs), including observing for clonus, every 4 hours. If the woman is on medications to decrease her blood pressure, monitor for the effectiveness of the medications and observe for side effects or toxic levels of the medications.

Ensure that any lab work that is ordered is drawn in a timely manner and report the values to the RN and the health care provider. Lab values of importance to monitor include liver enzymes and platelets. Assist with any fetal surveillance tests that are ordered.

Nursing Care Focus

When selecting the focus of nursing care for the woman with preeclampsia, consideration should be given to the safety of the woman and the fetus and prevention of any injury. As preeclampsia can be a frightening experience for the woman, reinforcing teaching done by the RN is also a priority.

Outcome Identification and Planning

Major goals for the woman include that she and the fetus do not suffer any harm from the elevated blood pressure. Also, a major goal is that the preeclampsia does not progress into eclampsia. If the woman's condition does worsen, a major goal is that the woman and the fetus do not experience harm from a seizure. As the woman can experience warning signs that indicate the preeclampsia is worsening, providing the woman with information about these warning signs is important. Planning of nursing activities is based upon these goals.

Nursing Care Focus

- Hypertension risk

Goal

- The woman will have blood pressures that are 140/90 or below and are not increasing.

Implementations for Monitoring for and Preventing Hypertension

Collect data on the woman frequently. Data include vital signs, central nervous system (CNS) observations, urine output, weight gain, and edema.

Monitor the woman's vital signs every 4 hours, or more frequently, as ordered. Report any blood pressure over 140/90 mm Hg or as ordered. A highly elevated blood pressure can interfere with blood flow to major body organs and extremities. Check deep tendon reflexes (DTRs) and observe for clonus. Monitor neurologic status (level of responsiveness). Determine if the woman is having any visual changes. The CNS is sensitive to increase in fluid volume. The retina responds with the woman reporting blurred or double vision or seeing spots. Changes in levels of consciousness may indicate the presence of cerebral edema.

Perform strict intake and output measurements. Monitor urinary output every 4 hours or as ordered; report outputs totaling less than 30 mL/hour, or 120 mL per 4-hour time period. An indwelling urinary catheter may be ordered to help monitor urinary output and to assist the woman with maintain bed rest. Dipstick the urine to check for proteinuria. Send urine samples or 24-hour urine collections to the lab as ordered. Reduced urinary output can indicate decreased blood flow to the kidneys, which should be treated promptly to prevent kidney damage. Protein in the urine indicates inability of the kidneys to function properly.

Weigh the woman daily. Use the same scale at the same time each day with the same amount of clothing. Report any sudden weight gain to the RN and the health care provider. Monitor for edema, especially periorbital edema. Sudden weight gain and edema indicates that fluid is being retained. Although the woman has more overall body water, the fluid is trapped in tissues so that less fluid is in the blood, a condition that leads to decreased perfusion.

Have the woman maintain bed rest in side-lying position as ordered (strict or with bathroom privileges). Bed rest in a side-lying position improves blood flow to the placenta, kidneys, and other vital organs. Have the woman avoid lying supine to prevent supine hypotension syndrome.

Administer medications as ordered. If the woman is on magnesium sulfate, monitor for symptoms of toxic levels including decreased DTRs and respiratory depression. Monitor lab values being drawn. Blood may be drawn to measure liver enzymes and platelets. Changes in liver perfusion can cause changes in liver enzymes.

Evaluation of Goal/Desired Outcome

The woman:

- remains alert, awake, and responsive.
- has a blood pressure of 140/90 mm Hg or lower.
- has a urinary output of at least 30 mL/hour.
- exhibits peripheral edema +1 or less.
- has a stable weight without sudden increases.

Nursing Care Focus

- Injury risk

Goal

- The woman remains seizure and injury free.

Implementations for Preventing Seizures and Injury

The woman with preeclampsia is at risk for seizures. While it is not possible to predict which woman will become eclamptic and have a seizure, there are some indications that she might be more prone to have a seizure. Also, there are nursing activities that can be implemented to help reduce conditions that can cause seizures. Additionally, the health care provider may order medication to help reduce the woman's risk for seizures.

Observe the woman frequently. Monitor her vital signs every 4 hours at a minimum and observe for increasing blood pressure. Increasing blood pressure indicates a worsening of status. The woman is then at risk for seizure activity. Monitor her deep tendon reflexes and observe for any increase in activity or clonus. Report these findings to the RN and the health care provider immediately.

Provide a quiet, stimulation-free room. Dim the lights, have the TV and radio off, have the woman silence her phone and avoid looking at screens (e.g., electronic readers, looking at/working on computer, playing games on her phone). Limit visitors. Instruct visitors to speak in soft voices and avoid excess conversation. Reinforce to the woman and her visitors the rationale for the decreased stimuli and the nursing procedures performed to increase compliance.

Have woman's room away from high-activity areas such as by elevators or waiting areas. To aid observation of the woman, her room should be close to the nurses' desk but far enough away to avoid overstimulation from noise. A noisy, stimulating environment increases the risk for the woman to have a seizure.

Monitor her for signs that her condition is worsening. These include headache, blurred vision, epigastric pain, hyperreactive reflexes, and presence of clonus. Institute seizure precautions, which include side rails up and padded; airway, suction, and oxygen equipment are set up at the woman's bedside. If the woman does have a seizure, these measures will all be needed to prevent serious injury from the seizure (e.g., aspiration).

Assist the RN to administer magnesium sulfate, as ordered. Monitor for magnesium toxicity. Monitor the woman's respiratory status and DTRs frequently. Monitor serum magnesium levels that are drawn. Report these findings to the RN and the health care provider immediately, even if they are within normal limits. Magnesium sulfate is a muscle relaxant and a CNS depressant that can prevent eclamptic seizures.

Prepare for delivery of infant if woman does experience a seizure. Notify the newborn intensive care unit (NICU) of the woman's status. If the woman is on magnesium sulfate prior to delivery, the newborn will need to be observed for respiratory depression after birth.

Evaluation of Goal/Desired Outcome

The woman:

- does not experience a seizure.
- does not experience injury from any seizure activity.

Nursing Care Focus

- Altered tissue perfusion

Goal

- The fetus will demonstrate signs of adequate tissue perfusion.

Implementations for Monitoring and Maintaining Tissue Perfusion

Alteration in the woman's blood pressure affects the fetus. To aid fetal oxygenation, it is important to maintain placental perfusion. Help the woman maintain a side-lying position, or with a wedge under one hip. A side-lying position increases perfusion to the placenta.

Perform frequent fetal heart rate (FHR) and contraction monitoring. Observe for contractions, decreased FHR, decelerations, or a decrease in variability. Report any changes in the fetal baseline status immediately to the RN and the health care provider. Monitoring is done to determine fetal status. Administer oxygen to the woman as ordered. An increase in maternal oxygen levels increases available oxygen to fetus.

Instruct the woman to monitor fetal movement (kick) count after each meal (see Chapter 7). If the fetus is moving as often as expected, there is reassurance the fetus is doing well. A decrease in fetal movement is an ominous sign. Assist the RN with performing NSTs, as ordered. Serial NSTs may be ordered to closely monitor fetal status. A non-reactive NST indicates the fetus may be in distress.

Evaluation of Goal/Desired Outcome

The fetus:

- maintains a heart rate between 110 and 160 bpm.
- remains active with normal fetal movement (kick) count.
- demonstrates well-being with reactive NSTs.

MULTIPLE GESTATION

A multiple gestation refers to a pregnancy in which the woman is carrying more than one fetus. (Singleton gestation is the term used for a pregnancy with one fetus.) Twins are the most common manifestation of multiple gestation. In the general population, naturally occurring twins (two fetuses) occur once in 250 deliveries, triplets (three fetuses) occur once in 8,000 deliveries, and quadruplets (four fetuses) occur once in 600,000 pregnancies (Fletcher, 2019). Most pregnancies resulting in more than two fetuses are the result of fertility treatments.

Twins can be identical (monozygotic), resulting from one ovum fertilized by one sperm, or fraternal (dizygotic), the result of two ova fertilized by two sperms (see Chapter 5 for review). A woman has an increased chance of conceiving dizygotic twins if she has one or more of the following risk factors: older maternal age, multiparity, or family history of dizygotic twins. Monozygotic twins may have one or two placentas and one or two amniotic sacs. The best situation occurs when monozygotic twins each have their own placenta and amniotic sac.

When twins share a placenta, a serious condition called twin-to-twin transfusion syndrome can occur. In this situation, one twin (called the recipient) receives more blood from the placenta than their sibling. The recipient twin gets too much blood, which can overload the cardiovascular system and result in polycythemia and heart failure. The other twin, called the donor, does not get enough blood from the placenta. This twin can become severely anemic and experience intrauterine growth restriction (IUGR).

The woman with multifetal pregnancy is at increased risk for hyperemesis gravidarum, pyelonephritis, preterm labor, placenta previa, and preeclampsia–eclampsia. The fetuses are at risk, as well. They may be conjoined, experience growth restriction, or be born prematurely. During labor, there is a higher risk for umbilical cord prolapse. During the postpartum period, the woman is at risk for postpartum hemorrhage.

A multifetal pregnancy also increases fetal nutrient demands. The woman carrying a multifetal pregnancy has increased nutritional needs as compared to a singleton pregnancy. This situation can easily lead to maternal anemia. Insufficient iron leads to iron-deficiency anemia, whereas insufficient folic acid may result in megaloblastic anemia.

Clinical Manifestations

The woman carrying multiple fetuses usually presents with a uterus that is large for dates. She is more likely than a woman carrying one fetus to experience anemia, fatigue, severe nausea and vomiting, and hyperemesis gravidarum. The health care provider performs an ultrasound examination to date the pregnancy and to rule out polyhydramnios, fibroid tumors (leiomyomas), and molar pregnancy.

Treatment

Management of a multifetal pregnancy often includes consultation with a perinatologist. There is increased emphasis on the woman's diet, multivitamin and iron supplements, and rest. Obstetric ultrasounds are done every 4 to 6 weeks after diagnosis to monitor fetal growth, presentation, and placental location. After 24 weeks' gestation, prenatal visits increase in frequency to every 2 weeks. The health care provider checks the cervix at every visit. Weekly NSTs begin after 32 weeks.

The provider must choose (or recommend) a mode of delivery. In general, a cesarean delivery is indicated if twin A (the first twin) is not in a vertex presentation. If twin A is vertex, the health care provider may opt to try a vaginal delivery. This method has a higher chance of success if both twins are vertex. If twin B (the second twin) is breech, the provider may schedule a cesarean delivery or attempt a vaginal delivery but only if twin B is not larger than twin A. If twin B experiences fetal distress or if there is difficulty delivering twin B vaginally, a cesarean delivery may be performed for twin B.

Nursing Care

Assist the health care provider in performing diagnostic tests to detect complications throughout the pregnancy. Instruct the woman regarding symptoms of preterm labor (Chapter 18). Inform the woman to perform fetal movement counts daily after 32 weeks' gestation. Encourage the woman to get adequate rest and a well-balanced diet.

> ### TEST YOURSELF
> ✔ List four categories of high blood pressure during pregnancy.
> ✔ What is the underlying process that causes most of the problems associated with preeclampsia?
> ✔ HELLP is an acronym for _____.
> ✔ List three complications for which a multiple gestation is at risk.

Remember **Shakeba Winters** from the start of the chapter. How would you know if her condition was worsening? If you were to see these symptoms, what would be the nursing measures you would want to implement, and why would you want to do so?

KEY POINTS

- Nursing care of the woman with hyperemesis gravidarum focuses on decreasing trigger factors and assisting the woman with regaining fluid balance and obtaining nutrition needed for healthy fetal development.

- Rh and ABO incompatibilities can cause hemolytic disease of the fetus/newborn. The goal of therapy for Rh incompatibility is to prevent isoimmunization of the woman. This is done by administering anti-D immune globulin to the Rh-negative woman within 72 hours of early pregnancy loss, birth, or invasive procedures, such as amniocentesis. If the woman is isoimmunized, the focus of nursing care becomes the fetus, who may require exchange transfusions.

- Signs and symptoms of ectopic pregnancy include missed menstrual period, nausea and vomiting, abdominal pain, shoulder pain, and vaginal spotting or bleeding. If the fallopian tube ruptures, the woman experiences hemorrhage into the abdominal cavity and may develop hypovolemic shock.

- Early pregnancy loss (also referred to as a spontaneous abortion or miscarriage) occurs before the fetus is able to survive outside the uterus on their own (before viability, usually 20 weeks' gestation). Spontaneous abortions are classified according to whether or not the uterus is emptied, or for how long the products of conception are retained. The six types of spontaneous abortion are threatened, inevitable, incomplete, complete, missed, and habitual (recurrent).

- Cerclage is the surgical procedure used to treat cervical insufficiency. A suture closes the cervix with the goal that the woman will be able to carry the pregnancy to near term.

- For the woman with a molar pregnancy, provide client information regarding follow-up care, including the importance of frequent obstetrical visits, monitoring of serum hCG levels, avoiding pregnancy for at least 1 year, and reporting any symptoms of metastasis (e.g., severe persistent headache, cough or bloody sputum, or unexpected vaginal bleeding).

- Placenta previa causes painless, bright red bleeding during pregnancy because of an abnormally implanted placenta that is too close to, or covers, the cervix. Abruptio placentae is associated with dark red, painful bleeding caused by the premature separation of the placenta from the wall of the uterus at any time before the end of labor.

- The focus of nursing care for the woman with a bleeding disorder is maintaining placental perfusion and fluid volume, avoiding maternal and fetal injury (dealing with decreased perfusion and hypoxia), preventing maternal injury (dealing with isoimmunization), and reducing anxiety and pain.

- Hypertensive disorders are classified according to when in relation to the pregnancy the high blood pressure is first diagnosed, the presence or absence of proteinuria, and whether or not the condition resolves spontaneously after delivery. The four categories of hypertension are gestational hypertension, preeclampsia/eclampsia, chronic hypertension, and preeclampsia superimposed on chronic hypertension.

- Priority nursing interventions for the woman with preeclampsia–eclampsia include maintaining bed rest in a side-lying position; monitoring neurologic status, blood pressure, urinary output, and daily weights; maintaining a minimally stimulating environment; instituting seizure precautions; observing for signs of an impending seizure (headache, blurred vision, epigastric pain, hyperactive reflexes, and presence of clonus); assisting the RN with administering magnesium sulfate; and monitoring the fetus (fetal movement [kick] count, FHR, and NSTs).

- A multiple gestation (multifetal pregnancy) is an at-risk pregnancy. The woman is more likely to experience hyperemesis gravidarum, pyelonephritis, preterm labor, placenta previa, preeclampsia–eclampsia, and postpartum hemorrhage. Close observation of the pregnancy with special attention to diet and fetal well-being is recommended. The mode of delivery is dependent on several factors, the most important of which is the presentation of each twin.

INTERNET RESOURCES

Hyperemesis Gravidarum

http://americanpregnancy.org/healthy-pregnancy/
pregnancy-complications/hyperemesis-gravidarum-880/

Early Pregnancy Loss

https://www.babycenter.com/pregnancy/health-and-safety/
miscarriage-signs-causes-and-treatment_252

Ectopic and Molar Pregnancy

https://www.mayoclinic.org/diseases-conditions/ectopic-pregnancy/
symptoms-causes/syc-20372088

https://www.mayoclinic.org/diseases-conditions/molar-pregnancy/
symptoms-causes/syc-20375175

Preeclampsia

https://www.whattoexpect.com/pregnancy/preeclampsia/

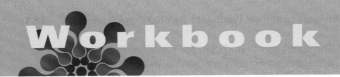
NCLEX-STYLE REVIEW QUESTIONS

1. A 28-year-old gravida 4, para 0 is at the prenatal clinic for complaints of lower abdominal cramping and spotting at 12 weeks' gestation. The nurse-midwife performs a pelvic examination and finds that the cervix is closed. What does the nurse suspect is the cause of the cramps and spotting?

   a. Ectopic pregnancy
   b. Habitual abortion
   c. Cervical insufficiency
   d. Threatened abortion

2. A 32-year-old gravida 1, para 0 at 36 weeks' gestation comes to the obstetric department reporting abdominal pain. Her blood pressure is 164/90 mm Hg, her pulse is 100 beats per minute, and her respirations are 24 breaths per minute. She is restless and slightly diaphoretic with a small amount of dark red vaginal bleeding. What should the nurse's next intervention be?

   a. Check deep tendon reflexes.
   b. Measure fundal height.
   c. Palpate the fundus and check FHR.
   d. Obtain a voided urine specimen and determine blood type.

3. Which data collection finding best correlates with a diagnosis of hydatidiform mole?

   a. Bright red, painless vaginal bleeding
   b. Brisk deep tendon reflexes and shoulder pain
   c. Dark red, "clumpy" vaginal discharge
   d. Painful uterine contractions and nausea

4. Which instruction is appropriate to give to a woman with hyperemesis gravidarum?

   a. Eat mainly high-fat foods to supply sufficient calories.
   b. Limit fluids with meals to increase retention of food.
   c. Do all your own cooking so you will build up a tolerance for food odors.
   d. Take your antinausea medicine after meals to help control the nausea.

5. The nurse is performing data collection on a woman at the pregnancy clinic. Which of the following should be reported to RN? (Select all that apply.)

   a. The pregnant woman states that her mother had preeclampsia during her first pregnancy.
   b. The pregnant woman states her previous health care provider prescribed antihypertensives for her to take.
   c. The pregnant woman is 25 years old.
   d. The pregnant woman identified her race as Asian.
   e. The pregnant woman states she is hoping to have a male baby.
   f. The pregnant woman is G1P0.

STUDY ACTIVITIES

1. Fill in the table to indicate how ectopic pregnancy, threatened abortion, inevitable abortion, and cervical insufficiency are alike and how they are different according to the signs and symptoms listed.

	Pain	Bleeding	Nausea and Vomiting	Cervical Dilatation
Ectopic pregnancy				
Threatened abortion				
Inevitable abortion				
Cervical insufficiency				

2. Think of an experience you, a relative, or a friend has had that involved a miscarriage. Be ready to share your story with your clinical group. Discuss interventions the nurse can use to help the parents cope after a miscarriage.

3. Do an internet search on women's personal stories with having preeclampsia. What are some common feelings these mothers express? What challenges did they face during their pregnancy, delivery, and recovery? What challenges or concerns did their families experience? How can the nurse address these feelings or concerns?

CRITICAL THINKING: WHAT WOULD YOU DO?

Apply your knowledge of hypertensive disorders of pregnancy to the following situation.

1. Maria, a 38-year-old primigravida, presents to the health care provider's office for a scheduled prenatal visit at 28 weeks' gestation. During the data collection, Maria comments that she must be eating more than she thought because she gained 5 lb (2.3 kg) during the course of 2 days. Her blood pressure is 150/92 mm Hg while sitting.

   a. What should the nurse ask next? Why?
   b. What additional information should be collected?
   c. Based on these data, what management plan is the health care provider likely to implement?

2. Maria is admitted to the hospital to rule out preeclampsia. The doctor's orders include bed rest with bathroom privileges, regular diet, private room, limit visitors, 24-hour urine specimen for protein and creatinine clearance, complete blood count, blood urea nitrogen and creatinine levels, liver profile, and coagulation studies.

   a. How should the nurse prepare the room for Maria? What supplies are needed? Why?

   b. If Maria has preeclampsia, what results does the nurse anticipate to see on the laboratory report for each test?

   c. Why did the health care provider write an order for a private room and to limit visitors?

3. Maria receives a diagnosis of mild preeclampsia. She is to remain in the hospital on bed rest.

   a. What fetal diagnostic tests should be done? How frequently?

   b. What special instructions and recurring observations should be included on the care plan?

   c. Maria asks the nurse, "Since my condition is mild, why can't I just go home? I could stay in bed there, and I'd be so much more comfortable." How should the nurse reply?

4. The nurse is doing the morning data collection and exam. Maria says, "I woke up with a terrible headache, and I can't seem to wake up enough to see well this morning. Everything looks blurry." Maria's blood pressure is 164/110 mm Hg.

   a. How is Maria's condition classified now?

   b. What other data should the nurse collect? What should be the nurse's priority intervention?

   c. How does the nurse expect the treatment plan will change?

Labor at Risk

Learning Objectives

At the conclusion of this chapter, you will:

1. Explain labor dystocia and describe appropriate nursing interventions.
2. Discuss the different types of fetal malpresentation and nursing interventions during each one.
3. Compare and contrast prelabor rupture of membranes (PROM) with preterm PROM.
4. Describe symptoms that may indicate preterm labor (PTL).
5. Discuss treatment options for PTL.
6. Apply the nursing process to the care of a woman in PTL.
7. Discuss potential complications, medical management, and nursing care for the woman with a postterm pregnancy.
8. Describe nursing interventions for the woman experiencing fetal demise.
9. Compare and contrast obstetric emergencies according to symptoms, treatment, and nursing care.

Bernadette Howard presents to the labor unit stating she thinks she is in labor. While gathering information from her, you learn that she is 34 weeks pregnant, this is her first pregnancy, and she started leaking amniotic fluid about 1 hour ago. As you read this chapter, think about what the causes of Bernadette's preterm labor (PTL) might be. Also, think about what interventions the health care provider might order to stop her PTL. How would this differ from the woman who was 42 weeks pregnant presenting to the labor unit with the same symptoms?

During labor, some situations may arise that put the woman and her fetus at risk. It is for this reason that many women prefer to deliver in a hospital setting. The following discussion describes complications that the nurse sometimes encounters during care of the laboring woman. Although you may not be directly responsible for the laboring woman, it is helpful to know the signs of labor complications to be able to summon help when needed.

DYSFUNCTIONAL LABOR (DYSTOCIA)

Labor dystocia is an abnormally slow progression of labor. Dystocia occurs because of a malfunction in one or more of the "four Ps" of labor that were discussed in Chapter 8: passageway, passenger, powers, and psyche. Passageway problems that may be encountered include that the pelvis may be small or contracted because of disease or injury. Passenger problems included the fetus being malpositioned, excessively large (macrosomic), or having an anomaly, such as hydrocephalus, which may not allow them to fit through the birth canal. Problems related to powers include uterine contractions that may be of insufficient quality or quantity, or that the woman may be unable to push effectively during the second stage of labor because of exhaustion. Psyche problems may include the woman "fighting" the contractions because of fear or pain. Frequently a combination of factors results in dysfunctional labor.

Complications

Difficult labor is associated with increased maternal and fetal morbidity and mortality. The risk for infection increases during prolonged labor, particularly in association with ruptured membranes. Bacteria can ascend the birth canal, resulting in fetal or maternal bacteremia and sepsis. Neonatal pneumonia can result from the fetus aspirating infected amniotic fluid. Uterine rupture can occur, which can be lethal for the woman and her fetus. Labor dystocia is the most common reason cited for performing a primary cesarean delivery.

Some complications of labor dystocia affect the woman after delivery. Fistula formation is more common in prolonged labor because the presenting part exerts pressure for prolonged periods on maternal soft tissue, a situation that can result in tissue necrosis and subsequent fistula development. Pelvic floor injury is more common for the woman who experiences a difficult labor or delivery.

Clinical Manifestations and Diagnosis

Before the birth attendant can diagnose abnormal labor, they must first be aware of what constitutes normal labor. Table 18-1 compares expected rates of labor progress for the primipara and multipara. For additional review of normal labor, refer to Chapters 8 and 10. Labor dystocia can occur in any stage of labor, although it occurs most commonly once the woman is in active labor (4- to 7-cm dilation) or when she reaches the second stage of labor (10-cm dilation to birth of fetus).

Causes of Labor Dysfunction

Labor dysfunction can occur because of problems with the uterus, maternal pelvis, or situations involving the fetus.

TABLE 18-1 Expected Labor Progress

	PRIMIPARA	MULTIPARA
Expected length of the latent phase of labor	<20 hours	<14 hours
Expected rate of dilation during active labor	At least 1.2 cm/hour	At least 1.5 cm/hour
Expected rate of fetal descent during active labor	At least 1 cm/hour	At least 2 cm/hour

Uterine Dysfunction

There are two types of uterine dysfunction: hypotonic and hypertonic. The most common is hypotonic dysfunction. This dysfunctional labor pattern manifests by uterine contractions that lack the quantity or strength to dilate the cervix, regardless of the regularity of the contraction pattern.

Hypertonic dysfunction presents in two different ways. The most common is frequent, but ineffective, contractions. Some birth attendants refer to this syndrome as uterine "irritability." The underlying problem with this disorder is that the uterine muscle cells do not contract in a coordinated fashion. The result is an increased resting uterine tone with small, short, frequent contractions.

The other type of hypertonic dysfunction manifests as increased frequency and intensity of uterine contractions. This type of hypertonic dysfunction often results in **precipitous labor**—labor that lasts less than 3 hours from the start of uterine contractions to birth. The maternal complication that most frequently results from a precipitous labor is soft tissue damage such as lacerations of the cervix, vaginal wall, and perineum. Newborn complications include bruising or other trauma to the infant from rapid descent through the birth canal. Additionally, the newborn is at risk for respiratory complications due to the fact they did not get much time to have the fetal lung fluid expelled from the lungs during labor.

Be Careful!
Do not confuse precipitous labor with precipitous delivery. Precipitous labor is an abnormally fast labor (lasting less than 3 hours), whereas a precipitous delivery refers to a delivery that is unattended by the health care provider.

Cephalopelvic Disproportion

Practitioners sometimes refer to the lack of labor progression as "failure to progress." If hypotonic labor is not the cause of failure to progress, the health care provider may suspect cephalopelvic disproportion (CPD). In this situation, the diameters of the fetal head are too large to pass through the birth canal. CPD can be due to an enlarged fetal head, such as in fetal macrosomia or hydrocephalus, or it can result from a small maternal pelvis.

Fetal Malposition

Fetal malposition can cause prolonged labor. When the back of the fetal head is toward the posterior portion of the maternal pelvis, the position is occiput posterior (OP) (see Chapter 8 for a review of fetal positions). A labor complicated by occiput posterior position is usually prolonged and characterized by maternal perception of increased intensity of back discomfort. The lay term for this type of labor is "back labor." Face presentation is another cause of prolonged labor. When the fetal face presents, the largest diameters of the fetal head present to the maternal pelvis, and labor is generally prolonged. Breech presentation, transverse lie, and compound presentations may also cause labor dystocia. Any of these fetal positions may result in the need for cesarean delivery, although vaginal delivery may be possible.

Treatment

Treatment depends on the cause of labor dystocia. However, because the cause is not always readily apparent, the birth attendant usually gives a "trial of labor." **Augmentation**, something added to labor in order to improve it, is usually the treatment for uterine hypofunction causing inadequate labor progress. This is done by artificial rupture of membranes, if they are still intact, or intravenous (IV) oxytocin infusion, or a combination of both. When oxytocin is ordered, the health care provider will use the same orders and precautions as when oxytocin is used for labor induction (see Chapter 11). Augmentation with oxytocin is the treatment of choice for uterine irritability. In this situation, oxytocin assists the uterus with contracting more effectively, causing the pattern to space out with individual contractions becoming stronger and more effective. Women on oxytocin often report more pain as compared to women in labor without oxytocin. Oxytocin is contraindicated when there is placental abruption.

Hypertonic labor, either increased uterine tone or more than five contractions in 10 minutes, may result from an increased sensitivity of uterine muscle to oxytocin, either from labor induction or augmentation. Treatment for this cause of hypertonic labor is to decrease or shut off the oxytocin infusion. If the hypertonic pattern causes the fetal heart rate to drop, the health care provider may order administration of a **tocolytic**, a substance that relaxes the uterine muscle.

If the cause of labor dystocia is fetal malposition, the health care provider may attempt to manipulate the fetus to a more favorable position. For occiput posterior position, the fetus may rotate unaided to an anterior position, although this process generally prolongs labor because the fetus must rotate 180 degrees, as compared with 90 degrees. If the woman completes the first stage of labor and the fetal head has not rotated, the health care provider may use the vacuum extractor or forceps to attempt to rotate the head to an anterior position. This requires that the fetal head be at +2 station or lower. It is possible for the fetus to deliver from an occiput posterior position. In this situation, the fetus is born face up.

Nursing Care

Fetal lie, presentation, and position are determined by the health care provider when the woman presents to the labor and delivery area. For the woman with labor dysfunction, monitor maternal vital signs and the contraction pattern every 30 minutes. Check frequency and intensity of uterine contractions. Note fetal response to uterine contractions. Perform a thorough pain evaluation every hour to include a pain scale to rate intensity. Ask the woman to describe her pain. Inquire regarding the presence of intense back pain.

Document cervical changes and fetal descent, as identified by the RN or the birth attendant, in the woman's medical record. Observe for slow progression or arrest of labor. Slow progression would be indicated if a primipara in active labor dilates slower than 1.2 cm/hour or if the fetal head descends at less than 1 cm/hour; or if a multipara in active labor dilates more slowly than 1.5 cm/hour or if the fetal head descends at less than 1.5 cm/hour over a period of several hours. Arrest of dilation occurs if no cervical change occurs during a 2-hour period and arrest of descent if no descent occurs during a 2-hour period.

Notify the RN and the health care provider if there is slow labor progression or descent. Check to see if the woman has a full bladder. Remember that a full bladder can interfere with the progress of labor. Next, determine if the contraction pattern is adequate. Contractions should occur every 2 to 3 minutes apart, last 60 to 90 seconds, and be of moderate-to-strong intensity during the active phase of labor.

If the woman's bladder is empty and the contraction pattern is adequate, inquire regarding the character of her pain. Suspect occiput posterior position if the woman complains of severe lower back pain. In some cases, having the woman on a hands and knees or Sims position may decrease her discomfort and help to reposition the fetus.

Determine if the woman might benefit from pain relief measures. The health care provider may order the RN to administer IV pain medication or sedation or to prepare the woman for epidural anesthesia. If the woman is "fighting" the contractions, pain control might help her relax and allow the cervix to dilate.

Don't Underestimate the Value of Comfort Measures!

Counterpressure applied to the lower back with a fisted hand or a tennis ball sometimes helps the woman cope with the "back labor" that is characteristic of occiput posterior positioning.

Notify the RN of your findings. Assist the RN with any ordered interventions, such as sedation, anesthesia, or oxytocin augmentation. Continue to monitor the woman's labor progress. Notify the RN if interventions do not result in decreased discomfort and progression of labor or if signs of fetal distress occur.

FETAL MALPRESENTATION

In the majority of pregnancies at term, the fetus presents head down. Malpresentation occurs when the fetus is not in the vertex presentation. The two most common malpresentations are breech and shoulder presentations. Shoulder presentation is more commonly known as transverse lie. Factors that predispose the fetus to malpresentation include multiparity, placenta previa, hydramnios, small pelvis, and uterine anomalies.

In a breech presentation, the fetal buttocks or the feet present to the birth canal (refer to Chapter 8 for pictures of breech presentation). Frequently the preterm fetus is breech because there is room to turn and maneuver in the uterus. At term, approximately 3% to 4% of fetuses are breech

(Hofmeyr, 2019). Breech presentation can cause several birth problems. Labor progress can be slow because the soft buttocks do not provide as much pressure on the cervix as does the head in a vertex presentation. There is an increased risk for umbilical cord prolapse, cervical spine injury, or the fetal head can become trapped during delivery.

Transverse lie (shoulder presentation) occurs once in approximately 300 deliveries (Strauss and Herrera, 2021). As with breech presentation, transverse lie is more common early in pregnancy with most fetuses turning to vertex presentation before term.

Clinical Manifestations and Diagnosis

There are three types of breech presentation: (1) frank (hips flexed, knees extended; also known as pike position); (2) complete (hips and knees flexed; also known as tailor position); and (3) footling or incomplete (one or both hips extended with the foot or feet presenting) (see Fig. 8-6). Frank breech is the preferred breech position for vaginal delivery (Hofmeyr, 2021a).

The most common method the health care provider uses to diagnose fetal malpresentation is Leopold maneuvers (see Fig. 10-3) followed by ultrasound. Sometimes transverse lie is noted by looking at the contour of the abdomen, which tends to be in the shape of a football, wider side to side than top to bottom.

Treatment

For breech presentation, most health care providers prefer to do a cesarean birth without labor or attempting a vaginal delivery. The health care provider may use **external cephalic version**, a process of manipulating the position of the fetus while in utero, to try to turn the fetus to a cephalic presentation (Fig. 18-1). Approximately half of the time this procedure is effective; however, sometimes the fetus turns back to a breech presentation before labor ensues. The woman may be permitted to labor with the fetus in a breech presentation and attempt a vaginal delivery, although this practice is not very common because of successful version techniques and the high risk for fetal and maternal complications during a breech vaginal birth.

For a transverse lie (shoulder presentation), there are two options. The health care provider will either use external cephalic version to try to turn the fetus to a cephalic presentation or deliver the fetus by cesarean. If a transverse lie persists, the fetus cannot deliver vaginally.

This is a Good Preparation!

When you prepare a table in anticipation of a vaginal breech delivery, be sure to include a set of Piper forceps. These special forceps can help deliver the head after the rest of the body has been born in a breech presentation.

Nursing Care

You may need to assist with the external cephalic version procedure, which is done only in facilities that have the capability to do emergency cesarean deliveries. Prior to the procedure, it is important to monitor the woman and

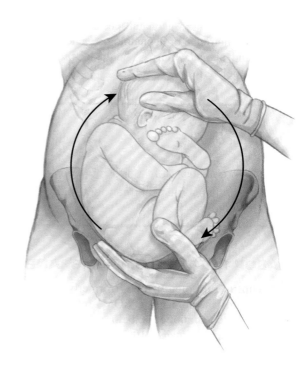

FIGURE 18-1 External cephalic version. One, or two, health care providers manipulate the fetus through the abdominal wall to coax the fetus to turn to a vertex presentation.

the fetus to obtain baseline data. A nonstress test (NST) or biophysical profile (BPP) is done along with fetal heart rate evaluation. Maternal vital signs are also taken. The woman should empty her bladder. Position her supine with a pillow or wedge under one hip. If ordered, the RN administers tocolytic drugs to relax the uterus. Sometimes intravenous access and a decrease in maternal oral intake is ordered preprocedure. The external cephalic version is mildly uncomfortable; assist the woman with relaxation techniques as appropriate. The health care provider may use cornstarch or transducer gel to help their hands glide easier over the woman's scan.

After the procedure, it is very important to monitor both the woman and the fetus as there are some risks to an external cephalic version. Monitor the fetal heart rate (FHR) and evaluate the fetal heart rate pattern for 20 to 40 minutes. Report any decrease in FHR or changes in the FHR pattern to the RN and the health care provider. Monitor the maternal vital signs. Observe for any vaginal bleeding or contractions. Administer anti-D immune globulin to the Rh-negative woman as ordered after the external cephalic version.

If the fetus in breech presentation is to deliver vaginally, expect to see passage of thick meconium. This normally occurs as the buttocks are squeezed during labor and does not usually cause a problem because the meconium does not mix with the amniotic fluid. Assist the RN to prepare for a difficult delivery. Check that all neonatal resuscitation supplies are available and in working order. Have Piper forceps available on the delivery table, and be prepared to assist the birth attendant. A neonatal specialist team (usually made up by a pediatrician or neonatologist, a neonatal nurse practitioner, and neonatal nurse) should be present at all vaginal breech deliveries.

TEST YOURSELF

✔ Name four complications associated with labor dystocia.

✔ Identify three causes of labor dysfunction.

✔ What is the usual medical treatment for uterine hypofunction?

PRELABOR RUPTURE OF MEMBRANES

Prelabor rupture of membranes (formerly called premature rupture of membranes) (PROM) refers to spontaneous rupture of the amniotic sac before the onset of labor. PROM occurs in approximately 10% of pregnancies at term (Jazayeri, 2018a). This condition is different from preterm labor (PTL), which is the onset of labor before the end of 37 weeks gestation.

PROM is also different from preterm PROM (PPROM), which refers to rupture of the amniotic sac before the onset of labor in a woman who is less than 37 weeks gestation. Complications of preterm PROM include maternal and neonatal infection, placental abruption (abruptio placentae), umbilical cord compression or prolapse, fetal pulmonary hypoplasia, and fetal/neonatal death.

Preterm PROM occurs in approximately 3% of all pregnancies and is a leading cause of preterm delivery. Infection is the most common cause of preterm PROM (Duff, 2020). Risk factors for preterm PROM are similar to those for preterm birth and include cigarette smoking, previous preterm delivery, vaginal bleeding, low socioeconomic conditions, sexually transmitted infections, and conditions causing uterine distention (e.g., polyhydramnios, multifetal pregnancy). Some procedures, such as a cervical cerclage or amniocentesis, can result in preterm PROM. The closer to term that PROM occurs, the better the chance for a healthy outcome. Most women with preterm PROM deliver within 1 week after the amniotic sac ruptures. PROM before the age of viability greatly increases the chance of neonatal mortality.

Clinical Manifestations and Diagnosis

The woman with PROM usually presents to the delivery suite with reports of a large gush or continuous leaking of fluid from the vagina. She may report vaginal discharge or bleeding and pelvic pressure. However, she does not present with regular uterine contractions because she is not in labor.

Sometimes the diagnosis is obvious when large amounts of amniotic fluid are visible. A speculum examination may be performed to look for pooling of amniotic fluid. The fluid is tested to see if it is amniotic fluid (instead of urine) by means of either Amnisure ROM test, nitrazine paper, or a fern test. See Chapter 10 for a discussion of these methods under "Immediate Assessments—Risk Assessment."

Treatment

The primary problem for the woman with PROM at term is increased risk for infection, specifically **chorioamnionitis**, which is a bacterial or viral infection of the amniotic fluid and membranes. Fortunately, most women go into spontaneous labor within 24 hours of PROM. Sometimes the labor is induced with oxytocin rather than wait for it to start on its own. Current research indicates that induction of labor for term PROM results in fewer maternal infections and fewer neonatal intensive care admissions (Scorza, 2020). Hospitalization is required for both treatment options, expectant management ("wait and see" method) and induction of labor.

Management of preterm PROM is more complicated. If there are signs of infection, such as elevated maternal temperature; maternal tachycardia; cloudy, foul-smelling amniotic fluid; and uterine tenderness, the health care provider obtains cultures, starts antibiotics, and facilitates delivery regardless of gestational age.

However, if there is no infection, the health care provider may choose expectant management ("wait and see" method). The goal is to allow the fetus time to mature and achieve delivery before the woman or her fetus becomes infected. Prophylactic antibiotics (usually ampicillin and erythromycin) may be ordered for preterm PROM. The usual practice is to administer 7 days of antibiotic therapy. Some studies indicate that prophylactic antibiotics do not change the infection rate and increases the risk for development of resistant strains of bacteria.

For preterm PROM between 24 and 34 weeks, intramuscular corticosteroids are given to the mother to reduce the risk of neonatal respiratory distress syndrome, intraventricular hemorrhage, and necrotizing enterocolitis (Jazayeri, 2018b). Current recommendations are to administer a tocolytic drug to prolong the pregnancy long enough for the corticosteroid injections to work but to avoid long-term tocolytic therapy. The presence of infection is a contraindication for tocolytic administration.

Pelvic rest, a situation in which nothing is placed in the vagina (including tampons or the health care provider's fingers to perform a cervical examination), is instituted because the risk for infection increases whenever the cervix is manipulated. A periodic sterile speculum examination to check for cervical changes may be performed instead. A digital examination of the cervix is not necessary unless signs of labor, such as pelvic pressure, cramping, regular contractions, or bloody show, are present.

Fetal surveillance is done at least daily. Generally, the woman performs kick counts after every meal. Daily nonstress tests may also be ordered. Frequent ultrasound examinations to measure the amount of amniotic fluid and fetal growth are also done.

Nursing Care

Perform thorough data collection on the woman who presents with reports of PROM. Ask the woman to describe the sequence of events that occurred in association with the rupture of the amniotic sac. Check for visible signs of PROM—pooling of fluid and positive Amnisure ROM test, nitrazine paper, or fern test.

Once the diagnosis is established, follow the health care provider's orders for management of PROM. If the woman is at term, expect continuous fetal heart rate monitoring. Watch for the sudden onset of deep variable decelerations, which may indicate umbilical cord prolapse. Take her temperature at least every 2 hours. Promptly report temperature elevation, prolonged maternal or fetal tachycardia, and cloudy or foul-smelling amniotic fluid. The health care provider will observe for the natural onset of labor or induce labor.

Always Give a Thorough Report!

The length of time from when the membranes rupture until delivery is an important part of the report to the newborn's nurse or health care provider. They will monitor the newborn closely for signs of sepsis in the event of prolonged rupture of membranes.

PRETERM LABOR

Preterm labor (PTL) is labor that occurs after 19 weeks and before the end of 37 weeks' gestation. PTL often leads to preterm birth. Preterm birth is the second leading cause for infant death and in 2019, almost 1 in 10 births were preterm (Centers for Disease Control and Prevention, 2020).

The top risk factors for PTL are history of previous preterm birth, current multiple gestation pregnancy (e.g., twins or triplets), infection, high blood pressure during pregnancy, and uterine or cervical abnormalities. Although history of previous preterm birth is one of the better predictors, this association is not helpful for predicting PTL for the primigravida. Box 18-1 lists selected risk factors for PTL. Dehydration can cause PTL. Sometimes the cause of PTL is not readily apparent.

Clinical Manifestations and Diagnosis

The presence of painful uterine contractions does not by itself indicate that the woman is in PTL, because pain is a subjective phenomenon affected by many variables. The definitive diagnosis of PTL is made when uterine contractions result in cervical change. The earlier the diagnosis is made, the greater the likelihood that treatment will be effective. If the health care provider makes the diagnosis after the cervix has dilated to greater than 3 cm, it is unlikely that labor will stop, and it is highly likely that the fetus will be born prematurely.

The woman in PTL often presents with signs that include uterine contractions, which may be painless; pelvic pressure; menstrual-like cramps; vaginal pain; and low, dull backache accompanied by vaginal discharge and bleeding. The membranes may be intact or ruptured. The most frequent examinations used to diagnose PTL include evaluation of contraction frequency, fetal fibronectin test (Box 18-2), and measurement of cervical length. Short cervical length with a positive fetal fibronectin test (meaning there was fetal fibronectin in the vaginal secretions) indicates that

---

BOX 18-1   Risk Factors for Preterm Labor and Birth

Obstetric and Gynecologic Risk Factors
- Multifetal pregnancy (twins, triplets)
- History of preterm birth
- Uterine or cervical abnormalities:
  - Uterine fibroids (uterine myomas)
  - Bicornuate uterus (a uterus with two separate cavities, looks heart shaped in appearance)
  - Cervical insufficiency
- Preterm PROM
- Placenta previa
- Retained intrauterine device
- Short time period (less than 6 to 9 months) between pregnancies
- Poor pregnancy weight gain
- In vitro fertilization
- Polyhydramnios

Demographic and Lifestyle Risk Factors
- Extremes of maternal age (under 17 years of age or over 35 years of age)
- Member of an ethnic minority
- Low socioeconomic status

- Late or no prenatal care
- Smoking
- Alcohol or illicit drug use
- Intimate partner violence
- Lack of social support
- High levels of stress
- Long working hours with long periods of standing

Medical Risk Factors
- Infection
  - Chorioamnionitis
  - Bacterial vaginosis
  - Bacteriuria
  - Acute pyelonephritis
  - Sexually transmitted infections
- High blood pressure
- Diabetes
- Clotting disorders
- Entering the pregnancy underweight
- Obesity
- Dehydration

BOX 18-2 Fetal Fibronectin Test

Fetal fibronectin is a protein that acts as a cellular adhesive (glue) to help the placenta and fetal membranes adhere to the uterus during pregnancy. It is normally absent between weeks 22 and 37 of gestation.

Testing
The health care provider uses a cotton swab to collect a sample of cervical secretions and sends the sample to a laboratory for analysis. It takes approximately 6 to 36 hours to get the results.

Interpreting Results
A negative result (absence of fetal fibronectin) is a reliable indicator that delivery is unlikely to occur within the 2 weeks following the test. A positive test (presence of fetal fibronectin) is a less reliable indicator. A positive test may or may not mean that the woman is in PTL.

the woman has an increased chance of delivering prematurely (Ross, 2018).

Treatment

Standard obstetric care includes evaluation of risk factors for preterm delivery at each office visit. If there are risk factors for PTL, the health care provider examines the cervix for evidence of injury and performs a workup to detect asymptomatic bacteriuria, sexually transmitted infections, and bacterial vaginosis. Antibiotics may be prescribed to treat these infections if present. At 20 and 26 weeks' gestation, cervical length may be measured using transvaginal ultrasound. A cervical length of less than 2.5 cm is associated with PTL (Ross, 2018). The woman receives education regarding

signs and symptoms of PTL. Weekly telephone contact with a nurse and regular prenatal visits are encouraged.

Once PTL is diagnosed, the health care provider must determine how best to treat it. The traditional treatment of bed rest is no longer recommended because of the increased risk of thromboembolism with prolonged bed rest. The health care provider must decide if tocolytics (Table 18-2) are appropriate. Although the medication may not prevent preterm birth, tocolytics often buy enough time to allow for corticosteroid injections to help mature the fetal lungs, treatment of group B streptococcal infections, if present, or to allow transfer to a facility with a higher level of neonatal intensive care. All of these interventions have consistently improved perinatal outcomes. A fetus less than 23 weeks gestation has almost no chance of surviving outside of the womb, so tocolytics generally are not used below this gestational age.

Another treatment is for weekly progesterone to be administered to the pregnant woman with a history of preterm delivery or short cervix (Norwitz, 2020). However, progesterone is not effective in stopping PTL once it has begun. If dehydration is the cause, once the woman receives a fluid bolus the contractions will subside and then stop, usually without the use of tocolytics.

Nursing Process and Care Plan *for the Woman With Preterm Labor*

The nursing care plan for the woman with preterm labor needs to focus on the safety of both the woman and the fetus. Nursing care should also focus on relieving the woman's discomfort and helping her cope with any anxiety she may have related to the preterm labor.

TABLE 18-2 Tocolytic Agents

MEDICATION	ROUTE OF ADMINISTRATION	CONTRAINDICATIONS	MATERNAL SIDE EFFECTS	FETAL/NEONATAL SIDE EFFECTS
Nifedipine	Oral	Use carefully concurrently with magnesium sulfate (increased rate of respiratory depression)	Flushing, headache, dizziness, nausea, transient hypotension	None known—reduction in adverse neonatal outcomes
Terbutaline	Subcutaneous or intravenous (IV)	Injectable not recommended for use >72 hours	Tachycardia, palpitations, anxiety, hypokalemia, hyperglycemia, hypotension, and hyperglycemia	Tachycardia, hyperglycemia
Magnesium sulfate	IV	Contraindicated in women with myasthenia gravis and some cardiac conditions	*At therapeutic levels:* Flushing, feelings of warmth, diaphoresis, lethargy, pulmonary edema *At toxic levels:* Respiratory depression, tetany, paralysis, profound hypotension, cardiac arrest	*At therapeutic levels:* Slight decrease in baseline fetal heart rate level and variability *At toxic levels:* Nonreactive NST; decreased fetal breathing movements
Indomethacin	*Loading dose:* Rectal suppository or oral dose *Maintenance dose:* Oral	Contraindicated in hepatic and renal dysfunction	Nausea, heartburn, gastritis, and emesis	Premature closure of the ductus arteriosus, oligohydramnios, neonatal necrotizing enterocolitis, and intraventricular hemorrhage

Assessment (Data Collection)

Collect a thorough history, including history of previous preterm birth, multifetal pregnancy, infections, cigarette smoking, and other risk factors for preterm labor (PTL) (see Box 18-1). Inquire if the woman is experiencing symptoms of PTL, such as uterine contractions; uncontrollable leaking of fluid from the vagina; backache; menstrual-like cramps; and vaginal pain, discharge, or bleeding.

Monitor for infection. Monitor vital signs, especially the maternal temperature. Observe for foul-smelling amniotic fluid or for fetal or maternal tachycardia.

Data collection includes testing the fluid to see if it is amniotic fluid or not. Place the woman on the fetal monitor. Observe for uterine irritability or contractions. Palpate the uterus carefully.

Observe the woman's emotional response. The threat of PTL may cause apprehension, fear, and anxiety. The woman and her partner may be concerned for the well-being of the fetus. Once the diagnosis is established, the woman may be concerned about the side effects of tocolytic therapy or fear of a preterm birth.

Nursing Care Focus

When selecting the focus of nursing care for the woman with preterm labor, safety is a priority. The woman's discomfort and her level of anxiety are also important to plan care for. The knowledge level of the woman's partner and support she has available during this timeframe is also to be considered when planning her care as this can impact her anxiety.

Outcome Identification and Planning

Major goals for the woman include being free from infection, that she remains free from injury, and that she reports her discomfort and anxiety are manageable. Planning of nursing activities is based upon these goals.

Appropriate safety goals include that the woman will remain free from injury from tocolytic therapy and free from infection. Additional goals and interventions are planned according to the individual needs and situation of the woman.

Nursing Care Focus

● Infection risk

Goal

● The woman will have no signs of infection.

Implementations for Monitoring for and Preventing Infection

The nurse should practice proper and consistent hand hygiene. Instruct the woman on the importance of her performing hand hygiene prior to and after toileting.

Monitor the woman's temperature at least every 4 hours. Monitor the fetal heart rate every 2 hours. Observe for any decrease or increase in variability and for fetal tachycardia (fetal heart rate above 160 bpm). Observe for any amniotic fluid. If it is present, note the color is clear or cloudy and for any foul odor. Encourage fluid intake as dehydration can increase the woman's temperature which can make detecting a fever due to infection difficult. Document your findings in the woman's medical record. Report any abnormal findings to the RN and to the health care provider.

Reinforce to the woman to maintain pelvic rest. She should avoid placing anything in her vagina including tampons and douching. Cervical checks should be avoided unless absolutely necessary. If cervical checks are done, they should be done with sterile technique.

Evaluation of Goal/Desired Outcome

The woman:

● remains afebrile.
● is not tachycardic.
● has amniotic fluid that is clear and not foul smelling.

The fetus:

● has a heart rate between 110 and 160 with moderate variability.

Nursing Care Focus

● Safety

Goal

● The woman will remain free from injury.

Implementations for Preventing Injury

If the woman is receiving magnesium sulfate therapy to stop PTL, observe her at least once per hour. Report dyspnea, tachycardia, productive cough, or adventitious breath sounds to the RN and health care provider. Monitor respiratory status every hour. Report bradypnea or periods of apnea. Check deep tendon reflexes at least hourly. Report decreased or absent reflexes immediately. Refer to Chapter 17 for other nursing actions necessary for magnesium infusion.

Monitor serum potassium and glucose levels, as ordered, if the woman is receiving terbutaline. Report low potassium or elevated glucose levels to the RN and health care provider.

Monitoring fluid status is an important nursing function for the woman in PTL. Monitor the IV site and the rate of infusion. If ordered, the RN may administer a fluid bolus of 500 to 1,000 mL and then reduce the IV to an ordered maintenance rate. Whenever a client receives a fluid bolus, it is important to monitor vital signs, lung sounds, and urine output.

Monitor vital signs. A normal blood pressure in conjunction with a rising pulse upon moving from a recumbent to a sitting or standing position is associated with low fluid volume. Hypotension is associated with severe dehydration. Monitor urinary output. Document urine characteristics.

Concentrated urine with a high specific gravity may indicate dehydration.

Watch for signs of fluid overload. Normally, a healthy pregnant woman can withstand high fluid volumes; however, if she is receiving tocolytics, watch closely for signs of developing pulmonary edema, such as dyspnea, tachycardia, productive cough, and adventitious breath sounds.

Monitor for and report any significant changes in the vital signs, in particular tachycardia or hypotension. The health care provider usually leaves orders detailing the pulse and blood pressure parameters that require reporting. Observe for shortness of breath, anxiety, and palpitations. Immediately report any complaints of chest pain. Monitor for signs of pulmonary edema.

Continue ongoing fetal assessments because a prolapsed umbilical cord can happen anytime after the woman has ruptured, or leaking, membranes. Monitor for an increase in bleeding or for a hard uterus with sharp, unrelenting pain. These could be signs of a labor complication. Report these findings immediately to the RN and health care provider.

Evaluation of Goal/Desired Outcome

The woman:

- has a stable blood pressure and heart rate.
- is without dyspnea or adventitious breath sounds.
- does not exhibit signs of respiratory depression or diminished deep tendon reflexes.

Nursing Care Focus

- Acute pain

Goal

- The woman will state her discomfort is manageable.

Implementations for Managing Pain

Determine the woman's pain using a standardized pain scale. Ask the woman at what level the pain is tolerable. Be sure to ask about and record pain location, characteristics, and intensity. Administer pain medication as ordered by the health care provider. Keep in mind that a sudden increase in pain intensity or pain that does not relent may be the sign of a developing complication. Report any changes in the character or intensity of pain.

Assist the woman with nonpharmacologic pain management including repositioning, effleurage, back rubs, distraction, and guided imagery. Provide distraction techniques as appropriate. Be aware of how the woman's culture affects her reporting and expression of pain. Evaluate the woman's anxiety level. Increased anxiety can increase the woman's pain. Be aware of noise and conversation. Increased stimuli can also increase the woman's pain.

Evaluation of Goal/Desired Outcome

- The woman will verbalize or demonstrate relief of pain.

Nursing Care Focus

- Acute anxiety

Goal

- The woman will display decreased signs and symptoms of anxiety.

Implementations for Reducing Anxiety

Observe the woman for signs of anxiety. Symptoms of anxiety can be expressed in elevated vital signs, sleep disturbances, difficulty concentrating, or changes in eating habits. Use therapeutic communication techniques to develop a trusting relationship with the woman and her support person. Provide care in a calm and reassuring manner. Provide the woman with quiet time and decreased environmental stimulation.

Answer questions honestly and to the best of your ability. If you do not know the answer, say so, and explain that you will find the answer as soon as possible. Make certain that the woman and her partner know the treatment plan. Explain procedures before performing them. With anxiety the woman may not remember prior explanations and plans. Patiently repeat instructions as needed.

Encourage the woman and her partner to verbalize their fears and concerns. She may not be able to voice her exact concerns. Reassure her this is a normal reaction. Allow the woman to ventilate her feelings. With the RN, explore coping strategies with the woman. Assist the woman with using positive coping strategies whenever possible. Explore therapies that reduce anxiety such as music therapy, aromatherapy, or hand or foot massage. The woman may have concerns that she does not share that adds to her anxiety (e.g., child care concerns for other children at home, having to take unexpected time off from work, or concerns related to the safety of the fetus). The woman may benefit from a social service or pastoral care consult.

Evaluation of Goal/Desired Outcome

The woman:

- utilizes positive strategies to reduce anxiety.
- has periods of uninterrupted sleep.
- has vital signs that are within her normal limits.
- verbalizes her concerns.

TEST YOURSELF

✔ What is the difference between PROM and preterm PROM?

✔ Describe four nursing interventions appropriate for the woman with PROM.

✔ List three treatment options that reduce neonatal morbidity and mortality for the woman in PTL.

Remember **Bernadette Howard** from the start of the chapter. What other signs besides the leaking amniotic fluid would indicate Bernadette is in preterm labor? What nursing measures would you perform and what medical interventions would you expect to be implemented? What interventions would be implemented to stop her preterm labor?

POSTTERM PREGNANCY AND LABOR

A postterm pregnancy, sometimes called prolonged pregnancy, is one that lasts longer than 2 weeks after the due date, (i.e., 42 weeks). Approximately 6% of pregnancies deliver at >41 weeks, with less than 1% delivered at >42 weeks (Norwitz, 2021). Miscalculation of gestational age can lead to an incorrect diagnosis of postterm pregnancy. When the woman seeks late prenatal care or is unsure of her last menstrual period, miscalculation of gestational age occurs more frequently. This is true because early sonograms are the most accurate tool to determine gestational age.

A postterm pregnancy is at risk for increased perinatal mortality, particularly during labor. This is due to insufficiency of the aging placenta (placental insufficiency) to nourish the fetus adequately. Oligohydramnios and meconium staining of the amniotic fluid are common complications of postterm pregnancy. Oligohydramnios increases the incidence of cord compression, which can lead to fetal distress during labor. Thick meconium-stained fluid increases the risk for meconium aspiration syndrome (discussed in Chapter 20). The risk for birth of an unusually large infant increases as the gestation advances. The woman in labor with a large infant is at higher risk for shoulder dystocia. A postterm pregnancy that is also complicated by intrauterine fetal growth restriction is particularly at risk for perinatal mortality (Ringer, 2020).

Clinical Manifestations and Diagnosis

If the woman has not had early prenatal care that documents a reliable due date, the health care provider will attempt to use several methods to determine fetal age. Examples include when the fetal heart rate was first heard by Doppler or by fetoscope, early ultrasound measurements, and recorded fundal height measurements.

Other findings associated with a postterm pregnancy such as decreased amniotic fluid volume on ultrasound, fetal macrosomia (birth weight over 4,000 grams), and meconium staining of the amniotic fluid are frequently noted.

Treatment

There are two basic treatment plans for the woman who is carrying a postterm pregnancy. One plan is expectant management. This treatment protocol involves frequent testing for fetal well-being. The health care provider instructs the woman to report decreased fetal movement immediately. The woman must have NSTs and ultrasounds to measure amniotic fluid volume at least twice weekly. Other testing may include biophysical profiles. The second strategy for managing a postterm pregnancy is induction of labor at 41 to 42 weeks' gestation. (Chapter 11 discusses labor induction.)

One intrapartum treatment that might be ordered for the postterm pregnancy is **amnioinfusion**, infusion of sterile isotonic fluid into the uterine cavity during labor. In the postterm pregnancy, amnioinfusion may be done to relieve persistent deep variable decelerations associated with cord compression from oligohydramnios. Some health care providers order amnioinfusion to dilute thick meconium-stained amniotic fluid in an effort to decrease morbidity and mortality from meconium aspiration syndrome; however, current evidence is that amnioinfusion for reducing neonatal morbidity from thick meconium is not beneficial (Goldfarb, 2020). Possible complications from amnioinfusion include polyhydramnios from trapped amniotic fluid, increased intrauterine pressures, and chorioamnionitis (from diluting the amniotic fluid as it has bacteriostatic properties).

Nursing Care

Instruct the woman who is postterm to monitor fetal movements daily. Explain the importance of reporting decreased fetal movement immediately. She may be anxious regarding the well-being of her fetus. Provide realistic reassurances. Be certain that the health care provider has answered all her questions and concerns adequately. If you identify a knowledge deficit or if the woman has questions, reinforce prior teaching or refer her to the RN or health care provider for clarification.

During labor, observe the fetal monitor strip closely for signs of fetal distress. Report these immediately to the RN. Carefully note and record the color and amount of amniotic fluid when the membranes rupture. No amniotic fluid is a concern because it may indicate oligohydramnios. Also observe the amniotic fluid for meconium staining. Document the characteristics of the amniotic fluid in the woman's medical record and notify the RN of your findings.

The RN is responsible for assisting with the amnioinfusion and monitoring the woman. The nurse connects the appropriate solution (either normal saline or Lactated Ringers without dextrose) to the IV tubing, primes the tubing, and then assists the health care provider to insert the intrauterine catheter. After the catheter is in place, the nurse attaches the IV tubing to the infusion port and slowly administers a fluid bolus of 250 mL and then connects the tubing to an IV pump and sets the rate as ordered. Slow gravity infusion can also be done. Usually no more than 1,000 mL is infused to avoid increased intrauterine pressure or causing polyhydramnios.

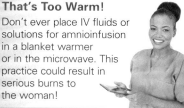

That's Too Warm!
Don't ever place IV fluids or solutions for amnioinfusion in a blanket warmer or in the microwave. This practice could result in serious burns to the woman!

The RN monitors the resting tone of the uterus at least every 30 minutes. The resting tone should not exceed

25 mm Hg. You may help monitor the resting tone and assist the woman with perineal care. Note and record the amount, color, and odor of the fluid expelled onto the under-buttocks pad. If no fluid is returning at all, notify the RN immediately.

INTRAUTERINE FETAL DEATH

Fetal death is death of the fetus in utero (as evidenced by lack of cardiac activity) at 20 weeks or greater gestation or a weight of 500 grams (some states use 350 grams) or more. This definition distinguishes fetal death from early pregnancy loss (miscarriage).

Causes of fetal death fall into four general types: fetal, placental, maternal, and unknown. Examples of fetal causes include genetic or congenital abnormalities and infection. The most common cause of fetal demise is placental abruption, which is usually categorized under placental causes; however, preeclampsia and other maternal disorders can increase the risk for placental abruption. Cord accidents (such as prolapse or true knot), prelabor rupture of membranes (PROM), and twin-to-twin transfusion syndrome are other placental causes. Maternal causes include advanced maternal age; medical disorders, such as diabetes and hypertension; and pregnancy-related complications such as preeclampsia–eclampsia, Rh isoimmunization, uterine rupture, and infection.

Clinical Manifestations and Diagnosis

Often the woman presents for treatment when she cannot detect fetal movements. Inability to find the fetal heart rate leads the health care provider to suspect fetal death. Ultrasound confirms fetal death.

Treatment

The current recommendation is to induce labor as soon as possible after diagnosis of fetal death to avoid the complication of a coagulopathy (e.g., disseminated intravascular coagulation [DIC]) (Mattingly, 2016). If the woman is at, or near, term the decision is usually made to induce labor. If the gestational age is less than 28 weeks, the cervix is rarely favorable for induction. In these cases, the health care provider may prescribe prostaglandin E_2 vaginal suppositories or oral or intravaginal misoprostol to prepare the cervix for labor induction.

Nursing Care

Physical care of the woman is similar to that for other women having labor induced. Pay careful attention to the history because the woman with a uterine scar from previous surgery is at risk for rupture. For the woman at term, use the tocodynamometer to monitor uterine contractions during labor. Postpartum care is the same as for other women.

Emotional care of the woman is more complex. She may experience shock, denial, anger, and depression. Remember that grief responses vary from individual to individual. Allow the woman and her family space to comfort one another, but do not avoid her. Offer to call a pastor or other spiritual leader. Be sure to determine whether the woman would like any religious sacraments or rituals. Most facilities provide postpartum care in a unit or room away from the nursery.

Be sure that mementos are collected. Take pictures as dictated by institutional policy. Pictures are usually taken even if the woman refuses them. The chaplain or social worker may keep the pictures on file for a year or more. Inform the woman that she can change her mind and come get the pictures at any time. Collect a lock of hair, footprints, and other reminders of the baby. Refer to Chapter 19 for further discussion of how to care for the grieving woman.

> **Don't Forget the Golden Rule!**
> A woman who has just received a diagnosis of fetal death is experiencing a significant loss. Be available to her without intruding. Answer her questions honestly. Encourage her to hold and name her baby if she is able. Avoid statements such as "It wasn't the baby's time to be born" which are nontherapeutic and hurtful to the grieving parent.

> **TEST YOURSELF**
> ✔ Name five complications for which the postterm pregnancy is at risk.
> ✔ List four categories of causes of fetal death.
> ✔ Describe at least three ways you can provide support for the woman with a fetal demise.

EMERGENCIES ASSOCIATED WITH LABOR AND BIRTH

Although most births occur without major complications, true emergencies can rapidly develop. The two goals of treatment in any obstetric emergency are prompt recognition of the problem and timely team intervention. Good communication skills are essential for team functioning. It is important for you to recognize risk factors for obstetric emergencies in order to anticipate possible complications. You must also be knowledgeable and skillful in responding to emergent situations.

Amniotic Fluid Embolism

Amniotic fluid embolism (AFE) is a rare obstetric emergency that happens during labor or within the 30 minutes after the placenta delivers. Research indicates that AFE more resembles anaphylaxis and septic shock than it does pulmonary embolism. AFE frequently results in maternal death and the majority of those that do survive AFE have neurologic damage due to cerebral hypoxia (Baldisseri, 2020).

Clinical Manifestations and Diagnosis

In most cases, symptoms of AFE occur suddenly during or immediately after delivery. The woman usually develops symptoms of acute respiratory distress, cyanosis, and hypotension. Sudden cardiorespiratory arrest can occur.

The diagnosis of AFE is based on the clinical symptoms and laboratory studies. Arterial blood gases demonstrate acidosis and hypoxemia. Bleeding times are usually prolonged. Disseminated intravascular coagulation (DIC) occurs in the majority of women with AFE (Baldisseri, 2020). With DIC, the woman has abnormal bleeding from puncture or incision sites or excessive bruising. Report any abnormal bleeding to the RN. The chest x-ray may initially look normal, but as AFE progresses it may show evidence of pulmonary edema or acute respiratory distress syndrome.

Treatment

Unfortunately, there is currently no curative therapy; therefore, treatment aims to support vital functions. An immediate response to the woman's initial complaint of respiratory distress is necessary to increase the woman's chances of survival. The woman often progresses quickly to full cardiopulmonary arrest and requires advanced cardiac life support, including mechanical intubation and ventilation. Typically, DIC is treated with massive fluid resuscitation and blood product replacement therapy. Once the woman is in stable condition, she requires care in an adult intensive care unit. If the fetus is not delivered soon after the event starts, there are also poor neonatal outcomes.

Nursing Care

Respond promptly, and summon for immediate assistance if a laboring or postpartum woman reports dyspnea.

 A Personal Glimpse

My wife Sally had just delivered our daughter. We had waited to have a child until we were in our 30s, and then it had taken us 2 years to get pregnant. I was so awed by the whole birth experience. I was taking pictures of my daughter when I heard Sally say to the nurse, "I can't breathe!" I looked over and saw that she was very pale, almost gray. In the blink of an eye, she stopped breathing and one of the nurses started helping her breathe. The other nurse took the baby and me to the nursery. The nursery nurse was very kind. She let me stay with the baby as long as I wanted; however, I couldn't concentrate on the baby because I was so worried about my wife. I went to the waiting room and I was pacing up and down. After what seemed like an eternity, the doctor came to talk to me. He said that he thought Sally had an embolism. He told me that she had a breathing tube and was connected to a machine that was helping her breathe. The nurse came out and took me to the ICU. I felt so frightened by all the tubes and machines that were connected to my wife. I felt very helpless. I also felt guilty for putting my wife through this. I didn't know if I could forgive myself if she didn't make it. Slowly, over the next week, Sally started to get better. I have never felt more thankful in my life than on the day I was able to take Sally home. She was very weak, but she was alive. It was such a joy to see her finally able to hold our little Jessica.

Bill

Learning Opportunity: *What could the nurses in this situation have done to help the husband cope with his wife's severe illness? What interventions could the nurse use to help promote attachment between the newborn and the woman when the woman who has been critically ill begins to get better?*

Administer oxygen via facemask. Measure the vital signs frequently, particularly the blood pressure and pulse. Hypotension, tachycardia, and other signs of shock are usually evident. Initiate CPR if needed, and be prepared to assist with a cesarean delivery if needed. Be prepared to assist the RN during fluid resuscitation and blood product administration. Anticipate transfer to the intensive care unit.

Shoulder Dystocia

Shoulder dystocia is an obstetric emergency. In shoulder dystocia, the fetal head delivers, but the shoulders become stuck in the bony pelvis, preventing delivery of the body. The fetus can suffer permanent brain damage because their chest cannot expand, limiting the first breath. Although macrosomia (fetal weight greater than 4,000 grams) and maternal diabetes are the two risk factors known to be associated with shoulder dystocia, shoulder dystocia cannot be predicted. Therefore, this complication should be anticipated at every delivery.

Shoulder dystocia puts the woman and the fetus at risk. Even if correct maneuvers are used, maternal and fetal injury and fetal death can still result. The woman is at increased risk for postpartum hemorrhage because of cervical or vaginal lacerations or uterine atony (failure of the uterus to contract effectively to stop bleeding). The fetus is at increased risk for brachial plexus injuries and fractures of the humerus and clavicle.

Clinical Manifestations and Diagnosis

The "turtle sign" is the classic sign that alerts the birth attendant to the probability of shoulder dystocia. The fetal head delivers, but then retracts similar to a turtle (Rodis, 2019). The birth attendant is unable to deliver the infant using the normal maneuvers including gentle downward pressure on the fetal head in an attempt to deliver the anterior shoulder.

Treatment

Several maneuvers are available to the birth attendant to relieve shoulder dystocia. Two of them require the direct assistance of the nurse or another health care provider:

- *McRoberts maneuver* (Fig. 18-2A). This intervention is frequently successful and is often tried first. McRoberts requires the assistance of two individuals. Two nurses are ideal; however, a support person or a technician can serve as the second assistant. With the woman in lithotomy position, each nurse holds one leg and sharply flexes the leg toward the woman's shoulders. This opens the pelvis to its widest diameters and allows the anterior shoulder to deliver in almost half of the cases (Rodis, 2019).
- *Suprapubic pressure* (Fig. 18-2B). In addition to McRoberts maneuver, one nurse can use a fist to apply suprapubic pressure. This will sometimes dislodge the impacted shoulder.

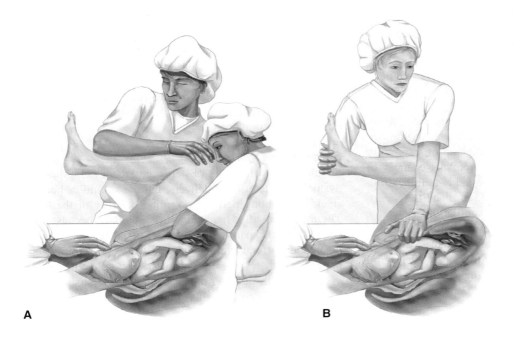

FIGURE 18-2 Maneuvers to relieve shoulder dystocia. **A.** McRoberts maneuver. **B.** Suprapubic pressure.

A

B

The birth attendant can try other maneuvers, such as placing a hand in the vagina and attempting to push one of the shoulders in a clockwise or counterclockwise motion. Intentionally fracturing a clavicle may help dislodge the fetus. In some cases, the fetal head may be pushed back in the birth canal and an emergency cesarean delivery performed. This maneuver, called Zavanelli maneuver, has been successful, but is associated with increased risk of trauma.

Nursing Care

Because shoulder dystocia often cannot be predicted, be prepared at every delivery for this emergency. Ensure that the woman's bladder is empty before every delivery. If she cannot void, you may need to use an in-and-out catheter to drain the bladder. Make sure that a hard surface is available, such as a CPR backboard, to place under the mattress or bed linens beneath the woman's hips when shoulder dystocia is diagnosed. Make certain that all neonatal resuscitation supplies are present and working before every delivery. Call for the neonatal specialist team and extra nurses to attend the delivery as soon as the diagnosis is made.

Assist the birth attendant with maneuvers as described above. Be prepared to go for an emergency cesarean delivery if the body does not deliver. If maneuvers are successful and a vaginal delivery is accomplished, the newborn must be observed carefully. Check for crepitus in the area of the clavicle, which might

This is Important!

Don't EVER apply pressure to the fundus (fundal pressure). The shoulder can become more impacted, and the woman has an increased chance of uterine or bladder rupture when fundal pressure is applied with shoulder dystocia.

indicate the bone is broken. Check for spontaneous movements of both arms. Sometimes the newborn will move only one arm, which may indicate Erb palsy. This injury involves nerve damage (usually temporary) and inability to move the arm. When edema subsides, full function normally returns, although injury can persist.

Umbilical Cord Prolapse

Umbilical cord prolapse occurs when the umbilical cord slips down in front of the presenting part. Factors that increase the risk of a prolapsed cord include fetal malpresentation, multiple gestation, multiparity, prematurity, polyhydramnios, and rupture of the membranes with the fetus at a high station (i.e., the fetus is not engaged).

Clinical Manifestations and Diagnosis

Prolapse of the umbilical cord can occur at any time during labor (Fig. 18-3). Sometimes the woman presents with a cord prolapse. The cord may be visible at the introitus or it may be palpable in the vaginal vault. An occult prolapse results in cord compression, but the cord is not easily palpable. The woman may report feeling "something coming out" when the membranes rupture. The majority of cases of cord prolapse happen immediately after spontaneous or artificial rupture of the membranes. The fetal heart rate drops precipitously. Vaginal examination typically confirms the diagnosis.

Treatment

When the fetal presenting part compresses the umbilical cord against the bony pelvis, it can compromise fetal circulation and result in fetal death unless the health care team intervenes quickly. Immediate cesarean delivery is the treatment of choice to save the fetus's life. The examiner who discovers the condition should push upward on the presenting part with the fingers to move the

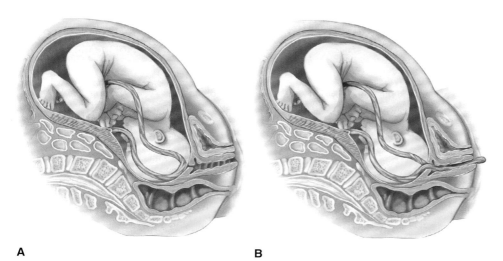

FIGURE 18-3 Prolapsed cord. **A.** Prolapse within the uterus (occult prolapse). **B.** Prolapse with the cord visible at the vulva.

A   B

fetus away from the cord. Emptying the bladder with an indwelling catheter is another method that can temporarily relieve cord compression while the woman is prepared for delivery.

Nursing Care

Always check fetal heart tones after spontaneous or artificial rupture of the membranes. If the fetal heart rate drops, the RN performs a vaginal examination and palpates for the umbilical cord. If you discover a visible prolapse, quickly place the woman in the knee–chest position, call for help, and gently palpate the cord for pulsations to verify fetal viability. Then use your fingers to press upward on the presenting part. Continue to hold the presenting part off the cord until delivery of the infant. You will be transported with the woman to the operating room. The sterile drapes will be placed over you. If another nurse is holding the presenting part off the cord, move quickly to prepare the woman for emergency cesarean delivery.

Uterine Rupture

Uterine rupture occurs when the uterus tears open, leaving the fetus and other uterine contents exposed to the peritoneal cavity. Rarely is this a spontaneous occurrence. It is usually associated with a uterine scar from previous uterine surgery. Often the scar results from a prior cesarean delivery; however, any surgery that requires an incision into the uterus can place the woman at risk for uterine rupture. Traumatic rupture can occur in connection with blunt trauma, such as that occurs in an automobile collision or intimate partner violence. Some medical interventions increase the woman's risk for uterine rupture such as medications given to induce labor.

Clinical Manifestations and Diagnosis

A nonreassuring fetal heart rate pattern is often the most significant sign associated with uterine rupture (Landon and Frey, 2020). Other signs are complaints of pain in the abdomen, shoulder, or back in a laboring woman who had previously efficient pain relief from epidural anesthesia. Falling blood pressure and rising pulse may be associated with hypovolemia caused by occult bleeding. A vaginal examination may demonstrate a higher fetal station than was present previously. There may or may not be changes in the contraction pattern (Landon and Frey, 2020).

Treatment

As soon as uterine rupture is recognized, the treatment is immediate cesarean delivery. This action is necessary to save the woman's life and, it is hoped, that of the fetus as well, although uterine rupture is associated with a high incidence of fetal death. This is true because the fetus can withstand only approximately 20 minutes in utero after uterine rupture. This time can be even shorter if the cord prolapses through the tear in the uterine wall and becomes compressed.

Nursing Care

Recognizing the signs of uterine rupture is critical for the obstetric nurse because the complication requires quick recognition and action to avoid fetal and maternal deaths. In cases of trial of labor after cesarean, the RN should monitor the woman during labor, particularly if oxytocin is infusing to induce or augment the labor. If signs of rupture occur, immediately prepare the woman for cesarean delivery and institute interventions to treat hypovolemic shock.

Placental and Umbilical Cord Abnormalities

Although, technically, abnormalities of the placenta and umbilical cord are not obstetric emergencies, they can lead to emergencies and can have dire outcomes for the woman and her fetus. Table 18-3 lists selected conditions that can result in maternal and fetal complications.

TABLE 18-3 Placental Abnormalities and Umbilical Cord Issues

CONDITION	DESCRIPTION	RISK FACTORS	MATERNAL AND FETAL IMPLICATIONS
Placental Abnormalities			
Placenta accreta	Abnormal adherence of the placenta to the uterine wall. It may invade the uterine muscle (called placenta increta) or even penetrate through the uterine muscle (called placenta percreta)	History of previous uterine surgery, such as the following: • Cesarean delivery (risk increases with each subsequent cesarean birth) • Myomectomy • Dilation and curettage • Induced abortion (medical abortion) Other risk factors include the following: • Age older than 35 • Placenta previa	*Maternal implications:* Interferes with normal placental separation in the third stage of labor, resulting in hemorrhage, which may require hysterectomy to control. May also cause uterine rupture during pregnancy or labor *Fetal implications:* Fetal death may occur if the condition results in uterine rupture
Velamentous insertion of the umbilical cord	The umbilical cord is attached to the side (vs. the center) of the placenta, and the fetal vessels separate in the membranes before reaching the placenta	Low-lying placenta, antepartum hemorrhage, in vitro fertilization (IVF) pregnancy	*Fetal implications:* Exsanguination (the fetus may bleed out) resulting in fetal death may occur if the cord tears away from the placenta

Washington Manual of Surgical Pathology

TABLE 18-3 Placental Abnormalities and Umbilical Cord Issues (Continued)

CONDITION	DESCRIPTION	RISK FACTORS	MATERNAL AND FETAL IMPLICATIONS
Umbilical Cord Issues			
Nuchal cord	The umbilical cord is wrapped once (or more) around the fetus's neck	This condition occurs frequently in normal pregnancies with no identifiable risk factors	*Fetal implications:* Moderate-to-deep variable decelerations may occur during labor. Rarely, a tight nuchal cord can lead to fetal death

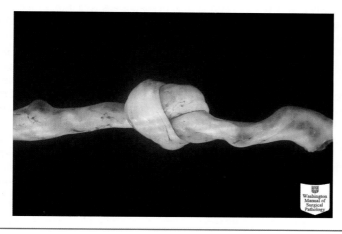

CONDITION	DESCRIPTION	RISK FACTORS	MATERNAL AND FETAL IMPLICATIONS
True knot	A true knot occurs when the umbilical cord is tied in a knot	This condition can occur in an active fetus with a long cord	*Fetal implications:* A true knot sometimes results in fetal death

Figure Sources: From (1) Pfeifer J. D., Humphrey P. A., Ritter J. H., & Dehner L. P. (2020). *The Washington manual of surgical pathology* (3rd ed.). Wolters Kluwer, (2) Creason C. (Ed.). (2011). *Stedman's medical terminology: Steps to success in medical language.* Wolters Kluwer Health | Lippincott Williams & Wilkins, (3) Humphrey P. A., Dehner L. P., & Pfeiffer J. D. (Eds.). (2008). *The Washington manual™ of surgical pathology.* Wolters Kluwer Health | Lippincott Williams & Wilkins.

TEST YOURSELF

✔ Describe three clinical manifestations of AFE.

✔ Describe two maneuvers with which the nurse can assist when shoulder dystocia complicates delivery.

✔ Describe three conditions affecting the placenta and umbilical cord and how each one can affect the fetus or mother.

Remember **Bernadette Howard** from the beginning of the chapter. She presented in labor at 34 weeks with leaking of amniotic fluid. If Bernadette was postterm at 42 weeks and presented with leaking amniotic fluid, what interventions would be ordered that would be similar to those for preterm labor? What interventions would be different?

KEY POINTS

- Labor dystocia is an abnormally slow progression of labor. Nursing interventions include carefully monitoring the woman's labor pattern. Compare the woman's progress with expected norms, and notify the RN and the health care provider when progress deviates from the expected. Assist the woman in repositioning and keeping her bladder empty, frequently monitor the adequacy of the contraction pattern, and administer pain relief interventions.

- Two types of fetal malpresentation are breech and transverse lie (shoulder presentation). For breech presentation, the health care provider may use external cephalic version, allow the woman to attempt vaginal delivery, or perform a cesarean delivery. For transverse lie, external cephalic version or cesarean delivery is needed.

- Prelabor rupture of membranes (PROM) is spontaneous rupture of the amniotic sac before the onset of labor in a full-term fetus; preterm PROM (PPROM) is PROM in a pregnancy that is less than 37 weeks gestation. In both cases, the woman presents to the labor and delivery unit with leaking of fluid from the vagina. Monitor the woman's temperature frequently to detect early signs of infection.

- Clinical manifestations of preterm labor (PTL) include uterine contractions, with or without pain; pelvic pressure; cramping; backache; and vaginal discharge and bleeding.

- For preterm labor (PTL), if the membranes are not ruptured and cervical dilation is less than 3 cm, tocolytics and injectable steroids may be ordered to stop the labor long enough to allow the fetal lungs to mature.

- Complications associated with postterm pregnancy include oligohydramnios which can lead to cord compression, meconium staining of the amniotic fluid that can lead to meconium aspiration syndrome, macrosomia, and fetal death.

- For the woman carrying a postterm pregnancy, labor is often induced. Frequent fetal movement (kick) counts and nonstress tests (NSTs) are used to monitor fetal well-being. Instruct the woman to report decreased fetal movement immediately.

- The labor of a woman with a fetal demise is often induced. Spontaneous labor can take 1 to 2 weeks to occur if the woman chooses to wait for labor to start on its own. Monitor the woman with a retained fetal demise for signs of disseminated intravascular coagulopathy. Provide emotional care for the woman and her family during and after the stillbirth. Do not pressure the woman to hold or look at the fetus but allow it if she desires.

- Amniotic fluid embolism occurs suddenly during labor or in the immediate postpartum period. The woman becomes acutely dyspneic, apprehensive, hypotensive, and cyanotic. Treatment is supportive, and the woman requires care in the intensive care unit.

- Shoulder dystocia occurs when the fetal head is born but the shoulders fail to deliver. McRoberts maneuver and suprapubic pressure are two interventions that require the active involvement of the nurse. Carefully observe the newborn for signs of birth injury.

- Umbilical cord prolapse occurs when the umbilical cord slips down in front of the presenting part. Unless pressure is immediately relieved, the fetus will die or will experience permanent brain injury from lack of oxygen. An immediate cesarean delivery is required.

- History of a previous uterine scar increases the risk of uterine rupture during labor. Ominous fetal heart rate patterns on the fetal monitor are usually the most significant sign of rupture. Prompt cesarean delivery is necessary to save the fetus and the woman.

INTERNET RESOURCES

Complications in Labor and Delivery
https://www.merckmanuals.com/professional/gynecology-and-obstetrics/abnormalities-and-complications-of-labor-and-delivery/introduction-to-abnormalities-and-complications-of-labor-and-delivery

Breech Birth
https://medlineplus.gov/ency/patientinstructions/000623.htm

Preterm Labor
https://www.marchofdimes.org/complications/preterm-labor-and-premature-birth-are-you-at-risk.aspx

Fetal Demise
https://www.compassionatefriends.org

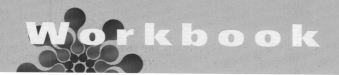

NCLEX-STYLE REVIEW QUESTIONS

1. A 35-year-old gravida 1 delivered after 24 hours of labor. Her membranes ruptured 4 hours after she started labor. Two hours before she delivered, she spiked a temperature of 101°F (38.3°C). For which of the following complications is her newborn most at risk?
   a. ABO incompatibility
   b. Fistula formation
   c. Pelvic floor injury
   d. Pneumonia

2. A 26-year-old primigravida is attempting natural childbirth. Her doula has been supporting her through the past 16 hours of labor. The laboring woman is now 6 cm dilated. She continues to report severe pain in her back with each contraction. She finds it comforting when her doula uses the ball of her hand to put counterpressure on her lower back. What is the likely cause of the woman's back pain?
   a. Breech presentation
   b. Fetal macrosomia
   c. Occiput posterior position
   d. Nongynecoid pelvis

3. A 31-year-old gravida 3 para 1 calls the clinic. She is at 29 weeks' gestation. She says that she has been having uterine contractions every 10 minutes for the past 2 hours. She also feels "heaviness" in her vaginal area. Her first baby was born prematurely at 28 weeks' gestation. What advice by the nurse is best for this woman?
   a. "Come into the hospital immediately. These signs strongly indicate that you may be in premature labor."
   b. "Drink two large glasses of water. Lie down on your left side. If the contractions don't stop in an hour, come in to the hospital."
   c. "Monitor your contractions for one more hour. If they increase in frequency, or get stronger, come in right away."
   d. "It is not likely that you will deliver a second baby prematurely. Don't panic. If you continue to have contractions, come in to be checked."

4. The nurse is assisting in a delivery that is complicated by shoulder dystocia. Which nursing action is indicated?
   a. Give fundal pressure.
   b. Start rescue breathing.
   c. Assist the RN to flex the woman's thighs.
   d. Watch the fetal monitor for signs of fetal distress.

5. Which of the following findings from your data collection should be reported to the RN? (Select all that apply.)
   a. The woman's pain is 6 out of 10 two hours after pain medication given.
   b. The woman states, "It feels like something is falling out of my vagina."
   c. The woman suddenly complains of sharp abdominal pain and her abdomen is rigid.
   d. The woman's temperature is 99.0°F (37.2°C).
   e. The woman's respirations become labored and tachypnic.
   f. The woman receiving magnesium sulfate complains of being warm and her face is reddened.

STUDY ACTIVITIES

1. Use the table provided to compare fetal and maternal causes of labor arrest.

Fetal Causes of Labor Arrest	Maternal Causes of Labor Arrest

2. Interview your local March of Dimes representative to see what is being done in your community to learn more about and prevent PTL. Share your findings with your clinical group.

3. Develop an education plan for a woman with a postterm pregnancy that is being managed expectantly.

CRITICAL THINKING: WHAT WOULD YOU DO?

Apply your knowledge of labor at risk to the following situations.

1. Julia, a gravida 2 para 0, just found out that her fetus is in a breech position at 36 weeks' gestation. Julia is afraid that she will have to have a cesarean delivery. What options does Julia have in this situation?

2. Julia's pregnancy proceeds to 39 weeks' gestation. She presents to labor and delivery because her "water bag broke." After the midwife confirms that the membranes have ruptured, she explains to Julia that the plan is for Julia and her husband to wait in the hospital until labor begins. Julia wants to know why she and her husband can't just go home to wait for contractions to begin.
   a. How do you reply to Julia?
   b. What nursing interventions will you plan for Julia during the wait before labor begins?
   c. How would your care be different if Julia were at 30 weeks' gestation with ruptured membranes versus 39 weeks?

3. Kimberly has been receiving tocolytic terbutaline for the past 12 hours. You are taking Kimberly's vital signs at the beginning of your shift. You notice that her pulse is 130 and blood pressure is 88/50 mm Hg. When you ask her how she is feeling, she replies, "I feel out of breath, and I have a feeling of pressure in my chest." What should you do?

Postpartum Woman at Risk

Key Terms

deep vein thrombosis (DVT)
endometritis
exudate
hematoma
hypovolemic shock
malattachment
mastitis
pulmonary embolism
uterine atony
uterine subinvolution
venous thromboembolism (VTE)

Learning Objectives

At the conclusion of this chapter, you will:

1. Identify major conditions that place a woman at risk during the postpartum period.
2. Differentiate between early and late postpartum hemorrhage.
3. Describe nursing interventions for the woman with postpartum hemorrhage.
4. Compare and contrast four types of infection that may occur in the postpartum period.
5. Identify factors that place a postpartum woman at risk for venous thromboembolism (VTE).
6. Explain treatment and nursing care for the postpartum woman experiencing VTE (deep vein thrombosis and pulmonary embolism).
7. Describe two major mental health issues that can complicate the postpartum period.
8. Discuss the nurse's role when caring for a postpartum woman who is grieving.
9. Identify behaviors that would suggest malattachment.

AmberLeigh Garcia is a 20-year-old gravida 3 para 2 who delivered 24 hours ago. When you enter her room, you notice that she is quietly crying. What other information would be helpful to know about her delivery at this time? As you start your beginning-of-shift routine, what physical symptoms would you need to pay attention to that would indicate that AmberLeigh is having complications during her postpartum period?

Often considered the "fourth trimester of pregnancy," the postpartum period encompasses the first 6 weeks after childbirth. After delivery, the woman begins to experience physiologic and psychological changes that return her body to the prepregnancy state. These changes usually occur without difficulty. However, factors such as blood loss, trauma during delivery, infection, or fatigue can place the postpartum woman at risk. As the licensed practical/vocational nurse (LPN/LVN), you play a key role in identifying the woman at risk for complications to ensure early detection and prompt intervention. You may be the person who identifies the problem and alerts the registered nurse (RN) or primary health care provider of the findings. Interventions for the postpartum woman at risk focus on treating the complication and thereby minimizing the effects on the woman's return to her prepregnant state, promoting adaptation to her role as mother of a new infant, and supporting and enhancing maternal–infant bonding.

This chapter addresses major complications associated with the postpartum period, including hemorrhage, infection, venous thromboembolism (VTE), and specific postpartum mental health issues. The chapter emphasizes priority aspects of care for each complication. This chapter also describes special postpartum situations, such as postpartal grieving and malattachment.

POSTPARTUM HEMORRHAGE

Postpartum hemorrhage is one of the top five causes of maternal deaths (Belfort, 2021). It can occur early, within the first 24 hours after delivery, or late, any time after the first 24 hours through the 6-week postpartum period. The woman is most vulnerable to hemorrhage during the first 24 hours after delivery, with the greatest risk occurring in the first hour after delivery.

Traditionally, postpartum hemorrhage was defined as any blood loss in an amount greater than 500 mL after a vaginal delivery or greater than 1,000 mL after a cesarean birth. However, because blood loss estimates during delivery are often inaccurate and the amount of blood loss that can be tolerated varies from woman to woman, the definition has been broadened. Most authorities accept the definition of postpartum hemorrhage as blood loss resulting in hemodynamic changes (e.g., change in the quality or rate of the pulse or blood pressure) or blood loss of greater than 1,000 mL (Belfort, 2021).

The four major causes of postpartum hemorrhage are the following: **uterine atony** (the inability of the uterus to contract effectively); trauma (caused by lacerations, uterine rupture, or surgical incisions); platelet dysfunction; and retained placental fragments (Belfort, 2021). Box 19-1 lists factors identified that increase the risk for postpartum hemorrhage. It is important to monitor all postpartum women for excessive bleeding because the risk factors do not always predict which woman will have a postpartum hemorrhage. Early detection and prompt intervention are necessary to control the hemorrhage. Otherwise, the woman can progress to shock, renal failure, and ultimately death from the loss of blood.

Early Postpartum Hemorrhage

Early postpartum hemorrhage occurs within the first 24 hours after delivery. Early postpartum hemorrhage usually results from one of the three following conditions:

- Uterine atony
- Lacerations
- Hematoma

Most cases of early postpartum hemorrhage result from uterine atony. With this condition, the uterus does not contract as it should. The muscles of the uterus remain relaxed and exert no compression on the open uterine blood vessels at the former placental site. As a result, the vessels continue

---

BOX 19-1 Risk Factors for Postpartum Hemorrhage

Risk factors are listed by cause.

Uterine Atony
- Multiparity
- Intrauterine infection
- Previous uterine surgery
- Prolonged or difficult labor
- History of postpartum hemorrhage
- Placenta previa or abruptio placentae
- Use of oxytocin for labor stimulation or augmentation
- Use of agents during labor that relax the uterus (tocolytics), such as:
  - Magnesium sulfate
  - Terbutaline
  - Certain anesthetics
  - Nitroglycerin
- Overdistention of the uterus, such as occurs with:
  - Multiple gestation
  - Polyhydramnios
  - Fetal macrosomia

Lacerations and Hematomas
- Episiotomy
- Macrosomia
- Precipitous labor
- Traumatic delivery
- Use of forceps or vacuum extraction for delivery

Placental Issues
- Retained placental fragments
- Abruptio placentae
- Placenta accreta
- Prolonged third stage of labor

Disruption in Maternal Clotting Abilities
- Fetal demise
- Thrombocytopenia
- Preeclampsia

---

to bleed. This blood loss can be extensive and rapid. Lacerations can be located on the perineal tissue, vaginal sidewall, or cervix; can be small or large; and can be caused by tears or cuts from the delivery. A **hematoma** is a collection of blood within tissues; the blood loss is concealed.

Regardless of the cause, the woman is at risk for developing hypovolemia, a system-wide decrease in blood volume from too much blood loss. If the blood loss continues, the woman may develop **hypovolemic shock**, which is characterized by a weak, thready, rapid pulse; drop in blood pressure; cool, clammy skin; a decrease in urine output (less than 30 mL/hour); and changes in level of consciousness. These findings may occur abruptly and be dramatic if the blood loss is large and occurs quickly. However, with bleeding of a more gradual onset, these signs and symptoms may be subtle because of the body's ability to compensate for the blood loss over time. With continued bleeding, the woman's body eventually is overwhelmed and is no longer able to compensate for the loss. At that point, she exhibits the typical signs and symptoms of shock.

The woman who experiences postpartum hemorrhage is also at risk for developing anemia from the blood loss and may require blood transfusions. The woman may require surgical intervention, which can prolong her postpartum recovery. A potential outcome of severe postpartum hemorrhage may include hysterectomy with loss of childbearing capability. Rare complications associated with uncontrolled postpartum hemorrhage include further bleeding, which may occur if clotting factors are used up or if disseminated intravascular coagulation (DIC) develops, and multiple organ failure.

Clinical Manifestations

Clinical manifestations of early postpartum hemorrhage differ according to the cause of the hemorrhage.

Hemorrhage Caused by Uterine Atony

If the underlying cause of hemorrhage is uterine atony, the woman's fundus may be difficult to palpate. With uterine atony, the fundus on palpation is soft (boggy), relaxed, and located above the level of the umbilicus. If the woman has a distended bladder, this condition further interferes with uterine contraction. A full bladder may cause the uterus to deviate to one side, rather than being at the midline. Vaginal bleeding (lochia) typically is moderate to heavy, possibly with numerous large clots.

Hemorrhage Caused by Lacerations

When lacerations are the cause of bleeding, the fundus is firm on palpation. However, the bleeding continues in a steady trickle. Characteristically, the bleeding is bright red in color, in contrast to the typical dark red color of lochia, and typically there are not clots present.

Hemorrhage Caused by Hematoma

Unlike uterine atony and lacerations, the bleeding associated with hematoma formation may not be apparent. A blood vessel ruptures and leaks into the surrounding tissue. This causes pressure, pain, swelling (edema), and dark red or purple discoloration, most commonly on one side of the perineum (Fig. 19-1). Initially, the area may feel soft. However, as leakage into the tissues continues, the area becomes firm to the touch. The area is tender on palpation.

> **Watch Out For Epidurals**
>
> A woman who has had an epidural may not feel the pain from a hematoma or laceration until the epidural wears off. Do not rely solely on the woman reporting pain as a symptom. Be sure to include visual inspection of the woman's perineum.

A hematoma can also form deep in the pelvis, where it is much more difficult to identify. The primary symptom is deep pain unrelieved by comfort measures or medication and accompanied by vital sign instability. Regardless of where the hematoma occurs, the woman's lochia is usually within expected parameters. However, if the hematoma is large, she may experience a significant loss of blood into the tissues, leading to signs and symptoms of hypovolemic shock.

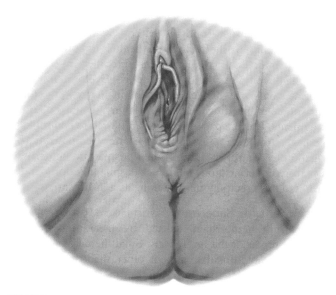

FIGURE 19-1 Perineal hematoma. Note the bulging, swollen mass.

Diagnosis

Clinical signs and changes in laboratory values point to the cause of bleeding. Common symptoms of hemorrhage include pallor, lightheadedness, weakness, palpitations, diaphoresis, restlessness, and changes in level of consciousness. With extensive blood loss, the woman's hemoglobin and hematocrit levels are decreased from her prelabor (baseline) levels, approximately 1 to 1.5 g/dL and 2% to 4%, respectively. Clotting times are increased, whereas platelet and prothrombin levels decrease, which leads to impaired coagulation.

Treatment

The goals of treatment for postpartum hemorrhage are to correct the underlying cause while attempting to control the hemorrhage and reduce its effects. If the woman is exhibiting signs and symptoms of hypovolemic shock, emergency measures are instituted to support vital functions. These include rapid intravenous (IV) fluid replacement, blood transfusions, oxygen administration, and frequent close monitoring of all vital functions. Insertion of an indwelling urinary catheter may be necessary to monitor the urine output hourly.

Treatment for Uterine Atony

If uterine atony is present, fundal massage is initiated (see Nursing Procedure 12-1: Fundal Palpation and Massage). Massage may help the uterus contract, which compresses the blood vessels and ultimately decreases the bleeding. Once the uterus contracts, use firm, steady, gentle fundal pressure to help express any clots that may have collected in the uterus. The woman's bladder must be empty; otherwise, the uterus will not remain contracted once the massage stops. Avoid overmassaging the fundus, as it may cause it to become overstimulated and fail to contract.

Drug therapy may be necessary if fundal massage fails to maintain the uterus in a contracted state. Typical medications include oxytocic agents, such as oxytocin, ergonovine, methylergonovine, carboprost, and misoprostol. If drug therapy is ineffective, the health care provider may need to intervene. The health care provider may perform bimanual compression of the uterus. Exploration of the uterine cavity may be the next option in an attempt to locate the source of bleeding and remove, if any, retained placental fragments. Uterine packing may be required to control hemorrhage. Another option is uterine artery embolization or ligation to control bleeding. When postpartum hemorrhage because of uterine atony continues despite all efforts to control it, a hysterectomy may be done as a last resort.

Treatment for Lacerations and Hematomas

Postpartum hemorrhage caused by lacerations requires surgical repair of the lacerations. Small hematomas usually require no additional treatment other than application of ice and analgesics to control pain. In most instances, small hematomas absorb spontaneously, usually during a period of 4 to 6 weeks. Surgical incision with drainage and evacuation of clots and ligation of the bleeding vessel may be required if the hematoma is large.

Late Postpartum Hemorrhage

Late postpartum hemorrhage refers to blood loss occurring after the first 24 hours after delivery and at any time throughout the 6-week postpartum period. Most cases of late postpartum hemorrhage result from retained placental fragments or **uterine subinvolution**, a condition in which the uterus returns to its prepregnancy shape and size at a rate that is slower than expected. Subinvolution is usually the result of retained placental fragments or an infection. The woman who has had uterine surgery, including a previous cesarean birth or an abortion, is at high risk for retained placental fragments along the site of the surgical scar.

 Concept Mastery Alert

Uterine atony is a common cause of early postpartum hemorrhage, whereas retained placental fragments are the most common cause of late postpartum hemorrhage.

Clinical Manifestations

As with early postpartum hemorrhage, the woman with late postpartal hemorrhage notices an increase in bleeding. This increase usually occurs abruptly several days after discharge. Along with an abrupt onset of bleeding, the woman's uterus is not well contracted. On palpation, the uterus is not descending at the usual rate of 1 cm or fingerbreadth per postpartum day. Lochia is heavier than expected. The woman may report episodes of intermittent, irregular, or excessive vaginal bleeding. In addition, the woman may report backache, fatigue, and general malaise. She may also report pelvic pain or heaviness. Her temperature may be elevated slightly, and lochia may be foul smelling if an infection is present.

Diagnosis

Similar to the findings of early postpartum hemorrhage, the woman's hemoglobin and hematocrit levels are low. If retained placental fragments are the cause, the woman's serum human chorionic gonadotropin levels remain elevated. Ultrasound may reveal evidence of placental fragments. An elevated white blood cell (WBC) count may indicate infection. However, this result may not be conclusive because a postpartal woman's WBC count is typically elevated in the early postpartum period.

Treatment

Treatment of late postpartum hemorrhage focuses on correcting the underlying cause of the hemorrhage. Oxytocic therapy, similar to that used for uterine atony, may assist the uterus to contract. Often, uterine contraction aids in removing any fragments from the uterus. If necessary, surgery, specifically dilation and curettage (D&C), may be done to remove the fragments from the myometrium. Surgical intervention is a last resort when other treatment measures have been ineffective because it can traumatize the uterus further, leading to additional bleeding. Antibiotic therapy treats an infection, if present.

Nursing Care

Most cases of late postpartum hemorrhage occur after the woman leaves the healthcare or birthing facility. Therefore, providing client information before discharge about expected changes and danger signs and symptoms of hemorrhage is crucial. Instruct the woman to call her health care provider if she experiences any signs of infection, such as fever greater than 100.4°F (38°C), chills, or foul-smelling lochia. She should also report lochia that increases in amount (instead of decreasing) or reversal of the pattern of lochia (i.e., moves from serosa back to rubra).

TEST YOURSELF

✔ What is the definition of postpartum hemorrhage?

✔ Name the most common cause of early postpartum hemorrhage.

✔ Name three nursing actions appropriate for the woman who is bleeding because of uterine atony.

Nursing Process and Care Plan *for the Woman With Postpartum Hemorrhage*

The LPN/LVN provides an important role in monitoring the woman's status, assisting with measures to control bleeding, providing support to the woman and her family, and updating the woman about her condition. Maintaining the woman's safety is paramount. Reinforce discharge teaching about signs and symptoms that might indicate late postpartum hemorrhage.

Assessment (Data Collection)

As with any client, thorough, frequent observation is necessary to allow for early detection and prompt intervention should hemorrhage occur. Be aware of the woman's history, labor and delivery details, and risk factors for postpartum hemorrhage. Note the use of any analgesia or anesthesia during labor and delivery or the use of oxytocin for labor induction or augmentation. Additionally, note if there were any interventions during labor (e.g., forceps or vacuum extraction). This information helps identify potential factors that would place the woman at risk for hemorrhage.

Ask the woman about the onset of the bleeding, if appropriate. For example, "Did the bleeding seem to increase suddenly, or have you noticed a constant trickling?" Ask about any associated symptoms, such as "Do you have any pain or pressure?" These types of questions help provide information about the possible cause of the hemorrhage. Ask the woman how frequently she is changing her perineal pads, how saturated they appear, and when she changed the pad last. The bleeding of a woman who has changed her perineal pads twice in the last hour with each pad containing approximately a half-dollar–sized amount of lochia is far different from that of a woman who has changed her perineal pads twice in the last hour because they were saturated. Additional data collection is necessary when the woman reports saturation of perineal pads. In this case, notify the RN and the health care provider of the findings.

Palpate the fundus for consistency, shape, and location. Remember that the uterus should be firm, be midline, and decrease 1 cm below the umbilicus each postpartum day. Inability to locate the fundus suggests that it is not firm and contracting. Displacement of the fundus to one side suggests that the woman has a distended bladder. Determine when the woman last urinated. Remember that a full bladder can impede uterine contraction, predisposing her to hemorrhage.

Observe lochia for color, amount, odor, and character, including evidence of any clots. When evaluating the lochia, turn the woman to her side and look under the buttocks for any pooling of blood that may occur while she is in bed. Note amount and characteristics of the bleeding. Dark red is the normal color of lochia in the first few postpartum days. A bright red color is associated with fresh bleeding, such as that from a laceration. Note whether bleeding decreases with fundal massage.

Inspect the woman's perineal area closely for evidence of lacerations or hematomas. Do not mistake an episiotomy for a laceration. Typically, an episiotomy is approximately 1 to 2 inches in length and has clean, regular sutured edges, whereas a laceration varies in length and its edges appear irregular and somewhat jagged. Evaluate pain and other associated symptoms. Severe pain and pressure that are unrelieved by ordinary pain control measures may indicate the presence of a hematoma. The woman may try to sit on one buttock in order to ease discomfort from a perineal hematoma.

Obtain the woman's vital signs to document a baseline, and then monitor vital signs as ordered, noting any changes suggesting hypovolemic shock. Note the color and temperature of the woman's skin and her level of consciousness. Recall that cool, clammy skin and decreasing level of consciousness may indicate hypovolemic shock. Table 19-1 highlights data collection findings for the major causes of early or late postpartum hemorrhage.

 Cultural Snapshot

For people of color (e.g., African American, Hispanic, and Asian), monitor skin color (pale, red, cyanotic, jaundiced) by looking at the mucous membranes of the mouth, tongue, and gums. The unpainted nail bed also gives a clear, nonpigmented view of color.

Nursing Care Focus

When selecting the focus of nursing care for the woman with early or late postpartum hemorrhage, it is important to help her return to a stable hemodynamic state and promote her safety.

Outcome Identification and Planning

Appropriate safety goals for the woman experiencing postpartum hemorrhage include that the woman will not experience harm from hypovolemia, will remain free of any injury, and will exhibit signs of adequate tissue perfusion.

Nursing care for the woman experiencing postpartum hemorrhage focuses on stopping the bleeding, restoring fluid balance, preventing injury, and promoting adequate tissue perfusion. As with any postpartal complication, be sure to provide emotional support to the woman and her family, explaining all events, laboratory tests, and procedures as well as any signs of improvement. These measures will help to minimize anxiety and fear. Allow the partner and family to discuss feelings, which may be intense. Fear, frustration, anger, blame, disbelief, and sorrow are common emotions. Listen, be calm, be present, and acknowledge that this is a difficult time.

Nursing Care Focus

● Hypovolemia related to hemorrhage

Goal

● The woman will maintain adequate fluid balance with no signs of hypovolemia.

Implementations for Preventing Hypovolemia

The most important factor in restoring fluid balance is stopping the bleeding. First, try fundal massage to contract the uterus and stop the bleeding (see Nursing Procedure 12-1: Fundal Palpation and Massage). Make sure the woman's bladder is empty before beginning massage. Be aware that the uterus may relax quickly when massage stops, placing the woman at risk for continued hemorrhage.

Don't Do It

Never attempt uterine massage without first placing one hand over the symphysis pubis. Neglecting to do so could cause the uterus to turn inside out (inversion) and lead to massive hemorrhage that can quickly lead to death.

TABLE 19-1 Sources and Symptoms of Postpartum Hemorrhage

	SOURCES OF EARLY POSTPARTUM HEMORRHAGE			SOURCES OF LATE POSTPARTUM HEMORRHAGE	
	UTERINE ATONY	LACERATIONS	HEMATOMA	RETAINED PLACENTAL FRAGMENTS	SUBINVOLUTION OF THE UTERUS
Occurrence	Early	Early	Early	Early or late	Late
Condition/ placement of uterus	Fundus is boggy and high. If bladder is full, fundus is displaced to one side	Normal	Normal	Fundus is slightly boggy but often becomes firm when massaged	Fundus may be firm when palpated but boggy a short time later
Characteristics of lochia	Moderate to heavy lochia (i.e., a perineal pad fills up with blood in under an hour)	Bleeding is heavy, bright red, and continues in a steady trickle or flow	Normal	Lochia contains intermittent clots	Initially, lochia flow is normal. Then lochia increases over what is expected and reverts to an earlier type of flow (e.g., the lochia becomes rubra after it has changed to serosa)
Characteristics of pain	May be absent	May be constant	Pressure and severe pain at the site (perineal hematoma). Deep pain unrelieved by comfort measures or medication (deep pelvic hematoma)	May be intermittent or heavier than normal cramping	May be absent or there may be constant cramping. Backache may be present
Other signs and symptoms	Tachycardia, hypotension, and other signs of hypovolemic shock if blood loss is severe	Bruising may be apparent	Swelling (edema) and dark red or purple discoloration (perineal hematoma). Accompanied by unstable blood pressure, pulse, and hemoglobin and hematocrit (deep pelvic hematoma)	Portions of maternal surface of placenta are missing at birth	Dizziness, light-headedness, and fatigue when changing positions or doing simple self-care tasks. Fever and other signs of infection may be present

If the woman is breast-feeding, encourage her to breast-feed the infant if she is able. This will cause her body to release oxytocin, which will aid in uterine contraction.

Administer oxytocics, as ordered. If an IV line with oxytocin is present, the RN may increase the rate of flow. Monitor the woman's response to the medications. Prepare the woman for surgical intervention if initial measures do not control bleeding or in cases of late postpartum hemorrhage when there are retained placental fragments. If the woman is going to surgery, withhold all food and fluids. If the woman continues to hemorrhage, anticipate transfer to the intensive care unit for closer, more frequent monitoring.

When a woman experiences postpartum hemorrhage, fluid is lost. Encourage her to increase her oral fluid intake, if allowed. If the woman is not able to drink oral fluids, or if fluid loss is significant, expect IV fluids to be administered by the RN. For fluid replacement therapy, the health care provider will order an isotonic IV solution, such as normal saline or lactated Ringer solution. Assist with IV catheter insertion, if the woman does not have one already, and monitor the IV site. Monitor the woman receiving IV fluids for signs of circulatory overload from too rapid an infusion or too much fluid.

Continue to monitor the woman's fundus and lochia frequently for changes indicating continuation or resolution of the hemorrhage. If uterine atony is causing the bleeding and the woman received IV oxytocin, fundal checks are crucial. Although oxytocin helps contract the uterus and this effect is immediate, the drug has a short duration of action, placing the woman at risk for hemorrhage secondary to recurrence of atony once the IV rate of administration slows or stops.

Inspect the perineum closely for evidence and amount of bleeding. Monitor perineal pad count to help determine the amount of blood lost. Be sure to turn the woman on her side and inspect the area under the buttocks because blood can pool.

Monitor the woman's hourly intake and output closely to determine the effectiveness of the interventions, and document progression or resolution of the fluid imbalance. Urine output should be at least 30 mL/hour, indicating adequate renal function. Encourage the woman to void frequently to prevent bladder distention from interfering with uterine contraction. If the woman has difficulty voiding, try measures such as running warm water over the perineum, placing the woman's hand in a basin or sink of warm water, or having the woman hear running water at the sink. If all else fails and the woman is unable to void, anticipate the need for insertion of an indwelling urinary catheter.

Expect to assist with obtaining blood specimens for laboratory testing, such as complete blood count (CBC), electrolyte levels, coagulation studies, and type and cross-matching for blood. If ordered, blood component therapy will be administered by the RN to aid in replacing fluid and blood loss. Monitor the woman receiving a blood product transfusion. Document and inform the RN and the health care provider of your observations.

Continue to monitor the woman's vital signs frequently for changes. Be alert for a rising pulse rate, pulse characteristics changing to rapid and thready, or decreasing blood pressure, which may indicate hypovolemic shock. Assess her capillary refill time. Prolonged capillary refill time indicates a decrease in circulating blood volume. Administer oxygen, as ordered, and monitor the woman's response.

Evaluation of Goal/Desired Outcome

The woman:

- has a urine output of at least 30 mL/hour.
- has a firm fundus with small to moderate amount of lochia without clots.
- has vital signs within normal limits.

Nursing Care Focus

- Injury risk

Goal

- The woman will remain free from injury.

Implementations for Preventing Injury

A postpartum woman who is hemorrhaging is at risk for injury. Reduction in blood supply to the brain can lead to changes in the woman's level of consciousness, placing her at risk for injury from lightheadedness, disorientation, and falls. Therefore, safety measures are necessary.

Keep the call light close by, and urge the woman to remain in bed. Check on her frequently, and encourage a family member to stay with her, if necessary. If the woman has bathroom privileges, instruct her to sit at the side of the bed for a short time before rising to prevent orthostatic hypotension and then assist her to ambulate and stay nearby in the event that she complains of lightheadedness or dizziness. If she is too unsteady to ambulate to the bathroom, have the woman use a bedpan or a bedside commode.

Continue to monitor the woman's vital signs for changes. If she reports dizziness or lightheadedness when getting up, obtain her blood pressure while lying, sitting, and standing, noting any change of 10 mm Hg or more. Should the woman's blood pressure drop with position changes, notify the RN and health care provider.

Evaluation of Goal/Desired Outcome

The woman:

- maintains vital signs within acceptable parameters.
- remains alert and oriented.
- remains free of falls.

Nursing Care Focus

- Altered tissue perfusion

Goal

- The woman will exhibit signs of improved tissue perfusion.

Implementations for Monitoring Tissue Perfusion

A decrease in circulating blood volume secondary to hemorrhage affects tissue perfusion (blood reaching the tissues of the body) and can cause hypoxia (a decrease in the amount of oxygen to the tissues). Both consequences need to be addressed. To minimize the effect of decreased tissue perfusion, the woman needs measures to correct the fluid imbalance (see previous section on controlling and restoring fluid balance).

Continue to observe the woman's skin color and temperature for changes. Cold, clammy skin may indicate constriction of the peripheral vessels, suggesting that the woman is developing hypovolemic shock or that her condition is worsening. Check nail beds for color and capillary refill. Keep in mind that a capillary refill greater than 3 seconds suggests impaired blood flow.

Monitor the woman's level of consciousness for changes. A woman who is alert and oriented is exhibiting adequate cerebral perfusion. However, confusion, disorientation, or deteriorating levels of consciousness suggest diminished blood flow and inadequate cerebral perfusion.

When adequately perfused, the kidneys function to produce urine. Urine output of at least 30 mL/hour demonstrates adequate renal function. Therefore, monitor the woman's urine output for changes. Report decreased urine output immediately.

To minimize the effect of hypoxia, the woman needs oxygen supplementation. Administer oxygen therapy via nasal cannula or facemask as ordered. Monitor oxygen saturation levels with continuous pulse oximetry. Notify the RN and health care provider if the oxygen saturation falls below 95%. However, do not rely solely on the oxygen saturation level as an indication of adequate tissue oxygenation; continue to monitor other symptoms such as level of consciousness. Arterial blood gas studies may be performed to evaluate the woman's acid–base balance and provide a more definitive evaluation of the woman's status. The health care provider may order changes to the oxygen flow rate based on the arterial blood gas findings.

Evaluation of Goal/Desired Outcome

The woman:

- is alert and oriented to person, place, and time.
- has warm, dry skin with quick capillary refill.
- maintains vital signs within acceptable parameters.
- maintains an oxygen saturation above 95%.
- has urine output of at least 30 mL/hour.

POSTPARTUM INFECTION

Postpartum infection, also called puerperal infection, refers to any infection that occurs after delivery. Most commonly, the infection involves the reproductive tract, but it can also involve other areas, such as the breast, a wound, or the urinary tract.

A postpartum infection is suspected when the postpartum woman develops a fever of 100.4°F (38°C) or greater. Various organisms are associated with postpartum infections, including but not limited to *Staphylococcus*, *Streptococcus*, *Escherichia coli*, and *Chlamydia*. Risk factors for a postpartum infection can be present antepartum, intrapartum, or postpartum. Box 19-2 lists examples of these risk factors. The major risk factor for postpartum infection is a nonelective cesarean birth.

Use of poor aseptic technique and inadequate handwashing by healthcare personnel or the woman increase the risk. A woman who experiences postpartum hemorrhage has a greater risk for postpartal infection because of her compromised state and reduced ability to fight off the infection.

Although postpartal infection usually remains localized, it can progress and spread to nearby structures such as the peritoneum, causing peritonitis, or to the blood, causing septicemia and posing a significant risk to the woman's well-being. Most postpartal infections occur once the woman goes home from the healthcare facility. Therefore, informing the woman about possible signs and symptoms is crucial to ensuring early detection and prompt intervention.

Endometritis

Endometritis refers to an infection of the uterine lining. It is the most common postpartal infection and occurs more frequently after a cesarean birth. The use of prophylactic antibiotics during a cesarean birth helps to decrease the risk of endometritis. Bacteria, frequently normal vaginal flora,

---

BOX 19-2 **Risk Factors for Postpartum Infection**

Antepartum Risk Factors
- History of infection
- History of a chronic condition
  - Diabetes
  - Hypertension
  - Anemia
  - Poor nutrition
- Infections of the genital tract
- Smoking
- Obesity
- Immunosuppression, including treatment with corticosteroids

Intrapartal Risk Factors
- Nonelective cesarean birth
- Urinary catheterization
- Episiotomy or lacerations
- Frequent vaginal examinations
- Retained placenta or one requiring manual removal
- Prolonged labor or rupture of membranes (usually over 24 hours)
- Chorioamnionitis (infection/inflammation of the fetal membranes)
- Birth with instruments
  - Forceps
  - Vacuum extractor
- Use of invasive procedures
  - Multiple cervical examinations
  - Internal fetal monitoring
  - Fetal scalp sampling
  - Amnioinfusion

Postpartum Risk Factors
- Postpartum hemorrhage
- Manual exploration of uterus for retained placental fragments
- Development of a hematoma

---

gain entrance to the uterus during birth or the immediate postpartum period.

Endometritis is a serious complication because the infection can spread to nearby organs, such as the fallopian tubes (causing salpingitis), ovaries (causing oophoritis), and occasionally the peritoneum (causing peritonitis).

Clinical Manifestations

The postpartum woman should be evaluated for endometritis if she has a fever ≥100.4°F (38°C), uterine tenderness, tachycardia that increases as the fever increases, and midline lower abdominal pain (Chen, 2020). There are other signs and symptoms of endometritis, but these may also be attributed to other conditions than endometritis. These signs include chills, anorexia, and general malaise; abdominal cramping and pain; uterine subinvolution; and tenderness. Lochia typically increases in amount and is dark, purulent, and foul smelling. However, with certain microorganisms, her lochia may be scant or absent.

Diagnosis

A CBC reveals an elevated WBC count with a left shift and rising neutrophil count. A urine culture, done to rule out a urinary tract infection (UTI), is often negative. Vaginal and blood cultures, if done, confirm the diagnosis and reveal the offending organisms. Often the diagnosis is made based on signs and symptoms and not laboratory tests. Pelvic ultrasound may reveal an abscess or possible retained placental fragments.

Pay Close Attention

The WBC count of a postpartal woman is normally elevated, ranging up to 20,000 to 30,000/mm^3. Before you report a high WBC count, observe for other signs of infection. This will help the health care provider make an accurate diagnosis.

Treatment

The standard treatment is antibiotic therapy. Typically, the woman is admitted to the healthcare facility for IV therapy. Until culture and sensitivity reports are available, broad-spectrum IV antibiotic therapy is started and continues until the woman has been afebrile longer than 24 hours. If bacteria is present in the blood, treatment may continue for longer (Chen, 2020).

The health care provider may prescribe oxytocic agents to aid in uterine involution and promote uterine drainage. Analgesics are appropriate for strong afterpains or abdominal discomfort. Hydration with IV and oral fluids and adequate nutrition are also important treatment measures.

Nursing Care

The woman with endometritis is visibly ill. Therefore, nursing care focuses on administering drug therapy to combat the infection, promoting physical and emotional comfort, alleviating anxiety, and informing the woman about measures used to treat the infection and to prevent recurrence, including proper perineal care and handwashing.

Managing Antibiotic Therapy

The RN will administer prescribed broad-spectrum IV antibiotics as ordered. Monitor the IV site and report any signs of edema, redness, or complaints of pain to the RN. Monitor the woman's vital signs every 2 to 4 hours, or more often if indicated. Expect to see a reduction in temperature and a return of the pulse rate to preinfection levels as the infection resolves. Monitor for a decrease in abdominal pain and tenderness and a change in the woman's lochia to normal color (based on the postpartum day) and amount. Palpate the fundus for position and firmness as well as if tenderness is present. Expect to administer oxytocic agents, as ordered, to promote uterine involution. As with any medication, check with the health care provider or lactation specialist to determine whether the woman can continue to breast-feed. In the instance the

antibiotic prescribed is contraindicated with breast-feeding, instruct the woman to pump her breasts (to maintain the milk supply) and discard the pumped milk until the antibiotic course is completed.

Keep in Mind

Many antibiotics are nephrotoxic (damaging to the kidneys). Encourage liberal fluid intake preferably to 3,000 mL/day. Report urine output less than 30 mL/hour.

The semi-Fowler position promotes uterine drainage and prevents the infection from spreading. Encourage frequent ambulation to promote drainage, unless contraindicated. Be alert for signs and symptoms of peritonitis, such as pronounced abdominal pain with distention, a rigid, boardlike abdomen, and absent bowel sounds. Monitor for tachycardia, tachypnea, hypotension, changes in level of orientation, and decreased urine output. These suggest septic shock, a rare but serious and possibly fatal complication.

Encourage frequent changing of perineal pads to remove infected drainage. Remind the woman to remove the pad using a front-to-back motion to avoid contaminating the perineal area. Reinforce the need to wash her hands before and after each change. Offer perineal care every 2 hours or as necessary. Be sure to wear gloves and utilize strict handwashing technique when handling soiled perineal pads to prevent infection transmission.

Providing Comfort Measures

The woman needs comfort care during this time. Provide cool washcloths and frequent linen changes, especially if she is febrile and diaphoretic. If she reports chills, add extra blankets to keep her warm; however, be careful that she does not become overheated. Keep the room calm and quiet to promote rest.

Administer analgesics, as ordered, for reports of abdominal pain. Encourage frequent position changes. Keep the head of the bed elevated. Fatigue is common during an infection. Allow for frequent rest periods so that she does not overexert herself. Assist with personal hygiene measures, including perineal care.

Alleviating Anxiety

The woman with endometritis typically develops symptoms after discharge. She may become anxious and upset when readmission is necessary because this causes separation from her newborn. Allow her to verbalize her feelings. Provide support and guidance as necessary. Enlist the aid of the woman's support system to help in alleviating her anxiety.

If the woman is breast-feeding, have her pump her breasts every 4 hours if the infant is not present to nurse or if she is prescribed antibiotics that are contraindicated with breast-feeding. Arrangements with the facility and/or the health care provider may allow the woman and her baby to be together for feedings. If not, encourage the family to bring in pictures of the baby for the woman to keep in her room. Encourage her to increase her fluids if she is breast-feeding, as a decrease in fluids can decrease or stop her milk supply.

Reinforcing Client Teaching

Reinforcement of teaching is a major focus of nursing care. One key area is reinforcing information about medication therapy, especially if she is to continue medications at home. Other areas to address include proper handwashing techniques, perineal care, expected changes in lochia, signs and symptoms of a recurrent infection, and danger signs to notify the health care provider. Tips for Reinforcing Family Teaching: Endometritis outlines the major discharge information points.

Wound Infection

Postpartal wound infections typically involve infections of the perineum that develop at the site of an episiotomy or laceration. Wound infection can also occur at the site of the abdominal incision after a cesarean birth. Perineal wound infections, although rare, commonly develop on the third or fourth postpartum day. Factors increasing the risk of perineal wound infections include infected lochia, fecal contamination of the wound, and inadequate hygiene measures. Refer to Box 19-2 for risk factors for a postpartum wound infection.

Clinical Manifestations

The woman with a perineal wound infection most likely will report pain out of proportion to what is expected. Inspection of the perineum reveals redness of the area and edema of the surrounding tissue. The wound edges may be separated (Fig. 19-2A). Often there is a foul-smelling, possibly purulent, vaginal drainage. The area is tender on palpation. Fever and general malaise may also be present.

The woman with an infected incision after a cesarean birth frequently has endometritis before the wound becomes infected. When this happens, she continues to be febrile, even with antibiotic treatment. Inspection of the abdominal wound reveals erythema and induration (area of hardened tissue). In addition, the wound edges may be separated (Fig. 19-2B). **Exudate** (drainage) may be present and may be purulent. The area surrounding the wound is typically warm and tender on palpation, and the woman reports pain. One potential complication of an incision is wound dehiscence, where part or all of the incision separates. A wound that is dehiscing (separating) is at high risk for an infection.

Diagnosis

A CBC with differential may reveal an elevation in WBC count. A culture, with sensitivity, of the area reveals the causative organism and guides treatment. If the health care provider suspects sepsis, blood cultures may be drawn. Ultrasound can locate abscesses that may require draining.

Treatment

Antibiotic therapy is used to treat the infection, regardless of location. Supportive therapy appropriate for perineal infections includes analgesics, local anesthetic sprays, warm compresses, and sitz baths. An infected incision requires regular cleansing and often a wound dressing. Surgical intervention may become necessary. This involves opening the wound for drainage, irrigation, débridement, and possibly packing. The goal of débridement is to clean the wound and promote granulation.

Nursing Care

For the woman with a perineal infection, place warm compresses to the wound site several times each day, as ordered. Assist with sitz baths to provide comfort. These measures aid the healing process by increasing circulation to the area.

TIPS FOR REINFORCING FAMILY TEACHING

Endometritis

- Be sure to complete all of your antibiotics, even though you are feeling better.
- Call your health care provider if you have any of the following symptoms of recurrent infection:
  - Temperature higher than 100.4°F (38°C)
  - Chills
  - Abdominal pain that does not go away with pain medication
  - Vaginal discharge that smells bad
- You should do the following things to prevent additional infection:
  - Wash your hands thoroughly before and after eating, using the restroom, or touching your vaginal area.
  - Wipe from front to back after using the restroom.
  - Rinse the perineum with a peri bottle after using the restroom.
  - Remove soiled sanitary pads from front to back. Fold the pad so that the discharge is contained in the middle section

of the pad, and then wrap it in toilet paper, or preferably a plastic bag. Dispose in the trash.
  - Wash hands before applying a new pad. Apply the pad from front to back. Do not touch the middle section of the pad. This part should remain very clean because it will be touching your vaginal area.
- You will heal faster and be less likely to get sick again if you do the following things:
  - Get at least 8 hours of sleep every night.
  - Rest frequently. Take naps when the baby is napping.
  - Eat a nutritious diet.
  - Gradually increase your activity as you are able to tolerate it.
  - Drink plenty (1 to 2 liters) of fluids each day.
- Be sure to attend your scheduled follow-up visits with your health care provider.

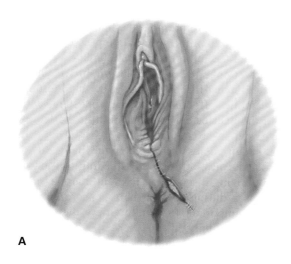
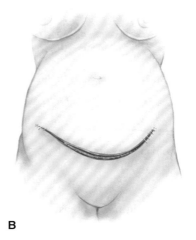

FIGURE 19-2 Postpartum wound infections. **A.** Infected episiotomy site. **B.** Dehiscence of cesarean birth incision.

A   B

Instruct the woman on the benefit of sitz baths and care of the equipment so as to prevent further infection.

Keeping the perineal area clean is important. Encourage the woman to change her perineal pads and to perform perineal care frequently. She should use a front-to-back motion when removing perineal pads and when cleaning the perineum after elimination. Remind her to wash her hands before and after performing any perineal care and using the bathroom. Although always important, thorough handwashing is essential when the woman cares for an infected wound at home to prevent transmitting the infection to the newborn.

For the woman with an incisional infection, perform wound care as ordered. This may include dressing changes, irrigations, débridement, or possibly wound packing. Always use aseptic technique when performing wound care. With each dressing change or procedure, inspect the wound for signs and symptoms indicating resolution of the infection and evidence of healing. Document measurements of the wound to aid in evaluating progress. If wound care will continue after discharge, show the woman or another family member how to perform the care. The woman or family member should be able to detect signs and symptoms of increasing infection and know the signs that indicate the wound is healing. Have the person perform a return demonstration of any procedure.

Mastitis

Mastitis refers to an infection of the connective tissue of the mammary gland (breast). Typically, only one breast is affected. Although the infection can occur at any time when the woman is breast-feeding, it is most common during the second and third weeks after delivery. Of breast-feeding mothers, 2% to 10% will develop mastitis but they rarely require hospitalization (Dixon, 2020).

Mastitis occurs when organisms are transferred from the woman's hands, staff's hands, or newborn's mouth to the breast and enter the breast tissue through a small, often microscopic, crack, fissure, or injured area on the nipple or breast tissue. The risk for mastitis can be increased because of some factors. These include the following:

- Milk stasis related to incomplete breast emptying during feeding or lack of frequent feedings
- Engorgement or oversupply of milk
- Clogged milk ducts
- Cracked, excoriated, or bleeding nipples
- Nipple piercing
- Pressure on breast from a too tight-fitting bra or underwire bra

If left untreated, mastitis can progress to an abscess, which may require surgical drainage.

Clinical Manifestations

The woman usually develops mastitis after discharge. Common complaints include general flu-like symptoms that occur suddenly, such as fever of 101°F (38.3°C) or greater, malaise, and possibly chills. In addition, the woman reports tenderness, pain, and heaviness in her breast. Inspection reveals erythema and edema in an area localized to one breast, often in a pie-shaped wedge (Fig. 19-3). The area is hard, warm, and tender on palpation.

Diagnosis

No specific tests are done to confirm the diagnosis of mastitis. Typically, signs and symptoms form the basis for diagnosis.

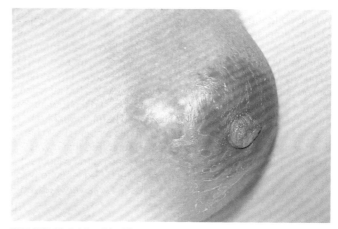

FIGURE 19-3 Mastitis. The woman with mastitis usually has a reddened, painful area on one breast that is warm to palpation.

Treatment

Supportive care in conjunction with antibiotic therapy is the treatment for mastitis. Therapy usually continues for 10 days. The woman may need analgesics for comfort. Warm compresses may also

> **Did You Know?**
>
> Antibiotic-resistant organisms are increasing in the cause of mastitis. Meticulous handwashing by both the mother and hospital staff is the best prevention.

provide comfort for the woman. The woman does not need to stop breast-feeding during treatment.

Nursing Care

Nursing care focuses on supporting continued breast-feeding, preventing milk stasis, and administering ordered antibiotics. Milk stasis is an important cause of discomfort and extension of the infection with possible abscess formation. Encourage the woman to breast-feed every 1.5 to 2 hours. Frequent feeding enhances complete emptying of the breast. It may be more comfortable for her to start the feeding session on the unaffected breast as the vigorous sucking of the infant may cause increased discomfort. If the woman is unable to breast-feed, for example because the affected breast is too sore or antibiotic therapy contraindicates breast-feeding, encourage the woman to manually express breast milk or use a breast pump to empty her breasts which will maintain her milk supply until she is able to resume breast-feeding. The woman does not need to stop breast-feeding when diagnosed with mastitis as the infection is in the tissues of the breast and not in the milk supply.

 A Personal Glimpse

Breast-feeding my daughter was a challenge from the very beginning. She didn't want to latch on, she arched her back and cried, and she fussed at the breast. It took us several months to finally get a good pattern down. When she was about 6 months old, she and I were visiting my grandmother at the beach. One morning I woke up and felt awful. I had a hard, red spot on my breast, and I felt both hot and cold and exhausted. I took my temperature and it was 103°F. The only option I had was to go to the emergency room. I knew it had to be mastitis, and the emergency room doctor verified this. All I wanted was the prescription for antibiotics so that I could get back to my daughter. When writing the prescription, the doctor said to me, "You know you should really stop breast-feeding." I must have looked at him rather strangely because he said, "The infection and the antibiotics aren't good for the baby." I did not want to stop nursing my daughter after all we had been through. As soon as I got home, I called a friend who is a nurse. I told her what antibiotic I was taking, and she assured me that it was perfectly fine for me to continue breast-feeding my daughter. In fact, she told me that I should breast-feed frequently to help unclog the blocked milk duct in my breast. I was very relieved.

Jill

Learning Opportunity: Why is it important for breast-feeding to continue while the woman is being treated for mastitis? What can the nurse do to help a woman with mastitis continue breast-feeding?

Recommend the use of warm compresses or a warm shower before feeding to promote the letdown reflex and stimulate the flow of milk. Warm compresses are also soothing and increase blood flow to the area to stimulate healing. Suggest that the woman begin breast-feeding on the affected breast first, if possible, so that the breast completely empties. If this is too painful, suggest that she start on the unaffected breast until after the letdown reflex, then switch to the affected breast. This strategy should result in less pain when the baby latches. Administer analgesics before breast-feeding or pumping to aid in minimizing discomfort. Explain that massaging the affected area during feeding helps ensure complete emptying. It is important for her to empty the breast to maintain the milk supply.

Provide support and encouragement for continuing breast-feeding. Encourage liberal fluid intake to ensure adequate milk formation. Review proper techniques for breast-feeding and proper infant positioning (refer to Chapter 15). A lactation specialist is a valuable resource for the woman with mastitis.

Urinary Tract Infection

A urinary tract infection (UTI) involves an infection of the bladder (cystitis) or the kidneys (pyelonephritis). Trauma during birth and inadequate bladder emptying during labor or postpartum may lead to urinary stasis, which increases the risk for developing a UTI. Frequent vaginal examinations during labor, urinary catheterizations, and delivery involving instrumentation further increase the risk for a postpartum UTI.

Clinical Manifestations

The signs and symptoms of cystitis differ from those of pyelonephritis. Typically, those associated with pyelonephritis are more dramatic and severe. The woman with cystitis characteristically reports burning and pain on urination. She reports urgency and frequency and voids only small amounts at a time. The woman usually has a low-grade fever and possibly suprapubic pain.

In addition to burning, pain, urgency, and frequency, the woman with pyelonephritis presents with a high, spiking fever that rises and falls abruptly as well as hematuria (blood in the urine). Often she has shaking chills and reports nausea and vomiting. Flank pain and tenderness are common. Tenderness at the costovertebral angle (the area on the back just above the waistline) is present on palpation.

Diagnosis

A urinalysis and clean-catch urine for culture and sensitivity provide evidence of an infection. The urinalysis typically reveals WBCs, protein, blood, and presence of bacteria. The clean-catch urine specimen reveals greater than 10^5 colony-forming units. A CBC may reveal an elevated WBC count.

Treatment

Antibiotic therapy is the treatment of choice based on the urine culture and sensitivity results. For the woman with cystitis, oral antibiotics are appropriate. For the woman with pyelonephritis, IV antibiotic therapy is the treatment of choice. Typically, therapy begins with a broad-spectrum antibiotic and is later adjusted based on the urine culture and sensitivity reports.

In addition to antibiotic therapy, antipyretics and analgesics, such as acetaminophen; antispasmodics; urinary analgesics, such as phenazopyridine hydrochloride; and antiemetics may be ordered. Hydration and good perineal hygiene are also important.

Nursing Care

Nursing care focuses on promoting comfort, ensuring adequate hydration, and reinforcing client teaching. The woman with cystitis typically does not require admission to a healthcare facility for treatment. However, the woman with pyelonephritis usually requires hospitalization for IV hydration and antibiotic therapy.

Providing Comfort

The woman with a UTI typically has pain and burning on urination, which can make voiding difficult. The discomfort can prevent the woman from emptying her bladder completely, resulting in urinary stasis. Urinary stasis provides a good medium for organism growth, further compounding her risk for infection and possibly increasing her risk for extension of the infection, for example from the bladder to the kidneys. Therefore, assist the woman with comfort measures such as running warm water over the perineum or using a sitz bath when attempting to urinate. Administer analgesics (e.g., acetaminophen) as ordered. A urinary analgesic (e.g., phenazopyridine hydrochloride) can also provide relief.

Consider This

The woman with a UTI may not drink enough fluid, fearing that she will need to void more frequently and thus increase her pain. Explain that an increased urinary output often decreases the pain associated with UTI.

Promoting Adequate Hydration

Adequate hydration is necessary to dilute the bacterial concentration in the urine and aid in clearing the organisms from the urinary tract. Encourage the woman to drink at least 3,000 mL of fluid a day. Suggest she drink one glass per hour to ensure adequate intake. Monitor intake and output.

Advise the woman to drink fluids that make the urine acidic, deterring organism growth. Fluids such as cranberry, plum, prune, or apricot juices are examples. Tell the woman to avoid carbonated beverages because they increase the alkalinity of urine, which promotes organism growth. If the woman has pyelonephritis, expect to administer IV fluids in addition to oral fluid to ensure adequate hydration.

Reinforcing Client Teaching

Reinforcement of teaching is essential for ensuring compliance with therapy and preventing a recurrence of cystitis or pyelonephritis. Remind the woman to complete the full-drug

regimen, which can range from 5 to 10 days. The woman with pyelonephritis receives IV antibiotic therapy initially. The health care provider may order oral antibiotics for the woman to continue after discharge (depending on her length of stay in the healthcare facility). If the woman is breast-feeding, provide instruction concerning the safety of continued breast-feeding based on the particular antibiotic she is taking. Other important topics include hydration measures; comfort measures; perineal care; and preventive measures, including signs and symptoms of a recurrence.

> ### TEST YOURSELF
> ✔ List five risk factors for postpartum infection.
> ✔ Name five signs and symptoms of endometritis.
> ✔ Describe four nursing interventions for the woman diagnosed with mastitis.

Nursing Process and Care Plan *for the Woman With a Postpartum Infection*

While there are different locations a postpartum infection can occur, the infectious process and nursing care focus remain very similar. The difference in the care plan is the nursing implementations.

Assessment (Data Collection)

Frequent observations of the postpartum woman help to monitor her for the onset of an infection. If the woman has been already diagnosed with a postpartum infection, frequent observations help to monitor the effectiveness of the medical and nursing interventions.

Note any risk factors that might predispose the woman to an infection. Ask her if she is experiencing any flu-like symptoms. Inquire about any other symptoms she might be experiencing such as dysuria, urgency, or flank or costovertebral angle pain or tenderness.

Monitor her temperature for fever greater than 100.4°F (38°C) and for tachycardia. Monitor intake and output. Obtain urine and wound specimens as ordered. Report the results of the laboratory tests, including CBC and blood cultures, to the RN and the health care provider.

Observe the woman's lochia. Note if there is a foul odor. Observe any wounds or incisions. Note if the wound edges are approximated (intact) or separated. Look for presence of excess redness, pain, or exudate. Observe the woman's breasts for any swelling, pain, excess warmth, or redness, especially a unilateral pie shaped wedge.

Monitor for the effectiveness of any antipyretics or analgesics the woman is taking. Monitor the woman while she is receiving antibiotics. If she is receiving them intravenously observe the IV insertion site during the infusion. Observe for any side effects of the medication.

If the woman is breast-feeding, monitor her technique including positioning and the newborn's ability to latch and maintain effective sucking. Observe the woman's nipples for any cracks or fissures.

Nursing Care Focus

When selecting the nursing care focus for the woman with a postpartum infection, it is important to take into consideration her symptoms, as not all infections present with the same symptoms. Also take into consideration the woman's support system and whether she is in the hospital or at home. Additionally, her knowledge level about both the infection and self-care measures is important to include in the plan of care.

Outcome Identification and Planning

Major goals for the woman with a postpartum infection include that her fever and discomfort will be managed and at an acceptable level for her. Goals also focus on her ability to care for herself and the newborn.

Perform a thorough physical assessment at least once a shift. Monitor vital signs every 4 hours. Perform a pain assessment with each set of vital signs. Perform extra assessments if the woman reports new onset of pain or other complaints of discomfort. Document your findings and report them to the RN and health care provider.

Obtain laboratory specimens as ordered and monitor results of the tests. Administer medications as ordered. Monitor antibiotic levels if ordered. If the woman is on oral antibiotics, remind her to complete the course of antibiotics as prescribed. Administer antipyretics and analgesics as ordered and monitor for effectiveness. Document the results of these interventions.

Help the woman with self-care. Cluster care to allow for periods of uninterrupted rest. Encourage the woman to increase her fluid intake. Place a pitcher near her and encourage her to drink frequently. Have her avoid caffeinated and sugary beverages that can contribute to a urinary tract infection. Monitor her intake and output. Encourage her to eat a nutritious diet. Emphasize the importance of handwashing before and after using the toilet and when handling sanitary pads.

When selecting nursing implementations for the woman with a postpartum infection, it is important to take into consideration if she is breast-feeding or not. Knowing this information is also important when carrying out nursing actions related to medication administration as certain antibiotics can pass through the breast milk to the newborn. Encourage her to continue to breast-feeding. If any medications that are prescribed for her are contraindicated with breast-feeding, the woman should be taught how to pump and dump her breast milk. Have the lactation consultant visit the woman if needed. Place warm compresses on the affected breast or have the woman take a warm shower.

Nursing Care Focus

- Hyperthermia related to infection

Goal

- The woman's temperature will be below 100.4°F (38°C).

Implementations for Monitoring and Maintaining Body Temperature

Monitor vital signs, including temperature, every 4 hours until it has been under 100.4°F (38°C) for at least 24 hours without antipyretics. Monitoring the vital signs will allow tracking of temperature spikes and overall response to therapy. Heart rate increases with hyperthermia. Monitor CBC values as ordered. The WBC count will begin decreasing as the infection resolves.

Administer an antipyretic, such as acetaminophen, as ordered. Antipyretics control body temperature and provide comfort. Administer antibiotics as ordered to treat the infection that is causing the elevated temperature.

Place a pitcher of water at the bedside, and refill it frequently as needed. Offer juices, popsicles, and other liquids every 1 to 2 hours. Avoid caffeinated beverages as they have a diuretic effect, which increases fluid loss. Temperature elevation can result in fluid loss due to the increased metabolic workload and tachypnea. Also, dehydration can elevate the temperature and interfere with temperature assessment. Adequate hydration is needed so that the body can effectively fight infection.

Evaluation of Goal/Desired Outcome

The woman:

- has a temperature less than 100.4°F (38°C) without antipyretics.
- has a pulse rate below 100 bpm.
- has a fluid intake of at least 3,000 mL/day.

Nursing Care Focus

- Acute pain

Goal

- The woman will verbalize or demonstrate relief of pain.

Implementations for Managing Pain

Administer analgesics as ordered. In the first 24 to 48 hours of the infection, administer the medication around the clock versus prn. Around-the-clock dosing prevents acute pain from becoming severe. Once pain becomes severe, it is more difficult to treat. An anti-inflammatory analgesic, such as ibuprofen, will further help reduce pain.

Assist the woman in applying warm compresses or a heating pad to the wound site. Encourage her to take warm showers, or sitz baths if indicated. Warmth helps decrease pain and increases blood flow to the area, which helps with healing. Assist her to a position of comfort.

Instruct the woman to start breast-feeding on the unaffected breast first if her affected breast is too uncomfortable, and have her pump her affected breast immediately after the feeding. Vigorous sucking by the newborn may cause excess discomfort. Having the newborn start on the unaffected breast will decrease the vigorous sucking on the affected side. Having the woman pump the affected side after the feeding session will empty the breast completely to avoid milk stasis.

Evaluation of Goal/Desired Outcome

The woman:

- verbalizes adequate relief from pain after interventions.
- empties affected breast without excessive pain.

Nursing Care Focus

- Fatigue

Goal

- The woman will demonstrate decreased symptoms of fatigue.

Implementations for Managing Fatigue

Encourage the woman to take frequent rest periods to promote healing. Rest periods should avoid screen time, television, and visitors as these distract from rest. Limit visitors as appropriate. Decreased stimuli (including dimmed lights, closed doors, and decreased sounds) promote rest. The nurse should group nursing interventions and care activities. Cluster care avoids unnecessary interruptions and promotes rest.

Encourage wakefulness during the early evening hours to promote sleep during the night, which provides the most restful sleep. Encourage her to use bedtime rituals, preferably ones she uses at home, and reduce light and noise stimuli at bedtime. These interventions promote sleep and a sense of routine.

Encourage adequate nutrition and hydration. This promotes healing of the tissues and provides an energy source. Wound infections need adequate protein and fluids in the diet to heal. Encourage the woman to avoid sugar-rich snacks and drinks. Healing of wounds helps increase energy levels. Have the woman consume a majority of her fluids by early evening so she isn't up frequently during the night to urinate.

Encourage a family member to assist with caring for the newborn (other than feedings) during the night. Promote periods of uninterrupted sleep. Having the family member help with diapering and bringing the newborn to her in bed is helpful.

Evaluation of Goal/Desired Outcome

The woman:

- verbalizes feeling rested.
- reports increased energy levels.
- performs self and newborn care without signs or complaints of fatigue.

Nursing Care Focus

- Knowledge deficiency

Goal

- The woman will demonstrate knowledge retention related to treatment and prevention of recurrent infections.

Implementations for Reinforcing Teaching

Ask questions to determine the woman's current knowledge level regarding her infection and any barriers to learning. Use the teach-back method to help evaluate the woman's understanding of fluid, nutrition, and rest needs to promote healing. Reinforce information about medications (including analgesics, antipyretics, and antibiotics) she is prescribed. Information to reinforce includes frequency of medication administration, indications for use, expected effects, and side effects to report.

Remind the woman about the importance of handwashing. Encourage frequent handwashing at appropriate times. Talk with her about wound care, the use of a peri bottle, and handling sanitary pads only by the edges. Doing this helps prevent the spread and recurrence of infection.

Encourage the woman to continue breast-feeding. Proper breast-feeding techniques decrease the likelihood that mastitis will recur. Suggest she let her nipples air dry and avoid plastic-lined breast pads. If her nipples are cracked, suggest the use of a lanolin-based product after nursing.

These measures help promote drying and prevent cracking of the nipples, which provide an entryway for pathogens. If the woman is prescribed an antibiotic that is contraindicated with breast-feeding, instruct her on the pump-and-dump method to help maintain her milk supply. Consult with a lactation specialist as appropriate.

Discuss with the woman conditions that increase her risk for mastitis including breast engorgement, nipple soreness or cracking, or a painful lump in one breast (which is a sign of a plugged duct, which increases her chance for mastitis). If the woman initiates interventions when a mastitis warning sign is present, she may be able to prevent a recurrence of mastitis. Interventions include:

- Rest in bed if possible
- Breast-feed frequently from the affected breast
- Put a warm compress on the affected breast
- Gently massage lump prior to and while the newborn is feeding
- Call her health care provider if she develops a fever of 100.4°F (38°C) or higher or if she does not get better within 24 hours or has flu-like symptoms

These measures encourage the flow of milk, help prevent milk stasis, and prevent early mastitis from becoming more severe.

Evaluation of Goal/Desired Outcome

The woman:

- verbalizes understanding of her plan of care including medications.
- washes her hands before and after using the restroom, eating, and touching the breasts.
- breast-feeds the newborn or pumps every 2 to 3 hours.

Remember **AmberLeigh Garcia** from the start of the chapter. What assessments would you have made to determine if she was experiencing a postpartum complication? What physical symptoms would you note that might indicate postpartum complications? When you investigate AmberLeigh's crying, what statements would you want to avoid saying, and why would you not want to use those statements? Remember therapeutic communication techniques.

VENOUS THROMBOEMBOLISM

Venous thromboembolism (VTE) is the umbrella term for deep vein thrombosis (DVT) and pulmonary embolism. The risk is greatest in the first few weeks of the postpartum period, and by 12 weeks postpartum the risk is equal to the woman's nonpregnancy risk (Berens, 2021). VTE is seen more often in women who have had a cesarean birth than women who have had a vaginal birth. VTE can lead to maternal death.

Risk Factors

The pregnant and postpartal woman is at risk for VTE for three reasons:

1. Clotting factors increase during pregnancy and remain elevated in the early postpartum period to promote blood clotting.
2. Pressure of the pregnant uterus on lower extremity veins leads to venous dilation and pooling of blood (venous stasis), which increase the risk for clots to form.
3. Vascular trauma during childbirth (particularly during forceps-assisted or cesarean delivery) and prolonged periods in the lithotomy position also cause venous stasis, resulting in risk for clot formation.

Box 19-3 lists factors that further increase the postpartum woman's risk for VTE.

Deep Vein Thrombosis

Deep vein thrombosis (DVT) is the formation of a blood clot (thrombus) in the deeper veins of the calf, thigh, or pelvis. These deep veins carry the majority of venous return from the legs to the heart. If part of the thrombus breaks off and travels to the lungs, it is now a **pulmonary embolism**.

BOX 19-3 Risk Factors for Postpartum Venous Thromboembolism

Medical Risk Factors
- Thrombophilia
- Hypertension
- Personal or family history of venous thromboembolism
- Obesity
- Smoking
- Older than 35 years
- Severe varicose veins
- Bed rest or immobility for over 3 days
- Dehydration

Obstetrical Risk Factors
- History of three or more pregnancies
- Prolonged labor
- Stillbirth
- Use of forceps
- Cesarean birth
- Eclampsia

Clinical Manifestations

The woman with DVT may exhibit typical signs, including edema, warmth, redness, and calf pain or tenderness in the affected leg. The woman may be observed walking and will avoid putting direct weight bearing on the affected leg. In extreme cases where the edema compromises circulation and the arterial blood flow, the leg may appear visibly pale or white with diminished pedal pulses (Chaar, 2020).

Diagnosis

The health care provider may order several diagnostic tests, such as venous compression ultrasonography, venography with a contrast medium, or Doppler flow studies. These tests reveal altered blood flow, confirming the presence of blood clots. Other tests may include D-dimer blood levels, computed tomography, or magnetic resonance venography.

Treatment

The primary goals of treatment for DVT are to prevent further thrombus formation and to prevent pulmonary embolism, a potentially fatal complication. Anticoagulation therapy is the treatment of choice. The health care provider may order subcutaneous, IV, or oral anticoagulants depending upon the woman's symptoms and severity of DVT and the presence of other risk factors (such as obesity or history of previous DVTs). Anticoagulant therapy may continue for 6 weeks and in some women for up to 12 months.

Nursing Care

Nursing care for the woman with DVT includes ambulation when pain and edema are under control, applying compression stockings as ordered, and elevating the affected extremity to promote venous return. Inspect the lower extremities for changes in color, temperature, and size, and palpate pedal pulses. Measure the circumference of each lower extremity and compare the results bilaterally to determine the degree of edema. Assist the woman with removing the compression stockings for an hour every 8 to 12 hours.

Apply warm compresses as ordered. When applying the compresses, ensure that they are at the proper temperature. Altered blood flow may diminish the woman's ability to sense temperature extremes, placing her at risk for a burn injury. Make sure that the weight of the compresses does not rest on the leg, compromising blood flow. Check the woman's bed linens and change them as necessary because the linens may become damp or wet from the moist heat applications. If possible, use a waterproof pad to protect the linens. Warm moist compresses can cool quickly. Provide the woman with extra blankets if necessary to prevent chilling. Medical warming pads may be used instead of warm compresses; however, the cautions for use remain the same.

It is important to monitor the woman's vital signs closely for slight elevations in temperature, possibly to 101°F (38.3°C), and to report this finding. Because the woman with DVT is at risk for developing a pulmonary embolism, be alert for and immediately report any sudden onset of breathing difficulties.

Administer anticoagulant therapy as ordered. When giving heparin, always have the antidote, protamine sulfate, readily available. Place the woman on bleeding precautions, which include monitoring for evidence of bleeding, applying 5 to 10 minutes of pressure to injection or venipuncture sites, avoiding unnecessary injections, and having her use a soft bristle toothbrush. Additionally, the woman should avoid medications that impact bleeding times (such as aspirin and nonsteroidal anti-inflammatory drugs (NSAIDS) like ibuprofen) unless directed to do so by the health care provider. Inform the woman to report any increase in vaginal bleeding, saturation of perineal pads or evidence of bruising, oozing at IV sites, or gingival bleeding.

The woman typically goes home on oral anticoagulant therapy. Therefore, give her information about the drug and signs and symptoms to report immediately. Tips for Reinforcing Family Teaching: Anticoagulant Therapy outlines information for the client who is prescribed anticoagulants.

Pulmonary Embolism

Pulmonary embolism occurs when a clot (thrombus) or part of the clot breaks free from the vessel wall (becoming an embolus), travels to the heart, and then moves through the pulmonary circulation, where it lodges and interrupts the blood flow to the lungs. The clot that migrates and creates a blockage is called a pulmonary embolus. If a large area of lung tissue is deprived of blood flow, cardiovascular collapse ultimately occurs, which can be fatal.

Clinical Manifestations

The postpartum woman who develops a pulmonary embolism typically exhibits a sudden onset of dyspnea, pleuritic chest pain, and an impending sense of severe apprehension or doom. If the woman experiences any of these, report them immediately to the RN and the health care provider. In addition, the woman may be tachypneic, tachycardic, and hypotensive. She may have a cough with bloody sputum (hemoptysis) and report abdominal pain. Cyanosis and changes in level of consciousness may also occur.

Diagnosis

Arterial blood gases reveal a decrease in the partial pressure of oxygen and partial pressure of carbon dioxide. A chest x-ray may show atelectasis, infiltrates, or pleural effusions, all of which suggest a pulmonary embolism. A ventilation/perfusion scan demonstrates a mismatching between lung tissue perfusion and ventilation, that is, a decrease in or absence of perfusion in parts of the lung to which ventilation is normal. Pulmonary angiography reveals decreased or absent blood flow at the location of the embolus.

Treatment

Pulmonary embolism is a life-threatening emergency requiring immediate treatment. Treatment is supportive therapy and includes oxygen via facemask and medications to treat the symptoms. For example, if the woman is hypotensive, the health care provider may order dopamine to raise her

---

 ## TIPS FOR REINFORCING FAMILY TEACHING

Anticoagulant Therapy

While you are on anticoagulant therapy, you are at risk for excessive bleeding. Look for the following signs of bleeding:

- Bruising
- Bleeding gums
- Nosebleed
- Oozing from scratches and scrapes
- Blood in the urine
- Black or tarry stools
- Increased vaginal bleeding

Notify the health care provider of any change in level of consciousness, decreased ability to follow commands, or decreased sensation or ability to move extremities. These signs may indicate a cerebral bleed. This emergency requires immediate intervention.

The following precautions will help prevent excessive bleeding:

- Use a soft toothbrush.
- Avoid using razor blades (use an electric razor to shave).
- Avoid aspirin-containing products (including baby aspirin, some migraine products, and bismuth subsalicylate).
- Check with the health care provider before taking any over-the-counter medications (including nonsteroidal anti-inflammatory agents like ibuprofen and naproxen).
- Notify your dentist and any other health care provider that you are on anticoagulant therapy.
- Apply pressure for 5 to 10 minutes after any injections, after blood is drawn, or if you accidentally cut or scrape yourself.

blood pressure. Heparin therapy prevents further clot formation. The provider may consider thrombolytic agents to dissolve the existing clot; however, this therapy is not used routinely in the postpartum period. Continuous electrocardiogram monitoring is necessary. Because of the woman's critical status, she usually receives care in the intensive care unit.

Nursing Care

Immediate action is crucial for the woman who develops a pulmonary embolism. Immediately raise the head of the bed to at least 45 degrees to facilitate breathing. Stay with the woman. Notify the RN and the health care provider immediately. Monitor vital signs closely. The health care provider will order oxygen therapy at 8 to 10 L/minute via facemask. Assist with obtaining specimens for arterial blood gas analysis and prepare the woman for diagnostic testing. Provide emotional support and explain all procedures and treatments to the woman, who is most likely apprehensive about what is happening. Prepare the woman for transfer to the intensive care unit if indicated.

TEST YOURSELF

✔ What three factors put the postpartum woman at risk for thrombus formation?

✔ Name four nursing interventions appropriate for the woman with DVT.

✔ What symptoms are associated with pulmonary embolism?

POSTPARTUM MENTAL HEALTH DISORDERS

Three mental health conditions manifest themselves during the postpartum period. These include postpartum blues (also known as "baby blues"), postpartum depression, and postpartum psychosis. Of these three conditions, postpartum blues is the most common and least serious. Studies show many women experience this transitory phase of sadness and crying, which starts about 2 to 3 days after delivery and resolves by about 2 weeks postpartum (Viguera, 2019). (See Chapter 12 for more discussion of this condition.)

Postpartum depression and postpartum psychosis are different than postpartum blues and are distinct disorders from each other. Depression affects the woman's ability to function; however, her perception of reality remains intact. This is different than the woman with postpartum psychosis, who experiences a severe distortion in her view of reality, often accompanied by hallucinations and delusions. Both disorders respond well to treatment if caught early.

The exact cause of these disorders is unknown. Researchers believe that multiple factors are responsible for their development. These factors may include hormonal changes, genetics, and major life and role changes (Viguera, 2021).

The nurse plays a key role in providing the woman with information about the signs and symptoms of each disorder, which can facilitate early detection, intervention, and treatment as indicated. It is important that the information regarding postpartum blues, depression, and psychosis be given to both the woman and her support system. Her support system may be the ones who recognize the symptoms before the woman does. Also, the woman may think her symptoms are common to being a new mother, that is, fatigue and sleep issues. Additionally, many women are reluctant to report these symptoms to the health care provider because of the myth that new mothers are always happy.

Postpartum Depression

Postpartum depression is a nonpsychotic depressive disorder. The symptoms can start during pregnancy or labor, or within 12 months after giving birth. Postpartum depression occurs in about 8% to 15% of postpartum women (Viguera, 2021). Box 19-4 lists risk factors for postpartum depression.

The incidence for men with depression in the United States is 4%; however, approximately 8% to 10% of fathers evaluated have depression in the postpartum period, with the peak incidence occurring at 6 to 12 months postpartum. The fathers who are diagnosed with depression in this time frame often have a history of depression or a partner with postpartum depression (Viguera, 2021).

Consequences of untreated postpartum depression include difficulty with normal maternal–infant attachment, marital discord, and maternal suicide (Viguera, 2021).

Clinical Manifestations

The woman with postpartum depression commonly demonstrates strong feelings of sadness, irritability, and anxiety. She is frequently tearful. She may have a lack of interest in her surroundings and have trouble motivating herself to do normal activities. She may show disinterest in others and a lack of enjoyment of life. Intense feelings of inadequacy, inability to cope, ambivalence, guilt, and unworthiness are often noted. The woman often reports problems sleeping, loss of libido, decreased appetite, inability to concentrate,

---

BOX 19-4 Risk Factors for Postpartum Depression

- Previous episode of depression (either prepregnancy or during the pregnancy)
- Stressful life events such as loss of employment, change in family situation, serious illness, or loss of family member
- Problems in relationship with partner or spouse
- Inadequate or lack of social support from family, friends, or partner
- Unplanned or unwanted pregnancy
- Family history of psychological problems
- History of physical or sexual abuse
- Intimate partner violence
- Miscarriage, stillbirth, or neonatal death
- Neonate with congenital malformation or serious health issues (e.g., preterm infant)

overwhelming fatigue, and obsessive thinking. She may contemplate harming herself (suicide) or the infant.

Diagnosis

Signs and symptoms are the basis for diagnosis. Depressive symptoms must be present on most days for at least 2 weeks for the diagnosis to apply. The Edinburgh Postnatal Depression Scale (Cox, Holden, & Sagovsky, 1987) may be used by the provider to screen the woman for depression. The health care provider usually screens the woman for medical conditions such as hypothyroidism and anemia that can cause symptoms similar to depression.

Treatment

Usually treatment for postpartum depression occurs on an outpatient basis, although severe cases may require hospitalization in a mental health facility. A trained mental health professional guides the treatment plan, which includes the woman's family.

Antidepressant therapy is the mainstay of treatment. Agents such as selective serotonin reuptake inhibitors (SSRIs), including paroxetine, fluoxetine, and sertraline, are first-line drugs in the treatment of postpartum depression. Current research indicates that these agents are safe for use in women who are breast-feeding. Additionally, if the woman had taken an antidepressant prior to or during pregnancy, it is recommended she be placed on that medication postpartum if it was effective in treating her symptoms (Kimmel & Meltzer-Brody, 2020). Electroconvulsive treatment is effective for women with severe postpartum depression that does not respond to medications, especially if the woman has thoughts of suicide (Viguera, 2021).

Nursing Care

Early detection and treatment are critical because the disorder can disrupt the woman's life and frequently interferes with interpersonal relationships. Therefore, all postpartum women and their families need information regarding the warning signs and symptoms. This should be part of routine postpartum discharge instructions. In fact, some states mandate that every pregnant woman receive written information about postpartum depression along with a list of local resources as a part of prenatal care and again before discharge from the hospital after giving birth. Other states have made screening for postpartum depression mandatory.

It is normal for the postpartum woman to be reluctant to verbalize any feelings of sadness or lack of enthusiasm about motherhood or child caring and rearing because of fear of rejection or feelings of guilt. As the nurse, you play a key role in dispelling the myth that happiness automatically occurs after the birth of a child.

Instruct the woman and her family that postpartum depression can occur at any time after delivery. Therefore, the family needs to keep a listening ear to the woman's concerns. Instruct the family to be especially alert for complaints about problems sleeping, lack of energy or lack of interest in daily activities, or fatigue out of proportion to the woman's status. It is especially important the woman understand that she should seek help immediately if she has thoughts of harming herself or her baby.

Explain the importance of the treatment plan. If the woman is hesitant to take antidepressants because she is breast-feeding, help her understand the possible consequences of not taking the medication (e.g., potential adverse effects on bonding with the baby and potential long-term negative effects on the baby's cognitive, emotional, and behavioral growth and development, etc.).

Acknowledge any feelings that the woman with postpartum depression expresses. Avoid statements that provide false reassurance or that discount the woman's feelings, such as "Don't worry, you'll feel better soon," or "Your baby is so cute. You shouldn't feel so sad!" Assist the woman in obtaining support as necessary. Contact with others in a support group can help alleviate feelings of isolation.

 A Personal Glimpse

When I gave birth to our oldest daughter, my husband and I were living away from our families and friends. I remember bringing our daughter home from the hospital and feeling completely overwhelmed and anxious. Our daughter was fussy and didn't nurse well. I had no mother, sister, or girlfriend nearby with whom I could talk or get advice. My husband was calm and very supportive, but he worked in a full-time shift. I remember feeling so lonely and depressed. I kept thinking that these feelings would go away after a few weeks. But they didn't. I wasn't eating or sleeping well, and I know I was miserable to be around. I felt completely inadequate as a mother. Finally, after 8 weeks of this, my husband suggested we go see the doctor. Reluctantly, I made an appointment. When we first got to the doctor's office, the nurse sat down with us to ask us questions. When she asked why we were there, I started crying but managed to explain what I had been feeling since the birth of our daughter. She handed me some tissues and put her hand on my arm. She assured me that she and the doctor would work with me to help me feel better and return to my normal emotional state.

I am so glad that my husband suggested I get help. The doctor gave me a prescription for paroxetine, and the nurse gave me all sorts of great suggestions, like joining a new mom support group and making sure that I got daily exercise. In just a few weeks, I felt so much better and had much more confidence in my ability to be a mother to our daughter.

Lynne

Learning Opportunity: What clues did this woman give that indicate she was suffering from postpartum depression versus the "baby blues"? What specific actions can the nurse take to quickly recognize and provide support for the woman who has postpartum depression?

Postpartum Psychosis

Postpartum psychosis is a rare mental health disorder with severe consequences for the woman, the newborn, and family if left untreated. The disorder mimics severe bipolar disorder in that the woman exhibits symptoms of mania, depression, confusion, abnormal behavior, and psychosis (i.e., hallucinations and delusions). Agitation and insomnia are often present. Symptoms appear abruptly during the first few months postpartum. The disorder may have its onset as early as 48 hours after delivery, although the typical onset is within the first 2 weeks after delivery (Payne, 2018). Postpartum psychosis is an emergency that requires inpatient treatment in a mental health facility.

Women who have a diagnosis of postpartum psychosis often have been, or will be, diagnosed with bipolar disorder. A history of schizophrenia increases the woman's risk for postpartum psychosis. However, about 50% of women who are diagnosed with postpartum psychosis have not had a mental health diagnosis prior to the event (Payne, 2018).

Clinical Manifestations

The onset of psychotic symptoms is sudden and usually occurs within 2 weeks after delivery. See Box 19-5 for symptoms of postpartum psychosis. Because of the woman's misperception of reality, suicide and infanticide are possible.

Treatment

Postpartum psychosis is a mental health emergency requiring immediate hospitalization. The woman is unable to care for the infant during the time of psychosis. Antipsychotic agents are the treatment of choice, although the treatment plan may also include antidepressants. The mental health care provider may consider electroconvulsive therapy, especially if the woman is suicidal (Payne, 2019). Psychotherapy will also be used in conjunction with the other treatments.

Nursing Care

Caring for the woman with postpartum psychosis requires specialized mental health training beyond the scope of practice for the obstetric nurse. However, you need to be aware of the signs and symptoms of postpartum psychosis so that early detection and prompt intervention can occur.

BOX 19-5 Symptoms of Postpartum Psychosis

- Delusions (she may express the belief that the infant is dead or defective)
- Hallucinations (she may hear voices telling her to kill herself or her child)
- Severe agitation, restlessness, or irritability
- Hyperactivity, euphoria, or little concern for self or infant (manic phase of bipolar disorder)
- Depression including preoccupation with guilt, feelings of worthlessness and isolation, extreme overconcern for the infant's health, and sleep disturbances
- Poor judgment and confusion

SPECIAL POSTPARTUM SITUATIONS

In addition to complications that can occur in the postpartum period, two other situations may require nursing intervention. These include grief and malattachment.

Grief in the Postpartal Period

Typically, the postpartum period is a happy time of celebrating the birth of a newborn. However, not all pregnancies conclude in a happy family taking home a healthy newborn. These situations may include the woman who is placing her newborn for adoption, the family faced with a newborn with congenital anomalies, or the family dealing with the death of the fetus or newborn. Other events may cause grief reactions in families, but may not be identified as a grief-provoking situation. Some of these events may include the family with a preterm infant, a cesarean birth when a vaginal birth was highly desired, or when the gender of the infant is different from what the woman or family desired.

Grief is a universal process that each individual experiences uniquely. Grief is a natural response to a loss, whether the loss is the result of a choice, such as occurs with adoption, or when the situation is completely out of the individual's control, such as when the newborn has a congenital anomaly or dies. Shock and disbelief are often the first feelings expressed. This feeling of numbness or unreality may last hours, days, or weeks. Anger, even to the point of rage, bargaining, and depression are natural expressions of the grieving process. It is normal for individuals to demonstrate many emotions as they work through their feelings.

Men and women may differ in their responses to grief. Common grief responses include tearfulness, isolation, or immersion in an activity such as work. These differences can cause a rift between the woman and her spouse unless the couple receives intervention to help them work through the differences. The woman may misperceive that her spouse "doesn't care" or that they "isn't grieving." Counseling can be beneficial.

The Woman Placing the Newborn for Adoption

Giving the newborn up for adoption is a complicated and difficult choice some women face. Each woman's circumstances are unique, and responses to this challenge are individualized. The woman often enters into a very somber period of grief and detachment. She may express intense emotions and need to discuss the dreams and hopes that she is releasing with this decision, or she may be withdrawn and quiet. In all cases, the woman requires support, personal care, and comfort through the early postpartum period.

The woman placing her newborn for adoption requires nonjudgmental support. It is critical for you to be aware of your own attitudes and avoid the temptation to influence the outcome toward your beliefs. Your role is to be an advocate for the woman, which involves keeping her informed of her rights and options and supporting her in whatever decision she makes. It is important for you to recognize that each state has laws that govern the rights of each party in the adoption process. Be knowledgeable of your institution's policies regarding handling of the adoption process.

The Family Whose Newborn Has Congenital Anomalies

Helping parents adjust to a newborn with congenital anomalies is a challenge for the postpartum nurse. The woman and her family must grieve the loss of the "dream" child and learn to accept one that is not as they had imagined (see Chapters 20 and 21).

Encourage frequent interaction with the newborn. Point out positive features. Role model healthy behaviors by talking and playing with the baby as you would with any newborn. When the family goes home, they may benefit by participation in a parent support group.

The Family Whose Fetus or Newborn Has Died

Death often forces individuals to face core issues and personal values; it leaves emotions raw, while people struggle for meaning. When a newborn or fetus dies, the parents are often unprepared to deal with their new reality. They frequently voice questions to which there are no good answers.

Coping with the death of the fetus or newborn can be stressful for the nurse as well as for the family. The nurse may feel inadequate to help and be tempted to withdraw from the situation. It is important for the nurse to recognize their feelings so that these feelings do not interfere with the nurse's ability to care for the woman and her family. It may be helpful for the nurse to talk through their feelings with a friend or coworker. The nurse should not let personal beliefs and values overshadow the family's beliefs and values, but should instead allow the family to experience their own grief process. Assistance and support should be provided in ways that are meaningful and helpful to the family.

Several measures can help provide meaning to the family during this difficult time. The baby who died is a part of a family and has a place with them. Encourage the family to name their newborn, even if it was stillborn. Memory items, such as footprints and handprints, a name record, blessing, souvenir birth record, receiving blanket, lock of hair, and identification bracelet, identify this baby as a member of a particular family. Parents have identified photos of the newborn as a precious memory. Keep in mind that the photos must be comforting photos, that is, ones with the baby clothed, washed, and positioned comfortably. Allow the family or mother to assist with clothes, bathing, animal toys, or blankets. Some families are not ready at the time of discharge to accept these memory items. Many hospitals secure these memory items for a time frame for families who come back for them after discharge.

Avoid saying phrases that are nontherapeutic or even potentially hurtful to the family. Statements such as "You have an angel in heaven," "It wasn't his time," or "You can always have another baby" may be perceived as thoughtless and hurtful by grieving families.

The Family Which Experiences Other Grief-Provoking Events

Grief is not only seen with death. Other events can also cause grief. These include the loss of an ideal such as when the infant is born preterm, the route of delivery is different from what the mother desired, or the infant's gender is different from what the family desired. Often these families may not realize that they are experiencing grief reactions and may feel guilty for not feeling "as happy as they should." Monitor the mother for symptoms of grief. Encourage her to discuss her feelings. Avoid patronizing statements such as "It will be OK" or "There is no reason to feel this way." These statements, instead of comforting the family, may increase feelings of guilt and grief. Be available to listen to the woman.

Malattachment in the Postpartum Period

Attachment is an enduring emotional bond between the baby and primary caregiver. The relationship of attachment begins when a women first finds out that she is pregnant. Through the prenatal visits, information about the well-being of her baby reinforces this attachment. As she hears the heartbeat, sees the baby's movements on ultrasound, and feels the movement inside her uterus, the woman begins to perceive this something inside her body as a "someone" other than herself. Preparations of the nursery and choosing names continue this bonding process.

Many things influence the degree of attachment. A stable relationship, good prenatal course, and positive anticipation of a healthy infant help a woman begin an internal relationship with her baby before it is born. However, difficulties during the pregnancy, immaturity on the part of the woman, or an unreliable support system may put the family at risk for **malattachment**, emotional distancing in the maternal–infant relationship. Pregnancy complications or difficult relationships with the father of the baby can also adversely affect attachment. In addition, alcohol and drug abuse can contribute to malattachment and infant neglect.

Key signs of malattachment include lack of eye contact, lack of verbal stimulation, and a lack of response to the newborn's cries or cues. Table 19-2 lists behaviors that may indicate malattachment. If you observe any of these signs, report them to the RN. Lack of bonding between the mother and her newborn can be serious if the woman goes home without proper support. Therefore, interventions include involving the whole family in the bonding process. Discharge planning includes a predischarge consult with a clinical psychologist or clinical social worker who will assess support systems available for the mother. A referral for home care may be appropriate.

TABLE 19-2 Comparing Attachment and Malattachment

ATTACHMENT	MALATTACHMENT
Uses endearments and pet names	Speaks of the newborn as an object, "it"
Speaks softly and uses "baby talk"	Makes no eye contact with the newborn
Often calls newborn by name	Does not use the newborn's name
Becomes involved in routine care of diapering, bathing, and feeding	Shows disinterest in daily care and feeding of the newborn
Holds newborn close to body or in direct face-to-face contact	Places newborn in crib or lays newborn on lap facing away from mother
Responds to crying, smiling, feeding, and elimination with positive reinforcement	Ignores crying and newborn cue behaviors; reacts negatively to elimination needs
Easily calms upset newborn	Does not perceive newborn's needs; newborn is frustrated and nervous

Note: The woman's culture must be taken into consideration when assessing for malattachment.

 Cultural Snapshot

In the United States, fathers take a more active role in the direct care of their newborns shortly after birth. Families from different cultures may incorporate other relatives in newborn care. Be careful not to misinterpret lack of the father's involvement as malattachment. Family cultural beliefs may prescribe that only female members, such as the woman's sisters, mother, or mother-in-law, are allowed to handle the baby until the child is older. In some cultures, the woman is expected to remain secluded at home for approximately 4 to 6 weeks after delivery. Ask the family directly about who will be attending to the needs of the woman and infant once they go home.

In traditional Vietnamese families, members may not name or make eye contact or show excessive attention toward the infant to avoid drawing attention to the infant by evil spirits. As another example, Native Americans may not name the infant until a naming ceremony or certain waiting period has occurred. These seemingly "detached" behaviors may be appropriate for the family's culture and should not be interpreted as malattachment.

TEST YOURSELF

✔ What signs indicate that the woman may be experiencing postpartum depression versus the "baby blues"?

✔ List three things you can do to help a family cope with the birth of a newborn with a congenital anomaly.

✔ Name three ways you can create memories for parents whose newborn has died.

Recall **AmberLeigh Garcia** from the start of the chapter. From your readings, what information would you want to know about AmberLeigh's delivery? Why would this information be useful? How will this information help you identify postpartum complications? What teaching would you want to reinforce in her discharge teaching related to postpartum complications?

KEY POINTS

- Hemorrhage, infection, VTE, and mental health disorders are conditions that put the postpartum woman at risk.
- Early postpartum hemorrhage occurs in the first 24 hours after birth and is most frequently caused by uterine atony. Late postpartum hemorrhage can occur any time after the first 24 hours. Frequent causes are infection, subinvolution, and retained placental fragments.
- Nursing interventions for the woman with postpartum hemorrhage are focused on identifying the cause and stopping the bleeding. Establishing an IV line, if not already in place, and frequent monitoring of vital signs and urinary output are critical actions. For uterine atony, massage the uterus and administer ordered oxytocics. For lacerations and hematomas, notify the RN and the health care provider.
- Endometritis, infection of the uterine lining, is the most common postpartal infection. IV antibiotics are necessary for serious infections.
- Wound infection can involve the episiotomy, laceration, or cesarean incision. Antibiotic therapy and drainage of the wound may be required.
- Mastitis is a localized infection of breast tissue caused by stasis in a milk duct and/or infection with organisms that enter the breast through a crack or fissure in the nipple. Treatment involves antibiotics, emptying the breasts

(preferably by breast-feeding), and warm compresses. A diagnosis of mastitis does not prevent the woman for breast-feeding.

- The postpartum woman is at an increased risk for urinary tract infections (UTIs) because of the urinary tract dilation, decrease in peristalsis, and urinary stasis that is common in pregnancy. UTI symptoms include frequency, urgency, and burning upon urination. Pyelonephritis (kidney infection) is a more serious infection than cystitis (bladder infection). High, intermittent fever with flank tenderness accompanies pyelonephritis. Antibiotics are the therapy of choice.

- All postpartum women are at risk for venous thromboembolism (VTE) because of increased clotting factors that remain elevated after birth. Stasis and pooling of blood in the extremities can be caused by pressure of the gravid uterus on the veins of the lower extremities during pregnancy, the length of time in labor and delivery, being inactive, or use of stirrups during labor. VTE includes deep vein thrombosis (DVT) and pulmonary embolism.

- Treatment for DVT includes anticoagulants and compression stockings. Treatment for a pulmonary embolism focuses on supportive measures, including oxygen, and is usually carried out in an intensive care setting.

- The two common mental health issues that can affect the woman in the postpartum period include postpartum blues and postpartum depression. Postpartum depression is a major mood disorder that interferes with the woman's ability to function in daily life and requires treatment by a mental health professional.

- Postpartum psychosis is a mental health emergency. The woman is unable to care for her infant during the psychosis and may harm herself or the infant. This condition requires inpatient treatment by a mental healthcare professional. Treatment consists of antipsychotics, electroconvulsive therapy (ECT) and psychotherapy.

- The nurse's role in the care of the grieving postpartum woman is to provide support. Listen, and be accepting of her feelings. Encourage the use of a support group and counseling for the couple. If the fetus or newborn dies, help the family make memories by encouraging them to hold the fetus or newborn and say goodbye, by taking pictures, and by giving them a memento box with clothes the newborn wore or blankets, and so on.

- Monitor for malattachment if the woman does not interact with or hold the newborn, or if she turns away or does not talk to the newborn or call them by name. Notify the RN if you notice any of these symptoms.

INTERNET RESOURCES

Postpartum Hemorrhage
https://www.marchofdimes.org/pregnancy/postpartum-hemorrhage.aspx

Mastitis
https://www.mayoclinic.org/diseases-conditions/mastitis/symptoms-causes/syc-20374829

Postpartum Depression
https://www.womenshealth.gov/mental-health/mental-health-conditions/postpartum-depression
https://www.helpguide.org/articles/depression/postpartum-depression-and-the-baby-blues.htm
https://www.postpartum.net

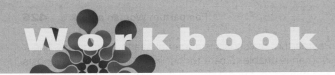

NCLEX-STYLE REVIEW QUESTIONS

1. A woman is in for her postpartum checkup. She has a fever of 101°F (38.3°C) and reports abdominal pain and a "bad smell" to her lochia. The nurse recognizes that these symptoms are associated with which condition?
   a. Mastitis
   b. Endometritis
   c. Chorioamnionitis
   d. Infection of the episiotomy

2. The nurse enters the room of a woman who delivered 12 hours ago. The woman is leaning forward in bed and is obviously having difficulty breathing. The area around her mouth is blue. What should the nurse do first?
   a. Administer oxygen by nasal cannula.
   b. Obtain arterial blood for blood gas analysis.
   c. Raise the head of the bed.
   d. Tell the woman that she doesn't need to worry.

3. A woman delivered a healthy baby girl 2 days ago. Which observation by the nurse indicates the need for additional data collection and follow-up?
   a. The woman actively participates in the care of her baby.
   b. The woman comments that her baby has red hair like her grandmother.
   c. The woman reports that she will be happy to get home because she does not like hospital food.
   d. The woman tells a friend about her baby stating, "It just cries all the time."

4. When caring for a postpartum woman who exhibits a large amount of bleeding, which areas would the nurse need to collect data on before the woman ambulates?
   a. Attachment, lochia color, complete blood cell count
   b. Blood pressure, pulse, complaints of dizziness
   c. Degree of responsiveness, respiratory rate, fundus location
   d. Height of fundus, level of orientation, support systems

5. The nurse reviews the medical record of a postpartum woman. Which of the following information would put the woman at risk for postpartum hemorrhage? (Select all that apply.)
   a. 26 years old
   b. G5 P4
   c. Received oxytocin for delivery of third child
   d. Infant weighs 4,200 grams
   e. Delivery was assisted with vacuum extraction
   f. Postpartum tubal ligation performed

STUDY ACTIVITIES

1. Use the following table to compare deep vein thrombosis and pulmonary embolism.

	Deep Vein Thrombosis	Pulmonary Embolism
Clinical manifestations		

	Deep Vein Thrombosis	Pulmonary Embolism
Diagnosis		
Treatment		
Nursing care		

2. Do an Internet search on postpartum depression. What resources for a woman experiencing postpartum depression are available in your community? How many of these are available at no charge to the woman? How can the woman find out about these resources? Share your findings with your clinical group.

3. Develop an education plan for a young teenage mother to help her decrease the chances for developing a postpartum infection.

CRITICAL THINKING: WHAT WOULD YOU DO?

Apply your knowledge of postpartum complications to the following situation.

1. Josie is an outgoing 15-year-old girl who delivered a baby girl 24 hours ago. You walk in because you hear the newborn crying. Josie is talking to a friend on the telephone about the football game next week. When you check on the newborn in the crib beside Josie's bed, the newborn is jittery and red in the face.
   a. What is your impression of this situation? What data collection will you do to evaluate this situation?
   b. What do you need to do for the newborn? Which individuals do you need to involve in the discharge planning process?

2. You just admitted Tiffany to the postpartum unit. She gave birth to a healthy female newborn after a normal delivery. Her fundus is slightly firm, above the umbilicus, and positioned to the right. Her sanitary pad is full, but the L&D nurse reported that she received perineal care just before transport.
   a. What is the likely source of the heavy lochia? What nursing interventions should be done?
   b. If the fundus remains firm and in the midline, but a steady flow of lochia is noted despite fundal massage, what do you suspect is causing the problem? What nursing interventions should be done in this instance?

3. A woman who had a cesarean birth 3 days ago asks you to look at her incision, which is red and warm to touch with amount of yellow drainage along the edges.
   a. What conclusions do you reach as a result of your observation? What additional data should be collected? What interventions are appropriate in this situation?
   b. What if the woman reported hardness in an area of one of her breasts? What data should be collected? What instructions would you give her?

The Newborn at Risk: Gestational and Acquired Disorders

Key Terms

acute bilirubin encephalopathy (kernicterus)
apnea
appropriate for gestational age (AGA)
Erb palsy
extremely low birth weight (ELBW)
gestational age
intrauterine growth restriction (IUGR)
large for gestational age (LGA)
low birth weight (LBW)
macroglossia
polycythemia
polyhydramnios
postterm
preterm
small for gestational age (SGA)
term
very low birth weight (VLBW)

Learning Objectives

At the conclusion of this chapter, you will:

1. Define the classifications used to describe a newborn based on size, gestational age, or weight.
2. Explain the various components of the gestational age assessment.
3. Describe the most common underlying condition that causes a newborn to be small for gestational age (SGA), and explain the reason this condition occurs.
4. Differentiate between symmetric and asymmetric growth restriction in infants.
5. List factors that contribute to a newborn being large for gestational age (LGA).
6. List possible contributing factors for preterm birth.
7. Compare characteristics of the preterm newborn with those of the term newborn.
8. Identify complications commonly associated with preterm newborns.
9. Describe the goals of care for the preterm newborn.
10. Describe major aspects of nursing care for the postterm newborn.
11. Give details of care for three acquired respiratory disorders associated with newborns.
12. Describe hemolytic disease of the newborn.
13. Explain important features of treatment, clinical manifestations, and nursing considerations for the newborn of a mother with diabetes.
14. Discuss the clinical manifestations of and nursing care for a newborn of a chemically dependent mother.
15. Differentiate causes of and care for newborns with congenitally acquired infections.

Kierra Jones was born at 35 weeks gestation. Her mother, Ella, is diabetic and had difficulty controlling her diabetes while she was pregnant. Kierra weighed 2,400 g at birth. As you read this chapter, think about what characteristics you would expect to note in Kierra.

Considering all that can go wrong, it is a wonder that the majority of babies are born healthy. However, for the 10% who are born ill or who develop health problems shortly after birth, the beginning of life can be a struggle. These fragile newborns need specialized care in the neonatal intensive care unit (NICU). Many Level III NICUs do not hire licensed practical/vocational nurses because the care of sick newborns can be complex and falls outside the scope of practical nursing. However, licensed practical/vocational nurses often work in Level II NICUs because these babies are more stable and have predictable needs. It is important for you to understand the major disorders and principles of care for newborns with these disorders. If you work in a newborn nursery, you must be able to identify when the newborn's condition is deteriorating so that you can get help quickly.

This chapter focuses on newborn conditions that result when the newborn differs in size from the norm or is born earlier or later than expected. It also discusses disorders that the newborn acquires as a result of factors present during the pregnancy or birth.

VARIATIONS IN SIZE AND GESTATIONAL AGE

The majority of newborns are born around 40 weeks' gestation, weighing from 5.5 to 10 lb (2,500 to 4,600 g) and measuring 18 to 23 in. (45 to 55 cm) in length. However, there are variations in birth size and **gestational age**, the length of time between fertilization of the egg and birth, that increase the newborn's risk for perinatal problems.

Terminology that describes newborns based on their size or gestational age is useful to facilitate communication. Size classifications consider the newborn's weight, length, and head circumference; these classifications include the following:

- **Small for gestational age (SGA)** describes a newborn whose weight, length, or head circumference falls below the 10th percentile for gestational age.
- **Appropriate for gestational age (AGA)** describes a newborn whose weight, length, or head circumference falls between the 10th and 90th percentiles for gestational age.
- **Large for gestational age (LGA)** describes a newborn whose weight, length, or head circumference is above the 90th percentile for gestational age.

There are three classifications that describe a newborn's size based on weight: **Low birth weight (LBW)**, weight less than 2,500 g; **very low birth weight (VLBW)**, weight less than 1,500 g; and **extremely low birth weight (ELBW)**, weight less than 1,000 g.

Newborn classification based on gestational age includes the following:

- **Preterm**, or premature, a newborn born at less than 37 weeks' gestation
- **Postterm**, or postmature, a newborn born at greater than 42 weeks' gestation
- **Term**, a newborn born between 37 and 42 weeks' gestation

Gestational Age Assessment

Assessment of gestational age is a critical evaluation. The registered nurse (RN) is ultimately responsible for performing the gestational age assessment. However, you should be familiar with the instruments used and be able to differentiate characteristics of the full-term newborn from those of the premature or postterm newborn. Although prenatal estimates of gestational age, particularly the sonogram, yield reliable information, the most precise way to assess gestational age is through direct evaluation of the newborn in the first few hours after birth.

The Ballard scoring system (Fig. 20-1) is a common gestational age assessment tool used in newborn nurseries. Gestational age assessment involves evaluation of two main categories of maturity: neuromuscular and physical maturity. The RN rates each category on a scale of 1 to 5, with 5 being the highest or most completed development. Table 20-1 compares gestational assessment findings in a term, preterm, and postterm newborn.

Neuromuscular Maturity

Six categories determining neuromuscular maturity are as follows:

1. Posture
2. Square window (measurement of wrist angle with flexion toward forearm until resistance is met)
3. Arm recoil (extension and release of arm after arm is completely flexed and held in position for approximately 5 seconds)
4. Popliteal angle (measurement of knee angle on flexion of thigh with extension of lower leg until resistance is met)
5. Scarf sign (arm pulled gently in front of and across top portion of body until resistance is met)
6. Heel to ear (movement of foot to as close to the head as possible)

Physical Maturity

Six categories determining physical maturity are as follows:

1. Skin
2. Lanugo
3. Plantar creases (surface)
4. Breast buds
5. Eye-ear
6. Genitals

The Small-for-Gestational Age (Growth-Restricted) Newborn

SGA describes an infant who is born smaller than the average size (in weight, length, or head circumference) for the number of weeks gestation at the time of delivery. The criteria are that the SGA newborn's weight falls below the 10th percentile of that expected for their gestational age, or that two of the three categories (weight, length, and head circumference) fall below the 10th percentile. Early identification of the SGA fetus with ultrasound is ideal.

Although some SGA newborns are small because their parents are small (genetics), most are small because of circumstances that occurred during the pregnancy, causing limited fetal growth. This condition is **intrauterine growth restriction (IUGR)** or fetal growth restriction (FGR). It occurs when

NEUROMUSCULAR MATURITY

NEUROMUSCULAR MATURITY SIGN	SCORE							RECORD SCORE HERE
	−1	0	1	2	3	4	5	
POSTURE								
SQUARE WINDOW (Wrist)	>90°	90°	60°	45°	30°	0°		
ARM RECOIL		180°	140°–180°	110°–140°	90°–110°	<90°		
POPLITEAL ANGLE	180°	160°	140°	120°	100°	90°	<90°	
SCARF SIGN								
HEEL TO EAR								
						TOTAL NEUROMUSCULAR MATURITY SCORE		

SCORE

Neuromuscular ____
Physical ____
Total ____

MATURITY RATING

Score	Weeks
−10	20
−5	22
0	24
5	26
10	28
15	30
20	32
25	34
30	36
35	38
40	40
45	42
50	44

PHYSICAL MATURITY

PHYSICAL MATURITY SIGN	SCORE							RECORD SCORE HERE
	−1	0	1	2	3	4	5	
SKIN	sticky, friable, transparent	gelatinous, red, translucent	smooth, pink, visible veins	superficial peeling and/or rash, few veins	cracking pale areas, rare veins	parchment, deep cracking, no vessels	leathery, cracked, wrinkled	
LANUGO	none	sparse	abundant	thinning	bald areas	mostly bald		
PLANTAR SURFACE	heel-toe 40–50 mm:−1 <40 mm:−2	>50 mm no crease	faint red marks	anterior transverse crease only	creases ant. 2/3	creases over entire sole		
BREAST	impercep-tible	barely perceptible	flat areola no bud	stippled areola 1–2 mm bud	raised areola 3–4 mm bud	full areola 5–10 mm bud		
EYE-EAR	lids fused loosely: −1 tightly: −2	lids open pinna flat stays folded	sl. curved pinna; soft; slow recoil	well-curved pinna; soft but ready recoil	formed and firm instant recoil	thick cartilage, ear stiff		
GENITALS (Male)	scrotum flat, smooth	scrotum empty, faint rugae	testes in upper canal, rare rugae	testes descending, few rugae	testes down, good rugae	testes pendulous, deep rugae		
GENITALS (Female)	clitoris prominent and labia flat	prominent clitoris and small labia minora	prominent clitoris and enlarging minora	majora and minora equally prominent	majora large, minora small	majora cover clitoris and minora		
						TOTAL PHYSICAL MATURITY SCORE		

FIGURE 20-1 Ballard's gestational age assessment tool, including neuromuscular and physical assessment criteria. (From Ballard J. L. (1991). New Ballard score expanded to include extremely premature infants. *Journal of Pediatrics*, 119, 417-423.)

the fetus does not receive adequate amounts of oxygen and nutrients necessary for the proper growth and development of organs and tissues. Intrauterine growth restriction (IUGR) can begin at any time during the pregnancy. The discussion for the remainder of this section focuses on the newborn who is small for gestational age (SGA) because of IUGR.

Contributing Factors

IUGR, the most common underlying condition leading to small for gestational age (SGA) newborns, results from interference in the supply of nutrients to the fetus. Inadequate maternal nutrition may be a contributing factor. If the mother is unable to meet the increased nutritional demands of pregnancy, the fetus does not receive the necessary nutrients for growth. Another factor may involve an abnormality in the placenta or its function. Placental damage, such as when the placenta separates prematurely, or a decrease in blood flow to the placenta, reduces its ability to transport nutrients. Maternal conditions that interfere with adequate blood flow to the placenta, such as preeclampsia/

TABLE 20-1 Comparing Gestational Age Assessment Findings

ASSESSMENT PARAMETER	TERM NEWBORN	PRETERM NEWBORN	POSTTERM NEWBORN
Neuromuscular Maturity			
Posture	Flexed position with good muscle tone	Hypotonic with extension of the extremities	Full flexion of arms and legs
Square window	Flexible wrists with a small angle, usually ranging from 0 to 30 degrees	Angle greater than 45 degrees	Similar to that for term newborn
Arm recoil	Quick recoil with angle at elbow less than 90 degrees	Slowed recoil time with angle greater than 90 degrees	Similar to that for term newborn
Popliteal angle	Resistance to extension with knee angle 90 degrees or less	Decreased resistance to extension with large angle at knee	Similar to that for term newborn
Scarf sign	Increased resistance to movement with elbow unable to reach midline	Increased flexibility with elbow extending past midline	Similar to that for term newborn
Heel to ear	Moderate resistance to movement	Little to no resistance to movement	Similar to that for term newborn
Physical Maturity			
Skin	Cracking of the skin and few visible veins	Very thin with little subcutaneous fat and easily visible veins	Leathery, cracked, and wrinkled
Lanugo	Thinning of lanugo with balding areas	Abundance of fine downy hair up to 34 weeks gestation	Almost absent lanugo with many balding areas
Plantar creases (surface)	Creases covering at least the anterior two thirds of foot	Smooth feet with few creases	Creases covering entire foot
Breast buds	Raised areola with 3- to 4-mm breast bud	Flat areola with little to no breast bud	Full areola with 5- to 10-mm breast bud
Eye-ear	Cartilage present within pinna with ability for natural recoil when folded	Little cartilage, allowing shape to be maintained when folded	Cartilage thick; pinna stiff
Genitals	Male with pendulous scrotum covered with rugae; testicles descended. Female with large labia majora covering minora	Male with smooth scrotum and undescended testicles. Female with prominent clitoris; labia minora not covered by majora	Male with pendulous scrotum with deep rugae. Female with clitoris and labia minora completely covered by labia majora

eclampsia or uncontrolled diabetes, contribute to placental malfunction. Maternal smoking interferes with placental blood flow and is the most common preventable cause of IUGR. In some situations, placental functioning may be normal, but the fetus is unable to use the supplied nutrients, such as when the fetus develops an intrauterine infection. Box 20-1 lists factors that contribute to IUGR.

Clinical Manifestations

The two classifications of IUGR are symmetric growth restriction and asymmetric growth restriction. Approximately 20% to 30% of newborns with IUGR have symmetric growth restriction (Mandy, 2021). These newborns have not grown at the expected rate for gestational age on standard growth charts, but the growth pattern is symmetric. In other words, both head and body parts are in proportion but are below normal size for gestational age. Generally, all three growth measurements (weight, length, and head circumference) fall below the 10th percentile when plotted on a standard growth chart. Symmetric growth

restriction is the more serious of the two types because it begins earlier in the pregnancy, frequently has a genetic cause, and the condition is generally chronic.

The majority (70% to 80%) of newborns with IUGR have asymmetric growth restriction. The asymmetrically growth-restricted newborn's head is large in comparison with the body. For this reason, asymmetric growth restriction is described as "head sparing." When the three growth measurements (weight, length, and head circumference) are plotted on a standard growth chart, one or two of the measurements fall below the 10th percentile. These newborns typically have normal measurements for head circumference and length but demonstrate a comparatively low birth weight (LBW).

The newborn with intrauterine growth restriction (IUGR) typically appears pale, thin, and wasted. The skin is loose and peeling with very little vernix. The face has a shrunken or "wizened" appearance. Skull sutures may overlap or be too wide, and the abdomen may be sunken. The umbilical cord appears thin and dull, compared with the

BOX 20-1 Contributing Factors to Intrauterine Growth Restriction (IUGR) and Preterm Birth

Maternal Factors

Lifestyle
- Smoking
- Alcohol use
- Substance abuse (e.g., narcotics, heroin, cocaine)
- Severe malnutrition during pregnancy

Chronic Diseases
- Heart disease
- Chronic hypertension
- Diabetes
- Anemia
- Connective tissue disorders (e.g., lupus)

Genetics and Demographics
- Race/ethnicity (African Americans have higher incidence; Latino Americans have lower incidence when compared to whites)

- Extremes of age (under 16 or over 40)
- Short stature

Pregnancy-Related
- Prior history of IUGR or other poor pregnancy outcomes (e.g., stillbirth or preterm delivery)
- Multiple pregnancy (e.g., twins, triplets)
- Preeclampsia/eclampsia
- Intrauterine infections
- Umbilical cord defects
- Placenta previa
- Placental abruption (abruptio placentae)

Fetal Factors
- Chromosomal abnormalities
- Congenital defects
- Congenital infections (TORCH)
- Hemolytic disease

---

shiny, plump cord of a normal newborn. Meconium staining is a frequent finding. Compared with the appropriate for gestational age (AGA) newborn, breast buds are smaller, ear cartilage is less developed, and female genitalia appear less mature.

The newborn with intrauterine growth restriction (IUGR) may have neurologic involvement. The cry may be shrill. The infant may have a wide-eyed expression and appear hyperalert. They may be irritable, jittery, and difficult to soothe with an exaggerated Moro reflex. The newborn may have difficulty sleeping and startle easily.

According to **Kierra Jones's** gestational age and weight at birth, into what categories would Kierra fall? What may have contributed to Kierra's presence in these categories? What characteristics would you expect to see in Kierra's physical and neuromuscular maturity?

Complications

Harsh conditions in utero can lead to a decrease in oxygen available to the fetus (hypoxia), causing the fetus to experience chronic fetal distress. Unable to meet the demands of normal labor and birth, the fetus may gasp in utero or with the first breaths at delivery, resulting in aspiration (breathing foreign matter into the lungs) of amniotic fluid. If the aspirated fluid contains meconium (the first stool), the newborn can develop meconium aspiration syndrome (MAS) (see the section Meconium Aspiration Syndrome).

The growth-restricted fetus is at increased risk for cesarean delivery because of fetal distress. They may be born prematurely with all the complications that accompany preterm birth. The newborn may have a difficult cardiopulmonary transition.

The newborn with intrauterine growth restriction (IUGR) has difficulty with thermoregulation for several reasons. This newborn has very little subcutaneous tissue and brown fat because they consumed stores in utero. Compared to the appropriate for gestational age (AGA) infant, the newborn with IUGR has a large ratio of body surface area to weight. As a result, the newborn may develop hypothermia. In addition, the newborn with IUGR typically experiences hypoglycemia (low blood sugar) because of a high metabolic rate in response to heat loss and low glycogen stores. Hypothermia and hypoglycemia can each lead to respiratory distress.

In response to chronic hypoxia in utero, the fetus increases red blood cell (RBC) production, leading to **polycythemia** (excess number of RBCs) and hyperviscosity of the blood. This newborn often has impaired immune function that continues throughout childhood. The newborn with IUGR has a much higher mortality rate compared to the AGA infant. Symmetrically growth-restricted newborns have the highest mortality rate.

Nursing Care

The RN is responsible for assessing gestational age, identifying potential complications, and initiating the plan of care. As the licensed practical/vocational nurse, you play an important role in carrying out interventions identified in the plan of care.

Review the maternal history and note any factors that might contribute to the infant being small for gestational age (SGA) or to having an intrauterine growth restriction (IUGR). Be alert for potential complications and risk factors related to respiratory distress, hypothermia, hypoglycemia, polycythemia, and altered parental interaction with the newborn. Conduct and document routine nursing care with special emphasis on the following:

- Monitor respiratory status, including respiratory rate and pattern, and observe for signs and symptoms of respiratory distress, such as cyanosis, nasal flaring, and expiratory grunting.

- Maintain a neutral thermal environment so that the skin temperature remains between 97.7°F and 99.5°F (36.5°C and 37.5°C).
- Monitor blood glucose levels as ordered and more frequently if symptoms develop. Maintain levels greater than or equal to 50 mg/dL.
- Monitor results of other blood studies, such as hematocrit (less than 65%), hemoglobin (less than 22 g/dL), and bilirubin (less than 12 mg/dL).
- Observe feeding tolerance, including amounts taken and any difficulties or problems encountered, such as inability to suck at breast, fatigue, excessive spitting up, or diarrhea.
- Monitor intake and output and daily weights.
- Observe for jaundice.
- Encourage family caregivers to visit frequently and care for their infant.

The Large-for-Gestational Age Newborn

An LGA newborn is one whose size (weight, length, or head circumference) is above the 90th percentile when plotted on a standard growth chart. The full-term LGA newborn weighs more than 4,000 g, or two of the three categories (weight, length, and head circumference) lie above the 90th percentile for gestational age. Generally, the newborn's overall body size is proportional, but both head and weight fall in the upper limits of growth charts. Most LGA infants are genetically and nutritionally adequate. The newborn could receive an incorrect designation of LGA because of miscalculation of the due date. A postbirth gestational age assessment is essential.

Size Can Be Misleading

A large-for-gestational age (LGA) newborn may look mature because of their size. However, they could be developmentally immature because of gestational age.

Contributing Factors

In the majority of cases, the underlying cause of a newborn being LGA is unknown. However, certain factors contribute. Maternal diabetes, particularly if it is poorly controlled, is the strongest known contributing factor. Genetic makeup may be a factor. For example, parents of large stature (height or weight) have an increased tendency to reproduce LGA newborns. Obesity is a strong contributing factor. Latino women have a higher incidence of LGA newborns. Newborn boys are also typically larger than newborn girls. In addition, multiparous women have two to three times the number of LGA newborns than do primiparous women.

Congenital disorders play a role in LGA newborns. Beckwith–Wiedemann syndrome, a rare genetic disorder, causes hormonally induced excessive weight gain and **macroglossia** (abnormally large tongue), which can cause feeding difficulties. Transposition of the great vessels, a congenital heart disease (see Chapter 21), is associated with LGA newborns. Other factors include umbilical abnormalities such as omphalocele, hypoglycemia, and hyperinsulinemia of the newborn.

Potential Complications

Most commonly, LGA newborns develop complications associated with the large body size. This newborn is more than twice as likely to deliver by cesarean birth as their appropriate for gestational age (AGA) counterpart is. The increased size is a leading cause of breech presentation and shoulder dystocia, which results in an increased incidence of birth injuries and trauma from a difficult extraction. Subsequent problems include fractured skull or clavicles, cervical or brachial plexus injury, and **Erb palsy** (a facial paralysis resulting from injury to the cervical nerves).

Nursing Care

Identifying the newborn at risk for being LGA is important for anticipating the plan of care. Carefully review the maternal history for any risk factors that would contribute to an LGA newborn. Note any prenatal ultrasound reports, such as fetal skull size measurement. Assist the RN with performing a gestational age assessment. Conduct and document routine nursing care with a special emphasis on the following:

- Monitor vital signs frequently, especially respiratory status for changes indicating respiratory distress.
- Observe for signs and symptoms of hypoglycemia, including monitoring results of blood glucose levels.
- Document and report any signs of birth trauma or injury.
- Help family caregivers verbalize feelings about any bruising or trauma they notice, including their fears of causing their newborn more pain.
- Encourage parent–newborn bonding by providing interaction and support, such as showing how to rouse a sleepy newborn, console a fussy newborn, and offer feedings.

> **TEST YOURSELF**
> ✔ What two major areas does a gestational age assessment evaluate?
> ✔ What is the underlying factor commonly associated with most small for gestational age (SGA) newborns?
> ✔ Large for gestational age (LGA) newborns are at an increased risk for what complications associated with their size?

The Preterm Newborn

The preterm (premature) newborn is any infant born at less than 37 weeks gestation. The preterm newborn's needs and care differ with the level of prematurity. Micropreemies are the tiniest newborns, weighing less than 1,000 g. The late preterm newborn is at the more mature end of the spectrum, born between 34 and 37 weeks' gestation. Determining the gestational age of the preterm newborn is crucial (see earlier discussion of gestational age assessment and Fig. 20-1).

The preterm infant's untimely departure from the uterus may mean that various organs and systems are not sufficiently mature to adjust to extrauterine life. Often, small community hospitals or birth centers are not equipped to adequately care for the preterm infant. When preterm delivery is expected, transport of the pregnant woman to a facility with a NICU is ideal. However, if delivery occurs before transport, then transportation of the newborn may be necessary. A team of specially trained personnel may come from the NICU to transport the neonate by ambulance, van, or helicopter. The newborn travels in a self-contained, battery-powered unit that provides warmth and oxygen. Intravenous (IV) fluids, monitors, and other emergency equipment are available during the transport.

Preparation is Vital

Because so many things can go wrong during a preterm birth, make sure that neonatal health care providers know about the impending birth so that equipment for resuscitation and emergency care is ready.

Contributing Factors

The underlying cause of preterm birth, in most cases, is unknown. The discovery and use of tocolytic drugs (medications that relax the uterus) brought hope that the incidence of preterm delivery would decrease. Tocolytic drugs have brought about better outcomes because they delay the delivery long enough for corticosteroids to enhance lung maturity, but they have had a negligible effect on the rate of occurrence of preterm births.

Prior preterm deliveries, maternal age extremes, and poor nutritional status are maternal factors that may contribute to preterm births. Multiple births are often a cause of preterm birth because of **polyhydramnios** (excessive amniotic fluid), a larger than average intrauterine mass, and early cervical dilation. Another common contributing factor is preterm prelabor rupture of membranes. This may occur due to various underlying conditions, particularly infection of the membranes, which is an indication for immediate delivery. The increased number of pregnant women with diabetes is another major contributor. All of the factors that contribute to intrauterine growth restriction (IUGR) also increase the risk of preterm birth (Box 20-1).

Characteristics of the Preterm Newborn

Compared with the term infant, the preterm infant is tiny, scrawny, and red. The extremities are thin with little muscle or subcutaneous fat. The head and abdomen are disproportionately large, and the skin is thin, relatively translucent, and usually wrinkled. Veins of the abdomen and scalp are more visible. Lanugo is plentiful over the extremities, back, and shoulders. The ears have soft, minimal cartilage and thus are extremely pliable. The soft bones of the skull tend to flatten on the sides, and the ribs yield with each labored breath. Testes are undescended in the male; the labia and clitoris are prominent in the female. The soles of the feet and the palms of the hands have few creases. Many of the typical newborn reflexes are weak or absent. Figure 20-2 shows several typical physical characteristics of the preterm newborn.

The preterm newborn's physiologic immaturity causes many difficulties involving virtually all body systems, the most critical of which is the respiratory system. Typically, respirations are shallow, rapid, and irregular with periods of **apnea**, absence of breathing that lasts for at least 20 seconds or that causes cyanosis or bradycardia. Retractions of the chest wall and sternum indicate labored respirations.

Thermoregulation and maintaining fluid and electrolyte balance are major problems for the preterm newborn because they lose heat and fluids more quickly and have fewer compensatory mechanisms than does the term newborn. Rapid heat and water loss occur because the preterm newborn does not have the insulation provided by subcutaneous and brown fat that is available to the term newborn, water and heat can escape through the thin skin, and this newborn has an increased surface area to body mass ratio. The preterm newborn cannot shiver to produce heat and cannot assume a flexed posture to conserve heat and water. Immaturity of the central nervous system (CNS) and the lack of integrated reflex control of peripheral blood vessels (to cause vasodilation or vasoconstriction) also affect the preterm newborn's ability to maintain body temperature.

The preterm newborn has high caloric needs but has a digestive system that may be unprepared to receive and digest food. The stomach is small, with a capacity that may be less than 1 to 2 oz. The sphincters at either end of the stomach are immature, causing regurgitation or vomiting if feedings distend the stomach. The immature liver cannot manage all the bilirubin produced by hemolysis (destruction of RBCs with the release of hemoglobin), making the infant prone to jaundice and high blood bilirubin levels (hyperbilirubinemia) that may result in brain damage.

The preterm infant does not receive enough antibodies from the mother and cannot produce them. This characteristic makes the infant particularly vulnerable to infection.

Muscle weakness in the premature infant contributes to nutritional and respiratory problems and to a posture distinct from that of the term infant (Fig. 20-3). The infant may not be able to change positions and is prone to fatigue and exhaustion, even from eating and breathing. Skilled, gentle intensive care is needed for the newborn to survive and develop. The family caregivers also need supportive, intensive care.

Treatment of Complications

The preterm newborn is at risk for a variety of complications. The most vulnerable body systems are respiratory, gastrointestinal, and central nervous systems. The most frequent complications include hypothermia, hypoglycemia, patent ductus arteriosus, jaundice, infection, respiratory distress syndrome (RDS), intraventricular hemorrhage (IVH), retinopathy of prematurity (ROP),

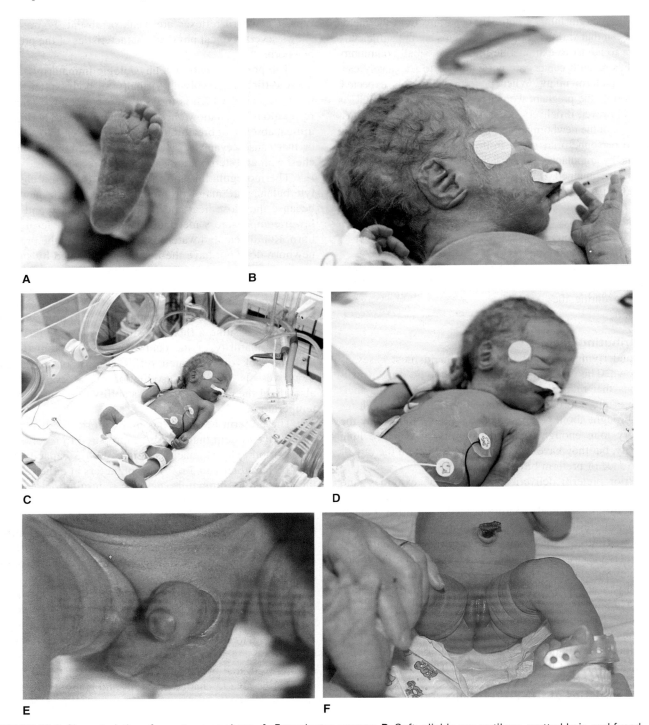

FIGURE 20-2 Characteristics of a preterm newborn. **A.** Few plantar creases. **B.** Soft, pliable ear cartilage, matted hair, and fused eyelids. **C.** Lax posture with poor muscle development. **D.** Breast and nipple area barely noticeable. **E.** Male genitalia. Note the minimal rugae on the scrotum. **F.** Female genitalia. Note the prominent labia and clitoris.

and necrotizing enterocolitis (NEC). Treatment of the preterm newborn and their complications is individualized because each newborn responds to the challenge of preterm transition to extrauterine life in their unique way. This section discusses treatment and special considerations of some of the more common conditions associated with prematurity.

Respiratory Distress Syndrome

Respiratory distress syndrome (RDS), also known as hyaline membrane disease, is a common problem in the preterm newborn. The lower the gestational age, the higher the risk of RDS. The risk is highest in neonates below 28 weeks' gestation, though RDS still occurs in neonates born after 28 weeks' gestation (Martin, 2021).

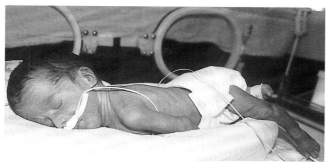

FIGURE 20-3 Typical resting posture of preterm newborn. Note the lax position and immature muscular development.

RDS occurs in the preterm newborn because the lungs are too immature. Normally, the lungs remain partially expanded after each breath because of surfactant, a biochemical compound that reduces surface tension inside the air sacs. The premature infant's lungs are deficient in surfactant and thus collapse after each breath, greatly increasing the work of breathing. The complex interplay of disease process and treatments (in particular oxygen therapy) causes damage to the lung cells. These damaged cells combine with other substances present in the lungs to form a hyaline membrane. This fibrous membrane lines the alveoli and blocks gas exchange.

The preterm newborn with respiratory distress syndrome (RDS) may exhibit problems breathing immediately or a few hours after birth. Typically, respirations increase to greater than 60 breaths per minute. Nasal flaring and retractions may be noted. Mucous membranes may appear cyanotic. As respiratory distress progresses, the newborn exhibits seesawlike respirations in which the chest wall retracts, the abdomen protrudes on inspiration, and then the sternum rises on expiration. Breathing is labored, the respiratory rate continues to increase, and expiratory grunting occurs. Breath sounds usually diminish, and the newborn may develop periods of apnea.

Surfactant replacement therapy is a treatment that has dramatically increased survival rates. Other therapy advances include the use of antenatal steroids, appropriate resuscitation techniques, immediate use of nasal continuous positive airway pressure (nCPAP), and gentle (vs. aggressive) ventilation procedures (Martin, 2021).

Treatment begins shortly after birth with synthetic or naturally occurring surfactant, obtained from animal sources or extracted from human amniotic fluid. The newborn receives surfactant as an inhalant through a catheter inserted into an endotracheal tube. The therapy may be preventive (rescue) treatment to avoid the development of RDS in the newborn at risk.

Did You Know?

Too much oxygen is toxic to tiny lungs and eyes. Research demonstrates that newborns with respiratory distress syndrome (RDS) have decreased incidence of chronic lung and eye conditions when oxygen saturation levels remain between 90% and 95% versus the 96% to 98% levels targeted in times past.

Newborns with RDS usually receive additional oxygen through nCPAP, using intubation or a plastic hood. This helps the lungs remain partially expanded until they begin producing surfactant, usually within the first 5 days of life. The preterm newborn that develops RDS requires supportive care to promote adequate oxygenation and prevent complications.

Intraventricular Hemorrhage

Intraventricular hemorrhage (IVH), bleeding into the brain's ventricles, is a complication of preterm birth that occurs more often in the newborn of less than 32 weeks' gestation. In addition to early gestational age, other factors commonly associated with IVH include birth asphyxia, low birth weight (LBW), respiratory distress, and hypotension. Ultrasonography, computed tomography, and magnetic resonance imaging screen for and provide the basis to diagnose the condition.

Two factors place the extremely premature infant at risk for IVH. First, the developing brain has a fragile capillary network that ruptures easily with cerebral pressure changes. Second, the preterm newborn may be unable to autoregulate cerebral pressure, which leaves the newborn with little protection from pressure fluctuations. In addition, too much stimulation and abrupt movements during care increase the risk.

Many infants who develop IVH are without symptoms or have subtle symptoms, such as a sudden drop in hematocrit levels, pallor, and poor perfusion. Therefore, the primary health care provider orders screening examinations to identify bleeding. Signs that may accompany IVH include hypotonia, apnea, bradycardia, a full (or bulging) fontanelle, cyanosis, and increased head circumference. Neurologic signs such as twitching, convulsions, and stupor may be noted.

Supportive care is the foundation for medical intervention. The focus is on preventing, diagnosing, and correcting acid–base imbalances, fluid and electrolyte imbalances, respiratory compromise, and cardiovascular disturbances. Nursing intervention focuses on prevention (see the nursing process and care plan section that follows for further discussion of preventative interventions).

Retinopathy of Prematurity

Retinopathy of prematurity (ROP) is a form of retinopathy (degenerative disease of the retina) commonly associated with the preterm newborn, particularly infants born at less than 28 weeks' gestation. Immature retinal blood vessels grow abnormally, often resulting in retinal scarring or detachment. These events lead to varying degrees of blindness. Wide fluctuations in oxygen levels and oxygen saturation limits maintained above 94% are major causes.

Prevention is the best treatment. The nursing process and care plan section that

A Simple Calculation

To calculate the corrected age, add the weeks since birth to the gestational age at birth. For example, if the birth occurred at 26 weeks' gestation, then the newborn would be 31 weeks corrected age at the chronologic age of 5 weeks.

follows discusses prevention strategies. It is not always possible to prevent retinopathy of prematurity (ROP), so treatment begins with early identification. An ophthalmologist with special training performs a screening examination at 31 weeks' corrected age to detect the changes associated with developing ROP. Laser surgery is the current treatment of choice. This therapy has proved more effective and less damaging to surrounding eye tissues than cryosurgery.

Necrotizing Enterocolitis

Necrotizing enterocolitis (NEC) is an acute inflammatory necrotic disease of the intestine. This devastating condition has a mortality rate of 23%, and surviving newborns often face lifelong health challenges and disability (Kim, 2021). The incidence is highest in small preterm newborns. The cause is unknown; however, the key risk factor is prematurity. Precipitating factors include formula feeding, bowel ischemia, and bacterial invasion of the intestine.

Initial clinical manifestations may be subtle and are not specific to NEC. The newborn feeds poorly and may experience lethargy, temperature instability, and vomiting of bile. Other findings include abdominal distention and occult blood in the stool. Abdominal x-rays confirm the diagnosis. Abdominal ultrasound is a useful diagnostic tool.

Initially, oral feedings are discontinued and nasogastric suction is applied to rest the bowel. IV fluids, including total parenteral nutrition, and antibiotics are given. Bowel perforation or necrosis necessitates surgical intervention to repair, bypass, or remove parts of the intestine.

Because NEC can lead to devastating outcomes, preventing preterm birth is a major goal to reduce the incidence of NEC. The use of probiotics continues to be researched as a preventive measure, but currently is not routinely recommended (Kim, 2021).

> **Nurses Definitely Make a Difference**
>
> Your observation skills are critical to detecting early and subtle changes associated with necrotizing enterocolitis (NEC). The sooner the newborn receives treatment for NEC, the better the outcomes.

> **TEST YOURSELF**
>
> ✔ Describe three characteristics of a preterm newborn.
>
> ✔ Which complication associated with preterm newborns is due to a surfactant deficiency?
>
> ✔ What factors increase the risk for retinopathy of prematurity (ROP)?

Nursing Process and Care Plan *for the Preterm Newborn*

The complex needs of a preterm newborn require skilled nursing care. Priorities of care include maintenance of adequate oxygenation, continuous electronic cardiac and respiratory monitoring, frequent manual monitoring of vital signs, thermoregulation, infection control, hydration, provision of adequate nutrition and developmental care for the newborn, and emotional support for the family caregivers.

Assessment (Data Collection)

Assessment of the preterm newborn is similar to that for any newborn, but the initial assessment focuses on the status of the respiratory, circulatory, and neurologic systems to determine the immediate needs of the infant. Although monitoring equipment provides a continual reading of the heart rate, take apical pulses periodically, listening to the heart through the chest using a stethoscope for one full minute so as not to miss an irregularity in rhythm. Note the pulse rate, rhythm, and strength. The pulse rate is normally rapid (110 to 160 beats per minute [bpm]) and unstable. Premature newborns are subject to dangerous periods of bradycardia (as low as 60 to 80 bpm) and tachycardia (as high as 180 to 200 bpm). Your observations of the pulse rate, rhythm, and strength are essential to determining how the infant is tolerating treatments, activity, feedings, and the temperature and oxygen concentration of the environment.

> **Don't Check Out**
>
> Although sophisticated monitoring equipment is available in the modern NICU, do not rely on monitors in place of careful assessment and data collection. Observe the equipment, make sure it is functioning properly, and systematically collect data about the infant.

Nursing Care Focus

Nursing care focuses that may be appropriate for the preterm newborn include respiratory issues and temperature regulation, which may be affected because of the immature development of the premature newborn. The risk for infection or injury should be considered. Dehydration, the risk for electrolyte imbalances, and malnutrition are concerns in caring for the preterm newborn. Because of prematurity and some treatments, care to maintain skin integrity is important. The weakened condition of the preterm newborn may cause the newborn to have a decreased ability to tolerate activity; thus, the potential for alterations in normal growth and development may occur. Having a seriously ill newborn with an unpredictable prognosis can create anxiety as well as psychosocial needs for the family and the family caregivers.

Outcome Identification and Planning

The major goals for the preterm newborn include improving respiratory function, maintaining body temperature, preventing infection, protecting neurologic status, maintaining fluid and electrolyte balance, maintaining adequate nutrition, preserving skin integrity, conserving energy, and supporting growth and development. Goals for the family include reducing anxiety and improving parenting skills and family functioning.

Nursing Care Focus

- Altered breathing pattern related to immature respiratory system

Goal

- The preterm newborn's respiratory function will improve.

Implementations for Improving Respiratory Function

Not all preterm newborns need extra oxygen, but many do. Isolettes have oxygen inlets and humidifiers for raising the oxygen concentration inside from 20% to 21% (room air) to a higher percentage. An oxyhood, a clear plastic hood placed over the infant's head, is another way to supply humidified oxygen for infants with mild respiratory distress. For newborns who require a little more help, continuous positive airway pressure (CPAP) is the preferred modality. This therapy does not allow the alveoli to collapse at the end of respiration, which greatly reduces the work of breathing and improves oxygenation. There are several ways to administer CPAP including nasal prongs, face masks, and nasopharyngeal or endotracheal tubes. The preterm newborn with severe respiratory distress syndrome (RDS) will likely need mechanical ventilation.

Pulse oximetry continuously monitors blood oxygen saturation. The RN programs the pulse oximeter to alarm when oxygen saturation levels fall below 85% or rise higher than 94%. If the alarm rings, respond immediately, and adjust the oxygen concentration as ordered to maintain the oxygen saturation within the prescribed limits. Clarify with the family caregivers and all staff (e.g., unit secretaries, housekeepers) to report alarms immediately so that action can be taken to limit the occurrence of retinopathy of prematurity (ROP) and intraventricular hemorrhage (IVH).

Observe the preterm newborn's respirations carefully. Observe for changes in respiratory effort, rate, depth, breath sounds, and regularity of respirations. Note any expiratory grunting or chest retractions (substernal, suprasternal, intercostal, subcostal), including severity, and nasal flaring to determine the newborn's ability to maintain respirations. Assist the RN in ensuring that oxygen support or ventilator settings and endotracheal tube placement, if present, are as prescribed to ensure adequacy of ventilation and respiratory assistance.

Reposition the newborn every 2 hours to reduce the risk for pneumonia and atelectasis. Frequent suctioning may be necessary to prevent airway obstruction, hypoxia, and asphyxiation. If not contraindicated, elevate the head of the bed as needed to maintain a patent airway. Organize care and promote rest times between procedures to conserve the newborn's energy and reduce oxygen consumption.

One of the more hazardous characteristics of the preterm newborn is the tendency to stop breathing periodically (apnea). The hypoxia caused by apnea and general respiratory difficulty may lead to long-term neurologic disability, such as cerebral palsy or intellectual disability. Monitors with apnea alarms alert the caregiver when an episode of apnea occurs. Electrodes positioned on the infant's chest with leads to the apnea monitor provide a continuous reading of the respiratory rate. Visual and audio alarms go off when the rate goes too high or too low or if the infant waits too long to take a breath.

Don't Succumb to Temptation

You may want to lower the sound when false alarms occur frequently. This highly unsafe practice can lead to tragedy if you miss a newborn's distress because the alarms are off. Instead, troubleshoot and fix the problem causing the false alarms.

Place, check, and replace the apnea monitor leads on the newborn. Each day, remove electrodes and reapply them in a slightly different location to protect the infant's sensitive skin from damage by the electrode paste and adhesive. Cleanse the skin carefully between applications of the electrodes. When an episode of apnea occurs, first try gentle tactile stimulation, such as wiggling a foot. Sometimes this is enough to remind the newborn to breathe. If not, the newborn may require respiratory assistance with a bag and mask.

Evaluation of Goal/Desired Outcome

The newborn:

- maintains a respiratory rate less than 60 breaths per minute with symmetric chest expansion.
- does not grunt or retract with breathing.
- has clear breath sounds.
- maintains oxygen saturation levels between 85% and 94%.
- remains free of episodes of apnea.

Nursing Care Focus

- Altered temperature regulation related to immaturity and transition to extrauterine life

Goal

- The preterm newborn's temperature will remain stable.

Implementations for Maintaining Body Temperature

Monitor the preterm newborn's body temperature closely. Observe for signs of cold stress such as low temperature, body cold to touch, pallor, and lethargy.

Protect the newborn from heat loss. If the newborn becomes wet, be sure to dry them quickly and remove wet linen to avoid heat loss via evaporation. Avoid positioning the preterm newborn on cold surfaces or placing cold objects (e.g., a cold stethoscope) on the newborn. Protect the infant from drafts. Be sure to expose as little of the newborn's skin as possible during procedures to minimize heat loss. Conversely, the preterm newborn must not be overheated because this causes increased consumption of oxygen and calories, possibly jeopardizing the newborn's status.

An isolette or a radiant warmer prevents heat loss and helps control other aspects of the premature infant's environment (Fig. 20-4). A heat-sensing probe attached to the newborn's skin controls the temperature of the isolette or the radiant warmer. The isolette has a clear Plexiglas top that allows a full view of the newborn from all aspects. The isolette maintains ideal temperature, humidity, and oxygen concentrations and isolates the infant from infection. Portholes at the side allow access to the newborn with minimal temperature and oxygen loss. Open units with overhead radiant warmers allow maximum access to the infant when sophisticated equipment or frequent manipulation for treatment and assessment is necessary.

Evaluation of Goal/Desired Outcome

- The newborn maintains temperature between 97.7°F and 99.5°F (36.5°C and 37.5°C).

Nursing Care Focus

- Infection risk related to an immature immune system and environmental factors

Goal

- The preterm newborn remains free of infection.

Implementations for Preventing Infection

Infection control is an urgent concern in the care of the preterm newborn. The preterm infant cannot resist bacterial invasions, so caregivers must provide an atmosphere that protects the infant from such attacks. The primary means of preventing infection is handwashing. All persons must practice good handwashing immediately before touching the newborn and when moving from one newborn to another.

Other important aspects of infection control include regular cleaning or changing of humidifier water; IV tubing; and suction, respiratory, and monitoring equipment. The NICU is separate from the normal newborn nursery and usually has its own staff. This separation helps eliminate sources of infection. Personnel in this area usually wear hospital-provided scrub uniforms, and personnel from other departments (radiology, respiratory therapy, or laboratory) put a cover gown over their uniforms while working with these newborns.

Signs of infection are nonspecific and subtle. Report signs and symptoms of infection including the following:

- Temperature instability (decrease or increase)
- Glucose instability and metabolic acidosis
- Poor sucking
- Vomiting
- Diarrhea
- Abdominal distention
- Apnea
- Respiratory distress and cyanosis
- Hepatosplenomegaly
- Jaundice
- Skin mottling
- Lethargy

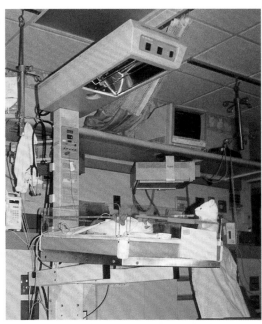
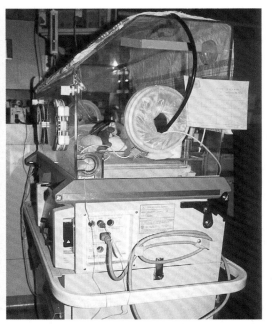

A   B

FIGURE 20-4 Maintenance of thermoregulation. **A.** Newborn under a radiant warmer. **B.** Newborn in an isolette.

- Hypotonia
- Seizures

Close observation allows for successful intervention if infection occurs. Laboratory tests used to diagnose and treat infections include blood cultures, cerebral spinal fluid analysis, urinalysis and urine cultures, tracheal aspirate culture, and skin cultures. Obtain diagnostic laboratory work as ordered, and report results that indicate the source and treatment of infection. Expect antibiotics to be ordered to treat suspected or confirmed bacterial infections.

Evaluation of Goal/Desired Outcome

The newborn:

- maintains vital signs within normal limits.
- has no signs or symptoms of infection.

Nursing Care Focus

- Injury risk related to cerebral bleeding secondary to premature status

Goal

- The preterm newborn's neurologic status remains stable.

Implementations for Protecting Neurologic Status

Because the preterm newborn is at risk for intraventricular hemorrhage (IVH), protecting neurologic status is critical. Neuroprotection involves avoiding activities that could cause wide fluctuations of cerebral blood pressures. Assist the RN to assess fluid volume status and prevent fluid overload. Ensure that the head and body remain in alignment when moving and turning the newborn (i.e., avoid twisting the head at the neck). Minimal stimulation is a necessary precaution to minimize pain and stress. Reduce procedures that cause crying, such as routine suctioning. Avoid painful procedures and disturbances when possible. Use narcotics, as ordered, to treat pain when avoidance is not possible. Control noise level in the environment.

Little Things Make a Big Difference

Because excessive noise can overstimulate and increase the risk for intraventricular hemorrhage (IVH), speak gently and softly around the preterm newborn. Do not tap on the sides of the isolette, and avoid frequent opening and closing of portholes.

Evaluation of Goal/Desired Outcome

- The newborn has a normal and stable neurologic status.

Nursing Care Focus

- Dehydration and electrolyte imbalance risk related to insensible water loss secondary to premature skin that favors evaporation, and therapies, such as overhead warmers and phototherapy, that also promote fluid loss

Goal

- The preterm newborn's fluid and electrolyte balance will be maintained.

Implementations for Maintaining Fluid and Electrolyte Balance

Maintaining fluid and electrolyte balance is a major challenge for the preterm newborn. In many instances, an IV "life line" is necessary immediately after delivery. Fluids infuse through a catheter placed in the umbilical vein in the stump of the umbilical cord. IV fluids may infuse through other veins, particularly the peripheral veins of the hands, feet, or scalp. Extremely small amounts of fluid are needed, perhaps as little as 5 to 10 mL/hr or even less. An infusion pump is critical to measure accurately and administer fluids at a steady rate. Keep accurate, complete records of IV fluids and frequently observe for signs of infiltration or overhydration.

Monitor laboratory values, as ordered. Serum electrolytes, blood urea nitrogen, creatinine, and plasma osmolarity levels are the most common tests. Report abnormal values. Ensure that the appropriate IV fluids are infusing and that the proper amounts of supplemental sodium, potassium, chloride, and other additives are included, as ordered.

Observe and record the number of voidings and the color of the urine, and note any edema. Keep strict intake and output records. Measure and record all urinary output by weighing the diapers before and after they are used. Urinary output should be at least 0.5 to 1.0 mL/kg/hr.

This is How It's Done

One gram equals approximately 1 mL. Weigh the wet diaper, and then subtract the weight of the dry diaper. The difference in grams is the output in mL.

Evaluation of Goal/Desired Outcome

The newborn's:

- intake is sufficient to produce a urine output of at least 0.5 to 1.0 mL/kg/hr.
- lab values are within normal range.

Nursing Care Focus

- Malnutrition risk related to ineffective infant feeding pattern related to inability to suck

Goal

- The preterm newborn's nutritional status will remain adequate.

Implementations for Maintaining Adequate Nutrition

At birth, a preterm newborn may be too weak or sick to suck. Commonly, the preterm newborn has difficulty coordinating sucking, swallowing, and breathing so that they can breast- or bottle-feed. Other problems that may inhibit oral feedings include limited stomach capacity, contributing to distention and inadequate intake; poor muscle tone of the cardiac sphincter, leading to regurgitation with secondary apnea and bradycardia; and muscle weakness, which leads to exhaustion. Premature newborns are likely to have problems with aspiration because the gag reflex does not develop until about the 32nd to 34th week of gestation, which predisposes them to distention and regurgitation. As a result, alternative feeding methods may be needed.

At first, some preterm newborns receive all their fluid, electrolyte, vitamin, and calorie needs by the IV route (usually with total parenteral nutrition); others can start with a nipple and bottle. However, many require gavage feeding (feeding by a tube passed from the nose or mouth to the stomach; see Fig. 30-6 in Chapter 30). It is important for the preterm newborn to receive enteral feedings as soon as possible after birth. Enteral feedings keep the gastrointestinal system functioning and healthy. Lack of food in the gut leads to atrophy of the mucosa. It then becomes more difficult to initiate feedings.

There are other feeding methods available if the preterm newborn cannot tolerate either gavage or nipple-feeding and if IV fluids are inadequate. Some preterm newborns do better if fed with a rubber-tipped medicine dropper. Others may require gastrostomy feedings (feeding by a tube passed through the abdominal wall into the stomach; see Fig. 30-7 in Chapter 30). Whatever the alternate method used, the preterm newborn who is not receiving nipple-feedings should receive nonnutritive sucking opportunities, such as with a pacifier.

It is important to monitor the nutritional health of the preterm newborn. Perform daily weights. Weight gain or loss patterns give an indication of overall health and indicate whether the newborn is consuming enough calories. Weigh the newborn with the same clothing, using the same scale, and at the same time each day to help ensure accurate, comparable data. Other indicators of nutritional health include skin condition, hair growth, and achievement of adequate growth patterns and developmental milestones.

Sources of Nutrition

Breast milk, the preferred source of nutrition for the preterm newborn, offers many benefits. Breast milk stimulates the newborn's immune system and provides immunoglobulins from the woman. Human milk protects from necrotizing enterocolitis (NEC), infections, cancers, metabolic disorders, and certain childhood disorders. Mothers can pump their breast milk and freeze it to use for bottle or gavage feedings until the preterm newborn is strong enough to breastfeed. Providing food which only she can supply to nourish her newborn provides a tremendous boost to the emotional satisfaction of the mother.

If the woman chooses not to breastfeed, human donor breast milk is a satisfactory substitute. A centralized milk bank collects pumped breast milk for distribution to NICU newborns, as needed. Before accepting and storing the donated milk, the milk bank screens the lactating donor for communicable diseases and other conditions that could adversely affect milk composition.

If the newborn is to receive formula, then a preterm formula with 20 cal/oz is the typical type chosen. Preterm formula has a different nutrient mix than formula for term newborns. This is because the preterm newborn has specialized nutritional needs. For example, if the formula is too rich (too high in carbohydrates and fats), vomiting and diarrhea may occur. Some preterm newborns require higher-density caloric formula. These formulas provide 22 or 24 cal/oz.

Gavage Feeding

When the preterm newborn is not able to receive oral feedings, gavage feedings through an orogastric or nasogastric tube may be necessary (see Chapter 30). The frequency and quantity of gavage feedings are individualized. Usually, feeding frequency is every 2 hours to allow for small amounts at frequent intervals. Preterm infants have a difficult time tolerating large amounts at one time due to limited stomach capacity, and if the feeding takes too long, the infant may tire. Figure 20-5 shows a nurse assisting a mother to gavage feed her newborn.

Check prefeed gastric residuals (aspiration of gastric contents before a feeding). If the stomach is not empty by the next feeding, allow more time between feedings or give smaller feedings. The newborn's tolerance level dictates the quantity. Increase the amount of formula or breast milk slowly (milliliter by milliliter) as quickly as tolerated. The feeding is too large if the newborn's stomach distends so that it causes respiratory difficulty, vomiting, or regurgitation and if there is formula left in the stomach by the next feeding. See Chapter 30 for more information on gavage feeding.

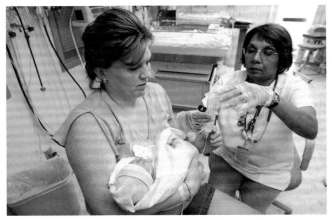

Pay Attention

Immediately report gradually increasing residuals and abdominal girth, or return of more than 2 mL of undigested formula. These signs indicate feeding intolerance and could herald the onset of necrotizing enterocolitis (NEC).

FIGURE 20-5 The nurse helps the family caregiver administer a gavage feeding to her premature infant.

Nipple (Bottle) Feeding

When a preterm newborn who is being gavage fed begins to suck vigorously on the fingers, hands, pacifier, or gavage tubing and demonstrates evidence of a gag reflex, it is time to introduce bottle feeding, and in some cases, breast-feeding. The infant who can take the same quantity of formula or breast milk by bottle that they took by gavage feeding without becoming too tired is ready for oral feeding. Alternating gavage and nipple-feedings may be necessary in some cases to assist the preterm newborn in making the transition. Special nipples and smaller bottles prevent too much liquid from flowing into the newborn's mouth. The nipple for a preterm newborn is usually made of softer rubber than is a regular nipple. It is also smaller, but no shorter, than the regular nipple.

To nipple-feed, hold the newborn in your arms or on your lap at a 45-degree angle. Be careful to prevent aspiration throughout the feeding. Make sure that oxygen is available, as needed. Burp the preterm newborn often, during and after feedings. Sometimes simply changing the infant's position is enough assistance; at other times, it may help to gently rub or pat the infant's back.

Evaluation of Goal/Desired Outcome

The infant:

- ingests increased amounts of oral nutrition.
- gains weight daily.

Nursing Care Focus

- Altered skin integrity risk related to prematurity and exposure to phototherapy light

Goal

- The preterm newborn will remain free of skin breakdown.

Implementations for Preserving Skin Integrity

Frequently collect data related to skin integrity (at least every shift) for changes in color, turgor, texture, vascularity, and signs of irritation or infection. Pay special attention to areas in which equipment is attached or inserted. Frequent skin monitoring allows for early detection and prompt intervention.

A preterm newborn's skin is extremely fragile and injures easily, so handle the infant gently. Reposition the preterm newborn every 2 to 4 hours and as needed. Preterm infants have a knack for wriggling into corners and cracks from which they cannot extract themselves, so close observation is necessary.

Keep the skin clean and dry, but avoid excessive bathing, which further dries the skin. Use water only or mild soaps when bathing twice weekly. Change the diaper as soon as possible after soiling to help prevent breakdown in the perineal area. Pad pressure-prone areas by using sheepskin blankets, waterbeds, pillows, or egg crate mattresses to help prevent additional skin breakdown to these areas. Monitor intake and output and avoid dehydration and overhydration. Box 20-2 outlines interventions to prevent preterm skin breakdown.

BOX 20-2 Interventions to Protect Preterm Skin

- Keep the infant's skin clean with water.
- Modify typical newborn bathing.
  - Schedule twice weekly.
  - Between baths, clean visibly soiled areas, face, and perineum as needed with water.
  - Use water only for infants less than 32 weeks' gestation.
  - For infants greater than 32 weeks' gestation, mild nonalkaline soap may be used at bath time only.
- Avoid alcohol on the skin.
- Avoid creams and ointments unless specifically ordered.
- Use water or mineral oil to help remove adhesives. Avoid adhesive remover.
- Use iodine or benzoin with caution because the newborn's skin readily absorbs these products.
- Use transparent dressings such as Tegaderm or OpSite to protect IV sites and over bony prominences as needed to prevent breakdown.

Evaluation of Goal/Desired Outcome

- The newborn maintains adequate skin turgor.
- The newborn's skin remains intact and free of redness, rashes, and irritation.

Nursing Care Focus

- Activity intolerance related to poor oxygenation and weakness

Goal

- The preterm newborn will show improved tolerance to activity.

Implementations for Promoting Energy Conservation

The preterm newborn uses most of their energy to breathe and maintain vital functions. Plan ahead and cluster care activities to avoid exhaustion from constant handling and movement. Energy conservation does not include ignoring or avoiding the newborn or discouraging the contact essential to establishing a normal relationship. Gentle touch and newborn massage are therapeutic.

Evaluation of Goal/Desired Outcome

The newborn:

- has stable vital signs.
- requires supplemental oxygen in decreasing amounts until oxygen is no longer necessary.

Nursing Care Focus

- Growth and development concerns related to prematurity and excess environmental stimuli

Goal

- The preterm newborn will demonstrate appropriate development.

Implementations for Supporting Growth and Development

All NICU newborns need developmental care, including preterm newborns. Interventions include decreasing environmental noise and stress, maintaining flexed positioning, and clustering care to conserve energy. Providing opportunities for nonnutritive sucking helps develop feeding skills. Skin-to-skin (kangaroo) care assists with keeping the newborn warm and promotes parental bonding.

As the preterm infant grows, they increasingly need sensory stimulation. Mobiles hung over the isolette and toys placed in or on the infant unit may provide visual stimulation. A radio with the volume turned low, a music box, or a wind-up toy in the isolette may provide auditory stimulation. An excellent form of auditory stimulation comes from the voices of the infant's family, health care providers, and nurses talking and singing. Being bathed, held, cuddled, and fondled provides needed tactile stimulation. Contact is essential to the infant and the family. Some NICUs have "foster grandparents" who regularly visit long-term NICU infants and provide them with sensory stimulation, cuddling, loving, and talking. These programs have proven beneficial to both the infants and the volunteer grandparents.

Evaluation of Goal/Desired Outcome

The newborn:

- responds appropriately to stimuli.
- achieves developmental milestones.
- increasingly interacts with the environment and caregivers.

Nursing Care Focus

- Acute family caregiver anxiety related to a seriously ill newborn with an unpredictable prognosis

Goal

- The family caregivers will demonstrate a reduction in anxiety level.

Implementations for Reducing Family Caregiver Anxiety

Birth of a preterm newborn creates a crisis for the family caregivers. Often their long-awaited baby is whisked away from them, sometimes to a distant neonatal center, and hooked up to a maze of machines. They cannot share the early, sensitive attachment period. It may take weeks to establish touch and eye contact, ordinarily achieved in 10 minutes with a term infant. Sometimes the woman's condition inhibits early contact with the preterm newborn. If the birth was by cesarean, or if the labor was difficult or prolonged, she may not have the strength to go to the NICU and to become involved with the infant. The parents of a preterm newborn often leave the hospital empty-handed, without the perfect, healthy infant of their dreams. How can they learn to know and love the strange, scrawny creature that now lives in that plastic box?

Parents may feel anxiety, guilt, fear, depression, and perhaps anger. These feelings are normal. Accept and encourage the parent(s) to express their feelings. If the parents ignore these feelings, long-term damage to the parent–child relationship can result. Unfortunately, unresolved negative feelings can even lead to child neglect or abuse.

Nurses who work with high-risk infants can do much to help families cope with the crisis of prematurity and early separation. To ease some of the apprehension of the family caregivers, transport teams prepare the newborn for transportation, then take the newborn in the transport incubator into the mother's room so that the parents may see (and touch, if possible) the newborn before the child is whisked away. In many cases, instant photos provide the family some concrete reminder of the newborn until they can visit in person.

 A Personal Glimpse

My son was born 8.5 weeks before his expected due date. I was unable to hold him until 12 hours after his birth. I was discharged from the hospital with a Polaroid snapshot of him and the phone number of the hospital's NICU.

For 2 weeks I visited him, learning new medical terms and gaining an understanding of all the obstacles he would have to overcome before being released. These days were an emotional roller coaster filled with feelings of joy over being blessed with a son, enormous concern over his condition, and a great deal of guilt. The thing I wanted most in the world was to take him home, healthy and without the IVs, equipment, monitors, and the hard hospital chairs. When I left him each day, I was leaving a part of myself, and I felt as though I would not be whole until he was home with me.

Looking back, I really appreciated that the staff was optimistic when informing me of things, but not overly so. Unmet expectations can be devastating! There is not a moment that I am not thankful for my son and his health and not a night that I don't sleep better after I have checked on him sleeping in bed.

Kerry

Learning Opportunity: *Give specific examples of what the nurse could do to support this mother and help decrease her fears and anxieties.*

Explain what is happening to the newborn in the NICU, and periodically report on their condition (by phone if the NICU is not in the same hospital) to reassure the family that the child is receiving excellent care and to keep them informed. Listen to the family, and encourage them to express their feelings and support one another. As soon as possible, the family should see, touch, and help care for the newborn. Most NICUs do not restrict visiting hours for family caregivers or support persons, and they encourage families to visit as often as possible. Many hospitals offer 24-hour phone privileges to families so that they are never out of touch with their newborn's caregivers.

Evaluation of Goal/Desired Outcome

Family caregivers:

- express feelings and anxieties concerning the newborn's condition.
- visit and establish a relationship with the newborn.
- demonstrate interaction with the newborn, holding and helping to provide care.

Nursing Care Focus

- Psychosocial needs related to family caregiver separation from the newborn, difficulty accepting loss of ideal newborn, and effect of prolonged hospitalization on the family

Goal

- The parents will demonstrate appropriate parenting skills, and the family will adapt to the crisis and function at an appropriate level.

Implementations for Improving Parenting Skills and Family Functioning

Ideally, before the woman goes home from the hospital, she is able to visit the preterm newborn and begin participating in the infant's care. The family caregivers need to feel that the newborn belongs to them, not to the hospital. To help foster this feeling and strengthen the attachment, encourage activities that help them take on the parenting role. Pumping her milk to feed the newborn is an excellent way to promote assumption of the maternal role. Encouraging the partner to provide skin-to-skin (kangaroo) care is one way to help them feel close and attached to the newborn.

Siblings should be included in the visits to see the preterm newborn (Fig. 20-6). The monitors, warmers, ventilators, and other equipment may be frightening to siblings

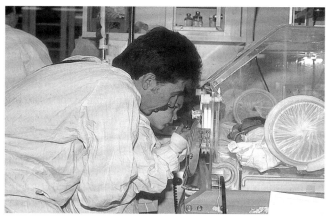

FIGURE 20-6 Encouraging sibling interaction with the preterm newborn.

and family caregivers. Help the family feel welcome and comfortable when they visit. A primary nurse assigned to care for the infant gives the family a constant person to contact, increasing their feelings of confidence in the care the newborn is receiving.

Support groups for families who have experienced the crisis of a preterm newborn are of great value. Members of these support groups can visit the families in the hospital and at home, helping the parents and other family members deal with their feelings and solve the problems that may arise when the infant is ready to come home or if the infant does not survive.

As the time for discharge of the infant nears, the family is understandably apprehensive. The NICU nurses must reinforce teaching with the parents and support persons the skills they need to care for the infant. This knowledge gives them confidence that they can take care of the infant. Some hospitals allow caregivers to stay overnight before the infant's discharge so that they can participate in around-the-clock care. The knowledge that they can telephone the health care provider and nurse at any time after discharge to have questions answered is reassuring.

In addition to feeding, bathing, and general care of the infant, many families of premature newborns need to learn infant cardiopulmonary resuscitation and the use of an apnea monitor before the infant is discharged. Some preterm infants go home with oxygen, gastrostomy feeding tubes, and many other kinds of sophisticated equipment. This helps place the infant in the home much earlier, but it requires intensive training and support of the family members who care for the infant. Support from a home health nurse may be required in this situation.

After the infant goes home, a nurse, usually a community health nurse, visits the family to check on the health of the mother and the infant. The nurse provides additional support, reinforces teaching about the infant's care, and answers any questions the family might have.

Evaluation of Goal/Desired Outcome

Family caregivers:

- learn how to care for the newborn in the hospital and at home.
- hold, cuddle, talk to, and feed the preterm newborn.
- demonstrate knowledge of appropriate infant care.
- have an adequate support system and use it.
- contact a support group for families of high-risk infants.

The Postterm Newborn

When pregnancy lasts longer than 42 weeks' gestation, the infant is postterm (postmature) regardless of birth weight.

Contributing Factors

The causes of delayed birth are unknown. However, some predisposing factors include first pregnancies between the ages of 15 and 19 years, the woman being older than 35 years with multiple pregnancies, prior postterm pregnancy, maternal obesity, and certain fetal anomalies.

Characteristics of the Postterm Newborn

Some postterm newborns have an appearance similar to term infants, but others look like infants 1 to 3 weeks old. They have a wide-eyed, hyperalert expression. Little lanugo or vernix remains, scalp hair is abundant, and fingernails are long. The skin is dry, cracked, wrinkled, peeling, and whiter than that of the normal newborn. The infant has little subcutaneous fat and appears long and thin.

These infants are at risk for intrauterine hypoxia during labor and delivery due to failing placental function. Thus, it is customary for the health care provider to induce labor or perform a cesarean delivery before the baby is markedly overdue. Many health care providers do not allow a pregnancy to continue beyond the end of 42 weeks' gestation.

Potential Complications

In the last weeks of gestation, the infant relies on glycogen for nutrition. This depletes the liver glycogen stores and may lead to neonatal hypoglycemia. Polycythemia may develop in response to intrauterine hypoxia. Polycythemia puts the infant at risk for cerebral ischemia, thrombus formation, and respiratory distress because of hyperviscosity of the blood. Often, the postterm infant expels meconium in utero. At birth, they may aspirate meconium into the lungs, obstructing the respiratory passages and irritating the lungs, resulting in meconium aspiration syndrome (MAS) (see later discussion).

Treatment

Prevention of postterm birth is the mainstay of treatment. Early ultrasounds are done routinely because these establish the most accurate dating of the pregnancy. Later in the pregnancy (after 42 weeks), ultrasound is used to evaluate fetal development, weight, the amount of amniotic fluid, and the placenta for signs of aging. This information allows the health care provider to make an informed decision regarding the safest form and timing of delivery.

Nursing Care

Typically, postterm newborns are ravenous eaters at birth. If the newborn is free from respiratory distress, offer feedings at 1 or 2 hours of age, and remain observant for potential aspiration and possible asphyxia. Monitor blood glucose levels. The newborn may require IV glucose infusions to stabilize the glucose level.

Provide a thermoneutral environment to promote thermoregulation. A radiant heat warmer or isolette may be helpful. Use measures to minimize heat loss, such as reducing drafts and drying the skin thoroughly after bathing.

Draw venous and arterial hematocrit levels, as ordered, to evaluate for polycythemia. If polycythemia is present, a partial exchange transfusion may be done to prevent or treat hyperviscosity.

Anticipate that the stressed postterm newborn will not tolerate the labor and delivery process well. Observe and monitor the newborn's cardiopulmonary status closely. Administer supplemental oxygen therapy as ordered for respiratory distress.

Postterm newborns can appear very different from what parents expect. Help facilitate a positive parent–newborn bond by explaining the newborn's condition and reasons for treatments and procedures. Point out positive features. Encourage them to express their feelings and to participate in their newborn's care, if possible, to alleviate their stresses and fears about the newborn's condition.

TEST YOURSELF

✔ Name three alternatives to breast-feeding or bottle feeding for a preterm newborn who cannot tolerate oral feedings.

✔ List three ways you can encourage the parents to take on the parental role for the preterm newborn.

✔ Name three potential complications associated with the postterm newborn.

ACQUIRED DISORDERS

Respiratory Disorders

A newborn is at risk for developing respiratory disorders after birth as the newborn adapts to the extrauterine environment. The risk for these disorders increases when the newborn experiences a gestational age variation.

Transient Tachypnea of the Newborn

Transient tachypnea of the newborn (TTN) involves the development of mild respiratory distress. It typically occurs within a few hours after birth, with the greatest degree of distress occurring at approximately 36 hours of life. TTN commonly disappears spontaneously around the third day.

TTN results from a delay in absorption of fetal lung fluid after birth. In utero, the lungs are filled with fluid. As the fetus passes through the birth canal during delivery, some of the fluid squeezes out as the thoracic area is compressed. After birth, the newborn breathes and fills the lungs with air, thus expelling additional lung fluid. The newborn typically absorbs any remaining fluid into the bloodstream or expels it by coughing. However, this process is incomplete for newborns that develop TTN.

Contributing Factors

TTN commonly occurs in newborns born by cesarean delivery. The newborn does not experience the compression of the thoracic cavity that occurs with passage through the birth canal, so they retain some fluid in the lungs. Other contributing factors include prematurity, being small for gestational age, maternal diabetes, and maternal smoking during pregnancy.

Clinical Manifestations and Diagnosis

A newborn who develops TTN typically exhibits mild respiratory distress, with a respiratory rate greater than 60 breaths per minute. Mild retractions, nasal flaring, and some expiratory grunting may be noted. However, cyanosis usually does not occur. Often the newborn has difficulty feeding because they are breathing at such a rapid rate and are therefore unable to suck and breathe at the same time.

Arterial blood gases may reveal hypoxemia and decreased carbon dioxide levels. A chest x-ray usually indicates some fluid in the central portion of the lungs with adequate aeration.

Treatment

Treatment depends on the newborn's gestational age, overall status, history, and extent of respiratory distress. Unless an infection is suspected, medication therapy is not typically required. IV fluids and gavage feedings may meet the newborn's fluid and nutritional requirements until the condition resolves. Supplemental oxygen is often ordered.

Nursing Care

Care for the newborn with TTN is supportive. Monitor the newborn's vital signs and oxygen saturation levels closely. Remain alert for changes that would indicate that the newborn is becoming fatigued from the rapid breathing. Administer IV fluids and supplemental oxygen as ordered. Assist the family caregivers in understanding what their newborn is experiencing. Help allay any fears or anxieties that they may have by explaining that the condition typically resolves without long-term consequences.

Meconium Aspiration Syndrome

Meconium aspiration syndrome (MAS) refers to a condition in which the fetus or newborn develops respiratory distress after inhaling meconium mixed with amniotic fluid. Meconium is a thick, pasty, greenish black substance that is present in the fetal bowel as early as 10 weeks' gestation. Meconium staining of amniotic fluid usually occurs as a reflex response that allows the rectal sphincter to relax. Subsequently, the fetus expels meconium into the amniotic fluid. The fetus may aspirate meconium while in utero or with their first breath after birth. The meconium can block the airway partially or completely and can irritate the newborn's airway, causing respiratory distress.

Contributing Factors

Typically, MAS is associated with fetal distress during labor. The fetus may experience hypoxia, causing peristalsis to increase and the anal sphincter to relax. The fetus then gasps or inhales the meconium-stained amniotic fluid. Other factors that contribute to the development of MAS include a maternal history of diabetes or hypertension, difficult delivery, advanced gestational age, and poor intrauterine growth.

Clinical Manifestations and Diagnosis

MAS is suspected whenever amniotic fluid is stained green to greenish black. Meconium staining may be seen on the newborn. Other manifestations include the following:

- Difficulty initiating respirations after birth
- Low Apgar score
- Tachypnea or apnea
- Retractions
- Grunting
- Nasal flaring
- Cyanosis

The health care provider suspects the diagnosis when the newborn develops respiratory distress after a delivery in which the amniotic fluid is meconium stained. Typically, a chest x-ray confirms the diagnosis.

Treatment

If the amniotic fluid is meconium stained, the nose and pharynx are suctioned before the newborn takes the first breath to decrease the likelihood of aspiration. The newborn is monitored closely for respiratory distress, and supportive care is given. Oxygen therapy and assisted ventilation may be used to support the newborn's respiratory status. If necessary, the health care provider may order tracheal and bronchial suctioning. In severe cases, extracorporeal membrane oxygenation (ECMO) is used to meet the newborn's oxygen requirements. Broad spectrum antibiotics are sometimes administered.

Nursing Care

Newborns with meconium aspiration syndrome (MAS) are extremely ill and require care in the NICU. Nursing care focuses on observing the neonate's respiratory status closely and ensuring adequate oxygenation. Measures to maintain thermoregulation are key factors in reducing the body's metabolic demands for oxygen. Be prepared to administer respiratory support and medication therapy as ordered.

Sudden Infant Death Syndrome

The term "sudden unexpected infant death" (SUID) is often used to describe all unexpected infant deaths. SUID can then be subdivided into explained SUID and unexplained SUID. Unexplained SUID cases are referred to as sudden infant death syndrome (SIDS). SIDS is defined as the sudden death of an apparently healthy infant, younger than 1 year of age, which remains unexplained after investigation, autopsy, examination of the death scene, and review of the clinical history. Previously referred to as "crib death," SIDS has caused much grief and anxiety among families for centuries. SIDS is the leading cause of death in infants between 30 and 365 days of age (Corwin, 2021).

The term SIDS is not a diagnosis but rather a description of the syndrome. Varying theories have been suggested about the cause of SIDS. Despite much research over the years, no single cause has been identified.

Contributing Factors

Infants who die of SIDS are usually 2 to 4 months old, although some deaths have occurred during the first and second weeks of life. Few infants older than 6 months of age die of SIDS. It is a greater threat to low birth weight (LBW) and preterm infants. It affects more male infants than female infants, as well as more infants from minority and lower socioeconomic groups. Infants born to mothers younger than 20 years of age and infants whose mothers smoked or used drugs or alcohol during pregnancy are also at greater risk. Prone sleeping position, sleeping on soft surfaces with blankets, pillows, or stuffed animals, sleeping in parents' beds and overheating are risk factors.

The American Academy of Pediatrics recommends placing infants in a supine position rather than a prone position for sleep until the infant is 6 months old. The incidence of SIDS has decreased since newborns have been put on their backs to sleep (Corwin, 2021).

Clinical Manifestations

SIDS is rapid and silent and occurs at any time of the day. There is no evidence of a struggle. People who have been nearby claim that they heard no unusual sounds before the death was discovered. The infant frequently appears in excellent health before the death.

A closely related syndrome is one called an apparent life-threatening event (ALTE). The infant is found in distress but responds immediately to stimulation. This infant recovers with no lasting problems. The health care provider may order a home apnea monitor for this infant (Fig. 20-7). The apnea monitor is set to sound an alarm if the infant does not take a breath within a given number of seconds. Family caregivers learn infant cardiopulmonary resuscitation so that they can respond quickly if the alarm sounds. Infants who have had an episode of an ALTE are at risk for additional episodes and may be at risk for SIDS. The infant stays on home apnea monitoring until they are 1 year old.

Nursing Care

The effects of SIDS on family caregivers are devastating. Grief coupled with guilt is a frequent response. Disbelief, hostility, and anger are common reactions. Even though the family caregivers are told that they are not to blame, it is difficult for most not to keep searching for evidence of some possible neglect on their parts. Prolonged depression usually follows the initial shock and anguish over the infant's death.

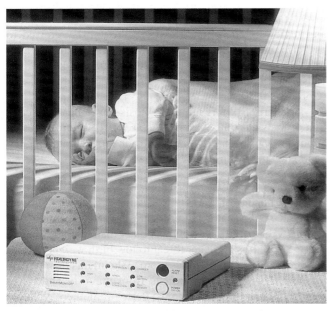

FIGURE 20-7 An apnea monitor for home monitoring.

The immediate response of the emergency department staff should be to allow the family to express their grief, encouraging them to say goodbye to their infant and providing a quiet, private place for them to do so. Compassionate care of the family caregivers includes help finding someone to accompany them home or to meet them there. Immediately refer the family to the local chapter of the National SIDS Foundation. Sudden Infant Death Syndrome Alliance (also known as First Candle) is another resource for help. Community health nurses can provide written materials, as well as information, guidance, and support in the family's home. They maintain contact with the family as long as necessary and provide support in a subsequent pregnancy.

Family caregivers are particularly concerned about subsequent infants. Studies have indicated that the risk for these infants is no greater than that for the general population. Many health care providers, however, continue to recommend monitoring these infants for the first few months of life to help reduce the family's stress. Monitoring continues until the new infant is past the age at which the infant with SIDS died.

Hemolytic Disease of the Newborn

Hemolytic disease of the newborn, also known as *erythroblastosis fetalis*, is a condition in which the infant's RBCs are broken down (hemolyzed) and destroyed, producing severe anemia and hyperbilirubinemia. In severe cases, heart failure, brain damage, and death can result.

Causes

There are two main causes of hemolytic disease of the newborn. One cause of hemolytic disease is Rh incompatibility. The use of immune globulin has markedly reduced the incidence of this disorder (see Chapter 17 for administration criteria). Today, hemolytic disease is principally the result of ABO incompatibility, which is generally much less severe than the Rh-induced disorder.

Rh Incompatibility

Rh factor is a protein substance (antigen) found on the surface of RBCs of individuals who are Rho(D)-positive. Individuals whose blood cells do not carry the Rh antigen are Rho(D)-negative. If an individual who is Rho(D)-negative encounters Rho(D)-positive blood, that individual's immune system views the Rh factor as foreign and produces anti-D antibodies that attack and destroy the antigen. This becomes a problem for the Rho(D)-positive fetus whose mother has developed the anti-D antibodies. The antibodies easily cross the placenta, enter the fetal circulation, and attack fetus RBCs. The result is hemolysis (destruction) of the fetal RBCs, which leads to severe

Think About This

If the fetus is Rho(D)-negative, their RBCs do not carry the antigen. Therefore, even if their mother is sensitized, the fetus will not experience hemolysis because the anti-D antibodies do not have anything to attack.

fetal anemia. The Rho(D)-positive fetus is vulnerable to hemolytic disease only if his mother is Rho(D)-negative and has been sensitized to Rho(D)-positive blood (i.e., she has anti-D antibodies).

The firstborn child does not usually develop hemolytic disease for two reasons. First, in response to the initial exposure to the Rho(D) antigen, the woman's body produces a large antibody that does not cross the placenta. Subsequent exposures induce production of the small anti-D antibody that crosses the placenta. Second, most sensitization occurs at birth when fetal blood cells escape into the woman's blood stream as the placenta separates from the uterine wall. This puts subsequent pregnancies at risk.

With the next pregnancy, the small maternal antibodies enter the fetal circulation and begin to hemolyze (destroy) the fetus's RBCs. The fetus makes a valiant attempt to replace the destroyed RBCs by releasing large amounts of immature RBCs (erythroblasts) into the bloodstream (thus the name erythroblastosis fetalis). As the rapid destruction of the fetus's RBCs continues, anemia develops. If the anemia is severe enough, the fetus develops heart failure and hydrops fetalis (extensive fetal edema), which can lead to fetal death.

Rapid destruction of the fetus's RBCs releases bilirubin, which is not usually a problem in utero because the woman's body processes and excretes the excess bilirubin. After birth, the newborn's immature liver cannot handle the high levels of bilirubin, and they develop pathologic jaundice. This condition can lead to **acute bilirubin encephalopathy (kernicterus)**, a disorder in which excess bilirubin stains neurons in the brain and spinal cord leading to irreversible injury or death.

ABO Incompatibility

The major blood groups are A, B, AB, and O, and each has antigens that may be incompatible with those of another group. The most common incompatibility in the newborn occurs between a woman with type O blood and an infant with type A or B blood. The reactions are usually less severe than in Rh incompatibility.

Diagnosis

When titers show the presence of anti-D antibodies, the health care provider monitors fetal well-being. Because direct sampling of fetal blood increases the risk of fetal loss, the health care provider usually uses indirect means to measure disease severity.

Traditionally, amniocentesis established the diagnosis (see Chapter 7 for discussion of amniocentesis). Analysis of a sample of amniotic fluid shows the amount of bile pigments (bilirubin) present. Thus, it can be determined if the fetus is mildly, moderately, or severely affected. Now, Doppler velocimetry is the diagnostic method of choice. It has the advantage of being noninvasive and yields more sensitive data about the fetal condition.

After birth, the following tests help determine presence of disease and severity.

- Direct Coombs test detects the presence of maternal antibodies
- Rh and ABO typing help identify the cause
- Hemoglobin levels and RBC counts determine severity of anemia
- Plasma bilirubin levels help determine disease severity

A positive direct Coombs test indicates that maternal anti-D antibodies are present on the surface of the infant's RBCs. Conversely, a negative direct Coombs test indicates that there are no antibodies on the infant's RBCs.

Clinical Manifestations

The initial examination for infants with known incompatibility (either Rh or ABO) includes evaluation for pallor, edema, jaundice, and an enlarged spleen and liver. If prenatal care was inadequate or absent, a severely affected infant may be stillborn or have hydrops fetalis, a condition marked by extensive edema, marked anemia and jaundice, and enlargement of the liver and spleen. If untreated, infants with hydrops are at risk for severe brain damage from acute bilirubin encephalopathy (kernicterus). Death occurs in about 75% of infants with acute bilirubin encephalopathy (kernicterus); those who survive may have an intellectual disability or develop spastic paralysis or nerve deafness.

Treatment

Because ABO incompatibilities are typically milder than are Rh incompatibilities, treatment during pregnancy is not required. For the severely affected fetus with an Rh incompatibility, the health care provider may perform an intrauterine transfusion of Rho(D)-negative blood. If the fetus is beyond 32 weeks gestation, delivery by labor induction or cesarean is the best treatment option.

After delivery, a positive Coombs test indicates the presence of the disease but not the degree of severity. If bilirubin and hemoglobin levels are within normal limits, the health care provider orders close observation and frequent laboratory tests. A newborn who has mild-to-moderate disease usually receives hydration and phototherapy after birth. Phototherapy involves the use of special lights to help reduce bilirubin levels. The lights work by converting fat-soluble unconjugated bilirubin, which the body cannot expel, to water-soluble conjugated bilirubin that the body excretes via the gastrointestinal and renal routes. A severely affected newborn requires care in a NICU and usually receives an exchange transfusion immediately after birth.

Nursing Care

Nursing care for the newborn with risk factors for hemolytic disease involves initial and ongoing monitoring for jaundice. Always report jaundice to the RN. Jaundice found within the first 24 hours after birth is always pathologic. Report this finding immediately.

For the newborn receiving phototherapy, place the lights above the isolette at an appropriate height (Fig. 20-8). If the lights are too far away from the newborn, the therapy will not work. If they are too close, the newborn may receive burns. The infant is nude, except for a small covering over the genitalia, to maximize the skin surface area exposed to the light. A pad or diaper is placed under the perineal area to collect urine and feces. Turn the newborn every 2 hours to rotate the area of exposure. Do not turn off the lights except to feed and to change the diaper.

Always shield the newborn's eyes from the ultraviolet light. Carefully apply eye patches to avoid eye irritation. If the eye patch is too loose, it can slip down and obstruct the nares or lead to retinal damage from the light. Remove the patches every 4 hours to cleanse the eyes and examine for irritation, inflammation, and dryness. Clean and change the patches daily.

The light may cause the infant to have skin rashes; sunburn or tanning; loose, greenish stools; hyperthermia; an increased metabolic rate; increased evaporative water loss; and priapism (a prolonged erection of the penis). Infants undergoing phototherapy need as much as 25% more fluids to prevent dehydration. Monitor the serum bilirubin levels routinely when the infant is receiving phototherapy.

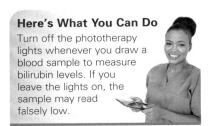

Here's What You Can Do

Turn off the phototherapy lights whenever you draw a blood sample to measure bilirubin levels. If you leave the lights on, the sample may read falsely low.

Phototherapy may also be administered using a fiber-optic blanket consisting of a pad attached to a halogen light source with illuminating plastic fibers. A disposable protective cover protects the blanket that wraps around the infant to disperse therapeutic light. These blankets are appropriate

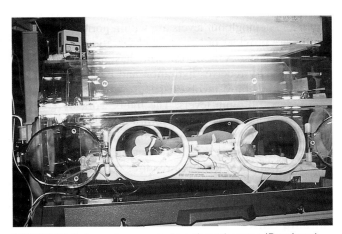

FIGURE 20-8 A newborn receiving phototherapy. (Reprinted with permission from Ricci S., Kyle T., & Carman S. (2021). *Maternity and pediatric nursing* (4th ed., p. 904, Figure 24.7). Wolters Kluwer.)

for home use, which can cut hospitalization costs and reduce the family separation time. The neonate's eyes do not require protection when the fiber-optic blanket is used. The blanket can stay on all the time without interfering with newborn care.

Remain sensitive to parental feelings of guilt and anxiety. Give them the opportunity to ventilate their feelings.

Newborn of a Mother With Diabetes

Maternal diabetes places the fetus and newborn at risk for serious complications. Perinatal outcome has a direct relationship with the severity and control of the mother's diabetes (see Chapter 16). The woman with diabetes who closely controls her blood glucose level before conception and throughout pregnancy, particularly in the early months, decreases her risk of having an infant with congenital anomalies. Fetal death is less likely with excellent control.

Clinical Manifestations

Infants of mothers with poorly controlled type 2 or gestational diabetes have a distinctive appearance. They are large for gestational age (LGA), plump and full faced with bulky shoulders, and coated with vernix caseosa. Both the placenta and the umbilical cord are oversized. In contrast, infants of mothers with poorly controlled, long-term, or severe type 1 diabetes actually may suffer from intrauterine growth restriction (IUGR).

Consistently elevated fetal insulin levels cause the distinctive growth pattern. Because maternal glucose levels are elevated and glucose readily crosses the placenta, the fetus responds by increasing insulin production. Because insulin acts as a fetal growth hormone, consistently high levels cause fetal *macrosomia*, birth weight of greater than 4,500 g (9 lb, 14 oz). Insulin also causes disproportionate fat buildup to the shoulders and upper body, increasing the risk for shoulder dystocia and birth trauma.

Newborns of mothers with diabetes are at risk for hypoglycemia in the first few hours after birth. In utero, the fetal pancreas adapts to the high blood glucose levels by producing and secreting more insulin. After birth, the glucose source is abruptly cut off when the umbilical cord is cut. The newborn's pancreas cannot readjust quickly enough, so it continues to produce insulin, leading to neonatal hypoglycemia. This condition may cause permanent brain damage or death unless health care providers detect it quickly and treat the newborn with oral or IV glucose. See Chapter 13 for an in-depth discussion of neonatal hypoglycemia.

High insulin levels can also delay fetal lung maturity; therefore, newborns of mothers with diabetes have a higher incidence of respiratory distress syndrome (RDS) and other respiratory difficulties. These infants are subject to many other hazards, including congenital anomalies, preterm delivery, difficult cardiopulmonary transition at birth, and an enlarged heart. Other issues include hypocalcemia, hypomagnesemia, polycythemia with hyperviscosity, and hyperbilirubinemia. This infant is at increased risk for developing early onset diabetes in adolescence or early adulthood.

Nursing Care

Newborns of mothers with diabetes require especially careful observation. Perform early (as soon as possible after birth) and frequent blood glucose checks. Administer early feedings, or if the newborn has respiratory distress or is otherwise ill, give IV glucose as ordered. Hypoglycemia can return after treatment, so watch for signs and symptoms. Watch for signs of respiratory distress. Anticipate supplemental oxygen and surfactant therapy. Some infants need ventilator support. Monitor electrolyte levels, especially magnesium and calcium, as ordered. Assist the RN with performing a gestational age assessment, as these infants can be deceptively large and still be preterm. Watch for and report any heart murmurs or other signs of cardiac dysfunction. Check carefully for signs of birth trauma.

TEST YOURSELF

✔ What respiratory disorder is associated with a delay in the absorption of fetal lung fluid after birth?

✔ List three signs that may indicate the infant is suffering from meconium aspiration.

✔ What medication has dramatically reduced the incidence of hemolytic disease of the newborn?

Newborn of a Mother With Substance Abuse

Alcohol use or prescription or illicit drug use by the mother during pregnancy can lead to many problems in the newborn. The newborn of a woman who uses alcohol is at risk for fetal alcohol syndrome (FAS). The newborn of a chemically dependent woman may be small for gestational age (SGA) or experience withdrawal symptoms.

Unfortunately, identifying the pregnant woman who abuses alcohol or drugs is often difficult. Many of these women have no prenatal care or only infrequent care. They may not keep appointments or may not follow prenatal guidelines. As a result, many of these infants suffer prenatal insults that result in intrauterine growth restriction (IUGR), congenital abnormalities, and premature birth.

Fetal Alcohol Syndrome

Alcohol is one of the many teratogenic substances that readily cross the placenta to the fetus. Fetal alcohol spectrum disorder (FASD) is a term used to describe the range of effects that can occur in an individual who was exposed to alcohol prenatally and who may have lifelong concerns from the alcohol exposure. One of the conditions included in FASD is fetal alcohol syndrome (FAS). Many newborns exposed to alcohol in utero exhibit withdrawal symptoms during the first few hours after delivery. FAS is often apparent in newborns of mothers with chronic alcoholism and sometimes appears in newborns whose mothers are low to moderate consumers of alcohol. Because we do not know exactly how much alcohol is safe, the woman should stop drinking at least 3 months before she plans to become pregnant and abstain from using any alcohol use during pregnancy.

Clinical Manifestations

The newborn who is withdrawing from alcohol is typically hyperactive and irritable, has trouble sleeping, and may have tremors or seizures. Characteristics of FAS include low birth weight (LBW), small height and head circumference, short palpebral fissures (eyelid folds), reduced ocular growth, and a flattened nasal bridge. This newborn is prone to respiratory difficulties, hypoglycemia, hypocalcemia, and hyperbilirubinemia. Growth during infancy and childhood continues to fall below average growth rates. Unfortunately, the brain damage that occurs during fetal development is permanent, resulting in intellectual disability.

Nursing Care

FAS is highly preventable. Societal interventions, of which nurses can be a part, include increasing the public's awareness of the detrimental effects of alcohol use during pregnancy. Other helpful interventions include screening women of reproductive age for alcohol problems and encouraging women to obtain adequate prenatal care and use appropriate resources to abstain from using alcohol during pregnancy.

Nursing care for the newborn who is withdrawing from alcohol includes the supportive interventions of swaddling, decreasing sensory stimulation, and ensuring adequate nutrition. Keep the newborn's environment quiet and dark during the first few days of withdrawal. Administer benzodiazepine or other anticonvulsants, as ordered, to prevent or treat seizure activity. Adequate nutrition is key to supporting weight gain. The newborn's sucking reflex may be weak, and they may be too irritable to feed. Give small amounts of formula or breast milk frequently. Monitor the newborn's daily weight, intake, and output. Encourage the parents to feed the newborn, which helps promote bonding.

Neonatal Abstinence Syndrome

The newborn of the woman with a substance use disorder such as an addiction to cocaine, heroin, methadone, or other drugs is born dependent upon these substances. Newborns may also be born dependent on a certain class of antidepressants, serotonin reuptake inhibitors. Many of these infants suffer withdrawal symptoms during the early neonatal period. However, the time of onset varies widely. For example, the newborn experiencing withdrawal from opioids typically experiences withdrawal symptoms within 24 to 48 hours after birth. However, it may take up to 2 weeks before the newborn exhibits any symptoms.

Clinical Manifestations

Withdrawal symptoms commonly include irritability, tremors, restlessness, hyperactivity, disorganized or hyperactive reflexes, increased muscle tone, sneezing, sweating, tachypnea, vomiting, diarrhea, disturbed sleep patterns, and a shrill high-pitched cry (Fig. 20-9). Ineffective sucking and swallowing reflexes create feeding problems, and regurgitation and vomiting occur often after feeding.

Nursing Care

Care of the newborn experiencing substance withdrawal focuses on providing physical and emotional support. Medications such as morphine, methadone, clonidine, or phenobarbital may ease the withdrawal and prevent complications, such as seizures.

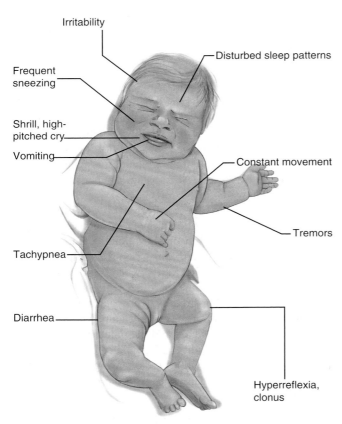

Irritability
Frequent sneezing
Shrill, high-pitched cry
Vomiting
Tachypnea
Diarrhea
Disturbed sleep patterns
Constant movement
Tremors
Hyperreflexia, clonus

FIGURE 20-9 Manifestations of a newborn with substance withdrawal.

Because of neuromuscular irritability, many of these newborns respond favorably to gentle rocking movements while in close bodily contact with their caregivers. Therefore, some nurseries place the newborns in special carriers that hold them close to the nurse's chest while the nurse moves about the nursery. Swaddling the infant (wrapping securely in a small blanket) with arms across the chest also is a method of quieting the agitated newborn. Keep the newborn's environment dimly lit to minimize stimulation. Maintain the airway and monitor respiratory status closely. Provide small frequent feedings. Keep the newborn's head elevated to promote effective sucking and reduce the risk of aspiration. Vomiting and diarrhea may lead to fluid and electrolyte imbalances. Monitor intake and output closely, and give supplemental fluids as ordered. Use a nonjudgmental approach when interacting with the newborn and their mother.

Newborn With a Congenitally Acquired Infection

All newborns are at increased risk for infections because their immune systems are immature, and they cannot localize infection. At-risk newborns are even more susceptible than are normal newborns. The newborn may acquire an infection prenatally from the mother (through the placenta), during the intrapartum period (during labor and delivery) from maternal vaginal infection or inhalation of contaminated amniotic fluid, and after birth from cross-contamination with other infants, healthcare personnel, or contaminated equipment.

A variety of organisms can cause newborn infection. Table 20-2 summarizes several prominent neonatal infections. (See Chapter 16 for a detailed discussion of congenitally acquired infections.) The newborn that develops an infection often does not have any specific signs of illness. The clue that alerts you to a possible problem may be signs such as cyanosis, pallor, thermal instability (difficulty keeping temperature within normal range), convulsions, lethargy, apnea, jaundice, or just "not looking right." Blood, urine, cerebrospinal fluid cultures, and other laboratory and x-ray tests necessary to isolate the specific organism confirm the diagnosis. Treatment consists of intensive antibiotic therapy, IV fluids, respiratory therapy, and other supportive measures.

Remember **Kierra Jones** from earlier in the chapter. As Kierra's nurse, what complications will you anticipate seeing, and what will you include in her nursing care?

TABLE 20-2 Neonatal Infections

INFECTIOUS AGENT	MODE OF TRANSMISSION TO FETUS OR NEONATE	ONSET	CLINICAL MANIFESTATIONS/ COMPLICATIONS	PREVENTION/ TREATMENT	NOTES
Chlamydia trachomatis (chlamydia) or *Neisseria gonorrhoeae* (gonorrhea)	Birth canal during vaginal birth	Variable	Ophthalmia neonatorum, a serious form of conjunctivitis that can lead to blindness	Prevention: routine ophthalmic administration of erythromycin ointment after birth	
Group B streptococcus (GBS)	In utero or via the birth canal during vaginal delivery	Early onset is within the first 24 hours of life. Late onset is up to 7 days of life	Septicemia (blood infection) and meningitis	Prevention: antibiotics to GBS-positive women during labor	The woman does not have an infection; GBS colonizes the vagina and gastrointestinal tracts of healthy women. GBS is the most common cause of neonatal sepsis; however, neonatal GBS infection is a rare event
Hepatitis B virus	Contact with infected blood during birth	Variable	Most infants with hepatitis B become chronic carriers, which puts them at risk for cirrhosis and liver cancer	Prevention: Newborns of mothers with hepatitis B receive hepatitis B immune globulin within 12 hours of birth. All newborns receive the first in a series of hepatitis B vaccines before discharge from the hospital	Incidence has decreased dramatically since newborns began receiving the vaccine
Herpes simplex virus type 1 or 2	Contact with vaginal secretions during birth (mother with active lesions is the most common mode); in utero infection when virus crosses the placenta to the fetus	At about 1 week of age	Initial signs and symptoms are nonspecific, such as irritability, lethargy, fever, or failure to feed. Later manifestations: skin, eye, or mouth disease; central nervous system disease with encephalitis; or disseminated disease with multiple major organ involvement	Prevention: suppressive therapy for the mother with acyclovir beginning at 36 weeks' gestation; cesarean delivery for women with active lesions at term	Neonatal herpes infection is rare
Human immunodeficiency virus (HIV)	In utero across the placenta; contact with infected blood in the birth canal; and breast-feeding	Commonly between 4 months and 1 year of age	Bacterial infections, such as pneumonia, meningitis, and bacteremia; thrush, mouth sores, and severe diaper rash	Prevention: antiretroviral therapy during pregnancy to suppress maternal viral load; and sometimes antiretroviral therapy to the newborn during the first 6 weeks of life	Very poor prognosis for infants who develop symptoms before 1 year of age

Continued

TABLE 20-2 Neonatal Infections (Continued)

INFECTIOUS AGENT	MODE OF TRANSMISSION TO FETUS OR NEONATE	ONSET	CLINICAL MANIFESTATIONS/ COMPLICATIONS	PREVENTION/ TREATMENT	NOTES
Methicillin-resistant *Staphylococcus aureus* (MRSA)	In NICUs due to overcrowding, lack of adequate cleaning procedures, poorly trained staff, or cross-contamination from a parent or family member visiting an infant; can also be transmitted during breast-feeding	Variable	Symptoms range from pustules or eye discharge to septicemia, pneumonia, and infant death	Prevention: screening at-risk pregnant women on admission to the hospital; careful adherence to infection control measures, such as handwashing and environmental cleanliness	
Rubella virus	In utero across the placenta	In utero	Spontaneous abortion, stillbirth, preterm delivery, and congenital anomalies; hearing impairment is the single most common defect followed by eye disorders, heart defects, and neurologic abnormalities, including intellectual disability	Prevention: rubella vaccine. There is no cure; treatment is supportive	
Treponema pallidum (*T. pallidum*) causes syphilis	In utero across the placenta	In utero, at birth, or months later	Intrauterine growth restriction, hydrops fetalis, fetal death, preterm birth, congenital infection, neonatal death, blindness, deafness, or other deformities; Hutchinson triad and snuffles (bloody discharge) are characteristic symptoms	Prevention: Treat maternal infection during pregnancy; Treatment: penicillin for the infected newborn	

KEY POINTS

- Newborns are classified by size as small for gestational age (SGA), appropriate for gestational age (AGA), and large for gestational age (LGA). Based on weight, newborns may be classified as low birth weight (LBW), very low birth weight (VLBW), or extremely low birth weight (ELBW). Classifications by gestational age are preterm, postterm, or term.

- A gestational age assessment evaluates two major categories of maturity: neuromuscular maturity and physical maturity.

- Intrauterine growth restriction (IUGR) is the most common underlying condition leading to SGA newborns. It occurs when the fetus does not receive adequate amounts of oxygen and nutrients

necessary for the proper growth and development of organs and tissues.

- Neither the symmetrically growth-restricted newborn nor the asymmetrically growth-restricted newborn has grown at the expected rate for gestational age on standard growth charts. When plotted on a standard growth chart, the symmetrically growth-restricted newborn's weight, length, and head circumference fall below the 10th percentile; the asymmetrically growth-restricted newborn falls below the 10th percentile on one or sometimes two of the measurements. For the asymmetrically growth-restricted infant, the birth weight is most commonly affected.

- The underlying cause of a newborn being LGA is unknown. Contributing factors may include maternal diabetes; genetic factors, such as parent size and male sex of the newborn; congenital disorders; or the number of pregnancies the mother has had with multiparous women having two to three times the number of LGA newborns.

- Preterm births may result from maternal factors, such as prior preterm deliveries, maternal age extremes, and poor nutritional status. Multiple births are a frequently seen cause of preterm births. One of the more common factors in preterm births is preterm prelabor rupture of membranes, due to underlying conditions such as infection of the membranes. The pregnant woman with diabetes is another major contributor. Factors that contribute to intrauterine growth restriction (IUGR) also increase the risk of preterm birth.

- Characteristics of the preterm newborn as compared to the term newborn include little muscle or subcutaneous fat; thin, translucent skin; visible veins on abdomen and scalp; plentiful lanugo; extremely pliable ears due to minimal cartilage; undescended testes in the male and prominent labia minor and clitoris in the female; very few creases in the soles of the feet or palms of the hands; and weak or absent newborn reflexes.

- Common complications associated with preterm newborns include hypothermia, hypoglycemia, patent ductus arteriosus, jaundice, infection, respiratory distress syndrome (RDS), intraventricular hemorrhage (IVH), retinopathy of prematurity (ROP), and necrotizing enterocolitis (NEC).

- Care of the preterm newborn focuses on improving respiratory function, maintaining body temperature, preventing infection, protecting neurologic status, maintaining fluid and electrolyte balance, maintaining adequate nutrition, preserving skin integrity, conserving energy, and supporting growth and development. Goals for the family include reducing anxiety and improving parenting skills and family functioning.

- Potential complications seen in the postterm newborn are hypoglycemia, polycythemia due to intrauterine hypoxia, and meconium aspiration. Polycythemia puts the infant at risk for cerebral ischemia, thrombus formation, and respiratory distress because of hyperviscosity of the blood. These are focus areas for nursing care.

- Common acquired respiratory disorders of the newborn include transient tachypnea of the newborn (TTN), meconium aspiration syndrome (MAS), and sudden infant death syndrome (SIDS). TTN occurs in the first few hours of life and is caused by retained lung fluid. MAS occurs when the newborn inhales meconium into the respiratory passages, often with the first breath; this leads to pneumonia. SIDS is the sudden, unexpected and unexplained death of an apparently healthy infant in whom investigation, clinical history and the postmortem examination fails to reveal a cause.

- Hemolytic disease of the newborn, a condition in which the infant's RBCs are broken down and destroyed, may be the result of Rh or ABO incompatibility. Hyperbilirubinemia occurs and may be treated by phototherapy or exchange transfusions.

- Characteristics in the appearance of the newborn of a mother with diabetes include being LGA, plump, full faced with bulky shoulders, and coated with vernix caseosa. These newborns are at risk for hypoglycemia; delayed fetal lung maturity resulting in respiratory disorders; and other concerns including congenital anomalies, preterm delivery, difficult cardiopulmonary transition at birth, and an enlarged heart.

- The newborn of a mother who is chemically dependent on alcohol may develop fetal alcohol syndrome (FAS). The newborn is prone to respiratory difficulties, hypoglycemia, hypocalcemia, hyperbilirubinemia, slowed growth, and intellectual disability. Nursing care for the newborn with FAS is supportive and focuses on preventing complications, such as seizures.

- The newborn of a mother with a substance use disorder may experience withdrawal symptoms. These include irritability, tremors, restlessness, hyperactivity, disorganized or hyperactive reflexes, increased muscle tone, sneezing, sweating, tachypnea, vomiting, diarrhea, disturbed sleep patterns, and a shrill high-pitched cry. Ineffective sucking and swallowing reflexes create feeding problems. Nursing care for the newborn focuses on providing physical and emotional support.

- Group B beta-hemolytic streptococcus is the major cause of congenitally acquired infections in the newborn. Other causes include rubella virus, *Chlamydia trachomatis (C. trachomatis)* or *Neisseria gonorrhoeae (N. gonorrhoeae)* (leading to ophthalmia neonatorum), hepatitis B, herpes virus types 1 and 2, *Treponema pallidum (T. pallidum)* that causes syphilis, human immunodeficiency virus, and methicillin-resistant *Staphylococcus aureus (MRSA)*.

INTERNET RESOURCES

Human Milk Bank
www.hmbana.org

Prematurity
www.marchofdimes.com/prematurity

SIDS
www.sids.org

First Candle
www.firstcandle.org

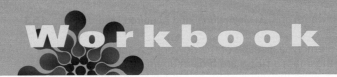

NCLEX-STYLE REVIEW QUESTIONS

1. The nurse is assisting in a newborn assessment of gestational age using the Ballard scoring system. What physical characteristics are associated with a newborn with the oldest gestational age?
   a. Abundant lanugo, flat areola, and pinna flat
   b. Anterior transverse plantar crease, soft ear recoil, and few scrotal rugae
   c. Transparent skin, no lanugo, and prominent clitoris
   d. Bald areas, plantar creases over 2/3 of sole area, and 3- to 4-mm breast bud

2. A newborn is considered large for gestational age (LGA) when the newborn is larger than the average baby is. What most likely would be a contributing factor in a newborn that is LGA?
   a. The mother of the newborn has no other children.
   b. The mother of the newborn has gained little weight during pregnancy.
   c. The mother of the newborn has a diagnosis of diabetes.
   d. The mother of the newborn has a history of smoking during pregnancy.

3. The nurse is caring for a preterm newborn. When creating a plan of care for the preterm newborn, what nursing intervention would be the most important to include?
   a. Repositioning at least every 2 hours
   b. Monitoring body temperature
   c. Promoting rest periods between procedures
   d. Recording urinary output

4. The nurse is caring for the newborn of a mother who abused cocaine during her pregnancy. What characteristic would the nurse most likely see in this newborn?
   a. The newborn weighs above average when born.
   b. The newborn sleeps for long periods of time.
   c. The newborn cries when touched.
   d. The newborn has facial deformities.

5. The preterm newborn has specific characteristics that differ from those of the term newborn. Which of the following are preterm characteristics? Select all that apply.
   a. Extremities are thin, with little muscle or subcutaneous fat.
   b. Skin is thickened and without wrinkles.
   c. Head and abdomen are disproportionately large.
   d. Veins of the abdomen and scalp are visible.
   e. Lanugo is not evident on the back and shoulders.
   f. Ears have soft, minimal cartilage and are pliable.

STUDY ACTIVITIES

1. Research your community to find sources of help for families who have lost children to sudden infant death syndrome (SIDS). What support groups and organizations are available that you might recommend to families who have lost a child because of SIDS? Discuss with your peers what you found, and make a list of resources to share.

2. Go to www.kidshealth.org. Type "When Your Baby's Born Premature" in the search box.
   a. What are the two basic needs of a premature infant discussed on this site?
   b. What are the common health problems often seen in premature infants?
   c. What suggestions does this site offer to families of children who have a premature infant?

CRITICAL THINKING: WHAT WOULD YOU DO?

1. The health care provider just told Andrea, the mother of Andrew, a newborn, that her son's bilirubin level is elevated, and he is going to be given phototherapy. Andrea appears concerned and anxious and looks as if she is about to cry.
   a. What is the first thing you would do and say to Andrea?
   b. What would you explain to Andrea regarding the purpose of the phototherapy for Andrew?
   c. What will you tell this mother in regard to what she might expect while Andrew is under the light?

2. You are leading a nutrition class for a group of pregnant women. One of the women says that she heard it was not a problem to drink a little alcohol while she was pregnant. Another member of the group says she has heard about something called fetal alcohol syndrome.
   a. What will you reinforce with this group regarding the use of alcohol during pregnancy?
   b. What is fetal alcohol syndrome?
   c. What are the characteristics of infants with fetal alcohol syndrome?
   d. What are the possible long-term complications of fetal alcohol syndrome?

The Newborn at Risk: Congenital Disorders

Learning Objectives

At the conclusion of this chapter, you will:

1. Differentiate the three types of spina bifida.
2. Discuss the two types of hydrocephalus, including the symptoms, treatment, and nursing care.
3. Describe the five common types of congenital heart defects, tracing the blood flow in each defect and discussing the treatment and nursing care.
4. Differentiate between cleft lip and cleft palate, including treatment and nursing care.
5. Discuss esophageal atresia and tracheoesophageal fistula.
6. Explain what occurs when an infant has an imperforate anus.
7. List and describe the four types of hernias that newborns may have.
8. Describe hypospadias, epispadias, exstrophy of the bladder, and ambiguous genitalia.
9. Discuss congenital talipes equinovarus.
10. Explain developmental dysplasia of the hip, including signs and symptoms, treatment, and nursing care.
11. Compare phenylketonuria, congenital hypothyroidism, galactosemia, and maple syrup urine disease.
12. Discuss Down syndrome, including common characteristics, treatment, and nursing care.
13. Differentiate Turner and Klinefelter syndromes.

Adrian Simmer was born with a cleft lip and a cleft palate. He is now 2 months old and has been admitted for repair of the cleft lip and the first stage of the repair of the cleft palate. As you read this chapter, think about what concerns Adrian's parents have been dealing with since he was born.

Chapter 20 discussed variations in size and gestational age as well as acquired disorders of the newborn. This chapter discusses congenital disorders, which are problems that occur during fetal development and are present in the infant at birth. Congenital disorders include malformations, or *congenital anomalies*, which can often be corrected during the first months or years of life. Congenital disorders also include inborn errors of metabolism and hereditary disorders (chromosomal abnormalities).

The birth of a newborn with a congenital defect (anomaly) is traumatic for parents and family caregivers. Depending on the defect, immediate or early surgery may be necessary. Early, continuous, skilled observation and nursing care are required. Rehabilitation of the newborn and education of the family caregivers in the newborn's care are essential. The emotional needs of the newborn and the family must be integrated into nursing care plans. Many of these newborns have a brighter future today as a result of increased diagnostic and medical knowledge and advances in surgical techniques.

Family caregivers experience a grief response whether the newborn's defect is a result of abnormal intrauterine development or a chromosomal abnormality. They mourn the loss of the perfect child of their dreams, question why it happened, and may wonder how they will show the newborn to family and friends without shame or embarrassment. This grief may interfere with the process of parent–newborn attachment. Parents need to understand that their response is normal and that they are entitled to honest answers to their questions about the newborn's condition. Other children in the family should be informed gently but honestly about the newborn and should be allowed to visit the newborn when accompanied by adult family members. Sufficient time and attention must be devoted to the older siblings to avoid jealousy toward the newborn.

CONGENITAL MALFORMATIONS

Congenital anomalies or malformations may be caused by genetic or environmental factors. Approximately 2% to 4% of all infants born have major malformations (Bacino, 2021). These anomalies include defects of the central nervous, cardiovascular, gastrointestinal, genitourinary, and skeletal systems. Defects such as cleft lip and severe neural tube defects are apparent at birth, but others may be discovered only after a complete physical examination. Congenital anomalies account for a large percentage of the health problems seen in newborns and children.

Central Nervous System Defects

Central nervous system defects include a range of disorders resulting from malformations of the neural tube during embryonic development. These are referred to as neural tube defects and are the most common central nervous system congenital anomaly. These defects vary from mild to severely disabling. The cause of neural tube defects is unknown, but supplementation of folic acid in women of childbearing age and during pregnancy has decreased the incidence of these defects. Other disorders are caused by an imbalance of cerebrospinal fluid (CSF) (as in hydrocephalus).

Spina Bifida

Caused by a defect in the neural arch, generally in the lumbosacral region, spina bifida is a failure of the posterior laminae of the vertebrae to close; this leaves an opening through which the spinal meninges and spinal cord may protrude (Fig. 21-1).

Clinical Manifestations

A bony defect that occurs without soft tissue involvement is called *spina bifida occulta*. In most instances, it is without symptoms and presents no problems. A dimple in the skin or a tuft of hair over the site may cause one to suspect its presence, or it may be overlooked entirely.

When part of the spinal meninges protrudes through the bony defect and forms a cystic sac, the condition is termed *spina bifida with meningocele*. No nerve roots are involved, so no paralysis or sensory loss below the lesion appears. However, the sac may rupture or perforate, introducing infection into the spinal fluid and causing meningitis. For this reason, as well as for cosmetic purposes, surgical removal of the sac with closure of the skin is indicated. In *spina bifida with myelomeningocele*, there is a protrusion of the spinal cord and the meninges, with nerve roots embedded in the wall of the cyst (Fig. 21-2).

The effects of this defect vary in severity from sensory loss or partial paralysis below the lesion to complete flaccid paralysis of all muscles below the lesion. Complete paralysis involves the lower trunk and legs, as well as bowel and bladder sphincters.

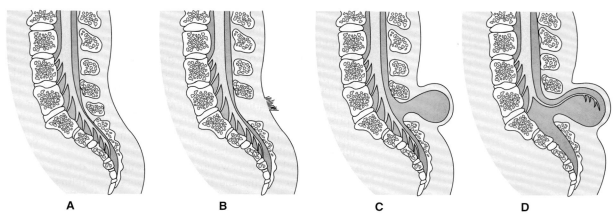

FIGURE 21-1 Degrees of spinal cord anomalies. **A.** The normal spinal closure. **B.** Spina bifida occulta. **C.** Spina bifida with meningocele. **D.** Spina bifida with myelomeningocele, clearly showing the spinal cord involvement.

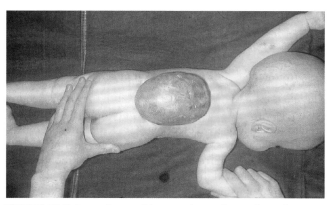

FIGURE 21-2 A newborn with a myelomeningocele and hydrocephalus.

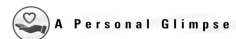

A Personal Glimpse

A child with "special needs." I never thought I would have to understand just what that really means. Courtney was our second child. A perfect pregnancy. Absolutely no problems. I didn't drink, never smoked, so I planned on a perfectly healthy baby. Until the alpha-fetoprotein (AFP) test. I will never forget that test now. I was 4 months' pregnant and went in for the routine test. A few days later the results were in. A neurotube defect—what in the world was that?

I have been asked many times if I was glad I knew before I had Courtney that she would have problems. I've thought a lot about it, and even though it made the last several months of the pregnancy a little (well, maybe more than a little) worrisome, yes, I'm very glad we knew. Courtney was born C-section at a regional medical center that is about 60 miles from home. She was in surgery just a few hours after she was born.

Words like spina bifida, hydrocephalus, VP shunt, catheterizations, glasses, walkers, braces, kidney infections, all became everyday words at our home. We have learned a lot in the last 5 years. Courtney has frequent doctor visits to all her specialists. She is the only 5-year-old concerned if her urine is cloudy and making sure her mom gives her medication on time.

A little over 5 years ago, a "special" child was born, and we feel very blessed she was given to us!

Rhonda

Learning Opportunity: *What reactions do you think the nurse might anticipate in working with a pregnant woman who finds her child will be born with "special needs?" In what ways could the nurse encourage this mother to share with other parents in similar situations?*

Making a clear-cut differentiation in diagnosis between a meningocele and a myelomeningocele on the basis of symptoms alone is not always possible. *Spina bifida cystica* is the term used to designate either of these protrusions. "Spina bifida" is the term commonly used to refer to myelomeningocele.

Diagnosis

Elevated maternal alpha-fetoprotein (AFP) levels followed by ultrasound examination of the fetus may show an incomplete neural tube. An elevated AFP level in the maternal serum or amniotic fluid indicates the probability of central nervous system abnormalities. Additional examination may confirm this and allow the pregnant woman the opportunity to consider terminating the pregnancy. The best time to perform these tests is between 13 and 15 weeks' gestation, when peak levels are reached. Most obstetric health care providers recommend doing AFP testing.

Diagnosis of the newborn with spina bifida is made from clinical observation and examination. Additional evaluation of the defect may include magnetic resonance imaging (MRI), ultrasonography, computed tomography, and myelography. The newborn needs to be examined carefully for other associated defects, particularly hydrocephalus, genitourinary defects, and orthopedic anomalies.

Treatment

Many specialists are involved in the treatment of these newborns, especially in the case of myelomeningocele. These specialists may include neurologists, neurosurgeons, orthopedic specialists, pediatricians, urologists, and physical therapists. After a thorough evaluation of the newborn, a plan of surgical repair and treatment is developed.

Highly skilled nursing care is necessary in all aspects of the newborn's care. The child requires years of ongoing follow-up and therapy. Surgery is required to close the open defect but may not be performed immediately, depending on the surgeon's decision. Waiting a few days does not seem to cause additional problems, and this period gives the family an opportunity to adjust to the initial shock and become involved in making the necessary decisions.

Nursing Process and Care Plan *for the Newborn With Myelomeningocele*

Assessment (Data Collection)

A routine newborn examination is conducted with emphasis on neurologic impairment. When collecting data during the examination, observe the movement and response to stimuli of the lower extremities. Carefully measure the head circumference and examine the fontanels (fontanelles). Thoroughly document the observations made. When handling the newborn, take great care to prevent injury to the sac.

The family needs support and understanding during the newborn's initial care and for the many years of care during the child's life. Determine the family's knowledge and understanding of the defect as well as their attitude concerning the birth of a newborn with such serious problems.

Nursing Care Focus

When selecting nursing care focuses for the newborn with myelomeningocele, the concerns related to infection, impaired skin integrity, and neuromuscular issues are included. In caring for the family, recognize that coping might be compromised. There is a need for reinforcing teaching related to the care of the newborn with neurologic and musculoskeletal defects.

Outcome Identification and Planning: Preoperative Care

The preoperative goals for care of the newborn with myelomeningocele include preventing infection, maintaining skin integrity, preventing trauma related to disuse, increasing family coping skills, education about the condition, and support.

Nursing Care Focus

- Infection risk related to vulnerability of the myelomeningocele sac

Goal

- The newborn will be free from signs and symptoms of infection.

Implementations for Preventing Infection

Monitor the newborn's vital signs, neurologic signs, and behavior frequently to observe for any deviations from normal that may indicate an infection. Prophylactic antibiotics may be ordered. Carry out routine aseptic techniques with conscientious handwashing, gloving, and gowning, as appropriate. Until surgery is performed, the sac must be covered with a sterile dressing moistened in a warm sterile solution (often sterile saline). Moisten the dressing every 2 hours; do not allow it to dry to avoid damage to the covering of the sac. The dressings may be covered with a plastic protective covering. Maintain the newborn in a prone position so that no pressure is placed on the sac. After surgery, continue this positioning until the surgical site is well healed.

Diapering is not advisable with a low defect, but the sac must be protected from contamination with fecal material. Placing a protective barrier between the anus and the sac may prevent this contamination. If the anal sphincter muscles are involved, the newborn may have continual loose stools, which adds to the challenge of keeping the sac free from infection.

Evaluation of Goal/Desired Outcome

The newborn:

- has vital and neurologic signs that are within normal limits.
- shows no signs of irritability or lethargy.

Nursing Care Focus

- Altered skin integrity risk related to exposure to urine and feces

Goal

- The newborn will have no evidence of skin breakdown.

Implementations for Promoting Skin Integrity

The nursing interventions discussed in the previous section on infection are also necessary to promote skin integrity around the area of the defect and the diaper area. As mentioned, leakage of stool and urine may be continual. This leakage causes skin irritation and breakdown if the newborn is not kept clean and the diaper area is not free of stool and urine. Scrupulous perineal care is necessary.

Evaluation of Goal/Desired Outcome

The newborn's skin:

- remains clean, dry, and intact.
- has no areas of reddening or signs of irritation.

Nursing Care Focus

- Injury risk related to neuromuscular impairment

Goal

- The newborn will remain free from injury.

Implementations for Preventing Contractures of Lower Extremities

Newborns with spina bifida often have clubfoot (talipes equinovarus) and developmental dysplasia of the hip (DDH) (dislocation of the hip), both of which are discussed in the "Skeletal System Defects" section later in this chapter. If there is loss of motion in the lower limbs because of the defect, perform range-of-motion exercises to prevent contractures. Position the newborn so that the hips are abducted and the feet are in a neutral position. Massage the knees and other bony prominences with lotion regularly, then pad them, and protect them from irritation. As stated, avoid putting pressure on the sac during care activities.

Evaluation of Goal/Desired Outcome

- The newborn's lower limbs show no evidence of contractures.

Nursing Care Focus

- Family coping impairment related to the perceived loss of the perfect newborn

Goal

- The family caregivers will show positive signs of beginning coping.

Implementations for Promoting Family Coping

The family of a newborn with such a major anomaly is in a state of shock on first learning of the problems.

Be especially sensitive to their needs and emotions. Encourage family members to express their feelings and emotions as openly as possible. Recognize that some families express emotions much more freely than others do, and adjust your responses to the family with this in mind. Provide privacy as needed for the family to mourn together over their loss, but do not avoid the family because this only exaggerates their feelings of loss and depression. If possible, encourage the family members to cuddle or touch the newborn using proper precautions for the safety of the defect. With the permission of the health care provider, the newborn may be held in a chest-to-chest position to provide closer contact.

Evaluation of Goal/Desired Outcome

The family members:

- verbalize their anxieties and needs.
- hold, cuddle, and soothe the newborn as appropriate.

Nursing Care Focus

- Knowledge deficiency of the family caregivers related to the complexities of caring for a newborn with serious neurologic and musculoskeletal defects

Goal

- The family caregivers will learn to care for the newborn.

Implementations for Reinforcing Family Teaching

Give family members information about the defect, and encourage them to discuss their concerns and ask questions. Provide information about the newborn's present state, the proposed surgery, and follow-up care. Remember that anxiety may block understanding and processing knowledge, so information may need to be repeated. Provide information in small segments to facilitate learning.

After surgery, the family needs to be prepared to care for the newborn at home. Encourage the family to hold the newborn's head, neck, and chest slightly raised in one hand during feeding. Also, remind them that stroking the newborn's cheek helps stimulate sucking. Showing the family how to care for the newborn, allowing them to participate in the care, and guiding them in performing return demonstrations are all methods to use in reinforcing family teaching.

For long-term care and support, refer the family to the Spina Bifida Association (http://spinabifidaassociation.org). Give them materials concerning spina bifida. These children need long-term care involving many aspects of medicine and surgery. Although children with spina bifida have many long-term problems, their intelligence is not affected; many of these children grow into productive young adults who may live independently.

Evaluation of Goal/Desired Outcome

The family:

- demonstrates competence in performing care for the newborn.
- verbalizes understanding of the signs and symptoms that should be reported.
- has information about support agencies.

Hydrocephalus

Hydrocephalus is a condition characterized by an excess of cerebral spinal fluid (CSF) within the ventricular and subarachnoid spaces of the cranial cavity. Normally, a delicate balance exists between the rate of formation and absorption of CSF; the entire volume is absorbed and replaced every 12 to 24 hours. In hydrocephalus, this balance is disturbed.

CSF is formed mainly in the lateral ventricles by the choroid plexus and is absorbed into the venous system through the arachnoid villi. CSF circulates within the ventricles and the subarachnoid space. It is a colorless fluid consisting of water with traces of protein, glucose, and lymphocytes.

In the *noncommunicating* type of congenital hydrocephalus, an obstruction occurs, and CSF is not able to pass between the ventricles and the spinal cord. The blockage causes increased pressure on the brain or spinal cord. One of the most common causes of noncommunicating hydrocephalus occurs when there is a narrowing in the aqueduct of Sylvius (Fig. 21-3).

In the *communicating* type of hydrocephalus, no obstruction of the free flow of CSF exists between the ventricles and the spinal theca; rather the condition is caused by defective absorption of CSF, which increases pressure on the brain or spinal cord. Congenital hydrocephalus is most often the obstructive or noncommunicating type.

 Concept Mastery Alert

In communicating hydrocephalus, there is defective absorption of the CSF. In noncommunicating hydrocephalus, an obstruction occurs, and CSF is not able to pass between the ventricles and the spinal cord.

Hydrocephalus may be recognized at birth, or it may not be evident until after a few weeks or months of life. The condition may not be congenital but instead may occur during later infancy or during childhood as the result of a neoplasm, a head injury, or an infection such as meningitis.

When hydrocephalus occurs early in life before the skull sutures close, the soft, pliable bones separate to allow head expansion. This condition is manifested by a rapid increase in head circumference. The fact that the soft bones can yield to pressure in this manner may partially explain why many of these newborns fail to show the usual symptoms of brain pressure and may exhibit little or no damage

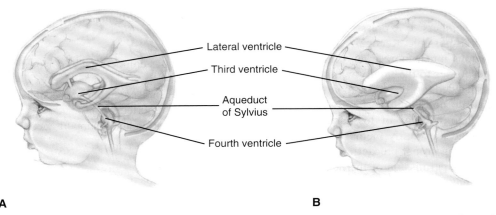

Lateral ventricle

Third ventricle

Aqueduct of Sylvius

Fourth ventricle

A   **B**

FIGURE 21-3 A. Infant *without* hydrocephalus. Note the ventricles of the brain and channels for the normal flow of cerebrospinal fluid. **B.** Infant *with* hydrocephalus. Note broadening of the forehead and large head size.

in mental function until later in life. Other newborns show severe brain damage, which has often occurred before birth.

Clinical Manifestations

An excessively large head at birth is suggestive of hydrocephalus. Rapid head growth with widening cranial sutures is also strongly suggestive and may be the first manifestation of this condition. An apparently large head in itself is not necessarily significant. The newborn's head is measured at birth, and the rate of growth is checked at subsequent examinations. If a newborn's head appears to be abnormally large at birth or appears to be enlarging, it should be measured frequently.

As the head enlarges, the suture lines separate and the spaces may be felt through the scalp. The anterior fontanel (fontanelle) becomes tense and bulging, the skull enlarges in all diameters, and the scalp becomes shiny and its veins dilate (Fig. 21-4).

If pressure continues to increase without intervention, the eyes appear to be pushed downward slightly with the sclera visible above the iris—the so-called setting sun sign.

If the condition progresses without adequate drainage of excessive fluid, the head becomes increasingly heavy, the neck muscles fail to develop sufficiently, and the newborn

has difficulty raising or turning the head. Unless hydrocephalus is arrested, the newborn becomes increasingly helpless and symptoms of increased intracranial pressure (IICP) develop. These symptoms may include irritability, restlessness, personality change, high-pitched cry, ataxia, projectile vomiting, failure to thrive, seizures, severe headache, changes in level of consciousness, and papilledema.

Diagnosis

Positive diagnosis of hydrocephalus is made with computed tomography and MRI. Echoencephalography and ventriculography may also be performed for further definition of the condition.

Treatment

Surgical intervention is the only effective means of relieving brain pressure and preventing additional damage to the brain tissue. If minimal brain damage has occurred, the child may be able to function within a normal mental range. Motor function is usually lagging. In some instances, surgical intervention may remove the cause of the obstruction, such as a neoplasm, a cyst, or a hematoma, but most children require placement of a shunting device that bypasses the point of obstruction, draining the excess cerebral spinal fluid (CSF) into a body cavity. This procedure arrests excessive head growth and prevents additional brain damage.

Many shunt procedures use a silicone rubber catheter that is radiopaque so that its position may be checked by x-ray examination. The silicone rubber catheter reduces the problem of tissue reaction. A valve or regulator is an essential part of each catheter that prevents excessive buildup of fluid or too-rapid decompression of the ventricle. The most common procedure, particularly for newborns and small children, is **ventriculoperitoneal shunting** (VP shunt). In this procedure, the CSF is drained from a lateral ventricle in the brain; the CSF runs through the subcutaneous catheter and empties into the peritoneal cavity (Fig. 21-5).

This procedure allows the insertion of some excess tubing to accommodate growth. As the child grows, the catheter needs to be revised and lengthened.

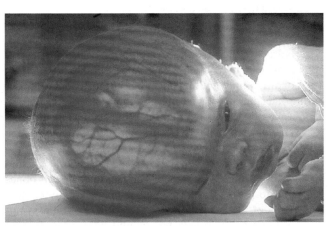

FIGURE 21-4 A newborn with hydrocephalus. Note the pull on the eyes giving the "setting sun" appearance.

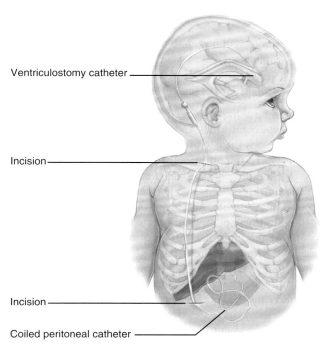

FIGURE 21-5 Ventriculoperitoneal shunting to drain excess cerebrospinal fluid in hydrocephalus.

Other pathways of drainage have been used with varying degrees of success. All types of shunts may have problems with kinking, blocking, moving, or shifting of tubing. The danger of infection in the tubing is a constant concern. Children with shunts must be observed constantly for signs of malfunction or infection.

The long-term outcome for a child with hydrocephalus depends on several factors. If untreated, the outcome is very poor, often leading to death. With shunting, the outcome depends on the initial cause of the increased fluid, the treatment of the cause, the brain damage sustained before shunting, complications with the shunting system, and continued long-term follow-up. Some of these children can lead relatively normal lives if they have follow-up and revisions as they grow.

Nursing Process and Care Plan *for the Postoperative Newborn With Hydrocephalus*

Assessment (Data Collection)

Obtaining accurate vital and neurologic signs is necessary before and after surgery. Measurement of the newborn's head is essential. If the fontanels (fontanelles) are not closed, carefully observe them for any signs of bulging. Observe, report, and document all signs of increased intracranial pressure (IICP). If the child has returned for revision of an existing shunt, obtain a complete history before surgery from the family caregiver to provide a baseline of the child's behavior.

Determine the level of knowledge family members have about the condition. For the family of the newborn or young infant, the diagnosis will probably come as an emotional shock. Conduct the interview and examination of the newborn with sensitivity and understanding.

Nursing Care Focus

When selecting nursing care focuses in the postoperative care of the newborn with hydrocephalus, keeping the infant safe from concerns of increased intracranial pressure (IICP) is included. Decreased mobility and the presence of a shunt require care to prevent skin breakdown and infection. Meeting growth and development needs of the newborn is important. Family caregiver anxiety as well as reinforcing family teaching is incorporated into nursing care.

Outcome Identification and Planning

The goals for the postoperative care of the newborn with shunt placement for hydrocephalus include preventing injury, maintaining skin integrity, preventing infection, promoting growth and development, and reducing family anxiety. Family goals include increasing knowledge about the condition and providing loving, supportive care to the newborn.

Nursing Care Focus

- Injury risk related to increased intracranial pressure (IICP)

Goal

- The newborn will be free from injury related to complications of excessive cerebral spinal fluid (CSF).

Implementations for Preventing Injury

At least every 2 to 4 hours, monitor the newborn's level of consciousness. Check the pupils for equality and reaction, monitor the neurologic status, and observe for a shrill cry, lethargy, or irritability. Measure and record the head circumference daily, Carry out appropriate procedures to care for the shunt as directed. To prevent a rapid decrease in ICP, keep the newborn flat. Observe for signs of seizure, and initiate seizure precautions. Keep suction and oxygen equipment convenient at the bedside.

Evaluation of Goal/Desired Outcome

The newborn:

- has no signs of IICP, such as lethargy, irritability, and seizure activity.
- has a stable level of consciousness.

Nursing Care Focus

● Altered skin integrity risk related to pressure from physical immobility

Goal

● The newborn's skin will remain intact.

Implementations for Promoting Skin Integrity

After a shunting procedure, keep the newborn's head turned away from the operative site until the health care provider allows a change in position. If the newborn's head is enlarged, prevent pressure sores from forming on the side where the child rests. Reposition the newborn at least every 2 hours as permitted. Inspect the dressings over the shunt site immediately after the surgery, every hour for the first 3 to 4 hours, and then at least every 4 hours.

This is Important!

Always support the head of a newborn with hydrocephalus when picking up, moving, or positioning. Using egg crate pads, lamb's wool, or a special mattress can prevent pressure and breakdown of the scalp.

Evaluation of Goal/Desired Outcome

● The newborn's skin shows no evidence of pressure sores, redness, or other signs of skin breakdown.

Nursing Care Focus

● Infection risk related to the presence of a shunt

Goal

● The newborn will remain free of infection.

Implementations for Preventing Infection

Infection is the primary threat after surgery. Closely observe for and promptly report any signs of infection, which include redness, heat, or swelling along the surgical site; fever; and signs of lethargy. Perform wound care thoroughly as ordered. Administer antibiotics as prescribed.

Evaluation of Goal/Desired Outcome

The newborn:

● shows no signs of infection.
● has stable vital signs.
● has no redness, drainage, or swelling at the surgical site.

Nursing Care Focus

● Risk for delayed growth and development related to impaired ability to achieve developmental tasks

Goal

● The newborn will have age-appropriate growth and development.

Implementations for Promoting Growth and Development

Every newborn has the need to be picked up and held, cuddled, and comforted. An uncomfortable or painful experience increases the need for emotional support. A newborn perceives such support principally through physical contact made in a soothing, loving manner.

The newborn needs social interaction and needs to be talked to, played with, and given the opportunity for activity. Provide toys appropriate for their physical and mental capacity. If the child has difficulty moving about the crib, place toys within easy reach and vision; a cradle gym, for example, may be tied close enough for the newborn to maneuver its parts.

Unless the newborn's nervous system is so impaired that all activity increases irritability, the newborn needs stimulation just as any child does. If repositioning from side to side means turning the newborn away from the sight of activity, the crib may be turned around so that vision is not obstructed.

A newborn who is given the contact and support that all newborns require develops a pleasing personality because they are nourished by emotional stimulation. Use the time spent on physical care as a time for social interaction. Talking, laughing, and playing with the newborn are important aspects of the newborn's care. Make frequent contacts, and do not limit them to the times when physical care is being performed.

Evaluation of Goal/Desired Outcome

The newborn:

● has social and developmental needs met.
● interacts and plays appropriately with toys and surroundings.

Nursing Care Focus

● Caregiver anxiety related to fear of surgical outcome

Goal

● The family caregiver's anxiety will be reduced.

Implementations for Reducing Family Anxiety

Explain to the family the condition and the surgical procedure in terms they can understand. Discuss the overall prognosis for the child. Encourage family members to express their anxieties and ask questions. Giving accurate, nontechnical answers is extremely helpful. Give the family information about support groups, such as the

National Hydrocephalus Foundation (www.nhfonline.org), and encourage them to contact the groups.

Evaluation of Goal/Desired Outcome

The family:

- expresses fears and concerns.
- interacts appropriately with the newborn.

Nursing Care Focus

- Knowledge deficiency related to the family's understanding of the child's condition and home care

Goal

- The family will learn how to care for the child.

Implementations for Reinforcing Family Teaching

Demonstrate care of the shunt to the family caregivers and have them perform a return demonstration. Provide them with a list of signs and symptoms that should be reported. Review these with the family members and make sure they understand them. Discuss appropriate growth and developmental expectations for the child, and stress realistic goals.

Evaluation of Goal/Desired Outcome

The family:

- participates in the care of the newborn.
- asks appropriate questions.
- lists signs and symptoms to report.

Cardiovascular System Defects: Congenital Heart Disease

Cardiovascular system defects range from mild to severe. They may be detected immediately at birth or may not be detected for several months. When a newborn is suspected of having a heart abnormality, the family is understandably upset. The heart is *the* vital organ; a person can live without a number of other organs and appendages, but life itself depends on the heart. The family caregivers will have many questions. The nurse may answer some; the health care provider must answer others. Many answers will not be available until after various evaluation procedures have been conducted.

Technologic advances have progressed rapidly in this field, making earlier detection and successful repair much more likely. However, heart defects are still the leading cause of death from congenital anomalies in the first year of life. A brief review of the development and function of the embryonic heart is useful to understanding the malformations that occur.

Development of the Heart

The heart begins beating early in the third to eighth week of intrauterine life. When first formed, the heart is a simple tube receiving blood from the placenta and pumping it out into its developing body. During this period, the heart rapidly develops into its normal, but complex, four-chambered structure.

Fetal circulation is unique. The fetal lungs are inactive, requiring only a small amount of blood to nourish their tissues. Blood is circulated through the umbilical arteries to the placenta, where waste products and carbon dioxide are exchanged for oxygen and nutrients. The blood is then returned to the fetus through the umbilical vein.

At birth, the umbilical cord is cut, and the newborn's own independent circulatory system is established. Certain circulatory bypasses, such as the *ductus arteriosus*, the *foramen ovale*, and the *ductus venosus*, are no longer necessary (see Chapter 5). They close during the first several weeks after birth. In addition, the pressure in the heart, which has been higher on the right side during fetal life, now changes so that the left side of the heart has the higher pressure (Fig. 21-6).

During this period of complex development, any error in formation may cause serious circulatory difficulty. The incidence of cardiovascular malformations is about 9 in 1,000 live births. Some abnormalities are slight and allow the person to lead a normal life without correction. Others cause little apparent difficulty but need correction to improve the chance for a longer life and for optimal health. Some severe anomalies are incompatible with life for more than a short time; others may be helped but not cured by surgery.

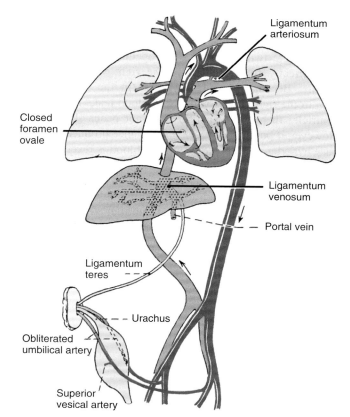

FIGURE 21-6 Normal blood circulation in the newborn. Highlighted ligaments indicate pathways that should close at or soon after birth. *Arrows* indicate normal flow of blood.

Common Types of Congenital Heart Defects

Traditionally, congenital heart defects have been described as cyanotic or acyanotic conditions. **Cyanotic heart disease** implies an oxygen saturation of the peripheral arterial blood of 85% or less. This condition occurs when a heart defect allows any appreciable amount of oxygen-poor blood in the right side of the heart to mix with the oxygenated blood in the left side of the heart (*right-to-left shunting*). Defects that permit right-to-left shunting may occur at the atrial, ventricular, or aortic level. However, because defects are often complex and occur in various combinations, this is an inadequate means of classification. A more clear-cut classification system is based on blood flow characteristics.

● Increased pulmonary blood flow (e.g., ventricular septal, atrial septal, and patent ductus arteriosus).
● Obstruction of blood flow out of the heart (e.g., coarctation of the aorta).
● Decreased pulmonary blood flow (e.g., tetralogy of Fallot).
● Mixed blood flow, where saturated and desaturated blood mix in the heart, aorta, and pulmonary vessels (e.g., transposition of the great arteries).

Because defects often occur in combination, they give rise to complex situations. Most nurses may never see many of the complex defects and most of the rare, isolated defects. The conditions discussed here are common enough that you need to be familiar with their diagnosis and treatment.

Ventricular Septal Defect

Ventricular septal defect is the most common intracardiac defect. It consists of an abnormal opening in the septum between the two ventricles. The opening allows blood to pass directly from the left to the right ventricle during systole. Because pressure is higher in the left ventricle than in the right, no unoxygenated blood leaks into the left ventricle; therefore, cyanosis does not occur (Fig. 21-7). However, if pulmonary vascular resistance produces pulmonary hypertension, then the shunt of blood is reversed from the right to the left ventricle, resulting in cyanosis.

Small, isolated defects are usually without symptoms and are often discovered during routine physical examinations. A characteristic loud, harsh murmur associated with a systolic thrill is occasionally heard on examination. A history of frequent respiratory infections may occur during infancy, but growth and development are unaffected. The child leads a normal life.

Corrective surgery may be postponed until the age of 18 months to 2 years, when the surgical risk is less than that for newborns. However, improved surgical techniques enable the repair to be made in the first year of life with high rates of success. The child is closely observed and may be prescribed a regimen of prophylactic antibiotics to prevent frequent respiratory infections. If pulmonary involvement becomes a problem, the repair is done without further delay. Repairs in children who are at high risk are done by the use of cardiac catheterization procedures.

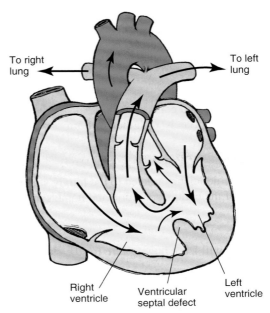

FIGURE 21-7 A ventricular septal defect is an abnormal opening between the right and the left ventricles. Ventricular septal defects vary in size and may occur in the membranous or muscular portion of the ventricular septum.

Atrial Septal Defect

An **atrial septal defect** is an abnormal opening between the right and left atria. The opening may be the result of an incompetent foramen ovale or incorrect development of the atrial septum (Fig. 21-8). In general, left-to-right shunting occurs in all true atrial septal defects. However, many healthy people have a patent foramen ovale that normally causes no problems because its valve is anatomically structured to withstand left chamber pressure, rendering it functionally closed.

True atrial septal defects are common heart anomalies and may occur as isolated defects or in combination with other heart anomalies. Atrial septal defects are amenable to surgery with a low surgical mortality risk. The surgical repair may be performed in a dry field using a heart–lung bypass machine. The opening is closed with sutures or a Dacron patch.

Patent Ductus Arteriosus

In fetal circulation, the ductus arteriosus is a vascular channel between the left main pulmonary artery and the descending aorta. It allows blood to bypass the nonfunctioning lungs and go directly from the pulmonary artery to the aorta and into the systemic circuit. After birth, the duct normally closes, eventually becoming obliterated and forming the ligamentum arteriosum. However, if the ductus arteriosus remains patent after birth, the higher pressure in the aorta reverses the direction of blood flow in the ductus. Blood is then shunted from the aorta into the pulmonary artery. This situation results in a flooding of the lungs and an overloading of the left heart chambers (Fig. 21-9).

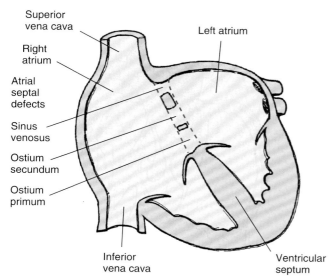

FIGURE 21-8 An atrial septal defect is an abnormal opening between the right and the left atria that allows left-to-right shunting of blood. The defect occurs most commonly because of an incompetent foramen ovale. The three types of atrial septal defects are identified based on the location of the opening: (1) a sinus venosus defect; (2) an ostium secundum defect, an opening in the middle of the septum that results from abnormal development of the septum secundum; and (3) an ostium primum defect, an opening at the lower end of the septum that results from improper development of the septum primum.

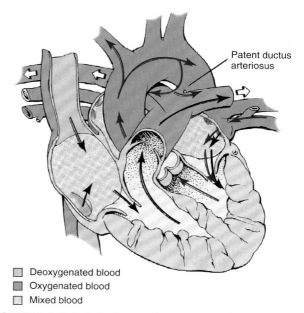

□ Deoxygenated blood
■ Oxygenated blood
□ Mixed blood

FIGURE 21-9 Patent ductus arteriosus occurs when the ductus arteriosus fails to close soon after birth. If the ductus fails to close, the blood is shunted from the aorta to the pulmonary artery rather than going into the systemic circulation.

Normally, the ductus arteriosus is nonpatent after the first or second week of life and should be obliterated by the fourth month. Why it fails to close is unknown. Patent ductus arteriosus is common in newborns who exhibit the rubella syndrome, but most newborns with this anomaly have no history of exposure to rubella during fetal life. It is also common in preterm newborns and in newborns with Down syndrome.

Symptoms of patent ductus arteriosus are often absent during childhood. Growth and development may be lagging in some children, with an easy fatigability and dyspnea on exertion. The diagnosis may be based on a characteristic machine-like murmur over the pulmonary area, a wide pulse pressure, and a bounding pulse. An echocardiogram shows the extent of the abnormal opening and confirms the diagnosis. Cardiac catheterization is also diagnostic but is not required in the presence of classic clinical features.

Indomethacin (Indocin), a prostaglandin inhibitor, may be administered with some success to premature newborns to promote closure of the ductus arteriosus. If this fails to close the ductus, surgery is indicated in all diagnosed cases, even if they are without symptoms. Some people live normal life spans without correction, but the risks of the defect far outweigh the surgical risks. Surgical correction consists of closure of the defect by ligation or by division of the ductus. Division is the method of choice if the child's condition permits because the ductus occasionally reopens after ligation. The optimal age for surgery is before the age of 2 years, with earlier surgery for severely affected newborns. Prognosis is excellent after a successful repair.

Coarctation of the Aorta

Coarctation of the aorta is a constriction or narrowing of the aortic arch or the descending aorta usually adjacent to the ligamentum arteriosum (Fig. 21-10). The constriction obstructs blood flow through the aorta, increasing left ventricular pressure and workload.

Most children with this congenital condition have no symptoms until later childhood or young adulthood. This delay of symptoms occurs because in the average child, blood is able to bypass the constricted portion of the aorta by way of collateral circulation (chiefly through the branches of the subclavian and carotid arteries that arise from the arch of the aorta). Eventually, however, the enlarged collateral arteries erode the rib margins, and the rib notching may be visualized by x-ray examination. A few newborns do have severe symptoms in their first year of life; they show dyspnea, tachycardia, and cyanosis, which are all signs of developing **congestive heart failure (CHF)**.

In older children, the condition is easily diagnosed based on hypertension in the upper extremities and hypotension in the lower extremities. The radial pulse is readily palpable, but the femoral pulses are weak or even impalpable. Blood pressure is normal or elevated in the arms and is low or undetectable in the legs. A high-pitched systolic murmur is usually present and heard over the base of the heart and in the suprasternal notch. The diagnosis may be confirmed by echocardiogram which shows the extent of the narrowing.

Uncorrected coarctation may cause hypertension and cardiac failure later in life. The optimal age for elective surgery is before the age of 2 years. Early surgery may be necessary for a gravely ill newborn who presents with severe CHF, especially if other congenital heart problems are present.

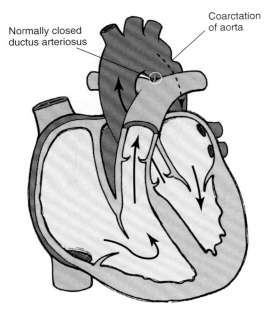

FIGURE 21-10 Coarctation of the aorta is characterized by a narrowed aortic lumen. It exists as a preductal or postductal obstruction, depending on the position of the obstruction in relation to the ductus arteriosus. The defect obstructs blood flow through the aorta, causing an increased left ventricular pressure and workload.

Surgery consists of resection of the coarcted area with an end-to-end anastomosis of the proximal and distal ends of the aorta. Occasionally, a long defect may necessitate an end-to-end graft using tubes of Dacron or similar material. Prognosis is excellent for the restoration of normal function after surgery.

Tetralogy of Fallot

Tetralogy of Fallot is a fairly common congenital heart defect. It consists of a grouping of heart defects (tetralogy denotes four abnormal conditions): (1) **pulmonary stenosis**, (2) **ventricular septal defect**, (3) **overriding aorta**, and (4) **right ventricular hypertrophy**. The pulmonary stenosis is usually seen as a narrowing of the upper portion of the right ventricle and may include stenosis of the valve cusps. Pulmonary stenosis results, in turn, in right ventricular hypertrophy (increase in size). The aorta appears to straddle the ventricular septum, overriding the ventricular septal defect. This defect allows a shunt of unsaturated blood from the right ventricle into the aorta or into the left ventricle (Fig. 21-11).

Tetralogy of Fallot is the most common defect causing cyanosis. The child with this defect may be precyanotic in early infancy, with the cyanotic phase starting at 4 to 6 months of age. However, some severely affected newborns may show cyanosis earlier. As long as the ductus arteriosus remains open, enough blood apparently passes through the lungs to prevent cyanosis.

The severity of symptoms depends on the degree of pulmonary stenosis, the size of the ventricular septal defect, and the degree to which the aorta overrides the septal defect.

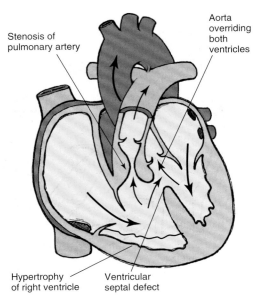

FIGURE 21-11 Tetralogy of Fallot is characterized by the combination of four defects: (1) pulmonary stenosis, (2) ventricular septal defect, (3) overriding aorta, and (4) hypertrophy of the right ventricle.

The infant presents with feeding difficulties and poor weight gain, resulting in slowed growth and development. Dyspnea and easy fatigability become evident. Exercise tolerance depends in part on the severity of the disease; some children become fatigued after little exertion. In the past, on experiencing fatigue, breathlessness, and increased cyanosis, the child was described as assuming a squatting posture for relief. Squatting apparently increased the systemic oxygen saturation. However, squatting is rarely seen today because these newborns' defects usually are repaired by the time they are 2 years old.

Attacks of paroxysmal dyspnea are common during infancy and early childhood. An anoxic spell is heralded by sudden restlessness, gasping respiration, and increased cyanosis that lead to a loss of consciousness and possibly convulsions. These attacks, called "tet spells," last from a few minutes to several hours and appear to be unpredictable, although stress does seem to trigger some episodes.

The history and clinical manifestations are usually sufficient to make a diagnosis. However, echocardiogram, cardiac catheterization, electrocardiography, chest radiography, and laboratory tests to determine polycythemia and arterial oxygen saturation may be performed for additional definition.

The preferred repair of these defects is total surgical correction. This procedure requires the use of a cardiopulmonary bypass machine. The heart is opened, and extensive resection is done. The repair relieves the pulmonary stenosis, and the septal defect is closed by the use of a patch. Successful total correction transforms a grossly abnormal heart into a functionally normal one. A valve-sparing approach is usually attempted; however, some of these children are left without a pulmonary valve.

In infants who cannot withstand the total surgical correction until they are older, the Blalock–Taussig procedure is performed. This procedure is an end-to-end anastomosis of a vessel arising from the aorta, usually the subclavian artery, to the corresponding right or left pulmonary artery. These shunts are now seen only occasionally because total surgical repair has much greater success and lower mortality rates.

Transposition of the Great Arteries

In **transposition of the great arteries**, the aorta arises from the right ventricle instead of the left, and the pulmonary artery arises from the left ventricle instead of the right. These newborns are usually cyanotic from birth. This severe defect was once almost always fatal. However, advancements in diagnosis and treatment have increased the survival rate.

TEST YOURSELF

✔ What is the difference between spina bifida with meningocele and spina bifida with myelomeningocele?

✔ What does the newborn have an excess of in the condition of hydrocephalus? How is hydrocephalus treated?

✔ List the five common types of congenital heart defects.

Risk Factors

The preterm newborn has a high risk of having congenital heart disease. Maternal alcoholism, smoking and ingestion of certain drugs during pregnancy, maternal diabetes, and advanced maternal age (older than 40 years) increase the incidence of heart defects in newborns. Rubella in the expectant mother during the first trimester can also cause cardiac malformations. Maternal malnutrition and heredity may be contributing factors. Offspring of mothers who had congenital heart anomalies have a much higher risk of having congenital heart anomalies. If one child in the family has a congenital heart abnormality, later siblings have a very high risk for such a defect.

Clinical Manifestations

The newborn with a severe cardiovascular abnormality, such as a transposition of the great vessels, is cyanotic from birth and requires oxygen and special treatment. A less seriously affected child, whose heart can compensate to some degree for the impaired circulation, may not have symptoms severe enough to call attention to the difficulty until they are a few months older and more active. Others may live a fairly normal life and not be aware of any heart trouble until a murmur or an enlarged heart is discovered during physical examination in later childhood.

A cardiac murmur discovered early in life necessitates frequent physical examinations. This murmur may be a functional, "innocent" murmur that may disappear as the child grows older, or it may be the chief manifestation of an abnormal heart or an abnormal circulatory system. The most common parental concern is that of feeding difficulties. Newborns with cardiac anomalies severe enough to cause circulatory difficulties have a history of being poor eaters, tiring easily from the effort to suck, and failing to grow or thrive normally. These manifestations of CHF may appear during the first year of life in newborns with conditions such as large ventricular septal defects, coarctation of the aorta, and other defects that place an increased workload on the ventricles.

Treatment and Nursing Care

Advances in medical technology have enabled heart repairs to be performed in newborns as young as less than 1-day old. Earlier diagnosis through the use of improved diagnostic techniques and sophisticated monitoring techniques have contributed to these advances.

Most health care providers now think it is important to operate as early as possible to repair defective hearts. Inadequate circulation may prevent adequate growth and development and cause permanent, irreparable physical, mental, and emotional damage. If the child receives a diagnosis early and correction or repair is possible, congestive heart failure (CHF) may be avoided.

In cases in which the child has CHF, it is important that the CHF be treated. The primary goals in the treatment of CHF are to reduce the workload of the heart and to improve the cardiac functioning, thus increasing oxygenation of the tissues. This is done by removing excess sodium and fluids, slowing the heart rate, and decreasing the demands on the heart. See Chapter 37 for a complete discussion of CHF and its treatment.

Care at Home Before Surgery

A child with congenital heart disease may show easy fatigability and slowed growth. If the child has a cyanotic type of heart disease, clubbing of the fingers or toes, periods of cyanosis, and reduced exercise tolerance are evident. This young child may assume a squatting position, which reduces the return flow to the heart, thus temporarily reducing the workload of the heart.

Such a child should be allowed to lead as normal a life as possible. Families are naturally apprehensive and find it difficult not to overprotect the child. They often increase the child's anxiety and cause fear in the child about participating in normal activities. Children are rather sensible about finding their own limitations and usually limit their activities to their capacity if they are not made unduly apprehensive.

Some families can adjust well and provide guidance and security for the sick child. Others may become confused and frightened and show hostility, disinterest, or neglect; these families need support, guidance, and counseling. The primary nursing goal is to reduce anxiety in the child and family. This goal may be accomplished through open communication and ongoing contact.

Routine clinic visits become a way of life, and the child may come to feel different from other people. Health care providers and nurses have a responsibility both to the family caregivers and to the child to give clear explanations of the defect, using readily understandable terms and diagrams, pictures, or models. A child who knows what is happening can accept a great deal and can continue with the business of living.

Cardiac Catheterization

Cardiac catheterization may be performed before heart surgery to obtain more accurate information about the child's condition. The child or newborn is sedated or anesthetized for this process, and a radiopaque catheter is inserted through an artery or vein into the right atrium. In the newborn or young child, the femoral vein is often used. Close observation of the child after the procedure is essential. Carefully monitor the site used and check the extremity for pulses, edema, skin temperature and color, and any other signs of poor circulation or infection. A pressure dressing is used over the catheterization site and left in place until the day after the procedure. The dressing should be snug and intact and monitored closely for any signs of bleeding from the site. The child is kept flat in bed with the extremity straight for as long as 6 hours after the procedure. Monitor vital signs closely.

Preoperative Preparation

When a child enters the hospital for cardiac surgery, it is seldom a first admission; generally, it has been preceded by cardiac catheterization or perhaps other hospitalizations. The child may be admitted before surgery to allow time for preparation, or more often, preoperative procedures are done on an outpatient basis. Preoperative teaching should be given and reinforced for the family and the child at an age-appropriate level. They should understand that blood might be obtained for typing and cross-matching and for other laboratory tests. Additional diagnostic studies may be done.

The equipment to be used after surgery should be described with drawings and pictures. If possible, the family caregivers and the child should have the opportunity to see chest tubes and oxygen equipment. They should meet the nursing personnel and see the general appearance of the unit. Of course, use good judgment about the timing and the extent of such preparation; nothing is gained by arousing additional anxiety with premature or excessively graphic descriptions. The child should be given the opportunity to become familiar with the surgical clothing worn by personnel, oxygen and other equipment, and perhaps even use a stethoscope to listen to a heartbeat. The child should learn how to cough and should practice coughing. They should understand that coughing is important after surgery and must be done regularly, even though it may hurt.

Cardiac Surgery

Open-heart surgery using the heart–lung machine (cardiopulmonary bypass machine) has made extensive heart correction possible. Machines have been refined for use with newborns and small children. Heart transplants may be performed when no other treatment is possible.

Inducing **hypothermia**—reducing the body temperature to 68°F to 78.8°F (20°C to 26°C)—is a technique sometimes used in surgery. A reduced body temperature increases the time that the circulation may be stopped without causing concerns. The blood temperature is reduced by the use of cooling agents in the heart–lung machine. This also provides a dry, bloodless, motionless field for the surgeon.

Postoperative Care

At the end of surgery, the child is taken to the pediatric intensive care unit, where they are cared for and managed for several days.

By the time the child returns to the regular pediatric unit, chest drainage tubes usually have been removed, and the child has started taking oral fluids and is ready to sit up in bed or in a chair. The child probably feels weak and helpless after such an experience and needs encouragement and reassurance. However, with recovery, a child is usually ready for activity. Family caregivers usually need to reorient themselves and accept their child's new status. This may not be easy for the family caregiver after what seemed like a long period of anxious watching. The surgeon makes necessary recommendations regarding resumption of the child's activities. Plans should be made for follow-up and supervision, as well as counseling and guidance.

Gastrointestinal System Defects

Most gastrointestinal system anomalies are apparent at birth or shortly thereafter. The anomalies are often the result of interruption of embryonic growth at a crucial stage. Many of these anomalies interfere with the normal nutrition and digestion essential to the newborn's normal growth and development. Many anomalies require immediate surgical intervention.

Cleft Lip and Cleft Palate

Cleft lip and cleft palate are the most common facial malformations. Cleft lip occurs in about 3 in 10,000 live births and is more common in males. Cleft palate occurs in 6 in 10,000 live births, more often in females. Their causes are not entirely clear; they appear to be genetically influenced, but they sometimes occur in isolated instances with no genetic history. Although a cleft lip and a cleft palate often appear together, either defect may appear alone.

The cleft lip and cleft palate defects result from failure of the primary and secondary palates to fuse. If the maxillary processes do not fuse during the fifth to eighth weeks of intrauterine life, a cleft (fissure) occurs, resulting in a cleft lip. The secondary palate closes later in embryonic development, and the failure to close occurs for different reasons. In an 8-week-old embryo, there is still no roof to the mouth; the tissues that are to become the palate are two shelves running from the front to the back of the mouth and projecting vertically downward on either side of the tongue. The shelves move from a vertical position to a horizontal position; their free edges meet and fuse in midline. Later, bone forms within this tissue to form the hard palate, normally by the 10th to 12th week of fetal life. Exactly what happens to prevent this closure is not known for sure. The incidence of cleft palate is higher in the close relatives of people with the defect than it is in the general population, and some evidence indicates that environmental and hereditary factors play a part in this defect.

Clinical Manifestations

The cleft lip may be a simple notch in the vermilion line, or it may extend up into the floor of the nose (Fig. 21-12). It may be either **unilateral** (one side of the lip) or **bilateral** (both sides). The cleft palate may be a small opening or it may involve the entire palate (Fig. 21-13). The cleft palate occurs with a cleft lip about 50% of the time, most often with bilateral cleft lip. The child born with a cleft palate but with an intact lip does not have the external disfigurement that may be distressing to the new parent. However, the problems are more serious. The cleft palate is often accompanied by nasal deformity and dental disorders, such as deformed, missing, or **supernumerary** (excessive in number) teeth.

Diagnosis

The physical appearance of the newborn confirms the diagnosis of cleft lip. The diagnosis of cleft palate is made at birth with the close inspection of the newborn's palate. To be certain that a cleft palate is not missed, the examiner must insert a gloved finger into the newborn's mouth to feel the palate to determine that it is intact. If a cleft is found, consultation is set up with a health care provider specializing in cleft palate repair.

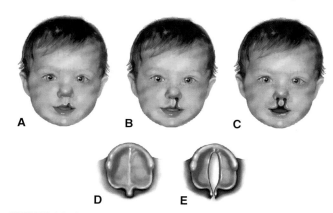

FIGURE 21-13 The cleft lip may be (**A**) a simple notch, (**B**) unilateral, or (**C**) bilateral. The cleft palate may (**D**) be a small opening or (**E**) involve the entire palate.

Treatment

Surgery, usually performed by a plastic surgeon, is a major part of the treatment of a newborn with a cleft lip, palate, or both. Total care involves many specialists, including pediatricians, nurses, orthodontists, prosthodontists, otolaryngologists, speech therapists, and occasionally psychiatrists. Long-term, intensive, multidisciplinary care is needed for newborns with major defects.

Plastic surgeons' opinions differ as to the best time for repair of the cleft lip. Some surgeons favor early repair, before the newborn is discharged from the hospital. They believe that early repair can alleviate some of the family's feelings of rejection of the newborn. Other surgeons prefer to wait until the newborn is 1 or 2 months old, weighs about 10 lb (4,536 g), and is gaining weight steadily. Newborns who are not born in medical centers with specialists on the staff are referred to a center or health care provider specializing in cleft lip and palate repair.

The goal in repairing the cleft palate is to give the child a union of the cleft parts to allow intelligible and pleasant speech and to avoid injury to the maxillary development. The timing of cleft palate repair is individualized according to the size, placement, and degree of deformity. The surgery may need to be done in stages over a period of years to achieve the best results. The optimal time for surgical repair of the cleft palate is considered to be between 6 months and 5 years of age. Earlier correction is preferred because the child cannot make certain sounds when starting to talk and undesirable speech habits are formed that are difficult to correct. If surgery must be delayed beyond the third year, a dental speech appliance may help the child develop intelligible speech.

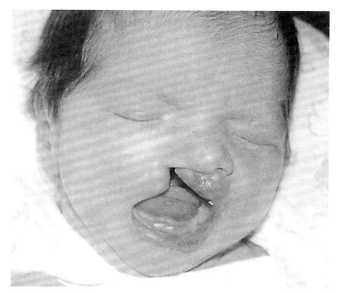

FIGURE 21-12 A cleft lip may extend up into the floor of the nose.

Nursing Process and Care Plan *for the Newborn With Cleft Lip and Cleft Palate*

The birth of a newborn with a facial deformity may change the atmosphere of the delivery from one of the joyous anticipation to one of the awkward tension. Although a facial deformity will often have been seen on a fetal ultrasound, it still may be a shock for the family seeing the facial disfigurement of a cleft lip. Their emotional reaction to such an obvious malformation is usually much stronger than to a "hidden" defect, such as congenital heart defect. They need encouragement and support, as well as considerable instruction about the newborn's feeding and care.

Assessment (Data Collection)

One primary concern in the nursing care of the newborn with a cleft lip with or without a cleft palate is the emotional care of the newborn's family. In interviewing the family and collecting data, explore the family's acceptance of the newborn. Practice active listening with reflective responses, accept the family's emotional responses, and demonstrate complete acceptance of the newborn.

The family caregivers who return to the hospital with their infant for the beginning repair of a cleft palate have already faced the challenges of feeding their infant. Conduct a thorough interview with the family caregiver that includes a question about the methods they found to be most effective in feeding the infant.

Physical examination of the infant includes temperature, apical pulse, and respirations. Listen to breath sounds to detect any pulmonary congestion. Observe skin turgor and color, noting any deviations from normal. In addition, observe the infant's neurologic status, noting alertness and responsiveness. Document a complete description of the cleft.

Nursing Care Focus (Preoperative)

Nursing care focuses for the newborn before cleft lip and cleft palate surgery include the nutritional needs of the infant. The cleft lip creates an inability for the infant to suck and may cause feeding issues. In caring for the family, recognize that coping might be compromised. The infant's condition and surgical outcome may cause anxiety for family caregivers. There is a need for reinforcing teaching related to the care of the child before surgery and to the surgical procedure itself.

Outcome Identification and Planning: Preoperative Care

Goal setting and planning must be modified to adapt to the surgical plans. If the newborn is to be discharged from the birth hospital to have surgery 1 to 2 months later, nursing care may focus on preparing the family to care for the newborn at home and helping them cope with their emotions. The major goals include maintaining adequate nutrition, increasing family coping, reducing the parents' anxiety and guilt regarding the newborn's physical defect, and preparing parents for the future repair of the cleft lip and palate.

Nursing Care Focus

- Malnutrition risk related to inability to suck secondary to cleft lip

Goal

- The newborn will show appropriate weight gain.

Implementations for Maintaining Adequate Nutrition

The newborn must be in good nutritional condition before surgery can be scheduled. However, feeding the newborn with a cleft lip or palate before repair is a challenge. Feeding may be time consuming and tedious because the newborn's ability to suck is inadequate. Breast-feeding may be successful because the breast tissue may mold to close the gap. If the newborn cannot breastfeed, the mother's breast milk may be expressed and used instead of formula until after the surgical repair heals. Various nipples and feeding devices may be tried to find the method that works best. A soft nipple with a crosscut made to promote easy flow of milk or formula may work well. A large nipple with holes that allow the milk to drip freely makes sucking easier. If the cleft lip is unilateral, the nipple should be aimed at the unaffected side. Sometimes an eyedropper or Asepto syringe with soft rubber tubing is used to drip formula slowly into the infant's mouth. The infant has high risk for aspiration, so the infant should be kept in an upright position during feeding to facilitate swallowing (Fig. 21-14).

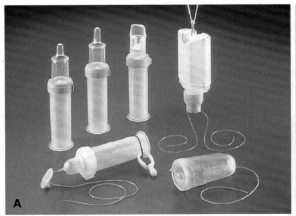
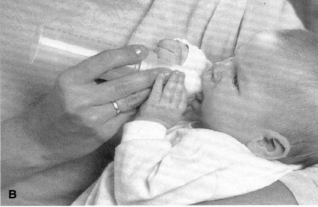

FIGURE 21-14 Specialty feeding devices used for the newborn with a cleft lip or palate include **(A)** special nipples and devices and **(B)** a special feeder.

If the infant does not have a cleft lip or if the lip has had an early repair, sucking may be learned more easily, even though the suction generated is not as good as in the infant with an intact palate. Special cleft palate nipples molded to fit into the open palate area to close the gap have been used with success.

As the newborn learns to eat, coughing, sputtering, and choking may occur. Be alert for signs of aspiration when feeding the newborn, and remind family caregivers to be alert as well.

Whatever feeding method is used, the experience may be frustrating for both the feeder and the newborn. Have family caregivers practice the feeding techniques under supervision. During the learning process, give them ample opportunity to ask questions so they feel able to care for the newborn (see Tips for Reinforcing Family Teaching: Cleft Lip/Cleft Palate).

Evaluation of Goal/Desired Outcome

- The newborn's weight increases at a predetermined goal of 1 oz or more per day.

TIPS FOR REINFORCING FAMILY TEACHING

Cleft Lip/Cleft Palate

- Sucking is important to speech development.
- Holding the baby upright while feeding helps avoid choking.
- Burp the baby frequently because a large amount of air is swallowed during feeding.
- Don't tire the baby. Limit feeding times to 20 to 30 minutes maximum. If necessary, feed the baby more often.
- Feed strained foods slowly from the side of the spoon in small amounts.
- Don't be alarmed if food seeps through the cleft and out the nose.
- Have baby's ears checked any time they have a cold or upper respiratory infection.
- Talk normally to baby (no "baby talk"). Talk often; repeat baby's babbling and cooing. This helps in speech development.
- Try to understand early talking without trying to correct the infant.
- Good mouth care is very important.
- Early dental care is essential to observe teething and prevent caries.

Nursing Care Focus

- Family caregiver's coping impairment and anxiety related to visible physical defect

Goal

- The family will demonstrate acceptance of the newborn. Family caregiver anxiety will be reduced.

Implementations for Promoting Family Coping and Reducing Anxiety

Encourage family members to verbalize their feelings regarding the defect and their disappointment. Convey to the family that their feelings are acceptable and normal. While caring for the newborn, demonstrate behavior that clearly displays acceptance of the newborn. Serve as a model for the family caregivers' attitudes toward the child.

Give the family caregivers information about cleft repairs. Pamphlets are available that present photographs of before and after corrections that will answer some of their questions. Encourage them to ask questions, and reassure them that any question is valid.

Evaluation of Goal/Desired Outcome

Family caregivers:

- verbalize their feelings about the newborn.
- cuddle and talk to the newborn.
- ask appropriate questions about surgery and openly discuss their concerns.
- voice reasonable expectations.

Cultural Snapshot

In some cultures, genetic defects are blamed on the mother—something she did or ate, stress or trauma that occurred during pregnancy, viewing a child with a defect caused her child to have the same defect. The mother may have feelings of guilt or fears of being an unacceptable mother and need nursing support.

Nursing Care Focus

- Knowledge deficiency of family caregivers related to the care of the child before surgery and the surgical procedure

Goal

- The family will learn how to care for the newborn and will have an understanding of surgical procedures.

Implementations for Reinforcing Family Teaching

Reinforcing teaching with the family caregivers regarding caring for the newborn and especially concerns with maintaining the newborn's nutritional status occurs from the infant's birth. By the time the infant is actually admitted for the repair, the family will have received a great amount of information, but all families need additional support throughout the procedure. Explain the usual routine of preoperative, intraoperative, and postoperative care. Written information is helpful, but be certain the parents understand the information. Simple things are important; show families where they may wait during surgery, inform them how long the surgery should last, tell them about the postanesthesia care unit procedure, and let them know where the surgeon will expect to find them to report on the surgery.

Evaluation of Goal/Desired Outcome

Family caregivers:

- demonstrate how to feed the newborn before surgery.
- ask appropriate questions.
- describe the surgical procedures.

Remember **Adrian Simmer.** What concerns did you determine that Adrian's parents have been dealing with? What nursing responsibilities will be important in Adrian's care preoperatively?

Nursing Care Focus (Postoperative)

Nursing care focuses applicable to the newborn after the surgical repair of a cleft lip or cleft palate include respiratory concerns related to a risk for aspiration and keeping the airway clear. Hydration and nutritional needs are important considerations since feeding is difficult following surgery. Pain, injury risk, and infection risk must be addressed in caring for the infant. Meeting growth and development needs of the newborn are important. Reinforcement of family teaching is incorporated into nursing care.

Outcome Identification and Planning: Postoperative Care

Major goals for the postoperative care of the infant who is hospitalized for surgical repair of cleft lip or palate include preventing aspiration, improving respiration, maintaining adequate fluid volume and nutritional requirements, relieving pain, preventing injury and infection of the surgical site, promoting normal growth and development, and increasing the family caregivers' knowledge about the child's long-term care.

Nursing Care Focus

- Ineffective airway clearance and risk of aspiration related to reduced level of consciousness after surgery

Goal

- The infant's respiratory tract will remain clear, the infant will breathe easily, and the respiratory rate will be within normal limits.

Implementations for Preventing Aspiration and Improving Respiration

To facilitate drainage of mucus and secretions, position the infant on the side, never on the abdomen, after a cleft

lip repair. The infant may be placed on the side or in an upright position after a cleft palate repair. Monitor the infant closely for any respiratory concerns in the immediate postoperative period. Do not put anything in the infant's mouth to clear mucus because of the danger of damaging the surgical site, particularly with a palate repair.

Immediately after a palate repair, the infant must change from a mouth-breathing pattern to nasal breathing. This change may frustrate the infant, so put the infant in an upright position to ease breathing. Given support, the infant should be able to adjust quickly.

Evaluation of Goal/Desired Outcome

The infant:

- has clear lung sounds with no aspiration.
- has a respiratory rate that stays within normal range.
- adjusts and breathes nasally with little stress.

Nursing Care Focus

- Dehydration risk related to NPO status after surgery

Goal

- The infant will show signs of adequate hydration during NPO period.

Implementations for Maintaining and Monitoring Fluid Volume

In the immediate postoperative period, the infant needs parenteral fluids. Follow all the usual precautions: check placement, discoloration of the site, swelling, and flow rate every 2 hours. Document the intake and output accurately. Parenteral fluids are continued until the infant can take oral fluids without vomiting.

Evaluation of Goal/Desired Outcome

The newborn:

- shows no evidence of parenteral fluid infiltration.
- has good skin turgor and moist mucous membranes.
- has adequate urine output.

Nursing Care Focus

- Malnutrition risk related to difficulty in feeding after surgery

Goal

- The infant will have adequate caloric intake and retain and tolerate oral nutrition.

Implementations for Maintaining Adequate Nutrition

As soon as the infant is no longer nauseated (vomiting should be avoided if possible), the surgeon usually permits clear liquids. After the cleft lip repair, no tension should be placed on the suture line to prevent the sutures from pulling apart and leaving a scar. A specialized feeder may need to be used because bottle feeding or breast-feeding may increase the tension on the suture line.

For an infant who has had a palate repair, no nipples, spoons, or straws are permitted; only a drinking glass or a cup is recommended. A favorite cup from home may be reassuring to the older infant. Offer clear liquids such as flavored gelatin water, apple juice, and synthetic fruit-flavored drinks. Red juices should not be given because they may conceal bleeding. Infants do not usually like broth. The diet is increased to full liquid, and the infant is usually discharged on a soft diet. When permitted, foods such as cooked infant cereals, ice cream, and flavored gelatin are often favorites. The surgeon determines the progression of the diet. Nothing hard or sharp should be placed in the infant's mouth. After each feeding, clear water is used to rinse the mouth and suture line.

Evaluation of Goal/Desired Outcome

The infant:

- does not experience nausea or vomiting.
- gains 0.75 to 1 oz/day (22 to 30 g/day) if younger than 6 months or 0.5 to 0.75 oz/day (13 to 22 g/day) if older than 6 months.

Nursing Care Focus

- Acute pain related to surgical procedure

Goal

- The infant's pain and discomfort will be minimized.

Implementations for Relieving Pain

Observe the infant for signs of pain or discomfort from the surgery. Administer ordered analgesics as needed. Relieving pain not only comforts the infant, but may also prevent crying, which is important because of the danger of disrupting the suture line. Make every effort to prevent the infant with a lip repair from crying to prevent excessive tension on the suture line.

Evaluation of Goal/Desired Outcome

- The infant rests quietly, does not cry, and is not fretful.

Nursing Care Focus

- Injury risk to the operative site related to the infant's desire to suck thumb or fingers

Goal

- The surgical site will remain free of injury.

Implementations for Preventing Postoperative Injury

Continuous, skilled observation is essential. Swollen mouth tissues cause excessive secretion of mucus that is handled poorly by a small infant. For the first few postoperative hours, never leave the infant alone because aspiration of mucus occurs quickly and easily. Because nothing is permitted in the infant's mouth, particularly the thumb or finger, elbow restraints are necessary. The thumb, although comforting, may quickly undo the repair or cause undesirable scarring along the suture line. The infant's ultimate well-being must take precedence over immediate satisfaction. Accustoming the infant to elbow restraints gradually before admission is helpful.

Elbow restraints must be applied properly and checked frequently (see Fig. 30-2 in Chapter 30). Place the restraints firmly around the arm and pin to the infant's shirt or gown to prevent them from sliding down below the elbow. The infant's arms can move freely but cannot bend at the elbows to reach the face. Apply the restraint snugly, but do not allow the circulation to be hindered. The older infant may also need to be placed in a jacket restraint. The use of restraints must be documented and circulation monitored closely.

Remove restraints at least every 2 hours; remove them only one at a time, and control the released arm so that the thumb or fingers do not pop into the mouth. Inspect and massage the skin, apply lotion, and perform range-of-motion exercises. Replace restraints when they become soiled. Explore various means of distracting and comforting the infant. Talk to the infant continuously while providing care.

> **Some Nurses Find This Approach Helpful**
> Playing "Peek-a-Boo" and other infant games will help to comfort and entertain the infant in restraints; however, "Patty Cake" does not work well with an infant in elbow restraints!

Evaluation of Goal/Desired Outcome

The infant:

- has an intact surgical site.
- puts nothing into the mouth such as thumb, fingers, straws, or sharp objects.

Nursing Care Focus

- Infection risk related to surgical incision

Goal

- The infant's incision site will remain free of signs and symptoms of infection.

Implementations for Preventing Infection

Aseptic technique is important while caring for the infant undergoing lip or palate repair. Good handwashing technique is essential. Instruct the family caregivers about the importance of preventing anyone with an upper respiratory infection from visiting the infant. Observe for signs of otitis media that may occur from drainage into the eustachian tube.

Care of Lip Suture Line

The lip suture line is left uncovered after the surgery and must be kept clean and dry to prevent infection and subsequent scarring. A wire bow called a Logan bow or a butterfly closure is applied across the upper lip and attached to the cheeks with adhesive tape to prevent tension on the sutures caused by crying or other facial movements (Fig. 21-15). Gently clean the infant's mouth with tepid water or clear liquid after feeding to clear the suture area of any food or liquids. Carefully clean the sutures after feeding and as often as necessary to prevent collection of dried formula or serum. Clean the sutures gently with sterile cotton swabs and saline or the solution of the surgeon's choice. Application of an ointment, such as bacitracin, may also be ordered. The care of the suture line is extremely important because it has a direct effect on the cosmetic appearance of the repair. Frequent gentle cleaning is essential as long as the sutures are in place. Reinforce teaching with the family about how to care for the suture line because the infant will most likely be discharged before the sutures are removed (7 to 10 days after surgery). The infant probably will be allowed to suck on a soft nipple at this time.

Evaluation of Goal/Desired Outcome

- The incisional site is clean with no redness or drainage.
- The infant's temperature is within normal limits.
- The caregivers and family members practice good hand-washing and aseptic techniques.

Nursing Care Focus

- Risk for delayed growth and development related to hospitalizations and surgery

Goal

- The infant will show evidence of normal growth and development.

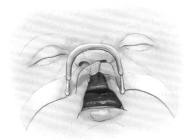

FIGURE 21-15 Logan bow for easing strain on sutures.

Implementations for Providing Sensory Stimulation

The infant needs stimulating, safe toys in the crib. Nurses and family caregivers must use every opportunity to provide sensory stimulation. Talking to the infant, cuddling and holding them, and responding to cries are important interventions. Provide freedom from restraints within the limitations of safety as much as possible. Family caregivers and healthcare personnel must encourage the older child to use speech and help enhance the child's self-esteem. An infant experiences emotional frustration because of restraints, so satisfaction must be provided in other ways. Rocking, snuggling, and other soothing techniques are important parts of nursing care and family caregiving.

Evaluation of Goal/Desired Outcome

The infant:

- is content most of the time and responds appropriately to the nurse and the family caregivers.
- engages in age- and development-appropriate activities within the limits of restraints.

Nursing Care Focus

- Knowledge deficiency of family caregivers related to long-term aspects of cleft palate

Goal

- The family will learn how to care for the infant's long-term needs.

Implementations for Reinforcing Family Teaching

After effective surgery and skilled, careful nursing care, the appearance of the infant's face should be improved greatly. The scar fades in time. Family caregivers need to know that the baby will probably need a slight adjustment of the vermilion line in later childhood, but they can expect a repair that is barely, if at all, noticeable.

Cleft lip and cleft palate centers have teams of specialists who can provide the services that these children and their families need through infancy, preschool, and the school years. Explain to the family caregivers the services offered by the healthcare professionals. These professionals can give explanations and counseling about the child's diet, speech training, immunizations, and general health. Encourage family caregivers to ask them any questions they may have. Be alert for any evidence that the caregivers need additional information, and arrange appropriate meetings.

Dental care for the deciduous teeth is even more important than usual. The incidence of dental caries is high in children with a cleft palate. Preservation of the deciduous teeth is important for the best results in speech and appearance.

Evaluation of Goal/Desired Outcome

The family caregivers:

- ask appropriate questions and respond appropriately to staff queries.
- describe services available for the child's long-term care.

Esophageal Atresia and Tracheoesophageal Fistula

Atresia is the absence of a normal body opening or the abnormal closure of a body passage. Esophageal atresia (EA) with or without fistula into the trachea is a serious congenital anomaly and is among the most common anomalies causing respiratory distress. This condition occurs in about 1 in 4,000 live births. Several types of EA occur; in more than 90% of affected newborns, the upper, or proximal, end of the esophagus ends in a blind pouch, and the lower, or distal, segment from the stomach is connected to the trachea by a fistulous tract (Fig. 21-16). This is referred to as a tracheoesophageal fistula.

Clinical Manifestations

Any mucus or fluid that a newborn swallows enters the blind pouch of the esophagus. This pouch soon fills and overflows, usually resulting in aspiration into the trachea. Few other conditions depend so greatly on careful nursing observation for early diagnosis and therefore improved chances of survival. The newborn with this disorder has frothing, excessive drooling, and periods of respiratory distress with coughing, choking, and cyanosis. Many newborns have difficulty with mucus, but be alert to the possibility of an anomaly and report such difficulties immediately. No feeding should be given until the newborn has been examined.

This newborn's life may depend on your careful observation. If early signs are overlooked and feeding is attempted, the newborn chokes, coughs, and regurgitates as the food enters the blind pouch. The newborn becomes deeply cyanotic and appears to be in severe respiratory distress. During this process, some of the formula may be aspirated, resulting in aspiration pneumonia. If there is a fistula of the distal portion of the esophagus into the trachea, the gastric contents may reflux into the lungs and could also cause aspiration pneumonia.

Treatment and Nursing Care

Aspiration of mucus must be prevented, and continuous, gentle oro- or nasogastric suction may be used. Elevate the head of the bed to prevent reflux and aspiration. The newborn needs intravenous fluids to maintain optimal hydration. Surgical intervention is necessary to correct the defect. Timing of the surgery depends on the surgeon's preference, the anomaly, and the newborn's condition. If the repair is complex, surgery may need to be done in stages. The first stage of surgery may involve placing a gastrostomy tube and a method of draining the proximal esophageal pouch. Total parenteral nutrition

(TPN) may be given to support the nutritional status of the infant. An end-to-end anastomosis is sometimes possible.

Often these defects occur in premature newborns, so additional factors may complicate the surgical repair and prognosis. If there are no other major problems, the long-term outcome should be good. Regular follow-up is necessary to observe for and dilate esophageal strictures that may be caused by scar tissue.

Imperforate Anus

Early in intrauterine life, the membrane between the rectum and the anus should be absorbed, and a clear passage from the rectum to the anus should exist. If the membrane remains and blocks the union between the rectum and the anus, an **imperforate anus** results. In a newborn with imperforate anus, the rectal pouch ends blindly at a distance above the anus; there is no anal orifice. A fistula may exist between the rectum and the vagina in females or between the rectum and the urinary tract in males.

Clinical Manifestations

In some newborns, only a dimple indicates the site of the anus (Fig. 21-17A). When the initial rectal temperature is attempted, it is apparent that there is no anal opening. However, a shallow opening may occur in the anus, with the rectum ending in a blind pouch some distance higher (Fig. 21-17B). Thus, being able to pass a thermometer into the rectum does not guarantee that the rectoanal canal is normal. More reliable presumptive evidence is obtained by watching carefully for the first meconium stool. If the newborn does not pass a stool within the first 24 hours, the health care provider should be notified. Abdominal distention also occurs. Definitive diagnosis is made by x-ray studies.

Treatment

If the rectal pouch is separated from the anus by only a thin membrane, the surgeon may repair the defect from below. For a high defect, abdominoperineal resection is indicated. In these newborns, a colostomy is performed, and extensive abdominoperineal resection is delayed until 3 to 5 months of age or later.

Nursing Care

When the newborn goes home with a colostomy, the family must learn how to give colostomy care. Reinforce teaching with family caregivers to keep the area around the colostomy clean with soap and water and to diaper the baby in the usual way. A protective ointment is useful to protect the skin around the colostomy.

Hernias

A **hernia** is the abnormal protrusion of a part of an organ through a weak spot or other abnormal opening in a body wall. Complications occur depending on the amount of circulatory impairment involved and how much the herniated organ impairs the functioning of another organ. Most hernias can be repaired surgically.

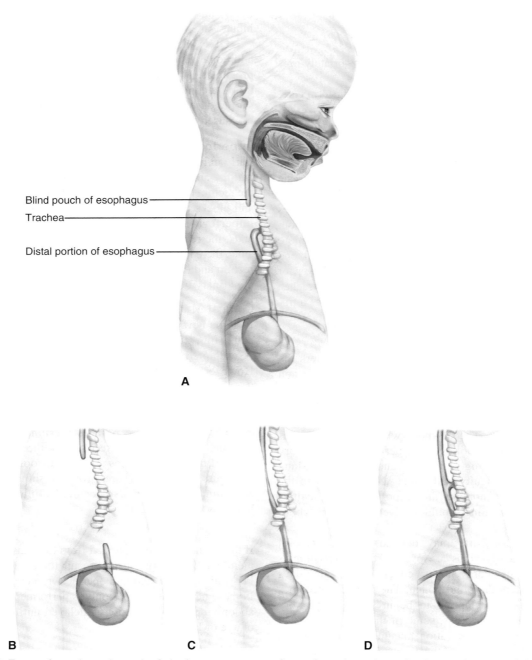

Blind pouch of esophagus

Trachea

Distal portion of esophagus

A

B   **C**   **D**

FIGURE 21-16 Types of esophageal atresia. **A.** In the most common form of esophageal atresia, the esophagus ends in a blind pouch, and a fistula connects the trachea with the distal portion of the esophagus (tracheoesophageal fistula). **B.** Both segments of the esophagus are blind pouches. **C.** The esophagus is continuous but with a narrowed segment. **D.** The upper segment of the esophagus opens into the trachea via a fistula.

Diaphragmatic Hernia

In a congenital hernia of the diaphragm, some of the abdominal organs are displaced into the left chest through an opening in the diaphragm. The heart is pushed toward the right, and the left lung is compressed. Rapid, labored respirations and cyanosis are present on the first day of life, and breathing becomes increasingly difficult. Surgery is essential and may be performed as an emergency procedure. During surgery, the abdominal viscera are withdrawn from the chest and the diaphragmatic defect is closed.

This defect may be minimal and repaired easily or so extensive that pulmonary tissue has failed to develop normally. The outcome of surgical repair depends on the degree of pulmonary development. The prognosis in severe cases is guarded.

Omphalocele

Omphalocele is a relatively rare congenital anomaly. Some of the abdominal contents protrude through into the root of the umbilical cord and form a sac lying on the abdomen. This

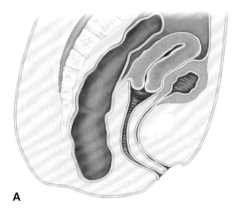
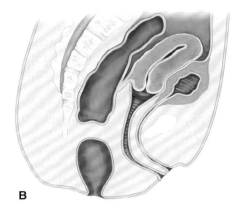

A   **B**

FIGURE 21-17 Imperforate anus. **A.** Membrane between anus and rectum. **B.** Rectum ending in a blind pouch at a distance above the perineum.

sac may be small, with only a loop of bowel, or large and containing much of the intestine and the liver (Fig. 21-18). The sac is covered with peritoneal membrane instead of skin.

These defects may be detected during prenatal ultrasound so that prompt repair may be anticipated. At birth, the defect should be covered immediately with gauze moistened in sterile saline, which then may be covered with plastic wrap to prevent heat loss. Surgical replacement of the organs into the abdomen may be difficult with a large omphalocele because there may not be enough space in the abdominal cavity. Other congenital defects are often present.

With large omphaloceles, surgery may be postponed and the surgeon will suture skin over the defect, creating a large hernia. As the child grows, the abdomen may enlarge enough to allow replacement.

Umbilical Hernia

Normally, the ring that encircled the fetal end of the umbilical cord closes gradually and spontaneously after birth. When this closure is incomplete, portions of omentum and intestine protrude through the opening. More common in preterm and African-American newborns, umbilical hernia is largely a cosmetic problem (Fig. 21-19). Although upsetting to parents, umbilical hernia is associated with little or no morbidity. In rare instances, the bowel may strangulate in the sac and require immediate surgery. Almost all of these hernias close spontaneously by the age of 3 years; hernias that do not close should be surgically corrected before the child enters school.

> **Did You Know?**
> Some people believe that taping a coin on an umbilical hernia will help reduce the hernia. This can actually result in a serious problem for the newborn and should not be done.

Inguinal Hernia

Primarily seen in males, inguinal hernias occur when the small sac of peritoneum surrounding the testes fails to close off after the testes descend from the abdominal sac into the scrotum. This failure allows the intestine to slip into the inguinal canal, with resultant swelling (Fig. 21-20). If the intestine becomes trapped (incarcerated) and the circulation to the trapped intestine is impaired (strangulated), surgery is necessary to prevent intestinal obstruction and gangrene of the bowel. As a preventive measure, inguinal hernias are normally repaired as soon as they are diagnosed.

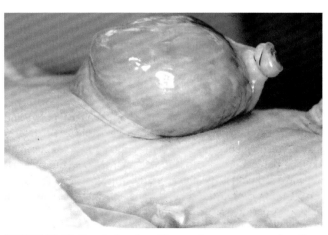

FIGURE 21-18 Omphalocele with membrane sac covering the organs.

> ### TEST YOURSELF
> ✔ What are the two major concerns for the newborn with a cleft lip or a cleft palate?
> ✔ What is the potential complication for the newborn who has esophageal atresia (EA)?
> ✔ How are hernias most often treated?

Genitourinary Tract Defects

Most congenital anomalies of the genitourinary tract are not life-threatening but may present social problems with lifelong implications for the child and family. Thus, early recognition and supportive, understanding care are essential.

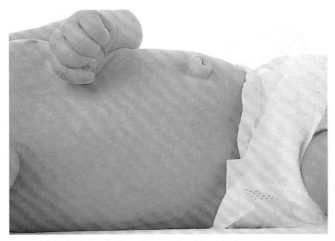

FIGURE 21-19 Small umbilical hernia in newborn.

Hypospadias and Epispadias

Hypospadias is a congenital condition affecting males in which the urethra terminates on the ventral (underside) surface of the penis, instead of at the tip. A cordlike anomaly (a **chordee**) extends from the scrotum to the penis, pulling the penis downward in an arc. Urination is not affected, but the boy cannot void while standing in the normal male fashion. Surgical repair is desirable between the ages of 6 and 18 months, before body image and castration anxiety become problems. Microscopic surgery makes early repair possible. Surgical repair is often accomplished in one stage and is often done as an outpatient surgery. These newborns should not be circumcised because the foreskin is used in the repair. Severe hypospadias may require additional surgical procedures.

In **epispadias**, the opening is on the dorsal (top) surface of the penis. This condition often occurs with exstrophy of the bladder. Surgical repair is indicated.

Exstrophy of the Bladder

Exstrophy of the bladder is a urinary tract malformation and is usually accompanied by other anomalies, such as epispadias, cleft scrotum, cryptorchidism (undescended testes), a shortened penis, and cleft clitoris. It is also associated with malformed pelvic musculature, resulting in a

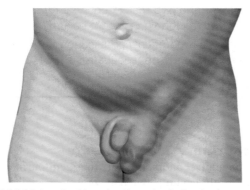

FIGURE 21-20 Inguinal hernia. Note the bulge in the groin area.

prolapsed rectum and inguinal hernias. Children with this defect have a widely split symphysis pubis and rotated hip sockets, causing a waddling gait.

In this condition, the anterior surface of the urinary bladder lies open on the lower abdomen (Fig. 21-21). The exposed mucosa is red and sensitive to touch and allows direct passage of urine to the outside. This condition makes the area vulnerable to infection and trauma. Surgical closure of the bladder is preferred within the first 48 hours of life. Final surgical correction is completed before the child goes to school. If bladder repair is not done early in the child's life, the family caregivers must be taught how to care for this condition and how to deal with their feelings toward this less-than-perfect child. Their emotional reaction may be further complicated if the malformation is so severe that the sex of the child may be determined only by a chromosome test (see the following section "Ambiguous Genitalia").

Nursing care of the newborn with exstrophy of the bladder should be directed toward preventing infection, preventing skin irritation around the seeping mucosa, meeting the newborn's need for touch and cuddling, and educating and supporting the family.

Ambiguous Genitalia

If a child's external sex organs did not follow a normal development in utero, at birth it may not be possible to determine by observation if the child is a male or female. The external sexual organs are either incompletely or abnormally formed. This condition is called ambiguous genitalia. Although rare, the birth of a newborn with ambiguous genitalia presents a highly charged emotional climate and has possible long-range social implications.

Regardless of the cause, it is important to establish the genetic sex and the sex of rearing as early as possible so that surgical correction of anomalies may occur before the child begins to function in a sex-related social role. Authorities believe that the newborn's anatomic structure, rather than the genetic sex, should determine the sex of rearing. It is possible to construct a functional vagina surgically and to administer hormones to offer an anatomically incomplete female a somewhat normal life. Currently, it is less possible to offer comparable surgical reconstruction to males with an inadequate penis. Parents may feel guilt, anxiety, and confusion about their child's condition and need understanding and support to help them cope.

Skeletal System Defects

Skeletal system defects in the newborn may be noted and treatment begun soon after birth. Some skeletal system defects may not be evident until later in the child's life. Two common skeletal defects are clubfoot (congenital talipes equinovarus) and developmental dysplasia of the hip (dislocation of the hip). Children with these conditions and their parents often face long periods of exhausting, costly treatment; therefore, they need continuing support, encouragement, and education.

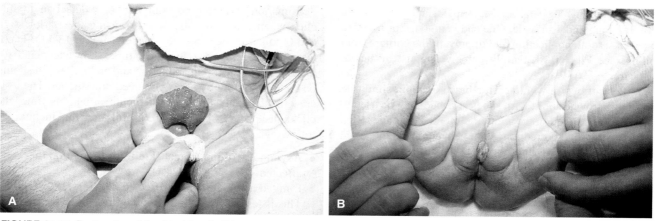

FIGURE 21-21 Exstrophy of the bladder. **A.** Prior to surgery, note the bright red color of the bladder. **B.** Following surgical repair.

Congenital Talipes Equinovarus

Congenital clubfoot is a deformity in which the entire foot is inverted, the heel is drawn up, and the forefoot is adducted. The Latin word *talus*, meaning ankle, and *pes*, meaning foot, make up the word *talipes*, which is used in connection with many foot deformities. *Equinus*, or plantar flexion, and *varus*, or inversion, denotes the kind of foot deformity present in this condition. The equinovarus foot has a clublike appearance, thus the term "clubfoot" (Fig. 21-22A). This defect is usually seen in utero in an ultrasound and evident at birth.

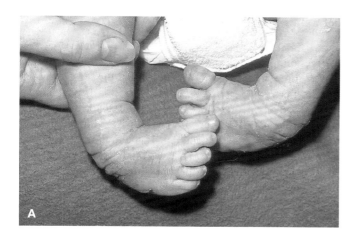

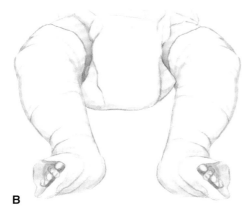

FIGURE 21-22 A. Bilateral clubfoot. **B.** Casting for clubfoot in typical overcorrected position.

Congenital talipes equinovarus is the most common congenital foot deformity, occurring in about 1 in 1,000 births. It appears as a single anomaly or in connection with other defects, such as myelomeningocele. It may be bilateral (both feet) or unilateral (one foot). The cause is unclear, although a hereditary factor is observed occasionally. One hypothesis is that it results from an arrested embryonic growth of the foot during the first trimester of pregnancy.

Clinical Manifestations

Talipes equinovarus is detected easily in a newborn but must be differentiated from a persisting "position of comfort" assumed in utero. The positional deformity may be corrected easily by the use of passive exercise, but the true clubfoot deformity is fixed and not corrected by exercise. The positional deformity should be explained to the family caregivers immediately to prevent anxiety.

Treatment

Nonsurgical Treatment. If treatment is started during the neonatal period, correction can usually be accomplished by manipulation and taping the foot to a plastic splint or by application of a cast. The cast is often applied while the newborn is still in the neonatal nursery. While the cast is applied, the foot is first moved gently into as nearly normal a position as possible. Force should not be used. If the family caregiver can be present to help hold the newborn while the cast is applied, the caregiver will have the opportunity to understand what is being done. The newborn gets satisfaction from sucking, so a pacifier helps prevent squirming while the cast is applied.

The cast is applied over the foot and ankle (and usually to midthigh) to hold the knee in right-angle flexion (Fig. 21-22B). Casts are changed frequently to provide gradual, atraumatic correction—every few days for the first several weeks, then every week or two. The treatment is usually continued for a matter of months until x-ray and clinical observation confirm complete correction.

Any cast applied to a child's body should have some type of waterproof material protecting the skin from the cast's sharp plaster edges. One method is to apply strips of adhesive vertically around the edges of the cast in a manner called "petaling." To petal a cast, strips of adhesive are cut 2 or 3 in long and 1 in wide. One end is notched or rounded to aid in smooth application and to prevent the corners from rolling (see Fig. 40-6). Family caregivers must be taught cast care.

After correction with a cast, a brace or splint similar to the Denis Browne splint with shoes attached may be used to maintain the correction for another 6 months or longer (Fig. 21-23). After overcorrection has been attained, the child should wear a special clubfoot shoe, which is a laced shoe whose turning out makes it appear that the shoe is being worn on the wrong foot. The brace still may be worn at night, and the caregivers should carry out passive exercises of the foot. The older infant may resist wearing the brace, so family caregivers must be taught the importance of gentle but firm insistence that the brace be worn.

Surgical Treatment. Children who do not respond to nonsurgical measures, especially older children, need surgical correction. This approach involves several procedures, depending on the age of the child and the degree of the deformity. It may involve lengthening the Achilles tendon and operating on the bony structure for the child older than 10 years. Prolonged observation after correction by either means should be carried out at least until adolescence; any recurrence is treated promptly.

Development Dysplasia of the Hip

Developmental dysplasia of the hip (DDH) results from defective development of the acetabulum, with or without dislocation. The malformed acetabulum permits dislocation, with the head of the femur becoming displaced upward and backward. The condition is difficult to recognize during early infancy. When there is a family history of the defect, increased observation of the young newborn is indicated. The condition is often bilateral and about six times more common in girls than in boys.

Clinical Manifestations

Early recognition and treatment before an infant starts to stand or walk are extremely important for successful correction. The first examination should be a part of the newborn examination. Experienced examiners may detect an audible click when examining the newborn using the Barlow sign and Ortolani maneuver (see Chapter 13, Fig. 13-11). These tests, used together on one hip at a time, show a tendency for dislocation of the hip in adduction and abduction and should be conducted only by an experienced practitioner. The tests are effective only for the first month; after this time, the clicks disappear. Signs that are useful after this include the following:

- Asymmetry of the gluteal skin folds (higher on the affected side) (Fig. 21-24A).
- Limited abduction of the affected hip (Fig. 21-24B). This is tested by placing the infant in a dorsal recumbent position with the knees flexed, then abducting both knees passively until they reach the examination table without resistance. If dislocation is present, the affected side cannot be abducted more than 45 degrees.
- Apparent shortening of the femur (Fig. 21-24C).

After the child has started walking, later signs include lordosis, swayback, protruding abdomen, shortened extremity, duck-waddle gait, and a positive Trendelenburg sign. To elicit this sign, the child stands on the affected leg and raises the normal leg. The pelvis tilts down, rather than up toward the unaffected side. X-ray studies are usually done to confirm the diagnosis in the older child. Uncorrected dislocation causes limping, easy fatigue, hip and low back discomfort, and postural deformities.

Treatment

Correction may be started in the newborn period by placing two or three diapers on the infant to hold the legs abducted in a froglike position. Cloth diapers work best for this purpose. Another treatment option when the dislocation is discovered during the first few months consists of manipulation of the femur into position and the application of a brace. The most common type of brace used is the Pavlik harness (Fig. 21-25). The health care provider assesses the infant weekly while the infant is in the harness and adjusts the harness to align the femur gradually. Sometimes, no additional treatment is needed.

If treatment is delayed until after the child has started to walk or if earlier treatment is ineffective, the child may be placed in Bryant traction (see Chapter 40, Fig. 40-8). The traction helps to stretch the tissue around the hip so the head of the femur can move back into the hip socket. After the child has been in traction for about 2 weeks, an open reduction is done followed by application of a spica cast. A spica or "hip spica cast," as it is often called, covers the lower part of the body from the waist down and either one or both legs, usually leaving the feet open. The cast maintains the legs in a froglike position, with the hips abducted. There may be a bar placed between the legs to help support the cast. After the cast is removed, a metal or a plastic brace is applied to keep the legs in wide abduction.

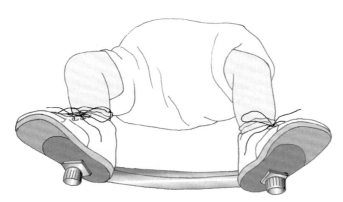

FIGURE 21-23 A Denis Browne splint with shoes attached is used to correct clubfoot.

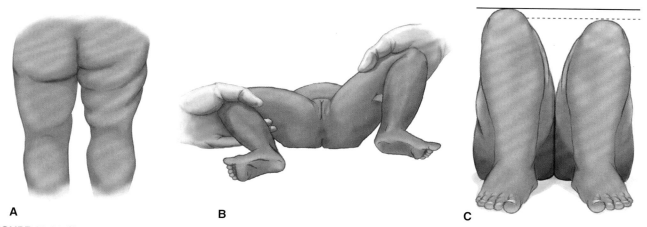

FIGURE 21-24 Signs of developmental dysplasia of the hip. **A.** Asymmetry of the gluteal folds of the thighs. **B.** Limited abduction of the affected hip. **C.** Apparent shortening of the femur.

Nursing Process and Care Plan *for the Infant in an Orthopedic Device or Cast*

Although the actual hospitalization of the infant is relatively short (if no other abnormalities require hospitalization), it is important to reinforce teaching with the family about cast care or care of the infant in an orthopedic device, such as a Pavlik harness. Determine the family caregiver's ability to understand and cooperate in the infant's care. Emotional support of the family is important.

Assessment (Data Collection)

The observation of the infant varies depending on the orthopedic device or cast used. Immediately after the application of a cast, observe for signs that the cast is drying evenly. Check the toes for circulation and movement. Check the skin at the edges of the cast for signs of pressure or irritation. If an open reduction has been performed, observe the child for signs of shock and bleeding in the immediate postoperative period.

Nursing Focus

When selecting nursing focuses for the infant in an orthopedic device or a cast, comfort and maintaining skin integrity are major concerns. Because of restricted mobility for the infant, it is important to meet the growth and development needs of the infant. Reinforcement of family teaching is incorporated into nursing care.

Outcome Identification and Planning

Goals include relieving pain and discomfort, and maintaining skin integrity. Promoting normal growth and development is important for this infant. Another goal is to increase the family caregivers' knowledge about the infant's home care.

Nursing Care Focus

- Acute pain related to discomfort of orthopedic device or cast

Goal

- The infant will show signs of being comfortable.

Implementations for Providing Comfort

The infant may be irritable and fussy because of the restricted movement caused by the device or cast. Useful methods of soothing the infant include nonnutritive sucking, stroking, cuddling, and talking. If irritability seems excessive, check the infant for signs of skin irritation from the device or cast. The infant in a cast may be held after the cast is completely dry. Do not remove the harness unless specific permission for bathing is granted by the health care provider. Show the family caregivers how to reapply the harness correctly. The infant in a Pavlik harness is not as difficult to handle as the infant in a cast.

Evaluation of Goal/Desired Outcome

The infant:

- is alert and content with no long periods of fussiness.
- interacts with caregivers with cooing, smiling, and eye contact.

 C u l t u r a l   S n a p s h o t

Cradleboards are devices used as baby carriers and to provide security for newborns in many Native American cultures. Using a cradleboard can sometimes aggravate hip dysplasia. Encourage the caregivers to use thick diapers, sometimes more than one, to help keep the hips in a slightly abducted position when the child is carried on a cradleboard. Cloth diapers work better than disposable diapers for this purpose.

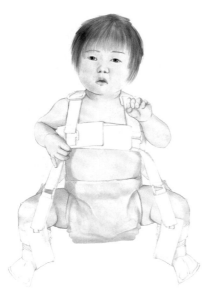

FIGURE 21-25 A Pavlik harness for the treatment of developmental dysplasia of the hip. The harness is composed of shoulder straps, stirrups, and a chest strap. It is placed on both legs, even if only one hip is dislocated.

Nursing Care Focus

- Altered skin integrity risk related to pressure of the cast on the skin surface

Goal

- The infant's skin will remain intact.

Implementations for Promoting Skin Integrity

For the first 24 to 48 hours after application of a cast, place the infant on a firm mattress, and support position changes with firm pillows. When handling the cast, use the palms of the hands to avoid excessive pressure on the cast. Carefully inspect the skin around the cast edges for signs of irritation, redness, or edema. Petal the edges of the cast around the waist and toes, and protect the cast with plastic covering around the perineal area. If the covering becomes soiled, remove it, wash and dry thoroughly, then reapply or replace it. With the Pavlik harness, monitor the skin under the straps frequently, and massage it gently to promote circulation. To relieve pressure under the shoulder straps, place extra padding in the area.

Diapering can be a challenge for the infant in a cast. Take great care to protect the diaper area from becoming soiled and moist. Urine and feces can cause irritation and skin breakdown. Disposable diapers are usually the most effective way to provide good protection of the cast and prevent leakage.

Avoid using powders and lotions because caking of the powder or lotion can cause areas of irritation. Daily sponge baths are important and must include close attention to the skin under the straps of the device or around the edge of the cast.

Observe the infant in a cast carefully for any restriction of breathing caused by tightness over the abdomen and lower chest area. Vomiting after a feeding may be an indication that the cast is too tight over the stomach. In either case, the cast may have to be removed and reapplied.

Prevent the older infant or child from pushing any small particles of food or toys down into the cast.

Evaluation of Goal/Desired Outcome

- The infant's skin around the edges of the cast shows no signs of redness or irritation.
- The diaper area is clean, dry and intact, and protected from soiling.

Nursing Care Focus

- Risk for delayed growth and development related to restricted mobility secondary to orthopedic device or cast

Goal

- The infant will attain appropriate developmental milestones.

Implementations for Providing Sensory Stimulation

Because the infant will be in the device or cast for an extended period when much growth and development occur, provide them with stimulation of a tactile nature. Provide mobiles, musical toys, and stuffed toys. Do not permit the infant to cry for long periods. Keep feeding times relaxed. Hold the infant if possible and encourage interaction. Provide a pacifier if the infant desires it. Encourage activities that use the infant's free hands. The older infant may enjoy looking at picture books and interacting with siblings. Diversionary activities should include transporting the infant to other areas in the home or in the car. Strollers and car seats may be adapted to allow safe transportation.

> **Here's an Idea**
> For older infants or toddlers in a hip spica cast, a wagon may provide a convenient and fun way to explore the environment, encourage stimulation, and promote independence.

Evaluation of Goal/Desired Outcome

The infant:

- responds positively to audio, visual, and diversionary activities.
- shows age-appropriate development.

Nursing Care Focus

- Knowledge deficiency of family caregivers related to home care of the infant in the orthopedic device or cast

Goal

- The family caregivers will learn home care of the infant.

Implementations for Reinforcing Family Teaching

Determine the family caregiver's knowledge, and help design a plan for caring for the infant at home. Use complete explanations, written guidelines, demonstrations, and return demonstrations. Provide the family with a resource person who may be called when a question arises and encourage them to feel free to call that person. Make definite plans for return visits to have the device or cast checked. The caregiver needs to understand the importance of keeping these appointments. Provide a home health nurse referral when appropriate.

Evaluation of Goal/Desired Outcome

- The family demonstrates care of the infant in the orthopedic device or cast, asks pertinent questions, and identifies a resource person to call.

TEST YOURSELF

✔ Why is it desirable for genitourinary tract defects such as hypospadias to be corrected by the time the child is 18 months old?

✔ How is congenital clubfoot treated?

✔ What three signs are seen in the infant with a developmental dysplasia of the hip?

✔ List five nursing interventions used to promote skin integrity for an infant in a cast.

INBORN ERRORS OF METABOLISM

Inborn errors of metabolism are hereditary disorders that affect metabolism. These disorders include phenylketonuria (PKU), galactosemia, congenital hypothyroidism, and maple syrup urine disease (MSUD). Nursing care for the newborn involves accurate observation of manifestations to aid in prompt diagnosis and initiation of treatment. Reinforcing family teaching might include dietary guidelines, information about the disorder, and genetic counseling. The family also needs support and information to prepare for the long-term care of a chronically ill child (see Chapter 32).

Phenylketonuria

Phenylketonuria (PKU) is a recessive hereditary defect of metabolism that, if untreated, causes severe intellectual disability in most but not all affected children. It is an uncommon defect. Children with this condition lack the enzyme that normally changes the essential amino acid phenylalanine into tyrosine.

As soon as the newborn with this defect begins to take milk (either breast or cow's milk), phenylalanine is absorbed in the normal manner. However, because the affected newborn cannot metabolize this amino acid, phenylalanine builds up in the blood serum to as much as 20 times the normal level. This buildup occurs so quickly that the increased levels of phenylalanine appear in the blood after only 1 or 2 days of ingestion of milk. Phenylpyruvic acid appears in the urine of these newborns between the second and sixth weeks of life.

Most untreated children with this condition develop severe and progressive mental deficiency. The high levels of phenylalanine in the bloodstream and tissues cause permanent damage to brain tissues. The newborn appears normal at birth but begins to show signs of mental arrest within a few weeks. Therefore, this disorder must be diagnosed as early as possible, and the child must be placed immediately on a low-phenylalanine formula.

Clinical Manifestations

Untreated newborns may experience frequent vomiting and have aggressive and hyperactive traits. Severe, progressive mental disability is characteristic. Convulsions may occur, and eczema is common, particularly in the perineal area. There is a characteristic musty smell to the urine.

Diagnosis

All states require newborns to undergo a blood test to detect the phenylalanine level. This screening procedure, the Guthrie inhibition assay test, uses blood from a simple heel prick. The test is most reliable after the newborn has ingested some form of protein. The accepted practice is to perform the test on the second or third day of life. If the newborn leaves the hospital before this time, the newborn is brought back to have the test performed. The test may be repeated in the third week of life if the first test was done before the newborn was 24 hours old. Health care providers caring for newborns not born in a hospital are responsible for screening these newborns. When screening indicates an increased level of phenylalanine, additional testing is done to make a firm diagnosis.

Treatment and Nursing Care

Dietary treatment is required. A formula low in phenylalanine (e.g., Lofenalac or Phenyl-free) should be started as soon as the condition is detected. Best results are obtained if the special formula is started before the newborn is 3 weeks of age. A low-phenylalanine diet is a very restricted one; foods to be omitted include most grains, meat, fish, dairy products, eggs, nuts, and legumes. A nutritionist should supervise the diet carefully. The child remains on the diet at least into early adulthood, and it may even be recommended indefinitely.

Maintaining the newborn on the restricted diet is relatively simple compared with the problems that arise as the child grows and becomes more independent. As the child ventures into the world beyond home, more and more dietary temptations are available, and dietary compliance is difficult. The family and the child need support and counseling throughout the child's developmental years.

If a woman who has PKU decides to have a child and is not following a diet low in phenylalanine, she should return to following the dietary treatment for at least 3 months before becoming pregnant. The diet is continued through the pregnancy to help in preventing the child from being born with mental impairment. Routine blood testing is done during pregnancy to monitor the serum phenylalanine level.

Galactosemia

Galactosemia is a recessive hereditary metabolic disorder in which the enzyme necessary to convert galactose into glucose is missing. Galactose is the primary sugar found in milk. The newborns generally appear normal at birth but experience difficulties after ingesting milk (breast, cow's, or goat's).

Clinical Manifestations

Early feeding difficulties with vomiting and diarrhea severe enough to produce dehydration and weight loss and jaundice are the primary manifestations. Unless milk is withheld early, other difficulties include cataracts, and mental disability, with a high mortality rate early in life. A screening test (Beutler test) can be used to test for the disorder.

Treatment and Nursing Care

Galactose must be omitted from the diet, which in the young infant means a substitution for milk. Nutramigen and Pregestimil are formulas that provide galactose-free nutrition for the newborn. The diet must continue to be free of lactose when the child moves on to table foods, but the diet allows more variety than does the phenylalanine-free diet.

Congenital Hypothyroidism

At one time referred to by the now unacceptable term "cretinism," congenital hypothyroidism is associated with either the congenital absence of a thyroid gland or the inability of the thyroid gland to secrete thyroid hormone.

Clinical Manifestations

The newborn appears normal at birth, but clinical signs and symptoms begin to be noticeable at about 6 weeks of life. The facial features are typical and include a depressed nasal bridge, large tongue, and puffy eyes. The neck is short and thick. The voice (cry) is hoarse, the skin is dry and cold, and the newborn has slow bone development. Two common features are chronic constipation and abdomen enlargement caused by poor muscle tone (Fig. 21-26). The newborn is a poor feeder and often characterized as a "good" baby by the family caregiver because they cry very little and sleep for long periods.

Diagnosis

Most states require a routine test for triiodothyronine (T_3) and thyroxine (T_4) levels to determine thyroid function in all newborns before discharge for early diagnosis of congenital hypothyroidism. This test is done as a part of the heel-stick screening, which includes the Guthrie screening test for PKU.

Treatment and Nursing Care

The thyroid hormone must be replaced as soon as the diagnosis is made. Levothyroxine sodium, a synthetic thyroid replacement, is the drug most commonly used. Blood levels

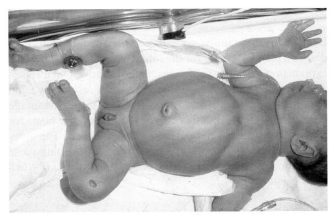

FIGURE 21-26 A newborn with congenital hypothyroidism. Note the short, thick neck and enlarged abdomen.

of T_3 and T_4 are monitored to prevent overdosage. Unless therapy is started in early infancy, intellectual disability and slow growth occur. The later the therapy started, the more severe the intellectual disability. The therapy must be continued for life.

Maple Syrup Urine Disease

MSUD is an inborn error of metabolism of the branched-chain amino acids. It is autosomal recessive in inheritance. It is rapidly progressive and often fatal.

Clinical Manifestations

The onset of MSUD occurs very early in infancy. In the first week of life, these newborns often have feeding problems and neurologic signs such as seizures, spasticity, and opisthotonos. The urine has a distinctive odor of maple syrup. Diagnosis is made through a blood test for amino acids. This is easily done at the same time the heel stick for PKU is performed.

Treatment and Nursing Care

Treatment of MSUD is dietary and must be initiated within 12 days of birth to be successful. The special formula is low in the branched-chain amino acids. The special diet must be continued indefinitely.

CHROMOSOMAL ABNORMALITIES

Chromosomal abnormalities are often evident at birth and frequently cause physical and cognitive challenges for the child throughout life. There are various forms of chromosomal abnormalities.

The most common abnormalities are nondisjunction abnormalities, which occur when the chromosomal division is uneven. Normally during cell division of the cells of reproduction, the 46 chromosomes divide in half, with 23 chromosomes in each new cell. Nondisjunction abnormalities occur when a new cell has an extra chromosome (e.g., 24) or not enough chromosomes (e.g., 22). When this defective chromosome joins with a normal reproductive cell having 23 chromosomes, an abnormality occurs. Down syndrome, the most common chromosomal abnormality, most often is a result of chromosomal nondisjunction with an extra chromosome on chromosome 21. Two other common chromosomal abnormalities are the Turner and Klinefelter syndromes, which are nondisjunction abnormalities occurring on the sex chromosomes.

Down Syndrome

Down syndrome is the most common chromosomal anomaly, occurring in about 1 in 700 to 800 births. Down syndrome has been observed in nearly all countries and races. Most people with Down syndrome have trisomy 21 (Fig. 21-27). A woman older than 35 years is at a greater risk of bearing a child with Down syndrome than is a younger woman, but children with Down syndrome are born to women of all ages. Increasing numbers of women are choosing to undergo screening during pregnancy with blood tests and ultrasound, looking for fluid behind the neck of the fetus, which indicate the possibility of Down syndrome. Amniocentesis and chorionic villus sampling are diagnostic tests that will confirm the blood test results. These screening and diagnostic tests give women the option of deciding whether to continue or terminate the pregnancy. If the choice is to continue the pregnancy, they can begin preparing themselves for the birth of a disabled child.

Clinical Manifestations

All forms of the condition show a variety of abnormal characteristics. Mental status is usually within the moderate to severe range of cognitive impairment, with most children being moderately impaired. The most common anomalies include the following:

- **Brachycephaly** (shortness of head)
- Short stature
- Upward and outward slanted eyes (almond-shaped) with an epicanthic fold at the inner angle
- Short, flattened bridge of the nose
- Thick, fissured, protruding tongue
- Dry, cracked, fissured skin that may be mottled
- Small hands with short broad fingers with a curved fifth finger
- A single deep crease on the palm of hand (palmar crease)
- Wide space between the first and second toes
- Lax muscle tone (often referred to as "double jointed" by others)
- Heart and eye anomalies
- Greater susceptibility to leukemia than that of the general population

Not all these physical signs are present in all people with Down syndrome. Some may have only one or two characteristics; others may show nearly all the characteristics (Fig. 21-28).

Treatment and Nursing Care

The physical characteristics of the child with Down syndrome determine the medical and nursing management. The child's relaxed muscle tone may contribute to respiratory complications as a result of decreased respiratory expansion. The

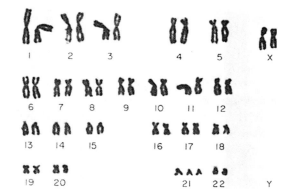

FIGURE 21-27 Karyotype showing trisomy 21. Note three chromosomes in the 21 position.

relaxed skeletal muscles contribute to late motor development. Gastric motility is also decreased, leading to problems with constipation. Congenital heart defects and vision or hearing problems add to the complexities of the child's care.

In infancy, the child's large tongue and poor muscle tone may contribute to difficulty breast-feeding or ingesting formula and can cause great problems when the time comes to introduce solid foods. The family caregivers need support during these trying times. As the child gets older, concern about excessive weight gain becomes a primary consideration.

The family caregivers of the child with Down syndrome need strong support and guidance from the time the child is born. Early intervention programs have yielded some encouraging results, but depending on the level of cognitive impairment, the family may have to decide if they can care for the child at home, or if other living arrangements need to be considered for the child. A cognitively impaired child who is undisciplined or improperly supervised may threaten the safety of others in the home and the neighborhood. Caring for the child may demand so much sacrifice from other family members that the family structure may be significantly affected. However, with consistent care, patience, and guidelines, families of children with Down syndrome often find joy and pleasure in the gentle and loving nature of the child.

TEST YOURSELF

✔ What is a serious outcome that can occur if phenylketonuria (PKU), congenital hypothyroidism, and galactosemia are not treated?

✔ What are the clinical manifestations often seen in the child with Down syndrome?

Turner Syndrome

The newborn with Turner syndrome has one less X chromosome than normal. The characteristics of Turner syndrome include short stature, low-set ears, a broad-based neck that appears webbed and short, a low-set hairline at the nape of the neck, broad chest, an increased angle of the arms, and

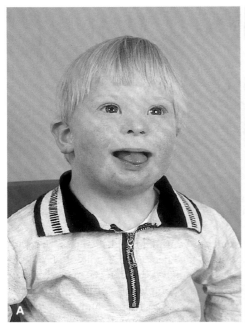
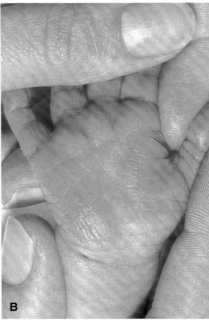

FIGURE 21-28 Typical features of a child with Down syndrome. **A.** Facial features. **B.** Horizontal palm crease (palmar crease).

edema of the hands and feet. These children frequently have congenital heart defects as well. Females are affected by Turner syndrome and with the exception of pubic hair, do not develop secondary sex characteristics.

Children with Turner syndrome have normal intelligence but may have visual–spatial concerns, learning disabilities, problems with social interaction, and may lack physical coordination. Growth hormones are given to increase the height, as well as the hormonal levels, but females with Turner syndrome can rarely become pregnant.

Klinefelter Syndrome

The presence of an extra X chromosome causes Klinefelter syndrome. The syndrome is most commonly seen in males. The characteristics are not often evident until puberty, when the child does not develop secondary sex characteristics. The testes are usually small and do not produce mature sperm. Increased breast size and a risk of developing breast cancer are frequently seen.

Boys with Klinefelter syndrome often have normal intelligence but frequently have behavior problems, show signs of immaturity and insecurity, and have difficulty with memory and processing. Hormone replacements of testosterone may be started in the early adolescence to promote normal adult development.

Adrian Simmer has just returned to the pediatric unit after having his cleft lip repaired. The first stage of repair for the cleft palate has also been completed. What data are important for you to collect as you care for Adrian? What are your priorities in caring for Adrian? What teaching will you reinforce with Adrian's parents related to caring for Adrian after his discharge?

KEY POINTS

- Spina bifida is caused when the spinal vertebrae fail to close and an opening is left where the spinal cord or meninges may protrude. In spina bifida occulta, soft tissue is not involved, and only a dimple in the skin may be seen. In spina bifida with meningocele, the spinal meninges protrude through and form a sac, and in spina bifida with myelomeningocele, both the spinal cord and meninges protrude. Myelomeningocele is the most difficult type to treat because of the concern of complete paralysis below the lesion.

- Noncommunicating hydrocephalus occurs when there is an obstruction in the circulation of CSF. With communicating hydrocephalus, absorption of CSF is defective. The most obvious symptom of hydrocephalus is the rapid increase in head circumference. Ventriculoperitoneal shunting (VP shunt) drains the CSF from the brain into the peritoneal cavity. Nursing care focuses on preventing injury, maintaining skin integrity, preventing infection, and maintaining growth and development.

- Ventricular septal defects allow the blood to pass from the left to the right ventricle; in the atrial septal defect the blood flows from the left to the right atria. With a patent ductus arteriosus, the blood is shunted from the aorta into the pulmonary artery. When coarctation of the aorta occurs, there is a narrowing of the aortic arch and an obstruction of blood flow.

- Tetralogy of Fallot is a group of heart defects including pulmonary stenosis, ventricular septal defect, overriding aorta, and right ventricular hypertrophy. The child with tetralogy of Fallot has cyanosis and low oxygen saturation. The severe and sometimes fatal defect, transposition of the great arteries, causes cyanosis and occurs because the aorta arises from the right ventricle instead of the left, and the pulmonary artery arises from the left ventricle instead of the right.

- A failure of the maxillary and premaxillary processes to fuse during fetal development can cause a cleft lip on one or both sides of the lip or a cleft palate, in which the tissue in the roof of the mouth does not fuse properly. Surgery is a major part of the treatment of either condition. Nursing care focuses on maintaining adequate nutrition, increasing family coping, and reducing the parents' anxiety and guilt. After surgery, nursing care focuses on preventing aspiration, improving respiration, maintaining adequate fluid volume and nutritional requirements, relieving pain, preventing injury and infection to the surgical site, and promoting normal growth and development.

- Esophageal atresia (EA) is the absence of a normal opening in or the abnormal closure of the esophagus. A tracheoesophageal fistula occurs when the upper, or proximal, end of the esophagus ends in a blind pouch, and the lower, or distal, segment from the stomach is connected to the trachea by a fistulous tract. Early signs of EA include frothing and excessive drooling and periods of respiratory distress with coughing, choking, and cyanosis. The newborn with tracheoesophageal fistula is at risk for aspiration, pneumonia, and respiratory distress. Surgical correction of the defect is necessary.

- If the membrane between the rectum and the anus remains after birth and blocks the union between the rectum and the anus, an imperforate anus results. If the newborn does not pass a stool within the first 24 hours, the health care provider should be notified. The infant requires surgery and may have a colostomy placed.

- A diaphragmatic hernia occurs when abdominal organs are displaced into the left chest through an opening in the diaphragm. A rare occurrence, an omphalocele is seen when the abdominal contents protrude through the umbilical cord and form a sac lying on the abdomen. If the end of the umbilical cord does not close completely and a portion of the intestine protrudes through the opening, an umbilical hernia forms. Inguinal hernias occur mostly in males when a part of the intestine slips into the inguinal canal.

- Hypospadias is a congenital condition in which the urethra terminates on the ventral (underside) surface of the penis, instead of at the tip. Epispadias occurs when the opening of the urethra is on the dorsal (top) surface of the penis. In the child with exstrophy of the bladder, the anterior surface of the urinary bladder lies open on the lower abdomen; surgical closure of the bladder is preferred within the first 48 hours of life. Ambiguous genitalia is a condition in which the external sexual organs are either incompletely or abnormally formed, and it may not be possible to determine by observation at birth if the child is a male or a female.

- Clubfoot (talipes equinovarus) and developmental dysplasia of the hip (DDH) are the most common skeletal deformities in the newborn. Clubfoot is treated by manipulation and taping or by application of a cast. Children who do not respond to nonsurgical measures need surgical correction. Signs and symptoms of developmental dysplasia of the hip include asymmetry of the gluteal skin folds, limited abduction of the affected hip, and apparent shortening of the femur. To treat hip dislocation, the femur is manipulated and a brace applied. A hip spica cast may be used after an open reduction, if necessary. Nursing care focuses on relieving pain and discomfort, maintaining skin integrity, promoting growth and development, and increasing family knowledge.

- Phenylketonuria (PKU) is a recessive hereditary defect of metabolism that, if untreated, causes severe intellectual disability. PKU is diagnosed with the Guthrie inhibition assay test to detect phenylalanine levels in the blood. Dietary treatment using a formula and diet low in phenylalanine is started and continued as the child gets older. Galactosemia is a hereditary metabolic disorder in which the enzyme necessary to convert galactose into glucose is missing. Galactose is omitted from the diet to treat the disorder. Congenital hypothyroidism is detected by performing tests for triiodothyronine (T_3) and thyroxine (T_4) levels to determine thyroid function. The thyroid hormone must be replaced to treat the disorder. Maple syrup urine disease (MSUD) is an inborn error of metabolism, which is autosomal recessive in inheritance. It is rapidly progressive and often fatal.

- If phenylketonuria (PKU), congenital hypothyroidism, and galactosemia are not treated, the newborn often has severe intellectual disability.

- Down syndrome is sometimes called trisomy 21 because of the three-chromosome pattern seen on the 21st pair of chromosomes. Signs and symptoms seen in children include brachycephaly (shortness of head); short stature; slanted (almond-shaped) eyes; short, flattened nose; thick, protruding tongue; dry, cracked, fissured skin; small hands with short, broad fingers and a curved fifth finger; single deep crease on the palm of hand (palmar crease); wide space between the first and second toes; lax muscle tone; heart and eye anomalies; and a greater susceptibility to leukemia.

- The newborn with Turner syndrome has one less X chromosome than normal. The presence of an extra X chromosome causes Klinefelter syndrome.

INTERNET RESOURCES

Spina Bifida
http://spinabifidaassociation.org/

Cleft Lip and Cleft Palate
www.cleft.org

Congenital Heart Defects
www.congenitalheartdefects.com
www.americanheart.org

Hydrocephalus
www.nhfonline.org

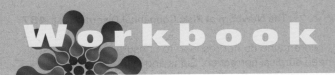

NCLEX-STYLE REVIEW QUESTIONS

1. The nurse is collecting data on a newborn with a diagnosis of hydrocephalus. If the following data were collected, which might indicate a common symptom of this diagnosis?
   a. Sac protruding on the lower back
   b. Respiratory rate of 30 breaths per minute
   c. Gluteal folds higher on one side than the other
   d. Head circumference of 18 inches

2. When collecting data during an admission interview and examination on a newborn, the nurse finds the newborn has cyanosis, dyspnea, tachycardia, and feeding difficulties. These symptoms might indicate the newborn has which condition?
   a. Spina bifida
   b. Tetralogy of Fallot
   c. Congenital rubella
   d. Development dysplasia of the hip

3. In caring for a newborn who has had a cleft lip/cleft palate repair, which nursing action is the *highest* priority?
   a. Document the time period the restraints are on and off.
   b. Observe the incision for redness or drainage.
   c. Teach the caregivers about dental care and hygiene.
   d. Provide sensory stimulation and age-appropriate toys.

4. In planning care for an infant who had a spica cast applied to treat a developmental dysplasia of the hip, which nursing intervention would be included in this infant's plan of care?
   a. Inspect skin for redness and irritation.
   b. Change bedding and clothing every 4 hours.
   c. Weigh every morning and evening using the same scale.
   d. Monitor temperature and pulse every 2 hours.

5. The nurse is caring for a newborn who has a myelomeningocele and has not yet had surgery to repair the defect. Which of the following measures will be used to prevent the site from becoming infected? (Select all that apply.)
   a. Give antibiotics as a prophylactic measure.
   b. Cover the sac with a saline-soaked sterile dressing.
   c. Maintain the newborn in a supine position.
   d. Place a plastic protective covering over the dressing.
   e. Change the dressing every 8 hours.

STUDY ACTIVITIES

1. Using a table like the one below, list the common types of congenital heart defects. Include the description of the defect (chambers and parts of the heart involved), the blood flow characteristics, symptoms, and treatment.

Defect	Description of Defect	Blood Flow Characteristics	Symptoms	Treatment

2. Make a list of the maternal risk factors that may cause congenital heart defects. For each of these risk factors, state what could be done to decrease the occurrence of these risks.

3. Develop a project by creating a mobile or gathering a collection of appropriate toys and activities that could be used for sensory stimulation with a newborn who is in an orthopedic cast. Present your project to your classmates and explain why and how these items would be appropriate to use for developmental stimulation.

4. Do an Internet search on "preparing your child for heart surgery."
   a. Make a list of some of the sites you discovered.
   b. What are some ways parents can prepare their child for heart surgery?
   c. What are some ways parents can prepare themselves when their child is having heart surgery?
   d. Make a list of resources available to parents of children who are having heart surgery.

CRITICAL THINKING: WHAT WOULD YOU DO?

1. Diane's baby was born with a bilateral cleft lip and cleft palate. When you bring the baby to her for feeding, she breaks down and sobs uncontrollably.
   a. Describe what your immediate response would be.
   b. What feelings and emotions do you think Diane is experiencing?
   c. Write out an example of a therapeutic response you could make.

2. Cody was born with hydrocephalus and has been admitted to the pediatric unit to have a ventriculoperitoneal (VP) shunt placed. You walk into Cody's room after the health care provider has discussed the procedure with Cody's parents. They seem anxious and begin asking you questions. How will you answer the following questions?

   a. What is hydrocephalus, and what caused Cody to have the disorder?

   b. Why does Cody need to have a shunt, and how does it work?

   c. What long-term problems will Cody have because of the disorder?

3. *Dosage calculation:* The nurse is preparing the preoperative medication of meperidine (Demerol) for an infant who is having a surgical procedure to correct a congenital heart defect. The infant weighs 9.9 lb (9 lb, 14.4 oz). The usual dosage range of this medication is 1 to 2.2 mg/kg. Answer the following:

   a. How many kilograms does the infant weigh?

   b. What is the low dose of meperidine (in milligrams) that this infant could be given?

   c. What is the high dose of meperidine (in milligrams) that this infant could be given?

UNIT 7
Health Promotion for Normal Growth and Development

Principles of Growth and Development

22

Key Terms

anticipatory guidance
archetypes
cephalocaudal
cognitive development
development
developmental tasks
ego
egocentric
growth
id
latchkey child
libido
maturation
proximodistal
sublimation
superego
temperament

Learning Objectives

At the conclusion of this chapter, you will:

1. Explain growth, development, and maturation.
2. Describe cephalocaudal and proximodistal patterns of growth.
3. Explain how length, height, and weight are used to monitor growth and development.
4. Discuss how tools for measuring standards of growth and development are used.
5. Describe genetic, nutritional, and environmental factors that can influence a child's growth and development.
6. List and discuss the six stages of psychosexual development according to Freud.
7. Identify and describe the eight stages of Erikson's theory of psychosocial development and the developmental tasks in each stage.
8. Identify and describe the four stages of Piaget's theory of cognitive development.
9. Discuss the ideas included in Kohlberg's theory of the development of moral reasoning.
10. Discuss the important aspects of communicating with children of various ages and family caregivers.
11. Discuss the role of the nurse in understanding growth and development.

Ethan Anderson comes to the clinic for his 2-month well-child check. As you are collecting data on Ethan, his mother says, "I have so many questions now that we have a baby." As you read this chapter, note the topics about which you think Ethan's mother will ask questions.

The process of growth and development continues from conception all the way to death. There are periods of time when growth is more rapid than others and times when development is slowed. Growth and development are influenced by many factors. Some basic foundations of growth and development are important to understand when working and communicating with infants, children, and adolescents.

FOUNDATIONS OF GROWTH AND DEVELOPMENT

Growth and development refers to the total growth of the child from birth toward maturity. **Growth** is the physical increase in the body's size and appearance caused by increasing numbers of new cells.

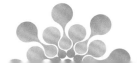

Development is the progressive change in the child toward maturity or **maturation**, completed growth and development. As children develop, their capacity to learn and think increases.

Growth of the child follows an orderly pattern starting with the head and moving downward. This pattern is referred to as **cephalocaudal**. The child is able to control the head and neck before being able to control the arms and legs. Growth also proceeds in a pattern referred to as **proximodistal**, in which growth starts in the center and progresses toward the periphery or outside (Fig. 22-1). Following this pattern, the child can control movement of the arms before being able to control movement of the hands. Another example of proximodistal growth is the ability to hold something in the hand before being able to use the fingers to pick up an object. The process of growth moves from the simple to complex.

 Concept Mastery Alert

Cephalocaudal and proximodistal growth patterns describe the way development normally occurs as children being to master new skills.

Developmental tasks or milestones are basic achievements associated with each stage of development. These tasks must be mastered to move successfully to the next developmental stage. Developmental tasks must be completed successfully at each stage for a person to achieve maturity.

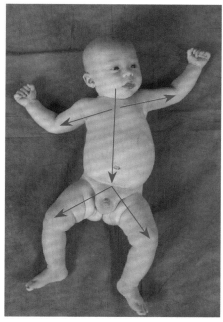

FIGURE 22-1 The pattern of growth starting with the head and moving downward is cephalocaudal. Proximodistal growth starts in the center and progresses outward.

Patterns of Growth

Each child has a unique pattern of growth. These patterns are related to height and weight. Monitoring these patterns and recognizing deviations from the child's normal pattern can be helpful in discovering medical issues and concerns.

Length and Height

As the child grows, the length or height, distance from the head to the feet, increases in a predictable pattern. The changes in a child's length and height provide a concrete measurement of the child's growth. Although predictable, the increases in length and height are not uniform but are often seen in growth spurts, or time periods during which there is rapid growth, and other periods of time when growth is slowed. The length of the infant and the increasing height of the child are measured routinely (see Chapter 28), and the patterns are monitored and plotted on a growth chart. The increase in length and height seen in children and adolescents results from the skeletal growth that is taking place.

Weight

The weight gain of the child also progresses in a predictable pattern. For many different reasons, there are variations in the weight of children of the same age, so the weight gain of each individual child is an important factor in the growth of the child. Patterns of weight increases are monitored and plotted on growth charts.

Body Proportions

From fetal life through adulthood, body proportions vary and change. As the fetus develops and the child grows, the development of body systems and organs affects and changes the body proportions (Fig. 22-2). In early fetal life, the head is growing faster than the rest of the body and is thus proportionately larger. During infancy, the trunk portion of the body grows significantly. The legs grow rapidly during childhood, again changing the body proportions. The trunk portion grows as the child grows into an adolescent, and the body proportions are those of an adult.

Standards of Growth

A growth chart with predictable patterns or growth curves is used to plot and monitor a child's growth through the years. These growth charts allow for comparison of children of the same age and sex. They also allow for comparison of the child's current measurements with the child's previous measurements. Standard growth charts are used to determine whether the child's pattern is appropriate or whether for some reason the child's growth is above or falls below a standardized normal range (see Appendix E). A growth chart is used for comparison only. It does not necessarily indicate that there is something of concern for that child, if a child does not fall into the "normal" range.

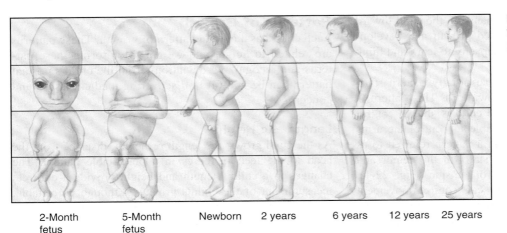

FIGURE 22-2 From fetal life through adulthood, the body proportions change.

2-Month fetus   5-Month fetus   Newborn   2 years   6 years   12 years   25 years

 A Personal Glimpse

Every time I had to take my baby to the pediatrician's office for his well-baby checkup, I would worry for days. The nurse would always weigh and measure him and look at the growth chart, then look at me with a curious look. Sometimes she would weigh him again and then just stare at me. I would ask what was wrong, and she would say in an accusing voice, "Well, he is in the 95th percentile for height and in the 5th percentile for weight." She would start asking me questions like was I feeding him often enough, did he cry all the time, did he have a babysitter who took care of him while I worked, or just why was he not gaining enough weight. I would get so upset because they acted like I was starving or neglecting my baby, and I knew I wasn't. Finally when he was 11 months old, it was discovered that he had a digestive problem and couldn't drink milk or eat wheat or oatmeal—his low weight didn't have anything to do with the way I was taking care of him. I started giving him soy milk, changed his diet, and right away he started gaining weight. I was so relieved that now finally he was in a higher percentile on the growth chart. I will never forget how bad I felt when I was treated as if I was a neglectful mother; that was so hard. I am glad the disorder was discovered—by the time he was 21, he was 6 ft and 3 in. tall and weighed 190 lb!

Diane

Learning Opportunity: *What were the benefits in this situation of plotting this child's growth on a growth chart? What do you think this mother was feeling when she was in the pediatrician's office? What could the nurse have done to support this mother?*

Standards of Development

Developmental screening is done by using standardized developmental tools, such as the Denver Developmental Screening Test. Development in children occurs in a range of time rather than at an exact time. Developmental screening identifies any delays in what is considered a standard or normal pattern. Although one child might develop at a faster rate than another child within a time range, both children will have mastered developmental tasks or milestones, thus following a normal and predictable pattern. It is important to recognize that developmental screening is used for the sake of comparison and does not automatically mean there is a concern if the child does not fit exactly into the standardized normal pattern.

A Word of Caution Is In Order!

Growth charts and developmental tools should be used only as a *guide*. Not every child, even though normal, follows the same growth and development pattern as other children of the same age.

TEST YOURSELF
✔ Define growth, development, and maturation.
✔ What do cephalocaudal and proximodistal mean?
✔ How do body proportions in the child differ from those in the adult?
✔ Why is the child's height and weight plotted on a growth chart?

INFLUENCES ON GROWTH AND DEVELOPMENT

There are many influences on the growth and development of a child. Prenatal factors that influence the child's growth and development include the mother's general health and nutrition, as well as her behaviors during pregnancy. These factors as well as genetic, nutritional, and environmental factors all affect the growth and development of the child.

Genetics

The science of genetics studies the ways in which normal and abnormal traits are transmitted from one generation to the next. The scientist Gregor Mendel did experiments that proved each parent's individual traits could reappear unchanged in later generations. Human cells contain 46 chromosomes, consisting of 23 essentially identical pairs. At conception, the union of the sperm and egg forms a single cell. This cell is made up of one member of each chromosome pair contributed by the father and one member of each pair contributed by the mother. This combination determines the sex and inherited traits of the new organism.

The genetic makeup of each child helps determine characteristics such as the child's eye color, height, weight, and other physical traits. Growth and development of the child is influenced by these factors. For example, each child is genetically programmed to grow to a certain height. Most children will attain this height with adequate nutrition and good health. Some diseases are genetically transmitted. If a child has a genetic predisposition to a certain disease, then that child might not grow and develop as completely as a healthy child would. Physical and mental disorders can occur as a result of a child's genetic factors.

 Cultural Snapshot

Some cultural groups are more prone to certain diseases and disorders. Many of these are genetically passed from generation to generation. It helps a nurse to remain supportive and objective when they are sensitive to the concerns, fears, and feelings of these people from various cultural backgrounds.

The child's heredity also influences personality characteristics, including **temperament**. Temperament is the combination of all of an individual's characteristics: the way the person thinks, behaves, and reacts to something that happens in their environment. Not all children react alike to the same situation. Depending on temperament, one child might react to a situation with a quiet, shy response, whereas another child might react with acting out or aggressive behavior in the same situation. Children with differing temperaments might adapt in different time frames to new situations. One child might quickly adapt to the new situation, whereas another child might adapt more slowly. Characteristics that evidence a child's temperament include their activity level; the development of regular patterns in daily life such as waking, eating, and elimination patterns; and how they approach and adapt to situations. Temperament also plays a part in a child's attention span and how easily they become distracted. All of these characteristics of temperament play a part in the child's development.

Nutrition

The quality of a child's nutrition during the growing years has a major effect on their overall health and development. The child needs adequate amounts of food and nutrients for the body to grow. Nutrition is also a factor in the child's ability to resist infection and diseases. Motor skill development is influenced by inadequate and excessive food intake. The child establishes nutritional habits and patterns early in life; these patterns are carried into adulthood, thusly influencing the individual's growth, development, and health throughout their life.

The U.S. Department of Agriculture has developed ChooseMyPlate on which daily dietary guidelines are based. These guidelines provide a healthy, balanced diet

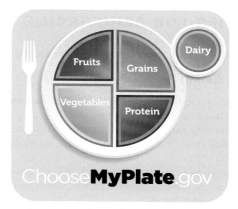

FIGURE 22-3 ChooseMyPlate. (Adapted from U.S. Department of Agriculture. (2021). *ChooseMyPlate*. http://www.choosemyplate.gov)

when followed. Foods from the main food groups necessary for good nutrition are included. Figure 22-3 shows the ChooseMyPlate graphic that includes each of the food groups. Fruits and vegetables should take up half the plate while grains like whole-grain cereal, bread, and pasta take up a quarter. Protein like low-fat meat and beans fills another quarter. Dairy should come in the form of low-fat milk, yogurt, and cheese. The U.S. Department of Agriculture also provides families with recommendations for healthy eating and physical activity (Tips for Reinforcing Family Teaching: Healthy Eating and Physical Activity).

Normal nutritional needs and daily requirements vary at each stage of development. In addition, eating patterns, skills, and behaviors vary at each stage. These aspects of nutrition are discussed in the chapters covering each of the stages of growth and development.

Environment

Many aspects of the child's environment affect growth and development. The family structures, including family size, sibling order, parent–child relationships, and cultural background, all affect the growth and development of the child (see Chapter 2). The socioeconomic level of the family can affect the child, especially if there are not sufficient funds to provide adequate nutrition, child care, and healthcare for the growing child. Living in a household in which family caregivers are addicted to drugs or alcohol can affect the child (see Chapter 33). Play and entertainment are important environmental aspects in the development of a child. Other environmental factors that can affect growth and development include family homelessness and divorce, a latchkey situation (in which children come home from school to an empty house each day), and running away from home.

Play and Entertainment

Play is an essential part of child development. Roles and types of play differ throughout the stages of growth and development. Various aspects of play, including the roles, types, and functions of play, are discussed in each of the chapters covering the stages of growth and development. Movies,

TIPS FOR REINFORCING FAMILY TEACHING

Healthy Eating and Physical Activity

Healthy Eating

- *Enjoy your food.* Follow the ChooseMyPlate recommendations. Balance calories and portions.
- *Focus on whole fruits.* Eat them at meals and at snack time, too. Choose fresh, frozen, canned, or dried, but go easy on fruit juice.
- *Vary your veggies.* Go dark green, red, and orange with your vegetables; eat spinach, broccoli, carrots, red peppers, tomatoes, and sweet potatoes.
- *Make half your grains whole.* Choose whole-grain foods more often: whole-wheat bread, oatmeal, brown rice, and low-fat popcorn.
- *Vary your protein routine.* Eat lean or low-fat beef, chicken, turkey, and fish. Also, change your tune with more dry beans and peas. Add chickpeas, nuts, or seeds to a salad; pinto beans to a burrito; or kidney beans to soup.
- *Get your dairy, calcium-rich foods.* To build strong bones, serve low-fat and fat-free milk, yogurt, cheese, and other dairy products every day.
- *Change your oil and eat less saturated fat.* We all need oil. Get yours from fish, nuts, and liquid oils, such as corn, soybean, canola, and olive oils.
- *Drink and eat less sodium.* Processed foods and drinks often contain high amounts of sodium. Choose fresh when possible. Use spices and herbs (dill, chili powder, paprika, cumin, lemon, or lime juice), rather than salt to add flavor.
- *Don't sugarcoat it.* Choose foods and beverages that do not have sugar and caloric sweeteners as one of the first ingredients listed on their nutrition labels. Added sugars contribute calories with few, if any, nutrients. Drink water!

Physical Activity

- *Set a good example.* Be active, and get your family to join you. Have fun together. Play with the kids or pets. Go for a walk, tumble in the leaves, or play catch.
- *Establish a routine.* Set aside time each day as activity time—walk, jog, skate, cycle, or swim. Adults need at least 30 minutes of physical activity most days of the week, and children need 60 minutes every day.
- *Have an activity party.* Make the next birthday party centered on physical activity. Try backyard Olympics or relay races. Have a bowling or skating party.
- *Set up a home gym.* Use household items, such as canned foods, as weights. Stairs can substitute for stair machines. There are also many exercises you can do without equipment like push-ups, yoga, squats, Pilates, etc. Look for some good ideas on the internet.
- *Move it!* Instead of sitting through TV commercials, get up and move. When you talk on the phone, lift weights or walk around. Remember to limit TV watching and computer time.
- *Give activity gifts.* Give gifts that encourage physical activity like active games or sporting equipment.

Adapted from U.S. Department of Agriculture. (2021). *ChooseMyPlate.* http://www.choosemyplate.gov

---

television, videogames, and the internet, while forms of entertainment for children of all ages, have both positive and negative influences on child development. These activities offer emotional enjoyment and educational opportunities, but are passive modes of play that do not always encourage a child to use their imagination. It is important to balance these activities with active modes of play that will encourage creativity and promote imagination.

"Playing" Is the Job of Every Child!

Children learn about themselves, the environments around them, and relationships with others through play.

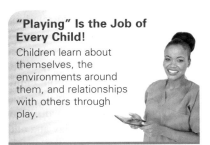

Be Aware!

When children participate in activities related to movies, television, videogames, computers, and the internet, it is important to carefully monitor or supervise what they are seeing and doing to ensure the activity is appropriate and healthy for the child's development.

The Homeless Family

A growing number of families are homeless in the United States. The causes of homelessness include job loss, loss of housing, drug addiction, insufficient income, domestic turmoil, and separation or divorce. Single mothers with children make up an increasing number of these families. Many of these homeless single mothers and their families have multiple problems. There are often higher rates of abuse, drug use, and mental health problems in homeless families. Many of these families lived with relatives for a time before being reduced to living in a car, an empty building, a welfare hotel, or perhaps a cardboard box. These families sometimes seek temporary housing in a shelter for the homeless. They often move from one living situation to another by living in a shelter for the time allowed and then moving elsewhere, only to return after a while to repeat the cycle.

Homelessness creates additional stresses for the family. Many homeless families have young children but have problems gaining entry into the healthcare system, even though these children are at high risk for developing acute and chronic conditions. Healthcare for these families commonly occurs as crisis intervention, instead of the more effective preventive intervention. Pregnant homeless women often receive little if any prenatal care, are poorly nourished, and bear low-birth-weight infants. Most of the children of homeless families do not have adequate immunizations. Homeless children often have chronic illnesses at a higher rate than that of the general population. These chronic conditions may include anemia, heart disease, peripheral vascular disease, and neurologic disorders. Many homeless children have developmental delays, perform poorly when they attend school, suffer from anxiety and depression, and exhibit behavioral problems.

Shelters available to the homeless are often overcrowded, lack privacy (the bathroom facilities are used by many people), have no personal bedding or cribs for infants, and have no facilities for cooking or refrigerating food. Many families must move from one shelter to another because of limits to the length of stay. This adds to the problems these families face by contributing to a lack of consistency in the services and programs available to them.

As a nurse, you can set the tone of the interaction between the homeless family and the healthcare facility. Establishing an environment in which the child's family caregiver feels respected and comfortable is important. Focusing initially on the positive factors in the family caregiver's relationship with the children alleviates some of the caregiver's guilt and fear of being criticized. Make every effort to offer down-to-earth suggestions and help the family in the most practical manner.

On the child's admission to the healthcare facility, the healthcare team performs a complete admission assessment. Ask the family caregiver about the family's living arrangements; such information will help in the care and planning for the child. During this interview, you may become aware of problems of other family members that need attention. Take care to supplement but not take over the family's functioning when giving assistance and guidance. For instance, tell the family how to go about getting a particular benefit and be certain they have complete and accurate information, but do not take the steps for them. These families need to feel self-reliant and in control, and they need realistic solutions to their problems.

Outreach programs for the homeless have been established in many major cities. These programs conduct screening, treat acute illnesses, and help families contact local healthcare services when needed. Provide information to the family about any assistance that is available.

TEST YOURSELF

✔ Name three influences on a child's growth and development.

✔ How does homelessness potentially influence a child's growth and development?

Divorce and the Child

Divorce has increased to the point that one in two marriages ends in divorce. About 50% of children experience the separation or divorce of their parents before they complete high school. Some children may experience more than one divorce because many people who remarry may divorce a second time. Divorce can be traumatic for children but may be better than the constant tension and turmoil that they have lived through in their homes.

Children often feel responsible for the breakup and believe that it would not have occurred if they had just done the right thing or been better. On the other hand, children may blame one of the parents for deciding to end the marriage and causing them grief and unhappiness. Counseling can help children acknowledge and understand their anger and their need to blame one or the other parent. This process may take a considerable amount of time to resolve. Both parents should make every effort to eliminate the child's feeling of guilt and should avoid placing the child in the middle of their divorce (e.g., using the child as a spy or go-between with the estranged spouse). Parents must avoid trying to buy the affection of the children. This is especially true for the noncustodial parent, who must not shower the children with special gifts, trips, and privileges when the children are visiting.

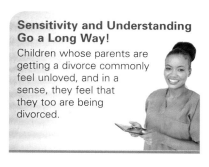

Sensitivity and Understanding Go a Long Way!

Children whose parents are getting a divorce commonly feel unloved, and in a sense, they feel that they too are being divorced.

Children should be encouraged to ask questions about the separation and divorce. A child who does not ask questions may be afraid to ask for fear of retaliation by one of the parents. Children should be discouraged from thinking that they might be able to do something that would get the parents back together again. They must be helped to recognize the finality of the divorce. Plans for the children should be made (e.g., where and with whom the children will live, where they will go to school) and shared with the children as soon as possible. This can give the child a sense of security in their chaotic personal world. Each child's confidence and self-esteem must be strengthened through carefully handling the transition (Fig. 22-4).

When a child of a divorce is hospitalized, be certain to have clear information about who is the custodial parent, as well as who may visit or otherwise contact the child. The custodial parent's instructions and wishes should be honored.

Encourage the child to express feelings of fear and guilt. Help the child understand that other children have divorced parents. The school nurse may function as an advocate for a counseling program in the school setting that brings together children of divorces. During counseling, children can voice their fears and concerns and begin to work through them with the help of an objective counselor in a protected environment. One of the most important aspects of such groups is the reassurance the children get that they are not alone in this crisis.

When the custodial parent begins to date and plans to remarry, the child may again have strong emotions that must be worked through. If the remarriage brings together a blended family of children from the previous marriages of both adults, the children may need extra support in accepting the new stepparent and stepsiblings. Adults who seek preventive counseling

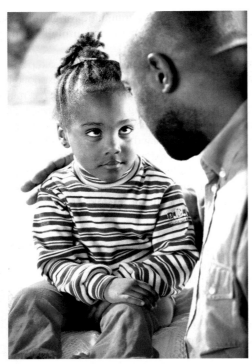

FIGURE 22-4 This father explains to his daughter that even though he and her mother will not be married and live in the same house anymore, he loves her and will see her often.

when planning to form a stepfamily have greater success than do those who seek help only after problems are overwhelming.

Children react in various ways to a parent's new marriage, depending in part on age. The new marriage may introduce additional problems of a new home, a new neighborhood, and a new school that can cause anxiety for any child. Although children should not be permitted to veto

the parent's choice of a new partner, every effort should be made to help them adjust to this new family member and view the change in a nonthreatening way.

The Latchkey Child

As a result of the increased number of families in which both parents work and the increase in single-parent families in which the parent must work, many children need after-school care and supervision; unfortunately, adequate or appropriate child care may not be readily available. A **latchkey child** is one who comes home to an empty house after school each day because the family caregivers are at work. The term was coined because this child often wears the house key around their neck. These children usually spend several hours alone before an adult comes home from work. The number of latchkey children may be as high as 12 million in the United States.

Latchkey children often have fears about being at home alone. When more than one child is involved and the older child is responsible for the younger one, conflicts can arise. The older child may have to assume responsibility that is beyond the normal expectations for the child's age. This can be a difficult situation for the family caregivers and the children. The caregivers must carefully outline permissible activities and safety rules (Fig. 22-5). A plan should be in place to help the older child solve any arising problems that involve both children. The older child should not feel that the complete responsibility is on their shoulders, but rather that it is a shared responsibility with the family caregiver. Some schools have after-school programs that provide safe activities for children. In addition, some communities have programs in which an adult calls the child regularly every day after school or there is a telephone hotline that the child can call (see Tips for Reinforcing Family Teaching: Tips for Family Caregivers of Latchkey Children).

TIPS FOR REINFORCING FAMILY TEACHING

Tips for Family Caregivers of Latchkey Children

- Remind the child to keep the key hidden and not show it to anyone.
- Remind the child not to enter house if something seems strange (open door, broken window, smoke).
- Establish a routine for the child to follow when they arrive home; work together to include something special for the child to do each day.
- Plan a telephone contact on the child's arrival home. Either have the child call you or you call the child. Texting can work as an alternative to calling, but remember to establish a security check of something that only you both know: what the child ate for breakfast, a security word, etc. You might even be able to hold a video chat or call. Check in with the child frequently.
- Always let the child know if you are going to be delayed.
- Have a code word that only family members know.
- Review safety rules with the child. Post them on the refrigerator as a reminder.
- Use a refrigerator chart to spell out daily responsibilities and have the child check off tasks as they are completed.

- Let the child know how much you appreciate their responsible behavior.
- Have a trusted neighbor for backup if the child needs help; be sure the child knows the telephone number and post it by the telephone. If the child is using a mobile phone, then make sure the neighbor is in their contacts list or that the child memorizes these numbers.
- Post telephone emergency numbers that the child can use; practice when to use them. Help them memorize these numbers.
- Remind the child to tell telephone callers that the caregiver is busy but never to say that the caregiver is not home.
- Remind the child not to open the door to anyone and to leave windows closed.
- Be specific about activities allowed and not allowed.
- Carefully survey your home for any hazards or dangerous temptations (e.g., guns, motorcycle, ATV, swimming pool, alcohol, medications). Eliminate them, if possible, or ensure that rules about them are clear.
- See if your community has a telephone friend program available for latchkey children.
- A pet can relieve loneliness, but give the child clear guidelines about care of the pet during your absence.

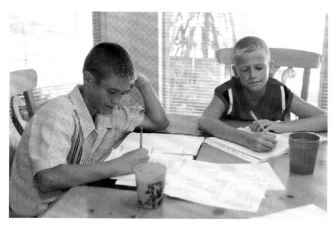

FIGURE 22-5 Latchkey children come home to an empty house after school. These boys have specific rules about activities to be done as they await the arrival of their family caregiver.

Despite concerns that latchkey children are more likely to become involved with smoking, stealing, or taking drugs, researchers have not found sufficient data to support this fear. Children who are given responsibility of this kind and who are recognized for their dependability usually live up to the expectations of the adults in their social environment.

Nurses must recognize the need for after-school services for these children and take an active role in the community to plan and support such services. Maintain a list of the facilities available to support families with latchkey children. Give family caregivers guidance in planning children's after-school activities and offer support to the caregivers in their attempts to provide for their children.

The Runaway Child

In the United States, as many as 750,000 to 2 million adolescents run away from home each year. A child can be considered a runaway after being absent from home overnight or longer without permission from a family caregiver. Most children who run away from home are 10 to 17 years of age.

A child may run away from home in response to circumstances that they view as too difficult to tolerate. Physical or sexual abuse, alcohol or drug abuse, divorce, stepfamilies, pregnancy, school failure, and truancy may contribute to a child's desire to escape. However, some adolescents are not runaways but rather *throwaways* who have been forced to leave home and are not wanted by the adults in the home. Often the throwaways have been forced out of the home because their behavior is unacceptable to family caregivers or because of other family stresses such as divorce, remarriage, and job loss.

Runaway or throwaway adolescents often turn to stealing, drug dealing, and prostitution to provide money for alcohol, drugs, food, and possibly shelter. Many of these adolescents live on the streets because they cannot pay for shelter. They may avoid going to public shelters for fear of being found by police. They may become victims of pimps or drug dealers who use the adolescents for their own gain.

There are numerous programs to help runaways, especially in urban areas. The 24-hour National Runaway Safeline (1-800-RUNAWAY, 1-800-786-2929) is available to give runaways information and referral (www.1800runaway.org). This service may help the runaway find a safe place to stay and may provide counseling, shelter, healthcare, legal aid, message relay to the family, and transportation home if desired. Runaways are not forced to go home but may be encouraged to inform their families that they are all right.

A sexually transmitted disease, pregnancy, acquired immunodeficiency syndrome, and drug overdose are the usual reasons that runaways are seen at healthcare facilities. When caring for such a child, be nonjudgmental. Any indication of being disturbed or disgusted by the adolescent's lifestyle may end any chance of cooperation and cause the adolescent to refuse to give any additional information. Try to build a trusting relationship with the child. Remember that the runaway viewed their problems as so great that escaping was the only way to resolve them. Counseling is necessary to begin to resolve the problems.

Health teaching for the runaway must be suited to their lifestyle and must be at a level the child can understand. Without prying excessively, try to find out the runaway's living circumstances and adjust the teaching plans accordingly. Remember that the child's problems did not come about overnight and they will not be resolved quickly. Caring for a runaway can be frustrating, challenging, and sometimes rewarding for the healthcare staff.

> ## TEST YOURSELF
> ✔ What are three commonly seen responses in children whose parents divorce?
> ✔ What are some concerns that might be expressed by family caregivers of "latchkey" children?
> ✔ Why is it especially important as a nurse to be nonjudgmental and develop a trusting relationship with the runaway child?

THEORIES OF CHILD DEVELOPMENT

How a helpless infant grows and develops into a fully functioning, independent adult has fascinated scientists for years. Four pioneering researchers whose theories in this area are widely accepted are Sigmund Freud, Erik Erikson, Jean Piaget, and Lawrence Kohlberg (Table 22-1). Their theories present human development as a series of overlapping stages that occur in predictable patterns. These stages are only approximations of what is likely to happen in children at various ages, and each child's development may differ from these stages.

TABLE 22-1 Comparative Summary of Theories of Freud, Erikson, Piaget, and Kohlberg

AGE (YEARS)	STAGE	FREUD (PSYCHOSEXUAL DEVELOPMENT)	ERIKSON (PSYCHOSOCIAL DEVELOPMENT)	PIAGET (INTELLECTUAL DEVELOPMENT)	KOHLBERG (MORAL DEVELOPMENT)
1	Infancy	Oral stage	Trust vs. mistrust	Sensorimotor phase	Stage 0—Do what pleases me
2–3	Toddlerhood	Anal stage	Autonomy vs. shame		Preconventional level Stage 1—Avoid punishment
4–6	Preschool (early childhood)	Phallic (infant genital) Oedipal stage	Initiative vs. guilt	Preoperational phase	Preconventional level Stage 2—Do what benefits me
7–12	School-age (middle childhood)	Latency stage	Industry vs. inferiority	Concrete operational phase	Conventional level Stage 3 (age 7–10)—Avoid disapproval Stage 4 (age 10–12)—Do duty, obey laws
13–18	Adolescence	Genital stage (puberty)	Identity vs. role confusion	Formal operational phase	Postconventional level Stage 5 (age 13)—Maintain respect of others Stage 6 (age 15)—Implement personal principles

Sigmund Freud

Most modern psychologists base their understanding of children at least partly on the work of Sigmund Freud. His theories focus primarily on the **libido** (sexual drive or development). Although Freud did not study children, his work focused on childhood development as a cause of later conflict. Freud believed that a child who did not adequately resolve a particular stage of development would have a fixation (compulsion) that correlated with that stage. Freud described three levels of consciousness: the **id**, which controls physical need and instincts of the body; the **ego**, the conscious self, which controls the pleasure principle of the id by delaying the instincts until an appropriate time; and the **superego**, the conscience or parental value system. These consciousness levels interact to check behavior and balance each other. The psychosexual stages in Freud's theory are the oral, anal, phallic, latency, and genital stages of development.

Oral Stage (Ages 0 to 2 Years)

The newborn first relates almost entirely to the mother (or someone taking a motherly role), and the first experiences with body satisfaction come through the mouth. This is true not only of sucking but also of making noises, crying, and breathing. It is through the mouth that the baby expresses needs, finds satisfaction, and begins to make sense of the world.

Anal Stage (Ages 2 to 3 Years)

The anal stage is the child's first encounter with the serious need to learn self-control and take responsibility. Toilet training looms large in the minds of many people as an important phase in childhood. Because elimination is one of the child's first experiences of creativity, it represents the beginnings of the desire to mold and control the environment.

The child has pride in the product created. Cleanliness and this natural pride do not always go together, so it may be necessary to help direct this pride and interest into more acceptable behaviors. Playing with such materials as modeling clay, crayons, and dough helps put the child's natural interests to good use, a process called **sublimation**.

Phallic (Infant Genital) Stage (Ages 3 to 6 Years)

In Freud's third stage, the child's interest moves to the genital area as a source of pride and curiosity. To the child's mind, this area constitutes the difference between boys and girls, a difference that the child is beginning to be aware of socially. The superego begins to develop during this stage.

During this stage, the child begins to understand what it means to be a boy or a girl. The child learns to identify with the parent of the same sex (Fig. 22-6). At about this time, a boy begins to take pride in being a male and a girl in being a female. In many families, a new brother or sister also arrives, arousing the child's natural interest in human origins. The family caregiver's reaction to the child's genital exploration may influence whether the child learns to feel satisfied with themselves as a sexual being or is laden with feelings of guilt and dissatisfaction throughout life.

Freud hypothesized that this awareness of genital differences also leads to a time of conflict in the child's emotional relationships with parents. The conflict occurs between attachment to and imitation of the parent of the same sex and the appeal of the other parent. The boy who for years has depended on his mother for all his emotional and physical needs now is confronted by his desire to be a man (Oedipus complex). The girl, who has imitated her mother, now finds her father a real attraction (Electra complex). It is through contact with parents that the child learns to relate

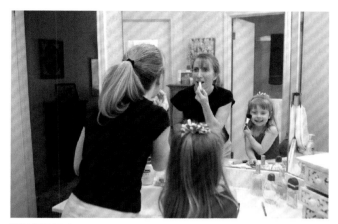

FIGURE 22-6 The preschool child learns to identify with the parent of the same sex.

to the opposite sex. The child learns the interests, attitudes, concerns, and wishes of the opposite sex.

Latency Stage (Ages 6 to 10 Years)

The latency stage is the time of primary schooling, when the child is preparing for adult life but must await maturity to exercise initiative in adult living. The child's sense of moral responsibility (the superego) develops, based on what has been taught through the parents' words and actions.

During this stage, the child is involved with learning, developing cognitive skills, and actively participating in sports activities with little thought given to sexual concerns. The child's main relationships are with peers of the same sex. Developing positive friendships at this stage helps the child learn about caring relationships.

When placed in an unfamiliar setting, children in this stage may become confused because they do not know what is expected of them. They need the sense of security that comes from approval and praise and usually respond favorably to a brief explanation of "how we do things here."

Genital Stage (Ages 11 to 13 Years)

Precocious puberty is occurring at an increasingly early age, and social puberty occurs even earlier, largely because of the influence of sexual frankness on television, in movies, and in the print media. At puberty, all of the child's earlier learning is concentrated on the powerful biologic drive of finding and relating to a mate. In earlier societies, mating and forming a family occurred at a young age. Our society delays mating for many years after puberty, creating a time of confusion and turmoil during which biologic readiness must take second place to educational and economic goals. This is a sensitive period during which privacy is important, and great uncertainty exists about relating to any member of the opposite sex. This development depends on a self-healing process that helps counterbalance the stresses created by natural and accidental crises. The self-healing process is delayed by any major crisis, such as hospitalization, that interrupts normal development. Interruptions may cause regression to an earlier stage, such as the older child who begins to wet the bed when hospitalized.

Erik Erikson

Building on Freud's theories, Erikson described human psychosocial development as a series of tasks or crises. According to Erikson and Senn (1958), "children 'fall apart' repeatedly, and unlike Humpty Dumpty, grow together again," if they are given time and sympathy and are not interfered with.

Erikson formulated a series of eight developmental tasks or crises with the first five pertaining to children and youth. To present a complete view of Erikson's theory, all eight tasks are presented. In each task, the person must master the central problem before moving on to the next one. Each task holds positive and negative counterparts, and each of the first five implies new developmental tasks for parents (Table 22-2).

TABLE 22-2 Child and Parent Developmental Tasks According to Erikson

DEVELOPMENTAL LEVEL	BASIC TASK	STAGE OF PARENTAL DEVELOPMENT	PARENTAL TASK
Infant	Trust	Learning to recognize and interpret infant's cues	To interpret cues and respond positively to the infant's needs; hold, cuddle, and talk to infant
Toddler	Autonomy	Learning to accept child's need for self-mastery	To accept child's growing need for freedom while setting consistent, realistic limits; offer support and understanding when separation anxiety occurs
Preschool-age	Initiative	Learning to allow child to explore surrounding environment	To allow independent development while modeling necessary standards; generously praise child's endeavors to build child's self-esteem
School-age	Industry	Learning to accept rejection without deserting	To accept child's successes and defeats, assuring child of acceptance to be there when needed without intruding unnecessarily
Adolescent	Identity	Learning to build a new life, supporting the emergence of the adolescent as an individual	To be available when adolescent feels need; provide examples of positive moral values; keep communication channels open; adjust to changing family roles and relationships during and after the adolescent's struggle to establish an identity

Trust Versus Mistrust (Ages 0 to 1 Year)

The infant has no way to control the world other than crying for help and hoping for rescue. During the first year, the child learns whether the world can be trusted to give love and concern or only frustration, fear, and despair. The infant who is fed on demand learns to trust that cries, communicating a need, will be answered. The baby fed according to the nurse's or family caregiver's schedule does not understand the importance of routine but only that these cries may go unanswered.

> **This Is Critical to Remember!**
> Trust has to be established and then reinforced at each stage of growth and development. Help the child build a trusting relationship by being consistent and responding appropriately to the child's needs at every age.

Autonomy Versus Doubt and Shame (Ages 1 to 3 Years)

Even the smallest child wants to feel in control and needs to learn to perform tasks independently, even when this takes a long time or makes a mess. The toddler gains reassurance from self-feeding, from crawling or walking alone where it is safe, and from being free to handle materials and learn about things in the environment (Fig. 22-7).

A toddler exploring the environment begins to explore and learn about their body, too. If family caregivers react appropriately to this normal behavior, the child will gain self-respect and pride. However, if caregivers shame the child for responding to this natural curiosity, the child may develop and sustain the belief that somehow the body is dirty, nasty, and bad.

Initiative Versus Guilt (Ages 3 to 6 Years)

During this period, the child engages in active, assertive play. Steadily improving physical coordination and expanding social skills encourage behavior to gain adult attention (showing off) and, the child hopes, approval. The preschool child is still self-centered and plays alone even though they are in the company of other children; interaction comes later. These children want to know what the rules are and enjoy being good and the adult approval that action gains. During this time, the child develops a conscience and accepts punishment for doing wrong because it relieves feelings of guilt.

Children in this phase of development generally do not have a concept of time. The child needs a familiar frame of reference to understand when something is going to happen. For example, the parent or caregiver may say, "I will be back when your lunch comes" or "I will be back when the cartoons come on TV." Explaining that it is time for "Mommy and Daddy to go to work" might help an unhappy child realize that they are not leaving because of any negative behavior of the child's.

> **Notice This Difference!**
> When working with children who have not fully developed a concept of time, explaining at the end of a shift that you must go home to your own family may help the child understand and realize you are not leaving because of any negative behavior of the child's.

Industry Versus Inferiority (Ages 6 to 12 Years)

Children begin to seek achievement in this phase. They learn to interact with others and sometimes to compete with them. They like activities they can follow through to completion and tangible results (Fig. 22-8).

Competition is healthy as long as the standards are not so high that the child feels there is no chance of winning. Praise, not criticism, helps the child build self-esteem and avoid feelings of inferiority. It is important to emphasize that everyone is a unique person and deserves to be appreciated for their own special qualities.

Identity Versus Role Confusion (Ages 12 to 18 Years)

Adolescents are confronted by marked physical and emotional changes and the knowledge that soon they will be

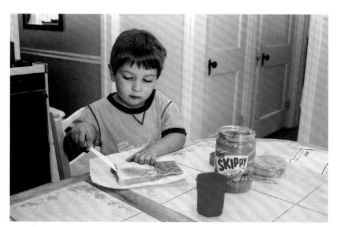

FIGURE 22-7 This toddler has a desire to do things independently.

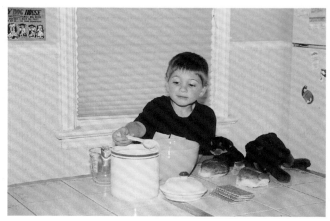

FIGURE 22-8 The school-aged child enjoys activities that produce tangible results.

responsible for their own lives. The adolescent develops a sense of being an independent person with unique ideals and goals and may feel that parents, caregivers, and other adults refuse to grant that independence. Adolescents may break rules just to prove that they can. Stress, anxiety, and mood swings are typical of this phase. Relationships with peers are more important than ever.

Intimacy Versus Isolation (Early Adulthood)
A person tries to establish intimate personal relationships with friends and an intimate love relationship with one person during early adulthood. Marriage and starting a family often occurs in this stage. Difficulty in establishing intimacy results in feelings of isolation.

Generativity Versus Self-Absorption (Young and Middle Adulthood)
For many people during this phase family and family life are most important. Others may find fulfillment in a profession, establishing a career, or in a religious vocation. Doing or producing something that makes a difference to society is an important part of this stage. The person who does not find this fulfillment becomes self-absorbed or stagnant and ceases to socially develop.

Ego Integrity Versus Despair (Old Age)
This final phase is often a period of reflection. Some look back and find their life was one of satisfaction and feel contented with themselves, their achievements, and their present condition without regret for the past or fear of the future. Others may have a sense of failure and despair.

Jean Piaget
Freud and Erikson studied psychosexual and psychosocial developments; Jean Piaget brought new insight into **cognitive development** or intellectual development—how a child learns and develops the quality called intelligence. He described intellectual development as a sequence of four principal stages made up of several substages (Piaget, 1967). All children move through these stages in the same order, but each moves at their own pace.

Sensorimotor Phase (Ages 0 to 2 Years)
The newborn behaves at a sensorimotor level linked entirely to desires for physical satisfaction. The newborn feels, hears, sees, tastes, and smells countless new things and moves in an apparently random way. Purposeful activities are controlled by reflexive responses to the environment. For example, a newborn gazes intently at the mother's face while nursing, grasps her finger, smells the nipple, and tastes the milk. This involves all senses.

As the infant grows, an understanding of cause and effect develops. When random arm motions strike the string of bells stretched across the crib, the newborn hears the sound made and eventually can manipulate the arms deliberately to make the bells ring.

In the same way, newborns cannot understand words or even the tone of voice; only through hearing conversation

directed to them can they pick out sounds and begin to understand (Fig. 22-9). As the infant produces verbal noises, the responses of those nearby are encouraging and eventually help the infant learn to talk.

Preoperational Phase (Ages 2 to 7 Years)
The child in this phase of development is **egocentric**. This means that they cannot perceive from another's point of view. The child's interpretation of the world is from a self-centered point of view and in terms of what is seen, heard, or otherwise experienced directly.

This child has no concept of quantity; if it looks like more, then it is more. Four ounces of juice poured into two glasses looks like more than 4 oz in one glass. A sense of time is not yet developed, so the preschool-aged or early school-aged child cannot always tell if something happened a day ago, a week ago, or a year ago.

Concrete Operations (Ages 7 to 11 Years)
During this stage, children develop the ability to begin problem solving in a concrete, systematic way. They can classify and organize information about their environments. Unlike in the preoperational stage, children begin to understand that volume or weight may remain the same even though the appearance changes. These children can consider another's point of view and can simultaneously deal with more than one aspect of a situation.

Formal Operations (Ages 12 to 15 Years)
The adolescent is capable of dealing with ideas, abstract concepts described only in words or symbols. The person in this stage begins to understand jokes based on double meanings and enjoys reading and discussing theories and philosophies. Adolescents can observe and then draw logical conclusions from their observations.

Lawrence Kohlberg
Each of the theorists focuses on one element in the development of children. Kohlberg's theory is about the development of moral reasoning in children. Moral development closely follows cognitive development because reasoning

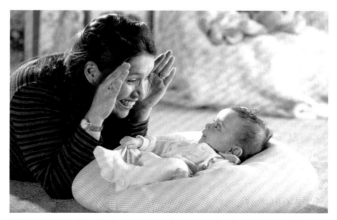

FIGURE 22-9 The infant responds to mother's voice and her facial expressions.

and abstract thinking (the ability to conceptualize an idea without physical representation) are necessary to make moral judgments. Kohlberg's theory is divided into three levels with two or three stages in each level.

Preconventional (Premoral) Level

During the first 2 years (stage 0), there is no moral sensitivity. This is a time of egocentricity where decisions are made with regard only to what pleases the child or makes them feel good and what displeases or hurts the child. The child is not aware of how their behavior may affect others. The child simply reacts to pleasure with love and to hurtful experiences with anger.

In stage 1, punishment and obedience orientation (ages 2 to 3 years), the child determines right or wrong by the physical consequence of a particular act. The child simply obeys the person in power with no understanding of the underlying moral principle.

In stage 2, naive instrumental self-indulgence (ages 4 to 7 years), the child views a specific act as right if it satisfies their needs. Children follow the rules to benefit themselves. They think, "I'll do something for you if you'll do something for me," and on the other hand, "If you do something bad to me, I'll do something bad to you." This is basically the attitude of equal reciprocity or "an eye for an eye."

Think About This!

When working with children who are in the process of developing a sense of right and wrong, it is important to understand that the child thinks if they are punished for doing something, then the action is wrong. If the child does not get punished, then they think the behavior is right or acceptable.

Conventional Level

As concrete operational thought develops, children can engage in moral reasoning. School-aged children become aware of the feelings of others. Living up to expectations is a primary concern, regardless of the consequences.

In stage 3, good-boy orientation (ages 7 to 10 years), being nice is very important. Children want to avoid a guilty conscience. Pleasing others is very important.

In stage 4, law and order orientation (ages 10 to 12 years), showing respect to others, obeying the rules, and maintaining social order are the desired behaviors. *Right* is defined as something that finds favor with family, teachers, and friends. *Wrong* is symbolized by broken relationships.

Postconventional (Principled) Level

The child usually achieves Piaget's formal operational stage by adolescence. The adolescent must have attained the formal operational stage of cognitive development in order to achieve the postconventional level of moral development. As a result, many people do not reach this level.

In stage 5, social contract orientation (ages 13 to 18 years), culturally accepted values define personal standards and personal rights. A person's rights must not be violated for the welfare of the group. The end no longer justifies the means. Laws are for mutual good, cooperation, and development.

Stage 6, personal principles, is not attained very frequently. The person who reaches this level does what they think is right without regard for legal restrictions, the cost to self, or the views of others. They would not do anything that would intentionally harm themselves or another because of their deep respect for life.

TEST YOURSELF

✔ What are the five stages of growth and development according to Freud?

✔ What are the tasks that must be mastered at each of the five stages of child development according to Erikson?

✔ How are Piaget and Kohlberg's theories of development similar?

Other Theorists

Freud, Erikson, Piaget, and Kohlberg are only four of the many researchers who have studied the development of children and families. Carl Jung's contribution to the study of child growth and development focused on the inner sequence of events that shape the personality. He emphasized that human development follows predetermined patterns called **archetypes**. These archetypes replace the instinctive behavior present in other animals. Interaction of the archetypes with the outside environment is evident throughout human life. For example, a normal child learns to suck, crawl, walk, and talk without any instruction, but the details of how the child does these things come from observation and imitation of others.

Jung believed that the first 3 years of a child's life are spent coordinating experiences and learning to make a conscious personality who is a distinct person separate from the rest of the environment. In the following years, the child learns to make sense of the environment by associating new discoveries to a general approach to the world. Dreams and nightmares help express personality developments that for some reason do not find a conscious outlet.

Jung points out that what happens to a child is not so critical to the child's development as the responses to these happenings. A hospital experience may permanently scar a child's personality if the child's natural feeling of terror is overlooked. Hospitalization may be accepted and even become a point of pride, however, if carried out in an atmosphere of assurance and support of the child's emotional concern and the need for love and acceptance.

The interaction between inner development and the environment is particularly clear in studies of young children who have been deprived in some way. John Bowlby's studies of children who were not held or loved and Bruno Bettelheim's studies of children given good physical care but little or no emotional satisfaction indicate how vital psychological interaction is.

In recent years, the theories of Erikson, Piaget, and Kohlberg have been criticized for being gender-specific to males and culturally specific to whites. In response, several theorists have conducted research on the growth and development of females and varying ethnic groups. Most notably, Carol Gilligan researched the moral development of males and females, and Patricia Green sought to construct a "truly universal theory of development through the empirical and theoretical understanding of cultural diversity" (Cocking & Greenfield, 1994).

DEVELOPMENTAL CONSIDERATIONS FOR COMMUNICATING WITH CHILDREN AND FAMILY CAREGIVERS

Communicating with children and family caregivers is a primary source of data collection during a well-child visit or in any health crisis situation. Communication occurs in all settings and focuses on data collection as well as information related to immunizations, developmental assessment, and reinforcing teaching. Offering **anticipatory guidance**, information that helps the caregiver understand and prepare for what to expect at a stage of growth and development, is important in communicating with family caregivers. Information about the child is derived from the child, the family caregivers, and observations of the child and family. Understanding the developmental level of the child and influences on the child's and caregiver's communication (e.g., family, culture, community, age, personality) is critical for communicating effectively.

Principles of Communication

Communication includes spoken and written words as well as the body language, facial expressions, voice intonations, and emotions behind the words. Listening is one of the most important aspects of communication. When listening, think about what the person is saying and *not* about how you are going to respond. Listening includes attending (giving the other person physical signs that you are listening) and following (encouraging the speaker to fully express what it is they need to say). Silence is also a form of communication, and it might indicate that the person is thinking, is unclear about what is being said, is having difficulty responding, is angry, and so on.

Always Remember!

Listening includes more than hearing. It includes tuning into the other person, being sensitive to the person's feelings, and concentrating on what the other person is trying to express.

Time management is an important aspect of communication. Communicate in a calm and unhurried manner, even though work demands and time constraints often make this difficult. It is important to gain skill in balancing communication needs of children and families with other nursing responsibilities.

Some nurses have difficulty accepting their own feelings while working with children. A nurse might feel anxious or inadequate when starting new relationships and beginning to communicate with children. Remember that this feeling is normal and that your communication skills will improve with experience over time.

To direct the focus of a conversation, use open-ended questions followed by guided statements. It is always important to clarify statements and feelings expressed by family caregivers and children. Reflective statements help indicate what you believe was expressed. For example, you might state, "You seem worried about Maria's loss of appetite."

One of the biggest challenges when several people are present is deciding to whom you should direct questions. Although eventually you will need information from the child and family caregivers, start with the child if they can talk. Even at age 3, some children can tell you about the specific problem. Good strategies when communicating with children include maintaining eye contact, playful engagement, and talking about what interests the child. Play is an important form of communication for children and can be an effective technique in communicating with children.

Avoid communication blocks, which include socializing, giving unsolicited advice, providing false assurances, being defensive, giving pat or cliché responses, being judgmental or stereotyping, not allowing issues to be fully explored, interrupting, and not allowing the person to finish a response.

Sometimes it is necessary to communicate through an interpreter because of language barriers or hearing impairments. A medical interpreter trained in the language of the child is preferable but not always available. When using an interpreter, ensure that the interpreter understands the goal of the conversation. Allow the interpreter and family to become acquainted, and then communicate directly with the family and the child, observing nonverbal responses. Pose questions to elicit one answer at a time, and do not interrupt the conversation between the interpreter and family. It is important not to talk about the family and child to the interpreter in English because the family might understand some information. Avoid medical jargon, and respect cultural differences. Follow up with the interpreter regarding their impression of the interaction and arrange for the interpreter to meet with the family on subsequent visits.

Communicating With Infants

Infants evaluate actions and respond to sensory cues. Infants cannot realize that a nurse who handles them abruptly and hurriedly may be rushed or insecure; they only feel that the nurse is frightening and unloving. To comfort the infant, hold, cuddle, and soothe them, or allow family caregivers to do so. Spending time in the beginning of an interaction to calm down and connect with the infant is helpful.

It is important to establish a relationship with the family caregiver up front. Begin by recognizing and praising the hard work of parenting. Allow the caregiver to hold the infant as you initiate conversation, and begin observing the infant, caregiver, and their interactions. When appropriate, ask the caregiver for permission to hold the infant yourself or to place them on an examination table or bed.

Sensory play activities, such as massaging the infant, stretching the arms and legs, looking at a colorful or moving object, and playing peek-a-boo and "this little piggy," can ease the child and convey a sense of safety and comfort.

During **Ethan Anderson**'s well-child check, his mother states, "I don't know how to communicate with an infant." What information will you reinforce with Ethan's mom regarding communicating with infants?

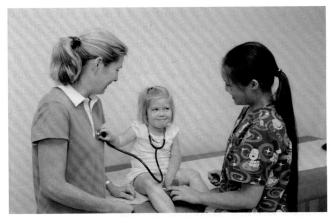

FIGURE 22-10 The nurse encourages the child to communicate by allowing her to play with the medical equipment.

Communicating With Young Children

Allow the family caregiver to hold the young child as you initiate conversation, and begin observing the child, caregiver, and their interactions. When appropriate, ask the caregiver permission to hold the child yourself or to place them on an examination table or bed.

Remember that according to normal stages of development, young children are egocentric. Explain to them how they will feel or what they can do. Experiences of others have no relevance. Use short sentences, positive explanations, familiar and nonthreatening terms, and concrete explanations.

Young children tend to be frightened of strangers. Sudden abrupt or noisy approaches signal danger. The child needs time to evaluate the situation while still in the arms of the caregiver. Do not rush the situation, but allow time for the child to initiate the relationship. Spending time calming down or connecting with the child is helpful. Conversation might be started through a doll, toy, or puppet. "What's doll's name?" "How does doll feel?" A casual approach with reluctant children is most effective. Games that pique the younger child's curiosity ("Which hand has the car?") might also help put them at ease. Children who show rejecting or aggressive behavior are putting up a defense. Ignore these behaviors unless they are harmful to the child or someone else.

Most Nurses Find This Approach Helpful!

Use your knowledge of growth and development to talk to the child at their level of development and understanding. Doing so will enable you to quickly establish rapport and begin a trusting relationship with the child.

Allow young children to handle or explore equipment that will come in contact with them. For example, have them touch the bell of a stethoscope, listen to their teddy bear's heart, or play a simple game with these objects (Fig. 22-10).

Such activities may communicate better than words because young children cannot yet understand abstract ideas.

Do not stand over and talk down to a young child when speaking with them. Instead, get down on eye level with them. Speak in a slow, clear, positive voice. Use simple words. Keep sentences short. Express statements and questions positively. Listen to the child's fears and worries and be honest in your answers. When possible, give the child choices so that they will feel a sense of having some control over the situation and often will be more cooperative. Choices should be simple and limited. Only offer choices if they exist. Do not ask, "Do you want medicine now?" if that is not an option. Do ask, "Would you like the red cup or the blue cup for your medicine?" Consult with the family caregiver about which choices are reasonable.

Young children tend to be literal and cannot separate fantasy from reality. Do not use analogies. For example, "This will be a little bee sting." Young children visualize a bee sting which might be traumatic.

Verbal skills are limited, so pay particular attention to nonverbal clues, such as pushing an object away, covering the eyes, crying, kicking, pointing, clinging, and exploring an object with the fingers.

Communicating With School-Aged Children

Remember to begin by calming down or connecting with the child. If family caregivers are present, briefly acknowledge them. Then, focus on the child. Include the child in the plan of care. School-aged children are interested in knowing the "what" and "why" of things. They will ask more questions if their curiosity is not satisfied. Provide simple, concrete responses using age-appropriate vocabulary. Complex or detailed explanations are not necessary. Provide explanations that help them understand how equipment works.

Be sensitive to the child's concern about body integrity. Children are particularly concerned about anything that poses a threat of injury to their bodies. Help reduce their anxieties by allowing them to voice concerns and by providing reassurances.

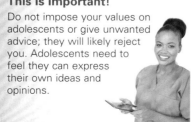

Here's a Helpful Hint!
When working with school-aged children, explain what is going to happen and why it is being done to *them* specifically. Charts, diagrams, and metaphors might be helpful. Elicit the child's cooperation by offering reasonable and limited choices.

Play, reenactment, or artwork can give insight into how well a child understands a procedure or experience. These activities can also reveal the child's perception of interpersonal relationships. Subsequent play can provide clues to the child's progress or changing feelings.

Communicating With Adolescents

Communicating with adolescents might be challenging. Adolescents waver between thinking like an adult and thinking like a child. Behavior is related to their developmental stage and not necessarily to chronologic age or physical maturation. Their age and appearance may fool you into assuming that they are functioning on a different level.

Adolescents respond positively to individuals who show a genuine interest in them. Show interest early and sustain a connection. Focus the interview on them rather than the problem. Build rapport by opening with informal conversation about friends, school, hobbies, and family. Once you have established rapport, return to more open-ended questions.

Adolescents might need to relate information they do not wish others to know, so they might not reveal much with family caregivers present. If adolescents and caregivers are to be interviewed, it might help to first interview the adolescent alone (thereby establishing relationship), then the adolescent and caregivers together, and then the caregivers separately. A discussion about confidentiality with both the family caregiver and adolescent might set concerns at ease. Explain to the caregiver and adolescent that some degree of independence will improve healthcare. Discuss why confidentiality is important, what will not be shared with caregivers, and what must be shared with caregivers (i.e., what the adolescent states is confidential unless the adolescent indicates that they intend to harm themselves or somebody else). Adolescents and caregivers might not always agree. In this case, clearly define the problem so an agreement might be reached. Encourage adolescents to discuss sensitive issues with caregivers.

This Is Important!
Do not impose your values on adolescents or give unwanted advice; they will likely reject you. Adolescents need to feel they can express their own ideas and opinions.

Let adolescents know that you will listen in an open-minded, nonjudgmental way. Avoid asking prying or embarrassing questions. Phrase questions regarding sensitive information in a way that encourages the adolescent to respond without feeling embarrassed. When feeling threatened, adolescents might not respond or only respond with monosyllabic answers. Reduce anxiety by confining conversations to nonthreatening topics until the adolescent feels at ease. Be aware of clues that they are ready to talk.

Make contracts with adolescents so that communication can remain open and honest and the plan of care may be more closely followed.

Communicating With Family Caregivers

Much of the information collected about the child comes from the family. In general, family members provide most of the care and are allies in promoting the health of the child. View the caregivers as experts in the care of the child and you as their consultant. Identify the child's family caregivers (not always mom or dad) and clarify roles. When the family structure is not immediately clear, you may avoid embarrassment by asking directly about other family members. "Who else lives in the home?" "Who is Jimmy's father?" "Do you live together?" Do not assume that because parents are separated that the other parent is not actively involved in care of the child. When talking with caregivers, observe how they interact with the child and how the child interacts with the environment. Watch how caregivers set limits or fail to set limits.

Include caregivers in providing information, problem solving, and planning of care (Fig. 22-11). Keep caregivers well informed of what is going on. Explain procedures and invite caregivers to help, but do not force them to participate if they are not comfortable doing so. Make the caregiver feel welcome and important. Encourage conferences between family caregivers and members of the healthcare team. Such meetings help caregivers form a clearer picture of the child and their behavior, condition, and health needs, and give them an opportunity to consider different types of treatments and relationships.

Pay attention to the verbal and nonverbal clues a family caregiver uses to convey concerns, worries, and anxieties about the child. Worries might be conveyed in an off-handed manner or referenced frequently. Remember the chief complaint might not relate to the real reason the caregiver has brought the child to the healthcare facility. Create a trusting atmosphere that allows caregivers to be open about all of their concerns. Ask facilitating questions: "Do you have any other concerns about Richie that you would like to tell me about?" "What did you hope I would be able to do for you today?" "Was there anything else that you wanted to tell or ask me about today?" When a caregiver introduces a concern or offers information without prompting, follow up with clarifying questions. Other times, it might be necessary to direct the conversation based on observations. When communicating with the caregiver, provide positive reinforcement and ask open-ended questions. This approach

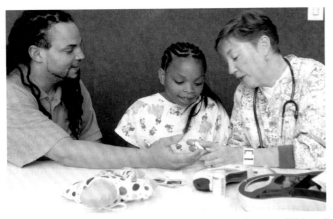

FIGURE 22-11 The nurse reinforces teaching with the child and caregiver together.

is nonthreatening and encourages description. Be supportive, not judgmental. "Why didn't you bring him sooner?" or "What did you do that for?" does not improve the relationship. Rather, acknowledge the hard work of parenting and praise successes.

To elicit information, it might be useful to compare what is actually happening with what the caregiver expects to be happening. If a mother says, "My 2-year-old son barely eats anything," it might be helpful to ask, "What do you think your child should be eating?" If the mother responds, "Three full meals a day, including green vegetables," you may interpret the problem differently from how the mother initially presented it to you.

Each individual in the room, including the health care provider, might have a different idea about the nature of the problem. Discover as many of these perspectives as possible. Family members who are not present may also have concerns. It is a good idea to ask about those concerns: "If Sally's father were here today, what questions or concerns would he have?" Agreement about a problem might not be mutual. Sometimes family caregivers might not perceive a problem you see; other times they might perceive a problem that you do not see. Explore what is behind the family caregiver perceptions and work toward a mutual agreement. Other members of the healthcare team might be needed.

Family caregiver concerns, anxieties, and negative attitudes might be conveyed to the child, which sometimes causes negative reactions from the child. Be alert to negative attitudes. Provide caregivers with opportunities to discuss and explore their anxieties, concerns, or problems. Demonstrate genuine care and concern to help ease these feelings. Some children might feel self-sufficient and view the caregiver's presence as being treated like a baby. However, it is often normal for the child to regress during illness, in which case the caregiver's presence may offer support.

Provide anticipatory guidance related to normal growth and development, nurturing childcare practices, and safety and injury prevention. In addition to providing information, help caregivers in using the information.

THE NURSE'S ROLE RELATED TO GROWTH AND DEVELOPMENT

As a pediatric nurse, it is important to have an understanding of factors and influences, as well as normal or expected patterns related to the growth and development of the infant, child, and adolescent. Knowledge of growth and development will help when working with the child in a well-child setting, during illness, or when a child is having surgery.

When interviewing the child and family caregiver, an understanding of growth and development will help you ask appropriate questions to determine whether the child's development is within the normal range or if there are variations or abnormalities present. Knowledge of growth and development helps you ask age-related questions, as well as answer caregiver questions regarding the child. In communicating with children, being aware of a child's language skills and development enables you to communicate at the child's level of understanding.

Much of your role as a pediatric nurse involves reinforcing teaching and working with family caregivers. Providing them with examples of normal growth and development and helping them think about safety and nutritional needs of their child are a vital aspect of anticipatory guidance. Anxiety and concerns of the family caregiver will be decreased by having an understanding of what to expect from the child in each stage of development.

When working with a sick child or one with a disease or disorder, be aware that the child's age and stage of growth and development can affect the way the child copes with the situation or responds to treatment. In developing a plan of care for any child, use knowledge of growth and development to provide the best care for the child.

> **This Advice Could be a Lifesaver!**
> An understanding of growth and development helps you offer suggestions to the caregivers about what behaviors to expect and what safety precautions to initiate for the child.

Remember Ethan from the beginning of the chapter. How will you answer these questions that Ethan's mother asks? "How do I know if Ethan is growing like he should be?" "What is important right now for Ethan's development?" "I am worried about keeping Ethan safe. How will I know what to do to keep him safe?"

KEY POINTS

- Growth is the physical increase in the body's size. Development is the progression of changes in the child toward maturity or maturation, which is completed growth and development.

- Growth following an orderly pattern from the head downward is called cephalocaudal. Proximodistal growth starts in the center and progresses outward.

- Length, height, and weight are monitored and plotted on growth charts to provide a comparison of measurements and patterns of a child's growth.

- Growth charts and developmental assessment tools are used to compare a child's growth to that of other children of the same age and sex. They are also used to compare the child's current measurements with their previous measurements.

- Genetic factors influence a child's physical characteristics such as the child's gender, race, eye color, height, and weight, as well as the child's overall growth and development. Some diseases as well as some physical and mental disorders are genetically transmitted. Personality characteristics, including temperament, are genetically influenced.

- The quality of a child's nutrition during the growing years has a major effect on the overall health and development of the child and throughout life. Nutrition is also a factor in the child's ability to resist infection and diseases.

- A lower socioeconomic level, decreased caregiver time and involvement, media exposure, and living in a household in which family caregivers are addicted to drugs or alcohol are environmental factors that may influence growth and development. Homelessness, divorce, latchkey situations, and running away from home are also environmental factors that influence a child's growth and development.

- According to Freud, in the oral stage of development, the newborn experiences bodily satisfaction through the mouth. During the anal stage, the child begins to learn self-control and taking responsibility. The child finds a source of pride and develops curiosity regarding the body in the phallic stage. Moral responsibility and preparing for adult life occur in the latency stage, and in the genital stage, puberty and the drive to find and relate to a mate occur.

- Erikson's theory of psychosocial development sets out sequential tasks that the child must successfully complete before going on to the next stage. His theory describes developmental tasks in eight stages as follows:

  - Trust versus mistrust—the infant learns that their needs will be met.

  - Autonomy versus doubt and shame—the toddler learns to perform independent tasks.

  - Initiative versus guilt—the child develops a conscience and sense of right and wrong.

  - Industry versus inferiority—the child competes with others and enjoys accomplishing tasks.

  - Identity versus role confusion—the adolescent goes through physical and emotional changes as they develop as an independent person with goals and ideas.

  - Intimacy versus isolation—the young adult develops intimate relationships.

  - Generativity versus self-absorption—the middle-aged adult finds fulfillment in life.

  - Ego integrity versus despair—the older adult is satisfied with life and the achievements attained.

- Piaget's four stages of cognitive development include the sensorimotor phase, in which the infant uses the senses for physical satisfaction. The young child in the preoperational phase sees the world from an egocentric or self-centered point of view. During the concrete operations phase, the child learns to problem-solve in a systematic way, and in the formal operations phase, the adolescent has their own ideas and can think in abstract ways.

- Kohlberg's theory relates to the development of moral reasoning in children. The child progresses from making decisions with no moral sensitivity to making decisions based on personal standards and values.

- Understanding the growth and development of the child and influences on the child and family caregivers is important for effective communication. Listening, maintaining eye contact, and playing with children can encourage communication. Infants evaluate actions and respond to sensory cues. Young children are egocentric and tend to be frightened of strangers. Use short sentences, positive explanations, familiar and nonthreatening terms, and concrete explanations. School-aged children are interested in knowing the *what* and *why* of things. Provide simple, concrete responses using age-appropriate vocabulary. Choices should be simple and limited. Let adolescents know that you will listen in an open-minded, nonjudgmental way. Phrase questions regarding sensitive information in a way that encourages the adolescent to respond without feeling embarrassed. Include caregivers in providing information, problem solving, and planning of care. Keep caregivers well informed.

- The nurse who understands normal growth and development is better able to develop an appropriate plan of care for the child, including the areas of communication, safety, and reinforcing family teaching. An understanding of growth and development helps the nurse offer appropriate anticipatory guidance to caregivers.

INTERNET RESOURCES

Runaway Children
http://www.missingkids.org/Runaway

Child Development
www.nacd.org (The National Association for Child Development)
www.piaget.org

Growth Charts
https://www.cdc.gov/growthcharts

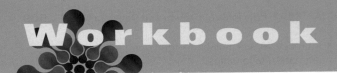
Workbook

NCLEX-STYLE REVIEW QUESTIONS

1. The nurse observes that during feeding, the newborn looks at the mother's face and holds her finger. According to Piaget, these observations indicate the child is in which phase of development?
  a. Sensorimotor
  b. Preoperational
  c. Concrete operations
  d. Formal operations

2. The nurse is caring for a toddler who has recently turned 2 years old. Of the following behaviors by the toddler, which would indicate the toddler is attempting to become autonomous? The toddler:
  a. cries when the caregiver leaves.
  b. walks alone around the room.
  c. "shows off" to get attention.
  d. competes when playing games.

3. In working with a preschool-aged child, which of the following statements made by the child's family caregiver would indicate an understanding of this child's stage of growth and development?
  a. "My child always wants her own way."
  b. "Why won't my child play with other children?"
  c. "I will tell my child I will be back after lunch."
  d. "She doesn't know when she has done something wrong."

4. In an interview, a 9-year-old child makes the following statement to the nurse: "I like to play basketball, especially when we win." This statement indicates this child is developing which basic task of child development?
  a. Trust
  b. Autonomy
  c. Initiative
  d. Industry

5. In discussing needs of adolescents with family caregivers, the nurse explains that to support the adolescent in developing their own identity, it would be *most* important for the adolescent caregiver to:
  a. respond to physical needs.
  b. praise the child's actions.
  c. accept the child's defeats.
  d. maintain open communication.

6. Using the growth charts in Appendix E, plot the measurements of a boy child who is 18 months old, 33 inches in length, and weighs 26 lb (1,179 g). What percentile is this child for length? Weight?

STUDY ACTIVITIES

1. Using the following table, compare the theories of Freud, Erikson, Piaget, and Kohlberg regarding children who are in the early elementary school years.

	Name of Theorist	Main Ideas and Similarities Between Theorist Ideas
Latency stage		
Industry stage		
Concrete opera-tional stage		
Conventional level		

2. Erikson identified trust as the development task for the first stage of life. Discuss why successful accomplishment of this task is essential to the person's future happiness and adjustment.

3. Go to http://www.cdc.gov/ncbddd/childdevelopment/screening.html.
  a. What is the main objective for doing developmental monitoring and screening?
  b. Standardized developmental and behavioral screening tests are most often done during well-child visits at what ages?
  c. What are some developmental delays or behavior concerns that might be detected during developmental screening?

4. Do an internet search on "safety for kids at home alone."
  a. Make a list of some of the sites you discovered.
  b. List two questions that family caregivers should ask themselves when considering leaving a child at home alone.
  c. List six factors that a family caregiver should consider before allowing a child to stay home alone.

CRITICAL THINKING: WHAT WOULD YOU DO?

1. The mother of a 4-month-old infant brings the baby to the healthcare clinic for her well-baby check. The baby is measured and weighed, and the measurements are plotted on a growth chart. The baby is in the 75th percentile for length and the 60th percentile for weight. When the health care provider examines the baby, the notion of doing a developmental screening on the child is discussed.

   a. What will you explain to this mother when she asks you the purpose of the growth chart?

   b. How often will the baby's measurements be plotted on the growth charts?

   c. What will you expect to see after the child has had several measurements plotted?

   d. What is the purpose of doing a developmental screening?

2. A group of family caregivers is participating in a class discussing influences on a child's growth and development. If you were the nurse leading this session, how would you answer the following questions?

   a. What influence does genetics have on growth and development?

   b. What are the effects of nutrition on a child's growth?

   c. What are some environmental factors that influence a child's development?

Growth and Development of the Infant: 28 Days to 1 Year

Learning Objectives

At the conclusion of this chapter, you will:

1. Explain the major developmental task of the infant according to Erikson.
2. Describe physical growth and development that occurs during the first year of life, including weight and height, head and skull, skeletal growth, teeth, circulatory system, respiratory rate, and neuromuscular development.
3. Describe the fear of strangers seen in the infant, including the age this usually appears, and the reason it occurs.
4. Discuss a useful purpose of the game *Peek-a-Boo*.
5. Discuss nutritional requirements and concerns of the infant.
6. Describe the process and challenge of adding solid foods to the infant's diet.
7. Discuss weaning: (a) the usual age when the infant becomes interested in a cup and (b) criteria to determine the appropriate time.
8. State the cause of early childhood caries, and discuss ways to prevent them.
9. List examples of foods to offer the infant who does not drink enough milk from a cup.
10. Discuss immunization of infants including (a) communicable diseases against which children are immunized, (b) schedule of immunizations, and (c) common side effects and treatments following immunization.
11. Outline family caregiver teaching to be reinforced during routine health maintenance visits for the infant.
12. Describe early dental care for the infant.
13. Discuss important safety issues for the infant, including anticipatory guidance.
14. Discuss the nurse's and family caregiver's roles related to the hospitalization of the infant.

Ella Sanderson weighed 7 lb 4 oz (3,289 g) when she was born. She is now 6 months old and weighs 15 lb 2 oz (6,861 g). As you read this chapter, think about Ella's growth and development and what changes will occur over the next 6 months of Ella's life.

The 1-month-old infant has a busy year ahead. During this year, the infant grows and develops skills more rapidly than they ever will again. In the brief span of a single year, this tiny, helpless bit of humanity becomes a person with strong emotions of love, fear, jealousy, and anger and gains the ability to rise from a supine to an upright position and move about purposefully.

Erikson's psychosocial developmental task for the infant is to develop a sense of trust. The development of trust occurs when the infant has a need and that need is met consistently. The infant feels secure when the basic needs are met. This stage creates the foundation for the developmental tasks of the next stages to be met. If the infant does not receive food, love, attention, and comfort, the infant learns to mistrust the environment and those who are responsible for caring for the child.

PHYSICAL DEVELOPMENT

Despite the many factors, such as genetic background, environment, health, gender, and race, that affect growth in the first year of life, the healthy infant progresses in a predictable pattern. By the end of the year, the dependent infant who at 1 month of age had no teeth and could not roll over, sit, or stand blossoms into an emerging toddler with teeth who can sit alone, stand, and begin to walk alone. The growth seen in the prenatal development of the fetus continues.

Weight and Height

In the first year, both weight and height increase rapidly. During the first 6 months, the infant's birth weight doubles, and height increases about 6 in. Growth slows slightly during the second 6 months but is still rapid. By 1 year of age, the infant has tripled their birth weight and has grown 10 to 12 in.

Thinking in terms of the "average" child is misleading. To determine if an infant is reaching acceptable levels of development, birth weight and height must be the standard to which later measurements are compared. An infant weighing 6 lb (2,721 g) at birth cannot be expected to weigh as much at 5 or 6 months of age as the infant who weighed 9 lb (4,082 g) at birth, but each is expected to double their birth weight at about this time. A growth graph is helpful for charting a child's progress (Fig. 23-1).

Head and Skull

Head Circumference

At birth, an infant's head circumference averages about 13.7 in. (35 cm) and is usually slightly larger than the chest circumference. The chest measures about the same as the abdomen at birth. At about 1 year of age, the head circumference has grown to about 18 in. (47 cm). The chest also grows rapidly, catching up to the head circumference at about 5 to 7 months of age. From then on, the chest can be expected to exceed the head in circumference.

Fontanels and Cranial Sutures

The posterior fontanel (fontanelle) is usually closed by the second or third month of life. The anterior fontanel may increase slightly in size during the first few months of life. After the sixth month, it begins to decrease in size, closing between the 12th and the 18th months. The sutures between the cranial bones do not ossify until later childhood.

Skeletal Growth and Maturation

During fetal life, the skeletal system is completely formed in cartilage at the end of 3 months of gestation. Bone ossification and growth occur during the remainder of fetal life and throughout childhood. The pattern of maturation is so regular that bone age can be determined by radiologic examination.

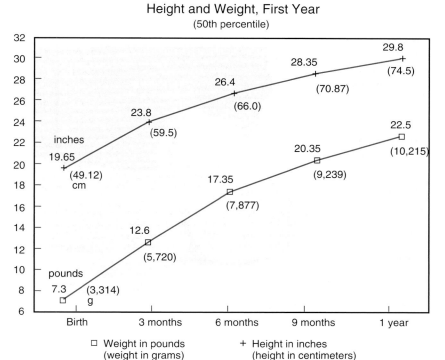

Height and Weight, First Year
(50th percentile)

FIGURE 23-1 Chart of infant growth representing an infant in the mid-range birth weight 7.3 lb (3,314 g) and birth length 19.65 in. (49.12 cm). Infants of different races vary in average size. Asian infants tend to be smaller, and African American infants tend to be larger.

When the bone age matches the child's chronologic age, the skeletal structure is maturing at a normal rate. To avoid unnecessary exposure to radiation, radiologic examination is performed only if a problem is suspected.

Eruption of Deciduous Teeth

Calcification of the primary or **deciduous teeth** starts early in fetal life. Shortly before birth, calcification begins in the permanent teeth that are the first to erupt in later childhood. The first deciduous teeth, usually the lower central incisors, usually erupt between 6 and 8 months of age (Fig. 23-2).

Babies in good health who show normal development may differ in the timing of tooth eruption. Some families show a tendency toward very early or very late eruption without having other signs of early or late development. Some infants may become restless or fussy from swollen, inflamed gums during teething. A cold teething ring may be helpful in soothing the infant's discomfort. Teething is a normal process of development and does not cause high fever or upper respiratory conditions.

Nutritional deficiency or prolonged illness in infancy may interfere with calcification of both the deciduous and the permanent teeth. The role of fluoride in strengthening calcification of teeth has been well documented. The American Dental Association recommends administration of fluoride to infants and children in areas where the fluoride content of drinking water is inadequate or absent.

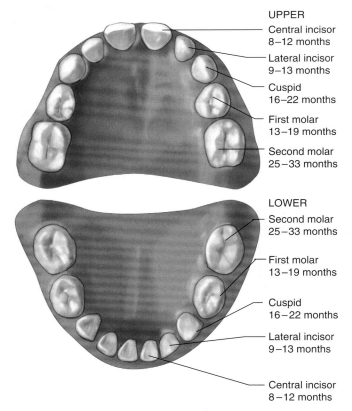

UPPER

Central incisor
8–12 months

Lateral incisor
9–13 months

Cuspid
16–22 months

First molar
13–19 months

Second molar
25–33 months

LOWER

Second molar
25–33 months

First molar
13–19 months

Cuspid
16–22 months

Lateral incisor
9–13 months

Central incisor
8–12 months

Figure 23-2 Approximate ages for the eruption of deciduous teeth.

> **TEST YOURSELF**
> ✔ When does an infant's birth weight double? Triple?
> ✔ When does the posterior fontanel close? Anterior fontanel?
> ✔ When do the first deciduous teeth erupt? Which teeth usually erupt first?

Circulatory System

In the first year of life, the circulatory system undergoes several changes. During fetal life, high levels of hemoglobin and red blood cells are necessary for adequate oxygenation. After birth, when the respiratory system supplies oxygen, hemoglobin decreases in volume, and red blood cells gradually decrease in number until 3 months of age. Thereafter, the count gradually increases until adult levels are reached.

Obtaining an accurate blood pressure measurement in an infant is difficult. Electronic or ultrasonographic monitoring equipment is often used (see Chapter 28). The average blood pressure during the first year of life is 85/55 mm Hg. However, variability is expected among children of the same age and body build.

An accurate determination of the infant's heartbeat requires an apical pulse count. Place a pediatric stethoscope with a small-diameter diaphragm over the left side of the chest in a position where the heartbeat can be clearly heard (Fig. 23-3).

Then, count the pulse for one full minute (see Chapter 28). During the first year of life, the average apical rate ranges from 90 (asleep) to 180 (awake) beats per minute and as high as 190 beats per minute while the infant is crying.

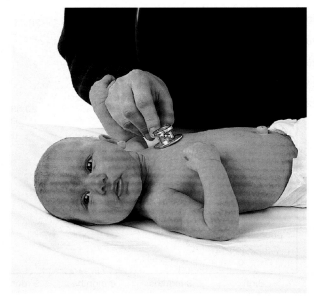

FIGURE 23-3 A pediatric stethoscope is used to clearly hear the heartbeat of the infant.

Body Temperature and Respiratory Rate

Body temperature follows the average normal range after the initial adjustment to postnatal living. Respirations average 30 breaths per minute, with a wide range (30 to 50 bpm) according to the infant's activity.

Neuromuscular Development

As the infant grows, nerve cells mature and fine muscles begin to coordinate in an orderly pattern of development. Naturally, the family caregivers are full of pride in the infant who learns to sit or stand before the neighbor's baby does, but accomplishing such milestones early means little. Each child follows their own unique pattern of progress within reasonable limits.

Average rates of growth and development are useful for purposes of making comparisons. Do not emphasize routine developmental tables with family caregivers; a small time lag may be insignificant. A large time lag may require greater stimulation from the environment or a watchful attitude to discover how overall development is proceeding.

Table 23-1 and Figure 23-4 summarize the accepted norms in physical, psychosocial, motor, language, and cognitive growth and development in the first year of life.

PSYCHOSOCIAL DEVELOPMENT

The infant who actively seeks food to fulfill feelings of hunger experiences the give-and-take of life. The infant begins to develop a sense of trust when fed on demand. However, the infant eventually learns that not every need is met immediately on demand. Slowly the infant becomes aware that something or someone separate from oneself fulfills one's needs. Gradually, as a result of the loving care of family caregivers, the infant learns that the environment responds to desires expressed through one's own efforts and signals. The infant is now aware that the environment is separate from self.

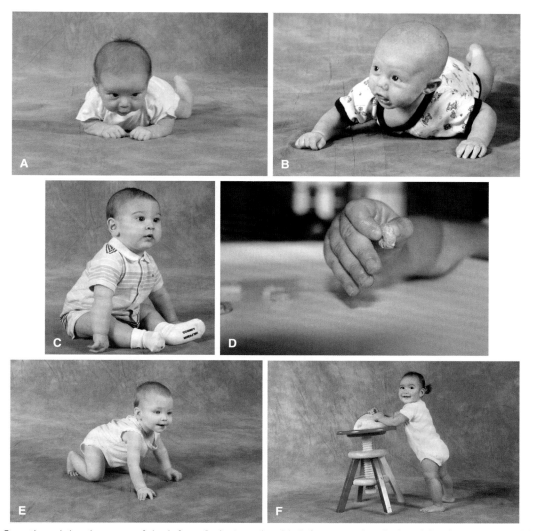

FIGURE 23-4 Growth and development of the infant. **A.** At 4 weeks, this infant turns head when lying in a prone position. **B.** At 12 weeks, this infant pushes up from a prone position. **C.** At 21 weeks, the infant sits up but tilts forward for balance. **D.** At 32 weeks, this infant uses the pincer grasp to pick up a piece of cereal. **E.** At 32 weeks, this infant is crawling around and on the go. **F.** At 43 weeks, this infant is getting ready to walk.

TABLE 23-1   Growth and Development: Birth to 1 Year

AGE	PHYSICAL	PERSONAL–SOCIAL	FINE MOTOR	GROSS MOTOR	LANGUAGE	COGNITIVE DEVELOPMENT
Birth–4 weeks	Weight gain of 5–7 oz (150–270 g) per weeks Height gain of 1 inch per month first 6 months Head circumference increases ½ in. per month Moro, Babinski, rooting, and tonic neck reflexes present	Some smiling begins Erikson's stage of "trust vs. mistrust"	Grasp reflex very strong Hands flexed	Catches and holds objects in sight that cross visual field Can turn head from side to side when lying in a prone position (Fig. 23-4A) When prone, body in a flexed position When prone, moves extremities in a crawling fashion	Cries when upset Makes enjoyment sounds during mealtimes	At 1 month, sucking activity with associated pleasurable sensations
6 weeks	Tears appear	Smiling in response to familiar stimuli Less flexion noted	Hands open Holds head up when prone	Tries to raise shoulders and arms when stimulated Smiles to familiar voices Less flexion of entire body when prone	Cooing predominant Begins to repeat actions Babbling sounds	**Primary circular reactions** (explores objects by touching or putting in mouth; infant unaware actions are what bring pleasure)
10–12 weeks	Posterior fontanel closes	Aware of new environment Less crying Smiles at significant others	No longer has grasp reflex Pulls on clothes, blanket, but does not reach for them Pumps arms, shoulders, and head from prone position (Fig. 23-4B)	No longer has Moro reflex Symmetric body positioning	Makes noises when spoken to	Beginning of coordinated responses to different kinds of stimuli
16 weeks	Moro, rooting, and tonic neck reflexes disappear; drooling begins	Responds to stimulus Sees bottle, squeals, and laughs Aware of new environment and shows interest	Grasps objects with two hands Eye–hand coordination beginning	Plays with hands Brings objects to mouth Balances head and body for short periods in sitting position	Laughs aloud Sounds *n, k, g,* and *b*	Likes social situations Fusses if bored or unattended, demands attention
20 weeks	May show signs of teething	Smiles at self in mirror Cries when limits are set or when objects are taken away	Holds one object while looking for another one Grasps objects voluntarily and brings them to mouth	Able to sit up (Fig. 23-4C) Can roll over	Cooing noises; squeals with delight Can bear weight on legs when held in a standing position Able to control head movements	Visually looks for an object that has fallen

TABLE 23-1 Growth and Development: Birth to 1 Year (Continued)

AGE	PHYSICAL	PERSONAL–SOCIAL	FINE MOTOR	GROSS MOTOR	LANGUAGE	COGNITIVE DEVELOPMENT
24 weeks	Birth weight doubles; weight gain slows to 3–5 oz (90–150 g) per week Height slows to ½ inches per month Teething begins with lower central incisors	Likes to be picked up Knows family from strangers Plays *Peek-a-Boo* Knows likes and dislikes Fear of strangers	Holds a bottle fairly well Tries to retrieve a dropped article	Tonic neck reflex disappears Sits alone in high chair, back erect Rolls over and back to abdomen	Makes sounds *guh, bah.* Sounds *p, m, b,* and *t* are pronounced Babbling sounds	**Secondary circular reactions** (realizes actions bring pleasure) Repeats actions that affect an object Beginning of **object permanence** (just because object cannot be seen does not mean it is gone)
28 weeks	Lower lateral incisors are followed in the next month by upper central incisors	Imitates simple acts Responds to *no* Shows preferences and dislikes for food	Holds cup Transfers objects from one hand to the other	Reaches without visual guidance Can lift head up when in a supine position	Babbling decreases Duplicates *ma-ma* and *pa-pa* sounds	
32 weeks	Teething continues	Dislikes diaper and clothing change Afraid of strangers Fear of separating from mother	Gradually palmar grasp reflex lessens and the **pincer grasp** (using thumb and index finger) develops (Fig. 23-4D) Adjusts body position to be able to reach for an object May stand up while holding on	Crawls around (Fig. 23-4E) Pulls toy toward self	Combines syllables but has trouble attributing meaning to them	
40 weeks–1 year	Birth weight tripled; has six teeth; Babinski reflex disappears Anterior fontanel closes between now and 18 months	Does things to attract attention Tries to follow when being read to Imitates parents Looks for objects not in sight	Holds tools with one hand and works on it with another Puts toy in box after demonstration Stacks blocks Holds crayon to scribble on paper	Stands alone; begins to walk alone (Fig. 23-4F) Can change self from prone to sitting to standing position	Words emerge Says, *da-da* and *ma-ma* with meaning	Coordination of secondary schemes (means to an end); masters barrier to reach goal,

Family caregivers who expect too much too soon from the infant are not encouraging optimal development. Rather than teaching the rules of life before the infant has learned to trust the environment, the caregivers are actually teaching that nothing is gained by one's own activity and that the world does not respond to one's needs.

Conversely, family caregivers who rush to anticipate every need give the infant no opportunity to test the environment. The opportunity to discover that through one's own actions the environment may be manipulated to suit one's own desires is withheld from the infant by these "smothering" caregivers. Tips for Reinforcing Family Teaching: Infants From Birth to 1 Year suggests healthy child-rearing patterns during infancy.

No one is perfect, and every family caregiver misinterprets the infant's signals at times. The caregiver may be

TIPS FOR REINFORCING FAMILY TEACHING

Infants from Birth to 1 Year

- *First 6 weeks:* Frequent holding of the infant gives the infant feeling of being loved and cared for. Rocking and soothing the baby are important.
- *6 weeks to 3½ months:* Continue to give the infant feeling of being loved and cared for; respond to cries; provide visual stimulation with toys, pictures, mobiles, and auditory stimulation by talking and singing to the baby; and repeat sounds that the infant makes to encourage vocal stimulation.
- *3½ to 5 months:* Play regularly with the baby; give the child a variety of things to look at; talk to the baby; offer a variety of items to touch—soft, fuzzy, smooth, and rough—to provide tactile stimulation; continue to respond to the infant's cries; move the baby around the home to provide additional visual

and auditory stimulation; and begin placing the infant on the floor to provide freedom of movement.
- *5 to 8 months:* Continue to give the infant feeling of being loved and cared for by holding, cuddling, and responding to needs; talk to the infant; put the infant on floor more often to roll and move about; fear of strangers is common at this age.
- *8 to 12 months:* Accident-proof the house; give the infant maximum access to living area; supply the infant with toys; stay close by to support the infant in difficult situations; and continue to talk to the infant to provide language stimulation. The baby at this age loves surprise toys like jack-in-the-box and separation games like *Peek-a-Boo*; loves putting-in and taking-out activities. The child is developing independence, and temper tantrums may begin.

---

tired, preoccupied, or responding momentarily to their own needs. The caregiver may not be able to ease the infant's pain or soothe the restlessness, but this also is a learning experience for the child.

As mentioned earlier, the infant's development depends on a mutual relationship with give and take between the infant and the environment in which the family caregivers play the most important role. Table 23-2 summarizes significant caregiver–infant interactions indicating positive behaviors.

During the first few weeks of life, actions such as kicking and sucking are simple reflex activities. In the next sequential stage, reflexes are coordinated and elaborated. For example, in early infancy, hand movements are random (Fig. 23-5A).

The infant finds that repetition of chance movements brings interesting changes, and in the latter part of the first year, these acts become clearly intentional (Fig. 23-5B). The infant expects that certain results follow certain actions.

The infant soon connects the smiling face looking down with the pleasure of being picked up, fed, or bathed. Anyone who smiles and talks softly to the infant may make that small face light up and cause squirming of anticipation. In only a few weeks, however, the infant learns that one particular person is the main source of comfort and pleasure.

An infant cannot apply abstract reasoning but understands only through the five senses. As the infant matures enough to recognize the mother or primary family caregiver, the infant may become fearful when this person disappears. To the infant, out of sight means out of existence, and the infant cannot tolerate this. For the infant, self-assurance is

necessary to confirm that objects and people do not cease to exist when out of sight. This is a learning experience on which the infant's entire attitude toward life depends.

NUTRITION

During the first year of life, the infant's rapid growth creates a need for nutrients greater than at any other time of life. The American Academy of Pediatrics Committee on Nutrition endorses breast-feeding as the best method of feeding infants. (See Chapter 15 for discussion of factors that influence the choice of a feeding method.)

Most of the infant's requirements for the first 4 to 6 months of life are supplied by either breast milk or commercial infant formulas. Nutrients that may need to be supplemented are vitamins C and D, iron, and fluoride. Breastfed infants need supplements of iron, as well as vitamin D, which can be supplied as vitamin drops. Most commercial infant formulas are enriched with vitamins C and D. Some infant formulas are fortified with iron. Infants who are fed home-prepared formulas (based on evaporated milk) need supplemental vitamin C and iron; however, evaporated milk has adequate amounts of vitamin D, which is unaffected by heating in the preparation of the formula. Vitamin C can be supplied in fruits, vegetables, or juices fortified with vitamin C.

Fluoride is needed in small amounts (0.25 mg/day) for strengthening calcification of the teeth and preventing tooth decay. Starting at 6 months of age, a supplement is recommended for breastfed and commercial formula-fed babies and for those whose home-prepared formulas are made with water that is deficient in fluoride. Vitamin preparations are available combined with fluoride.

Addition of Solid Foods

The time or order requirement for starting solid foods is not exact. However, at about 4 to 6 months of age, the infant's milk consumption alone is not likely to be sufficient to meet

Think About This!

The ancient game of *Peek-a-Boo* is a universal example of how the infant learns. It is one of the joys of infancy as the child affirms the ability to control the disappearance and reappearance of self. In the same manner by which the infant affirms self-existence, they confirm the existence of others, even when they are temporarily out of sight.

TABLE 23-2 Criteria of Positive Caregiver and Infant Interactions

AREA OF INTERACTION	POSITIVE CAREGIVER RESPONSE
Feeding	Offers infant adequate amounts and proper types of food and prepares food appropriately
	Holds infant in comfortable, secure position during feeding
	Burps infant during or after feeding
	Offers food at a comfortable pace for infant
Stimulation	Provides appropriate nonaggressive verbal stimulation to infant
	Provides a variety of tactile experiences and touches infant in caring ways.
	Provides appropriate toys and interacts with infant in a way satisfying to infant
Rest and sleep	Provides a quiet, relaxed environment and a regular, scheduled sleep time for infant
	Makes certain infant is adequately fed, warm, and dry before putting down to sleep
Understanding of infant	Has realistic expectations of infant and recognizes infant's developing skills and behavior
	Has realistic view of own parenting skills
Problem-solving initiative	Motivated to manage infant's problems; diligently seeks information about infant; thorough on plans involving infant
Interaction with other children	Demonstrates positive interaction with other children in home without aggression or hostility
Caregiver's recreation	Seeks positive outlets for own recreation and relaxation
Parenting role	Expresses satisfaction with parenting role; expresses positive attitudes

caloric, protein, mineral, and vitamin needs. In particular, the infant's iron supply becomes low, and supplements of iron-rich foods are needed. Table 23-3 provides guidelines for introducing new foods into an infant's diet.

Infant Feeding

The infant knows only one way to take food, namely to thrust the tongue forward as if to suck. This is called the **extrusion (protrusion) reflex** (Fig. 23-6) and has the effect of pushing solid food out of the infant's mouth. The process of transferring food from the front of the mouth to the throat for swallowing is a complicated skill that must be learned. The eager, hungry infant is puzzled over this new turn of events and is apt to become frustrated and annoyed, protesting loudly and clearly. Taking the edge off the very hungry infant's appetite by giving part of the formula is best before proceeding with this new experience.

If the family caregivers understand that pushing food out with the tongue does not mean rejection, their patience will be rewarded.

The infant's clothing (and the caregiver's as well) needs protection when the infant is held for a feeding. A small spoon fits the infant's mouth better than a large one and makes it easier to put food further back on the tongue, but not far enough to make the infant gag. If the food is pushed out, the caregiver must catch it and offer it again. The infant soon learns to manipulate the tongue and comes to enjoy this novel way of eating. To avoid the danger of aspiration, the caregiver must quiet an upset or crying infant before proceeding with feeding.

Foods are started in small amounts, 1 or 2 tsp daily. Infants like their food smooth, thin, lukewarm, and bland. The choice of mealtime does not matter. It works best, at first, to offer one new food at a time, allowing 4 or 5 days

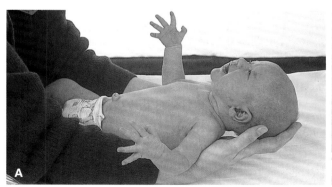

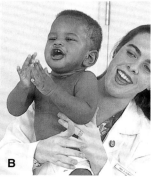

FIGURE 23-5 **A.** In the early stages of infancy, hand movements are random. **B.** Later in infancy, hand movements are coordinated and intentional.

TABLE 23-3 Suggested Feeding Schedule for the First Year of Life

AGE	FOOD ITEM	AMOUNT	RATIONALE
Birth–6 months	Human milk or iron-fortified formula	Daily totals 0–1 months: 18–24 oz 1–2 months: 22–28 oz 2–3 months: 25–32 oz 3–4 months: 28–32 oz 4–5 months: 27–39 oz 5–6 months: 27–45 oz	Infants' well-developed sucking and rooting reflexes allow them to take in milk and formula. Infants do not accept semisolid food because their tongues protrude when a spoon is put in their mouths. They cannot transfer food to the back of the mouth. Infant's size determines daily totals.
	Water	Not routinely recommended	Small amounts may be offered under special circumstances (e.g., hot weather, elevated bilirubin level, or diarrhea).
4–6 months	[a]Iron-fortified infant cereal[b]; begin with rice cereal (delay adding barley, oats, and wheat until sixth month)	4–8 tbsp after mixing	At this age, there is a decrease of the extrusion reflex, the infant can depress the tongue and transfer semi-solid food from a spoon to the back of the pharynx to swallow it.
	[a]Unsweetened fruit juices[b,c]; plain, vitamin C-fortified	2–4 oz	Cereal adds a source of iron and B vitamins; fruit juices introduce a source of vitamin C.
	Dilute juices with equal parts of water		Delay orange, pineapple, grapefruit, or tomato juice until sixth month.
	Human milk or iron-fortified formula	Daily totals 4–5 months: 27–39 oz 5–6 months: 27–45 oz	Do not offer water as a substitute for formula or breast milk, but rather as a source of additional fluids.
	Water	As desired	
7–8 months	[a]Fruits, plain strained; avoid fruit desserts [a]Yogurt[b]	1–2 tbsp	Teething is beginning; thus, there is an increased ability to bite and chew.
	[a]Vegetables,[b] plain strained; avoid combination meat and vegetable dinners	5–7 tbsp	Vegetables introduce new flavors and textures.
	[a]Meats,[b] plain strained; avoid combination or high-protein dinners	1–2 tbsp	Meat provides additional iron, protein, and B vitamins.
	[a]Crackers, toast, zwieback[b]	1 small serving	
	Iron-fortified infant cereal or enriched cream of wheat	4–6 tbsp	
	Fruit juices[c]	4 oz	
	Human milk or iron-fortified formula	24–32 oz	Iron-fortified formula or iron supplementation with human milk is still needed because the infant is not consuming significant amounts of meat.
	Water	As desired	May introduce a cup to the infant.
9–10 months	[a]Finger foods[b]—well-cooked, mashed, soft, bite-sized pieces of meat and vegetables	In small servings	Rhythmic biting movements begin; enhance this development with foods that require chewing.
	Iron-fortified infant cereal or enriched cream of wheat	4–6 tbsp	Decrease amounts of mashed foods as amounts of finger foods increase.
	Fruit juices[c]	4 oz	
	Fruits	6–8 tbsp	
	Vegetables	6–8 tbsp	
	Meat, fish, poultry, yogurt, cottage cheese	4–6 tbsp	Formula or breast milk consumption may begin to decrease; thus, add other sources of calcium, riboflavin, and protein (e.g., cheese, yogurt, and cottage cheese).

TABLE 23-3 Suggested Feeding Schedule for the First Year of Life (Continued)

AGE	FOOD ITEM	AMOUNT	RATIONALE
	Human milk or iron-fortified formula	24–32 oz	
	Water	As desired	
11–12 months	Soft table foods[b] as follows:		
	Cereal: iron-fortified infant cereal; may introduce dry, unsweetened cereal as a finger food	4–6 tbsp	Motor skills are developing; enhance this development with more finger foods.
	Breads: crackers, toast, zwieback	1 or 2 small servings	Rotary chewing motion develops; thus, child can handle whole foods that require more chewing.
	Fruit juice[c]	4 oz	
	Fruit: soft, canned fruits or ripe banana, cut up, peeled raw fruit as the infant approaches 12 months	½ cup	Infant is relying less on breast milk or formula for nutrients; a proper variety of solid foods (fruits, vegetables, starches, protein sources, and dairy products) will continue to meet the young child's needs.
	Vegetables: soft cooked, cut into bite-sized pieces	½ cup	
	Meats and other protein sources: strips of tender, lean meat, cheese strips, peanut butter	2 oz or ½ cup chopped	Delay peanut butter until 12th month.
	Mashed potatoes, noodles		
	Human milk or iron-fortified infant formula	24–30 oz	
	Water	As desired	

[a]Amounts listed are daily totals and goals to be achieved gradually. Intake varies depending on the infant's appetite.
[b]New food items for age group.
[c]The Committee on Nutrition of the American Academy of Pediatrics recommends that fruit juices be introduced when infant can drink from a cup.

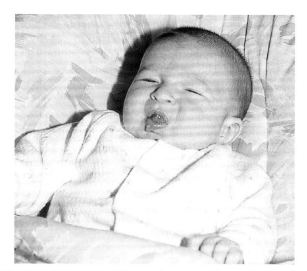

FIGURE 23-6 The infant thrusts the tongue forward using the extrusion reflex. This causes food to be pushed out of the mouth.

before introducing another so that the infant becomes accustomed to it. This method also helps determine which food is responsible if the infant has a reaction to a new food.

When teeth start erupting, anytime between 4 and 7 months of age, the infant may enjoy a teething biscuit or cookie to practice chewing and to offer comfort. At about 9 or 10 months of age, after a few teeth have erupted, chopped foods can be substituted for pureed foods. Breast milk or formula is given during the first 12 months of life. Whole milk is introduced as the infant learns to drink from a cup, usually between 12 and 13 months of age. This change takes some time because the infant continues to derive comfort from sucking at the breast or bottle. Infants need fat and should be given whole milk rather than reduced-fat milk (skim, 1%, or 2%).

Preparation of Foods

Various pureed baby foods, chopped junior foods, and prepared milk formulas are available on the market. These products save caregivers much preparation time, but many families cannot afford them. No matter which type of food is used, family caregivers should read food labels carefully to avoid foods that have undesirable additives, especially sugar and salt, or other unnecessary ingredients.

Point out that vegetables and fruits can be cooked and strained or pureed in a blender and are as acceptable to the infant as commercially prepared baby foods. Baby foods prepared at home should be made from freshly prepared foods, not canned, to avoid commercial additives. Caregivers should carefully check labels of frozen foods used because sugar and salt are commonly added. Excess blended food can be stored in the freezer in ice cube trays for future use. Caregivers can cook cereals and prepare formulas at home as well. Instead of purchasing junior foods, the caregiver can substitute well-cooked, unseasoned table foods that have been mashed or ground.

Preparation and storage of baby food at home require careful sanitary practices. All equipment used in the preparation of the infant's food must be carefully cleaned with hot, soapy water and rinsed thoroughly.

Some families prefer to spend more money for convenience and economize elsewhere, but no one should be made to feel that the infant's health or well-being depends on commercially prepared foods.

The healthy infant's appetite is the best index of the proper amount of food. Healthy babies enjoy eating and accept most foods, but they do not like strongly flavored or bitter foods. If the infant shows a definite dislike for any particular food, forcing it may develop into a battle of wills. A dislike for a certain food is not always permanent, and the rejected food may be offered again later. The important point is to avoid making an issue of likes or dislikes. The caregiver should also avoid introducing any personal attitudes about food preferences.

Self-Feeding

The infant has an overpowering urge to investigate and learn. At around 7 or 8 months of age, the infant may grab the spoon from the caregiver, examine it, and mouth it. The baby also sticks fingers in the food to feel the texture and to bring it to the mouth for tasting (Fig. 23-7). This is an essential, though messy, part of the learning experience.

After preliminary testing, the infant's next task is to try self-feeding. The baby soon finds that the motions involved in getting a spoon right side up into the mouth are too complex, so fingers become favored over the spoon. However, the infant returns to the spoon again until they eventually succeed in getting some food from spoon to mouth, at least part of the time. Help family caregivers understand that all this is not deliberate messiness to be forbidden but rather a necessary part of the infant's learning.

Weaning the Infant

Weaning, either from the breast or from the bottle, must be attempted gradually without fuss or strain. The infant is still testing the environment. The abrupt removal of a main source of satisfaction—sucking—before basic distrust of

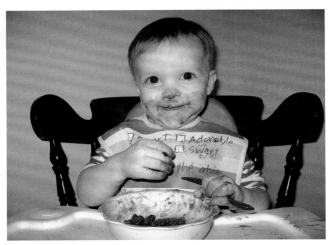

FIGURE 23-7 Eating by yourself is a messy business but so much fun!

the environment has been conquered may prove detrimental to normal development. The speed with which weaning is accomplished must be suited to each infant's readiness to give up this form of pleasure for a more mature way of life.

At the age of 5 or 6 months, the infant who has watched others drink from a cup usually is ready to try a sip when it is offered. The infant seldom is ready at this point, however, to give up the pleasures of sucking altogether. Forcing the child to give up sucking creates resistance and suspicion. Letting the infant set the pace is best.

An infant who takes food from a dish and milk from a cup during the day may still be reluctant to give up a bedtime bottle. However, the infant must never be permitted to take a bottle of formula, milk, or juice to bed. **Pedodontists** (dentists who specialize in the care and treatment of children's teeth) discourage the bedtime bottle because the sugar from formula or sweetened juice coats the infant's teeth for long periods and causes erosion of the enamel on the deciduous teeth, resulting in a condition known as **early childhood caries** (formerly referred to as baby bottle syndrome or nursing bottle caries). This condition can also occur in infants who sleep with their mothers and nurse intermittently throughout the night. In addition to the caries, liquid from milk, formula, or juice can pool in the mouth and flow into the eustachian tube, causing otitis media (ear infection) if the infant falls asleep with the bottle.

A few babies resist drinking from a cup. Milk needs (calcium, vitamin D) may be met by offering yogurt, custard, cottage cheese, and other milk products until the infant becomes accustomed to the cup. The caregiver should be cautioned not to use honey or corn syrup to sweeten milk because of the danger of botulism, which the infant's system is not strong enough to combat.

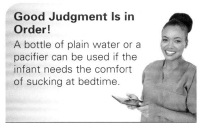

Good Judgment Is in Order!

A bottle of plain water or a pacifier can be used if the infant needs the comfort of sucking at bedtime.

Women, Infants, and Children Food Program

Women, Infants, and Children (WIC) is a special supplemental food program for pregnant, breast-feeding, or postpartum women; infants; and children as old as 5 years of age. This federal program provides nutritious supplemental foods, nutrition information, and healthcare referrals. It is available free of charge to people who are eligible based on financial and nutritional needs and who live in a WIC service area. The family's food stamp benefits or school children's breakfast and lunch program benefits are unaffected. The foods prescribed by the program include iron-fortified infant formula and cereal, milk, fruits and vegetables, whole wheat bread, fish (canned), dry beans, peanut butter, cheese, juice, and eggs. These foods may be purchased with vouchers or distributed through clinics. To encourage the use of WIC services, many healthcare facilities give WIC information to eligible mothers during prenatal visits or at the time of delivery.

HEALTH PROMOTION AND MAINTENANCE

Routine checkups, immunizations, family teaching, and education about accident prevention are important aspects of health promotion and maintenance. Immunizations and frequent well-child visits help ensure good health. Reinforcing family teaching and accident prevention help family caregivers provide the best care for the rapidly growing child.

Routine Checkups

During the first year of life, at least six visits to the healthcare facility are recommended. These are considered well-child visits and usually occur at 2 weeks, 2 months, 4 months, 6 months, 9 months, and 12 months. During these visits, the infant receives immunizations to guard against disease. Collect data regarding the infant's growth and development, nutrition, and sleep; the caregiver–infant relationship; and any potential problems. Document the infant's weight, height, and head circumference. Reinforcing family teaching, particularly for first-time family caregivers, is an integral part of health promotion and maintenance.

Immunizations

Every infant is entitled to the best possible protection against disease. Obviously, infants cannot take proper precautions, so family caregivers and healthcare professionals must be responsible for them. This care extends beyond the daily needs for food, sleep, cleanliness, love, and security to a concern for the infant's future health and well-being. Protection is available against a number of serious or disabling diseases, such as diphtheria, tetanus, pertussis, rotavirus, hepatitis A and B, polio, measles, mumps, German measles (rubella), varicella (chickenpox), *Haemophilus influenzae* meningitis, pneumococcal diseases, and meningococcal disease, making it unnecessary to take chances with a child's health because of inadequate immunization.

The American Academy of Pediatrics, through its committee on the control of infectious diseases and the Advisory Committee on Immunization Practices for the Centers for Disease Control and Prevention (CDC), recommends a schedule of immunizations for healthy children living in normal conditions (www.cdc.gov/vaccines). Additional recommendations are made for children who live in certain regions and areas or who have certain risk factors. Immunizations should be given within the prescribed time table unless the child's physical condition makes this impossible. An immunization need not be postponed if the child has a cold but should be postponed if the child has an acute febrile condition or a condition causing immunosuppression or if they are receiving corticosteroids, radiation, or antimetabolites.

Side effects vary with the type of immunization but usually are minor in nature. The most common side effect is a low-grade fever within the first 24 to 48 hours and possibly a local reaction, such as tenderness, redness, and swelling at the injection site. These reactions are treated symptomatically with acetaminophen for the fever and cool compresses to the injection site. The child may be fussy and eat less than usual. The child is encouraged to drink fluids, and holding and cuddling is comforting to the child. Encourage the family caregivers to call the health care provider if they are concerned, if there are any other reactions, or if these symptoms do not go away within about 48 hours.

Many children do not get their initial immunizations in infancy and may not get them until they reach school age, when immunizations are required for school entrance. Healthcare personnel should make every effort to encourage family caregivers to have their children immunized in infancy to avoid the danger of possible epidemic outbreaks. For instance, measles outbreaks resulting in the deaths of children have been increasing at an alarming rate because of inadequate immunization. Serious illnesses, permanent disability, and deaths from inadequate immunizations are senseless and tragic. Answer any questions the family caregiver may have about immunizations. Remember, however, that the caregiver has a right to refuse immunization if they have been fully informed about immunizations and any possible reactions. Maintain a nonjudgmental viewpoint throughout the discussion.

This Advice Could Save the Day!

Preparing family caregivers by giving information regarding common side effects following immunizations may help decrease caregiver anxiety and concerns. A written information sheet gives the caregiver something to refer to at home if the child has a side effect.

TEST YOURSELF

✔ Discuss the reasons immunizations are given.

✔ What are the diseases against which children can be immunized?

Ella Sanderson has just received the immunizations she needs to be up-to-date. Look up the most current immunization schedule at www.cdc.gov. Which immunizations would Ella have had by the time she was 6 months old in order for her to be up-to-date with immunizations?

Family Teaching

Mothers are discharged so early after giving birth, so use every opportunity to reinforce teaching and promote healthy baby care. Well-child visits provide an opportunity to ask the family caregiver about concerns and to reinforce teaching. During well visits, offer anticipatory guidance to help caregivers prepare for the many changes that occur with each developmental level. Discuss normal growth and development milestones but emphasize that these milestones vary from infant to infant. The infant's overall progress is the most important concern, not when they accomplish a given task as compared with another infant or a developmental table. Discuss any infant sleep and activity concerns that the family caregiver has. Encourage the caregiver to seek information about any other problems, worries, or anxieties they have. Provide ample time and opportunity for the caregivers to ask questions and gain information. It is not only wise to ask if the caregiver has concerns but also to suggest possible topics that may need to be reinforced. Some of those topics are discussed here.

Bathing the Infant

A daily bath is unnecessary but is desirable and soothing in very hot weather. Placing the baby into a small tub for a bath, rather than giving a sponge bath, may have a soothing and comforting effect as long as the infant is healthy and has no open skin areas. The small tub or large basin bath is described in the Tips for Reinforcing Family Teaching: Giving a Small Tub Bath.

The bathing procedure is essentially the same for the older infant. When old enough to sit and move about freely, the infant may enjoy the regular bathtub, but this is often frightening to them. Splashing about in a small tub may be more fun, especially with a floating toy. An infant in a tub should always be held securely (Fig. 23-8).

If possible, time should be scheduled so that bathing is a leisurely process, a time for the caregiver and baby to enjoy. As noted in Chapter 41, regular shampooing is important to prevent seborrheic dermatitis (cradle cap), which is caused by a collection of **seborrhea**, yellow crusty patches of lesions on the scalp.

Scented or talcum powder should not be used after the bath; powder tends to cake in skin creases causing irritation and may cause respiratory problems when inhaled by the

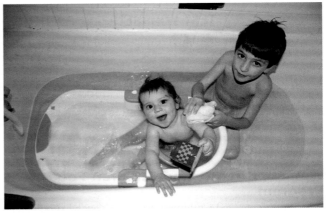

FIGURE 23-8 Bath time can be an enjoyable experience for the infant, especially when held securely in a bath seat.

infant. Scented powders and lotions cause allergic reactions in some babies. In any case, a clean baby has a sweet smell without the use of additional fragrances. Excessively dry skin may benefit from the application of lanolin or A+D Ointment, but oils are believed to block pores and cause infection. Various medicated ointments are available for excoriated skin areas.

After the bath, the infant's fingernails need to be inspected and cut, if long. Otherwise, the infant may scratch their face during random arm movements. The nails should be cut straight across with great care. While cutting, hold the arm securely and the hand firmly.

Caring for the Diaper Area

To prevent diaper rash, soiled diapers should be changed frequently. The caregiver should check every 2 to 4 hours while the infant is awake to see if the diaper is soiled. Waking the baby to change the diaper is not necessary. Cleanse the diaper area with water and a mild soap if needed (see Tips for Reinforcing Family Teaching: Preventing and Treating Diaper Rash in Chapter 41). Commercial diaper wipes may also be used, but they are an added expense (Fig. 23-9).

Diapers are available in various sizes and shapes. The choice of cloth versus disposable diapers is controversial. Disposable diapers have an environmental impact, but cloth diapers are inconvenient and associated with a higher risk of infection. Whatever the type, size, and folding method used, there should be no bunched material between the thighs. Two popular cloth diaper styles are the oblong strip fastened at the sides or the square diaper folded kite-fashion. The latter has the advantage of being useful for different ages and sizes. When folding a cloth diaper for a boy, the excess material is folded in the front, but for a girl, it is folded to the back. Many reusable cloth diaper products have an outside pocket or cover with an insert that helps absorb the urine. An advantage of these diapers is that plastic snap or Velcro closures reduce the concern of using safety pins. If safety pins are used, they must always be securely closed when they are used to fasten the diaper. When removed, they must be closed and placed out of the infant's reach.

For the older infant, the diaper must be fastened snugly at the hips and legs to prevent feces from running out of the

TIPS FOR REINFORCING FAMILY TEACHING

Giving a Small Tub Bath

Preparation

Make sure room is warm and draft-free. Wash hands, put on protective covering, and assemble the following equipment.

- Large basin or small tub
- Mild soap/shampoo
- Nonsterile protective gloves
- Clean cotton balls
- Soft washcloth
- Large soft towel or small cotton blanket
- Clean diaper and clothes for infant

Fill tub with several inches of warm water (95°F to 100°F [35°C to 37°C]). This is comfortably warm to the elbow. Place basin or tub in crib or other protected surface. *Never* turn from the baby during bathing. *Always* keep at least one hand holding the infant.

Bathing Procedure

Wash the infant's face and head at the beginning of the bath. Use clear water with no soap. Wash each eye with a separate cotton ball, from the inner canthus outward. Gently wash the outer folds of the ears and behind them. Wash the rest of the face. Hold the infant with your nondominant arm using the football hold. Lather the hair with a mild shampoo, intended for use with infants, and rinse thoroughly.

After drying the head, undress the infant and examine for skin rashes or excoriations. Wearing protective gloves, remove diaper and wipe any feces from diaper area.

Place the infant in the tub, and soap the body while supporting the infant's head and shoulders on your arm. If the infant's skin is dry, soap may be eliminated or a prescribed soap substitute used. If the baby is enjoying the experience, make it leisurely by engaging the infant in talk, paddling in the water, and playing for a few extra minutes. When finished, lift the infant from the tub, place on a dry towel and pat dry with careful attention to folds and creases (underarms, neck, perineal area).

After the bath, gently separate the female infant's labia and cleanse with moistened cotton balls and clean water, wiping from *front to back* to avoid bacterial contamination from the anal region. Circumcised male infants need only be inspected for cleanliness. Uncircumcised males may have the foreskin gently retracted to remove smegma and accumulated debris. The foreskin is gently replaced. Do not force foreskin if not easily retracted, but document and report this occurrence.

---

open spaces. Cleaning a soiled crib and a smeared baby once or twice serves as an effective reminder!

Dressing the Infant

Dressing an infant can sometimes create a dilemma, especially for the first-time caregiver. Sometimes merely getting clothes on the infant is difficult. For instance, babies tend to spread their hands when the caregiver is trying to put on

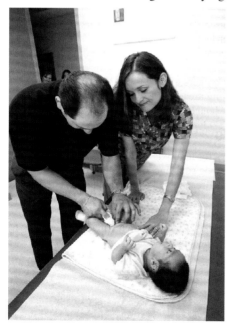

FIGURE 23-9 While the father changes his child's diaper, the nurse takes this opportunity to reinforce teaching on care of the diaper area.

a top with long sleeves. The easiest way to put an infant's arm into a sleeve is to work the sleeve so that the armhole and the opening are held together, then to reach through the armhole and pull the arm through the opening. Clothing should not bind but should allow freedom of movement and be appropriate for the weather.

One rule of thumb is to dress the infant with the same amount of clothing that the adult finds comfortable. Overdressing in hot weather can cause overheating and prickly heat (miliaria rubra; see Chapter 41). In very hot weather, a diaper may be sufficient. When the infant begins to crawl, long pants help protect the knees from becoming chafed from the rug or flooring. When dressing the infant to go outdoors in cold weather, a head covering is important because infants lose a large amount of heat through their heads. In hot, sunny weather, the infant should not spend much time in the direct sun because the infant's skin is tender and burns easily.

Choosing shoes for the infant can be a problem for the new caregiver. Infants do not need hard-soled shoes; in fact, health care providers often recommend that infants be allowed to go barefoot and wear shoes only to protect them from harsh surfaces. Shoes with stiff soles actually hamper the development of the infant's foot. Sneakers made with a smooth lining with no rough surfaces to irritate the infant's foot are a good choice. They should be durable and flexible and have ample room in the toe. Properly made moccasins also are a good choice. High-topped shoes are unnecessary. Socks should provide plenty of toe room. Shoes should be replaced frequently as the infant's feet grow.

Promoting Sleep

Most infants sleep 10 to 12 hours at night and take two to three naps during the day. Each child develops their own sleeping patterns, and these vary from child to child. Family caregivers often have concerns about their child's sleep needs and patterns. Infants should not have pillows placed in bed with them because of the possibility of suffocation. Sleep habits and patterns vary, but a consistent bedtime routine is usually helpful in establishing healthy sleeping patterns and in preventing sleep problems. Placing the child in the crib while awake and letting the child fall asleep in the crib creates good sleeping habits. In addition, this will often prevent the child from waking up when they are moved from the position or place they have fallen asleep. Using the crib for sleeping only, not for play activities, helps the child associate the bed with sleep rather than play. Sleep disturbances may be learned behaviors. Explore in depth any concern expressed by the family caregiver. With the older child, bedtime rituals, consistent limits, and use of a reward system may decrease bedtime and sleep concerns and problems.

Dental Care

When teething begins in the second half of the first year, the family caregiver can start practicing good dental hygiene with the infant. Initially the caregiver can rub the gums and newly erupting teeth with a clean, damp cloth while holding the infant in the lap. This time can be made pleasant by talking or singing to the infant. Brushing the teeth with a small, soft brush usually is not started until several teeth have erupted. Gentle cleansing with plain water is adequate. Toothpaste is not recommended at this stage because the infant will swallow too much of it.

Accident Prevention

Discussing safety issues with family caregivers is important. Provide information and anticipatory guidance about car safety, childproofing, and preventing aspiration, falls, burns, poisoning, and bathing accidents. Remind family caregivers that the infant is developing rapidly and safety precautions should stay one step ahead of the infant's developmental abilities. Caregivers should teach older children in the family to be watchful for possible dangers to the infant, and they must be alert to potential dangers that the older sibling may introduce, such as unsafe toys, rough play, or jealous, harmful behavior (see Tips for Reinforcing Family Teaching: Infant Safety).

 Cultural Snapshot

In some cultures, it is a common and accepted practice for some or all of the children in the family to sleep in the bed with the parents.

 TIPS FOR REINFORCING FAMILY TEACHING

Infant Safety
Be one step ahead of child's development and prepared for the next stage.

Aspiration/Suffocation

- Always hold bottle when feeding, *never* prop bottle.
- Crib and playpen bars should be spaced no more than 2 3/8 in apart.
- Check toys for loose or sharp parts or small buttons.
- Keep small articles (such as buttons, marbles, safety pins, lint, balloons) off the floor and out of infant's reach.
- Store products used in caring for the child out of child's reach.
- Keep plastic bags out of child's reach.
- Do not use pillows in a crib.
- Avoid giving child foods such as hot dogs, grapes, nuts, candy, and popcorn.
- Remove bibs at nap and bedtimes.
- Do not tie pacifier on a string around the child's neck.

Falls

- Never leave child unattended on a high surface such as a high chair, changing table, bed, couch, or countertop.
- Place gates at the tops and bottoms of stairways.
- Raise crib rails and be sure they are securely locked.

Motor Vehicle

- Place infant in an approved infant car carrier in the back seat when in a car. Follow the manufacturer's instructions regarding the age and size of the infant regarding placement of the carrier (rear- or front-facing).
- Never leave child unattended in a car.

Drowning

- Never leave child alone in the bathtub, or near any water, including toilets, buckets, or swimming pools.
- Fence and use locked gates around swimming pools.

Burns/Injuries

- Cover unused plugs with plastic covers.
- Keep electrical cords out of sight.
- Remove tablecloths or dresser scarves that child might grasp and pull.
- Pad sharp corners of low furniture or remove them from child's living area.
- Turn household hot water to a safe temperature—120°F (48.8°C).

Poisoning

- Check toys for nontoxic material.
- Move all toxic substances (cleaning fluids, detergents, insecticides) out of reach and keep them in locked areas.
- Remove any houseplants that may be poisonous.
- Protect child from inhaling lead paint dust (from remodeling) or chewing on surfaces painted with lead paint.
- Place medicines in locked cupboards; remind family and friends (especially those with grown children or no children) to do the same.

TEST YOURSELF

✔ List the areas of family teaching that are important to reinforce with family caregivers of infants.

✔ What are the areas of concern for the safety of an infant?

THE INFANT IN THE HEALTHCARE FACILITY

Hospitalization, however brief, hampers the infant's normal pattern of living. Disruption occurs even if a family caregiver stays with the infant during hospitalization. All or most of the sick infant's energies may be needed to cope with the illness. If given sufficient affection and loving care and if promptly restored to the family, however, the infant is not likely to suffer any serious psychological problems. Long-term hospitalization, though, may present serious problems, even with the best of care.

Illness itself is frustrating; it causes pain and discomfort and limits normal activity, none of which the infant can understand. If the hospital atmosphere is emotionally unresponsive and offers little if any cuddling or rocking, the infant may fail to respond to treatment, despite cleanliness and proper hygiene. Touching, rocking, and cuddling a child are essential elements of nursing care (Fig. 23-10).

Hospitalization may have other adverse effects. The small infant matures largely as a result of physical development. If hindered from reaching out and responding to the environment, the infant becomes apathetic and ceases to learn. This situation is particularly apparent when restraints are necessary to keep the child from undoing surgical procedures or dressings or to prevent injury. The child in restraints needs an extra measure of love and attention and the use of every possible method to provide comfort.

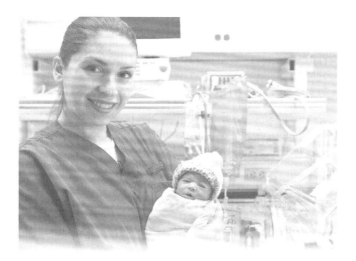

FIGURE 23-10 Holding and cuddling can ease the discomfort of the hospital experience.

A Personal Glimpse

By the time my second son Noah was 6 months old, my husband and I were relaxed and confident parents. Perhaps too much so! Noah had just begun crawling. "We need to dig out the gates," I said to my husband, Richard. He agreed. However, we didn't do it right away, being busy with two kids and work.

Shortly afterward, Richard was working in our upstairs office. Noah was playing underfoot. I opened the door to the office and walked in to put something away. On my way out, I carelessly left the door open. I went downstairs to the kitchen and began coloring with my older son Jacob. A few minutes later, Noah crawled past my husband and out into the hallway. Richard was reading e-mail and didn't notice.

Then I heard something heavy and hard tumbling down the stairs and knocking into the walls, followed by my husband's screaming. I ran to the foyer and found Noah wailing face down on the hardwood floors. I fell to the ground, scooped him up, rocked him, and began crying. Will he be OK? Did he break anything? How could I be so careless? Why didn't we put the gates up? Why am I such a bad parent? I should have known better.

In the end, Noah was fine. His cheek was bruised, and his arm was sore. My husband and I were shaken, but we were OK too. The gates went up that afternoon!

Darlene

Learning Opportunity: *What would you say to these parents to support and reassure them? What recommendations would you make to family caregivers regarding safety in the home?*

Spending time, playing music in the room, or encouraging someone to stay with the infant might help make the infant more comfortable. Provide age-appropriate sensory stimulation within the constraints of the infant's condition. Coo to and cuddle the infant, talk to them in warm and soft tones, and provide opportunities to fulfill sucking needs. Engage the infant in play. Singing songs, looking at picture books, reading stories, reciting rhymes, playing "Peek-a-Boo," and other activities are strongly recommended. Introduce toys that are safe and age-appropriate and that stimulate interest and responsiveness. Provide family caregivers with information about normal developmental activities appropriate for the infant, and encourage them to provide sensory and cognitive stimulation. This approach helps the infant build trust in the caregiver, which is a major developmental task, according to Erikson. It also helps family caregivers feel needed and useful.

As the nurse, your relationship with family caregivers is extremely important. The hospitalized infant needs continued stimulation, empathetic care, and loving attention from family caregivers. Encourage caregivers to feed, hold, diaper, and participate in their infant's care as much as they can. Through conscientious use of the nursing process, collect data regarding the needs of the caregivers and the infant and plan care with these needs in mind. Identify and acknowledge the caregiver's apprehensions and develop plans to resolve or eliminate them. Make arrangements for rooming-in for the family caregiver if possible. Family caregivers are often sensitive to changes in the infant that may help to identify discomfort, pain, or fear. Caregivers may sometimes assist during treatments and other procedures by stroking, talking to, and looking directly at the infant, thus helping to provide comfort during a time of stress. After the procedure, the infant may benefit from rocking, cuddling, singing, stroking, and other comfort measures that the family caregivers may provide. If the family caregivers are unavailable or can spend only limited time with the infant, the nursing staff must meet these emotional needs.

Think back to **Ella Sanderson**. She is now 1 year old. What would you expect Ella to weigh now? What are some developmental characteristics you would most likely see in Ella?

KEY POINTS

- According to Erikson, the developmental task for the infant is to develop a sense of trust, which happens when the needs of the infant are consistently met.
- An infant's birth weight doubles by age 6 months and triples by 1 year.
- At birth, an infant's head circumference is usually slightly larger than the chest circumference. The head and chest grow rapidly and after about 5 to 7 months of age, the chest can be expected to exceed the head in circumference.
- The posterior fontanel closes by the 2nd or 3rd month and the anterior fontanel closes between the 12th and 18th month.
- The first tooth to erupt is usually one of the upper or lower incisors. This occurs between 6 and 8 months of age in most children. Family history, nutritional status, and prolonged illness affect the eruption of teeth. Fluoride is recommended at 6 months of age to strengthen calcification of teeth and prevent tooth decay.
- The average apical rate ranges from 90 (asleep) to 180 (awake) beats per minute and as high as 190 beats per minute when the infant is crying.
- As the infant grows, nerve cells mature, and fine muscles begin to coordinate in an orderly pattern of development.
- Between the ages of 6 and 7 months, most children develop a fear of strangers. As the infant matures enough to recognize the mother or primary family caregiver, the infant becomes fearful when this person disappears. To the infant, out of sight means out of existence, and the infant cannot tolerate this. The game *Peek-a-Boo* is useful in affirming self-existence to the infant and that even when temporarily out of sight, others still exist.
- The infant's nutritional requirements for the first 4 to 6 months are supplied by either breast milk or commercial infant formulas. Nutrients that may need to be supplemented are vitamins C and D, iron, and fluoride.

At about 4 to 6 months of age, the infant's iron supply becomes low and supplements of iron-rich foods are needed. At around 7 or 8 months of age, the infant begins experimenting with finger foods and self-feeding.

- Infants have a tendency to push solid food out of their mouths with their tongue thrust forward because of the extrusion reflex.
- New foods are introduced one at a time to determine the food responsible if the infant has a reaction.
- An infant can be gradually weaned to a cup as their desire for sucking decreases, usually around the age of 12 to 13 months.
- Early childhood caries, formerly referred to as bottle mouth caries, can occur when an infant is given a bottle at bedtime; the sugar from the formula causes erosion of the tooth enamel. To prevent early childhood caries, a bottle of plain water or a pacifier for sucking can be given at bedtime.
- If an infant resists drinking milk from a cup, calcium and vitamin D needs can be met by giving foods such as yogurt, custard, and cottage cheese.
- Children are immunized against hepatitis B virus, diphtheria, tetanus, pertussis, rotavirus, *Haemophilus influenzae* type b, polio, measles, mumps, rubella, varicella (chickenpox), pneumococcal disease, and meningococcal disease. In addition, they may be immunized against the hepatitis A virus. Immunizations should be given according to the American Academy of Pediatrics recommended schedule. The most common side effect is a low-grade fever and possibly tenderness, redness, and swelling at the injection site. Acetaminophen is given for fever, and cool compresses are applied to the injection site. The child may be fussy and eat less than usual. The child is encouraged to drink fluids, and holding and cuddling is comforting to the child.
- During routine health maintenance visits, reinforce teaching to family caregivers regarding normal growth and development milestones, bathing, diapering, dressing, sleep patterns, dental care, and safety.
- Infant gums and teeth should be cleaned with a clean, damp cloth and plain water.
- Accident prevention for the infant includes closely watching the infant and monitoring the environment for safety hazards. Anticipatory guidance is given in regard to safety concerns.
- In addition to nursing care, touching, rocking, and cuddling are essential for the hospitalized infant. Age-appropriate sensory stimulation and play within the constraints of the infant's condition are important. When an infant is hospitalized, the family caregiver can give the child stimulation, care, and attention by feeding, holding, and diapering the infant.

INTERNET RESOURCES

General Resources
www.cdc.gov
www.kidshealth.org/en/parents/growth
www.drspock.com

Child Passenger Safety
www.nhtsa.gov

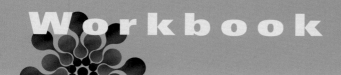

NCLEX-STYLE REVIEW QUESTIONS

1. The nurse would expect an infant who weighs 7 lb 2 oz (3,231 g) at birth to weigh approximately how many pounds at 6 months of age?

   a. 10 lb
   b. 14 lb
   c. 17 lb
   d. 21 lb

2. In caring for a 4-month-old infant, which of the following actions by the infant would the nurse note as appropriate for a 4-month-old infant?

   a. Grasping objects with two hands.
   b. Holding a bottle well.
   c. Trying to pick up a dropped object.
   d. Transferring an object from one hand to the other.

3. When assisting with a physical examination on an infant, the nurse would expect to find the posterior fontanel closed by what age?

   a. 1 week
   b. 3 weeks
   c. 7 weeks
   d. 12 weeks

4. In working with a group of parents of infants, the nurse would explain to the family caregivers that between 6 and 8 months of age, which of the following teeth usually erupt?

   a. First molars
   b. Upper lateral incisors
   c. Lower central incisors
   d. Cuspid

5. An infant had the following intake in the 12 hours after receiving immunizations. Calculate the 12-hour intake for this infant. Record your answer in milliliters (mL)

Pedialyte, 4 oz
Rice cereal, 4 tbsp
Dilute apple juice, 3 oz
Applesauce, 1½ cup
Iron-fortified formula, 8 oz
Yogurt, ¼ cup
Crackers, 4 small
Iron-fortified formula, 5 oz
Strained vegetables, 1 jar
Iron-fortified formula, 7 oz
12-hour intake _____ mL (milliliters)

STUDY ACTIVITIES

1. List and compare the fine motor and gross motor skills in each of the following ages.

	4 Weeks Old	24 Weeks Old	32 Weeks Old
Fine motor skills			
Gross motor skills			

2. Answer the following regarding immunizations.

   a. By the time the infant is 1 year old, immunizations should have been given to prevent which diseases?
   b. How many doses of the hepatitis B vaccine are recommended?
   c. What are the two most common side effects of immunizations? How are these treated?

3. List five safety tips important in the infant stage of growth and development.

4. Go to the following internet site: www.cdc.gov/vaccines/schedules. Click on the link to "Child and Adolescent Immunization Schedule (birth through 18 years)." Answer the following questions.

   a. What is the date of this immunization schedule?
   b. List the immunizations that would be given to a 2-month-old infant.
   c. If the recommended immunization schedule is followed, how many doses of each of the immunizations given at 2 months of age will have been given by the time the child is 18 months of age?

CRITICAL THINKING: WHAT WOULD YOU DO?

1. Tony Ricardo brings 6-month-old Essie for a routine checkup. You are responsible for formulating a plan for the visit.

   a. What characteristics would you observe for during the physical examination?
   b. What immunizations will the child need at this visit (assuming she is up-to-date)?
   c. What nutritional factors will you observe for? What guidelines related to nutrition will you reinforce with Essie's father?
   d. What other age-appropriate teaching will you reinforce with Essie's father?

2. As you review nutrition with Mr. Ricardo, he states that Essie loves her bedtime bottle.

   a. What information will you reinforce with Mr. Ricardo regarding this practice?
   b. What suggestions will you make to help prevent the problems that often result from bedtime bottles?

3. At Nicole's 6-month checkup, her mother tells you that Nicole does not like the baby food, and she just spits it out.

   a. What will you tell Nicole's mother to help her understand what is happening?
   b. What other information about feeding infants will you provide for this mother?

24

Growth and Development of the Toddler: 1 to 3 Years

Learning Objectives

At the conclusion of this chapter, you will:

1. Identify characteristics of the toddler age group.
2. Explain the major developmental task of the toddler according to Erikson.
3. Describe physical growth that occurs during toddlerhood.
4. Define the following terms as they relate to the psychosocial development of the toddler: (a) negativism, (b) ritualism, (c) dawdling, and (d) temper tantrums.
5. Discuss psychosocial development of the toddler in relationship to (a) play, (b) discipline, and (c) the addition of a sibling to the toddler's home situation.
6. Discuss nutritional concerns of the toddler and the progression of the toddler's self-feeding skills.
7. Describe routine checkups as an important part of health promotion and maintenance for the toddler.
8. Identify important aspects of family teaching to be reinforced with the caregivers of toddlers, including (a) bathing, (b) dressing, (c) dental care, (d) toilet training, and (e) sleep.
9. State why accident prevention is a primary concern when caring for a toddler.
10. Discuss the four leading causes of accidental death of toddlers and preventive measures.
11. Discuss important aspects of nursing care for the toddler in the healthcare facility.

Shira Chandra, age 2 years, is the first child of her parents Nila and Daha. Shira's parents are moving into a new home and are asking for information about things they might do to make their home a safer environment for Shira. As you read this chapter, think about the anticipatory guidance that will be appropriate to give Shira's parents, related to safety and other areas of growth and development of the toddler.

Soon after a child's first birthday, important and sometimes dramatic changes take place: physical growth slows considerably, mobility and communication skills improve rapidly, and a determined and often stubborn little person creates a new set of challenges for the family caregivers. *No*, *mine*, and *want* are favorite words. Temper tantrums appear.

During this transition from infancy to early childhood, the child learns many new physical and social skills. With additional teeth and better motor skills, the toddler's self-feeding abilities improve and

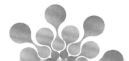

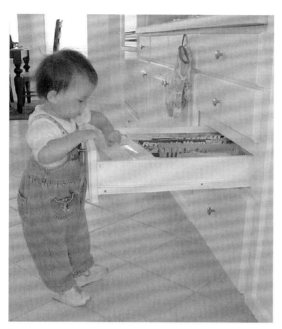

FIGURE 24-1 This curious toddler explores in a kitchen drawer while mom supervises closely.

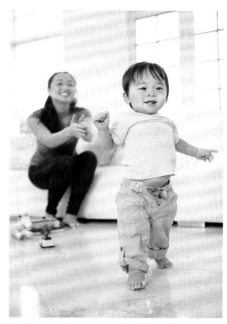

FIGURE 24-2 The toddler is proud of his ability to walk.

include the addition of a new assortment of foods. Left unsupervised, the toddler also may taste many nonfood items that may be harmful or even fatal.

This transition is a time of unpredictability. One moment, the toddler insists on "me do it"; the next moment, the child reverts to dependence on the mother or other family caregiver. While seeking to assert independence, the toddler develops a fear of separation. The toddler's curiosity about the world increases, as does their ability to explore. Family caregivers soon discover that this exploration can wreak havoc on orderly routine and a well-kept house and that the toddler requires close supervision to prevent injury to self or objects in the environment (Fig. 24-1). The toddler justly earns the title of explorer.

Toddlerhood can be a difficult time for family caregivers. Just as parents are beginning to feel confident in their ability to care for and understand their infant, the toddler changes into a walking, talking person whose attitudes and behaviors impacts the entire family. Accident-proofing, safety measures, and firm but gentle discipline are the primary tasks for caregivers of toddlers. Learning to discipline with patience and understanding is difficult but eventually rewarding. At the end of the toddlerhood stage, the child's behavior generally becomes more acceptable and predictable.

Erikson's psychosocial developmental task for this age group is **autonomy** (independence) while overcoming doubt and shame. In contrast to the infant's task of building trust, the toddler seeks independence, wavers between dependence and freedom, and gains self-awareness. Stubborn behavior asserting independence is so common that the stage is commonly referred to as the "terrible twos," but it is just as often referred to as the "terrific twos" because of the toddler's exciting language development, the exuberance with which they greet the world, and a newfound sense of accomplishment. Both aspects of being 2 years old are essential to the child's development, and family caregivers must learn to manage the fast-paced switching between anxiety and enthusiasm.

PHYSICAL DEVELOPMENT

Toddlerhood is a time of slowed growth and rapid development. Each year the toddler gains 4.5 to 6.0 lb (2.0 to 2.7 kg) and about 3 inches (7.62 cm). Continued eruption of teeth, particularly the molars, helps the toddler learn to chew food. The toddler learns to stand alone and to walk (Fig. 24-2) between the ages of 1 and 2 years. By the end of this period, the toddler may have learned partial or total toilet training.

The rate of development varies with each child, depending on the individual personality and the opportunities available to test, explore, and learn. Table 24-1 summarizes significant landmarks in the toddler's growth and development.

PSYCHOSOCIAL DEVELOPMENT

During this time, most children say their first words and continue to improve and refine their language skills. The toddler develops a growing awareness of the self as a being separate from other people or objects. Invigorated with newly discovered powers and lacking experience, the child tends to test personal independence to the limit.

TABLE 24-1 Growth and Development: The Toddler

AGE (MONTHS)	PERSONAL–SOCIAL	FINE MOTOR	GROSS MOTOR	LANGUAGE	COGNITIVE DEVELOPMENT
12–15	Begins Erikson's stage of "autonomy vs. shame and doubt" Seeks novel ways to pursue new experiences Imitations of people are more advanced	Builds with blocks; finger paints Able to reach out with hands and bring food to mouth Holds a spoon Drinks from a cup	Movements become more voluntary Postural control improves; able to stand and may take few independent steps	First words are not generally classified as true language. They are generally associated with the concrete and are usually activity-oriented	Begins to accommodate to the environment, and the adaptive process evolves
18	Extremely curious Becomes a communicative social being Parallel play Fleeting contacts with other children Make-believe play begins	Better control of spoon; good control when drinking from cup Turns pages of a book Places objects in holes or slots	Walks alone; gait may still be a bit unsteady Begins to walk sideways and backward	Begins to use language in a symbolic form to represent images or ideas that reflect the thinking process Uses some meaningful words such as *hi, bye-bye,* and *all gone* Comprehension is significantly greater	Demonstrates foresight and can discover solutions to problems without excessive trial-and-error procedures Can imitate without the presence of a model (deferred imitation)
24	Language facilitates autonomy Sense of power from saying *no* and *mine* Increased independence from mother	Turns pages of a book singly Adept at building a tower of six or seven cubes When drawing, attempts to enclose a space	Runs well with little falling Throws and kicks a ball Walks up and down stairs one step at a time	Begins to use words to explain past events or to discuss objects not observably present Rapidly expands vocabulary to about 300 words; uses plurals	Enters preconceptual phase of cognitive development State of continuous investigations Primary focus is egocentric
36	Basic concepts of sexuality are established Separates from mother more easily Attends to toilet needs	Copies a circle and a straight line Grasps the spoon between the thumb and index finger Holds cup by handle	Balances on one foot; jumps in place; pedals tricycle	Quest for information furthered by questions like *why, when, where,* and *how* Has acquired the language that will be used in the course of simple conversation during adult years	Preconceptual phase continues; can think of only one idea at a time; cannot think of all parts in terms of the whole

Behavioral Characteristics

Negativism, ritualism, dawdling, and temper tantrums are characteristic behaviors seen in toddlers.

Negativism

This age has been called an age of **negativism**. Certainly, the toddler's response to nearly everything is a firm *no*, but this is more an assertion of individuality than of an intention to disobey. Limiting the number of questions asked of the toddler and making a statement, rather than asking a question, is helpful in decreasing the number of negative responses from the child.

Here's a Helpful Hint!
Limiting the number of questions asked and offering a choice to the toddler will help decrease the number of *no* responses. For example, the question, "Are you ready for your bath?" might be replaced by saying, "It is bath time. Do you want to take your duck or your toy boat to the tub with you?"

Ritualism

Ritualism, employed by the young child to help develop security, involves following routines that make rituals of even simple tasks. At bedtime, all toys must be in accustomed places, and the caregiver must follow a habitual practice. This passion for a set routine is not found in every child to the same degree, but it does provide a comfortable base from which to step out into new and potentially dangerous paths. These practices often become more evident when a sitter is in the home, especially at bedtime. This gives the child some measure of security when the primary family caregiver is absent.

Dawdling

Dawdling, wasting time or being idle, serves the purpose of asserting independence. The young child must decide between following the wishes and routines of the family caregiver or asserting independence by following personal desires. The toddler compromises and tries both because they are incapable of making such a choice. If the task to be done is an important one, the caregiver with a firm and friendly manner should help the child follow along the way they should go; otherwise, dawdling can be ignored within reasonable limits.

Temper Tantrums

Temper tantrums, aggressive displays of temper during which the child reacts with rebellion to the wishes of the family caregiver, spring from the many frustrations that are natural results of a child's urge to be independent. Add to this a child's reluctance to leave the scene for necessary rest, and frequently the frustrations become too great. Even the best of caregivers may lose patience and show a temporary lack of understanding. The child reacts with enthusiastic rebellion, but this too is a phase that the family must live through while the child works toward becoming an individual.

Reasoning, scolding, or punishing during a tantrum is useless. A trusted person who remains calm and patient needs to be nearby until the child gains self-control. After the tantrum is over, diverting attention with a toy or some other interesting distraction can help the child relax. However, do not yield the point or give in to the child's whim. Giving in would tell the child that to get whatever they want, a person need only throw themselves on the floor and scream. The child would have to learn painfully later in life that people cannot be controlled in this manner.

These tantrums can be accompanied by head banging and breath holding. Breath holding can be frightening to the family caregiver, but the child will shortly lose consciousness and begin breathing. Head banging can cause injury to the child, so the caregiver needs to provide protection.

The family caregiver should try to be calm when dealing with a toddler having a tantrum. The child is out of control and needs help regaining control; the adult must maintain self-control to reassure the child and provide security.

> **Remaining Calm Is a Must!**
> It is not easy to handle a small child who drops to the floor screaming and kicking in rage in the middle of the supermarket or to deal with comments from onlookers. The best a caregiver can do is pick up the out-of-control child as calmly as possible and carry him or her to a quiet, neutral place to regain self-control. The family caregiver must ensure the child's safety by remaining nearby but ignoring the child's behavior.

Cultural Snapshot

A common cultural belief is that children are to respect their elders, be quiet and humble, and often to be seen and not heard. This may create a problem for the toddler who is attempting to express their independence and having a temper tantrum.

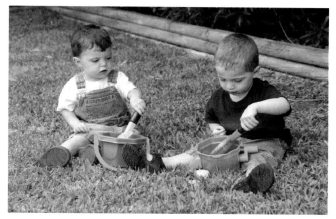

FIGURE 24-3 Toddlers engaged in parallel play.

Play

The toddler's play moves from the solitary play of the infant to **parallel play**, in which the toddler plays alongside other children but not with them (Fig. 24-3). Much of the playtime involves imitation of the people the child sees as role models: adults around him or her, siblings, and other children. Toys that involve the toddler's new gross motor skills, such as push–pull toys, rocking horses, large blocks, and balls, are popular. Fine motor skills develop through use of thick crayons, play dough, finger paints, wooden puzzles with large pieces, toys that fit pieces into shaped holes, and cloth books. Toddlers enjoy talking on a play telephone and like pots, pans, and toys, such as brooms, dishes, and lawn mowers that help them imitate the adults in their environment and promote socialization. The toddler cannot share toys until the later stage of toddlerhood, and adults should not make an issue of sharing at this early stage.

Adults should carefully check toys for loose pieces and sharp edges to ensure the toddler's safety. Toddlers still put things into their mouths; therefore, small pieces that may come loose, such as small beads and buttons, must be avoided.

For an adult, staying quietly on the sidelines and observing the toddler play can be a fascinating revelation of what is going on in the child's world. However, the adult must intervene if necessary to avoid injury.

> **TEST YOURSELF**
> ✔ What does autonomy mean? How does the toddler develop autonomy?
> ✔ What type of play is typically seen in the toddler?
> ✔ List examples of parallel play.

Discipline

The word *discipline* has come to mean punishment to many people, but the concepts are not the same. To **discipline** means to train or instruct in order to produce a particular behavior pattern, especially moral or mental improvement, and self-control. **Punishment** means penalizing someone for wrongdoing. Although all small children need discipline, the need for punishment occurs much less frequently.

The toddler learns self-control gradually. The development from an egotistic being whose world exists only to give self-satisfaction into a person who understands and respects the rights of others is a long, involved process. The child cannot do this alone but must be taught.

At age 2, children begin to show some signs of accepting responsibility for their own actions, but they lack inner controls because of their egocentricity. The toddler still wants the forbidden thing but may repeat "no, no, no" while reaching for a desired treasure, recognizing that the act is not approved. Although the child understands the act is not approved, the desire is too strong to resist. Even at this age, children want and need limits. When no limits are set, the child develops a feeling of insecurity and fear. With proper guidance, the child gradually absorbs the restraints and develops self-control or conscience.

Consistency and timing are important in the approach that the family caregiver uses when disciplining the child. The toddler needs a lot of help during this time. People caring for the child should agree on the methods of discipline, and they should all operate by the same rules so that the child knows what is expected. This need for consistency can cause disagreement for family caregivers who have experienced different types of child-rearing themselves. The caregivers may be confused by this child who had been a sweet, loving infant and now has turned into a belligerent little being who throws tantrums at will.

This period can be challenging to adults. The child needs to learn that the adults are in control and will help the child gain self-control while learning to be independent. When the toddler hits or bites another child, caregivers should calmly remove the offender from the situation. Negative messages, such as "You are a bad boy for hitting Jamal," or "Bad girl! You don't bite people," are not helpful. Instead, messages such as "Biting hurts—be gentle" do not label the child as bad but label the act as unacceptable.

Another useful method for a child who is not cooperating or who is out of control is to send the child to a time-out chair. This should be a place where the child can be alone but observed without other distractions. The duration of the isolation should be limited—1 minute per year of age is usually adequate. Caregivers should warn the child in advance of this possibility, but only one warning per event is necessary.

Extinction is another discipline technique effective with this age group. If the child has certain undesirable behaviors that occur frequently, family caregivers ignore the behavior. In this technique, adults do not react to the child as long as the behavior is not harmful to the child or others. Caregivers must be consistent and never react in any way to

that particular behavior. However, when the child responds acceptably in a situation in which the undesirable behavior was the usual response, it is important to compliment the child. Suppose, for example, that the child screams or makes a scene when the caregiver will not buy cookies in the grocery store. If, after the caregiver practices extinction, the child talks in a normal voice on another visit to the grocery store, caregivers should compliment the child's grown-up behavior.

Spanking or other physical punishment usually does not work well because the child is merely taught that hitting or other physical violence is acceptable, and the child who is spanked frequently becomes immune to it.

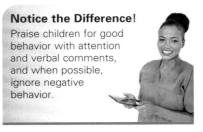

Notice the Difference!
Praise children for good behavior with attention and verbal comments, and when possible, ignore negative behavior.

Sharing With a New Baby

The first child has the family caregiver's undivided attention until a new baby arrives, often when the first child is a toddler. Preparing a child just emerging from babyhood for this arrival is difficult. Although the toddler can feel the mother's abdomen and understand that this is where the new baby lives, this alone does not give adequate preparation for the newborn's arrival. This real baby represents a rival for the mother's affection.

As in many stressful situations, the toddler frequently regresses to more infantile behavior. The toddler who no longer takes milk from a bottle may need or want a bottle when the new baby is being fed. Toilet training, which may have been moving along well, may regress with the toddler having episodes of soiling and wetting.

The new infant creates considerable change in the home, whether they are the first child or the fifth. In homes where the previous child is displaced by the newcomer, some special preparation is necessary. Moving the older child to a larger bed some time before the new baby appears lets the toddler take pride in being grown-up now.

Preparation of the toddler for a new brother or sister is helpful but should not be intense until just before the expected birth. Many hospitals have sibling classes for new siblings-to-be that are scheduled shortly before the anticipated delivery. These classes, geared to the young child, give the child some tasks to do for the new baby and discuss both negative and positive aspects of having a new baby in the home. Many books are available to help prepare the young child for the birth and that explore sibling rivalry.

Probably the greatest help in preparing the child of any age to accept the new baby is to help the child feel that this is "our baby," not just "mommy's baby" (Fig. 24-4). Helping to

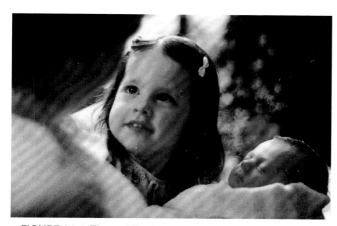

FIGURE 24-4 The toddler is meeting her new baby brother.

care for the baby, according to the child's ability, contributes to a feeling of continuing importance and self-worth.

The displaced toddler will almost certainly feel some jealousy. With careful planning, however, the mother can reserve some time for cuddling and playing with the toddler just as before. Perhaps the toddler may profit from a little extra parental attention for a time. The toddler needs to feel that parental love is just as great as ever and that there is plenty of room in the parent's lives for both children.

The child should not be made to grow up too soon. The toddler should not be shamed or reproved for reverting to babyish behavior but should receive understanding and a bit more love and attention. Perhaps the father or other family member can occasionally take over the care of the new baby while the mother devotes herself to the toddler. The mother may also plan special times with the toddler when the new infant is sleeping and the mother has no interruptions. This approach helps the toddler feel special.

NUTRITION

The toddler needs foods from the major food groups each day. The USDA guidelines found in the ChooseMyPlate in Figure 22-3 in Chapter 22 are appropriate for children beginning at age 2. Daily nutritional needs for the toddler, including caloric requirements and the appropriate number of servings per day, are listed in Table 24-2.

Eating problems commonly appear between the ages of 1 and 3 years. These problems occur for a number of reasons, such as the following:

- The child's growth rate has slowed; therefore, they may want and need less food than before. Family caregivers need to know that this is normal.
- The child's strong drive for independence and autonomy compels an assertion of will to prove their individuality, both to self and to others.
- A child's appetite varies. *Food jags*, the desire for only one kind of food for a while, are common.

To minimize these eating problems and ensure that the child gets a balanced diet with all the nutrients essential for health and well-being, caregivers should plan meals with an understanding of the toddler's developing feeding skills. Tips for Reinforcing Family Teaching: Feeding Toddlers offers guidance for toddler mealtimes. Messiness is to be expected and prepared for when learning begins; it gradually diminishes as the child gains skill in self-feeding. At 15 months, the toddler can sit through meals, prefers finger

 TIPS FOR REINFORCING FAMILY TEACHING

Feeding Toddlers

- Serve small portions, and provide a second serving when the first has been eaten. One or two teaspoonfuls is an adequate serving for the toddler. Too much food on the dish may overwhelm the child.
- There is no *one* food essential to health. Allow substitution for a disliked food. Food jags, during which toddlers prefer one food for days on end, are common and not harmful. If the child refuses a particular food such as milk, use appropriate substitutes such as pudding, cheese, yogurt, and cottage cheese. Avoid a battle of wills at mealtime.
- Toddlers like simply prepared foods served warm or cool, not hot or cold.
- Provide a social atmosphere at mealtimes; allow the toddler to eat with others in the family. Toddlers learn by imitating the acceptance or even the rejection of foods by other family members.
- Toddlers prefer foods that they can pick up with their fingers; however, they should be allowed to use a spoon or fork when they want to try.
- Try to plan regular mealtimes with small nutritious snacks between meals. Do not attach too much importance to food by urging the child to choose what to eat.
- Dawdling at mealtime is common with this age group and can be ignored unless it stretches to unreasonable lengths or becomes a play for power. Mealtime for the toddler should not exceed 20 minutes. Calmly remove food without comment.
- Do not make desserts a reward for good eating habits. It gives unfair value to the dessert and makes vegetables or other foods seem less desirable.
- Offer regularly planned nutritious snacks such as milk, crackers and peanut butter, cheese cubes, and pieces of fruit. Plan snacks midway between meals and at bedtime.
- Remember that the total amount eaten each day is more important than the amount eaten at a specific meal.

TABLE 24-2 Daily Nutritional Needs of the 1- to 3-Year-Old

For a 1,000- to 1,400-Calorie diet, the toddler needs the amounts below from each food group. Toddlers should play actively several times every day.

FRUITS	VEGETABLES	GRAINS	PROTEIN FOODS	DAIRY
1–1.5 cups	1–1.5 cups	3–5 oz	2–4 oz	2–2.5 cups

feeding, and wants to self-feed. They try to use a spoon but has difficulty with scooping and spilling. The 15-month-old grasps the cup with the thumb and forefinger but tilts the cup instead of the head. By 18 months, the toddler's appetite decreases. The 18-month-old has improved control of the spoon, puts spilled food back on the spoon, holds the cup with both hands, spills less often, and may throw the cup when finished if no one is there to take it. At 24 months, the toddler's appetite is fair to moderate. The toddler at this age has clearly defined likes and dislikes and food jags. The 24-month-old grasps the spoon between the thumb and forefinger, can put food on the spoon with one hand, continues to spill, and accepts no help ("Me do!"). By 30 months, refusals and preferences are less evident. Some toddlers at this age hold the spoon like an adult, with the palm turned inward. The cup, too, may be handled in an adult manner. The 30-month-old tilts their head back to get the very last drop.

HEALTH PROMOTION AND MAINTENANCE

Three important aspects of health promotion and maintenance for the toddler are routine checkups, family teaching, and accident prevention. Routine checkups help protect the toddler's health and ensure continuing growth and development. Use these opportunities to encourage good health through reinforcing family teaching, support of positive parenting behaviors, and reinforcement of the toddler's achievements. Toddlers need a stimulating environment and the opportunity to explore it. This environment, however, must be safe to help prevent accidents and infection. Give family caregivers anticipatory guidance and information regarding accident prevention and home safety.

Routine Checkups

The health care provider sees the child at 15 months of age for immunization boosters and at least annually thereafter. Routine physical checkups include assessment of growth and development, oral hygiene, toilet training, daily health-care, the family caregiver–toddler relationship, and parenting skills. Interviews with family caregivers, observations of the toddler, observations of the caregiver–toddler inter-action, and communication with the toddler are all effective means to elicit this information. Remember that family caregiver interpretations may not be completely accurate. Communicate with the toddler on their level, and offer only realistic options.

The child should receive current immunizations. Table 24-3 details nursing measures to ensure optimal health practices.

Reinforcing Family Teaching

The toddler is rapidly learning about the world in which they live. As part of that process, the toddler learns about everyday care needed for healthy growth and development. The toddler's urge for independence and the caregiver's response to that urge play an important part in everyday life

with the toddler. Some of these activities are included in the following discussion.

Bathing

Toddlers generally love to take tub baths. Setting a regular time for the bath helps give the toddler a sense of security about what to expect. Although the toddler can sit well in the tub, they should never be left alone. An adult must supervise the bath continuously to prevent an accident. The toddler enjoys having tub toys with which to play. Family caregivers should avoid using bubble bath, especially for young girls, because it can create an environment that encourages the growth of organisms that cause bladder infections. A bath is often relaxing and may help the toddler quiet down before bedtime.

Dressing

By the second birthday, toddlers take an active interest in helping to put on their clothes. They often begin around 18 months by removing their socks and shoes whenever they choose. This behavior can be frustrating to the caregiver, but if accepted as another small step in development, the family caregiver may feel less frustration. Between the ages of 2 and 3 years, the toddler can begin by putting on underpants, shirts, or socks. Often the clothing ends up backward, but the important thing is that the toddler accomplished the task. Encourage the family caregiver to take a relaxed attitude as the toddler learns to dress themselves. If clothes must be put on correctly, the caregiver should try to do it without criticizing the toddler's job. The caregiver should warmly acknowledge the toddler's accomplishment of putting on a piece of clothing that they may have struggled with for some time. Roomy clothing with easy buttons; large, smooth-running zippers; and Velcro are easier for the toddler to handle.

As in late infancy, shoes need to be worn primarily to protect the toddler's feet from harsh surfaces. Sneakers are still a good choice. Avoid hard-soled shoes. High-topped shoes are unnecessary.

Dental Care

Dental caries (cavities) are a major health problem in children and young adults. Sound teeth depend in part on sound nutrition. The development of dental caries is linked to the effect the diet has on the oral environment.

Bacteria that act in the presence of sugar and form a film, or dental plaque, on the teeth cause tooth decay. People who eat sweet foods frequently accumulate plaque easily and are prone to dental caries. Sugars eaten at mealtime appear to be neutralized by the presence of other foods and are therefore not as damaging as between-meal sweets and bedtime bottles. Foods consisting of hard or sticky sugars, such as lollipops and caramels that remain in the mouth for longer periods, tend to cause more dental caries than those eaten quickly. Sugarless gum or candies are not as harmful.

When the child is about 2 years of age, they should learn to brush the teeth or at least to rinse the mouth after each meal or snack. Because this is the period when the

TABLE 24-3   Guidelines for Health Promotion in the Toddler

DEVELOPMENTAL CHARACTERISTICS OF TODDLER (2–3 YEARS)	POSSIBLE DEVIATIONS FROM HEALTH	NURSING MEASURES TO ENSURE OPTIMAL HEALTH PRACTICES
Self-feeding (foods and objects more accessible for mouthing, handling, and eating)	Inadequate nutritional intake Accidental poisoning Gastrointestinal disturbances: Instability of gastrointestinal tract Infection from parasites (pinworm)	Reinforcing teaching about diet and nutrition Childproofing the home Careful handwashing (before meals, after toileting) Avoidance of rich foods Observe for perianal itching (Scotch tape test, administer anthelmintic)
Toilet training	Constipation (if training procedures are too rigid) Urinary tract infection (especially prevalent in girls due to anatomic structure and poor toilet habits)	Reinforce teaching about toileting procedures Urinalysis when indicated (e.g., burning) Reinforce teaching about hygiene practices (at the onset of training, instruct girls to wipe from front to back, and wash hands to prevent cross-infection)
Increased socialization	Increased prevalence of upper respiratory infections (immune levels still at immature levels)	Hygienic practices (e.g., use of tissue, handwashing, not drinking from same glass) Immunizations for passive immunity against communicable disease
Primary dentition	Caries with resultant infection or loss of primary teeth; caries can also cause concerns for permanent teeth	Oral hygiene, regular tooth brushing, dental examination by 2 years of age Proper nutrition to ensure dentition
Sleep disturbances	Lack of sleep may cause irritability, lethargy, decreased resistance to infection	Reinforce teaching regarding recommended amounts of sleep (12–14 hours in first year, decreasing to 10–12 hours by age 3); need for rituals to enhance transition process to bedtime; possibility of need for nap; setting bedtime limits

toddler likes to imitate others, the child learns best by example. Plain water should be used until the child has learned how to spit out toothpaste. An adult should also brush the toddler's teeth until the child becomes experienced (Fig. 24-5). One good method is to stand behind the

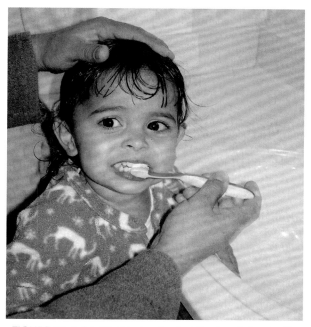

FIGURE 24-5 An adult helps the toddler brush her teeth.

child in front of a mirror and brush the child's teeth. In addition to cleaning adequately, this also helps the child learn how it feels to have the teeth thoroughly brushed. The use of fluoride toothpaste strengthens tooth enamel and helps prevent tooth decay, particularly in communities with unfluoridated water. An adult should supervise the use of fluoride toothpaste; the child should use only a small pea-sized amount. The health care provider may recommend supplemental fluoride, but families on limited incomes may find this difficult to afford. A fluoride supplement is a medication and should be treated and stored as such. Fluoride can also be applied during regular visits to the dentist, but the greatest benefit to the tooth enamel occurs before the eruption of the teeth.

The first visit to the dentist is recommended to occur soon after the child's first birthday so the child gets acquainted with the dentist, staff, and office. If there are older siblings, the toddler can go along on a visit with them to help overcome the fears of a strange setting. At a second visit, the child has a preliminary examination and is evaluated for any dental risks. The family caregivers are given anticipatory guidance regarding dental hygiene, diet and dietary habits, and the use of fluoride. Visits twice a year for checkups are recommended.

Children of low-income families often have poor dental hygiene and care, both because of the cost of care and lack of knowledge of the family caregiver about proper care and nutrition. Some family caregivers may believe it is unnecessary to take proper care of baby teeth because "they fall out anyway." However, the care and condition of the baby teeth affect the normal growth of permanent teeth, which are forming in the jaw under the baby teeth.

> **Pay Attention to the Little Details!**
> It is important to reinforce teaching with the family caregivers regarding the importance of proper care of the child's baby teeth.

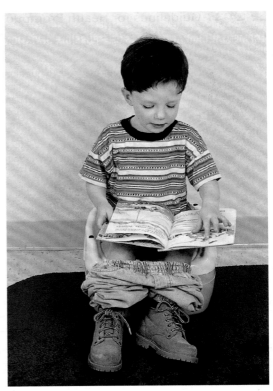

Toilet Training

Learning bowel and bladder control is an important part of the socialization process. In Western culture, a great sense of shame and disgust has been associated with body waste products. To function successfully in this culture, one must learn to dispose of body waste products in a place considered proper by society.

The toddler has been operating on the pleasure principle by simply emptying the bowel and bladder when the urge is present without thinking of anything but personal comfort. During toilet training, the child, who is just learning about control of the personal environment, finds that some of that control must be given up to please those most important people, the family caregivers. The toddler now must learn to conform not only to please those special loved ones, but also to preserve self-integrity.

Timing is an important aspect of toilet training. To be able to cooperate in toilet training, the child's anal and urethral sphincter muscles must have developed to the stage where the child can control them. Control of the anal sphincter usually develops first. The child must also be able to postpone the urge to defecate or urinate until reaching the toilet or potty and must be able to signal the need before the event. In addition, before toilet training can occur, the child must have a desire to please the caregiver by holding feces and urine, rather than satisfying their own immediate need for gratification. This level of maturation seldom takes place before the age of 18 to 24 months.

At the start of toilet training, the child does not understand the use of the potty chair but will sit there for a short time to please the family caregiver (Fig. 24-6). If the child's bowel movements occur at about the same time every day, one day a bowel movement will occur while the child is sitting on the potty. Although there is no sense of special achievement for this event itself, the child does like the praise and approval caregivers provide. Eventually the child will connect this approval with the bowel movement in the potty, and the child will be happy that the caregiver is pleased.

FIGURE 24-6 Toddlers will sit on the potty chair to please a caregiver.

on the Elmo chair and get a treat. "No," he'd say again. "Gimme back my diaper." Taking this as a sign that he wasn't ready, we decided to delay potty training. Then, one day, William followed our 5-year-old son, Jack, into the bathroom. From the other room I heard Jack say, "See, Will, this is how I use the potty." William, ever eager to please his brother, pulled up a step stool and mimicked Jack. Nothing happened, but William was starting to show interest. I praised them and gave them both small treats. I suggested to Jack that he ask William to sit on the little potty while he sat on the big potty to "pee," which would be easier for William. "Got it," Jack said with two thumbs up. We resumed potty training. Jack took the lead in our family effort. A week later, Jack and William came bounding out of the bathroom together. "We did it," Jack exclaimed. "We did it," William repeated. "I go pee-pee like Jack!" Upon further inspection, I found that William had in fact successfully used the little potty. "High-five," Jack said. "High-five," William dutifully repeated. "High-five all around," I giggled. We still have a long way to go, but we are making progress—all four of us together!

Melanie (and Joe)

Learning Opportunity: *What behavioral characteristics commonly seen in the toddler did this child show? What would you suggest these parents do to praise and support both of their children in the toilet training process?*

Generally, the first indication of readiness for bladder training is when the child makes a connection between the puddle on the floor and something they did. In the next

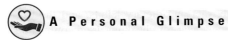 **A Personal Glimpse**

My husband and I decided it was time to potty train our near 3-year-old son, William. We started by introducing him to the potty. In the morning, my husband would casually ask William if he'd like to sit on the potty. "No," he'd assert. Before a bath, I'd ask William if he would like to sit

stage, the child runs to the family caregiver and indicates a need to urinate, but only after it has happened. Sometimes the child who is ready for toilet training will pull on a wet or soiled diaper

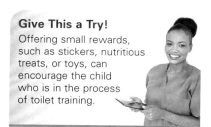

Give This a Try!
Offering small rewards, such as stickers, nutritious treats, or toys, can encourage the child who is in the process of toilet training.

or even bring a clean diaper to the caregiver to indicate they need a diaper change. A serious training program will have little benefit, however, until the child is sufficiently mature to control the urethral sphincter and reach the desired place. When the child stays dry for about 2 hours at a time during the day, this may indicate sufficient maturity.

The family caregiver should not expect perfection, even after control has been achieved. Each child follows an individual pattern of development, so no caregiver should feel embarrassed or ashamed because a child continues to have accidents. Lapses inevitably occur, perhaps because the child is completely absorbed in play or because of a temporary episode of loose stools. Occasionally a child feels aggression, frustration, or anger and may use this method to get even. As long as the lapses are occasional, caregivers should ignore them. If the lapses are frequent and persistent, the cause should be explored.

No one should expect the child to accomplish self-training, and family caregivers should be alert to the signs of readiness. Patience and understanding of the caregivers are essential. Tips for Reinforcing Family Teaching: Toilet Training offers suggestions for caregivers. Complete control, especially at night, may not be achieved until 4 or 5 years of age. Each child should be taught a term or phrase to use for toileting that is recognizable to others, clearly understood, and socially acceptable. This is especially true for children who are cared for outside the home.

Here's a Tip for Family Caregivers!
To help the child remember to use the toilet or potty chair, set a timer to sound at appropriate intervals. When the timer sounds, the child will be reminded to go to the bathroom.

Sleep

The toddler's sleep needs change gradually between the ages of 1 and 3 years. A total daily need for 12 to 14 hours of sleep is to be expected in the first year of toddlerhood, decreasing to 10 to 12 hours by 3 years of age. The toddler soon gives up a morning nap, but most continue to need an afternoon nap until sometime near the third birthday.

Bedtime rituals are common. A bedtime ritual provides structure and a feeling of security because the toddler

Check Out This Tip!
Bedtime routines, such as reading a story or having a quiet time, are helpful in providing a calming end to a busy day for the toddler.

TIPS FOR REINFORCING FAMILY TEACHING

Toilet Training

- A potty chair in which a child can comfortably sit with the feet on the floor is preferable.
- Leave the child on the potty chair for only a short time. Be readily available but do not hover anxiously over the child. If a bowel movement or urination occurs, approval is in order; if not, no comment is necessary.
- Have the child wash their hands after sitting on the toilet or potty chair to instill good hygiene practices.
- Dressing the child in clothes that are easily removed and in training pants or pull-up type diapers and pants increases the child's success with training.
- Children love to copy and imitate others, and often, observing a parent or an older sibling gives the toddler a positive role model for toilet training.
- During the beginning stages of training, the child is likely to have a bowel movement or wet diaper soon after leaving the potty. This is not willful defiance and need not be mentioned.
- Empty the potty chair unobtrusively after the child has resumed playing. The child has cooperated and produced the product desired. If it is immediately thrown away, the child may be confused and not so eager to please the next time. However, some children enjoy the fun of flushing the toilet and watching as the materials disappear.
- Be careful not to flush the toilet while the child is sitting on it, as this can be frightening to the child.
- The ability to feel shame and self-doubt appears at this age. Therefore, the child should not be teased about reluctance or inability to conform. This teasing can shake the child's confidence and cause feelings of doubt in self-worth.
- Do not expect perfection; even after control has been achieved, lapses inevitably occur.

knows what to expect and what is expected of them. The separation anxiety common in the toddler may contribute to some of the toddler's reluctance to go to bed. Family caregivers must be careful that the toddler does not use this to manipulate them and delay bedtime. Gentle, firm consistency by caregivers is ultimately reassuring to the toddler. Regular schedules with set bedtimes are important.

> ### TEST YOURSELF
> ✔ List the areas of teaching that are important to reinforce with the family caregivers of toddlers.
> ✔ What must develop in order for the toddler to be physically ready for toilet training? By what age are most children toilet-trained?

Accident Prevention

Toddlers are explorers who require constant supervision in a controlled environment to encourage autonomy and prevent injury. When supervision is inadequate or the environment is unsafe, tragedy often results; accidents are the leading cause of death for children between the ages of 1 and 4 years. Accidents involving motor vehicles, drowning, burns, and poisoning are the most common causes of death. The number of motor vehicle deaths in this age group is more than three times greater than the number of deaths caused by burns or drowning. Reinforcing family teaching can help minimize the risk for accident and injury.

Motor Vehicle Accidents

Many childhood deaths or injuries resulting from motor vehicle accidents can be prevented by proper use of restraints. Federally approved child safety seats are designed to give the child maximum protection if used correctly (Fig. 24-7). Adults must be responsible for teaching the child that seat belts are required for safe car travel and that they must be securely fastened in the car seat before the car starts. Adults in the car with a child should set the example by also using seat belts. Many toddlers are killed or injured by moving vehicles while playing in their own driveways or garages. Family caregivers need to be aware that these tragedies can occur and must take proper precautions at all times. See Tips for Reinforcing Family Teaching: Preventing Motor Vehicle Accidents.

Drowning

Although drowning of young children is often associated with bathtubs, the increased number of home swimming pools has added significantly to the number of accidental drownings. Often, these pools are fenced on three sides to keep out nonresidents but are bordered on one side by the family home, making the pool accessible to infants and toddlers. Even small plastic wading pools hold enough water to drown an unsupervised toddler. Any family living near a body of water, no matter how small, must not leave a mobile infant or toddler unattended, even for a moment. Even a small amount of water, such as that in a bucket, may be enough to drown a small child.

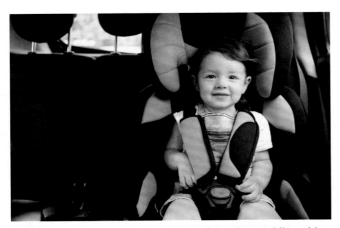

FIGURE 24-7 Car seats are used for safety when toddlers ride in a vehicle. (Africa Studio/Shutterstock.com).

TIPS FOR REINFORCING FAMILY TEACHING

Preventing Motor Vehicle Accidents

- Never start the car until the child is securely in the car seat.
- If the child manages to get out of the car seat or unfasten it, pull over to the curb or side of the road as soon as possible, turn off the car, and tell the child that the car will not go until they are safely in the seat. Children love to go in the car, and they will comply if they learn that they cannot go unless in the car seat.
- Never permit a child to stand in a car that is in motion.
- Remind the toddler to stop at a curb and wait for an adult escort to cross the street. An older child should be taught to look both ways for traffic. Start this as a game with toddlers, and continually reinforce it.
- Remind the child to cross only at corners.
- Begin in toddlerhood to instill awareness of traffic signals and their meanings. As soon as the child recognizes color, they can tell you when it is all right to cross.
- Never let a child run into the street after a ball.
- Remind the child to never to walk between parked cars.
- As a driver, always be on the alert for children running into the street when in a residential area or running in a parking lot.

Burns

Burn accidents occur most often as scalds from immersions and spills and from exposure to uninsulated electrical wires or live extension cord plugs. Children are also burned while playing with matches or while left unattended in a home where a fire breaks out. Whether the fire results from a child's mischief, an adult's carelessness, or some unforeseeable event, the injuries, even if not fatal, can have long-term or permanent effects. Burns can often be prevented by following simple safety practices (Tips for Reinforcing Family Teaching: Preventing Burns).

Ingestion of Toxic Substances

The curious toddler wants to touch and taste everything. Left unsupervised, the toddler may sample cosmetics, personal care products, household cleaners, prescription or over-the-counter drugs, kerosene, gasoline, peeling lead-based paint chips or dust particles, or nicotine (electronic cigarettes, gum, patches). Poisoning is still the most common medical emergency in children with the highest incidence between the ages of 1 and 4 years.

Family caregivers need continual reminders about the possibility of childhood poisoning. Even with precautionary labeling and child-resistant

Always Exercise Caution! The importance of careful, continuous supervision of toddlers and other young children cannot be overemphasized.

TIPS FOR REINFORCING FAMILY TEACHING

Preventing Burns

- Do not let electrical cords dangle over a counter or a table. Repair frayed cords. Newer small appliances have shorter cords to prevent dangling.
- Cover electrical wall outlets with safety caps.
- Turn handles of pans on the stove toward the back of the stove. If possible, place pans on back burners out of the toddler's reach.
- Place cups of hot liquid out of reach. Do not use overhanging tablecloths that toddlers can pull.
- Use caution when serving foods heated in the microwave; they can be hotter than is apparent.
- Supervise small children at all times in the bathtub so they cannot turn on the hot water tap.
- Turn thermostat on home water heater down so that the water temperature is no higher than 120°F.
- Place matches in metal containers and out of reach of small children. Keep lighters out of reach of children.
- Never leave small children unattended by an adult or a responsible adolescent.

packaging of medication and household cleaners, children display amazing ingenuity in opening bottles and packages that catch their curiosity. Mr. Yuk stickers are available from the nearest poison control center. The child can be taught that products are harmful if they have the Mr. Yuk sticker on them. However, labeling is not sufficient; all items that are in any way toxic to the child must be placed under lock and key or totally out of the child's reach.

Preventive measures that all caregivers of small children should observe are listed in Tips for Reinforcing Family Teaching: Preventing Poisoning.

The following medications are most commonly involved in cases of childhood poisoning.

- Acetaminophen
- Salicylates (aspirin)
- Laxatives
- Sedatives
- Tranquilizers
- Analgesics, such as ibuprofen, opioids
- Antihistamines
- Cardiac medications
- Cough/cold medicines
- Birth control pills

Stay Alert!

Batteries, especially button batteries (found in hearing aids, games and toys, watches, calculators, flashlights and remote control devices), can be a cause of poisoning as well as a choking hazard in children.

TIPS FOR REINFORCING FAMILY TEACHING

Preventing Poisoning

- Keep harmful products and household cleaning products (laundry and dishwashing detergent pods) locked up and out of a child's sight and reach.
- Use safety latches or locks on drawers and cabinets.
- Read labels with care before using any product.
- Replace child-resistant closures and safety caps immediately after using product.
- Never leave alcohol or electronic cigarettes/nicotine refill cartridges, gum, patches within a child's reach.
- Keep products in their original containers; never put nonfood products in food or drink containers.
- Remind children not to drink or eat anything unless it is given to them by a trusted adult.
- Do not take medicine in front of small children; children tend to copy adult behavior.
- Do not refer to medicine as candy; call medicine by its correct name.
- Check your home often for old medications and get rid of them following the U.S. FDA drug disposal guidelines (U.S. FDA, 2019).
- Keep button battery compartments on household products taped and secured, store batteries out of reach and sight of children, and do not allow children to play with batteries.
- Keep plants off floor and out of children's reach.
- Keep lotion, cream, powder, cosmetics, insect repellent out of children's reach.
- Post the Poison Help Line (formerly called the Poison Control Center) number near each telephone: (800) 222-1222.
- Program the Poison Help Line number into your cell phones and into your home phone.

TEST YOURSELF

✔ What are the major causes of accidents in the toddler?
✔ List the measures you can reinforce with family caregivers of toddlers to prevent accidents.

What anticipatory guidance will you give to **Shira Chandra**'s parents regarding safety in their new home? Make a list of things Shira's parents might do to make their home a safer environment for Shira.

THE TODDLER IN THE HEALTHCARE FACILITY

Although hospitalization is difficult and frightening for a child of any age, the developmental stage of the toddler intensifies these problems. When providing care, keep in mind the toddler's developmental tasks and needs. The toddler, engaged in trying to establish self-control and autonomy, finds that strangers seem to have total power; this eliminates any control on the toddler's part. Add these fears to the inability to communicate well, discomfort from pain, separation from family, the presence of unfamiliar people and surroundings, physical restraint, and uncomfortable or frightening procedures, and the toddler's reaction can be clearly understood.

Maintaining Routines

Part of the child's admission procedure includes a social assessment survey conducted by interviewing the family caregiver who has accompanied the child to the facility. Usually part of the standard pediatric nursing assessment form, the social assessment covers eating habits and food preferences, toileting habits and terms used for toileting, family members and the names the child calls them, the name the child is called by family members, pets and their names, favorite toys, sleeping or napping patterns and rituals, and other significant information that helps the staff better plan care for the toddler (Fig. 28-2 in Chapter 28). This information should become an indispensable part of the nursing care plan. The nursing care plan should provide opportunities for independence for the toddler whenever possible.

Separation anxiety is high during the toddler age. As discussed in detail in Chapter 29, the stages of protest and despair are common. Acknowledge these stages, and communicate to the child that it is acceptable to feel angry and anxious at being separated from the primary family caregiver, the person foremost in the child's life. Never interpret the toddler's angry protest as a personal attack. Many facilities encourage family involvement in the child's care to minimize separation anxiety. The mother is often the family member who stays with the child, but in many families, other members who are close to the child may take turns staying. Having a family caregiver with the toddler can be extremely helpful. However, do not neglect caring for the toddler who has a loved one present. In many families, it is impossible for the family caregiver to stay with the child for any of a number of reasons. These children need extra attention and care. All children should be assigned a constant health care provider while in the facility, but this is especially important for the toddler who is alone (Fig. 24-8).

As the nurse assigned to the toddler, you may become a surrogate parent while caring for the child. Maintaining as much as possible the pattern, schedule, and rituals that the toddler is used to helps to provide some measure of security to the child. This is a time when the toddler needs the security of a beloved thumb or other *lovey*, a favorite stuffed animal or blanket. It is important to recognize that the toddler uses this to provide self-comfort (Fig. 24-9).

The lovey may be well worn and dirty, but the toddler finds great reassurance in having it to snuggle or cuddle. Do

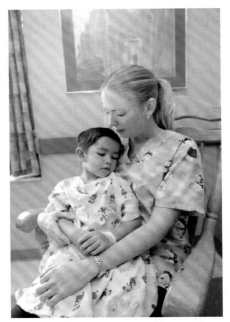

FIGURE 24-8 The nurse may become a surrogate family caregiver for the hospitalized toddler.

not ridicule the child for its unkempt appearance, and make every effort to allow the toddler to have it whenever desired.

When the family caregiver must leave the toddler, it may be helpful for the adult to give the child some personal item to keep until the adult returns. The family caregiver can tell the child that they will return "when the cartoons come on TV" or "when your lunch comes." These are concrete times that the toddler will probably understand.

Special Considerations

The busy toddler just learning to use the toilet, self-feed, and be disciplined presents a unique challenge to the nurse. Maintain control on the pediatric unit, promote safety, and help establish the toddler's sense of security while allowing the toddler's development to continue.

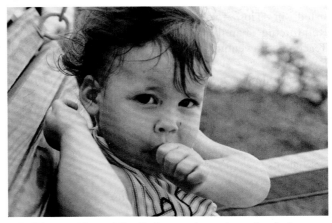

FIGURE 24-9 The toddler finds security and comfort in her beloved thumb.

The toddler learning sphincter control is still dependent on familiar surroundings and the family caregiver's support. For this reason, some pediatric personnel automatically put toddlers back in diapers when they are admitted. This practice should be discouraged. Under the right circumstances and especially with the caregiver's help, many of these children can maintain control. They at least should be given a chance to try. Potty chairs can be provided for the child when appropriate. The nursing staff must know the method and times of accomplishing toilet training used at home and must try to comply with them as closely as possible in the hospital.

Some limits are needed for the toddler, but be careful when setting them. Toddlers, like children of any age, need to feel that someone is in control and need limits set with love and understanding. A child who has been overindulged for a long time may need firm, calm statements of limits delivered in a no-nonsense but kind manner. Explaining what is going to be done, what is expected of the toddler, and what the toddler can expect from you as the nurse may be helpful. Sometimes giving some tactful guidance to the family caregiver may help to set limits for the toddler. This is an area in which nursing experience helps you solve difficult problems. Discipline on the pediatric unit is discussed in Chapter 29.

A toddler's eating habits may loom large in your mind as a potential problem. In the hospital or clinic, as at home, food can assume an importance out of proportion to its value and create unnecessary problems. Eating concerns for the pediatric client are fully discussed in Chapter 29. Some helpful hints to minimize potential problems are as follows:

- View mealtime as a social event.
- Encourage self-feeding.
- Do not push the child to eat.
- Allow others to eat with the child.
- Offer familiar foods.
- Provide fluids in small but frequent amounts.

Safety is a concern with all hospitalized children, but safety promotion for a toddler may be particularly challenging. The curious toddler needs to be watched with extra care, but the toddler should not be unnecessarily prohibited from exploring and moving about freely. Safety in the hospital setting is discussed in detail in Chapter 29.

Remember 2-year-old **Shira Chandra**. What other areas of anticipatory guidance in addition to safety for their toddler would be important to talk to Shira's parents about?

KEY POINTS

- The toddler tries to assert their independence, is curious about the world around them, and at times fears separation from family caregivers. Because of the toddler's new-found independence, parenting can be frustrating and a challenge, especially related to creating a safe environment and disciplining the child.

- Erikson's developmental task for the toddler is autonomy (independence) while overcoming doubt and shame. The toddler seeks independence, wavers between dependence and freedom, and gains self-awareness.

- The toddler's physical growth slows while motor, social, and language development rapidly increase. Each year the toddler gains 4.5 to 6.0 lb (2.0 to 2.7 kg) and about 3 inches (7.62 cm).

- Using negativism, the toddler often responds *no* to almost everything to assert individuality. To develop security, the toddler likes to follow specific sets of routines; this is referred to as ritualism. Dawdling occurs when toddlers follow their own desires, rather than the caregiver's wishes and routines. Temper tantrums are an aggressive display of temper, in which the child reacts with rebellion to the wishes of the caregiver.

- The toddler's play is often parallel play, in which the toddler plays alongside other children but not with them. Playtime involves imitation of the people the child sees as role models. The toddler learns self-control gradually, and the development from an egotistic being into a person who understands and respects the rights of others is a long, involved process, which the child must be taught.

- Toddlers want and need limits. Consistency and timing are important in the family caregiver's approach to disciplining the child.

- The toddler frequently regresses to more infantile behavior when a new sibling arrives. Special preparation and parental attention is necessary to show that there is room in the parent's lives for both children.

- Nutritional concerns and eating problems occur in the toddler because of a slower growth rate, a drive for independence, food jags, and variations in appetite. A balanced diet should be planned with an understanding of the toddler's developing feeding skills. The toddler progresses from finger feeding and tilting the cup to being able to hold a spoon and handle a cup in an adult manner.

- The toddler undergoes routine checkups at 15 months of age for immunization boosters and at least annually thereafter.

- Reinforcing family teaching includes aspects of everyday life with a toddler.
  - A regular time for a bath helps give the toddler a sense of security. Caregivers should avoid using bubble bath, especially for girls, because it can create an environment that encourages the growth of organisms that cause bladder infections.
  - Encourage the family caregiver to take a relaxed attitude as the toddler learns to dress themselves.
  - Bacteria forms dental plaque on teeth because of the presence of sugar in foods. The toddler should visit the dentist just after their first birthday to be introduced to the process of a dental checkup. By the age of 2 years, a toddler can be taught to brush their teeth by following the example of adults. Toilet training can be started

when the child's sphincter muscles have developed enough so the child can control them; this usually occurs at age 18 to 24 months. Perfection should not be expected. To aid in training, the caregiver leaves the child on the potty chair for only a short time. If the child has a bowel movement or urinates after leaving the potty, this is ignored. The child should not be teased, and the potty chair should not be emptied until the child has gone back to playing or other activities.

- A child needs a total of 12 to 14 hours of sleep daily in the first year of toddlerhood; this need decreases to 10 to 12 hours by 3 years of age. A bedtime ritual provides structure and a feeling of security.

- Supervision and prevention of accidents is especially important because of the exploring nature of the toddler.

- The leading causes of death in toddlers are accidents involving motor vehicles, drowning, burns, and poisons. Toddlers should always be secured in a car seat when in a motor vehicle. Supervision is important when toddlers are near motor vehicles, streets, bathtubs, and swimming pools. Toxic substances should be stored out of reach and in childproof containers. The most common medications involved in child poisonings are acetaminophen, aspirin, laxatives, sedatives, tranquilizers, analgesics, antihistamines, cardiac medications, cough/cold medicines, and birth control pills.

- Keep in mind the toddler's developmental tasks and needs. When the toddler is hospitalized, it is important to know their specific habits, terms used, patterns, and rituals. Maintaining as much as possible the pattern, schedule, and rituals that the toddler is used to helps to provide security. The curious toddler needs to be watched closely to maintain safety, but should not be unnecessarily prohibited from exploring.

INTERNET RESOURCES

Toddlers
www.babycenter.com/toddler

Poison Control
www.aapcc.org

Accident Prevention
www.safekids.org

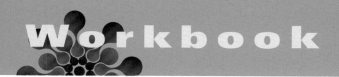

NCLEX-STYLE REVIEW QUESTIONS

1. The nurse is weighing a toddler who is 3 years old. If this child has had a typical pattern of growth and weighed 18 lb at the age of 1 year, the nurse would expect this toddler to weigh approximately how many pounds?
   a. 22 lb
   b. 30 lb
   c. 36 lb
   d. 42 lb

2. The nurse is observing a group of 2-year-old children. Which of the following actions by the toddlers would indicate a gross motor skill seen in children this age?
   a. Turns pages of a book
   b. Uses words to explain an object
   c. Drinks from a cup
   d. Runs with little falling

3. The toddler-aged child engages in parallel play. The nurse observes the following behaviors in a room where two children are playing with dolls and stuffed animals. Which of the following is an example of parallel play?
   a. Sharing stuffed animals with each other
   b. Sitting next to each other, each playing with their own doll
   c. Taking turns playing with the same stuffed animal
   d. Feeding the first doll, then feeding the second doll

4. In preparing snacks for a 15-month-old toddler, which of the following would be the *best* choice for this age child?
   a. Small cup of yogurt
   b. Five or six green grapes
   c. Handful of dry cereal
   d. Three or four cookies

5. The nurse is working with a group of family caregivers of toddlers. The nurse explains that accident prevention and safety are very important when working with children. Which of the following statements is true regarding accidents and safety for the toddler? Select all that apply.
   a. Child car restraints are required for children.
   b. Accidents are the leading cause of death in children up to age 4 years.
   c. At least 5 to 6 inches of water is necessary for drowning to occur.
   d. Touching and tasting substances in the environment is a concern.
   e. Poisonous items should be kept in a locked area.
   f. Child-resistant packaging keeps children from opening any bottle.

STUDY ACTIVITIES

1. List and compare the fine motor and gross motor skills in each of the following ages.

	15 Months	24 Months	36 Months
Fine motor skills			
Gross motor skills			

2. Discuss the development of language seen in toddlerhood. Compare the language development of the 15-month-old child to the language development of the 36-month-old child.

3. List the four leading causes of accidents in toddlers. For each of these causes state three prevention tips that you could share with family caregivers of toddlers.

4. Do an internet search on the topic "toilet training readiness checklist."
   a. What are the common physical, behavioral, and cognitive signs of toilet training readiness?
   b. After reading this information, what could you share with the family caregivers of a toddler regarding toilet training?

CRITICAL THINKING: WHAT WOULD YOU DO?

1. You are in the supermarket with your 2-year-old niece, Lauren. She is having a loud, screaming temper tantrum because you will not buy some expensive cookies she wants. As you are trying to talk with her, she is yelling, "No, I want them."
   a. What are the reasons toddlers have temper tantrums?
   b. What is the best way to respond to a toddler who is having a temper tantrum? Why?
   c. What would you say to Lauren in this situation?
   d. What actions would you take during the temper tantrum? After the temper tantrum?

2. Marti complains to you that 2-year-old Tasha is very difficult to put to bed at night. Marti often just gives up and lets Tasha fall asleep in front of the television.
   a. What are some of the factors that might be affecting Tasha at bedtime?
   b. What would you explain to Marti regarding bedtime rituals and routines for toddlers?
   c. What would you suggest Marti do with Tasha at her bedtime?

3. Jed is a 26-month-old child whose family caregivers work outside the home. He goes to a day care center 3 days a week and stays with his grandmother the other 2 days. Jed's mother asks you for advice in toilet training Jed.

a. What questions would you ask Jed's mother regarding his physical readiness for toilet training?

b. What suggestions will you offer regarding bowel training? Bladder training?

c. How might the variety of caregivers Jed has affect his toilet training?

d. What could Jed's mother do to provide consistency in toilet training for her child?

Growth and Development of the Preschool-Aged Child: 3 to 6 Years

Key Terms
associative play
cooperative play
dramatic play
magical thinking
noncommunicative language
onlooker play
solitary independent play
unoccupied behavior

Learning Objectives

At the conclusion of this chapter, you will:

1. State the major developmental task of the preschool-aged child according to Erikson.
2. Discuss the physical development of the preschool-aged child: (a) growth rate, (b) dentition, (c) visual development, and (d) skeletal growth.
3. Discuss the progression of language development in the preschool-aged child, including factors that delay or enhance progress.
4. Discuss the role of magical thinking and imagination in the preschool-aged child.
5. Discuss the nurse's role in helping parents understand the preschool-aged child's sexual curiosity and masturbation.
6. List six types of play in which preschool-aged children engage. Define each type.
7. Discuss aggression in the preschool-aged child and the family caregiver's role and response.
8. Discuss the role of discipline for the preschool-aged child and the effects of family caregiver behaviors when disciplining.
9. Discuss the special needs of the disadvantaged preschool-aged child and the value of Head Start programs.
10. Describe the nutritional needs of preschool-aged children, including (a) daily needs, (b) appetite variations, (c) suggested snacks, and (d) television commercials and other influences.
11. Discuss the recommended health maintenance checkup schedule for the preschool-aged child.
12. Identify important aspects of family teaching for the caregivers of preschool-aged children, including (a) bathing, (b) dressing, (c) dental care, (d) toileting, and (e) sleep.
13. List guidelines and anticipatory guidance for accident prevention in the preschool-aged population.
14. Discuss infection prevention in the preschool-aged child, describing the need for it and preventive measures to reinforce with the child.
15. Discuss important aspects of nursing care for the preschool child in the health care facility.

Lily Chang is a 4-year-old child. Her mother expresses concern about Lily's nutrition. Lily is at the 50th percentile for both height and weight on the growth chart. Her mother says, "One meal she will eat everything on her plate and then the next meal, she won't eat anything." She further expresses her concern that Lily is a picky eater and won't even try some foods. As you read this chapter think about the anticipatory guidance and information that would be appropriate to offer Lily's mother.

Preschool-aged children are fascinating creatures. As their social circles enlarge to include peers and adults outside the family, their language, play patterns, and appearance change markedly. Their curiosity about the world around them grows, as does their ability to explore that world in greater detail and see new meanings in what they find. It can be said that preschool-aged children soak up information like a sponge. *Why* and *how* are favorite words. This curiosity also means that accidents are still a serious concern.

At 3 years of age, the child still has the chubby, baby-face look of a toddler; by age 5, a leaner, taller, better-coordinated social being emerges. The child works and plays tirelessly, making things and telling everyone about them. In children of this age, exploring and learning go on continuously. They sometimes have problems separating fantasy from reality. According to Erikson, the developmental task of the preschool age is initiative versus guilt. Preschool-aged children often try to find ways to do things to help, but they may feel guilty if they extend themselves beyond their capabilities and fail, or disappoint the family caregiver because of inexperience or lack of skill.

PHYSICAL DEVELOPMENT

The physical development seen in the preschool-aged child includes a slowed growth rate, changes in dentition and visual development, and skeletal growth changes, especially in the feet and legs.

Growth Rate

The preschool period is one of slow growth. The child gains about 4 to 5 lb each year (1.8 to 2.3 kg) and grows about 2.5 to 3.0 in. (6.3 to 7.8 cm). Because the increase in height is proportionately greater than the increase in weight, the 5-year-old child appears much thinner and less babyish than the 3-year-old child does. Boys tend to be leaner than girls during this time. Gross and fine motor skills continue to develop rapidly (Fig. 25-1). Balance improves and confidence emerges to try new activities. By age 5, the child

generally can throw and catch a ball well, climb effectively, and ride a bicycle. Table 25-1 summarizes important milestones for growth and development.

Dentition

By 6 years of age, the child's skull is 90% of its adult size. The deciduous teeth have completely emerged by the beginning of the preschool period. Toward the end of the preschool stage, these teeth begin to be replaced by permanent teeth. This is an event that most children anticipate as an indication that they are growing up. Pictures of smiling 5- and 6-year-olds typically show missing front teeth (Fig. 25-2).

The age at which permanent teeth erupt varies with individual children and with various ethnic and economic groups. Permanent teeth of African-American children erupt at least 6 months earlier than those of American children of European ancestry. The central incisors are usually the first to go, just as they were the first to erupt in infancy.

Visual Development

Although the preschool-aged child's senses of taste and smell are acute, visual development is still immature at age 3. Eye–hand coordination is good, but judgment of distances generally is faulty, leading to many bumps and falls. During the preschool years, the child's vision should be checked to screen for amblyopia. Usually by age 6, the child achieves 20/20 vision, but mature depth perception may not develop in some children until 8 to 10 years of age.

Skeletal Growth

Between the third and sixth birthdays, the greatest amount of skeletal growth occurs in the feet and legs. This contributes to the change from the wide-gaited, potbellied look of the toddler into the slim, taller figure of the 6-year-old child. In addition, the carpals and tarsals mature in the hands and feet, which contributes to better hand and foot control.

TEST YOURSELF

✔ When do children start to lose their deciduous teeth?

✔ Give examples of fine motor skill development.

✔ Give examples of gross motor skill development.

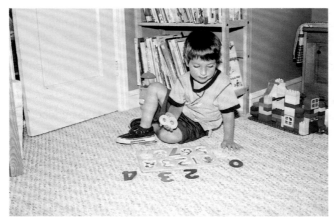

FIGURE 25-1 This 3-year-old child is developing fine motor skills, has good hand–eye coordination, and shows preference for using his right hand in putting a puzzle together.

PSYCHOSOCIAL DEVELOPMENT

The preschool age is characteristic of rapid language development. Imagination, sexual and social development, and a variety of types of play also characterize the preschool child's psychosocial development.

Language Development

Between the ages of 3 and 5 years, language development is generally rapid. Most 3-year-old children can construct simple sentences, but their speech has many hesitations

TABLE 25-1 Growth and Development: The Preschool-Aged Child

AGE (YEAR)	PERSONAL–SOCIAL	FINE MOTOR	GROSS MOTOR	LANGUAGE	COGNITIVE DEVELOPMENT
3	Begins Erikson's stage of "initiative vs. guilt." Conscience develops. Shy with strangers and inept with peers. Sufficiently independent to be interested in group experiences with age mates (e.g., preschool, day care)	Able to button clothes Copies *o* and + Uses pencils, crayons, paints Shows preference for right or left hand (Fig. 25-1)	Tends to watch others before attempting motor activities Can jump several feet Uses hands in broad movements Rides tricycle Negotiates stairs well	Vocabulary up to 1,000 words Articulates vowels accurately Talks a lot Sings and recites Asks many questions	Continues in pre-operational state (2–7 years) characterized by the following: 1. *Symbolic thinking,* making one object stand for something else (ability to imagine or pretend) 2. *Egocentricity,* or the inability to consider the perception of others
4	Boisterous and inflammatory Aggressive physically and verbally but developing behaviors to become socially acceptable Becomes socially acceptable Accepts punishment for wrongdoing because it relieves guilt	Can use scissors; copies a square Adds three parts to stick figures	Has some hesitation but tends to try feats beyond ability Greater powers of balance and accuracy Hops on one foot; can control movements of hands	Vocabulary of about 1,500 words Constant questions Sentences of four or five words Uses profanity Reports fantasies as truth	Reality and fantasy are not always clear Believes that words make things real— magical thinking
5	Initiates contacts with strangers and relates interesting little tales Interested in telling and comparing stories about self Peer relations are important ("best friends" abound) Responds to social values by assuming sex roles with rigidity	Ties shoelaces Copies a diamond and a triangle Prints a few letters or numbers May print first name Cuts food	Will not attempt feats beyond ability Throws and catches ball well Jumps rope Walks backward with heel to toe Skips and hops Adept on bicycle and climbing equipment	Vocabulary of 3,000 words Speech is intelligible Asks meanings of words Enjoys telling stories	Thinks feelings and thoughts can happen Intrusions into the body cause fear and anxiety (fear of mutilation and castration)

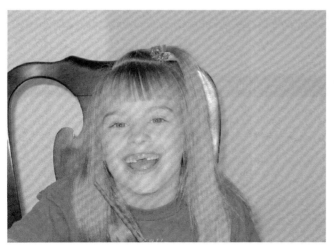

FIGURE 25-2 The smiling 6-year-old is often seen without front teeth.

and repetitions as they search for the right word or try to make the right sound. Stuttering can develop during this period but often disappears within 3 to 6 months. By the end of the fifth year, preschool-aged children use long, rather complex sentences; their vocabulary will have increased by more than 1,500 words since the age of 2 years.

The use of language changes during this period. Three-year-old children often talk to themselves or to their toys or pets without any apparent purpose other than the pleasure of using words. Piaget called this egocentric or **noncommunicative language**. By 4 years of age, children increase their use of communicative language, using words to transmit information other than their own needs and feelings.

Four- and 5-year-olds delight in using naughty words or swearing. Bathroom words become favorites and taunts such as "you're a big doo-doo" bring excitement to them.

Family caregivers may become concerned by this turn of events, but the child simply may be trying words out to test their impact.

Table 25-2 summarizes typical development of verbal abilities of preschool-aged children.

Delays or other difficulties in language development may result from one or more of the following factors.

- Hearing impairment or other physical problem
- Lack of stimulation
- Overprotection
- Lack of parental interest or rejection by parents

> **Here's a Helpful Hint!**
> By using a calm, matter-of-fact response when a preschool-aged child uses naughty or swear words, some of the power of using that type of language will be diffused. The child learns that this is not the language to use in the company of others.

Good language skills develop as the child regularly engages in conversation with family caregivers and others. The conversation should be on a level that the child can understand. Reading to the child is an excellent method of contributing to language development. Talking with the child about the pictures in storybooks can enhance this. Praise, approval, and encouragement are all part of supporting attempts at communication.

Family and cultural patterns also influence language development. Some children come from bilingual families and are trying to learn the rules of both languages. Others may come from geographic or social communities that have dialects different from the general population.

Development of Imagination

Preschool-aged children have learned to think about something without actually seeing it—to visualize or imagine. This normal development, sometimes called **magical thinking**, makes it difficult for them to separate fantasy from reality. Preschool-aged children believe that words or thoughts can make things real, and this belief can have either positive or negative results. For example, in a moment of anger, a child may wish that a parent or a sibling would die; if that person is hurt later, the child feels responsible and suffers guilt. The child needs reassurance that this is not so.

Imagination makes preschool-aged children good audiences for storytelling, simple plays, and television, as long as the characters and events are not too frightening or sad. When preschool-aged children see a television character die, they believe it is real and often cry. The child's television viewing should be supervised to avoid programs with negative impacts or overstimulation.

During this stage, children often have imaginary playmates who are very real to them. This occurs particularly with families with one child for whom imaginary playmates fill times of loneliness. The imaginary friend often has the characteristics that the child might wish for in a real friend. Sometimes the child blames the imaginary friend for breaking a toy or engaging in another act for which the child does not want to take responsibility. Family caregivers need assurance that this is normal behavior.

The preschool-aged child's active imagination often leads to a fear of the dark or nightmares. Consequently, problems with sleep are common (see the "Sleep" section later in this chapter).

A Personal Glimpse

We had just returned from a weekend visit to my parents' house. My 2-year-old was sleeping quietly. I was in the laundry room doing the laundry from our weekend trip, and my 5-year-old (Kayla) was playing in the family room (or so I thought). Suddenly I heard a loud crashing sound that came from the kitchen. I asked, "What was that?" "Nothing, Mom." I asked again, "What WAS that?" and headed toward the kitchen. When I got to the kitchen, I discovered what the sound had been—the entire sugar canister was empty—the canister on its side, rolling on the floor with the contents all over the cabinet and kitchen floor. Clearly, SOMETHING had happened. I called to Kayla to come to the kitchen. This time I said, "Kayla, tell me how this happened." She told me, "I was playing Legos and Sandy [her imaginary friend] was making cookies just like at Gramma's house, and Sandy was getting the sugar, and

TABLE 25-2 Verbal Mastery by Preschool-Aged Children

AGE (YEAR)	CHARACTERISTICS OF LANGUAGE USAGE	VOCABULARY SIZE, PATTERN, COMPREHENSION, RHYTHM
3–4	Loves to talk; talks a lot; makes up words; sings or recites own version of song; likes new words; asks many questions and wants answers. Not always logical in sentences and concepts. Uses four- or five-word phrases. Aggressive with words rather than actions.	Vocabulary of 900–1,500 words; at 3 years, understands up to 3,600 words; up to 5,600 words by 4 years. By 4 years, speech understandable even with mispronunciations. May have hesitations, repetitions, and revisions while trying to imitate adult speech. Stuttering may occur but often disappears within 3–6 months; may continue up to 2 years without being permanent.
4–5	Understands out-of-context words. Speech highly emotional. Difficulty finding right word; tells function rather than name of item. Changes subject rapidly. Boasts, brags, quarrels; loves naughty words. Relates fanciful tales.	Vocabulary of 3,000 words; understands up to 9,600 words by 5 years. Speech completely understandable.

then it was all over the floor." As I looked at the mess she continued, "Like last time Sandy got the toothpaste all over the wall, only this time it was in the kitchen." As upset as I was at having to clean the mess, I thought it was creative of Kayla to use her "imaginary friend" as the mess maker.

Ann

Learning Opportunity: *What would you tell this mother regarding preschool-aged children and imaginary friends? What would you suggest this mother should say to respond to her child in this situation?*

Sexual Development

The preschool period is the stage that Freud termed the oedipal or phallic (genital) period. During these years, children become acutely aware of their sexuality, including sexual roles and organs. They generally develop a strong emotional attachment to the parent of the opposite sex. Children's curiosity about their own genitalia and those of peers and adults may make parents uncomfortable and evoke responses that indicate to the child that sex is dirty and something about which to be ashamed and guilty.

Despite today's abundance of sexually oriented literature, many families find it difficult to deal with the young child's questions and actions. You can help family caregivers understand that the child's sexual curiosity is a normal, natural part of total curiosity about oneself and the surrounding world. The informed, understanding family caregiver can help the child develop positive attitudes toward sexuality and toward themselves as a sexual human being.

In addition to responsible teaching of sexual information, the family caregiver should also teach the child about "good touch" and "bad touch." The child needs to understand that no one should touch the child's body in a way that is unpleasant.

Exploration of the genitalia is as natural for the preschool-aged child as thumb sucking is for the infant. It is one way the child learns to perceive the body as a possible source of pleasure and is the beginning of the acceptance of sex as natural and pleasurable.

Family caregivers can be reassured that this is not uncommon behavior, and a calm, matter-of-fact response to the child found masturbating is the most effective approach. The child should be helped to understand that masturbation is not an activity that is appropriate in public. If the child seems to be masturbating excessively, counseling may be needed, especially if the child's life has been unsettled in other aspects.

Social Development

Preschool-aged children are outgoing, imaginative, social beings. They play vigorously and in the process, learn about the world in which they live. As they gain control over their environments, preschool-aged children try to manipulate them, and this may lead to conflict with family caregivers. Preschool children are delightful to watch as they go about the business of growing and learning.

Play

Play activities are one way that children learn. Normally by 3 years of age, children begin imitative play, pretending to be the mommy, the daddy, a policeman, a cowboy, an astronaut, or some well-known person or television character (Fig. 25-3). Family caregivers can gain good insight into the way the child interprets family behavior by watching the child play. Listening to a preschool-aged child scold a doll or a stuffed animal for "bothering me while I'm busy talking on the phone" lets the adults hear how they sound to the child.

Preschool-aged children engage in various types of play: dramatic, cooperative, associative, parallel, solitary independent, onlooker, and unoccupied behavior. **Dramatic play** allows a child to act out troubling situations and to control the solution to the problem. This is important to remember when reinforcing teaching with children who are going to be hospitalized. Using dolls and puppets to explain procedures makes the experience less threatening. In **cooperative play**, children play in an organized group with each other, as in team sports. **Associative play** occurs when children play together and are engaged in a similar activity but without organization, rules, or a leader, and each child does what they wish. In parallel play, children play alongside each other but independently. Although common among toddlers, parallel play exists in all age groups, for example, in a preschool classroom where each student is working on an individual project or craft. **Solitary independent play** means playing apart from others without making an effort to be part of the group or group activity. Watching television is one form of **onlooker play** in which there is observation without participation. In **unoccupied behavior**, the child may be daydreaming or fingering clothing or a toy without apparent purpose.

Watch Out!

Preschool-aged children love to imitate adults. Dressing up like Mommy or Daddy is a favorite play activity. Listening to a preschool-aged child gives adults an idea of how they sound to the preschool-aged child!

 Concept Mastery Alert

While children of this age sometimes engage in parallel play, they are much more likely to play together. Imitative play is a favorite activity.

Drawing is another form of play through which children learn to express themselves. During the preschool years, as fine motor skills improve, children's drawings become much more complex and controlled and can be revealing about the child's self-concept and perception of the environment.

Children need all types of play to aid in their total development. Too much of one kind may signal a problem;

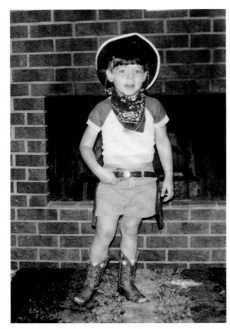

FIGURE 25-3 Imitative play is common. This preschool-aged child pretends to be a cowboy.

for example, a youngster who spends most of the time unoccupied may be troubled, depressed, or not stimulated. Cooperative play helps develop social interaction skills and often physical health.

Too much onlooker play, particularly television or internet viewing, means that children are missing the benefits of other kinds of play and may be forming strong, highly inaccurate impressions of people and their behaviors. Family caregivers should limit the amount of time that preschool-aged children spend watching television and electronic devices, and they should encourage interactive play.

TEST YOURSELF

✔ What is magical thinking? Why do preschool-aged children have imaginary friends?

✔ Who do preschool-aged children imitate when they are playing?

✔ List the types of play seen in the preschool-aged child.

Aggression

Temper tantrums are an early form of aggression. The preschool-aged child with newly developed language skills uses words aggressively in name calling and threats. Four-year-old children use physical aggression as well; they push, hit, and kick in an effort to manipulate the environment. The family caregiver's task during these years is to help the child understand that the anger and frustration that result in aggressive behavior are normal but need to be handled differently because aggressive behavior is not socially acceptable.

Children who come from unhappy home situations are likely to be more aggressive than children from comfortable family situations. Their family caregivers have served as role models, and their aggressive behavior toward each other has said to the child, "this is acceptable."

Discipline

Family caregivers need to remember that preschool-aged children are developing initiative and a sense of guilt. They want to be good and follow instructions, and they feel bad when they do not, even if they are not physically punished. Discipline during this time should strive to teach the child a sense of responsibility and inner control. All the child's family caregivers must understand and agree to the limits and discipline measures for the child. If one caregiver says *no* and another one says *yes*, the child soon learns to play one against the other, leading to confusion about limits. Spanking and other forms of physical punishment remove the responsibility from the child. Taking a privilege away from a child who has misbehaved until they can demonstrate that there has been an improvement in behavior is much more effective. Because the child's concept of time is not clear, the period should be comparatively brief (Fig. 25-4). Table 25-3 presents some examples of the effects of family caregiver's positive and negative responses.

Preschool or Day Care Experience

Group experiences with peers and adults outside the immediate family are important to a child's development. However, the transition to new experiences, new people, and new surroundings can be threatening to some preschool-aged children. Children vary in their willingness or ability to handle new situations. Gradually introducing children to the

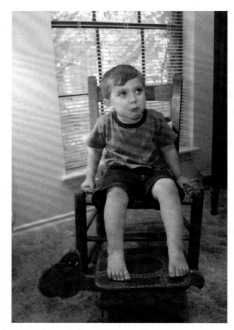

FIGURE 25-4 Although he may not like it, quiet solitude helps the preschool-aged child develop inner control.

TABLE 25-3 Effects of Positive and Negative Family Caregiver Behaviors

BEHAVIOR	EFFECT ON CHILD	EFFECT ON ADULT
Attending only to desired behaviors Calm reasoning with expression of dislike of behavior Isolation of child for a period of time equal to 1 minute per year of age Withholding of desired treats, outings, presents	Development of inner control	Feelings of adequacy as a parent
Yelling, screaming, and implying guilt and punishment Telling child that they are bad Physical punishment	Development of fears and compulsive behaviors	Feelings of guilt and inadequacy
Giving treats, presents, or food for lack of undesired behavior Physical punishment Threatening punishment from God or other authority figure	Development of control based on external forces	Feelings of being manipulated by child

new situation according to individual readiness produces the most satisfactory adjustment.

Some children spend only a few hours each week in a preschool or other day care program; others must spend a great deal more time away from home and family because the adult family members work outside the home. The family should understand that the child who spends more time away from home will probably demand more of their attention during the hours when they are together. As the child grows older and the attachment to peers becomes stronger, family caregivers sense a decrease in the need for adult attention and a greater sense of independence in the child.

The Disadvantaged Child

Discussions of normal growth and development assume that children come from secure, well-adjusted homes in which there is ample opportunity for social, cultural, and intellectual enrichment. Many children, however, are deprived of such backgrounds for many reasons. This population is the one most likely to have health problems and to need health services.

Children who have not been able to achieve a sense of security and trust, for whatever reason, need special understanding, warm acceptance, and guidance to grow into self-accepting people. Society is gradually awakening to the needs of these children and is trying to provide enriched day care, preschool, and kindergarten experiences for those whose home life cannot do this for them.

Recognition that environmental enrichment is often unavailable in families with limited social, cultural, and economic resources led to the establishment of Head Start programs. Head Start programs are funded by federal and local money and are free to the children enrolled. Children in such programs have an opportunity to broaden their horizons through varied experiences and to increase their understanding of the world in which they live. Family caregiver participation is a central component of the Head Start concept and often has a positive effect on other children in the household. In some programs, teachers go into the home to help the caregiver teach the young child motor, cognitive, self-help, and language skills. Counseling and referral services are also provided through Head Start programs.

Children who have had a background of Head Start enrichment are better prepared to enter kindergarten or first grade and compete successfully with their peers.

NUTRITION

The preschool period is not a time of rapid growth, so children do not need large quantities of food. Children do need foods from the major food groups each day. Protein needs continue to remain high to provide for muscle growth. Refer to the USDA guidelines found in the ChooseMyPlate in Figure 22-3 in Chapter 22. Daily nutritional needs including caloric requirements and the appropriate number of servings per day for the preschool child are listed in Table 25-4.

The preschool-aged child's appetite is erratic; at one sitting, the preschool-aged child may devour everything on the plate and at the next meal, they may be satisfied with just a few bites. Portions are smaller than adult-sized portions, so the child may need to have meals supplemented with nutritious snacks (Box 25-1). Note that certain snacks are recommended only for the older child to avoid any danger of choking. The preschool-aged child generally best accepts frequent, small meals with snacks in between.

Among the preschool-aged child's favorites are soft foods, grain and dairy products, raw vegetables, and sweets. Television commercials for sugar-coated cereals, snacks, and fast foods of questionable nutritional value have a powerful influence on the preschool-aged child and can make supermarket shopping an emotional struggle between the family caregiver and the child. Family caregivers should read labels carefully before making a purchase.

Lily Chang's mother described Lily as a picky eater. What explanations will you give Lily's mother regarding the preschool child's appetite and food requirements? What questions might you ask Lily's mother to better understand the family's eating practices? As you talk with Lily's mother, what will you suggest to her regarding food choices, portions, meals, and snacks?

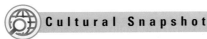

Cultural Snapshot

Food preferences, likes, and dislikes are seen in many cultures. Take these variations into consideration when helping family caregivers make nutritious food choices for snacks and meals.

Preschool-aged children need guidance in choosing foods and are strongly influenced by the example of family members and peers. Food should never be used as a reward or bribe; otherwise, the child will continue to use food as a means to manipulate the environment and the behavior of others.

Preschool-aged children have definite food preferences. They generally do not like highly spiced foods, often will eat raw vegetables but not cooked ones, and prefer plain foods, rather than casseroles. New foods may be accepted but should be introduced one at a time to avoid overwhelming the child.

The preschool-aged child shows growing independence and skill in eating. The 3-year-old child tries to mimic adult behavior at the table but often reverts to eating with the fingers, spilling liquids, and squirming. The 4-year-old is more skilled with the use of utensils, although an occasional misjudgment of abilities results in a mess. The 5-year-old uses utensils well, often can cut their own food, and can be taught to practice sophisticated table manners (Fig. 25-5). Rituals, such as using the same plate, cereal bowl, cup, or place mat, may become important to the child's mealtime happiness.

HEALTH PROMOTION AND MAINTENANCE

Routine checkups, reinforcing family teaching, and accident and infection prevention are important aspects of health promotion and maintenance for the preschool child.

Routine Checkups

Preschool-aged children with up-to-date immunizations need boosters of diphtheria-tetanus-pertussis vaccine, polio vaccine, measles-mumps-rubella (MMR) vaccine, and varicella vaccine between 4 and 6 years of age. These are required as preschool boosters for entrance into kindergarten.

TABLE 25-4 Daily Nutritional Needs of 3- to 6-Year-Olds

For a 1,200–1,800 calorie diet, the preschool-aged child needs the amounts below from each food group. Young preschool-aged children should play actively several times a day and by age 6 should be moderately active for 60 minutes every day.

FRUITS	VEGETABLES	GRAINS	PROTEIN FOODS	DAIRY
1–1.5 cups	1.5–2.5 cups	4–6 oz	3–5 oz	2.5 cups

BOX 25-1 Suggested Snacks for the Preschool-Aged Child[a]

Raw vegetables: Carrots, cucumbers, celery, green beans, bell peppers, mushrooms, turnips, broccoli, cauliflower, tomatoes
Fresh fruits: Apples, oranges, pears, peaches, grapes, cherries, melons, sliced bananas, berries
Unsalted whole-grain crackers
Whole-grain bread: Cut to finger-sized sticks; plain, toasted, or with peanut butter
Small sandwiches: Cut into quarters
Natural cheese: Cut into cubes
Cooked meat: Cut into small chunks or sliced thinly
Nuts
Sunflower seeds (shells removed)
Cookies: Made with lightly sweetened whole grains
Plain popcorn
Yogurt: Plain or with fresh fruit added

[a]Children younger than 2 years of age may choke on nuts, seeds, popcorn, grapes, celery strings, or carrot sticks. Avoid these until preschool years and then always cut into small, bite-sized pieces.

An annual health examination is recommended to monitor the child's growth and development and to screen for potential health problems. Children who attend preschool or day care programs may be required to have annual examination. An annual examination is suggested even for children who stay at home. Recommended screening procedures include urinalysis, hematocrit, lead level, tuberculin skin testing, and Denver Developmental Screening Test. The health care provider should pay particular attention to the child's vision and hearing so that any problems can be treated before they enter school at age 5 or 6. A semiannual dental examination is also recommended.

It is wise for the family caregiver to tell the preschool child in advance about the upcoming examination. The caregiver should use simple explanations and provide an opportunity for the child to ask questions and voice anxieties. A number of books available through public libraries are excellent for this purpose.

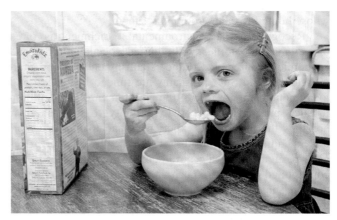

FIGURE 25-5 The 5-year-old can use a spoon well to feed herself.

Family Teaching

Use routine checkups and any other opportunities to reinforce teaching to family caregivers about common aspects of everyday life with a preschool-aged child. Preschool-aged children are busy learning and show initiative as they are involved in their day-to-day lives. Preschool-aged children are usually a pleasure to be around because they are so eager to learn anything new and are full of questions.

Bathing

Although preschool-aged children view themselves as grown up, they still need continual supervision while bathing. The caregiver should run the bath water. The hot water heater should be turned to no higher than 120°F (49°C), to avoid the danger of burns. Caregivers should teach children to leave the faucets alone. Preschool-aged children can generally wash themselves with supervision. Ears, necks, and faces are spots that often need extra attention. Hands and fingernails often get soaked clean in the tub, but fingernails do need to be checked by the family caregiver.

Preschool-aged children cannot wash their own hair, so this can be a time of tension between the child and the family caregiver. Shampooing in the tub with a nonirritating children's shampoo may work best. The child can lean the head back, look at the ceiling, and hold a washcloth on the forehead to keep water and soap from getting into the eyes. Shampoo protectors (clear plastic brims with no crowns) can be purchased if desired.

Bath time can be rather lengthy if the preschool-aged child gets involved in playing with bath toys. This is something the family caregiver can negotiate if limits need to be set. Some children of this age are interested in taking a shower and may do so with adult supervision.

When washing their hands before meals or before or after going to the bathroom, preschool-aged children often wash only the fronts while ignoring the backs. If not supervised, the child may use only cold water and no soap. Again, the family caregiver should turn the water on to a warm temperature to avoid burns.

Dressing

The preschool-aged child may have definite ideas about what they want to wear. Giving the child the opportunity to choose what to wear each day is an excellent way to begin fostering a sense of control and to help the child learn to make decisions. Preschool-aged children do not have very good taste in what matches, so some interesting outfits may result! Nevertheless, the child should be permitted to make these choices, and the caregivers (as well as older siblings and other adults) should accept the choices without negative comments. When it does matter—for the adults—how the child is dressed, the best plan is to give the child limited choices that will suit the occasion.

Dental Care

The family caregiver needs to supervise the preschool child in toothbrushing. Although the preschool-aged child can brush well, the caregiver should check the cleanliness of the child's teeth. The caregiver should be responsible for flossing because the preschool-aged child does not have the necessary motor skills. To help prevent tooth decay, the preschool-aged child should be encouraged to eat healthy snacks, such as fruits, raw vegetables, and natural cheeses, rather than candy, cakes, or sugar-filled gum. The preschool child should continue the use of fluoridated water, toothpaste, or fluoride supplements as recommended by the child's dentist.

Toileting

By the preschool years, almost all children have succeeded in toilet training, although an occasional accident may occur. When the child does have an accident, treating it in a matter-of-fact way and providing the child with clean, dry clothing is best. The preschool-aged child needs continual reminders to wash the hands before and after toileting. Little girls should be taught to wipe from front to back. Preschool-aged children may still need to be checked for careful wiping, especially after a bowel movement.

Bed-wetting is not uncommon for young preschool-aged children and is not a concern unless it continues past the age of 5 to 7 (see Chapter 39 for further discussion).

Sleep

Preschool-aged children are often ready to give up their nap. This may depend partially on if they go to a preschool program that has a rest time. Often preschool-aged children will just curl up and fall asleep on a chair, a couch, or the floor. Bedtime can still be a challenge, but leading up to it with a period of quiet activities or stories encourages the child to wind down for the day.

Dreams and nightmares are common during the preschool period. Caregivers need to explain that "it was only a dream" and offer love and understanding until the fear has subsided. Fear of the dark is another common problem during these years. Children may be afraid to go to sleep in a dark bedroom. These are very real fears to the child. A small night light may be reassuring to the child.

Creativity Can Be Useful!

One mother found a creative solution for her child's fear of going to sleep. The child was afraid of a monster in the closet or under the bed. The mother acknowledged the child's fears and purchased a spray can of room air freshener. At bedtime, she ceremoniously sprayed around the room, in the closet, and under the bed. She assured the child that it was a special spray to kill monsters, just like bug spray kills bugs. The reassured child slept without fear.

Accident Prevention

Adults caring for preschool-aged children need to be just as attentive as they are with toddlers because a child's curiosity at this stage still exceeds their judgment. Burns, poisoning, and falls are common accidents. Preschool-aged children are often victims of motor vehicle accidents either because they dart into the street or driveway or fail to wear proper restraints. All states have laws that define safety seat and restraint requirements for children. Adults must teach and reinforce these rules.

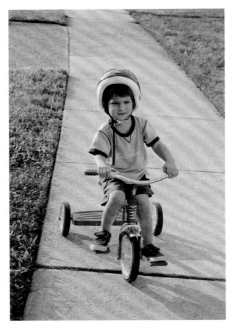

FIGURE 25-6 This preschool-aged child has learned to always wear a proper safety helmet.

One primary responsibility of adults is always to wear seat belts themselves and to make certain that the child always is in a safety seat or has a seat belt on when in a motor vehicle. Caregivers can calmly teach a child that the vehicle "won't go" unless the child is properly restrained.

By the age of 5, many preschool-aged children move from riding a tricycle to riding a bicycle. If the preschool-aged child is not already wearing a bicycle helmet, it is important to reinforce with family caregivers that safety helmets are a necessary safety precaution. Lightweight, child-sized safety helmets that fit properly can be purchased, and the child should be taught that the helmet must be worn when riding a bike (Fig. 25-6). Adults who wear helmets provide the best incentive to children. Safety rules for bicycle riding should be reinforced. The preschool child should be limited to protected areas for riding and should have adult supervision.

The preschool age is an excellent time to begin teaching safety rules. The rules for crossing the street and playing in an area near traffic are of vital importance. Adults who care for preschool children should be careful to serve as good role models. These safety rules should extend into all aspects of the child's life. See Tips for Reinforcing Family Teaching: Safety Suggestions for Preschool-Aged Children.

TIPS FOR REINFORCING FAMILY TEACHING

Safety Suggestions for Preschool-Aged Children

- Look both ways before crossing the street.
- Cross the street only with an adult.
- Watch for cars coming out of driveways.
- Never play behind a car or truck.
- Watch for cars or trucks backing up.
- Wear a safety helmet when bike riding.
- Learn your name, address, and phone number.
- Stay away from strange dogs.
- Stay away from any dog while it is eating.
- Take only medicine that your caregiver gives you.
- Do not play with matches or lighters.
- Stay away from fires.
- Do not run near a swimming pool.
- Only swim when with an adult.
- Do not go anywhere with someone you do not know.
- Do not let anyone touch you in a way you do not like.

Infection Prevention

Preschool-aged children who enjoy sound nutrition and adequate rest, exercise, and shelter usually are not seriously affected by simple childhood infections. Children who live in less than adequate economic circumstances, however, can be severely threatened by even a simple illness, such as diarrhea or chickenpox. Immunizations are available for many childhood communicable diseases, but some family caregivers do not have their children immunized until it is required for entrance to school. As a result, some children suffer unnecessary illnesses.

Preschool-aged children are just learning to share, and that can mean sharing infections with the entire family—and playmates as well. Teaching them basic precautions can help prevent the spread of infections. See Tips for Reinforcing Family Teaching: Preventing Infections.

TIPS FOR REINFORCING FAMILY TEACHING

Preventing Infections

- Cover your mouth with a tissue when coughing or sneezing.
- Throw away tissues in the trash after using and immediately wash your hands.
- Cough into your sleeve at the elbow.
- Wipe carefully after bowel movements (girls wipe front to back).
- Wash hands after going to the bathroom, coughing, or blowing your nose.
- Wash hands before eating.
- Do not share food that you have partly eaten.
- If an eating utensil falls on the floor, wash it right away.
- If food falls on the floor, do not eat it.
- Do not drink from another person's cup.
- Do not share a toothbrush with someone else.

TEST YOURSELF

✔ What are some of the reasons preschool-aged children need close supervision while bathing?

✔ What are the major causes of accidents in the preschool-aged child?

✔ List the measures preschool-aged children should be taught to prevent accidents.

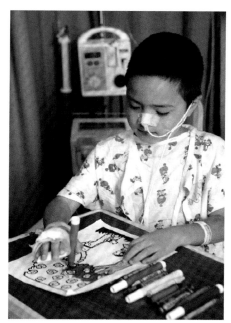

FIGURE 25-7 This hospitalized child can enjoy age-appropriate activities, even when on bed rest.

THE PRESCHOOL-AGED CHILD IN THE HEALTH CARE FACILITY

The preschool-aged child may view hospitalization as an exciting new adventure or as a frightening, dangerous experience, depending on the preparation by family caregivers and health care providers. As mentioned, play is an effective way to let children act out their anxieties and to learn what to expect from the hospital situation. Preschool-aged children are frightened about intrusive procedures; therefore, it is preferable to take the temperature with an oral or tympanic thermometer, rather than with a rectal one.

The hospitalized preschool-aged child may revert to bed-wetting but should not be scolded for it. Assure the family that this is normal. Explanations of where the bathrooms are and how to use the call light or bell to get help can help avoid problems with bed-wetting. If a child is afraid of the dark, a night light can be provided.

Hospital routines should follow home routines as closely as possible. Allow the child to participate in the care, even though this may take longer. Carefully explain all procedures to the child in words appropriate for the child's age, and repeat the information as necessary.

If the child is ambulatory and not on infection transmission precautions, the playroom can offer diversionary activities. If not, play materials can be provided for use in bed (Fig. 25-7).

Some Nurses Find This Approach Helpful!
Children are less anxious about procedures if they are allowed to handle equipment beforehand and perhaps use it on a doll or another toy.

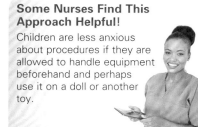

Think back to **Lily Chang** from the beginning of this chapter. What would you anticipate regarding Lily's growth during the preschool age? What are some areas of anticipatory guidance that you would reinforce teaching with Lily's mother?

KEY POINTS

• According to Erikson, the major developmental task for the preschool-aged group is initiative versus guilt. Preschool-aged children try to find ways to do things to help, but they may feel guilty if they extend themselves beyond their capabilities and fail, or disappoint the family caregiver because of inexperience or lack of skill.

• During the preschool years, physical growth slows. The child gains about 4 to 5 lb each year (1.8 to 2.3 kg) and grows about 2.5 to 3.0 in. (6.3 to 7.8 cm). Toward the end of the preschool stage, deciduous teeth begin to be replaced by permanent teeth. By the age of 6, children usually have achieved 20/20 vision. The greatest amount of skeletal growth in the preschool-aged child occurs in the feet and legs.

• Language develops rapidly during the preschool period. Reading to the child, engaging the child in conversation, and offering encouragement contribute to language development. Language development may be delayed because of hearing impairment or physical problems, lack of stimulation, overprotection, or lack of parental support.

• Magical thinking and imagination contribute to fears and anxieties of the preschool-aged child because these make it difficult for the child to separate fantasy from reality. Caregivers must acknowledge these concerns, be patient with explanations, and offer reassurance to the child.

• A preschool-aged child's sexual curiosity and exploration of their genitalia is normal. A calm, understanding family caregiver can help the child develop positive attitudes about themselves as a sexual being.

• Dramatic play allows for acting out troubling situations. Cooperative play is when children play in organized groups, and associative play occurs when children engage in similar activity but there is no organization or rules. When children play apart from others, it is solitary independent play. Watching TV is a form of onlooker play. In unoccupied behavior, the child is often daydreaming without specific purpose.

• The preschool-aged child may show verbal aggression by name calling and physical aggression by pushing, hitting, or kicking. Family caregivers need to help the child understand that aggressive behavior is not socially acceptable. Family caregivers also serve as role models.

• The family caregiver disciplines by setting limits and helping the child develop inner control and take responsibility for their actions.

• The disadvantaged child who has not been able to develop a sense of trust needs understanding, acceptance, and guidance to develop appropriately.

Programs such as Head Start give children opportunities to promote development.

- Even though the preschool child has a decreased and erratic appetite, adequate protein, nutritious snacks, and avoidance of foods that lack nutritional value are important.
- Preschool-aged children should have annual routine checkups to monitor growth, administer immunizations, and perform screening.
- Preschool-aged children need supervision while bathing and toothbrushing and need help with flossing. Fluoride supplements should be continued, as recommended. Preschool-aged children may want to dress themselves. Preschool-aged children need continual reminders to wash their hands before and after toileting. Girls should be taught to wipe from front to back. Dreams, nightmares, and fear of the dark are common, and caregivers need to be reminded to reassure and offer understanding to the child.
- Seat belt use, wearing bicycle safety helmets, and practicing street safety will help in prevention of accidents in the preschool-aged child. Stranger, fire, and swimming safety should also be taught.
- The preschool-aged child learns to share with family and playmates and the process often shares infections. To prevent infection, the child is taught to cover their mouth when coughing or sneezing, proper disposal of tissues, correct wiping after bowel movements, good handwashing, and to not share cups, utensils, food, or toothbrushes.
- Keep in mind the preschool-aged child's developmental tasks and needs. Play is an effective way to let children act out their anxieties and learn what to expect from the hospital situation. Explain procedures in words appropriate for the child's age.

INTERNET RESOURCES

Head Start Programs
http://www.acf.hhs.gov/ohs
www.earlychildhood.com

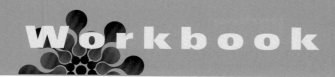

NCLEX-STYLE REVIEW QUESTIONS

1. The nurse is assisting with a well-child visit for a 5½-year-old child. This child's records show that at the age of 3 years, this child weighed 32 lb, was 35.5 in. tall, had 20 teeth, and slept 11 hours a day. If this child is following a normal pattern of growth and development, which of the following would the nurse expect to find in this visit?
   a. The child weighs 54 pounds.
   b. The child measures 38 inches tall.
   c. The child has two permanent teeth.
   d. The child sleeps 2 hours for a morning nap.

2. In working with a group of preschool children, which of the following activities would this age child *most* likely be doing?
   a. Pretending to be television characters.
   b. Playing a game with large balls and blocks.
   c. Participating in a group activity.
   d. Collecting stamps or coins.

3. The nurse is talking with a group of family caregivers of preschool-aged children. Which of the following statements made by a caregiver would require further data collection?
   a. "My child calls her sister bad names when she doesn't get her way."
   b. "She told me her imaginary friend broke my favorite picture frame."
   c. "My son always wants to eat cookies for lunch and for snacks."
   d. "Even when his friends are over to play, he wants to play by himself."

4. A family caregiver of a preschool-aged child says to the nurse, "My 4-year-old touches her genitals sometimes when she is resting." Which of the following statements would be appropriate for the nurse to respond?
   a. "Masturbation is embarrassing to the parents; scolding the child will stop the behavior."
   b. "When children are angry or upset, they often masturbate."
   c. "When this age child masturbates, it can be unhealthy and dangerous."
   d. "Masturbation is a normal behavior, so providing another activity for the child would be appropriate."

5. In working with the preschool-aged child and this child's family, reinforcing teaching regarding prevention of infection is important. Which of the following are true regarding prevention of infection? Select all that apply.
   a. Girls should be taught to wipe from front to back after a bowel movement.
   b. Sharing foods or utensils with family members is acceptable.
   c. It is important to wash hands after coughing, sneezing, or blowing your nose.
   d. Each person should have their own toothbrush and use only that one.
   e. When washing hands, cold water works as well as warm water.

STUDY ACTIVITIES

1. List and compare the fine motor skills, gross motor skills, and language development in each of the following ages.

	3 Years	4 Years	5 Years
Fine motor skills			
Gross motor skills			
Language development			

2. Describe the guidelines you would give a family to help children develop good eating habits and encourage the trying of new foods. Write a 1-day menu including snacks for a preschool-aged child.

3. You are working with the staff in a day care facility to help them develop activities for their preschool program. Using your knowledge of preschool growth and development, make a list of behaviors you would suggest the staff look for in the preschool-aged child. What activities would you suggest to encourage normal preschool growth and development?

4. Do an internet search on "child dental health."
   a. Make a list of three sites you find related to child dental health.
   b. What topics are discussed on these sites?
   c. What did you learn that you can share with peers, children, and family caregivers related to child dental health?

CRITICAL THINKING: WHAT WOULD YOU DO?

1. Clara has noticed her 5-year-old son Ted masturbating. She is upset and comes to you for help.

   a. What reactions and concerns might Clara express regarding masturbation in her preschool child?

   b. What will you tell Clara to help her understand preschool-aged children and masturbation?

   c. What actions would you suggest for Clara to do when she notices Ted is masturbating?

2. Jenny reports that her 3.5-year-old daughter, Krista, wakes up screaming in the middle of the night. This is causing the family to lose sleep.

   a. What concerns do you think Jenny might have regarding this situation?

   b. What characteristics of a preschool-aged child might be causing Krista to wake up at night screaming?

   c. What would you suggest Jenny do and say to Krista when this happens?

3. A group of family caregivers of 4-year-olds are discussing their children and the behaviors they are noticing. One of the caregivers states, "My child is so frustrating." Several of the other caregivers nod their heads in agreement.

   a. What characteristics of preschool-aged children might lead to these caregiver feelings of frustration?

   b. What explanations would you offer these caregivers as to the reasons they are seeing these behaviors in their children?

   c. How would you suggest these caregivers respond when they feel frustrated by these preschool-aged children?

Growth and Development of the School-Aged Child: 6 to 10 Years

Learning Objectives

At the conclusion of this chapter, you will:

1. State the major developmental task of the school-aged group according to Erikson.
2. Discuss the physical growth patterns during the school-aged years.
3. Describe dentition in school-aged children.
4. Discuss the psychosocial development of the school-aged child.
5. Explain the cognitive development seen in the school-aged child regarding (a) conservation, (b) decentration, (c) reversibility, and (d) classification.
6. Identify nutritional influences on the school-aged child, including (a) family attitudes, (b) mealtime atmosphere, (c) snacks, and (d) school's role.
7. List three factors that contribute to obesity in the school-aged child.
8. State two appropriate ways to help an obese child control weight.
9. Discuss recommended health promotion and maintenance for the school-aged child, including (a) scoliosis screening, (b) vision and hearing screening, (c) dental hygiene, (d) exercise, and (e) sleep.
10. Discuss the need for sex education in the school-aged group, and describe the role of the family, school, and others in this education.
11. Describe principles that a family caregiver can use to teach children about substance abuse.
12. Identify common inhalant products that children may use as deliriants.
13. Describe safety education appropriate for the school-aged group.
14. Identify factors that may influence the school-aged child in the healthcare facility.
15. Discuss the effects of the progression in the 6- to 10-year-old child's concept of biology, including the concepts of (a) birth, (b) death, (c) the human body, (d) health, and (e) illness.

Juan Gallegos, age 8, and his family have just moved to a new community. School for Juan will start in a few weeks. At his routine checkup, Juan weighs 51 lb and is 48 in. tall. As you read this chapter, think about Juan's size and expected growth over the next couple of years. Consider what anticipatory guidance you might give Juan's parents about this stage of development.

The first day of school marks a major milestone in a child's development, opening a new world of learning and growth. Between the ages of 6 and 10 years, dramatic changes occur in the child's thinking process, social skills, activities, attitudes, and use of language. The squirmy, boisterous 6-year-old child with a limited attention span bears little resemblance to the more reserved 10-year-old child who can become absorbed in a solitary craft activity for several hours.

Moving from the small circle of family into the school and community, children begin to see differences in their own lives and the lives of others. They constantly compare their families with other children's families and observe the way other children are disciplined, the foods they eat, the way they dress, and their homes. Every aspect of lifestyle is subject to comparison.

Most children reach school age with the necessary skills, abilities, and independence to function successfully in this new environment. They can feed and dress themselves, use the primary language of their culture to communicate their needs and feelings, and separate from their family caregivers for extended periods. They show increasing interest in group activities and in making things. Children of this age work at many activities that involve motor, cognitive, and social skills. Success in these activities provides the child with self-confidence and a feeling of competence. Erikson's developmental task for this age group is industry versus inferiority. Children who are unsuccessful in completing activities during this stage, whether from physical, social, or cognitive disadvantages, develop a feeling of inferiority.

The health of the school-aged child is no longer the exclusive concern of the family but of the community as well. Before admittance, most schools require that children have physical examinations and that immunizations meet state requirements. Generally, this is a healthy period in the child's life, although minor respiratory disorders and other communicable diseases can spread quickly within a classroom. Few major diseases have their onset during this period. Accidents still pose a serious hazard; therefore, safety measures are an important part of learning.

PHYSICAL DEVELOPMENT

The physical development of the school-aged child includes changes in weight and height, as well as changes in dentition and the eruption of permanent teeth. The school-aged child's skeletal growth and changes are evident during this period.

Weight and Height

Between the ages of 6 and 10 years, growth is slow and steady. Average annual weight gain is about 5 to 6 lb (2 to 3 kg). By age 7, the child weighs about seven times as much as at birth. Annual height increase is about 2.5 in. (6 cm). This period ends in the preadolescent growth spurt, in girls at about age 10 and in boys at about age 12.

Dentition

At about age 5 to 6, the child starts to lose the deciduous (baby) teeth, usually beginning with the lower incisors. At about the same time, the first permanent teeth, the 6-year molars, appear directly behind the deciduous molars (Fig. 26-1). These 6-year molars are of the utmost importance; they are the key or pivot

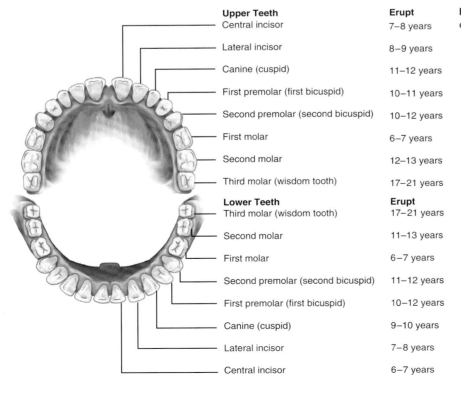

Upper Teeth	Erupt
Central incisor	7–8 years
Lateral incisor	8–9 years
Canine (cuspid)	11–12 years
First premolar (first bicuspid)	10–11 years
Second premolar (second bicuspid)	10–12 years
First molar	6–7 years
Second molar	12–13 years
Third molar (wisdom tooth)	17–21 years
Lower Teeth	**Erupt**
Third molar (wisdom tooth)	17–21 years
Second molar	11–13 years
First molar	6–7 years
Second premolar (second bicuspid)	11–12 years
First premolar (first bicuspid)	10–12 years
Canine (cuspid)	9–10 years
Lateral incisor	7–8 years
Central incisor	6–7 years

FIGURE 26-1 The usual sequence of eruption of permanent teeth.

PSYCHOSOCIAL DEVELOPMENT

A sense of duty and accomplishment occupies the years from ages 6 to 10. During this stage, the child enjoys engaging in meaningful projects and seeing them through to completion. The child applies the energies earlier put into play toward accomplishing tasks and often spends numerous sessions on one project (Fig. 26-3). With these attempts comes the refinement of motor, cognitive, and social skills and development of a positive sense of self. Some school-aged children, however, may not be ready for this stage because of environmental deprivation, a dysfunctional family, insecure attachment to parents, immaturity, or other reasons. Entering school at a disadvantage, these children may not be ready to be productive. Excessive or unrealistic goals set by a teacher or family caregiver who is insensitive to this child's needs will defeat such a child and possibly lead to the child's feeling inferior, rather than self-confident.

When environmental support is adequate, the child should complete several personality development tasks during these years. These tasks include developing coping mechanisms, a sense of right and wrong, a feeling of self-esteem, and an ability to care for oneself.

During the school-aged years, the child's cognitive skills develop; at about the age of 7 years, the child enters the concrete operational stage identified by Piaget. The skills of **conservation** (the ability to recognize that a change in shape does not necessarily mean a change in amount or mass) are significant in this stage. This begins with the conservation of numbers, when the child understands that the number of cookies does not change even though they may be rearranged, along with the conservation of mass, when the child can see that an amount of

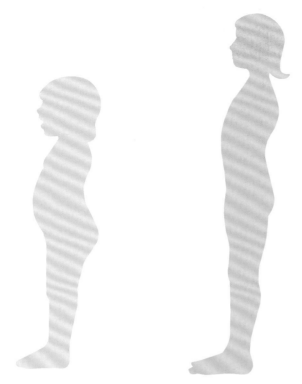

FIGURE 26-2 Left. Profile of a 6-year-old showing protuberant abdomen. **Right**. Profile of a 10-year-old showing flat abdomen and four curves of adultlike spine.

teeth that help to shape the jaw and affect the alignment of the permanent teeth. If these molars are allowed to decay so severely that they must be removed, the child will have dental problems later. (More information on care of the teeth is given later in this chapter.)

Skeletal Growth

The 6-year-old's silhouette is characterized by a flatter but still protruding abdomen and lordosis (sway-back). By the time the child has reached the age of 10 years, the spine is straighter, the abdomen flatter, and the body generally more slender and long-legged (Fig. 26-2). Bone growth occurs mostly in the long bones and is gradual during the school years. Cartilage is being replaced by bone at the **epiphyses** (growth centers at the end of long bones and at the wrists). Skeletal maturation is more rapid in girls than in boys, and in African American children, skeletal maturation is more rapid than in whites. Table 26-1 summarizes growth and development of the school-aged child.

TEST YOURSELF
✔ Why is the health of a child's first permanent molars important?
✔ What are the growth centers at the end of the long bones and wrist called?

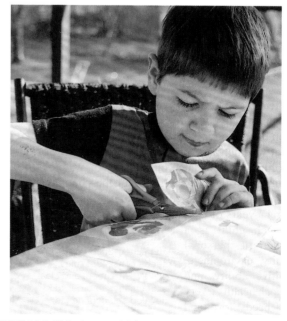

FIGURE 26-3 This 6-year-old focuses on cutting out shapes with safety scissors to complete a craft project.

TABLE 26-1 Developmental Milestones for the School-Aged Child

AGE (YEARS)	PHYSICAL	MOTOR	PERSONAL–SOCIAL	LANGUAGE	PERCEPTUAL	COGNITIVE DEVELOPMENT
6	Average height 45 in. (116 cm) Average weight 46 lb (21 kg) Loses first tooth (lower incisors) 6-year molars erupt Food jags Appetite increased	Ties shoes Can use scissors (see Fig. 26-3) Runs, jumps, climbs, skips Can ride bicycle Cannot sit for long periods Cuts, pastes, prints, draws with some detail	Increased need to socialize with same sex Egocentric—believes everyone thinks as they do Still in preoperational stage until age 7	Uses every form of sentence structure Vocabulary of 2,500 words Sentence length about five words	Knows right from left May reverse letters Can discriminate vertical, horizontal, and oblique Perceives pictures in parts or whole but not both	Recognizes simple words Conservation of number Defines objects by use Can group according to an attribute to form subclasses
7	Weight is seven times birth weight Gains 4.4–6.6 lb/year (2–3 kg) Grows 2–2.5 in./year (5–6 cm)	More cautious Swims Printing smaller than 6-year-old's Activity level lower than 6-year-old's	More cooperative Same-sex play group and friends Less egocentric	Can name day, month, season Produces all language sounds	b, p, d, q confusion resolved Can copy a diamond	Begins to use simple logic Can group in ascending order Grasps basic idea of addition and subtraction Conservation of substance Can tell time
8	Average height 49.5 in. (127 cm) Average weight 55 lb (25 kg)	Movements more graceful Writes in cursive Can throw and hit a baseball Has symmetric balance and can hop	Adheres to simple rules Hero worship begins Same-sex peer group	Gives precise definitions Articulation near adult level	Can catch a ball Visual acuity 20/20 Perceives pictures in parts and whole	Increasing memory span Conservation of length Can put thoughts in a chronologic sequence
9–10	Average height 51.5–53.5 in. (132–137 cm) Average weight 59.5–77 lb (27–35 kg)	Good coordination Can achieve the strength and speed needed for most sports	Enjoys team competition Moves from group to best friend Hero worship intensifies	Can use language to convey thoughts and look at others' points of view	Eye–hand coordination almost perfect	Classifies objects Understands explanations Conservation of area and weight Describes characteristics of objects Can group in descending order

cookie dough is the same whether in ball form or flattened for baking. This is followed by conservation of weight, in which the child recognizes that a pound is a pound, regardless of whether plastic or bricks are weighed. Conservation of volume (for instance, a half cup of water is the same amount regardless of the shape of the container) does not come until late in the concrete operational stage, at about 11 or 12 years of age.

Each child is a product of personal heredity, environment, cognitive ability, and physical health. Every child needs love and acceptance with understanding, support, and

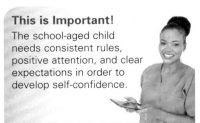

This is Important!
The school-aged child needs consistent rules, positive attention, and clear expectations in order to develop self-confidence.

concern when mistakes are made. Children thrive on praise and recognition and will work to earn them (see Tips for Reinforcing Family Teaching: Guiding Your School-Aged Child).

Development From Ages 6 to 7 Years

Children in the age group of 6 to 7 years are still characterized by magical thinking—believing in the tooth fairy, Santa Claus, the Easter Bunny, and others. Keen imaginations contribute to fears, especially at night, about remote, fanciful, or imaginary events. Trouble distinguishing fantasy from reality can contribute to lying to escape punishment or to boost self-confidence.

Children who have attended a day care center, preschool, kindergarten, or Head Start program usually make the transition into first grade with pleasure, excitement,

TIPS FOR REINFORCING FAMILY TEACHING

Guiding Your School-Aged Child

- Give your child consistent love and attention. Try to see the situation through your child's eyes. Do your best to avoid a hostile or angry reaction toward your child.
- Know where your child is at all times and who their friends are. Never leave your child home alone.
- Encourage your child to become involved in school and community activities. Become involved with your child's activities whenever possible. Encourage fair play and good sportsmanship.
- Show your children good examples by your behavior toward others.
- Never hit your children. Physical punishment shows them that it is all right to hit others and that they can solve problems in that way.
- Use positive nonphysical methods of discipline such as the following:
  - Time-out—1 minute per year of age is an appropriate amount of time.

- Grounding—do not permit them to play with friends or take part in a special activity.
- Take away a special privilege.
- Set these limits for brief periods only. Consistency is extremely important in setting these restrictions.
- Make a reasonable rule, let your child know the rule, and then stick with it. Be consistent. You can involve your children in helping to set rules.
- Treat your child with love and respect. Always try to find the positives and praise the child for those behaviors. Don't treat your child in a manner that you would not use with an adult friend.
- Let the child know what you expect of them. Children who have age-appropriate responsibilities learn self-discipline and self-control.
- When you have a problem with your child, try to sit down and solve it together. Help them figure out ways to solve problems nonviolently.

and little anxiety. Those without that experience may find it helpful to visit the school to experience separation from home and family caregivers and to try getting along with other children on a trial basis. Most 6-year-old children can sit still for short periods of time and understand taking turns. Those who have not matured sufficiently for this experience will find school unpleasant and may not do well.

Group activities are important to most 6-year-old children, even if the groups include only two or three children. They delight in learning and show an intense interest in every experience. Judgment about acceptable and

unacceptable behavior is not well developed and possibly results in name calling and the use of vulgar words.

Between the ages of 6 and 8 years, children begin to enjoy participating in real-life activities, such as helping with gardening, housework, and other chores. They love making things, such as drawings, paintings, and craft projects (Fig. 26-4).

Development From Ages 7 to 10 Years

Between the seventh and eighth birthdays, children begin to shake off their acceptance of parental standards as the ultimate authority and become more impressed by the behavior of their peers. Interest in group play increases, and acceptance by the group is tremendously important. These groups quickly become all-boy or all-girl groups and are often project-oriented, such as scout troops or athletic teams. Private clubs with homemade clubhouses, secret codes, and languages are popular. Individual friendships also form, and best friends are intensely loyal, if only for short periods. Table games, arts and crafts requiring skill and dexterity, computer games, school science projects, and science fairs are popular, as are more active pursuits. This period includes the beginning of many neighborhood team sports, including little league, softball, football, and soccer (Fig. 26-5). Both boys and girls are actively involved in many of these sports.

Even though family caregivers are no longer considered the ultimate authority, their standards have become part of the child's personality and conscience. Although the child may cheat, lie, or steal on occasion, they suffer considerable guilt if they learn that these are unacceptable behaviors.

Important changes occur in a child's thinking processes at about age 7, when there is movement from preoperational, egocentric thinking to concrete, operational, decentered thought. For the first time, children can see the world from someone else's point of view. **Decentration** means being

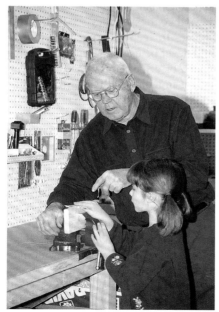

FIGURE 26-4 A 6-year-old works with her grandfather on a woodworking project.

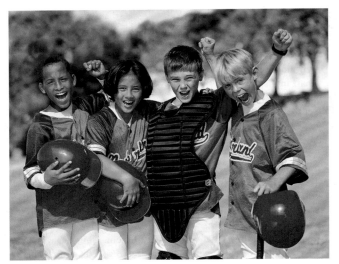

FIGURE 26-5 These 8-year-olds enjoy being part of a sports team.

able to see several aspects of a problem at the same time and to understand the relation of various parts to the whole situation. Cause-and-effect relations become clear; consequently, magical thinking begins to disappear.

During the seventh or eighth year, children have an increased understanding of the conservation of continuous quantity. Understanding conservation depends on **reversibility**, the ability to think in either direction. Seven-year-old children can add and subtract, count forward and backward, and see how it is possible to put something back the way it was. A 7- or 8-year-old can understand that illness is probably only temporary, whereas a 6-year-old may think it is permanent.

 Cultural Snapshot

In some cultures, children are pressured to achieve high scores in school, as well as on college entrance exams, to bring value and pride to the family and culture. These children sometimes are pushed to study rather than to play and have normal relationships with their peers.

Another important change in thinking during this period is **classification**, the ability to group objects into a **hierarchical arrangement** (grouping by some common system). Children in this age group love to collect sports cards, insects, rocks, stamps, coins, or anything else that strikes their fancy. These collections may be only a short-term interest, but some can develop into lifetime hobbies.

TEST YOURSELF

✔ How is the developmental task of industry attained in the school-aged child?

✔ What sex are most of the school-aged child's friends and play groups?

TABLE 26-2 Daily Nutritional Needs of the 6- to 10-Year-Old

For a 1,600–2,200-calorie diet, the school-aged child needs the amounts below from each food group. School-aged children should be moderately active for 60 minutes every day

FRUITS	VEGETABLES	GRAINS	PROTEIN FOODS	DAIRY
1.5–2 cups	2–3 cups	5–7 oz	5–6 oz	2.5–3 cups

NUTRITION

As coordination improves, the child becomes increasingly active and requires more food to supply necessary energy. The nutritional needs of the school-aged child should be met by choosing foods from all the food groups with the appropriate number of servings from each group in the child's daily diet (Table 26-2). (See also ChooseMyPlate in Fig. 22-3 in Chapter 22.) Increased appetite and a tendency to go on food jags (the desire for only one kind of food for a while) are typical of the 6-year-old child. This stage soon passes and is unimportant if the child generally gets the necessary nutrients. As the child's tastes develop, once-disliked foods may become favorites unless earlier battles have been waged over the food. Children are more likely to learn to eat most foods if everyone else accepts them in a matter-of-fact way.

Offering Choices Can Make a Difference!

Allowing the child to express food dislikes and permitting refusal of a disliked food item is usually the best way to handle the school-aged child.

Children learn by the examples that family caregivers and others set for them. They will more readily accept the importance of manners, calm voices, appropriate table conversation, and courtesy if they see them carried out consistently at home. To keep mealtime a positive and pleasant time, it should never be used for nagging, finding fault, correcting manners, or discussing a poor report card. Hygiene should be taught in a cheerful but firm manner, even if the child must leave the table more than once to wash their hands adequately.

Most children prefer simple, plain foods and are good judges of their own needs if they are not coaxed, nagged, bribed, rewarded, or influenced by television commercials. Disease or strong emotions may cause loss of appetite. Forcing the child to eat is not helpful and can have harmful effects.

Family caregivers must carefully supervise children's snacking habits to be sure that snacks are nutritious and not too frequent. Children should avoid junk food; continual nibbling can cause lack of interest at mealtime. Caregivers should encourage children to eat good breakfasts to provide the energy and nutrients needed to perform well in school. Children need clearly planned schedules that allow time for a good breakfast and toothbrushing before leaving for school.

Obesity can be a concern during this age. Some children may have a genetic tendency to obesity; environment and a sedentary lifestyle also play a part. In many families, caregivers urge children to "clean their plates." In addition, many families eat fast foods several times a week; fast foods tend to have high fat and calorie content and contribute to obesity. Other children, especially in the later elementary grades, can be unkind to overweight children by teasing them, not choosing them in games, or avoiding them as friends. The child who becomes sensitive to being overweight is often miserable.

Encouraging physical activity and limiting dietary fat intake to no more than 35% of total calories help control the child's weight. Popular fad diets must be avoided because they do not supply adequate nutrients for the growing child. Family caregivers must avoid nagging and creating feelings of inferiority or guilt because the child may simply rebel. The child who is pressured too much to lose weight may sneak food, setting up patterns that will be harmful later in life. In addition, anorexia nervosa (see Chapter 42) has become a problem for some children in the older school-aged group.

Health teaching at school should reinforce the importance of a proper diet. Family and cultural food patterns are strong, however, and tend to persist despite nutrition education. Some families are making positive efforts to reduce fat and cholesterol when preparing meals. Most schools have subsidized lunch programs for eligible children, and some have breakfast programs. These provide well-balanced meals, but often children eat only part of what they are offered. Some families post the school lunch menu on the refrigerator or kitchen bulletin board so that children can decide whether to eat the school's lunch or pack their own on any particular day. This way the child can avoid lunches they dislike or simply refuse to eat. School-aged children are old enough to be at least partially responsible for preparing their own lunches.

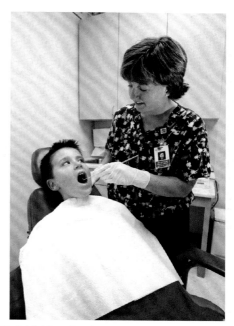

FIGURE 26-6 Visiting the dentist twice a year is important for school-aged children.

Routine Checkups

The school-aged child should have a physical examination by a health care provider every year. Additional visits are commonly made throughout the year for minor illness. The school-aged child should visit the dentist at least twice a year for a cleaning and application of fluoride (Fig. 26-6).

Most states have immunization requirements that must be met when the child enters school. A booster of tetanus–diphtheria–pertussis (Tdap) vaccine is recommended every 10 years throughout life. The human papillomavirus (HPV) vaccine is now recommended for adolescent males and females, and the first dose may be given as early as 9 years of age. During a physical examination at about the age of 10 to 11 years, the child undergoes initial examination for signs of **scoliosis** (lateral curvature of the spine). The child is monitored on an ongoing basis and reexamined during adolescence (Fig. 26-7; see Chapter 40). Vision and hearing screening should be performed before entrance to school and on a periodic basis (annual or biannual) thereafter. The school nurse often conducts these examinations.

Elementary school children are commonly healthy, with only minor illnesses that are usually respiratory or gastrointestinal in nature. The leading cause of death in this age group continues to be accidents.

Family Teaching

The school-aged child generally incorporates healthy habits into their daily routine but still needs reinforcement by family caregivers. Education for the care of the teeth with particular attention to the 6-year molars is important. Proper dental hygiene includes a routine inspection and conscientious brushing after meals. A well-balanced diet with plenty of calcium and phosphorus and minimal sugar is important

---

TEST YOURSELF

✔ List the factors that may contribute to obesity in the school-aged child.

✔ What can be suggested as ways to control a school-aged child's weight?

HEALTH PROMOTION AND MAINTENANCE

The school years are generally healthy years for most children. However, routine healthcare and health education, including health habits, safety, sex education, and substance abuse education, are very important aspects of well-planned health promotion and maintenance programs for school-aged children.

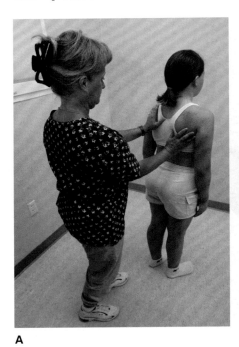
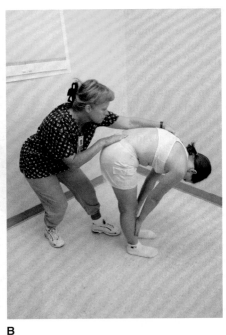

A

B

FIGURE 26-7 Scoliosis checkup. **A.** Viewing from the back, the examiner checks the symmetry of the girl's shoulders. She will also look for a prominent shoulder blade, an unequal distance between the girl's arms and waist, a higher or more prominent hip, and curvature of the spinal column. **B.** With the child bending over and touching her toes, the examiner checks for a curvature of the spinal column. She will also look for a rib hump.

to healthy teeth. Foods containing sugar should be eaten only at mealtimes and should be followed immediately by proper brushing (Fig. 26-8).

Exercise and sufficient rest are also important during this period. Family caregivers need to help school-aged children balance their rest needs and their extracurricular activities. Extracurricular activities help the child remain fit, bond with peers, and establish positive, lifelong attitudes toward exercise. The school-aged child needs

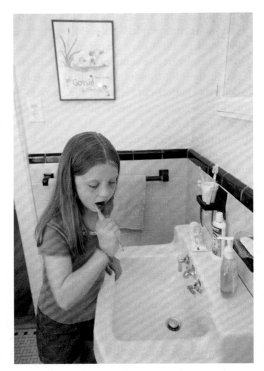

FIGURE 26-8 The school-aged child needs encouragement to brush teeth after meals and at bedtime as part of a good dental hygiene program.

10 to 12 hours of sleep per night. The 6-year-old needs 12 hours of sleep and should be provided with quiet time after school to recharge after a busy day in the classroom. Highlight these important aspects of daily healthcare to both the family caregivers and child.

Health Education

Health teaching in the home and at school is essential. Family caregivers have a responsibility to teach the child about basic hygiene, sexual functioning, substance abuse, and accident prevention. Schools must include these topics in the curriculum because many families are not informed well enough to cover them adequately. Some schools offer health classes taught by a health educator at each grade level. In other schools, health and sex education are integrated into the curriculum and taught by each classroom teacher. Nurses should become active in their communities to ensure that these kinds of programs are available to children.

Sex Education

Children learn about femininity and masculinity from the time they are born. Behaviors, attitudes, and actions of the men and women in the child's life, especially their actions toward the child and toward each other, form impressions in the child that last a lifetime. The proper time and place for formal sex education have been very controversial. Part of the problem seems to be that many people automatically think that sex education means just adult sexuality and reproduction. However, sex education includes helping children develop positive attitudes toward their own bodies, their own sex, and their own sexual role to achieve optimum satisfaction in being a boy or a girl.

In some schools, sex education is limited to one class, usually in the fifth grade, in which children watch films about menstruation and their developing bodies; schools often offer separate classes for boys and girls. Some health educators strongly recommend that sex education begin in kindergarten and develop gradually over the successive grades. Learning about reproduction of plants and animals, about birth and nurturing in other animals, and about the roles of men and women in family units can lead to the natural introduction of human reproduction, male and female roles, families, and nurturing. If all children grew up in secure, loving, ideal families, much of this could be learned at home. However, many children do not have this type of home, so they need healthy, positive information to help them develop healthy attitudes about their own sexuality. Feelings of self-worth woven into these lessons help children feel good about themselves and who they are.

Family caregivers who feel uncomfortable discussing sex with their children may find it helpful to use books or pamphlets available for various age groups. Generally, women family caregivers find it easier to discuss sex with a girl, and men family caregivers feel more comfortable with a boy. This can pose special problems for the single caregiver with a child of the opposite sex. Again, printed materials may be helpful. As a nurse, you may be called on to help a family caregiver provide information, and it is important to be comfortable with your own sexuality to handle these discussions well.

At a young age, children are exposed to a large amount of sexually provocative information through the media. Children who do not get accurate information at home or at school will learn what they want to know from their peers; this information is often inaccurate, which makes sex education even more urgent. In addition, the U.S. Centers for Disease Control and Prevention currently recommends that elementary school children be taught about human immunodeficiency virus and acquired immunodeficiency syndrome and how they are spread. Many school districts are working hard to integrate this information into the health curriculum at all grade levels in a sensitive, age-appropriate manner.

Substance Abuse Education

In addition to nutrition, health practices, safety, and sex education, school-aged children also need substance abuse education. Programs that teach children to "just say no" are one way that children can learn that they are in control of the choices they make regarding substance abuse.

Children as young as elementary school age may try cigarette smoking, chewing tobacco, using electronic cigarettes, alcohol, and other substances. Teaching children the unhealthy aspects of tobacco and alcohol use and drug abuse should begin in elementary school as a good foundation for more advanced information in adolescence.

Children may experiment with **inhalants** (substances whose volatile vapors can be abused) because they are readily available and may seem no more threatening than an innocent prank. Inhalants classified as **deliriants** contain chemicals that give off fumes that can produce symptoms of confusion, disorientation, excitement, and hallucinations. Many inhalants are commonly found in the home (Box 26-1). The fumes are mind-altering when inhaled. The child initially may experience a temporary high, giddiness, nausea,

BOX 26-1	Common Products Inhaled as Deliriants
Model glue	Hair spray
Rubber cement	Nail polish remover
Cleaning fluids	Shoe polish
Kerosene vapors	Computer keyboard cleaner
Gasoline vapors	Propellant in whipped
Butane lighter fluid	cream spray cans
Paint thinner	Aerosol spray paint
Varnish	Upholstery/fabric protec-
Shellac	tion spray cans

coughing, nosebleed, fatigue, lack of coordination, or loss of appetite. Overdose can cause loss of consciousness and possible death from suffocation by replacing oxygen in the lungs or depressing the central nervous system, thereby causing respiratory arrest. Permanent damage to the lungs, the nervous system, or the liver can result. Children who experiment with inhalants may proceed to abuse other drugs in an attempt to get similar effects. Addiction occurs in younger children more rapidly than in adults.

 A Personal Glimpse

When we had the program on drugs at school, I learned some things. Like when you take drugs, you can get sick or even die. In one part of the lesson, we watched a video where a kid took drugs and almost died, and during the other part, the school nurse showed us samples of drugs. Even though I learned about drugs from the program, I think that all children should be taught this subject by their parents.

Stephen, age 10 years

Learning Opportunity: *What do you think is the most effective way to teach school-aged children about the dangers of substance abuse? List some ways you can help reduce substance abuse among school-aged children.*

Family caregivers must work to develop strong, loving relationships with the children in the family, teach the children the family's values and the difference between right and wrong, set and enforce rules for acceptable behavior of family members, learn facts about drugs and alcohol, and actively listen to the children (see Tips for Reinforcing Family Teaching: Guidelines to Prevent Substance Abuse). An excellent reference for family caregivers is *Tips for Parents on Keeping Children Drug Free*, which is published by the U.S. Department of Education and is available for free (1-877-433-7827 or www2.ed.gov/parents/academic/involve/drugfree/index.html).

Accident Prevention

As stated, accidents continue to be a leading cause of death during this period. Even though school-aged children do

TIPS FOR REINFORCING FAMILY TEACHING

Guidelines to Prevent Substance Abuse

- Openly communicate values by talking about the importance of honesty, responsibility, and self-reliance. Encourage decision making. Help children see how each decision builds on previous decisions.
- Provide a good role model for the child to copy. Children tend to copy family caregivers habits of smoking and drinking alcohol and attitudes about drug use, whether they are over-the-counter, prescription, or illicit drugs.
- Avoid conflicts between what you say and what you do. For example, don't ask the child to lie that you are not home when you are or encourage the child to lie about age when trying to get a lower admission price at amusement centers.

- Talk about values during family times. Give the child what-if examples, and discuss the best responses when faced with a difficult situation. For example, "What would you do if you found money that someone dropped?"
- Set strong rules about using alcohol and other drugs. Make specific rules with specific punishments. Discuss these rules and the reasons for them.
- Be consistent in applying the rules that you set.
- Be reasonable; don't make wild threats. Respond calmly and carry out the expected punishment.
- Get the facts about alcohol and other drugs, and provide children with current, correct information. This helps you in discussions with children and also helps you recognize symptoms if a child has been using them.

TEST YOURSELF

- ✔ How is a child screened for scoliosis? At what age is a child usually initially examined for signs of scoliosis?
- ✔ List substances that school-aged children might abuse.

---

not require constant supervision, they must learn certain safety rules and practice them until they are routine (Fig. 26-9). They should understand the function of traffic lights. Family members should obey traffic lights; example is the best teacher for any child. Every child should know their full name, the caregivers' names, and their own home address and telephone number. Children should be taught the appropriate way to call for emergency help in their community (911 in a community that has such a system). Many communities have safe-home programs that designate homes where children can go if they have a problem on the way home from school. These homes are clearly marked in a way that children are taught to recognize. In many communities, local police officers or firefighters come into the classroom to help teach safety. Children benefit from meeting police officers and understanding that the officer's duty is to help children, not punish them. Safety rules should be stressed at home and at school. Tips for Reinforcing Family Teaching: Safety Topics for Elementary School-Aged Children summarizes important safety considerations for school-aged children.

Since **Juan Gallegos** now lives in a new community and will be going to a new school, what information would you encourage Juan's parents to talk to Juan about related to safety in the neighborhood and at school?

THE SCHOOL-AGED CHILD IN THE HEALTHCARE FACILITY

Increased understanding of their bodies, continuing curiosity about how things work, and development of concrete thinking all contribute to helping school-aged children understand and accept a healthcare experience better than younger children do. They can communicate better with health care providers, understand cause and effect, and tolerate longer separations from their family.

As a nurse caring for school-aged children, you should understand how concepts about birth, death, the body, health, and illness change between the ages of 6 and 10 years (Table 26-3). Explain all procedures to children and their families; showing the equipment and materials to be used (or pictures of them) and outlining realistic expectations of procedures

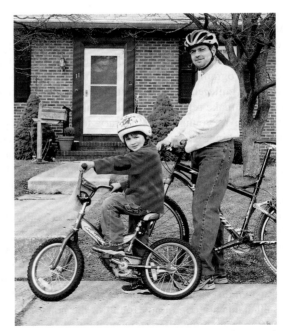

FIGURE 26-9 Helmets are an important aspect of bike safety. Family caregivers can be role models for their children by also wearing bike helmets.

TABLE 26-3 Children's Concept of Biology

CONCEPT	6–8 YEARS	8–10 YEARS	IMPLICATIONS FOR NURSING
Birth	Gradually see babies as the result of three factors: social and sexual intercourse and biogenetic fusion Tend to see baby as emerging from female only; many still see baby as manufactured by outside force—created whole Boys less knowledgeable about baby formation than girls	Begin to put three components together; recognize that sperm and egg come together but may not be sure why Fewer discrepancies in knowledge based on sex differences	Cultural and educational factors play a part in development of where babies come from Nurse should consider children's ideas about birth and if they can understand where babies come from and how before reinforcing teaching Explanations about roles of both parents can begin, but the idea of sperm and egg union may not be understood until 8 or 9 years of age
Death	May be viewed as reversible May think that natural things such as plants, rocks, thunder can influence human events; death viewed as a result of an outside force Experiences with death facilitate concept development	Considered irreversible Ideas about what happens after death unclear; related to concreteness of thinking and social or religious upbringing	Change from vague view of death as reversible and caused by external forces to awareness of irreversibility and bodily causes Fears about death more common at 8; adults should be alert to this Explanations about death, the fact that their thoughts will not cause a death, and they will not die (if illness is not fatal) are needed
Human body	Know body holds everything inside Use outside world to explain Aware of major organs Interested in visible functions of body	Can understand physiology; use general principles to explain body functions; interested in invisible functions of body	Cultural factors may play a part in ability and willingness to discuss bodily functions Educational programs can be very effective because of natural interest Evaluate knowledge of body by using diagrams before reinforcing teaching
Health	See health as doing desired activities List concrete practices as components of health Many do not see sickness as related to health; may not consider cause and effect	See health as doing desired activities Understand cause and effect Believe it is possible to be part healthy and part not at the same time; can reverse from health to sickness and back to health	Need assistance in seeing cause and effect Capitalize on positiveness of concept; health lets you do what you really want to do Young children who are sick may feel they will never get well again
Illness	Sick children may see illness as punishment; evidence suggests that healthy children do not see illness as punishment Highly anxious children more likely to view illness as disruptive Sickness is a diffuse state; rely on others to tell them when they are ill	Same as 6–8 years of age; can identify illness states, report bodily discomfort, recognize that illness is caused by specific factors	Social factors play a part in illness concept Recognize that some see illness as punishment Encourage self-care and self-help behavior, especially in older children

and treatments are helpful. It is important to answer children's questions, including those about pain, truthfully. Children of this age have anxieties about looking different from other children. An opportunity to verbalize these anxieties will help a child deal with them. School-aged children need privacy more than younger children do and may not want to have physical contact with adults; this wish should be respected. Boys may be uncomfortable having a female nurse bathe them, and girls may feel uncomfortable with a male nurse. These attitudes should be recognized and handled in a way that ensures as much privacy as possible.

Family caregivers may feel guilty about the child's need for hospitalization and, as a result, may overindulge the child. The child may regress in response to this, but this regression should not be encouraged. Sometimes the family needs as much reassurance as the child does.

Discipline and rules have a place on a pediatric unit. Inform families and children about the rules as part of the admission routine. Opportunities for interaction with peers,

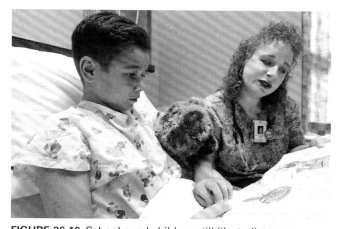

FIGURE 26-10 School-aged children still like to listen to stories, in either the hospital or the home setting.

learning situations, and doing crafts and projects can help make the child's experience more tolerable (Fig. 26-10).

TIPS FOR REINFORCING FAMILY TEACHING

Safety Topics for Elementary School-Aged Children

- Traffic signals and safe pedestrian practices
- Safety belt use for car passengers
- Bicycle safety
  - Wear a helmet.
  - Use hand signals.
  - Ride with traffic.
  - Be sure others see you.
- Skateboard and skating safety
  - Wear a helmet.
  - Wear elbow and knee pads.

- Skate only in safe skating areas.
- Swimming safety
  - Learn to swim.
  - Never swim alone.
  - Always know the water depth.
  - Do not dive head first.
  - No running or horseplay at a pool.
- Danger of projectile toys
- Danger of all-terrain vehicles
- Use of life jacket when boating

- Stranger safety
  - Who is a stranger?
  - Never accept a ride from someone you do not know.
  - If offered a ride, check the vehicle license number and try to remember it.
  - Never accept food or gifts from someone you do not know.
- Good touch and bad touch

Juan Gallegos, from the beginning of the chapter, has now completed his first month at his new school. What percentiles does Juan fit into on the growth charts for his height and weight (see Appendix E). What areas of anticipatory guidance will be important for you to discuss with Juan's parents? What activities might be helpful for Juan to participate in to promote development at this age?

KEY POINTS

- According to Erikson, the developmental task of school-aged children is industry versus inferiority. Success in activities using motor, cognitive, and social skills is necessary for the child to develop a sense of competency.
- Physical growth is slow and steady during the school-aged years. Average annual weight gain is about 5 to 6 lb (2 to 3 kg). The child begins to lose deciduous teeth and the first permanent teeth appear at about 6 years of age. Bone growth occurs mostly in the long bones and is gradual. By the time the child has reached the age of 10 years, the spine is straighter, the abdomen flatter, and the body generally more slender and long-legged.
- During this stage, the child is interested in engaging in meaningful projects and seeing them through to completion. Excessive or unrealistic goals defeat the child and possibly lead to feeling inferior, rather than self-confident. With positive support, the child develops a sense of right and wrong, a feeling of self-esteem, and an ability to care for oneself. Even though family is still a major influence, the school-aged child has a need to be accepted by groups of peers, often spends time in activities with children of the same sex, and enjoys team sports.
- The school-aged child develops the cognitive skills to understand *conservation* of numbers, mass, weight, and volume. The child can understand *decentration*, meaning they can see several aspects of a problem at the same time and understand the relation of various parts to the whole situation. Cause-and-effect relations become clear. They can think in either direction, so they learn to count forward and backward as well as add and subtract (the process of *reversibility*). Thinking also includes *classification*, the ability to group objects into a hierarchical arrangement (grouping by some common system).
- By allowing expression of food likes and dislikes and by setting good examples, family caregivers can help the

school-aged child develop good nutrition habits to be followed at home and school for meals as well as snacks.
- Obesity in the school-aged child can be related to genetic, environmental, or sedentary lifestyle factors. Appropriate physical activity, limiting fat intake, and positive family caregiver support can be helpful in decreasing obesity.
- At about the age of 10 to 11 years, the child is initially examined for signs of scoliosis (lateral curvature of the spine). Vision and hearing screening should be performed before entrance to school and on a periodic basis. Routine inspection, a well-balanced diet with adequate calcium and phosphorus, brushing after meals, and eating foods containing sugar only at mealtimes contribute to good dental health. Exercise and sufficient rest are important. The school-aged child needs 10 to 12 hours of sleep each night.
- Sex education regarding sexuality, reproduction, and positive attitudes toward sexuality are important roles that families and schools often share.
- Substance abuse is an ever-increasing concern in school-aged children, especially the use of products that can be inhaled and used as deliriants. Family caregivers must make every effort to develop strong, loving relationships; teach family values; set and enforce rules for acceptable behavior; learn facts about drugs and alcohol; listen to what the child is saying; and teach the child about the unhealthy aspects of tobacco, alcohol, and other substances. Also, family caregivers need to be alert to children's use of inhalants, deliriants, alcohol, or tobacco and to talk with the school-aged child about the abuse of substances.
- Children may use common inhalant products found in the home as deliriants.
- Safety issues for the school-aged child include reinforcing teaching regarding traffic safety, especially in bicycle riding and skateboarding, seat belt use, and stranger safety.
- The changes in a school-aged child's understanding of birth, death, the human body, health, and illness influence the child's view of their own healthcare. Understanding these concepts is necessary to plan nursing care for the school-aged child. The child in the healthcare facility needs explanations and privacy.

INTERNET RESOURCES

Substance Abuse
http://www.drugabuse.gov/

Family Support Groups
www.keepkidshealthy.com

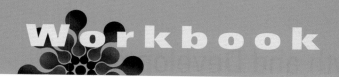

NCLEX-STYLE REVIEW QUESTIONS

1. The nurse is assisting with a well-child visit for a 7-year-old. This child's records show that at birth, this child weighed 7 lb 8 oz. At the age of 6 years, this child was 45 in. tall. If this child is following a normal pattern of growth and development, which of the following would the nurse expect to find in this visit?
   a. The child weighs 54 lb.
   b. The child measures 50 in. height.
   c. The child has four molars in the lower jaw.
   d. The child has an apical pulse of 60 beats a minute.

2. In working with a group of school-aged children, which of the following activities would this aged child most likely be doing?
   a. Pretending to be television characters
   b. Playing a game with large balls
   c. Participating in a group activity
   d. Telling stories about themselves

3. During the school-aged years, according to Erikson, the child is in the stage of growth and development known as industry versus inferiority. If the family caregivers of a group of children made the following statements, which statement reflects that the child is developing industry?
   a. "When my child falls down, he tries so hard to just get up and not cry."
   b. "My child was so excited when she finished her science project all by herself."
   c. "Every night my child follows the same routine at bedtime."
   d. "My child loves to make up stories about tall, big buildings."

4. In reinforcing teaching to caregivers of school-aged children, the nurse would reinforce that which of the following would be most important for this age group?
   a. Encouragement to brush teeth
   b. Basic sex education
   c. Screening for scoliosis
   d. Wearing a bicycle helmet

5. In working with the school-aged child and their family, reinforcing teaching is an important role of the nurse. Which of the following are important to reinforce with the child and family? Select all that apply.
   a. Food jags are common at this age.
   b. Eating foods that are disliked is important.
   c. Obesity can be a concern at this age.
   d. Scoliosis screening should be done.
   e. Foods containing sugar can be eaten as snacks.
   f. Sex education is best taught in the home.

STUDY ACTIVITIES

1. List and compare the motor skills, social skills, and cognitive development in each of the following ages.

	6 Years	7 Years	8 Years	9–10 Years
Motor skills				
Social skills				
Cognitive development				

2. Make a poster or visual aid to use in an elementary school classroom related to safety concerns. Perhaps you can make this a class project and donate the posters to your pediatric unit or nearby school.

3. Survey your home and make a list of all the products available that a child could use as an inhalant for a deliriant effect.

4. Research the internet for "tips on bicycle safety."
   a. Make a list of things you would suggest as a bike safety checklist.
   b. Describe how a bicycle helmet works.
   c. After reading this information, how would you answer the parent of a school-aged child who asks, "Does my child really need a bicycle helmet?"

CRITICAL THINKING: WHAT WOULD YOU DO?

1. Delsey, the mother of 6-year-old Jasmine, is upset because Jasmine is a picky eater and often does not want to eat what Delsey has prepared.
   a. What eating patterns are seen in most school-aged children?
   b. What information would you share with Delsey about the normal nutrition requirements for Jasmine?
   c. What suggestions would you give Delsey regarding what she might offer Jasmine at meal and snack times?
   d. How could Delsey involve Jasmine in developing good nutritional patterns?

2. Steve, the primary family caregiver of 8-year-old Rebekah, feels that he should offer her sex education and asks for your advice.
   a. What topics need to be included in sex education for the school-aged child?
   b. How would you suggest Steve go about giving his daughter the sex education she needs?
   c. What resources would you offer to Steve to help him in teaching his daughter?
   d. Why is it important for the family to be part of the sex education for a child?

3. You have been asked to present a program for school-aged children regarding substance abuse, including alcohol and tobacco use.
   a. What areas would you include in your presentation?
   b. What would be the most effective way to present this material to school-aged children?
   c. What questions and concerns would you anticipate from these children?

27

Growth and Development of the Adolescent: 11 to 18 Years

Key Terms

early adolescence
heterosexual
homosexual
malocclusion
menarche
nocturnal emissions
orthodontia
puberty
transgender

Learning Objectives

At the conclusion of this chapter, you will:

1. State the ages of the preadolescent and the adolescent.
2. Discuss the physical changes that occur in early or preadolescence.
3. List the secondary sexual characteristics that appear in adolescent boys and in adolescent girls.
4. Describe the psychosocial development of the adolescent.
5. Discuss (a) the major cognitive task of the adolescent according to Piaget and (b) the major developmental task according to Erikson.
6. Explain some problems that adolescents face when making career choices today.
7. Discuss the adolescent's need to conform to peers.
8. Discuss the influence of peer pressure on psychosocial development.
9. Explain the role of intimacy in adolescence in preparation for long-term relationships.
10. Discuss adolescent body image and associated problems.
11. Describe adolescent nutritional concerns, including (a) daily minimum needs and deficiencies, (b) habits and fads, (c) cultural influences, and (d) vegetarian diets.
12. Explain recommended health maintenance and promotion as well as health concerns for the adolescent.
13. Discuss the aspects of sexual maturity that affect the need for health education for the adolescent.
14. Discuss the issues that the adolescent faces in making decisions related to sexual responsibility, substance use, mental health, and accident prevention.
15. State factors that may influence the adolescent's hospital experience.

Madison Davis is having her 16th birthday soon. She has told her parents the only thing she wants for her birthday is to get a body piercing. She and her parents have been arguing about Madison getting a piercing, but after much discussion they have agreed to let her get one. As you read this chapter, think about the reasons Madison might want to get a body piercing.

A
dolescence comes from the Latin word meaning "to come to maturity," a fitting description of this stage of life. The adolescent is maturing physically and emotionally, growing from childhood toward adulthood, and seeking to understand what it means to be grown up.

Early adolescence (preadolescence, pubescence) begins with a dramatic growth spurt that signals the advent of **puberty** (reproductive

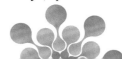

maturity). It is usually between ages 10 and 12 years. This early period ends, and true adolescence begins with the onset of menstruation in girls and the production of sperm in boys. Adolescence usually spans ages 13 to 18 years.

Adolescents are fascinated and sometimes fearful and confused by the changes occurring in their bodies and their thinking processes. Body image is critical. Health problems that threaten body image, such as acne, obesity, dental or vision problems, and trauma, can seriously interfere with development.

Adolescents begin to look grown up, but they do not have the judgment or independence to participate in society as an adult. These young people are strongly influenced by their peer groups and often resent parental authority. Roller coaster emotions characterize this age group, as does intense interest in romantic relationships.

The uncertainty and turmoil of adolescence often create conflict between family caregivers and children. If these conflicts are resolved, normal development can continue. Unresolved conflicts can foster delays in development and prevent the young person from maturing into a fully functioning adult.

Erikson describes the developmental task of adolescence as "identity versus role confusion." Adolescents confront marked physical and emotional changes and the knowledge that soon they will be responsible for their own lives. They must develop their own personal identities—a sense of being independent people with unique ideals and goals (Fig. 27-1). If parents, caregivers, and other adults refuse to grant that independence, adolescents may break rules just to prove that they can. Stress, anxiety, and mood swings are typical of this phase and add to the feelings of role confusion.

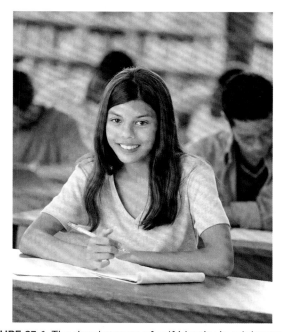

FIGURE 27-1 The development of self-identity in adolescence involves developing interests and goals and becoming emotionally independent.

PREADOLESCENT DEVELOPMENT

The rate of growth varies greatly in boys and girls between ages 10 and 12. This variability in growth and maturation can be a concern to the child who develops rapidly or the one who develops more slowly than their peers. Children of this age do not want to be different from their friends. The developmental characteristics of the preadolescent child in the late school-aged stage overlap with those of early adolescence; nevertheless, there are unique characteristics to set this stage apart (Table 27-1).

Physical Development

Preadolescence begins in girls between ages 9 and 11 years and is marked by a growth spurt that lasts for about 18 months. Girls grow about 3 inches each year until **menarche** (the beginning of menstruation), after which growth slows considerably. Early in adolescence, girls' bodies begin to develop adultlike contours, the pelvis broadens, and axillary and pubic hair begins to appear along with many changes in hormone levels. The variation between girls is great and is often a cause for much concern by the early or late *bloomer*. Girls who begin to develop physically as early as 9 years of age are often embarrassed by these physical changes. In girls, the onset of menarche marks the end of the preadolescent period.

 Concept Mastery Alert

Girls grow about 3 inches each year until menarche, after which growth slows.

Boys enter preadolescence a little later, usually between 11 and 13 years of age, and grow generally at a slower, steadier rate than do girls. During this time, the scrotum and testes begin to enlarge, the skin of the scrotum begins to change in coloring and texture, and sparse hair begins to show at the base of the penis. Boys who start their growth spurts later are often concerned about being shorter than their peers. In boys, the appearance of **nocturnal emissions** (or *wet dreams*) is often used as the indication that the preadolescent period has ended.

Preparation for Adolescence

Preadolescents need information about their changing bodies and feelings. Sex education that includes information about the hormonal changes that are occurring or will be occurring is necessary to help them through this developmental stage.

Girls need information that will help them handle their early menstrual periods with minimal apprehension. Most girls have irregular periods for the first year or so; they need to know that this is not a cause for worry. They have many questions about protection during the menstrual period and the advisability of using sanitary pads or tampons. They may fear that "everybody will know" when they have their first period and must be allowed to express this fear and be reassured.

TABLE 27-1 Growth and Development of the Preadolescent: 10 to 13 Years

PHYSICAL	MOTOR	PERSONAL–SOCIAL	LANGUAGE	PERCEPTUAL	COGNITIVE DEVELOPMENT
Average height 56.75–59 inches (144–150 cm) Average weight 77–88 lb (35–40 kg) Pubescence may begin Girls may surpass boys in height Remaining permanent teeth erupt	Refines gross and fine motor skills May have difficulty with some fine motor coordination due to the growth of large muscles before that of small muscle; hands and feet are first structures to increase in size; actions may appear uncoordinated during early preadolescence Can do crafts Uses tools increasingly well	Attends school primarily for peer association Peer relationships are of greatest importance Intolerant of violation of group norms Can follow rules of group and adapt to another point of view Can use stored knowledge to make independent judgments	Fluent in spoken language Vocabulary 50,000 words for reading; oral vocabulary of 7,200 words Uses slang words and terms, vulgarities, jeers, jokes, and sayings	Can catch or intercept ball thrown from a distance Possible growth spurts may cause myopia	Begins abstract thinking Conservation of volume Understands relations among time, speed, and distance Ability to sympathize, love, and reason are all evolving Right and wrong become logically clear

Boys also need information about their bodies. Erections and nocturnal emissions are topics they need to discuss, as are the development of other secondary sex characteristics of men.

Both boys and girls need information about changes in the opposite sex, including discussions that address their questions. This kind of information helps them increase their understanding of human sexuality. School programs may provide a good foundation for sex education, but each preadolescent needs an adult to turn to with particular questions. Even a well-planned program does not address all the needs of the preadolescent. The best school program begins early and builds from year to year as the child's needs progress (see Chapter 26).

Preadolescence is an appropriate time for discussions that will help the young teen resist pressures to become sexually active too early. Family caregivers may turn to a nurse acquaintance for guidance in preparing the child. Perhaps the most important aspect of discussions about sexuality is that honest, straightforward answers must be given in an atmosphere of caring concern. Children whose need for information is not met through family, school, or community programs will often get inaccurate information from peers, movies, television, the Internet, or other media.

ADOLESCENT DEVELOPMENT

Adolescence spans the ages of about 13 to 18 years. Some boys do not complete adolescence until they are 20 years old. The rate of development during adolescence varies greatly from one teen to another. It is a time of many physical, emotional, and social changes. During this period, the adolescent struggles to master the developmental tasks that lead to successful completion of this stage of development (Table 27-2). Completion of the developmental tasks of earlier developmental stages is a prerequisite for the completion of these new tasks.

Physical Development

Rapid growth occurs during adolescence. Girls begin growing more rapidly during the preadolescent period and achieve 98% of their adult height by the age of 16. Boys start their growth spurt, a period of rapid growth, around 13 years of age and may continue to grow until 20 years of age. The skeletal system's rapid growth, which outpaces muscular system growth, causes the long and lanky appearance of many teens and contributes to the clumsiness often seen during this age. The bone growth that began during intrauterine life continues through adolescence and is usually completed by the end of this period.

The adolescent's body begins to take on adultlike contours, the primary sex organs enlarge, secondary sexual characteristics appear, and hormonal activity increases. During the first menstrual cycles for girls, ovulation does not usually occur because increased estrogen levels are needed to produce an ovum mature enough to be released. However, at 13 to 15 years of age, the cycle becomes ovulatory, and pregnancy is possible. The girl's breasts take on an adult appearance by age 16, and pubic hair is curly and abundant.

By the age of 16 years, a boy's penis, testes, and scrotum are adult in size and shape, and mature spermatozoa are produced. Pubic hair is also adult in appearance and amount. After age 13, muscle strength and coordination develop rapidly. The larynx and vocal cords enlarge, and the voice deepens. The "change of voice" makes the teenage boy's voice vary unexpectedly, which occasionally causes embarrassment for the teen.

Psychosocial Development

Adolescence is a time of transition from childhood to adulthood. Between the ages of 10 and 18 years, adolescents move from Freud's latency stage to the genital stage, from Erikson's industry versus inferiority to identity versus role confusion, and from Piaget's concrete operational thinking

TABLE 27-2   Developmental Tasks of Adolescence

BASIC TASK	ASSOCIATED TASKS
Appreciate own uniqueness[a]	Identify interests, skills, and talents Identify differences from peers Accept strengths and limitations Challenge own skill levels
Develop independent internal identity[a]	Value self as a person Separate physical self from psychological self Differentiate personal worth from cultural stereotypes Separate internal value from societal feedback
Determine own value system[a]	Identify options Establish priorities Commit self to decisions made Translate values into behaviors Resist peer and cultural pressures to conform to their value system Find comfortable balance between own and peer/cultural standards, behaviors, and needs
Develop self-evaluation skills[a]	Develop basis for self-evaluation and monitoring Evaluate quality of products Assess approach to tasks and responsibilities Develop sensitivity to intrapersonal relationships Evaluate dynamics of interpersonal relationships
Assume increasing responsibility for own behavior[a]	Quality of work, chores Emotional tone Money management Time management Decision making Personal habits Social behaviors
Find meaning in life	Accept and integrate meaning of death Develop philosophy of life Begin to identify life or career goals
Acquire skills essential for adult living	Acquire skills essential to independent living Develop social and emotional abilities and temperament Identify and experiment with alternatives for facing life Acquire employment skills Seek growth-inducing activities
Seek affiliations outside of family	Seek companionship with compatible peers Affiliate with organizations that support uniqueness Actively seek models or mentors Identify potential emotional support systems Differentiate between acquaintances and friends Identify ways to express sexuality
Adapt to adult body functioning	Adapt to physical changes Refine balance and coordination Develop physical strength Consider sexuality and reproduction issues

[a]Tasks deemed crucial to continued maturation.

to formal operational thought. Adolescents develop a sense of moral judgment and a system of values and beliefs that will affect their entire lives. The foundation provided by family, religious groups, school, and community experiences is still a strong influence, but the peer group exerts tremendous power. Trends and fads among adolescents dictate clothing choices, hairstyles, music, and other recreational choices (Fig. 27-2). The adolescent whose family caregivers make it difficult to conform has more stress added to an already emotion-laden period. Peer pressure to experiment with potentially dangerous practices, such as drugs, alcohol, and reckless driving, can also be strong; adolescents may need careful guidance and understanding support to help resist this peer influence.

Personality Development

Erikson considered the central task of adolescence to be the establishment of identity. Adolescents spend a lot of time

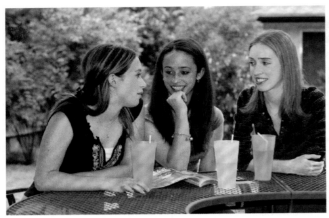

FIGURE 27-2 For many teens, hanging out with friends is an important way to share common interests and gain a sense of belonging.

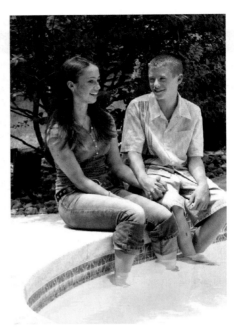

FIGURE 27-3 Intense interest in romantic relationships characterizes adolescence.

asking themselves, "Who am I as a person? What will I do with my life? Marry? Have children? Will I go to college? If so, where? If not, why not? What kind of career should I choose?"

Adolescents are confronted with a greater variety of choices than ever before. Gender role stereotypes are being reexamined to suit the need of the individual: Men are no longer required to be the sole financial provider for the family, and women are no longer required to assume all household and childrearing responsibilities. Transportation and remote working has made greater geographic mobility possible, so adolescents can spend summers or a full school year in a foreign country, plan to attend college thousands of miles from home, and begin a career in a remote location. Making decisions and choices is never simple. With such a tremendous variety of options, it is understandable that adolescents are often preoccupied with their own concerns.

When identity has been established, generally between the ages of 16 and 18 years, adolescents seek intimate relationships, usually with members of the opposite sex (Fig. 27-3). Intimacy, which is mutual sharing of one's deepest feelings with another person, is impossible unless each person has established a sense of trust and a sense of identity. Intimate relationships are a preparation for long-term relationships, and people who fail to achieve intimacy may develop feelings of isolation and experience chronic difficulty in communicating with others.

Intimate relationships during adolescence can be **heterosexual**, or between members of the opposite sex. Sometimes, however, young people form intimate attachments with members of the same sex in **homosexual** relationships. Because our culture is predominately heterosexual and is still struggling to understand homosexual relationships, these relationships can cause great anxiety for family caregivers and children. Although much of America is beginning to accept homosexual relationships, prejudice and discrimination still exist. So great a stigma has been attached to homosexuality that many adolescents fear they are homosexual if they are uncomfortable about

heterosexual intimacy. However, this discomfort is normal as adolescents move from same-sex peer group activities to dating peers of the opposite sex. Some adolescents struggle with gender identity. They are born with the anatomy of a man or woman but their internal sense is that they are in the wrong body, and they identify themselves as a person of the opposite sex and/or gender. The term used to describe this situation is **transgender**.

Body Image

Body image is closely related to self-esteem. Seeing one's body as attractive and functional contributes to a positive sense of self-esteem. During adolescence, the desire to not be different can extend to feelings about one's body and can cause adolescents to feel that their bodies are inadequate, even though they are actually healthy and attractive.

American culture tends to equate a slender figure with feminine beauty and acceptability and a lean, tall, muscular figure with masculine virility and strength. Adolescents, particularly boys, who feel that they are underdeveloped suffer great anxiety. Adolescent girls have even undergone plastic surgery to augment their breasts to relieve this anxiety. Girls in this age group often feel that they are overweight and sometimes try strange, nutritionally unsound diets to reduce their weight. Some literally starve themselves. Even after their bodies have become emaciated, they truly believe that they are still fat and therefore unattractive. This condition is called *anorexia nervosa* and is discussed further in Chapter 42.

Adolescents need to establish a positive body image by the end of their developmental stage. Because bone growth is completed during adolescence, a person's height will remain basically the same throughout adult life, even though weight can fluctuate greatly. Tall girls who long to be petite and shorter boys who would like to be 6 ft tall may need guidance and support to bring their expectations in line with reality and learn to have positive feelings about their bodies and accept them the way they are.

> ### TEST YOURSELF
> ✔ What are the secondary sex characteristics that develop in (a) adolescent boys and (b) adolescent girls?
> ✔ Why is body image so important for the adolescent?

NUTRITION

Adolescents need a balanced diet consisting of servings from each of the food groups (Table 27-3). (See also ChooseMyPlate in Fig. 22-3 in Chapter 22.) Nutritional requirements greatly increase during periods of rapid growth. Adolescent boys need more calories than do girls throughout the growth period. Appetites increase, and most teens eat frequently. Families with teenage children often jokingly say that they cannot keep the refrigerator filled. Nutritional needs are related to growth and sexual maturity rather than age.

Even though adolescents understand something about nutrition, they may not relate this understanding to their dietary habits. Their accelerated growth rate and increased physical activities, for some, mean that they need more food to meet their energy requirements. Because adolescents are seeking to establish their independence, their food choices are sometimes not wise and tend to be influenced by peer preference, rather than parental advice. Teens frequently skip meals (especially breakfast), snack on foods that provide empty calories, and eat a lot of fast foods. The era of fast food meals has given adolescents easy access to high-calorie, nutritionally unbalanced meals. Too many fast food meals and nutritionally empty snacks can result in nutritional deficiencies (Fig. 27-4).

Nutrients that are often deficient in the teen's diet include calcium; iron; zinc; vitamins A, D, and B_6; and folic acid. Calcium intake needs to increase during skeletal growth. Girls need additional iron because of losses during menstruation. Boys also need additional iron during this growth period (Table 27-4). When good nutritional habits have been established in early childhood, adolescent nutrition is likely to be better balanced than when nutritional teaching has been insufficient. Being part of a family that practices sound nutrition helps ensure that occasional lapses into sweets, fast foods, and other peer group food preferences will not create serious deficiencies.

In their quest for identity and independence, some adolescents experiment with food fads and diets. Adolescent girls, worried about being fat, may fall prey to a variety of fad diets. Athletes also may follow fad diets that may include supplements, in the belief that these diets enhance bodybuilding. These diets often include increased amounts of protein and amino acids that cause diuresis and calcium loss. Carbohydrate loading, which some practice during the week before an athletic event, increases the muscle glycogen level to two to three times the normal amount and may hinder heart function. A meal that is low in fat and high in complex carbohydrates eaten 3 to 4 hours before an event is much more appropriate for the teen athlete.

Adolescents often resist pressure from family members to eat balanced meals; all family caregivers can do is to provide nutritious meals and snacks at regular mealtimes. A good example may be the best teacher at this point. A refrigerator stocked with ready-to-eat nutritious snacks can be a good weapon against snacking on empty calories.

Families with low incomes may have difficulty providing the kinds of foods that meet the requirements for a growing teen. These families need help to learn how to make low-cost, nutritious food selections and plan adequate meals and snacks. As a nurse, you can be instrumental in helping them plan appropriate food purchases. For instance, you might recommend fruit and vegetable stores or farm stands that accept food stamps.

Culture also influences adolescent food choices and habits. For example, many Mexican Americans are accustomed to having their big meal at noon. When school lunches do not provide such a heavy meal, the Mexican American adolescent may supplement the lunch with sweets or fast foods. In the Asian American community, milk is not a popular drink; this can result in a calcium deficiency. Many Asian people are lactose intolerant; therefore, you can recommend other products high in calcium, such as tofu (soybean curd), soybeans, and greens to increase calcium intake.

TABLE 27-3 Daily Nutritional Needs of the 11- to 18-Year-Old Adolescent

Men (M) need 1,800–3,200 calories/day; women (W) need 1,600–2,400 calories/day. The moderately active adolescent needs the amounts below from each food group.

Fruits	Vegetables	Grains	Protein Foods	Dairy
M: 1.5–2.5 cups	M: 2.5–4 cups	M: 6–10 oz	M: 5–7 oz	M: 3 cups
W: 1.5–2 cups	W: 2–3 cups	W: 5–8 oz	W: 5–6.5 oz	W: 3 cups

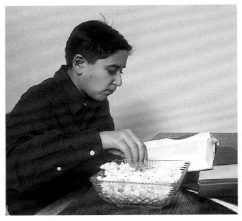

FIGURE 27-4 Teens are always hungry but often choose convenient junk foods, which lack nutritional value.

A person may follow a vegetarian diet for religious, ecologic, or philosophic reasons. If planned with care, vegetarian diets can provide needed nutrients. The most common types of vegetarian diets are the following:

- *Semivegetarian* includes dairy products, eggs, and fish but excludes red meat and possibly poultry.
- *Lacto-ovo-vegetarian* includes eggs and dairy products but excludes meat, poultry, and fish.
- *Lactovegetarian* includes dairy products and excludes meat, fish, poultry, and eggs.
- *Vegan* excludes all food of animal origin, including dairy products, eggs, fish, meat, and poultry.

Vegan diets may not provide adequate nutrients without careful planning. All vegetarians should include whole-grain products, legumes, nuts, seeds, and fortified soy substitutes if low-fat dairy products are unacceptable.

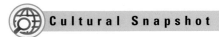

Cultural Snapshot

Be alert to cultural dietary influences on the adolescent; take these into consideration when helping the adolescent and the family devise an adequate food plan.

HEALTH PROMOTION AND MAINTENANCE

Adolescents have much the same need for regular health checkups, protection against infection, and prevention of accidents as do younger children. They also have special needs that can best be met by health professionals with in-depth knowledge and understanding of adolescent concerns. The number of adolescent clinics and health centers has increased along with innovative health services, such as school-based clinics, crisis hotlines, homes for runaways, and rehabilitation centers for adolescents who have been involved with alcohol or other drugs or with prostitution. Staff members in these programs provide teens with services needed for healthy growth.

Routine Checkups

A routine physical examination is recommended at least twice during the teen years, although annual physical examinations are encouraged. At this time, a complete history of developmental milestones, school problems, behavioral problems, family relationships, and immunizations should be completed. Immunizations that have not been administered at the recommended age should be administered in order to catch the adolescent up. A urine pregnancy screening is advisable before the rubella vaccine is administered to a girl of childbearing age because administration of the vaccine during pregnancy can cause serious risks to the developing fetus. Tuberculin testing is included in at least one visit and depending on the community may be recommended at both visits if there is an interval of several years between visits.

Measure and record height, weight, and blood pressure. Vision and hearing screening are done if they have not been part of a regular school screening program. Adolescents up to the age of 16 years need to be screened for scoliosis. Thyroid enlargement should be checked. Sexually active girls must have pelvic examinations, screening for sexually transmitted infections (STIs), and Papanicolaou smears. Urinalysis is performed on all adolescent girls, and a urine culture is performed if the girl has any symptoms of a urinary tract infection, such as urgency or burning and pain on

TABLE 27-4 Food Sources of Nutrients Commonly Deficient in Preadolescent and Adolescent Diets

COMMON NUTRIENT DEFICIENCIES	FOOD SOURCES
Vitamin A	Liver, whole milk, butter, cheese; sources of carotene such as yellow vegetables, green leafy vegetables, tomatoes, yellow fruits
Vitamin D	Fortified milk, egg yolk, butter
Vitamin B$_6$ (pyridoxine)	Chicken, fish, peanuts, bananas, pork, egg yolk, whole-grain cereals
Folate (folic acid)	Green leafy vegetables, enriched cereals, liver, dried peas and beans, whole grains
Calcium	Milk, hard cheese, yogurt, ice cream, small fish eaten with bones (e.g., sardines), dark-green vegetables, tofu, soybeans, calcium-enriched orange juice
Iron	Lean meats, liver, legumes, dried fruits, green leafy vegetables, whole-grain and fortified cereals
Zinc	Oysters, herring, meat, liver, fish, milk, whole grains, nuts, legumes

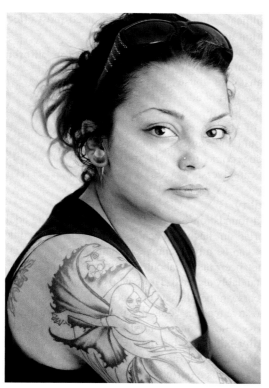

FIGURE 27-5 This adolescent expresses her identity with body piercings and tattoos.

urination. A routine physical is an excellent time for you to counsel the adolescent about sexual activity, STIs, and human immunodeficiency virus (HIV) infection.

Body piercing and tattoos are becoming more common in the adolescent population (Fig. 27-5). Piercings are seen in ears, eyebrows, noses, lips, tongues, chins, breasts, navels—in almost every part of the body. Tattoos of all designs are seen in the adolescent. The adolescent with piercings and tattoos needs to be aware of the signs and symptoms of infection (redness, swelling, warmth, drainage, discomfort) and that these must be reported immediately if they occur. Sharing needles for piercing or tattooing needs to be discussed, and the adolescent needs to be taught that sharing needles carries the same risks as sharing needles with IV drug users.

Madison Davis is getting a body piercing. What information would be important to share with Madison and her parents about the piercing?

Adolescents must be given privacy, individualized attention, confidentiality, and the right to participate in decisions about their healthcare. They may feel uncomfortable and out of place in a pediatrician's waiting room, where most of the clients are 3 ft tall, or in a waiting room filled with adults. Some clinics and health care providers specialize in adolescent healthcare, but many adolescents do not have these facilities available to them.

 A Personal Glimpse

Every year around our birthdays, my little brother and I always go to our pediatrician's office. After being called by the nurse, we both go down to a tiny room with bright walls, baby pictures, and the kind of mobiles hung over a crib, the same kind of decorations that cover the entire office. I suppose the room itself is comforting, but then I have to strip down to my underwear right in front of my 6-year-old brother. To make matters worse, I have to put on a skimpy little gown that hardly covers my underwear and wait in a room with huge windows and blinds that don't close, overlooking the next building's parking lot. It's so embarrassing, having to climb up onto the examining table with a gown falling down underneath me. Why can't the gowns be longer? It isn't just 6-year-olds who have to wear them!

Jessica, age 12 years

Learning Opportunity: *What do nurses and health care providers need to take into consideration regarding the privacy needs of adolescents? What specific things would you do in this situation to acknowledge and respect the needs of this adolescent girl?*

Continuity of care helps build the adolescent's confidence in the health care providers. Professionals dealing with teens should recognize that the physical symptoms offered as the reason for seeking care are often not the most significant problem about which the adolescent is concerned. An attitude of nonjudgmental acceptance on the part of healthcare personnel can often encourage the adolescent to ask questions and share feelings and concerns about troubling matters. Family members may accompany adolescents to the healthcare facility, but it is important to provide an opportunity to interview the adolescent alone (Fig. 27-6). Asking questions in a way that is concrete and specific will encourage the adolescent to give direct answers. The interviewer must be alert to verbal and nonverbal clues.

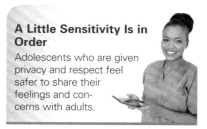

A Little Sensitivity Is in Order

Adolescents who are given privacy and respect feel safer to share their feelings and concerns with adults.

Dental Checkups

Adolescents need continued regular dental checkups every 6 months. Dental **malocclusion** (improper alignment of the teeth) is a common condition that affects the way the teeth and jaws function. Correction of the malocclusion with dental braces improves chewing ability and appearance. The treatment of the malocclusion with dental braces is called **orthodontia**. Braces have become very common among adolescents because many malocclusions can be corrected. Orthodontic treatment usually begins in early adolescence or late school age. The use of braces has become widespread, and braces are readily accepted among teens, although many

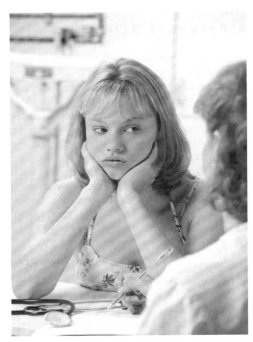

FIGURE 27-6 Interviewing the adolescent in private and conveying a nonjudgmental attitude will encourage her to ask questions and express concerns about a troubling matter. Adolescents need to be included in plans and decisions regarding their healthcare.

teens still feel awkward and self-conscious during their orthodontic treatment. Tongue piercing among adolescents has increased, and dental checkups provide a good time to discuss concerns of possible infections and tooth damage that can occur when an adolescent has a pierced tongue.

Family Teaching

The adolescent years are difficult for the maturing young person and often are just as difficult for the family caregiver. Family caregivers must allow the independent teen to flourish while continuing to safeguard them from risky and immature behavior. Family caregivers and adolescents struggle with issues related to sexuality, substance abuse, accidents, discipline, poor nutrition, and volatile emotions.

Learning about adolescent physical and psychosocial developments can help family caregivers struggling to understand their teen. Family caregivers will find information on sexuality and substance abuse enlightening and useful. Attending workshops or consulting counselors, teachers, religious leaders, or healthcare workers may enhance the family caregiver's communication skills. Good communication between adolescents and their family is essential to fostering healthy relationships between them. Family caregivers may need both anticipatory guidance in preparing their teen for adulthood and emotional support to feel successful in this difficult period. Take every opportunity to provide the family caregiver with information and support.

Health Education and Counseling

Before adolescents can take an active role in their own healthcare, they need information and guidance on the need for healthcare and how to meet that need most effectively. Education and counseling about sexuality, STIs, contraception, and substance abuse are a vital part of adolescent healthcare. Some of this teaching should and sometimes does come from family caregivers.

> **You Can Make the Difference**
> A family caregiver's lack of information or discomfort in discussing certain topics with adolescents sometimes means that the job will have to be done by healthcare professionals.

Sexuality

A good foundation in sex education can help the adolescent take pride in having reached sexual maturity; otherwise, puberty can be a frightening, shameful experience. Girls who have not been taught about menstruation until it occurs are understandably alarmed. Those who have been taught to regard it as a curse, rather than an entrance into womanhood, will not have positive feelings about this part of their sexuality.

Boys who are unprepared for nocturnal emissions may feel guilty, believing that they have caused these wet dreams by sexual fantasies or masturbation. They need to understand that this is a normal occurrence and simply the body's method of getting rid of surplus semen.

Assuming that adolescents are adequately prepared for the events of puberty, sex education during adolescence can deal with the important issues of responsible sexuality, contraception, and STIs. More adolescents today are sexually active than ever, resulting in an alarmingly rapid increase in teenage pregnancies and STIs. The incidence of HIV infection is particularly increasing among adolescents.

Girls need to learn the importance of regular pelvic examinations and Pap smears. Although breast self-examination is now considered optional in breast cancer detection, it is important for the adolescent girl to become aware of the normal nature of her breasts. The technique for the monthly breast self-examination (Tips for Reinforcing Family Teaching: Breast Self-Examination) helps to identify any breast changes that may occur. Boys need to learn that testicular cancer is one of the most common cancers in young men between the ages of 15 and 35 years and must be taught how and when to perform testicular self-examination (Tips for Reinforcing Family Teaching: Testicular Self-Examination).

An adolescent's growing awareness of their sexuality, sexually provocative material in the media, and lack of acceptable means to gratify sexual desires make masturbation a common practice during adolescence. Unlike young children's genital exploration, adolescent masturbation can produce orgasm in the adolescent girl and ejaculation in the adolescent boy. Generally, it is a private and solitary activity, but occasionally it occurs with other members of the peer group. Healthcare professionals recognize masturbation as a positive way to release sexual tension and increase one's knowledge of body sensations. Reassure adolescents that masturbation is common in both young men and women and is a normal outlet for sexual urges.

TIPS FOR REINFORCING FAMILY TEACHING

Breast Self-Examination

Instructions

The best time to do the breast self-examination is a week after your period ends. The breast is not as tender or swollen at this point in the menstrual cycle.

1. Lie down with a pillow under your right shoulder. Place your right arm behind your head (Fig. A).

A

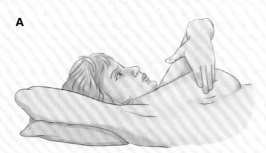

2. Use the sensitive finger pads (where your fingerprints are, not the tips) of the middle three fingers on your left hand to feel for lumps in the right breast (Fig. B). Use overlapping dime-sized circular motions of the finger pads to feel the breast tissue. Powder, oil, or lotion can be applied to the breast to make it easier for the fingers to glide over the surface and feel changes.

B

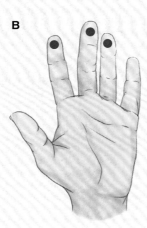

3. Use three different levels of pressure to feel the breast tissue. First, light pressure to just move the skin without jostling the tissue beneath, then medium pressure pressing midway into the tissue, and finally firm pressure to probe more deeply down to the chest and ribs or to the point just short of discomfort. Use each pressure level to feel the breast tissue before moving on to the next spot.

4. Move your fingers around the breast in an up-and-down pattern (called the vertical pattern), starting at an imaginary line drawn straight down your side from the underarm and moving across the breast to the middle of the chest bone (sternum or breastbone). Check the entire breast using each of the pressures described above. Completely feel all of the breast and chest area up under your armpit, up to the collarbone, and all the way over to your shoulder to cover breast tissue that extends toward the shoulder (Fig. C).

C

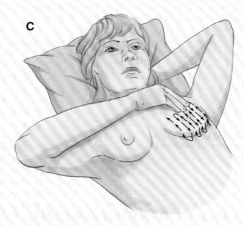

5. Repeat the examination on your left breast using the finger pads of your right hand, with a pillow under your left shoulder.

6. While standing in front of a mirror, with your hands pressing firmly down on your hips (this position shows more clearly any breast changes), look at your breasts for any change in size, shape, contour, dimpling of the skin, changes in the nipple, redness, or spontaneous nipple discharge (Fig. D).

D

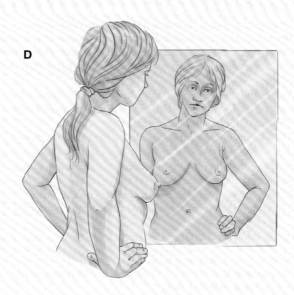

7. Examine each underarm while sitting or standing, with your arm only slightly raised (raising your arm straight tightens the tissue and makes it difficult to examine). The upright position makes it easier to check the upper and outer parts of the breasts (toward your armpits). You may want to do this part of the examination while showering. It is easy to slide soapy hands over your skin, and to feel anything unusual (Fig. E).

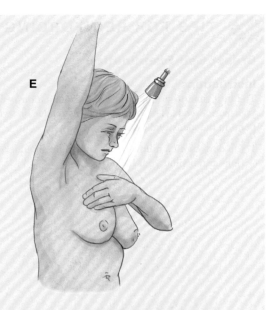

E

Adapted from National Breast Cancer Foundation, Inc. (n.d.). *Breast self-exam.* http://www.nationalbreastcancer.org/breast-self-exam.

 TIPS FOR REINFORCING FAMILY TEACHING

Testicular Self-Examination

Instructions
Perform the examination once a month after a warm bath or shower. The scrotum is relaxed from the warmth. Select a day that is easy to remember, such as the first or last day of the month.

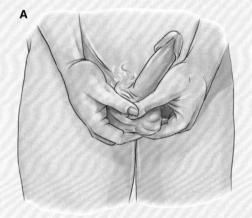

A

1. Stand in front of a mirror and look for any swelling on the skin of the scrotum.
2. Examine each testicle, one at a time, using both hands.
3. Place the index and middle fingers under the testicle and the thumbs on top. Roll each testicle gently between the thumbs and fingers (Fig. A). One testicle is normally larger than the other.
4. The epididymis is the soft, tubelike structure located at the back of the testicle that collects and carries sperm (Fig. B). This must not be mistaken for an abnormal lump.
5. Most lumps are found on the sides of the testicle, although they may also appear on the front. Look and feel for any hard lumps or nodules (smooth, rounded masses) or any change in the size, shape, or consistency of the testes.
6. Report any lump to your health care provider at once. Testicular cancer is highly curable when treated promptly.

Signs of Testicular Cancer

- Small, painless lump in a testicle.
- Enlargement of a testicle. It is normal for one testicle to be slightly larger than the other.
- Significant loss in size of a testicle.
- A feeling of scrotal heaviness.
- A dull ache in the lower abdomen or groin.
- Testicular or scrotal pain or discomfort.
- Sudden accumulation of blood or fluid in the scrotum.
- Enlargement or tenderness of the breasts.

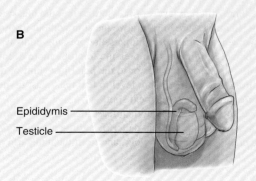

B

Epididymis ———
Testicle ———

Sexual Responsibility

Not all adolescents are sexually active, but the number of those who are increases with each year of age. Although abstinence is the only completely successful protection, all adolescents need to have information concerning safe sex practices to be prepared for the occasion when they wish to be sexually intimate with someone. Adolescents do not have a good record of using contraceptives to prevent pregnancy. Many teens give excuses and think sex should not be planned because if it is planned, then it is wrong or they feel guilty. They need to feel that it "just happened" in the heat of the moment, not because they really wanted or planned it. Many adolescents are beginning to realize that much more than pregnancy may be at risk, but their attitude of "it won't happen to me," which is typical of this developmental age, continues to contribute to their increasing sexual activity.

Some adults continue to resist providing contraceptive information to adolescents in school, believing that such information encourages teens to become sexually active. However, as human immunodeficiency virus (HIV) infections become a greater threat to every sexually active person, this argument becomes harder to defend. Adolescents need contraceptive information to prevent pregnancy, but more importantly, they need straightforward information about using condoms to protect them against HIV and other infections. Both adolescent girls and boys need this information. Adolescent boys and girls must be advised to carry their own condoms if they believe that there is any possibility of having sexual intercourse.

When condoms are used consistently and correctly, they are highly effective in preventing pregnancy and sexually transmitted infections (STIs). Condoms used with spermicidal foam have an even greater effective rate against pregnancy. The safest condom is one made of latex with a prelubricated tip or reservoir and pretreated with nonoxynol-9 spermicide. Tips for Reinforcing Family Teaching: Safe Condom Use and Figures 4-4 to 4-6, in Chapter 4, provide guidelines for natural contraceptive methods and for the use of condoms for men and women.

Other STIs that sexually active adolescents need to know about are syphilis, gonorrhea, genital herpes, genital warts, and chlamydial and trichomonal infections. Prevention of STIs is the primary aim of education for adolescents. If prevention proves ineffective, however, the most important factor is referral for treatment. Many adolescents are reluctant to seek treatment, fearing that their family caregivers will discover their activity. Crisis hotlines are valuable resources to assure adolescents that treatment is vital for them and their partners and that confidentiality is ensured.

Healthcare personnel who work with adolescents seeking treatment for an STI must be nonjudgmental, supportive, and understanding. Adolescents need treatment and information about preventing spread of the STI to others, as well as how to prevent contracting another STI. See Chapter 41 for a thorough discussion of STIs and related nursing care.

Many adolescents are not sexually active, but most spend time dating or socializing with peers. In recent years, the use of Rohypnol, also known as the date rape drug, has become a concern for the adolescent. Rohypnol is not sold legally in the United States, but it is brought in from countries where it is sold legally. The drug, especially in combination with alcohol, causes memory loss, blackouts, and an inability to resist sexual attacks. Often, the drug is secretly slipped into a person's drink. The drug has no taste or odor, but within a few minutes after ingesting the drug, the person feels dizzy, disoriented, and nauseated, and then rapidly passes out. After several hours, the person awakens and has no memories of what happened while under the influence of the drug. The adolescent needs to be encouraged to stay aware and alert to avoid becoming a victim of date rape. They should be taught to avoid using alcohol and never to leave any drink unattended.

Substance Abuse

As adolescents search for identity and independence, they are susceptible to many pressures from society and their peers. Adolescents may experiment with substances that may be habit-forming or addictive and ultimately will harm them. This may be done "just for kicks," to "go along with the crowd" (peer group), or to rebel against the authority of family caregivers or other adults. Some substances abused by adolescents are also abused by many adults; so to some adolescents, using these substances may appear sophisticated.

Alcohol and certain other drugs provide an escape, however brief, from pressures the adolescent may feel. Alcohol is the mind-altering substance most commonly abused by adolescents. Other substances that adolescents may abuse are tobacco (including smokeless tobacco), marijuana, cocaine or "crack," heroin, "ecstasy," other street drugs, and prescription drugs. (See Chapter 42 for further discussion of substance abuse.) Adolescents can often easily obtain tobacco products, despite federal legislation to enforce strict age limitations on their sale.

Programs developed to educate students about substance abuse meet with varying success. Healthcare personnel must stress to adolescents that use of alcohol or mind-altering chemicals is often accompanied by irresponsible sexual behavior that could further complicate their lives. Chapter 42 discusses these problems in more detail.

TEST YOURSELF

✔ What nutrients are often missing in the adolescent diet?

✔ List the topics of health education that should be discussed with the adolescent.

Mental Health

The turmoil that adolescents experience while searching for self-esteem and self-confidence can cause stress that may lead to depression, suicide, and conduct disorders. Academic and social pressures add to that stress. The family may also be under stress due to unemployment or economic difficulties, separation, divorce, or death of a family caregiver. Healthcare personnel must be sensitive to signs that the adolescent is having problems. Adolescents need the opportunity to express their fears, concerns, and frustrations. The rapport between family caregivers and teens may not be such that the adolescent can express these feelings to the family. Many schools have mental health personnel on staff that can provide counseling when needed. Adolescents need counseling to work through troublesome situations and to avoid chronic mental health problems. Mental health assessment is an important part of the adolescent's total health assessment.

With the increased use of computers and the Internet, Internet safety is an important aspect of adolescent mental health. Parents need to be aware of the adolescent's computer activities and the sites they access, especially communication sites with chat rooms. Discussions with adolescents regarding safety concerns on Internet sites help to increase their awareness and decrease potential dangers. See Tips for Reinforcing Family Teaching: Internet Safety.

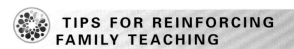

TIPS FOR REINFORCING FAMILY TEACHING

Internet Safety

Signs that might indicate online risks in a child or adolescent are the following:

- Spends large amounts of time online, especially at night
- Has pornography on computer
- Receives phone calls from adults you don't know
- Makes calls, especially long distance, to numbers you don't recognize
- Receives mail, gifts, and packages from someone you don't know
- Turns computer monitor off or changes screen when you enter room
- Becomes withdrawn from family
- Uses an online account belonging to someone else

Ways to minimize online concerns are as follows:

- Communicate and talk with your child; openly discuss concerns and dangers
- Spend time with your child online
- Keep computer in a common area in the house
- Set up accounts with special privileges to block content from your child
- Monitor the call log on your child's phone or family phone
- Maintain access to your child's online account and monitor activity

Adapted from U.S. Department of Justice Federal Bureau of Investigation (n.d.). *A parent's guide to Internet safety.* https://www2.fbi.gov/publications/pguide/pguidee.htm

Accident Prevention

In every part of society, increasing numbers of adolescents are dying as a result of violence, which includes motor vehicle accidents, homicide, suicide, and other causes. Unintentional injuries and homicide rank as the leading causes of death for 15- to 19-year-old youths, regardless of sex. Statistics regarding adolescents are difficult to interpret, but death among adolescents is often related to risky behaviors. These behaviors include the unintentional (those involving motor vehicles, fires) as well as the intentional (violence, suicide), alcohol and other drug use, sexual behaviors, tobacco use, and dietary behaviors. Alcohol and other drugs are often involved in fatal accidents. Death is not the only negative outcome of violence: Many adolescents are injured and hospitalized or treated in emergency departments, and many adolescents suffer psychological injury from being victims of violence.

Violence is also on the rise in schools—not just inner-city schools. Weapons are detected on students in schools all over the country. Guns and knives are the weapons most often found. The problem has become so serious that some schools have installed metal detectors to protect students.

Adolescents are also victims of violence in their own homes in greater numbers than any other age group of children. Rape and other violence in a dating relationship are common too.

Students have formed peer support groups such as Students Against Destructive Decisions (formerly known as Students Against Drunk Driving) with the mission to help their peers make good decisions related to drinking, drug use, risky and distracted driving, violence, and suicide (www.sadd.org). Many schools provide support groups that help students work through their grief after schoolmates have met with violent death.

Much work needs to be done to understand the reason for this increasing violence. One factor in adolescents is that they often act recklessly without the benefit of mature judgment. Adolescents have relatively easy access to guns and often use them as a means to solve problems. Efforts to control and regulate gun sales are nationally discussed topics. Acts of terror and violence in the world increase the confusion and anxiety that adolescents have regarding conflicts and conflict resolution.

Nurses who have any contact with adolescents must make every effort to help them work through their problems in nonviolent ways. As a nurse, you can become involved at the school or community level by becoming an advocate for adolescents and an educator to promote safe driving, as well as by wearing a helmet and safety practices when using a motorcycle, all-terrain vehicle, bicycle, skateboard, or in-line skates. You can also work with support groups that offer counseling to adolescents involved in date violence. As a community member and a healthcare worker, you can be a positive role model for adolescents.

THE ADOLESCENT IN THE HEALTHCARE FACILITY

When adolescents are hospitalized, it is usually because of a major health problem such as an injury from violence or from a motor vehicle accident, substance abuse, attempted suicide, or a chronic health problem intensified by the physiologic changes of adolescence. Adolescents must cope with the stress of hospitalization, possible dramatic alterations in body image, partial or total inability to conform to peer group norms, and an interrupted search for identity. They fear loss of control and loss of privacy. Provide opportunities for the adolescent to make choices, whenever possible. Providing screening and adequate covering during procedures helps protect the adolescent's privacy.

Adolescents may react with anger and refuse to cooperate when their privacy or feelings of control are threatened. Be aware of this possible reaction and avoid labeling such an adolescent as a difficult client.

The admission interview for an adolescent may be more successful if the family caregiver and the adolescent are interviewed separately. This provides the opportunity to gain information that the adolescent may not want to reveal in the presence of the family caregiver. It is important to thoroughly explore the adolescent's developmental level, listen carefully with empathy to their concerns, encourage maximum participation in self-care, and provide sufficient information to make this participation possible.

This is Critical to Remember

In working with adolescents, as with all clients, clear, honest explanations about treatments and procedures are essential.

During the admission interview, advise the adolescent of the unit's rules. Adolescents need to know what limits are set for their behavior while they are in the hospital. To share feelings and gain information, many find it helpful to discuss their own health problems with a peer who has had the same or a related problem.

Adolescents need access to a telephone to contact peers and keep up social contacts. Recreation areas are important. In settings specifically designed for adolescents, recreation rooms can provide an area where teens can gather to do school work, play games and cards, and socialize. In many hospitals with adolescent units, video games as well as a television are provided in each client room. Access to a computer and email might also help the teen stay connected to peers. Supervision is important to decrease misuse of computer privileges. Teens are encouraged to wear their own clothes. They can be encouraged to shampoo and style their hair, and can wear their usual makeup.

The adolescent's health problem may require a lengthy hospitalization and intense rehabilitation efforts. Adequate preparation and guidance can help make that difficult experience easier and less damaging to normal growth and development.

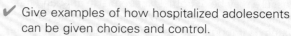

TEST YOURSELF

✔ What are the most frequent causes of accidents in adolescents?

✔ Give examples of how hospitalized adolescents can be given choices and control.

Remember **Madison Davis** from the beginning of the chapter. What characteristics of adolescent growth and development might lead Madison to want a body piercing? Madison had her tongue pierced. What would need to be monitored at each of Madison's dental checkups following her piercing? What are your thoughts about body piercing?

KEY POINTS

- The preadolescent period is between ages 10 and 12 years, and adolescence spans ages 13 to 18 years.

- In preadolescence, the child's body begins to take on adultlike contours, the primary sex organs enlarge, secondary sexual characteristics appear, and hormonal activity increases. This early period ends with the onset of menstruation in young women and the production of sperm in young men. The rapid growth of the skeletal system outpaces the growth of the muscular system, contributing to the clumsiness sometimes noted in the adolescent.

- During adolescence, children go through many psychosocial changes on their way to adulthood. They are fascinated and sometimes fearful of and confused by the changes occurring in their bodies and their thinking processes. The adolescent begins to look grown up but lacks the judgment or independence to participate in society as an adult. They are strongly influenced by their peer group and often resent parental authority. Roller coaster emotions characterize this age group, as does intense interest in romantic relationships.

- Secondary sexual characteristics seen in the adolescent boy include penis, testes, and scrotum reaching adult size and shape; pubic hair; increased strength; and a deepening of the voice. Adolescent girls develop breasts and pubic hair and begin ovulation and menstruation.

- According to Piaget, the adolescent moves from concrete operational thinking to formal operational thought. Erikson's stage of development in the adolescent is referred to as identity versus role confusion. The adolescent's task is to establish their own identity and to find a place in society.

- Changing sex role stereotypes, geographic mobility, and abundant career opportunities and options add to the adolescent's difficulties in making a career choice.

- Intimacy or mutual sharing of deep feelings with another person occurs when people have developed trust and their own sense of identity. Intimate relationships in adolescents help in preparation for long-term relationships.

- In trying to develop their own sense of self and identity, adolescents begin the process of separating from family caregivers. The peers exert influence, and the adolescent feels a need to conform and to fit in with peers. This peer pressure may be extremely influential in affecting the adolescent's attitudes and behaviors. A strong support system is important to help the adolescent through this stressful stage of development.

- Body image and self-esteem are closely related, and the adolescent struggles with wanting to be attractive and accepted. This drive can create anxiety in the adolescent, which can lead to unhealthy behavior, practices, and conditions.

- Appetites increase and most teens eat frequently. It is important for the adolescent to maintain a balanced diet with healthy food choices. Their food choices are sometimes not wise and tend to be influenced by peers. Adolescent diets are often deficient in calcium; iron; zinc; vitamins A, D, and B_6; and folic acid. Culture influences food choices and habits, as does the choice to follow a vegetarian diet.

- Routine physical examinations, including history of developmental milestones, school problems, behavioral problems, family relationships, and immunizations should be completed. Discussion of signs and symptoms of infection related to piercing and tattoos needs to be part of health promotion. Dental checkups every 6 months, correction of dental malocclusion with dental braces, and

discussion of tongue-piercing concerns are important. Adolescent girls need regular pelvic examinations, Pap smears, and reinforcement of teaching regarding breast self-examination. Adolescent boys must be taught how and when to perform testicular self-examination. Mental health assessment is an important part of the adolescent's total health assessment.

- Health education in the adolescent needs to include information regarding sexuality, sexual responsibility, sexually transmitted infections (STIs), and contraception, as well as teaching about substance abuse and mental health issues. Adolescents face peer pressure, personal values and beliefs, and societal influences in making decisions related to sexual responsibility, substance use, and other risk-taking behaviors.

- In the healthcare facility, the adolescent fears loss of control and loss of privacy. Be sensitive to the hospitalized adolescent's needs, provide supportive care, and encourage as much participation by the adolescent as possible. Health problems that threaten the adolescent's body image may threaten the satisfactory completion of developmental tasks.

INTERNET RESOURCES

Testicular Examination/Cancer
www.testicularcancerawarenessfoundation.org

Breast Self-Examination
www.nationalbreastcancer.org/breast-self-exam

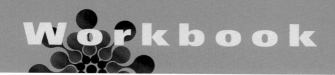
NCLEX-STYLE REVIEW QUESTIONS

1. The nurse is assisting with a physical examination of a 12-year-old girl. Her record indicates that at age 9, she was 51 inches tall and weighed 72 lb. Which of the following would the nurse *most likely* find if the child were following a normal pattern of growth and development?
   a. The adolescent weighs 98 lb.
   b. The adolescent measures 53 inches in height.
   c. The adolescent has a small amount of pubic hair.
   d. The adolescent has well-developed breasts.

2. The nurse is working with a group of family caregivers of adolescents who are discussing normal adolescent growth and development. Which of the following statements made by a caregiver would indicate a need for follow-up?
   a. "He wants to be a nurse after he finishes college."
   b. "She has her own money to spend now because she has a job."
   c. "My son has been spending at least half an hour to an hour in front of the mirror the last 3 months while getting ready for school."
   d. "My daughter is so slim and trim, she has lost 10 lb in the last 6 weeks."

3. The nurse is reinforcing teaching with a group of adolescent girls about good nutrition habits and eating foods that will help increase the deficient nutrients in the adolescent diet. Which of the following statements made by the girls in the group is correct?
   a. "Eating lots of broccoli will help increase the iron in my diet."
   b. "If I drink three glasses of milk each day, I will get plenty of vitamin C."
   c. "Even though I don't like eggs, if I eat four eggs a week I will get enough calcium."
   d. "I am sure I get enough vitamin A since I eat bread at every meal."

4. In working with adolescent children, the nurse would know that if the adolescents were following normal development patterns, the children would *most* likely be involved in which of the following activities?
   a. Working to establish a career
   b. Playing a board game with siblings
   c. Participating in activities with peers
   d. Volunteering in community projects

5. The nurse is reinforcing teaching with a group of adolescent girls about how to perform a breast self-examination. Which of the following actions should the nurse reinforce regarding the breast self-examination? Select all that apply.
   a. Perform the breast examination each month.
   b. Do the breast examination just before your period starts.
   c. Use the pads of the fingers to examine the breast.
   d. Use the same pattern to feel every part of the breast.
   e. Stand in front of a mirror to look for changes in breasts.
   f. Examine the breasts while in the bathtub.

STUDY ACTIVITIES

1. List and compare a 15-year-old girl and a 15-year-old boy in regard to physical development, psychosocial development, personality development, and their feelings about body image.

Area of Development	15-Year-Old Girl	15-Year-Old Boy
Physical development		
Psychosocial development		
Personality development		
Body image		

2. Mattie is the mother of 13-year-old Chantal. Chantal has decided she will not eat meat or poultry because animals had to be killed to obtain it. Mattie is concerned about Chantal's nutrition. Develop a menu for a day for Chantal. Be sure your menu provides nutrients often deficient in adolescents and that it supports Chantal in her choice to not eat meat and poultry.

3. You are working with a group of adolescents in a school-based clinic and plan to have a discussion about substance abuse and STIs. Make a list of questions you think the adolescents might want to ask but are uncomfortable asking. Discuss with your peers the answers you could give to each of these questions.

4. Do an Internet search on "body piercing."
   a. Why is it a concern to pierce the mouth or nose? Tongue? Lip?
   b. What specifically can make piercing safer?
   c. List 10 risks related to body piercing.

CRITICAL THINKING: WHAT WOULD YOU DO?

1. You have the opportunity to talk with a group of 16-year-old girls. The topics you have decided to focus on during this talk are breast self-examination and Pap smears.
   a. What are the reasons adolescent girls should do breast self-examinations and have routine Pap smears?
   b. What steps will you suggest these girls follow when doing breast self-examinations?
   c. What areas of concern would you anticipate these girls would have regarding breast self-examinations and Pap smears?
   d. What would your responses to these concerns be?

2. Jamal is an adolescent athlete. He has told you he is planning to use a carbohydrate-loading diet before a big track meet.

   a. What reasons do you think Jamal will give you for wanting to follow this diet before his track meet?

   b. What concerns would you share with Jamal about his plan?

   c. What alternate suggestions and guidance could you offer to Jamal that would be more appropriate for him to follow?

3. Fifteen-year-old Caitlin is in a group discussing condom use. She scornfully tells you that girls don't need to know anything about condoms.

   a. How would you respond to Caitlin?

   b. What are your ideas regarding what you think should and should not be part of health education in high school settings?

   c. What are your rationales for your ideas?

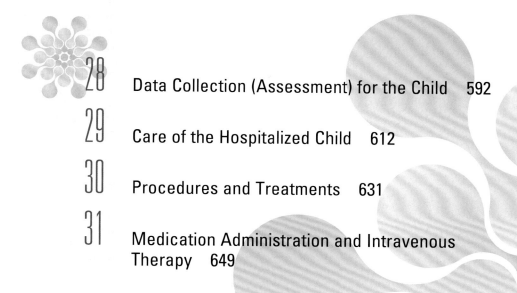

UNIT 8
Foundations of Pediatric Nursing

28

Data Collection (Assessment) for the Child

Learning Objectives

At the conclusion of this chapter, you will:

1. Describe the process for collecting subjective data from family caregivers and children.
2. Discuss what should be included when obtaining a client history.
3. Define chief complaint.
4. Explain the purpose of doing a review of systems when gathering data.
5. State how the family caregiver may be involved in the collection of objective data regarding the child.
6. Discuss how the collection of objective data regarding general appearance, psychological status, and behavior provides indicators of health or illness in children.
7. Discuss the reasons height, weight, and head circumference are measured on an ongoing basis.
8. Discuss the appropriate use of growth charts.
9. Explain the purpose and processes for obtaining vital signs, including (a) temperature, (b) pulse, (c) respirations, and (d) blood pressure.
10. List the types of clients on whom a rectal temperature should not be taken.
11. Identify the five types of respiratory retractions and the location of each.
12. State the purpose of pulse oximetry.
13. Describe the components of a physical examination.
14. Identify the purpose of using the Glasgow Coma Scale for neurologic assessment.

Isabella Daniels is 4½ years old and comes to the clinic with her mother Suzanne for her prekindergarten health examination. Suzanne tells you that she overheard Isabella talking with some of her friends about this examination and although she is excited about going to kindergarten, she told her friends she was afraid to have her "before-school checkup." As you read this chapter, think about the data you will be collecting during Isabella's visit. Review Chapter 25 and keep in mind Isabella's stage of growth and development.

Whether the setting is a hospital or other healthcare facility, it is important to gather information regarding the child's history and current status. Although data collection is continuous throughout a child's care, most data are collected during the interview, from the physical examination, and from the results of diagnostic tests and studies.

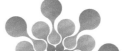

COLLECTING SUBJECTIVE DATA

Information spoken by the child or family is called *subjective data.* Interviewing the family caregiver and the child allows you to collect information that can be used to develop a plan of care for the child. Communicating with the child and the family caregiver requires knowledge of growth and development and an understanding of communication techniques (see Chapter 22).

Conducting the Client Interview

Most subjective data are collected through interviewing the family caregiver and the child. The interview helps you establish relationships with the child and the family. Listening and using appropriate communication techniques help promote a good interview (see Chapter 22). Using focused questions and allowing time for answering help the child and family feel comfortable. A private, quiet setting decreases distractions during the interview.

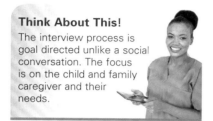

Think About This!
The interview process is goal directed unlike a social conversation. The focus is on the child and family caregiver and their needs.

When entering the room, knock on the door and wait for a response, the child may be playing on the other side of the door, thus potentially causing injury as you open the door. Introduce yourself to the child and family caregiver, and state the purpose of the interview. A calm, reassuring manner helps establish trust and comfort. Past experiences with healthcare may influence the interview. The family caregiver and the interviewer should be comfortably seated, and the child should be included in the interview process (Fig. 28-1). The child may sit on the caregiver's lap or, if a crib is available, the child can be placed in the crib with the side rails up. This positioning will help to ensure the safety of the infant or child during the interview. Maintain eye contact, face the child and family caregiver as much as possible, and offer your undivided attention.

Remember to Look!
Computers and electronic devices are often used to enter data collected during the interview process. Eye contact and acknowledging the child and family caregiver are especially valuable, even when using a device, to help establish a positive relationship.

Interviewing Family Caregivers

The family caregiver provides most of the information needed in caring for the child, especially the infant or toddler. Rather than simply asking the caregiver to fill out a form, it may be helpful to ask the questions and write down the answers; this process gives the opportunity to observe the reactions of the child and the caregiver as they interact with each other and answer the questions. In addition, this approach eases the problem of the family caregiver who cannot read or write. It is important to be nonjudgmental, being

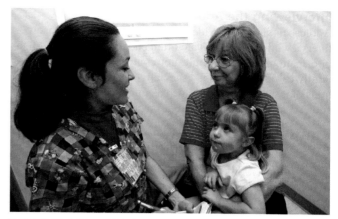

FIGURE 28-1 The child sits on the family caregiver's lap during the interview process.

careful not to indicate disapproval by verbal or nonverbal responses. While gathering information about the child's physical condition, allow the caregiver to express concerns and anxieties. If a certain topic seems uncomfortable for the family caregiver to discuss in front of the child, discuss that topic later when the child cannot hear what is being said.

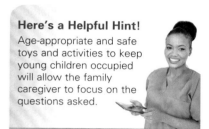

Here's a Helpful Hint!
Age-appropriate and safe toys and activities to keep young children occupied will allow the family caregiver to focus on the questions asked.

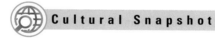

Cultural Snapshot

Be aware of the primary language spoken, and use an interpreter when needed to help in gaining accurate information. It is important to note and respect various cultural patterns, such as avoiding eye contact.

Interviewing the Child

Include the preschool child and the older child in the interview. Use age-appropriate questions when talking with the child. Showing interest in the child and what they say helps both the child and the family caregiver feel comfortable. Being honest when answering the child's questions helps establish trust with the child. Using stories or books written at a child's level helps with understanding what the child is thinking or feeling. Listen attentively to the child's comments, and make the child feel important in the interview.

Check Out This Tip!
Using a doll or a stuffed animal that the child is familiar with can help involve the child in the interview process.

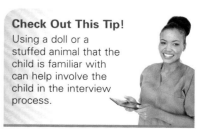

Interviewing the Adolescent

Adolescents can provide information about themselves. Interviewing them in private often encourages them to share information that they might not contribute in front of their family caregivers. This is especially true when asking questions of a sensitive nature, such as information regarding the adolescent's drug use or sexual practices.

> ### TEST YOURSELF
>
> ✔ Define subjective data. How are subjective data collected?
>
> ✔ Why is it important to interview the family caregiver when caring for children?
>
> ✔ In what ways does interviewing the adolescent differ from interviewing the child?

After reviewing common aspects of **Isabella's** stage of growth and development, what did you determine about how you can best gather data from Isabella? What are some things you can do to be supportive of Isabella through her prekindergarten examination? What are some things you think Isabella might be afraid of regarding her exam?

Obtaining a Client History

When a child arrives in any healthcare setting, it is important to gather information regarding the child's current condition, as well as past medical history. This information is used to develop a plan of care for the child. In obtaining information from the child and the family caregiver, you are developing a relationship, as well as noting what the child and family know and understand about the child's health. Observations of the caregiver–child relationship can also provide important information.

Biographical Data

To begin obtaining a client history, collect and record identifying information about the child, including the child's name, address, and phone number, as well as information about the family caregiver. This information is part of the legal record and should be treated as confidential. A questionnaire often is used to gather information, such as the child's nickname, feeding habits, food likes and dislikes, allergies, sleeping schedule, and toilet-training status (Fig. 28-2). Any special words the child uses or understands to indicate needs or desires, such as words used for urinating and bowel movements, are included on the questionnaire.

Chief Complaint

The reason for the child's visit to the healthcare setting is called the **chief complaint**. In a well-child setting, this reason might be a routine check or immunizations, whereas an illness or other condition might be the reason in another setting. The family caregiver's primary concern is their reason for seeking healthcare for the child. To best care for the child, it is important to get the most complete explanation of what brought the child to the healthcare setting. Repeating the family caregiver's statement regarding the child's chief complaint helps ensure a correct understanding of what the caregiver has said.

History of Present Health Concern

To help discover the child's needs, elicit information about the current situation, including the child's symptoms, when they began, how long the symptoms have been present, a description of the symptoms, their intensity and frequency, and treatments to this time. Ask questions in a way that encourages the family caregiver to be specific. This is also the time to ask the caregiver about any other concerns regarding the child.

Health History

Information regarding the mother's pregnancy and prenatal history is included in a health history for the child. Any occurrences during the delivery can contribute to the child's health concerns. The child's primary caregiver is usually the best source of this information. Other areas to ask questions about include common childhood, serious, or chronic illnesses; immunizations and health maintenance; feeding and nutrition; as well as hospitalizations and injuries.

Family Health History

Some diseases and conditions are seen in families and are important areas for prevention, as well as detection, for the child. The caregiver can usually provide information regarding family health history. Use this information to do preventative reinforcement teaching with the child and family. Certain risk factors in families contribute to the development of healthcare concerns; monitoring or changing risk factors early in a child's life can decrease the child's risk of getting these diseases or conditions.

> ### TEST YOURSELF
>
> ✔ Why is it important to collect biographical data when developing a plan of care for a child?
>
> ✔ Explain what is meant by the "chief complaint."
>
> ✔ What are the reasons it is important to ask about a child's present, past, and family health history?

Review of Systems for Current Health Problem

While collecting subjective data, ask the family caregiver or child questions about each body system. Gathering this information helps focus the physical examination and get an overall picture of the child's current status. Review the body system involved in the chief complaint in detail. As other body

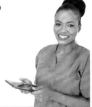

Pay Attention to the Details!

Using a head-to-toe approach is an organized way to gather subjective data.

PEDIATRIC NURSING ASSESSMENT FORM

1. Name _____ Date/Time of Admission _____ Via _____
2. Birth Date _____ Information obtained from:_____ Relationship to child _____
3. Child's legal guardian: _____ Child's Nickname: _____

VITAL SIGNS	Temp	Apical Pulse	Radial Pulse	Respirations	BP	Height	Weight	Head Circum

CURRENT CHIEF COMPLAINT/DIAGNOSIS:
Symptoms and Duration

Child's/Caregivers' Understanding of Condition:

PREVIOUS ILLNESS/INJURIES/DIAGNOSIS:
Illness, Symptoms, and Duration

Injuries or Surgery:

Anesthesia Complications?

Allergies and Reactions:	Immunizations	Dates:	Exposure to Infectious Disease	Date
	DTaP (DT)		(chicken pox, measles, etc.)	
	Polio			
	Hepatitis B			
	Hib (type)			
	MMR (measles, mumps, rubella)			
	TB skin test Result			

Medications: Name:	Dose	Frequency	Time of Last Dose

Child's reaction to previous hospitalizations: _____

Special fears of child about hospitalization? _____

Family History: (Check all that apply—indicate relationship to child)

_____ Cancer _____   _____ Seizures _____   _____ TB _____
_____ Heart disease _____   _____ Asthma _____   _____ Anesthesia complications_____
_____ Allergy _____   _____ Smoking _____   _____ Other (specify) _____
_____ Diabetes _____   _____ Hypertension _____

FIGURE 28-2 A sample pediatric nursing assessment form. *(continued)*

Living Facilities (check)

_____ House _____ Apartment _____ Trailer _____ Steps to travel?_____

Who does child live with? _____

Names, ages, of siblings in home_____

Names, ages of other children in home _____

Other persons in home _____

Special interests, toys, games, hobbies: _____

_____

Security object:_____ Was it brought to hospital? _____

Bowel/Bladder Habits:

Toilet Training(if applicable)

Started	_____ Yes	_____ No
Completed	_____ Yes	_____ No

Diapers:

Day	_____ Yes	_____ No
Night	_____ Yes	_____ No

Potty Chair:	_____ Yes	_____ No
Toilet:	_____ Yes	_____ No
Bedwetter:	_____ Yes	_____ No

Terms Used for:

Bowel Movement _____ Urination _____

Frequency of BM _____ Color _____ Consistency _____
Does child have problems with diarrhea or constipation?_____
_____

Does child have urinary frequency, burning, discomfort: _____ Yes _____ No
If yes, please explain:_____
_____
_____

Patterns of:

Sleep/rest:

Bedtime_____ Wakeup _____
Nap _____ Yes _____ No — When? _____

Activity:

Does infant roll over? _____
Does child stand/walk? _____
Does child climb? _____
Does child dress self? _____
Does child go up and down stairs? _____
Does child talk in formed sentences? _____

Eating Habits:

Does child: Feed self _____ Yes _____ No
Does child need help to eat? _____
Food and beverage:

Likes:_____
_____

Dislikes: _____
_____

Usual appetite? _____
Appetite now? _____
Last time child had food or beverage: _____

Items brought to hospital:

Glasses	_____ Yes	_____ No
Contacts	_____ Yes	_____ No
Hearing Aid	_____ Yes	_____ No
Dentures	_____ Yes	_____ No
Braces	_____ Yes	_____ No
Retainer	_____ Yes	_____ No

Special bottle	_____ Yes	_____ No
Own pacifier	_____ Yes	_____ No

Does child smoke or drink alcoholic beverages? _____ Yes _____ No
If yes, please give details _____

Does child use street drugs? _____ Yes _____ No
If yes, please give details_____
_____

Other behavior habits of the child (Please check)

Thumbsucking _____ ; Nailbiting _____ ; Headbanging _____
Rituals (Explain) _____
_____

Disposition (Describe)_____
_____

Skin Assessment:

_____ Jaundice _____ Cyanosis _____ Pallor _____ Redness
_____ Cool _____ Warm _____ Clammy _____ Dry
_____ Normal appearance

Describe: (Location and character)

Rash _____
Abrasions _____
Lacerations _____
Contusions _____

Respiratory Assessment:

_____ Clear _____ Stridor _____ Rales (___moist, ___ dry) _____ Wheezing
_____ Rhonchi _____ Retractions (type) _____
_____ Coughing, Sneezing _____ Nasal Discharge (describe) _____

Child/Caregiver oriented to unit? _____ Yes _____ No; understanding verbalized by child _____, caregiver _____
Reviewed safety measures with child _____, caregiver _____; understanding verbalized by child _____, caregiver _____
Additional information nursing staff should know:

FIGURE 28-2 _(Continued)_

TABLE 28-1 Review of Systems

AREAS TO BE REVIEWED	DATA TO BE NOTED
General	Calm, nervous, shy Weight gain or loss, over/underweight, malnourished Appearance—normal, ill-looking, neat, disheveled Activity—alert, active, sedate, fatigued Behavior—happy, sad, irritable
Skin	Itching, dryness, rash, color change, bruising
Head and neck	Headache, dizziness, injury, stiff neck, swollen neck glands
Eyes and vision	Drainage, pain, trouble focusing, reading, or seeing, rubbing, redness
Ears and hearing	Pulling, pain, drainage, difficulty hearing
Nose, mouth, throat	Nosebleeds, drainage, trouble breathing, nasal congestion, swollen gums, toothache, sore throat, trouble chewing, swallowing
Chest and lungs—respiratory	Coughing, wheezing, shortness of breath, pain, snoring, sputum, breast development
Heart—cardiovascular	Cyanosis, fatigue, anemia, heart murmurs
Abdomen—gastrointestinal	Nausea, vomiting, pain, cramping Increased thirst, appetite changes
Genitalia and rectum	Pain or burning when voiding, blood in urine or stool, constipation, diarrhea Males—undescended testicles, genital sores, discharge Females—vaginal discharge, itching, rash
Back and extremities—musculoskeletal	Back—stiffness, pain, posture, spinal curvatures Extremities—pain, difficult movement, swollen joints, broken bones, muscle sprains
Neurologic	Numbness, tingling, seizures, loss of consciousness, altered mood Cry—hardy, weak, listless, high-pitched

systems are discussed, reassure the family caregiver that the chief complaint has not been forgotten or ignored. Table 28-1 lists areas to be reviewed and data to be noted in doing a review of the body systems.

Allergies, Medications, and Substance Abuse

Discuss allergic reactions to any foods, medications, or any other known allergies to prevent the child being given any medications or substances that might cause an allergic reaction. Record medications the child is taking or has taken, whether prescribed by a health care provider or over the counter. This information will help avoid the possibility of overmedicating or causing drug interactions. It is important, especially with the adolescent, to gather information about the use of substances, such as tobacco, alcohol, or illegal drugs (substance abuse is discussed in Chapters 27 and 42).

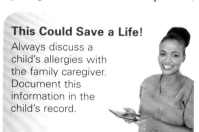

This Could Save a Life!
Always discuss a child's allergies with the family caregiver. Document this information in the child's record.

Lifestyle

School history includes information regarding the child's current grade level and academic performance, as well as behavior at school. The child's interactions with teachers and peers often give insight into areas of concern that might affect the child's health.

Social history offers information about the child's environment, including the home setting, family caregivers' occupations, siblings, family pets, religious affiliations, and economic factors. The people who live in the home and those who care for the child are important data, especially in cases of separation, divorce, and other living situations.

Personal history relates to data collected about such things as the child's hygiene, sleeping, and elimination patterns. Activities, exercise, special interests, and the child's favorite toys or objects are included. Questions about relationships and how the child emotionally handles certain situations can help in understanding the child. Discuss any behaviors such as thumb sucking, nail biting, or temper tantrums.

Nutrition history of the child includes information regarding eating habits and preferences, as well as nutrition concerns that might indicate illness.

Developmental Level

To gather information about the child's developmental level, ask questions directly related to growth and development milestones. These milestones are discussed in detail in the growth and development chapters (Chapters 23 to 27) of this text. Knowing normal development patterns will help you determine if there are concerns that should be explored further regarding the child's development.

COLLECTING OBJECTIVE DATA

Information you observe directly is called *objective data*. Objective data to collect include baseline measurements of the child's height, weight, temperature, pulse, respiration, and blood pressure. Data are also collected by examination of the body systems. Often the physical examination for a child does not proceed in a head-to-toe manner as in adults but rather in an order that takes the child's age and developmental needs into consideration. Aspects of the examination that might be more traumatic or uncomfortable for the child are done last.

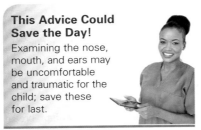

This Advice Could Save the Day!
Examining the nose, mouth, and ears may be uncomfortable and traumatic for the child; save these for last.

The procedure of the physical examination may be familiar from previous healthcare visits. If comfortable with helping, the family caregiver may help with the data collection. For example, the caregiver might help take a young child's temperature and obtain a urine specimen. Arrangements should be made so that the family caregiver may also be present, if possible, for tests or examinations that need to be performed. Included in this initial examination is an inspection of the child's body. Respect the child's privacy and allow them to be covered until each specific part of their body is examined. Record all observations and carefully describe in detail any finding that is not within normal limits.

Conduct or assist in conducting a complete physical examination with special attention to any symptoms that the family caregiver has identified. As the practical/vocational nurse, your primary role in the examination may be to support the child. All the information gathered is used to plan the child's care.

TEST YOURSELF

✔ What approach is used to do a review of systems in a child? Why is this approach used?

✔ What is included when collecting information about the child's lifestyle?

✔ Define objective data. How are objective data collected?

Noting General Status

Use knowledge of normal growth and development to note if the child appears to fit the characteristics of the stated age. Interactions the child has with family caregivers and siblings provide information about these relationships. Note the child's overall general appearance, facial expressions, speech, and behavior as you begin collecting information about the child.

General Appearance

Observing physical appearance and condition can give clues to the child's overall health. The infant or child's face and body should be symmetrical (i.e., well balanced). Observations provide information related to nutritional status, hygiene, mental alertness, and body posture and movements. Examine the skin for color, lesions, bruises, scars, and birthmarks. Observe hair texture, thickness, and distribution.

Psychological Status and Behavior

Carefully observing the child's behavior and recording those observations provide vital clues to a child's condition. When recording observed behavior, include factors that influence the behavior and how often the behavior is repeated. Note physical behavior as well as emotional and intellectual responses. Behavior may depend on the child's age and developmental level, the abnormal environment of the healthcare facility, and whether the child has been hospitalized previously, or otherwise separated from family caregivers. Note if the behavior is consistent or unpredictable and any apparent reasons for changed behavior.

Observation of the infant's behavior is critical because infants cannot articulate information regarding their health status. Table 28-2 compares characteristic behaviors of the healthy infant with behaviors that may indicate signs of illness. Be cautious when using the type of information shown in such a table because occasional evidence of one or more of the behaviors may not be significant.

Any instance of behavior indicating illness needs to be documented and further evaluated in light of the behavior frequency, as well as the child's usual behavior. If the family caregiver indicates in the interview or on further questioning that this behavior is not out of the ordinary for the child, it may not be indicative of a problem.

Measuring Weight, Height, and Length

The child's weight, height, and length are helpful indicators of growth and development. These should be measured and recorded each time the child has a routine physical examination, as well as at other healthcare visits. These measurements must be charted and compared with norms for the child's age (see Appendix E). Plotting the child's growth on a growth chart gives a good indication of the child's health status. This process gives a picture of how the child is progressing and often indicates wellness. Although the charts are indicators, the size of other family members, the child's illnesses, general nutritional status, and developmental milestones must also be considered.

In a hospital setting, weigh the infant or child at the same time each day on the same scales in the same amount of clothing. The scale should be calibrated and set to the zero "0" position before starting the procedure. The young child is weighed nude. The infant is weighed lying on an infant scale; the toddler who is able to sit can be weighed while sitting (Fig. 28-3A,B). Keep a hand within 1 inch of the child at all times to be ready

TABLE 28-2 Comparison of Observations of an Infant's Physical and Emotional Behavior

OBSERVATION	HEALTHY ACTIVITY	BEHAVIOR INDICATING ILLNESS[a]
Activity	Constantly active; some infants are more intense and curious than others	Lies quietly; little or no interest in surroundings; may stay in the same position
State of muscular tension	Muscular state is tense; grasp is tight; head is raised when prone; kicks are vigorous When supine, there is a space between the mattress and the infant's back	Lies relaxed with arms and legs straight and lax; makes no attempt to turn or raise head if placed in prone position; does not move about in crib
Constancy of reaction	Shows a constancy in reaction; does not regress in development; peppy and vigorous; interested in food; responds to family caregiver's presence or voice	Not as peppy as usual; responds to discomfort and pain in apathetic manner; turns away from food that had once caused interest; turns head and cries instead of usual response
Behavior indicating pain	Appreciates being picked up Activity is not restlessness Shows activity in every part of body	Cries or protests when handled; seems to want to be left alone. May cry when picked up, but settles down after being held for a time, indicating something hurts when moved Turns head fretfully from side to side; pulls ear or rubs head; turns and rolls constantly, seemingly to try to get away from pain
Cry	Strong, vigorous cry	Weak, feeble cry or whimper High-pitched cry; shrill cry may indicate increased intracranial pressure
Skin color	Healthy tint to skin; nail beds, oral mucosa, conjunctiva, and tongue are reddish-pink	Light-skinned babies may show unusual pallor or blueness around the eyes and nose. All babies may have dark or cyanotic nail beds; pale oral mucosa, conjunctiva, and tongue
Appetite or feeding pattern	Exhibits an eagerness and impatience to satisfy hunger	May show indifference toward formula; sucks half-heartedly; vomits feeding; habitually regurgitates. May exhibit discomfort after feeding
Bizarre behavior		Any behavior that differs from expected for level of development; unusually good, or passive when in strange surroundings; responds with rejection to every overture, friendly or otherwise; extremely clinging, never satisfied with amount of attention received

[a]Any *one* manifestation in itself may not be significant. The important thing is whether this behavior is consistent with this particular child or is a change from previous behavior. The significance depends greatly on the constancy of the behavior.

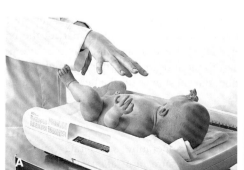 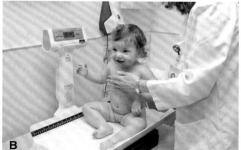 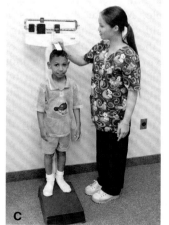

FIGURE 28-3 The nurse keeps a hand close while weighing **(A)** the infant or **(B)** the toddler. **C.** The nurse measures the older child for height and weight on a standing scale.

NURSING PROCEDURE 28-1 Weighing the Infant or Child

EQUIPMENT
Scale appropriate for child's age and ability to sit or stand
Disposable paper covering for scale
Paper and pen to record weight
Cleaning and disinfecting solution and equipment, according to facility policy

PROCEDURE
1. Explain procedure to the child and family caregiver.
2. Perform hand hygiene.
3. Place paper on scale.
4. Balance scale to a reading of "0."
5. Weigh the hospitalized child at the same time, using same scale, and same amount of clothing each time the child is weighed.
6. Weigh infant with no clothing, older child in underwear or lightweight gown; child should not wear shoes.
7. *Always* hold one hand within 1 inch of the child for safety.
8. Read the weight on the scale.
9. Record the weight on a paper to be transferred to permanent document.
10. Pick up the child or have older child step off scale.
11. Remove and discard paper scale cover.
12. Perform hand hygiene.
13. Clean and disinfect the scale according to the facility's policy.
14. Report weight as appropriate.

---

to protect the child from injury. Cover the scale with a clean sheet of examination paper as a means of infection control (Nursing Procedure 28-1). A child who can stand alone steadily is weighed without shoes on platform-type scales. Bed scales may be used if the child cannot get out of bed. If an infant or toddler scale is not available or the child is extremely active or fearful, a less accurate method of weighing the child is to weight the caregiver alone, then have the caregiver hold the child and record the weight of both of them. Subtract the weight of the caregiver alone from the weight of them together to get the child's weight measurement. Record weights in grams and kilograms or pounds and ounces.

The child who can stand is usually measured for height at the same time. The standing scales have a useful, adjustable measuring device (Fig. 28-3C). To measure the length of a child who is not able to stand alone steadily, usually younger than the age of about 2, place the child flat with the knees held flat on an examining table. Measure the child's length by straightening the child's body and measuring from the top of the head to the bottom of the foot. Sometimes examining tables have a measuring device mounted along the side of the table or have a measuring board attached (Fig. 28-4). If using a measuring board, place the child's head at the top of the board and the heels against the footboard. If not using a measuring device, make marks on the paper table covering and then measure between the marks. Record height or length in centimeters or inches according to the practice of the healthcare facility; it is important to know which measuring system is used.

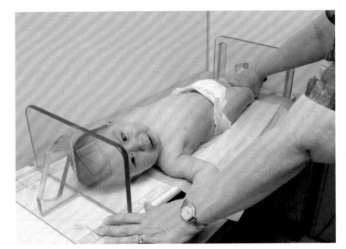

FIGURE 28-4 The measuring board is the most accurate method for obtaining the length of the infant or toddler.

Measuring Head Circumference
The head circumference is measured routinely in children up to the age of 3 years or in any child with a neurologic or developmental concern. Place a paper or plastic tape measure around the largest part of the head, just above the eyebrows, and around the most prominent part of the back of the head (Fig. 28-5). Record and plot this measurement on a growth chart to monitor the growth of the child's head. During childhood, the chest exceeds the head circumference by 2 to 3 inches.

Taking Vital Signs
Vital signs, including temperature, heart rate (pulse), respirations, and blood pressure, are taken at each visit and compared with the normal values for children of the same age, as well as to that child's previous recordings. In a hospital setting, closely monitor and record the vital signs, and report any changes. Keep in mind the child's developmental needs to increase your ability to take accurate vital sign

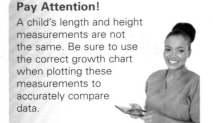

Pay Attention!
A child's length and height measurements are not the same. Be sure to use the correct growth chart when plotting these measurements to accurately compare data.

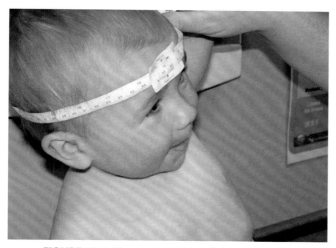

FIGURE 28-5 Measuring the head circumference.

measurements. It is usually less traumatic for the infant to count the respirations before disturbing the child and to then take the pulse and the temperature.

 A Personal Glimpse

I am 11 years old, and I have already been in the hospital for four surgeries. I think I could be a nurse. One time a student nurse and her teacher came to do my vital signs. The teacher left, and the student, named Joan, told me I was her first patient ever. She tried three of those electronic thermometers to take my temperature, but she said they were all broken. Then she tried to take my blood pressure with the blood pressure machine and she said it was broken. Then she used another blood pressure cuff, and this time she put it on backward. I knew it was wrong, but I just let her pump it up and up until it exploded off my arm. I laughed, but she almost cried. I showed her how to do it right, and she seemed pretty glad that she finally got it to work. I was kind of happy when she left because I didn't know if I could teach her everything. A little while later, she came back with her teacher and the teacher said, "Joan is going to give you your shot." "Uh oh!" I thought, "Here comes trouble." I just held my breath and hoped she wouldn't do that wrong too. It wasn't too bad. Later, before she went home, she brought me a pear. I am pretty sure she was relieved the day was over, and I was too.

Abigail, age 11 years

Learning Opportunity: What could this student nurse have done to be better prepared to take care of this child? What feelings do you think this child might have had when the nurse came in with the medication?

Temperature

The method of measuring a child's temperature is commonly set by the policy of the healthcare setting. The temperature can be measured by the oral, tympanic, temporal, rectal, or axillary method. Temperatures are recorded in Celsius or Fahrenheit, according to the policy of the healthcare facility. A normal oral temperature range is 97.6°F to 99.3°F (36.4°C to 37.4°C). A rectal temperature is usually 0.5°F to 1°F higher than the oral measurement. An axillary temperature usually measures 0.5°F to 1°F lower than the oral measurement. The temperature measurement taken by the tympanic method is in the same range as the oral method. Report any deviation from the normal range of temperature.

Accurately Document!
Temperatures vary according to the method by which they are taken, so it is important to record the method of temperature measurement, as well as the measured temperature.

Electronic thermometers have oral and rectal probes. Be careful to select the correct probe when using the thermometer. Mercury thermometers have been replaced by mercury-free glass thermometers, electronic, tympanic membrane, and digital devices, which accurately measure temperatures.

Be Alert for Patient Safety!
Some caregivers might still have a mercury thermometer at home. Advise them to replace it with a nonmercury thermometer, which can be easily purchased at many pharmacies or super stores.

Oral Temperatures

Oral temperatures are usually taken only on children older than 4 to 6 years of age who are conscious and cooperative. Place oral thermometers under the tongue, toward the side of the child's mouth. Do not leave the child unattended while any temperature is being taken. Recent intake of oral fluids and use of oxygen or nebulized medications can affect oral temperatures.

Tympanic Temperatures

Tympanic thermometers are now used in many healthcare settings (Fig. 28-6A). The tympanic thermometer records the temperature rapidly (registering in about 2 seconds), is noninvasive, and causes little disturbance to the child. A tympanic measurement often can be obtained without awakening a sleeping infant or child. Use tympanic thermometers according to the manufacturer's directions and the facility's policy. Use a disposable speculum for each child.

Temporal Temperatures

The temporal method of measuring temperature in the child uses an infrared sensor probe, which is scanned across the skin on the forehead (Fig. 28-6B). The sensor measures heat from blood flow in the temporal artery. This noninvasive procedure is often used as a screening tool and to detect rapid temperature changes. Sweating can affect the accuracy of the measurement.

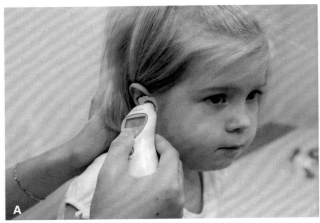
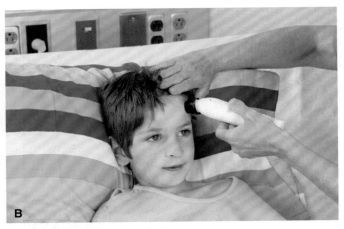
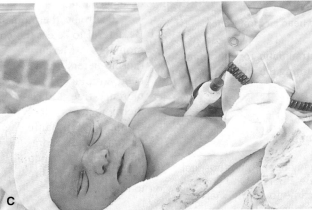

FIGURE 28-6 **A.** Many facilities use a tympanic thermometer sensor to take the child's temperature. **B.** Temporal thermometers are noninvasive and used on the child. **C.** Taking an axillary temperature on a newborn. (Photo © B. Proud.)

Rectal Temperatures

Rectal temperatures may be taken in children but because they are invasive and uncomfortable, they are used only if another method cannot be used. They are not desirable in the newborn because of the danger of irritation to the rectal mucosa or in children who have had rectal surgery, are immunosuppressed, or who have diarrhea or a bleeding disorder. When taking a rectal temperature, lubricate the end of the thermometer with a water-soluble lubricant. Place the child in a prone position, gently separate the buttocks with one hand, and gently insert the thermometer about ½ to 1 inch into the rectum. If you feel any resistance, remove the thermometer immediately, take the temperature by some other method, and notify the health care provider about the resistance. Keep one hand on the child's buttocks and the other on the thermometer during the entire time the rectal thermometer is in place. Remove an electronic thermometer as soon as it signals a recorded temperature.

Axillary Temperatures

Axillary temperatures are taken on newborns and on infants and children when other methods for measuring the temperature are contraindicated. When taking an axillary temperature on an infant or a child, be certain to place the thermometer tip well into the armpit and bring the child's arm down close to the body (Fig. 28-6C). Check to see that there is skin-to-skin contact with no clothing in the way.

Leave the thermometer in place until the electronic thermometer signals.

Heart Rate

Counting an apical pulse is the preferred method to determine the heart rate in an infant or a young child. Try to accomplish this while the child is quiet.

Count the apical pulse before the child is disturbed for other procedures. A family caregiver can hold the child on their lap for security for the full minute that the pulse is counted. Place the stethoscope between the child's left nipple and sternum. On an older child, a radial pulse may be taken and counted for 30 seconds and multiplied by two. If a pulse is unusual in quality, rate, or rhythm, count it for a full minute. Report any rate that deviates from the normal rate. Heart rates vary with age: From 100 to 180 beats per minute for a newborn to 55 to 95 beats per minute for the adolescent (Table 28-3). Pulses can be palpated in various sites throughout the body including the carotid, apical, brachial, radial, femoral, popliteal, posterior tibial, and the dorsalis pedis arteries (see Fig. 28-12 for location of these sites).

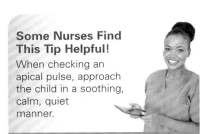

Some Nurses Find This Tip Helpful!
When checking an apical pulse, approach the child in a soothing, calm, quiet manner.

TABLE 28-3 Normal Pulse Ranges in Children

AGE	NORMAL RANGE (BPM)
Newborn	100–180
Infant	90–180
Toddler	80–140
Preschool-aged child	65–120
School-age	60–110
Adolescent	55–95

bpm, beats per minute.

Cardiac Monitors

Cardiac monitors are used to detect changes in cardiac function. Many of these monitors have a visual display of the cardiac actions. Electrodes must be placed properly to obtain accurate readings of the cardiac system. Cleanse the skin with soap and water or a skin preparation product to remove oil, dirt, lotions, and powder. Alarms are set to maximum and minimum settings above and below the child's resting heart rate. Check the electrode sites every 2 hours to detect any skin redness or irritation and to determine that the electrodes are secure. The child's cardiac status must be checked *immediately* when the alarm sounds. Sometimes the monitor used will monitor both cardiac and respiratory functions. Apnea monitors, which monitor respiratory function, are discussed later in this chapter.

Respirations

Respirations of an infant or a young child must also be counted during a quiet time. Observe the child while they are lying or sitting quietly. Infants are abdominal breathers; therefore, observe the movement of the infant's abdomen to count respirations. Observe the older child's chest, much as you would an adult's. The infant's respirations must be counted for a full minute because of normal irregularity. Observe the chest of the infant or young child for retractions that indicate respiratory distress. Note retractions as

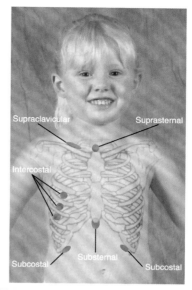

FIGURE 28-7 Sites of respiratory retraction.

supraclavicular (above the clavicle), suprasternal (above the sternum), intercostal (between the ribs), substernal (below the sternum), or subcostal (below the ribs) (Fig. 28-7).

Pulse Oximetry

Pulse oximetry measures the oxygen saturation of arterial hemoglobin. The probe of the oximetry unit can be placed on the finger, toe, or clipped on the ear lobe. In an infant, the foot or toe is often used (Fig. 28-8). Take the pulse oximetry and record it with other vital signs. In certain situations, the probe is left in place to continually monitor the oxygen saturation. Check the site every 2 hours to ensure that the probe is secure and tissue perfusion is adequate. Change the site at least every 4 hours to prevent skin irritation. Alarms can be set to sound when oxygen saturation registers lower than a predetermined limit. At the beginning of each shift and after transport of the patient, check that alarms are accurately set and have not been inadvertently changed. This is true for all types of monitors.

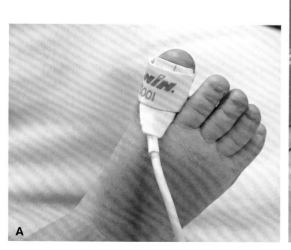

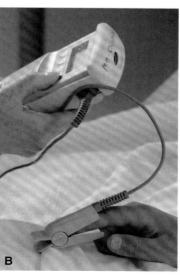

FIGURE 28-8 The pulse oximetry sensor measuring the oxygen saturation in the **(A)** infant and the **(B)** older child.

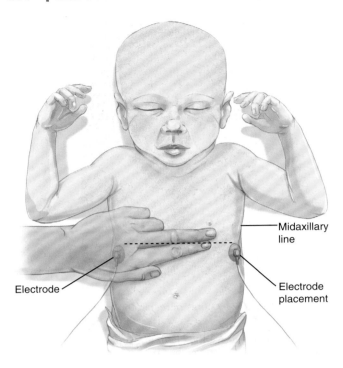

FIGURE 28-9 Placement of electrodes for apnea monitoring. Electrodes are placed two fingerbreadths below the nipple.

Apnea Monitor

An apnea monitor detects the infant's respiratory movement. Place the electrodes or belt on the infant's chest where the greatest amount of respiratory movement is detected; the electrodes are attached to the monitor by a cable (Fig. 28-9). Set the limits on the alarm to sound when the infant does not breathe for a predetermined number of seconds.

Warning, Be Alert for Patient Safety!

Respond *immediately* when the alarm on the apnea monitor sounds. The child must be observed to determine what caused the alarm to sound.

These monitors can be used in a hospital setting and may be used in the home for an infant who is at risk for apnea, respiratory failure, or who has a tracheostomy. Family caregivers learn to stimulate the infant when the monitor sounds and to perform cardiopulmonary resuscitation if the infant does not begin breathing.

Blood Pressure

For children 3 years of age and older, blood pressure monitoring is part of routine and ongoing data collection. Obtaining an accurate blood pressure in a child younger than 3 years of age is difficult and usually only done if the child has a risk factor for a condition such as heart or renal disease. Take a baseline blood pressure for a child who presents to a healthcare facility. Explain the procedure to the child in terms the young child can understand. First taking a blood pressure on a stuffed animal or a doll will further show the child the procedure is not to be feared.

Obtaining a blood pressure measurement in an infant or a small child is difficult, but the equipment of the proper size helps ease the problem. The most common sites used to obtain a blood pressure reading in children are the upper arm, lower arm or forearm, thigh, and calf or ankle (Fig. 28-10). When the upper arm is used, the cuff should be wide enough to cover about two thirds of the upper arm and long enough to encircle the extremity without overlapping. If other sites are used, the size of the cuff is determined by the size of the extremity; a smaller cuff is used on the forearm, whereas a larger cuff is used on the thigh or calf.

Try This Approach!

Referring to the blood pressure cuff as "giving your arm a hug" will help explain taking the blood pressure.

A more accurate reading is obtained if the child has been resting in a quiet environment for several minutes before taking the blood pressure. Take the blood pressure by auscultation, palpation, or automated device (Doppler

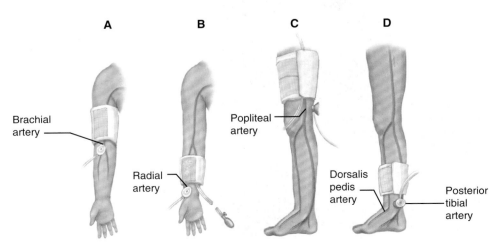

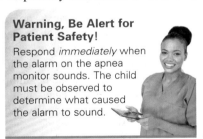

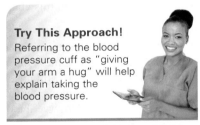

FIGURE 28-10 Various positions of cuff placement and auscultation site for obtaining blood pressure: **(A)** upper arm, **(B)** lower arm, **(C)** thigh, **(D)** calf/ankle.

NURSING PROCEDURE 28-2 Methods for Measuring Pediatric Blood Pressure

EQUIPMENT
Stethoscope, pediatric preferred
Blood pressure cuff, appropriate size for child
Wide enough to cover two thirds of child's upper arm
Long enough to encircle child's arm
Automated blood pressure device (Doppler or oscillometric)
Paper and pen to record blood pressure

PROCEDURE
1. Explain procedure to child and family caregiver.
2. Wash hands. Clean stethoscope bell with antiseptic wipe.
3. Allow child to handle equipment when appropriate.
4. Use terminology appropriate to child's age.
5. Encourage preschool- or school-aged child to use equipment to "take" blood pressure on a doll or a stuffed animal.
6. Record blood pressure on paper to be transferred to permanent document.
7. Report blood pressure as appropriate.

AUSCULTATION
1. Place the correct size of cuff on the infant's or child's bare arm.
2. Locate the artery by palpating the antecubital fossa.
3. Inflate the cuff until radial pulse disappears or about 30 mm Hg above expected systolic reading.
4. Place stethoscope lightly over the artery and slowly release air until pulse is heard.
5. Record readings as in adults.

PALPATION
1. Follow steps 1 and 2 above.
2. Keep the palpating finger over the artery and inflate the cuff as above.
3. The point at which the pulse is felt is recorded as the systolic pressure.

AUTOMATED BLOOD PRESSURE DEVICE (DOPPLER OR OSCILLOMETRIC)
1. Obtain the device, air hose, and proper size cuff.
2. If device is not on a mobile stand, be certain that it is placed on a firm surface.
3. Plug in device (unless battery operated) and attach hose if necessary.
4. Attach appropriate-size blood pressure cuff and wrap around child's limb. Stabilize extremity.
5. Turn on power switch. Record the reading.

TABLE 28-4 Normal Blood Pressure Ranges in Children (mm Hg)

AGE	SYSTOLIC (MM HG)	DIASTOLIC (MM HG)
Newborn	60–80	40–45
Infant	72–104	37–56
Toddler	86–106	42–63
Preschool-aged child	89–112	46–72
School-age	97–115	57–76
Adolescent	102–131	61–83

or oscillometric) methods (Nursing Procedure 28-2). The automated device method is used most often to monitor pediatric blood pressure. Check the blood pressure twice, at least 1 or 2 minutes apart. Normal blood pressure values gradually increase from infancy through adolescence (Table 28-4).

TEST YOURSELF
✔ How is comparing behaviors seen in a healthy child to behaviors that might indicate illness helpful in caring for the child?

✔ Why should weight and height or length be routinely measured and monitored in children?

✔ What is the purpose in doing pulse oximetry when obtaining vital signs?

✔ Describe the methods used to obtain a blood pressure measurement in a child.

Conducting or Assisting With a Physical Examination
Data are also collected by examining the body systems of the child. You may be responsible for performing the physical examination or assisting the health care provider in doing the physical examination.

Head and Neck
The head's general shape and movement should be observed. The features of the face and the head should have **symmetry** or balance. Observe the child's ability to control the head and the range of motion. To see full range of motion, ask the older child to move their head in all directions. Gently move the infant's head to observe for any stiffness in the neck. Feel the infant's skull to determine if the fontanels are open or closed and to check for any swelling or depression.

Eyes
Observe the eyes for symmetry and location in relationship to the nose. Note any redness, evidence of rubbing, or drainage. Observe pupils for equality, roundness, and reaction to light. When a light is quickly shined toward the eye, the pupil constricts. As the light is moved away, the pupil should expand. **Accommodation** occurs when the pupils constrict in order to bring an object into focus. When a bright object is held at a distance and then quickly moved toward the face, the pupil will constrict, and thus accommodate. Normal pupil reactions are recorded as PERRLA (pupils equal, round, react to light, and accommodation). Neurologic considerations are discussed later in this chapter. Routine vision screening occurs in school or clinic settings. Screening helps identify vision concerns in children; with early detection, appropriate visual aids can be provided.

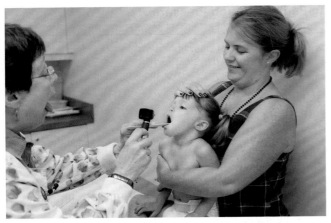

FIGURE 28-11 The young child may need to be gently restrained to safely observe the mouth and throat.

Ears

Note the alignment of the ears by drawing an imaginary line from the inner to the outer canthus of the eye and continuing past the ear; the top of the ear, known as the **pinna**, should be even with or above this line (see Fig. 13-8 in Chapter 13). Ears that are set low often indicate intellectual disability (see Chapter 35). Note the child's ability to hear during normal conversation. A child who speaks loudly, responds inappropriately, or does not speak clearly may have hearing difficulties that should be explored. Note any drainage or swelling.

Nose, Mouth, and Throat

The nose is in the middle of the face. If an imaginary line was drawn down the middle, both sides of the nose should be symmetrical. Flaring of the nostrils might indicate respiratory distress and should be reported immediately. Observe for swelling, drainage, or bleeding. To observe the mouth and throat, have the older child hold their mouth wide open and move the tongue from side to side. With the infant or toddler, use a tongue blade to see the mouth and throat. Gently place the tongue blade on the side of the tongue to hold it down (Fig. 28-11). A light will help visualize the mouth and throat. Observe the mucous membranes for color, moisture, and any patchy areas that might indicate infection. Observe the number and condition of the child's teeth. The lips should be moist and pink. Note any difficulty in swallowing.

Chest and Lungs

Chest measurements are done on infants and children to determine normal growth rate. Take the measurement at the nipple level with a tape measure. Observe the chest for size, shape, movement of the chest with breathing, and any retractions (see "Respirations" section in this chapter). In the older school-aged child or adolescent, note evidence of breast development. Evaluate respiratory rate, rhythm, and depth. Report any noisy or grunting respirations. Using a stethoscope, listen to breath sounds in each lobe of the lung, anterior and posterior, while the child inhales and exhales.

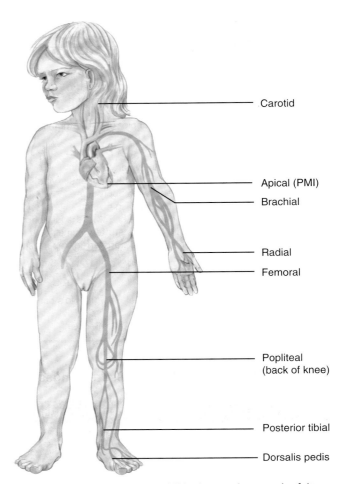

FIGURE 28-12 Sites in the child where pulses can be felt.

Describe, document, and report absent or diminished breath sounds, as well as unusual sounds, such as crackling or wheezing. If the child is coughing or bringing up sputum, record the frequency, color, and consistency of sputum.

Heart

In some infants and children, a pulsation can be seen in the chest that indicates the heartbeat. This point is called the **point of maximum impulse (PMI)**. This point is where the heartbeat can be heard the best with a stethoscope. Listen for the rhythm of the heart sounds, and count the rate for one full minute. Abnormal or unusual heart sounds or irregular rhythms might indicate the child has a heart murmur, heart condition, or other abnormality that should be reported. The heart is responsible for circulating blood to the body. Check the pulses in various parts of the body to determine the effectiveness of the heart function (Fig. 28-12). Other indicators of good cardiac function are included in this textbook's discussions of specific disorders.

Abdomen

The abdomen may protrude slightly in infants and small children. To describe the abdomen, divide the area into four sections, and label sections with the terms left upper quadrant (LUQ), left lower quadrant (LLQ), right upper quadrant (RUQ), and right lower quadrant (RLQ). Using a stethoscope, listen for bowel sounds or evidence of peristalsis in each section of the abdomen, and record what is heard. Observe the umbilicus for cleanliness and any abnormalities. Infants and young children sometimes have protrusions in the umbilicus or inguinal canal that are called hernias (see Chapter 21). Report a tense or firm abdomen or unusual tenderness.

Genitalia and Rectum

When inspecting the genitalia and rectum, it is important to respect the child's privacy and take into account the child's age and the stage of growth and development.

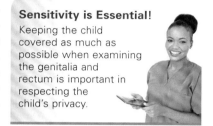

Sensitivity is Essential!
Keeping the child covered as much as possible when examining the genitalia and rectum is important in respecting the child's privacy.

While wearing gloves, inspect the genitalia and rectum. Observe the area for any sores or lesions, swelling, or discharge. In male children, the testes descend at varying times during childhood; if the testes cannot be palpated, report this information. Be aware that unusual findings, such as bruises in soft tissue, bruises with a clear outline of an object, or unexplained injuries, might indicate child abuse and should be further investigated (see Chapter 33).

Back and Extremities

Observe the back for symmetry and for the curvature of the spine. In infants, the spine is rounded and flexible. As the child grows and develops motor skills, the spine further develops. Screening is done in school-aged children to detect abnormal curvatures of the spine, such as scoliosis (see Chapter 40). Note gait and posture when the child enters or is walking in the room. The extremities should be warm, have good color, and be symmetrical. When observing the child's movements during the examination, note range of motion, movement of the joints, and muscle strength. In infants, examine the hips, and report any dislocation or asymmetry of gluteal skin folds. These could indicate a congenital hip dislocation (see Chapter 21).

Neurologic

Collecting data related to the neurologic status of the infant and child is the most complex aspect of the physical examination. All the body systems function in relationship to the nervous system. The health care provider in the healthcare setting assesses the neurologic status of the child by doing a complete neurologic examination. This examination includes detailed examination of the reflex responses as well as the functioning of each of the cranial nerves. The health care provider will perform a neurologic examination on a child after a head injury or seizure or on children who have metabolic conditions, such as diabetes, drug ingestion, severe hemorrhage, or dehydration, which might affect neurologic status. A neurologic assessment determines the level of the child's neurologic functioning.

As the nurse, when collecting data, you may be responsible for using neurologic assessment tool, such as the Glasgow Coma Scale, to monitor a child's neurologic status after the initial neurologic examination. The use of a standard scale for monitoring permits the comparison of results from one time to another and from one examiner to another. Use this tool to monitor various aspects of the child's neurologic functioning (Fig. 28-13). If a child is hospitalized with a neurologic concern, closely monitor the neurologic status, and use a neurologic assessment tool every 1 or 2 hours to observe for significant changes.

Assisting With Common Diagnostic Tests

Diagnostic tests and studies often are done to further evaluate the subjective and objective data collected. These diagnostic tests help the health care provider to more clearly determine the nature of the child's concern. The needs of the infant or child during these studies vary greatly from child to child. The role of the nurse in assisting with common diagnostic tests is discussed in Chapter 30.

TEST YOURSELF

✔ Explain the term symmetry and the importance of observing for symmetry when doing a physical examination on a child.

✔ What does the term *PMI* mean, and how does it relate to the physical examination in children?

✔ What is included when doing a neurologic examination on a child?

You have now completed collecting data during **Isabella Daniels's** prekindergarten examination. What subjective and objective data were gathered? As Isabella's nurse during this visit, what data did you collect, and how did you support Isabella? How did you relieve her fears as you gathered data?

GLASGOW COMA SCALES			MODIFIED COMA SCALE FOR INFANTS		
ACTIVITY	**BEST RESPONSE**		**ACTIVITY**	**BEST RESPONSE**	
Eye Opening	Spontaneous	4	Eye Opening	Spontaneous	4
	To speech	3		To speech	3
	To pain	2		To pain	2
	None	1		None	1
Verbal	Oriented	5	Verbal	Coos, babbles	5
	Confused	4		Irritable	4
	Inappropriate words	3		Cries to pain	3
	Nonspecific sounds	2		Moans to pain	2
	None	1		None	1
Motor	Follows commands	6	Motor	Normal spontaneous movements	6
	Localizes pain	5		Withdraws to touch	5
	Withdraws to pain	4		Withdraws to pain	4
	Abnormal flexion	3		Abnormal flexion	3
	Extend	2		Abnormal extension	2
	None	1		None	1

PUPIL SIZE:

6 mm ⬤ 5 mm ⬤ 4 mm ⬤

3 mm ● 2 mm · 1 mm ·

REACTION: **N**–normal, **S**–sluggish, **F**–fixed

		PUPIL SIZE		PUPIL REACTION		EXTREMITY MOVEMENT/ RESPONSE				GLASGOW COMA SCALE			VITAL SIGNS		
DATE	TIME	R	L	R	L	RA	LA	RL	LL	VERBAL RESP.	MOTOR RESP.	EYE OPENING	BP	PULSE	RESP.

GUIDE TO NEUROLOGIC EVALUATION

Pupils

Pupils should be examined in dim light

1. Compare each pupil with the size chart and record pupil size.
2. Use a bright flashlight to check the reaction of each pupil. Hold the flashlight to the outer aspect of the eye. While watching the pupil, turn the flashlight on and bring it directly over the pupil. Record the reaction. Repeat for the other eye. Report if either pupil is fixed or dilated.

Extremities

1. Observe the child for quality and strength of muscle tone in each upper extremity. Have child squeeze nurse's hand. Have child raise arms. Ask child to turn palms up, then palms down. Infant is observed for movement and position of arms when stroked or lightly pinched.
2. The child should be able to move each leg on command, and push against nurse's hands with each foot. Infant is observed for movement of legs and feet when stroked or lightly pinched.
3. Score the extremities using the motor scale appropriate for age (below).

Glasgow Coma Scale

Assess each response according to age

Eye opening

4 Opens eyes spontaneously when approached
3 Opens eyes to spoken or shouted speech

2 Opens eyes only to painful stimuli (nail bed pressure)
1 Does not open eyes in response to pain

Verbal

5 Oriented to time, place, person; infant responds by cooing and babbling, recognizes parent
4 Talks, not oriented to time, place, person; infant irritable, doesn't recognize parent
3 Words senseless, unintelligible; infant cries in response to pain
2 Responds with moaning and groaning, no intelligible words; infant moans to pain
1 No response

Motor

6 Responds to commands; infant smiles, responds
5 Tries to remove painful stimuli with hands; infant withdraws from touch
4 Attempts to withdraw from painful stimuli; infant withdraws from pain source
3 Flexes arms at elbows and wrists in response to pain (decorticate rigidity)
2 Extends arms at elbows in response to pain (cerebrate rigidity)
1 No motor response to pain

Check infant's fontanelle for bulging and record results

FIGURE 28-13 Neurologic flow sheet and neurologic evaluation guide.

KEY POINTS

- Interviewing the family caregiver and the child is important to collect subjective data regarding the child that can be used to develop a plan of care.

- Biographical data, chief complaint, history of the present health concern, and child and family health history are included in obtaining a client history. A review of each body system and related information gives an overall picture of the current status. Information related to allergies, medications being taken, or concerns of substance abuse are gathered. School, social, personal, and nutritional histories as well as observing aspects of the developmental level of the child add additional information for the health care provider.

- The chief complaint is the reason the child was brought to the healthcare setting and should be fully explored with the child and the family caregiver.

- When doing a review of systems, ask questions about each of the body systems, using a head-to-toe approach to gather data to get an overall picture of the child's current status.

- The family caregiver may be involved in collecting objective data by being a support to the child as well as assisting with tasks such as obtaining a temperature or urine specimen.

- Observing and recording the child's general appearance, behavior, and emotional and intellectual responses provides indications of overall health status. Possible indications of illness in children include the child being quieter or less active than usual, crying or acting uncomfortable, refusing to eat, exhibiting behaviors that are different from expected for the child's level of development, and having changes in skin coloration.

- Weight, height or length, and head circumference are monitored on an ongoing basis because they are good indicators of the child's growth and development, as well as the child's health status.

- Growth charts are used to establish a standard to compare an individual child's growth progress.

- Vital signs are taken and compared with normal values for children of the same age, as well as to that of child's previous recordings.

- Temperatures are taken by oral, tympanic, temporal, rectal, or axillary methods. A rectal temperature should not be taken on newborns, children who have had rectal surgery, are immunosuppressed, or who have diarrhea or a bleeding disorder.

- An apical pulse is taken on infants and small children to measure heart rate. Cardiac monitors may be used in some situations.

- Respirations are counted for a full minute when the child is lying or sitting quietly. Respiratory retractions are supraclavicular (above the clavicle), suprasternal (above the sternum), intercostal (between the ribs), substernal (below the sternum), or subcostal (below the ribs). Pulse oximetry is used to measure oxygen saturation levels. Apnea monitors are used when indicated.

- Blood pressure measurement can be obtained by auscultation, palpation, and automated device (Doppler or oscillometric) methods.

- To collect objective data, a physical examination is done on a child, using knowledge of normal growth and development as a basis for the examination. Unlike the head-to-toe examination in the adult, the physical examination in the child proceeds from the less traumatic areas to be examined to the areas that are more traumatic or uncomfortable to the child. Range of motion is observed in the head and neck, and facial features are noted for balance or symmetry. The chest is measured and respiratory characteristics noted. Heart sounds are listened to at the PMI, and pulses throughout the body are assessed. The abdomen is assessed for abnormalities. Bowel sounds in the four quadrants are noted. The genitalia and rectum are inspected as well as the back and extremities.

- The Glasgow Coma Scale is used as a tool for neurologic assessment and to consistently monitor the child's neurologic functioning.

INTERNET RESOURCES

National Institute of Child Health and Human Development
www.nichd.nih.gov

NCLEX-STYLE REVIEW QUESTIONS

1. The nurse is doing an admission interview with a toddler and the child's family caregiver. Which of the following statements that the nurse makes to the family caregiver indicates the nurse has an understanding of this child's growth and development needs?

   a. "You can sit in one chair, and your child can sit in the other chair."
   b. "It would be best if you let the child play in the play-room while we are talking."
   c. "If you would like to hold your child on your lap, that would be fine."
   d. "I can find someone to take your child for a walk for a while."

2. When interviewing an adolescent, which of the following is the *most* important for the nurse to keep in mind?

   a. The adolescent will be able to give accurate details regarding their history.
   b. The adolescent may feel more comfortable discussing some issues in private.
   c. The adolescent may have a better understanding if books and pamphlets are provided.
   d. The adolescent will be more cooperative if age-appropriate questions are asked.

3. In taking vital signs on a 6-month-old infant, the nurse obtains the following vital sign measurements. Which set of vital signs would the nurse be *most* concerned about?

   a. Pulse 94 beats per minute (bpm), temperature 36.9°C, blood pressure 80/50 mm Hg
   b. Pulse 118 bpm, temperature 37.6°C, blood pressure 88/60 mm Hg
   c. Pulse 134 bpm, temperature 38°C, blood pressure 92/62 mm Hg
   d. Pulse 152 bpm, temperature 38.9°C, blood pressure 96/56 mm Hg

4. When doing a physical examination on an infant, an understanding of this child's developmental needs is recognized when the examination is done by examining the:

   a. heart before the abdomen
   b. chest before the nose
   c. legs before the feet
   d. neurologic status before the back

5. The nurse is measuring an 18-month-old child's length and weight. Which of the following actions should the nurse implement? Select all that apply.

   a. Plot the measurements on a growth chart.
   b. Wear a gown and mask during the procedure.
   c. Keep a hand within 1 inch of the child.
   d. Encourage the family caregiver to gently hold the child's legs.
   e. Have the child wear the same amount of clothing each time the procedure is done.
   f. Cover the scale with a clean sheet of paper before placing the child on the scale.

6. The nurse is collecting data on a child who has a respiratory condition. Identify the area where the nurse will observe this child for substernal respiratory retractions by marking an X on the spot where substernal retractions are noted.

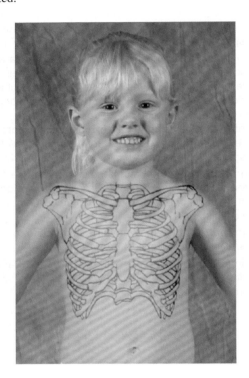

STUDY ACTIVITIES

1. Explain the step-by-step procedure you would follow to take vital signs on a 3-month-old infant. List the order in which you would take the vital signs, and explain why you would do them in that order.

2. For each of the following body parts or systems, write a question that would be appropriate to ask a child or family caregiver when doing a review of systems as part of an interview.

Body Part or System	Question to Ask
General	
Skin	
Head and neck	
Eyes and vision	
Ears and hearing	
Nose, mouth, throat	
Chest and lungs—respiratory	
Heart—cardiovascular	
Abdomen—gastrointestinal	
Genitalia and rectum	
Back and extremities—musculoskeletal	
Neurologic	

3. List five methods of taking a temperature and describe each method. Give an example of a reason that each method might be used to take a child's temperature.

CRITICAL THINKING: WHAT WOULD YOU DO?

1. You are conducting an interview with the family caregiver of a preschool-aged child.
   a. What would you discuss with the family caregiver?
   b. What would you say and do with the caregiver to get the important information you need to care for the child?
   c. What would you say to the preschool-aged child during the interview with the family caregiver?

2. As the nurse in a pediatric outpatient setting, you are responsible for obtaining the child's weight and height or length at each visit.
   a. What would you explain to the family caregiver when you are asked why the weight and height or length of a child are measured at each healthcare visit?
   b. What information would you record and document on the child's growth record?
   c. What is the purpose and significance of plotting weight and height or length on a pediatric growth chart?

3. You are assisting in doing a physical examination on a toddler.
   a. What is the process of doing a physical examination on a child?
   b. How does the examination on a child differ from that of an adult?
   c. What are the most important considerations to keep in mind when doing a physical examination on a child?

Care of the Hospitalized Child

Key Terms

anuria
child-life program
patient-controlled analgesia
play therapy
rooming-in
therapeutic play

Learning Objectives

At the conclusion of this chapter, you will:

1. List nine possible influences on the family's response to a child's illness.
2. Explain the family caregiver's role in educating the young child about hospitals.
3. Describe ways in which pediatric units differ from adult care settings.
4. Explain safety concerns in the pediatric hospital setting and why special precautions are needed in times of stress, such as hospitalization.
5. Identify four ways that pathogens are transmitted and give an example of each.
6. Differentiate standard precautions and transmission-based precautions, and state the role that handwashing and hand hygiene plays in infection control.
7. Describe how to help ease the feelings of isolation a child may have when segregated because of transmission-based precautions.
8. Identify and differentiate the three stages of a child's response to separation from family caregivers.
9. Explain why and how family caregivers participate in the care of the hospitalized child.
10. Explain how a planned admission with a preadmission visit differs from an emergency admission.
11. State the role of the family caregiver in the child's admission process.
12. Outline topics that should be covered when reinforcing family teaching before the child is discharged from the hospital.
13. Describe how healthcare professionals can help the adjustment of the child scheduled for surgery through preoperative teaching.
14. Discuss variations in preoperative preparation for children, including skin, gastrointestinal, urinary, and medication preparation.
15. Discuss postoperative care of the child.
16. Describe pain management in children and identify behavioral characteristics that may indicate an infant or a young child is in pain.
17. Discuss the role of play for the hospitalized child, including (a) play room or activity area, (b) play therapy, (c) therapeutic play, and (d) play materials.

The emergency department has notified the pediatric unit that **Kylem Williams**, age 8, is being admitted with a diagnosis of appendicitis and will be scheduled for surgery within a few hours. Kylem is admitted to the pediatric unit and you are his nurse. Since this is an emergency admission, think about what your nursing priorities for Kylem and his family are. Review normal growth and development of the school-aged child from Chapter 26.

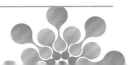

Healthcare is often provided in community settings such as outpatient clinics and offices, urgent care and surgical centers and even in the home. When a child is hospitalized, they are often acutely ill or in need of major surgery or treatment. Hospitalization may cause anxiety and stress at any age. Fear of the unknown is always threatening. The child who faces hospitalization is no exception. Children are often too young to understand what is happening or are afraid to ask questions. Short hospital stays occur more frequently than extended hospitalization, but even during a short stay, the child is often apprehensive. In addition, the child may pick up on the fears of family caregivers, and these negative emotions may hinder the child's progress.

The child's family suffers stress for a number of reasons. The cause of the illness, its treatment, guilt about the illness, past experiences of illness and hospitalization, disruption in family life, the threat to the child's long-term health, cultural or religious influences, coping methods within the family, and financial impact of the hospitalization all may affect how the family responds to the child's illness. Although some of these are concerns of the family and not specifically the child, they nevertheless influence how the child feels.

> **This is Important to Keep in Mind!**
> Children are tuned in to the feelings and emotions of their family caregivers. By supporting the caregiver, you are also supporting the child.

The child's developmental level also plays an important role in determining how they handle the stress of illness and hospitalization. When you understand the child's developmental needs, you may significantly improve the child's hospital stay and overall recovery (Fig. 29-1).

Many hospitals have **child-life programs** to make hospitalization less threatening for children and their families. These programs are usually under the direction of a child-life specialist whose background is in psychology and early childhood development. This person works with nurses, health care providers, students, and other health team members to help them meet the developmental, emotional, and intellectual needs of hospitalized children. One way to ease the stress of hospitalization is to ensure that the child has been well prepared for the hospital experience.

THE PEDIATRIC HOSPITAL SETTING

Early Childhood Education About Hospitals

Hospitals are part of the child's community, just as police and fire departments are. When the child is capable of understanding the basic functions of community resources and the people who staff them, it is time for an explanation. Some hospitals have regular open house programs for healthy children. Children may attend with family caregivers or in an organized community or school group. A room is set aside where children can handle equipment, try out call bells, try on masks and gowns, have their blood pressure taken to feel the squeeze of the blood pressure cuff, and see a hospital pediatric bed and compare it with their beds at home. Hospital staff members explain simple procedures and answer children's questions. A tour of the pediatric department, including the play room or activity area, may be offered (Fig. 29-2). Some hospitals have puppet shows, slideshows, or videos about admission and care. Child-life specialists, nurses, and volunteers help with these orientation programs.

Families are encouraged to help children develop positive attitudes about hospitals at an early age. The family should avoid negative attitudes about hospitals. Young children need to know that the hospital is more than a place where "mommies go to get babies"; it is also important to avoid fostering the view of the hospital as a place where

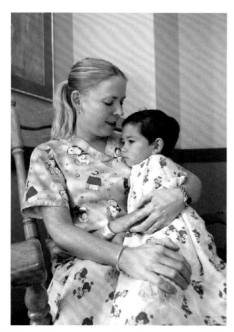

FIGURE 29-1 Holding and rocking the younger child helps alleviate the anxiety of hospitalization, especially when family caregivers are not able to be with the child.

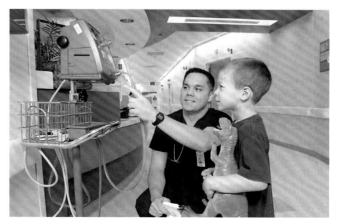

FIGURE 29-2 A nurse helps children learn what to expect from hospitalization during a prehospital program and tour of the facility.

people go to die. This is a particular concern if the child knows someone who died in the hospital. A careful explanation of the person's illness and simple, honest answers to questions about the death are necessary.

The Pediatric Unit Atmosphere

An effort by pediatric units and hospitals to create friendly, warm surroundings for children has produced many attractive, colorful pediatric settings. Walls are colorful, often decorated with murals, wallpaper, photos, and paintings specifically designed for children. Curtains and drapes in appealing colors and designs are often coordinated with wall coverings.

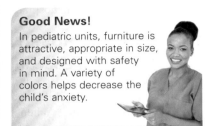

Good News!

In pediatric units, furniture is attractive, appropriate in size, and designed with safety in mind. A variety of colors helps decrease the child's anxiety.

The staff members of the pediatric unit often wear colorful uniforms or printed scrub suits. Children are encouraged to wear their own clothing during the day. Colorful printed gowns and pajamas are provided for children who need to wear hospital clothing.

Treatments are performed in a treatment room, not in the child's room. Using a separate room to perform procedures promotes the concept that the child's bed is a "safe" place. All treatments should be performed in the treatment room to reassure the child.

A play room or activity area is a vital part of all pediatric units (see later discussion of "The Hospital Play Program"). The playroom should be a place that is safe from any kind of procedures.

Most pediatric settings encourage family caregivers to visit as frequently as possible. This approach helps minimize the separation anxiety of the young child in particular. Family caregivers are involved in much of the young child's care.

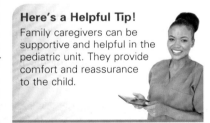

Here's a Helpful Tip!

Family caregivers can be supportive and helpful in the pediatric unit. They provide comfort and reassurance to the child.

Many pediatric units try to make nursing assignments so that the same nurse is with a child as much as possible. This approach provides the opportunity to establish a trusting relationship with the child.

Planning meals that include the child's favorite foods, within the limitations of any special dietary restrictions, may perk up a poor appetite. In addition, when space permits, several children may eat together at a small table. Younger children can be seated in high chairs or other suitable seats and should always be supervised by an adult. Meals should be served out of bed, if possible, and in a pleasant atmosphere. Some pediatric units use the play room or activity area to serve meals to ambulatory children.

♡ A Personal Glimpse

Hi, my name is Jenni. I am 15 years old and would like to tell you about my experience in the hospital.

I am an asthmatic. I have been since I was a little girl because of allergies to many things. Whenever I get a cold, it sometimes aggravates my asthma. I recently had an episode where I needed to be hospitalized because of an asthma attack.

I don't like hospitals. I could not wait until I was released. The intravenous (IV) hurt and needed to be put back in. The nurse had dry, scaly hands. It looked like she worked on a farm and then came to work at the hospital. The food was not too great either, not like Pizza Hut or McDonald's.

The person who made the whole ordeal better for me was the respiratory therapist. I needed regular nebulizer treatments, and it was a dream when he came into the room. Yes, he was good looking, but what made the difference was his personality and sense of humor. It makes a big difference when it seems like the staff person wants to be there and really cares, rather than being cared for by someone who is there just because it's a job and can't wait until the shift ends.

Jenni, age 15 years

Learning Opportunity: What do you think are three important behaviors by the nurse or healthcare professional that indicate to a client that they are cared about as a person?

Pediatric Intensive Care Units

A child's admission to a pediatric intensive care unit (PICU) may be overwhelming for both the child and the family, especially if the admission is unexpected. Highly technical equipment, bright lights, and the crisis atmosphere may be frightening. Visiting may be restricted. The many stressors present increase the effects on the child and the family. PICU nurses should take great care to prepare the family for how the child will look when they first visit. The family should be given a schedule of visiting hours so that they may plan permitted visits. The family can bring in a special doll or child's toy to provide comfort and security. The child's developmental level must be considered so that appropriate explanations and reassurances are given before and during procedures. Positive reinforcements, such as stickers and small badges, may provide symbols of courage. Interpret technical information for family members. To promote the relationship between the family caregiver and the child, encourage the caregiver to touch and talk to the child. If possible, the family caregiver may hold and rock the child; if not, they can comfort the child by caressing and stroking.

Safety

Safety is an essential aspect of pediatric nursing care. Accidents occur more often when people are in stressful situations; infants, children, and their family caregivers experience additional stress when a child is hospitalized. They are removed from a familiar home environment, faced with anxieties and fear, and must adjust to an unfamiliar schedule. Consciously looking at every situation for accident potential, you must have safety in mind at all times as a pediatric nurse.

The pediatric environment should meet all the safety standards appropriate for other areas of the facility, including good lighting, dry floors with no obstacles that may cause falls, electrical equipment and furniture checked for hazards, safe bath and shower facilities, and beds in low position for ambulatory clients.

Additional safety considerations depend on the child's age and developmental level. Toddlers are explorers whose developmental task is to develop autonomy. Toddlers love to put small objects into equally small openings, whether the opening is in their bodies, in equipment, or elsewhere in the pediatric unit. Careful observation to eliminate dangers may prevent the toddler from having access to small objects. Toddlers are also often climbers and must be protected from climbing and falling. Encourage family members to keep the crib sides up when not directly caring for the infant in the crib. One unguarded moment may mean that the infant falls out of a crib. Box 29-1 presents a summary of pediatric safety precautions.

Infection Control

Infection control is important in the pediatric hospital setting. The ill child may be especially vulnerable to pathogenic (disease-carrying) microorganisms. Precautions must be taken to protect the children, families, and personnel. Microorganisms are spread by contact (direct or indirect); droplet (coughing, sneezing, talking); vehicle (food, water, blood, or contaminated products); airborne (particles in the air); or vector (mosquitoes, vermin) means of transmission. Each type of microorganism is transmitted in a specific way, so precautions are tailored to prevent the spread of specific microorganisms.

The U.S. Centers for Disease Control and Prevention and the Healthcare Infection Control Practices Advisory Committee (HICPAC) publish guidelines for infection prevention and control practices. The guidelines include two levels of precautions: standard precautions and transmission-based precautions (see Appendix A). All healthcare facilities follow these guidelines.

Standard Precautions

Standard precautions blend the primary characteristics of universal precautions and body substance isolation.

BOX 29-1	Safety Precautions for Pediatric Units

- Cover electrical outlets; keep children away from electrical equipment, cords.
- Keep children away from heat sources (radiators, lamps, heat vents).
- If using heat as a therapy, closely monitor child's temperature and skin.
- Keep floor dry and free of clutter.
- Use tape or Velcro closures when possible.
- Always close safety pins when not in use.
- Inspect toys (child's or hospital's) for loose or small parts, sharp edges, dangerous cords, or other hazards.
- Use toys that can be disinfected and frequently clean and disinfect them, always between uses by different children.
- Do not permit friction toys where oxygen is in use.
- Supervise child when using pencils, pens, or scissors.
- Never leave scissors or other sharp instruments within a child's reach.
- Do not allow children to have or play with latex balloons.
- Do not leave child unattended in high chair or when eating.
- Keep crib sides up all the way except when caring for child.
- If the crib side is down, keep hand firmly on infant at all times.
- Use crib with top if child stands or climbs.
- Always check temperature of bath water to prevent burns.

- Never leave infant or child unattended in any amount of bath water.
- Keep beds of ambulatory children locked in low position.
- Turn off motor of electric bed if young children might have access to controls.
- Always use safety belts or straps for children in infant seats, feeding chairs, strollers, wheelchairs, or stretchers.
- Use restraints only when necessary.
- When restraints are used, remove and check for skin integrity, circulation, and correct application at least every hour or two.
- Never tie a restraint to the crib side; tie to bed frame only.
- Keep medications securely locked in designated area; children should never be permitted in this area.
- Set limits and enforce them consistently; do not let children get out of control.
- Place needles and syringes in sharps containers; make sure children have no access to these containers.
- Always pick up any equipment after a procedure.
- Be aware of facility policies for fire, severe weather, and other potential dangerous situations.
- Do not allow sleepy family caregivers to hold a sleeping child as they may fall asleep and drop the child.

Standard precautions apply to blood; all body fluids, secretions, and excretions, except sweat; nonintact skin; and mucous membranes. Standard precautions are intended to reduce the risk of transmission of microorganisms from recognized or unrecognized sources of infection in healthcare settings. Health care providers follow standard precautions in the care of all clients.

Transmission-Based Precautions

For clients documented or suspected of having highly transmissible pathogens, health care providers must follow transmission-based precautions. These precautions are in addition to the standard precautions. Transmission-based precautions include three types: contact precautions, droplet precautions, and airborne precautions. Certain diseases may require more than one type of precaution. See Nursing Process and Care Plan for the Child Placed on Transmission-Based Precautions.

> **This is Critical to Remember!**
>
> Handwashing and hand hygiene is the cornerstone of all infection control. Wash your hands or use alcohol-based hand disinfectant conscientiously between seeing each client, even when gloves are worn for a procedure.

Nursing Process and Care Plan
for the Child Placed on Transmission-Based Precautions

When a child has a known or suspected infection which can be spread to others, they are placed on transmission-based precautions. These infections include microorganisms that can be spread by contact, droplet, or airborne transmission. Specific guidelines and personal protective equipment (PPE) are used to decrease and prevent the spread of these pathogens.

Assessment (Data Collection)

The child placed on transmission-based precautions has a known infection, often highly infectious. Monitoring the child for signs and symptoms and treating the infection are aspects of the child's care. Exploring with the child and family caregiver their understanding of the precautions the child is on helps determine information they need reinforced. Asking questions about the child's normal daily activities helps the nurse recognize needs the child has in relationship to their stage of growth and development.

Nursing Care Focus

When developing evidence-based nursing care focuses for the child who is in transmission-based precautions, adhering to the precautions and preventing transmitting microorganisms to others is important. Psychosocial needs related to isolation, loneliness, anxiety, depression and the need for diversional activity are addressed. Reinforcing teaching with the child and family caregiver is included in the care of the child.

Outcome Identification and Planning

The major goals for the child include preventing the spread of infection and helping the child cope with the confinement of being in isolation and having to maintain transmission-based precautions. Goals for the child and family include learning about and following the guidelines of the transmission-based precautions.

Nursing Care Focus

- Infection risk related to possibility of transmitting microorganisms to others
- Nonadherence related to following transmission-based precautions

Goal

- The child's infection will not be spread to others.

Implementations for Preventing the Spread of Infection

Hand hygiene, handwashing with soap and water or the use of alcohol-based hand disinfectant, is key to helping decrease spread of infection and must be performed frequently. Appropriate personal protective equipment (PPE) is needed depending on the type of transmission precautions. Follow the guidelines and institution policies and ensure that everyone who has contact with the child follows them as well. Help the family caregivers with gowning and other necessary precaution procedures so that they become more comfortable in the situation. Family caregivers may need reminders about precaution measures, including handwashing and hand hygiene, gowning, gloving, and masking as necessary. Encourage the family to bring some of the child's toys, but remind them to only bring items that can be washed and disinfected. Follow institution policies regarding cleaning equipment and disposing of soiled linens and dressings.

Evaluation of Goal/Desired Outcome

The child's:

- infection is not spread to others.

Nursing Care Focus

- Psychosocial needs related to feelings of isolation and loneliness from being in transmission-based precautions
- Anxiety and depression related to separation resulting from required transmission-based precautions

Goal

- The child will have adequate social contact.
- The child will have control over some aspects of the situation.

Implementations for Reducing Feelings of Isolation, Loneliness, Anxiety, and Depression

The child who is segregated because of transmission-based precautions is subject to social isolation. No matter what precautions are necessary, always be alert to the child's loneliness and sadness and make every effort to help reduce these feelings. The child must not think that being in a room alone is a punishment. Arrange to spend extra time in the room when performing treatments and procedures rather than going quickly in and out of the room.

Identify ways in which the child can communicate with staff, family, and friends. Frequent contact with family and staff helps decrease the child's feeling of isolation. Facilitate the use of telephone and electronics to help the child feel connected with friends. Suggest family caregivers ask the child's friends to send notes and drawings. For the school-aged child, family caregivers might contact the child's teacher so that classmates can send cards and other school items to keep the child involved. Notes, photos, and drawings are concrete signs to the child that their friends are thinking of them.

Include the child in planning for daily activities such as bath routine, food choices, timing of meals and snacks, and other flexible activities. The child will feel some control over their life if they are included in ways that give them a choice. Maintain the schedule after making the plan. Keeping the schedule reinforces for the child that they do have some control. Plan a special activity with the child each day and keep your promise. Encourage family members to do the same.

Positioning the child's bed near a window may help reduce feelings of isolation. If masks or gloves are part of the necessary precautions, the child may experience even greater feelings of isolation. Before putting on the mask, allow the child to see your face; that process will help the child easily identify you. Gloves prevent the child from experiencing skin-to-skin contact; talk to the child to draw out any of the child's feelings about this. Explaining at the child's level of understanding why gloves are necessary may help the child accept them. If the child is upset by the fact that family caregivers must wear gowns, a careful explanation should help the child accept this.

Evaluation of Goal/Desired Outcome

The child:

- interacts with nursing staff and family.
- visits with friends and family via phone or electronic devices.
- makes choices about some of their daily routine.

The child's family caregivers:

- follow through with planned activities.

Nursing Care Focus

- Psychosocial need for diversionary activities related to monotony of restrictions

Goal

- The child will be engaged in age-appropriate activities.

Implementations for Promoting Age-Appropriate Development

A variety of activities can provide diversion and entertainment without boredom for the child in isolation and transmission-based precautions. Gather a collection of age-appropriate books, puzzles, and games. Consult with play therapist if available. Encourage family caregivers to engage the child in activities they enjoy. Family caregivers can use visiting time to help alleviate the monotony of isolation. Facilitate use of electronics to visit with friends (Zoom, Skype, FaceTime). Seeing and visiting friends via electronics helps promote socialization. Plan nursing care to include time for reading or playing a game with the child. Activities with a variety of persons (besides family caregivers) are welcome to the child. Encourage physical exercise within the restrictions of the child's condition. Physical activity helps to improve circulation and feelings of well-being.

Evaluation of Goal/Desired Outcome

- The child participates in age-appropriate activities.
- The child approaches planned activities with enthusiasm.

Nursing Care Focus

- Knowledge deficiency of child and family caregivers regarding transmission-based precautions

Goal

The child and family caregivers:

- will verbalize and follow guidelines for transmission-based precautions.

Implementations for Reinforcing Child and Family Teaching About Transmission-Based Precautions

Review and explain reasons the child is on transmission-based precautions to increase the family caregivers' understanding of the importance of following the precautions and to decrease anxiety they may have about the precautions. Help them put on the needed personal protective equipment (PPE) and clarify with them the correct way to remove and dispose of these. Discuss the timeframe the child will likely be in isolation assuring them that it will not always be necessary.

Evaluation of Goal/Desired Outcome

The child and family caregivers:

- follow guidelines for transmission-based precaution.
- verbalize an understanding of the necessary precautions.

Importance of Family Caregiver Participation

Research has shown that separating young children from their family caregivers, especially during times of stress, may have damaging effects. Young children have no concept of time, so separation from their primary caregivers is especially difficult for them to understand.

Children often go through three characteristic stages of response to the separation: protest, despair, and denial. During the first stage (*protest*), the young child cries, often refuses to be comforted by others, and constantly seeks the primary caregiver at every sight and sound. When the primary caregiver does not appear, the child enters the second stage (*despair*) and becomes apathetic and listless. Healthcare personnel often interpret this as a sign that the child is accepting the situation, but this is not the case; the child has given up. In the third stage (*denial*), the child begins taking interest in the surroundings and appears to accept the situation. However, when the family caregivers do visit, the child often turns away from them, showing distrust and rejection. It may take a long time before the child accepts them again. The child may have a memory of being "abandoned" at the hospital. Regardless of how mistaken they may be, childhood impressions can have a deep effect.

Most pediatric settings provide **rooming-in** facilities, where the family caregiver can stay in the room with the child (Fig. 29-3).

Rooming-in helps minimize the hospitalized child's separation anxiety and depression. Although separation from primary caregivers is thought to cause the greatest upset in children younger than 5 years, children of all ages should be considered when setting up a rooming-in system.

One advantage of rooming-in is the measure of security the child feels as a result of the family caregiver's care and attention. The family caregiver may participate in bathing, dressing, and feeding; preparing the child for bed; and providing recreational activities. If treatments are to be continued at home, rooming-in creates an excellent opportunity for the family caregiver to observe and practice before leaving the hospital.

Rules should be clearly understood before admission, and facilities for family caregivers should be clearly explained. The hospital may provide a foldout bed or reclining chair in the child's room. Provision for meals should be explained to the family caregiver.

Avoid creating a situation in which you appear to be expecting the family caregivers to perform as healthcare technicians. The family caregiver's basic role is to provide security and stability for the child.

> **Nursing Judgment is in Order!**
> Rooming-in should not be used to relieve staff shortage. The role of the family caregiver is to help the child feel safe and secure.

Many pediatric units also allow siblings to visit the ill child. This policy benefits both the ill child and the sibling. The sibling at home may be imagining a much more serious illness than is actually the case. Visiting policies usually require that a family adult accompany and be responsible for the sibling and that the visiting period is not too long. Visiting siblings must not have a fever, cold, or other illness and must have up-to-date immunizations.

While encouraging family caregiver participation, the nursing staff should also be aware of the caregiver's needs. The caregiver needs to be encouraged to take breaks, leave for meals, or occasionally go home, if possible, for a shower and rest. The family caregiver may give a personal possession to the child to help reassure them that the caregiver will return. Having a way to contact the family caregiver quickly gives the family freedom and reassurance. This is particularly useful during periods when the family caregivers must wait for procedures, surgery, or other activities.

> **This Advice Could Be a Lifesaver!**
> Having family caregivers' mobile phone numbers easily accessible is helpful in contacting them. Some hospitals provide pagers or mobile devices for family caregivers so that they can leave the immediate area of the child's room or waiting area but can be quickly contacted to return, if needed.

> **TEST YOURSELF**
> ✔ Why is infection control especially important in the pediatric setting?
> ✔ Explain the difference between standard precautions and transmission-based precautions.
> ✔ Why is family caregiver participation important in the pediatric hospital setting?

ADMISSION AND DISCHARGE PLANNING

Although admission may be a frightening experience, the child feels in much better control of the situation if the person taking the child to the hospital has explained where they are going and why and has answered questions truthfully.

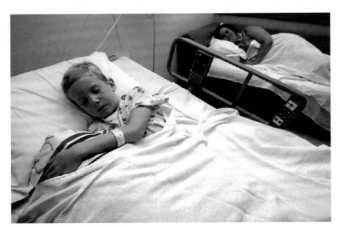

FIGURE 29-3 Rooming-in helps alleviate separation anxiety for both the child and the family caregiver.

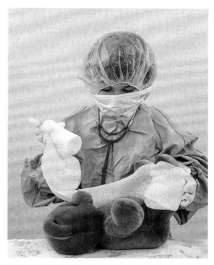

FIGURE 29-4 The child who is going to have surgery may act out the procedure on a doll, thereby reducing some of her fear. (© B. Proud.)

BOX 29-2 Guidelines to Orient Child to Pediatric Unit

1. Introduce the primary nurse.
2. Orient to the child's room.
   a. Demonstrate bed, bed controls, side rails.
   b. Demonstrate call light.
   c. Demonstrate television; include cost, if any.
   d. Show bathroom facilities.
   e. Explain telephone and rules that apply.
3. Introduce to roommate(s); include families.
4. Give directions to or show "special" rooms.
   a. Playroom—rules that apply, hours available, toys or equipment that may be taken to child's room.
   b. Treatment room—explain purpose.
   c. Unit kitchen—rules that apply.
   d. Other special rooms.
5. Explain pediatric rules; give written rules if available.
   a. Visiting hours, who may visit.
   b. Mealtimes, rules about bringing in food.
   c. Bedtimes, naptimes, or quiet time.
   d. Rooming-in arrangements.
6. Explain daily routines.
   a. Vital signs routine.
   b. Bath routine.
   c. Other routines.
7. Provide guidelines for involvement of family caregiver.

When the family caregiver and the child arrive on the nursing unit, they should be greeted in a warm, friendly manner and taken to the child's room or to a room set aside specifically for the admission procedure. The family caregiver and the child need to be oriented to the child's room, the nursing unit, and regulations (Box 29-2).

Planned Admissions

Preadmission preparation may make the experience less threatening and the adjustment to admission as smooth as possible. Children who are candidates for hospital admission may attend open house or other special programs that are more detailed and specifically related to the upcoming experience. Books, videos, and pictures are also valuable in helping the child understand and become familiar with the planned admission. It is important for family caregivers and siblings to attend the preadmission tour with the future client to reduce anxiety in all family members.

During the preadmission visit, children may be given surgical masks, caps, shoe covers, and the opportunity to "operate" or put a dressing on a doll or other stuffed toy specifically designed for teaching purposes (Fig. 29-4).

Many hospitals have developed special coloring books to help prepare children for specific surgical procedures. These books are given to children during the preadmission visit or they are sent to children at home before admission. During the visit, children and their families are often hesitant to ask questions or express feelings; be sensitive to this and discuss common questions and feelings. Children are told that some things will hurt, but that doctors and nurses will do everything they can to make the hurt go away. Avoid using terminology the child might not know or misinterpret, instead use terms that they will better understand. For instance, instead of referring to an "incision," use the words "a small opening." Be honest and specific to help establish trust with the child. Be sensitive to cultural and language differences and make adjustments whenever appropriate.

Emergency Admissions

Emergencies leave little time for explanation. The emergency itself is frightening to the child and the family, and the need for treatment is urgent. Even though a family caregiver tries to act calm and composed, the child often may sense the anxiety. If the hospital is still a great unknown, it will only add to the child's fear and panic. If the child has even a basic understanding about hospitals and what happens there, the emergency may seem a little less frightening.

In an emergency, physical needs assume priority over emotional needs. When possible, the presence of a family caregiver who can conceal their own fear is often comforting to the child; however, the child may be angry that the family caregiver does not prevent invasive procedures from being performed. Sometimes, however, it is impossible for the family caregiver to stay with the child. The family caregiver may provide a staff member with information about the child while the child receives treatment. This helps the family member feel involved in the child's care.

Emergency department nurses must be sensitive to the needs of the child and the family. Recognizing the child's cognitive level and how it affects the child's reactions is important. Explain procedures and maintain a caring, calm manner to reassure both the child and the family.

The Admission Interview

An admission interview is conducted as soon as possible after the child has been admitted. See Chapter 28 for specific information related to the client interview, history, and data to be collected. During the interview, an identification bracelet is placed on the child's wrist. If the child has allergies, an allergy bracelet must be placed on the wrist as well. The child must be prepared for even this simple procedure with an explanation of why it is necessary. When receiving the child on the pediatric unit, be friendly and casual, remembering that even a well-informed child may be shy and suspicious.

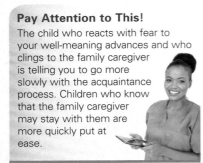

Pay Attention to This!
The child who reacts with fear to your well-meaning advances and who clings to the family caregiver is telling you to go more slowly with the acquaintance process. Children who know that the family caregiver may stay with them are more quickly put at ease.

Through careful questioning, the interviewer tries to determine what the family's previous experience has been with hospitals and health care providers. It is also important to ascertain how much the family caregiver and the child understand about the child's condition and their expectations of this hospitalization, what support systems are available when the child returns home, and any concerns on the part of the family caregiver or the child. These findings, in addition to the client history and physical examination (see Chapter 28), form the basis for the client's total plan of care while hospitalized.

The Admission Physical Examination

After the child has been oriented to the new surroundings by perhaps clinging to the family caregiver's hand or carrying a favorite toy or blanket, the family caregiver may undress the child for the physical examination. This procedure may be familiar from previous healthcare visits. If comfortable with helping, the caregiver may stay with the child during the physical examination (Fig. 29-5). See Chapter 28 for specific information related to the physical examination.

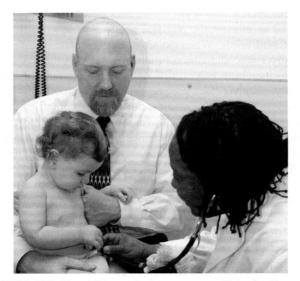

FIGURE 29-5 The child may feel more secure if the family caregiver stays with the child during the physical examination.

Discharge Planning

Planning for the child's discharge and care at home begins early in the hospital experience. Nurses and other healthcare team members must determine the levels of understanding of the child and family caregivers and their abilities to learn about the child's condition and the care necessary after the child goes home. Giving medications, using special equipment, and enforcing necessary restrictions must be discussed with the person who will be the primary family caregiver and with at least one other person, if possible. Specific, written instructions should be provided for reference at home; the anxiety and strangeness of hospitalization often limit the amount of information retained. Be certain the family caregiver can understand the written materials too. If the treatment necessary at home appears too complex for the family caregiver to manage, it may be helpful for a home health nurse to assist for a period of time after the child returns home.

Shortly before the child is discharged from the hospital, review information and procedures with the family caregivers. This information may or may not be given to child as well, depending on their age and cognitive level. Health care providers must approach questions and concerns honestly and offer a resource such as a telephone number or email access that the family caregiver can use to make a contact for questions that arise after discharge.

The return home may be a difficult period of adjustment for the entire family. The preschool child may be aloof at first, followed by a period of clinging, demanding behavior. Other behaviors, such as regression, temper tantrums, excessive attachment to a toy or blanket, night waking, and nightmares, may demonstrate fear of another separation. The older child may demonstrate anger or jealousy of siblings. The family may be advised to encourage positive behavior and avoid making the child the center of attention because of the illness. Discipline should be firm, loving, and consistent. The child may express feelings verbally or in play activities. Reassure the family that this is not unusual.

THE CHILD UNDERGOING SURGERY

Surgery frightens most adults, even though they understand why it is necessary and how it helps correct their health problems. Young children do not have this understanding and may become frightened of even a minor surgical procedure. If properly prepared, older children and adolescents are capable of understanding the need for surgery and what it will accomplish.

Many minor surgical procedures are performed in outpatient surgery facilities that permit the client to return home the day of the operation. These facilities reduce or eliminate the separation of family caregivers and children, one of the most stressful factors in surgery for infants and young children. Whether admitted for less than 1 day or for several weeks, the child who has surgery needs compassionate and thorough preoperative and postoperative care.

Preoperative Care

Specific physical and psychological preparation of the child and the family varies according to the type of surgery planned. General aspects of care include client and family teaching, skin preparation, preparation of the gastrointestinal and urinary systems, and preoperative medication.

Client and Family Teaching

The child admitted for planned surgery probably has had some preadmission preparation by the health care provider and family caregivers. Many families, however, have an unclear understanding of the surgery and what it involves, or they may be too anxious to be helpful. The healthcare professionals involved in the child's care must determine how much the child knows and is capable of learning, help correct any misunderstandings, and explain the preparation for surgery, what the surgery will "fix," and how the child will feel after surgery. This preparation must be based on the child's age, developmental level, previous experiences, and family caregiver support. All explanations should be clear, honest, and expressed in terms the child and the family caregivers can understand. Encourage questions to ensure that the child and the family caregivers correctly understand all the information. When the child is too young to benefit from preoperative teaching, direct explanations to family caregivers help relieve their anxiety and prepare them to participate in the child's care after surgery.

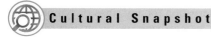

Balance is the Order of the Day!

If possible, offer preoperative information and reinforcement of teaching in short sessions, rather than trying to discuss everything at once.

Children need to be prepared for standard preoperative tests and procedures, such as radiographs and blood and urine tests. Explain the reason for withholding food and fluids before surgery, so children do not feel they are being neglected or punished when others receive meal trays.

Children sometimes interpret surgery as punishment and should be reassured that they did not cause the condition. They also fear mutilation or death and must be able to explore those feelings, while recognizing them as acceptable fears. Children deserve careful explanation that the health care provider is going to repair only the affected body part.

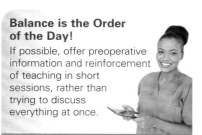

Cultural Snapshot

Surgery and surgical procedures are feared in some cultures. Anxiety over anesthesia and being "put to sleep" causes such concern in some cultures that surgery is refused. Careful explanations of procedures and the benefits to the client are important. Using an interpreter when language barriers exist is helpful.

Therapeutic play, discussed later in this chapter, is useful in preparing the child for surgery. Using drawings

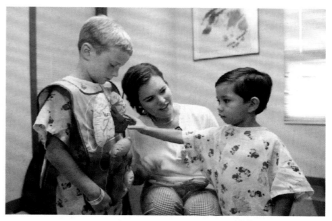

FIGURE 29-6 Before surgery, these children work with a child-life specialist using a model of the body organs.

to identify the area of the body to be operated on helps the child have a better understanding of what is going to happen. Role playing, adjusted to the child's age and understanding, is helpful. This approach may include a trip on a stretcher and pretending to go to surgery.

The older child or adolescent may have a greater interest in the surgery itself, what is wrong and why, how the repair is done, and the expected postoperative results. Models of a child's internal organs or individual organs, such as a heart, are useful for demonstration, or the child may be involved in making a drawing (Fig. 29-6).

Emphasize to the child that they will not feel anything during surgery because of the special sleep that anesthesia causes. Describing the postanesthesia care unit (PACU) (or wake-up room) and any tubes, bandages, or appliances that will be in place after surgery lets the child know what to expect. If possible, the child should see and handle the equipment that will be part of the operative experience. A preoperative tour of the ICU or PACU is also helpful.

A child needs to understand that several people will be involved in preoperative, surgical, and postoperative care. If possible, staff members from the anesthesia department and the operating room, recovery room, or the ICU should visit the child before surgery. Explaining what the people will be wearing (caps, masks, and gloves) and what equipment will be used (including bright lights) helps make the operating room experience less frightening.

Most clients experience postoperative pain, and children should be prepared for this experience. They also need to know when they may expect to be allowed to have fluids and food after surgery.

Children should practice coughing and deep-breathing exercises. Deep-breathing practice may be done with games that encourage blowing, such as blowing a cotton ball across a table using a straw. Encouraging children to splint the operative site with a pillow helps reassure them that the sutures will not break and allow the wound to open (Fig. 29-7).

Tell children where the family will be during and after surgery and make every effort to minimize separation.

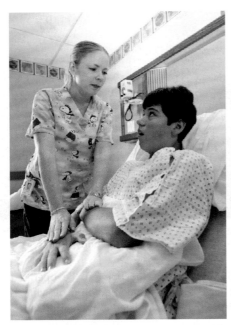

FIGURE 29-7 The preoperative reinforcement teaching this adolescent received helps him splint his abdomen after surgery.

Encourage family caregivers to be present when the child leaves for the operating room.

Skin Preparation

Depending on the type of surgery, skin preparation may include a tub bath or shower and includes special cleaning and inspection of the operative site. Any necessary shaving is usually performed in the operating room. If fingers or toes are involved, the nails are carefully trimmed. The operative site may be cleansed with a special antiseptic solution as an extra precaution against infection, depending on the health care providers' orders and the procedures of the hospital.

Gastrointestinal and Urinary System Preparation

The surgeon may order a cleansing enema the night before surgery (see Chapter 30). An enema is an intrusive procedure and must be explained to the child before it is given. If old enough, the child should understand the reason for the enema.

Children usually receive nothing by mouth (NPO) for a period of 4 to 12 hours before surgery because any food or fluids in the stomach may cause vomiting and aspiration, particularly during general anesthesia.

The NPO period varies according to the child's age; infants become dehydrated more rapidly than older children and thus require a shorter NPO period before surgery. Pediatric NPO orders are often accompanied by an IV fluid initiation order. Loose

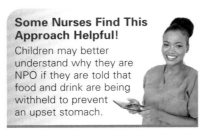

Some Nurses Find This Approach Helpful!
Children may better understand why they are NPO if they are told that food and drink are being withheld to prevent an upset stomach.

teeth are a potential hazard and should be counted and recorded according to hospital policy.

In some instances, urinary catheterization may be performed before surgery, but usually it is done while the child is in the operating room. The catheter is often removed immediately after surgery but can be left in place for several hours or days. Children who are not catheterized before surgery should be encouraged to void before the administration of preoperative medication.

Preoperative Medication

Depending on the health care providers' order, preoperative medications may be given in two stages: a sedative may be administered about 1.5 to 2 hours before surgery, and an analgesic–anticholinergic mixture may be administered immediately before the client leaves for the operating room. When the sedative has been given, dimming the lights and minimizing noise will help the child relax.

Bring preoperative medication to the child's room when it is time for administration. Tell the child that it is time for medication. Administer medication carefully and quickly because delays only increase the child's anxiety.

If hospital regulations permit, family caregivers should accompany the child to the operating room and wait until the child is anesthetized. If this is impossible, the nurse who has been caring for the child can go along to the operating room and introduce the child to personnel there.

What you will be doing preoperatively for **Kylem** and his family? What safety and infection control measures you will follow? Keeping his stage of growth and development in mind, what concerns do you think he might have and how will you support Kylem.

Postoperative Care

During the immediate postoperative period, the child receives care in the PACU or the surgical ICU. Meanwhile, the room in the pediatric unit should be prepared with appropriate equipment for the child's return. Depending on the type of surgery performed, it may be necessary to have suctioning, resuscitation, or other equipment at the bedside.

When the child returns to the room, nursing care focuses on careful observation for any signs or symptoms of complications: shock, hemorrhage, or respiratory distress. Monitor and record vital signs according to postoperative orders. Keep the child warm with blankets, as needed. Take note of any dressings, IV apparatus, urinary catheters, and any other appliances. An IV flow sheet is used to document the type of fluid, the amount of fluid to be absorbed, the rate of flow, any additive medications, the site, and the site's appearance and condition.

The first postoperative voiding is important to document because it indicates the adequacy of blood flow and urinary output. An inadequate amount of urine voided might indicate possible urinary retention. Also note any irritation or burning, and notify the health care provider if **anuria** (absence of urine) persists longer than 6 hours.

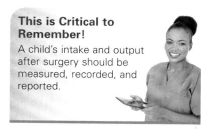

This is Critical to Remember!
A child's intake and output after surgery should be measured, recorded, and reported.

Postoperative orders may provide for ice chips or clear liquids. These may be administered with a spoon or in a small medicine cup. Frequent repositioning is necessary to prevent skin breakdown, orthostatic pneumonia, and decreased circulation. Coughing, deep breathing, and position changes are performed at least every 2 hours (Fig. 29-8).

Pain Management

Pain is a concern of postoperative clients in any age group. Most adult clients can verbally express the pain they feel, so they request relief. However, infants and young children cannot adequately express themselves and need help to tell where or how great the pain is. Beliefs that children do not have the same amount of pain that adults have or that they tolerate pain better than adults have contributed to under-medicating infants and children in pain. Research has shown that infants and children do experience pain.

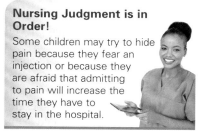

Nursing Judgment is in Order!
Some children may try to hide pain because they fear an injection or because they are afraid that admitting to pain will increase the time they have to stay in the hospital.

Be alert to indications of pain. Facial expressions are often an indicator of pain, especially in the infant. Careful observation is necessary—for example, noting changes in behavior such as rigidity, thrashing, loud crying or screaming, flexion of knees (indicating abdominal pain), restlessness, and irritability. Physiologic indications, such as changes in heart and respiratory rate and blood pressure, decreased oxygen saturation, sweating palms, dilated pupils, flushed or moist skin, and loss of appetite, may also indicate

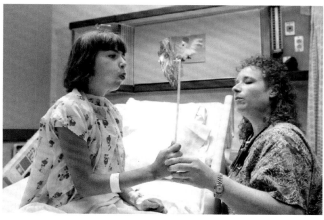

FIGURE 29-8 The nurse encourages this child to deep-breathe after surgery by using a pinwheel.

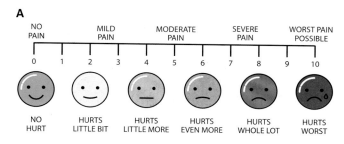
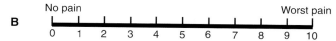

FIGURE 29-9 Pain scales: **(A)** pain faces measurement scale **(B)** numeric scale. (A. Oxy_gen/shutterstock.com).

pain. The toddler may be able to point to an area that hurts and use simple words such as "ouch" or "owie." Although the preschool-aged child might not report their pain and may have trouble describing it, they can indicate where the pain is and use tools to describe the severity. School-age children and adolescents can usually communicate the location, type, and intensity of their pain.

Various tools have been devised to help children express the amount of pain they feel. The tools also allow you to measure the effectiveness of pain management efforts. These tools include the pain faces measurement scale and the numeric scale, which are useful primarily with children 7 years of age and older (Fig. 29-9). Using the same tool consistently gives a more accurate comparison of the pain level and effectiveness of pain management interventions for the child.

Pain medication may be administered by oral, intramuscular, or IV routes, or by **patient-controlled analgesia**, a programmed infusion of narcotic analgesia that the child may control within set limits. A low-level dose of analgesia may be administered as a continuous infusion, or continuous with the child able to administer an additional bolus dose when needed, or it may be set so the child presses a button to administer only a bolus dose when pain medication is needed. Patient-controlled analgesia may be used for children 7 years of age or older who have no cognitive impairment and undergo a careful evaluation. Intramuscular injections are avoided if possible because they can be traumatic and painful for the child. Monitor vital signs and document the child's level of consciousness frequently, following the standards of the facility.

Nonpharmacologic comfort measures, such as position changes, massage, distraction, heat, cold, play, soothing touch, talk, coddling, and affection should be used along with the administration of analgesics. Activities provided for distraction must be appropriate for the child's age, level of development, and interests (Fig. 29-10).

Surgical Dressings

Postoperative care includes close observation of any dressings for signs of drainage or hemorrhage and reinforcing or

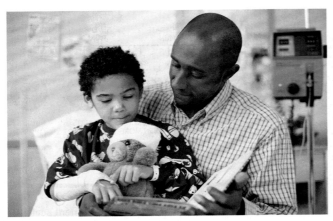

FIGURE 29-10 Distraction supplements pain control while a child is using patient-controlled analgesia.

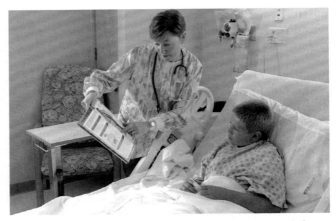

FIGURE 29-11 The nurse uses charts with pictures to reinforce teaching before the child goes home.

changing dressings as ordered. Wet dressings can increase the possibility of contamination; clean, dry dressings increase the child's comfort. If there is no health care providers' order to change the dressing, reinforce the moist original dressing by covering it with a dry dressing and taping the second dressing in place. If bloody drainage is present, draw around the outline of the drainage with a marker, and record the time and date. In this way, the amount of additional drainage can be determined when the dressings are inspected later.

> **Remember to Measure and Record!**
>
> When dressings are changed, record the amount of drainage on the output record by first weighing the dry dressing, then weighing the wet dressing and subtracting to get the difference. Record the difference as the output from the site.

Supplies needed for changing dressings vary according to the wound site and the health care providers' orders that specify the sterile or antiseptic technique to be used. Detailed procedures for these techniques and the supplies to be used can be found in the facility's procedures manual.

As with all procedures, explain to the child what will be done and why before beginning the dressing change. Some dressing changes are painful; if so, tell the child that it will hurt and offer praise for behavior that shows courage and cooperation.

Client and Family Teaching

Postoperative reinforcement of client teaching is as important as preoperative teaching. It is important to repeat some explanations and instructions given before surgery because the child's earlier anxiety may have prevented thorough understanding. Now that tubes, restraints, and dressings are part of the child's reality, they need to be discussed again—why they are important and how they affect the child's activities.

Family caregivers want to know how they can help care for the child and what limitations are placed on the child's activity. If family caregivers know what to expect and how to aid in their child's recovery, they will be cooperative during the postoperative period.

As the child recuperates, encourage the family caregivers and the child to share their feelings about the surgery, any changes in body image, and their expectations for recovery and rehabilitation.

When the sutures are removed, reassure the child that the opening has healed and the child's insides will not "fall out," which is a common fear.

Before the child is discharged from the hospital, reinforcement of teaching focuses on home care, use of any special equipment or appliances, medications, diet, restrictions on activities, and therapeutic exercise (Fig. 29-11).

Family caregivers should demonstrate the procedures or repeat the information to confirm that learning has occurred. Use the nursing process to determine the needs of the child and the family to plan appropriate postoperative care and reinforcement of teaching.

> ### TEST YOURSELF
> ✔ Why is preoperative teaching and reinforcement of teaching important for the child and family caregivers?
> ✔ What preparation procedures might the child have before surgery?
> ✔ What factors are important in pain management for the child after surgery?
> ✔ What might be included in postoperative reinforcement of teaching for the child and family?

THE HOSPITAL PLAY PROGRAM

Play is the business of children and a principal way in which they learn, grow, develop, and act out feelings and problems. Playing is a normal activity; the more it can be part of hospital care, the more normal and more comfortable this environment becomes.

Play helps children come to terms with the hurts, anxieties, and separation that accompany hospitalization. In the hospital playroom, children may express frustrations, hostilities, and aggressions through play without the fear of being scolded or corrected. Children who keep these negative emotions bottled up suffer much greater damage than do those who are allowed to express them where they may be handled constructively. Children must feel secure enough in the situation to express negative emotions without fear of disapproval.

Children, however, must not be allowed to harm themselves or others. Although it is important to express acceptable or unacceptable feelings, unlimited permissiveness is as harmful as excessive strictness. Children rely on adults to guide them and set limits for behavior because this means the adults care about them. When behavior correction is necessary, it is important to make it clear that the child's action, not the child, is being disapproved.

The Hospital Play Environment

An organized and well-planned play or activity area is important in the overall care of the hospitalized child. The area should be large enough to accommodate cribs, wheelchairs, IV poles, and children in casts. It should provide a variety of play materials suitable for the ages and needs of all children (Fig. 29-12). Play is usually unstructured; the child chooses the toy and the kind of play needed or desired. However, all children should participate, and the play leaders should ignore no one.

If possible, older children and adolescents should have a separate recreation room or area away from young children. Ideally, this is an area where adolescents may gather to talk, play pool or ping pong, watch television and movies, use a computer, and if permitted eat snacks. Tables and chairs

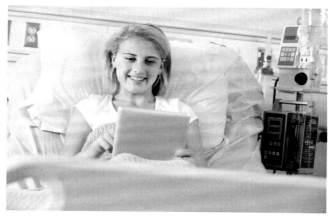

FIGURE 29-13 This adolescent enjoys using her tablet computer in her hospital room.

should be provided to encourage interaction among the adolescents. Rules may be clearly spelled out and posted. If a separate room is not available or the adolescents must stay in their room because they are on transmission-based precautions, the adolescents will need age-appropriate activities available in their room (Fig. 29-13).

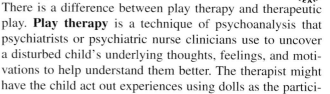

A Little Sensitivity is Important!
Even if older children and adolescents share the same room for recreation and activities with younger children, they will likely respond in a more positive way if the room is referred to an "activity center" or a name other than a "playroom."

Although a well-equipped playroom is of major importance in any pediatric department, some children cannot be brought to the playroom. In these situations, be creative in providing play opportunities for children. Children may act out their fantasies and emotions in their own cribs or beds if materials are brought to them and someone (a nurse, student, or volunteer) is available to give them needed support and attention. Children in isolation may be given play material, provided infection control precautions are strictly followed.

Therapeutic Play

There is a difference between play therapy and therapeutic play. **Play therapy** is a technique of psychoanalysis that psychiatrists or psychiatric nurse clinicians use to uncover a disturbed child's underlying thoughts, feelings, and motivations to help understand them better. The therapist might have the child act out experiences using dolls as the participants in the experience.

Therapeutic play is a play technique used to help the child have a better understanding of what will be happening to them in a specific situation. For instance, the child who will be having an IV started before surgery might be given the materials and encouraged to "start" an IV on a stuffed animal or doll. By observing the child, you can often note concerns, fears, and anxieties the child might express. Therapeutic play is a play technique that play therapists, nurses, or child-life specialists may use to help the child express feelings, fears, and concerns (Fig. 29-14).

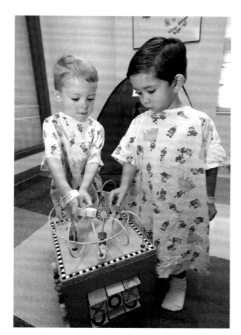

FIGURE 29-12 Children occupied in a hospital playroom. It is important to provide age-appropriate activities for children.

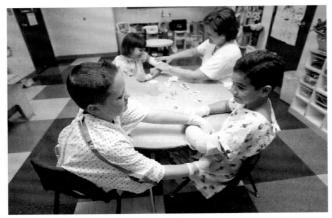

FIGURE 29-14 This group of children is involved in therapeutic play with the supervision of the child-life specialist.

The play leader should be alert to the needs of the child who is afraid to act independently. Even normally sociable children may carry their fears of the hospital environment into the playroom. It could be some time before timid, fearful, or nonassertive children feel free enough to take advantage of the play opportunities. Too much enthusiasm on the part of the play leader in trying to get the child to participate may defeat the purpose and make the child withdraw. The leader must decide carefully whether to initiate an activity for a child or let the child advance at a self-set pace.

Often other children provide the best incentive by doing something interesting, so that the timid child forgets their apprehensions and tries it, or another child says, "Come and help me with this," and soon the other child becomes involved. A fearful child may trust a peer before trusting an adult. The leader shows the child around the playroom, indicating that the children are free to play with whatever they wish and that the leader is there to answer questions and to help when a child wants help.

When initiating group play, the leader may invite but not insist that the timid child participate. The leader must give the child time to adjust and gain confidence.

Play Material

Play material should be chosen with safety in mind; there should be no sharp edges and no small parts that can be swallowed or aspirated. Toys and equipment should be inspected regularly for broken parts or sharp edges and cleaned and disinfected routinely.

One important playroom function is that it gives the child opportunities to dramatize hospital experiences. Providing hospital equipment, miniature or real, as play material gives the child an opportunity to act out feelings about the hospital environment

Be Alert for Client Safety!

Constant supervision of children while they are playing is necessary for safety.

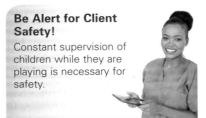

and treatments. Stethoscopes, simulated thermometers, stretchers, wheelchairs, examining tables, instruments, bandages, and other medical and hospital equipment are useful for this purpose.

Dolls or puppets dressed to represent the people with whom the child comes in contact daily—a boy, girl, infant, adult family members, nurses, health care providers, therapists, and other personnel—should be available. Hospital scrub suits, scrub caps, isolation-type gowns, masks, or other types of uniforms may be provided for children to use in acting out their hospital experiences. These simulated hospitals also serve an educational purpose: They may help a child who is to have surgery, tests, or special treatments understand the procedures and why they are done.

Hand puppets can be useful to orient or reassure a hospitalized child. The doctor or nurse puppet on the play leader's hand answers questions (and discusses feelings) that the puppet on the child's hand has asked. A child often finds it easier to express feelings, fears, and questions through a puppet than to verbalize them directly. The child can make believe that the puppet is really expressing things that they hesitate to ask.

Other useful play materials include clay, paints, markers, crayons, stamps, stickers, sand art, cut-out books, construction paper, puzzles, building sets, and board games. Tricycles, small sliding boards, and seesaws may be fun for children who can be more physically active. Books for all age groups are also important.

Sometimes only a little imagination is needed to initiate an interesting playtime. Table 29-1 suggests activities for various age levels, most of which may be played in the child's room. These are especially useful for the child who cannot go to the playroom.

TEST YOURSELF

✔ Why is play an important part of the hospitalization of children?

✔ Explain the difference between play therapy and therapeutic play.

✔ What is the most important factor to keep in mind when choosing play materials as well as other activities on the pediatric unit?

Think back to **Kylem Williams**. How did Kylem's admission differ from a routine scheduled admission? What postoperative care did you give Kylem? What did you use to collect data related to Kylem's pain after surgery? What activities did you incorporate to promote his stage of growth and development?

TABLE 29-1 Games and Activities Using Materials Available on a Nursing Unit

AGE	ACTIVITY
Infant	Make a mobile from roller gauze and tongue blades to hang over a crib
	Ask the pharmacy or central supply for different size boxes to use for put-in, take-out toys. (Do not use round vials from pharmacy; if accidentally aspirated, these can completely occlude the airway)
	Blow up a glove as a balloon; draw a smiling face on it with a marker. Hang it out of infant's reach
	Play "patty cake," "so big," "peek-a-boo"
Toddler	Ask central supply for boxes to use as blocks for stacking
	Tie roller gauze to a glove box for a pull toy
	Sing or recite familiar nursery rhymes such as "Peter, Peter, Pumpkin Eater"
Preschool	Play "Simon Says" or "Mother, May I?"
	Draw a picture of a dog; ask child to close eyes; add an additional feature to the dog; ask child to guess the added part; repeat until a full picture is drawn
	Make a puppet from a lunch bag or draw a face on your hand with a marker
	Cut out a picture from a newspaper or a magazine (or draw a picture); cut it into large puzzle pieces
	Pour breakfast cereal into a basin; furnish boxes to pour and spoons to dig
	Furnish paper and a marker for coloring
	Make modeling clay from 1 cup salt, 1/2 cup flour, 1/2 cup water from kitchen
	Play "Ring-Around-the-Rosy" or "London Bridge"
School age	Play "I Spy" or charades
	Make a deck of cards to play "Go Fish" or "Old Maid"; invent cards such as Nicholas Nurse, Doctor Dolittle, Irene Intern, Polly Patient
	Play "Hangman"
	Furnish scale or table paper and a marker for a hug drawing or sign
	Hide an object in the child's room and have the child look for it (have the child name places for you to look if the child cannot be out of bed)
Adolescent	Color squares on a chart form to make a checker board
	Have adolescent make a deck of cards to use for "Hearts" or "Rummy"
	Compete to see how many words the adolescent can make from the letters in their name
	Compete to guess whether the next person to enter the room will be a man or woman, next car to go by window will be red or black, and so forth
	Compete to see who can name the characters in current television shows or movies

KEY POINTS

- The cause of the illness, its treatment, guilt about the illness, past experiences of illness and hospitalization, disruption in family life, the threat to the child's long-term health, cultural or religious influences, coping methods within the family, and financial impact of the hospitalization may all affect how the family responds to the child's illness.

- The family caregiver's role in educating the child about hospitals includes helping the child develop a positive attitude about hospitals, hospitalization, and illness, and giving children simple, honest answers to their questions.

- Pediatric units are developed to create comfortable and safe atmospheres for children and are decorated with a variety of colors. Treatments are done in treatment rooms rather than the child's room. Play rooms and activity areas encourage activities for promoting normal age-related development.

- Safety is an essential aspect of pediatric care. The stress that infants, children, and their family caregivers experience when a child is hospitalized may increase the frequency of accidents. Understanding the growth and development levels of each age group helps you be alert to possible dangers for each child.

- Microorganisms are spread by contact (direct or indirect); droplet (coughing, sneezing, talking); vehicle (food, water, blood, or contaminated products); airborne (particles in the air); or vector (mosquitoes, vermin) means of transmission.

- Standard precautions reduce the risk of transmission of microorganisms from recognized or unrecognized sources of infection. Transmission-based precautions are used for clients documented or suspected of having highly transmissible pathogens that require additional precautions. Handwashing and hand hygiene is the cornerstone of all infection control. Wash hands or use alcohol-based hand disinfectant conscientiously between seeing each client, even when gloves are worn for a procedure.

- For a child placed on transmission-based precautions, preventing the spread of infection to others; encouraging compliance with the precautions; helping the child cope with feelings of isolation, loneliness, anxiety, and depression; and promoting normal development are important aspects of nursing care. Spending extra time in the room when performing treatments and procedures, reading a story, playing a game, or talking with the child can help comfort and support the child.

- The three stages of response to separation seen in the child include *protest* (the child cries, refuses to be comforted, and constantly seeks the primary caregiver); *despair* (the child becomes apathetic and listless when the caregiver does not appear); and *denial* (the child appears to accept the situation, but ignores the primary caregiver when they return).

- Family caregiver participation is important to relieve the child's separation anxiety. Rooming-in is encouraged to make the child feel more secure and to provide opportunities to reinforce teaching with family caregivers about how to care for the child after discharge. Encourage family caregivers to take breaks from the child when needed.

- In a planned admission, preadmission education helps prepare the child for hospitalization. There is time to explain procedures to the child and let the child play with equipment to become familiar with it. In an emergency admission, there may be little time for explanations because physical needs are the priority.

- The family caregiver is a vital participant in the care of an ill child. The caregiver participates in the admission interview and should be included in the planning of nursing care.

- Discharge planning includes reinforcing teaching with the child and the family about the care needed after discharge from the hospital. Written instructions should be provided. Also include information about how the child may respond after discharge. The family should encourage positive behavior, avoid making the child the center of attention, and provide loving but firm discipline.

- In reinforcing preoperative teaching, health professionals determine how much the child knows and is capable of learning, help correct any misunderstandings, explain the preparation for surgery, and explain how the child will feel after surgery. Information given must be based on the child's age, developmental level, previous experiences, and family caregiver support.

- Preoperative preparation for the child may include skin preparation, such as a tub bath or shower, shaving the surgical site, administering enemas, keeping the child NPO, urinary catheterization, and administering preoperative medications.

- Postoperative care of the child following surgery includes careful observation and looking for signs of complications; close monitoring of vital signs, dressings, intake, and output; following postoperative orders; and reinforcing client and family teaching.

- Gathering data and treatment of pain is important in caring for children. Use of pain assessment tools helps children express the amount of pain they are having. Behaviors such as rigidity, thrashing, facial expressions, loud crying or screaming, flexion of knees (indicating abdominal pain), restlessness, and irritability may indicate the child is in pain. Physiologic changes, such as a change in heart or respiratory rate or blood pressure, sweating palms, dilated pupils, flushed or moist skin, and loss of appetite, may also indicate pain.

- Play is the principal way in which children learn, grow, develop, and act out feelings and problems. In hospital play programs, children may express frustrations, hostilities, and aggressions through play without the fear of being scolded. A well-planned hospital play or activity area with safe play materials and activities for children of all ages is important. Play therapy is a technique used to uncover a disturbed child's underlying thoughts, feelings, and motivations to help understand them better. Therapeutic play is a play technique used to help the child have a better understanding of what will be happening to them in a specific situation.

INTERNET RESOURCES

Virtual Pediatric Hospital
www.virtualpediatrichospital.org

Hospitalization
http://kidshealth.org

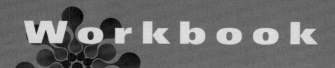

NCLEX-STYLE REVIEW QUESTIONS

1. When caring for a child in a pediatric setting, which action by the nurse indicates an understanding of standard precautions?
   a. Carrying used syringes immediately to the sharps container in the medication room
   b. Wearing one pair of gloves while doing all care for a client
   c. Leaving an isolation gown hanging inside the client's room to reuse for the next treatment or procedure
   d. Cleaning reusable equipment before using it for another client

2. When discussing postoperative pain management with a family caregiver of a school-aged child, which statement made by the caregiver indicates a need for further information?
   a. "My child can push the patient-controlled analgesia pump button without any help."
   b. "After the last surgery, they gave my child pain medicine shots in the leg."
   c. "Talking or singing seems to decrease the amount of pain medication my child needs."
   d. "I am relieved to know my child will have less pain than do adults."

3. A 5-year-old child is placed on transmission-based precautions and is in isolation. Which action by the nurse would best help the child cope with the loneliness the child may experience because of being in isolation?
   a. Talking to the child about how they feel being alone
   b. Answering the call light over the intercom immediately
   c. Encouraging the child to talk to friends on the telephone
   d. Providing age-appropriate activities that can be played alone

4. The hospitalized child away from their home and normal environment goes through stages of separation. Which behavior by the child might indicate the child is in the "denial" stage of separation?
   a. Crying loudly even when being held by the nurse
   b. Searching for the family caregiver to arrive
   c. Ignoring family caregivers when they visit
   d. Quietly lying in the crib when no one is in the room

5. After the discharge of a preschool-aged child from the hospital, which behavior by the child might indicate they are afraid of another separation?
   a. The child plays with siblings for long periods of time.
   b. The child carries a favorite blanket around the house.
   c. The child requests to go visit the nurses at the hospital.
   d. The child wakes up very early in the morning.

6. The nurse is following standard precautions when caring for a child on the pediatric unit when the nurse does which of the following? Select all that apply.
   a. Washes hands when gloves are removed
   b. Wears gloves when touching contaminated articles
   c. Cleans reusable equipment with hot water before using on another client
   d. Removes needle from syringe immediately after medication administration
   e. Wears protective eye covering when secretions are likely to splash
   f. Removes disposable gown promptly if soiling has occurred

STUDY ACTIVITIES

1. Design an ideal teen activity room. List all furniture and equipment you would have, and state the use(s) for each.

2. Discuss how rooming-in can be helpful in discharge planning.

3. Participate in an orientation tour of a pediatric unit in your local area. If not available, plan an orientation visit for a group of preschool-aged children and share with your classmates what you would include and what activities you would have the preschool-aged children participate in.

4. Do an internet search on "preparing children for surgery." After exploring some of the sites you find, answer the following:
   a. What are some of the sites you found?
   b. What books did you find that you think might help a family caregiver prepare a child who will be having a planned surgery?
   c. What other information on these sites do you think would be helpful in preparing a child for hospitalization?

CRITICAL THINKING: WHAT WOULD YOU DO?

1. Your neighbor's daughter, 3-year-old Angela, is going to be admitted to the pediatric unit for tests and possible surgery.
   a. What will you say to Angela to help prepare her for the tests that will be done?
   b. What activities will you suggest Angela's mother might do to prepare her daughter for this event?
   c. What will you tell Angela when she asks you what surgery is?

2. Edgar, the 4-year-old son of migrant workers, is hurt in a farming accident. You are working in the emergency department when he is brought in for treatment. His grandmother, who speaks little English, is with him.

   a. What will you include in Edgar's plan of care that will help both the child and his grandmother?

   b. What can you do to further communication between you, Edgar, and his grandmother?

3. On a playground, you hear a child's family caregiver say, "If you don't stop that, you're going to hurt yourself and end up in the hospital!"

   a. What are your feelings about this statement?

   b. What would you say if you had the opportunity to respond to this caregiver after this statement was made?

   c. What statement do you think would have been more appropriate for the family caregiver to say in this situation?

Procedures and Treatments

Learning Objectives

At the conclusion of this chapter, you will:

1. Describe nursing responsibilities when preparing the child for a procedure or treatment.
2. Describe nursing responsibilities after the child undergoes a procedure or treatment.
3. Explain different types of restraints, their uses, and safety measures to consider in children.
4. Describe appropriate positioning of the child for holding, transporting, and sleeping.
5. List methods of reducing an elevated body temperature in children.
6. Explain the reason for monitoring accurate intake and output measurements when caring for children.
7. Discuss the reasons and procedure for inserting an enteral feeding tube and administering a gavage feeding.
8. Explain the use of gastrostomy feeding in children and how it is different from gavage feeding.
9. Describe oxygen administration methods and safety considerations for children.
10. Describe nasal or oral suctioning to improve the child's respiratory function.
11. Explain basic components of tracheostomy care for the child.
12. Discuss the use of hot or cold therapy in children in relation to circulation.
13. Describe nursing care for three types of ostomies that are created in children with problems related to elimination.
14. Explain how and why nose and throat specimens may be collected from the child.
15. Describe four methods of urine specimen collection.
16. Explain the method of stool collection for the child.
17. Discuss the role of the nurse in assisting with procedures related to blood collection, lumbar puncture, and diagnostic tests and studies in children.

Reyna Vargas was born prematurely and is now 5 months old. Since Reyna was born, she has been hospitalized several times and has just been readmitted to the pediatric unit. She is being fed via a nasogastric tube, has an IV infusing, and is on oxygen via a nasal cannula. As you read this chapter, think about how you will administer her feedings, restraints that may need to be used to keep Reyna safe, and factors important in administering Reyna's oxygen.

NURSE'S ROLE IN PREPARATION AND FOLLOW-UP

As a pediatric nurse, your role in performing or assisting with procedures and treatments includes following guidelines set by the healthcare institution. These guidelines include the preparation before the procedure and the follow-up needed when the procedure is completed. You are also responsible for following facility policies and ensuring client safety before, during, and after all procedures and treatments.

Preparation for Procedures

An important role in preparation for pediatric procedures is supporting the child and family. It is also important to follow the facility's policies to ensure that legal requirements and safety precautions are met.

Psychological or Emotional Support

Many highly technologic procedures in healthcare facilities may be frightening and painful to children. You can be an important source of comfort to children who must undergo these procedures, even though it is difficult to assist with or perform procedures that cause discomfort or pain. Explain the procedure and its purpose to the family caregiver to help decrease anxiety.

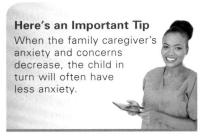

Here's an Important Tip
When the family caregiver's anxiety and concerns decrease, the child in turn will often have less anxiety.

Explain the procedure to the child in a manner appropriate for the child's age and level of development. If the child is old enough to understand, explain the purpose of the procedure and the expected benefit. Encourage the child to ask questions, and give complete answers (Fig. 30-1).

Toddlers require some explanation of procedures and what to expect, but their understanding will be limited. Even when toddlers grasp the words, they are not likely to fully understand the meaning. The reality is the pain that occurs. For infants, help soothe and comfort them before and after the procedure.

Sometimes children's interest can be diverted so that they may forget their fear. They must be allowed to cry if necessary, and they should always be listened to and have their questions answered. You learn with experience to know exactly which questions are stalling techniques and which call for firmness and action. Children need someone to take charge in a kind, firm manner that tells them the decision is not in their hands. They are too young to take this responsibility for themselves.

Legal and Safety Factors

When preparing to perform or assist with any procedures or treatments, there are certain steps to follow, no matter what the healthcare setting is. Most procedures require a written order before they are done. Clarify orders when needed. Always use two methods to identify the child before any treatment or procedure; check the child's identification band, and verify that information by having the child or family caregiver state the child's name and birthdate. Follow institution policies and if informed consent is needed, see that the form is completed, signed, and witnessed. As stated earlier, discuss the procedure with the child and family caregiver and answer any questions. Washing hands or using alcohol-based hand disinfectant before and after any procedure helps prevent or control the spread of microorganisms.

Gather the needed supplies and equipment, and review the steps for the procedure. Safety for the child (see Chapter 29) is a priority. Standard precautions are followed for all procedures (see Appendix A).

Keep it Legal
The health care provider doing the procedure explains, gives information, and answers questions before having the appropriate individual sign the informed consent.

Follow-Up for Procedures

When the procedure is completed, leave the child in a safe position with the side rails raised and the bed lowered. For the older child, place the call light within reach. Comfort and reassure the child, particularly if the procedure has been uncomfortable or traumatic. The family caregiver might have concerns or questions to discuss.

Remove equipment and supplies and dispose of them properly. Handle contaminated linens according to facility policy. If a specimen is to be taken to another department, label the specimen with the client's name, identifying information, and the type of specimen in the container. Follow the appropriate facility policies. Often paperwork must go with the specimen, and certain precautions are taken to prevent any exposure to the specimen. Documentation includes the procedure, the child's response, and the description and characteristics of any specimen obtained. If specimens are sent to another department in the facility, also record this information.

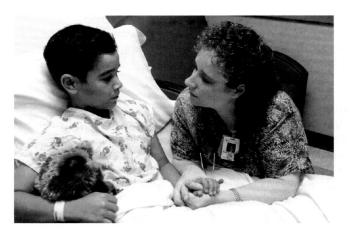

FIGURE 30-1 The nurse explains the procedure to the older child in a calm, reassuring manner and allows him to ask questions. This open communication helps minimize the child's stress related to the procedure.

There are con- flicting thoughts about the merit of giving the child some reward after a treatment. If a child receives a reward, it is not for being brave or good; it is simply a part of the entire treat- ment. The unpleasant

Good News

Children given a treat or a small toy after an uncomfortable procedure tend to remember the experience as not totally bad.

part is mitigated by the pleasant. An older person's reward is contemplating the improved health that the procedure may provide, but the child does not have sufficient reasoning ability to understand future benefits.

PERFORMING PROCEDURES RELATED TO POSITION

Safety is the most important nursing responsibility when performing procedures related to positioning a child. The child's safety and comfort must be a priority when using restraints or transporting children. Safety is also an import- ant factor when holding, transporting, or positioning chil- dren for sleep.

Using Restraints

Restraints are often needed to protect a child from injury during a procedure or an examination or to ensure the infant's or child's safety and comfort. Restraints are used as a last resort and should never be used as a form of pun- ishment. It is important to follow the healthcare facility's procedure and policy regarding restraints. In addition, the Joint Commission's guidelines and standards for the use of restraints must be followed. Most settings require a written order and have a set procedure of releasing the restraint at least every 2 hours, doing range of motion, monitoring circulation and neurovascular status, and documenting this and any findings. As well, orders for most restraints must be renewed every 24 hours. When possible, restraining by hand is the best method. However, mechanical restraints must be used to secure a child in certain situations such as during intravenous infusions; to protect a surgical site from

injury, for example, a cleft lip and cleft palate repair; or when restraint by hand is impractical. The most appropriate and least restrictive restraint is always used.

Be alert to family concerns when the child is in restraints. Explanations about the need for restraints help the family caregiver understand and be coopera- tive. The family care- giver may wish to restrain the child by hand to prevent the use of restraints, and this action is often possible. Each situ- ation must be judged individually.

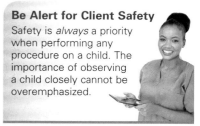

Be Alert for Client Safety

Safety is *always* a priority when performing any procedure on a child. The importance of observing a child closely cannot be overemphasized.

Various types of restraints may be used for children (Fig. 30-2). Whatever the type of restraint, close observation is a necessary part of nursing care.

Mummy Restraints and Papoose Boards

Mummy restraints are snug wraps used to restrain an infant or small child's body during a procedure. This device is effective when performing a scalp venipuncture, inserting a nasogastric tube, or performing other procedures that involve only the head or neck. Be sure the face is not covered and the airway is not restricted. **Papoose boards** are used with toddlers or preschoolers for similar purposes.

Clove Hitch Restraints

Clove hitch restraints are used occasionally to secure an arm or leg if motion needs to be limited in that extremity. They are most often used when a child is receiving an intra- venous infusion. The restraint is made of soft cloth formed in a figure-of-eight. Padding under the restraint is desirable if the child puts any pull on it. Loosen the restraint and check the site at least every 1 to 2 hours. Commercial restraints are also available for this purpose. Secure this restraint to the lower part of the crib or bed, not to the side rail, to avoid possibly causing injury when the side rail is raised or lowered. With the use of soft, pliable IV catheters and IV house devices (see Fig. 31-7A and 7B in Chapter 31), which decrease the movement of the IV catheter and decrease the risk of the IV becoming dislodged, there is less need to restrain and immobilize the extremity with the IV site.

Elbow Restraints

Elbow restraints are wrapped around the child's arm and tied securely to prevent the child from bending the elbow. They are often made of muslin or other materials in two layers. Pockets wide enough to hold tongue depressors are placed vertically in the width of the fabric. The top flap folds over to close the pockets. Care must be taken to ensure that the elbow restraints fit the child properly. They should not be too high under the axillae. They may be pinned to the child's shirt to keep them from slipping. Commercially made elbow restraints may also be used.

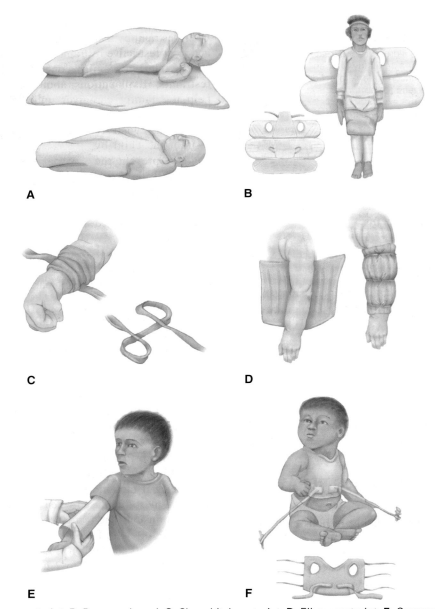

FIGURE 30-2 A. Mummy restraint. **B.** Papoose board. **C.** Clove hitch restraint. **D.** Elbow restraint. **E.** Commercial elbow restraint. **F.** Jacket restraint.

Jacket Restraints

Jacket restraints are used to secure the child from climbing out of bed or a chair or to keep the child in a horizontal position. The restraint must be the correct size for the child and is put on over clothing to decrease skin irritation. Monitor the child in a jacket restraint closely to prevent them from slipping and choking on the neck of the jacket. Ties must be secured to the bed frame, not the side rails, so that the jacket is not pulled when the side rails are moved up and down.

Crib Top Restraints

A crib top restraint is a clear plastic cover attached to the top of the crib. This type of restraint is used for older infants and toddlers who are able to stand and climb, to prevent them from climbing over the side of the bed and falling (Fig. 30-3).

> ### TEST YOURSELF
>
> ✔ What are the different types of restraints used in children?
>
> ✔ When are each of the different types of restraints used?

Holding

When a child is held, they need to be safe and feel secure. The three most common methods of holding a child are the cradle position, upright or over the shoulder position, or the

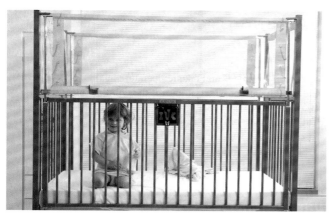

FIGURE 30-3 Crib top restraint. A clear plastic cover attached to the top of the crib keeps the older infant or toddler from climbing out of the crib. (Reprinted with permission from Ricci, S., Kyle T., & Carman, S. (2021). *Maternity and pediatric nursing* (4th ed., p. 1174, Fig. 33-6). Wolters Kluwer.)

football hold (Fig. 30-4). When holding an infant, always support the infant's head and back.

During and after feedings, hold the infant in a sitting position on the lap for burping. Lean the infant forward against one hand and use the thumb and finger to support the infant's head; this leaves the other hand free to gently pat the infant's back (Fig. 30-5).

Transporting

When moving infants and small children in a healthcare setting, the safety of the child is the biggest concern. It is best to carry the infant or place them in a crib or bassinet. The toddler may be transported in a crib with high side rails or one with a crib top restraint. Strollers or wheelchairs are used when the child is able to sit. Many pediatric settings use wagons with high sides to transport children.

Older children are placed in wheelchairs or on stretchers. They may be moved in their beds; often a hospitalized child who is in traction, which cannot be removed, can go to the playroom or other areas in the hospital in this manner.

Seat belts or safety straps should always be used when transporting the child.

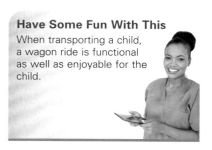

Have Some Fun With This

When transporting a child, a wagon ride is functional as well as enjoyable for the child.

Positioning for Sleep

Position infants on their backs for sleeping. This position seems to have decreased the incidence of crib death or sudden infant death syndrome (see Chapter 20) in infants. Reinforce this information with family caregivers.

PERFORMING PROCEDURES RELATED TO ELEVATED BODY TEMPERATURE

Significant alterations in body temperature can have severe consequences for children. "Normal" body temperature varies from 97.6°F (36.4°C) orally to 100.3°F (37.9°C) rectally. The body temperature should generally be maintained below 101°F (38.3°C) orally or 102°F (38.9°C) rectally, although the healthcare facility or health care provider may set lower limits. Methods used to reduce fever include maintaining hydration by encouraging fluids and administering antipyretics such as acetaminophen or ibuprofen. Because of their ineffectiveness in reducing fever and the discomfort they cause, tepid sponge baths are not recommended for reducing fever. Because many children get fevers but do not need hospitalization, family caregivers need instructions on fever reduction (see Tips for Reinforcing Family Teaching: Reducing Fever).

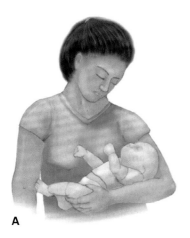
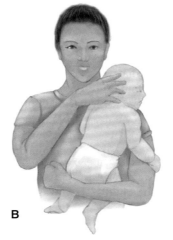
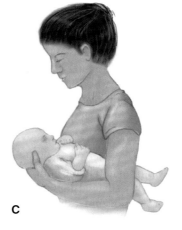

A **B** **C**

FIGURE 30-4 Positions to hold an infant or child: **(A)** cradle position, **(B)** upright or over the shoulder position, and **(C)** football hold.

TIPS FOR REINFORCING FAMILY TEACHING

Reducing Fever

- Do not overdress or heavily cover the child. Diaper, light sheet, or light pajamas are sufficient.
- Encourage the child to drink fluids.
- Keep room environment cool.
- Use acetaminophen or other antipyretics according to the health care provider's directions. Do not give aspirin.

- Wait for 30 minutes and take temperature again.
- Call health care provider at once if the child's temperature is 105°F (40.6°C) or higher.
- Call health care provider if the child has history of febrile seizures.

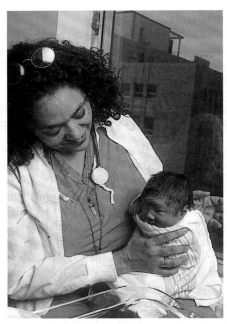

FIGURE 30-5 The nurse holds the infant in a sitting position to burp the baby.

Control of Environmental Factors

Removing excess coverings from the child with fever permits additional cooling through evaporation. Changing to lightweight clothes, removing clothes, using cotton sheets and blankets, lowering the room temperature, or applying cool compresses to the forehead may help to lower the child's temperature. If a child begins to shiver, whatever method is being used to lower the temperature should be stopped. Shivering indicates the child is chilling and will cause the body temperature to increase.

Cooling Devices

A cooling device, such as a hypothermia pad or blanket, can lower or maintain the child's body temperature. The blanket is always covered before being placed next to the child's skin so moisture can be absorbed from the skin. Closely monitor the child's temperature by checking it frequently with a regular thermometer. Document the child's baseline temperature and additional temperature measurements, as well as information regarding the child's response to the treatment.

PERFORMING PROCEDURES RELATED TO FEEDING AND NUTRITION

Monitoring the intake of fluids and nutrients is important in both maintaining and promoting appropriate growth in children. As the nurse, you are responsible for accurately documenting both a child's intake and output. If a child is unable to consume adequate amounts of fluid or foods, enteral feedings are administered to meet the child's nutrient needs and promote normal growth.

Intake and Output Measurements

Accurately measuring and recording intake and output are especially important in working with the ill or hospitalized child to monitor and maintain the child's fluid balance. In a well-child setting, the family caregiver can provide information about the child's usual patterns of intake and output. With the ill or hospitalized child, more exact measurements of fluid intake and output are required. In many settings, these measurements are recorded as often as every hour, and a running total is kept to closely monitor the child.

Oral fluids, enteral feeding intake, intravenous fluids, and foods that become liquid at room temperature (e.g., frozen foods such as popsicles) are all measured and recorded as intake. Urine, vomitus, diarrhea, gastric suctioning, and any other liquid drainage are measured and considered output. Describe and record the color and characteristics of the output.

To measure the output of an infant wearing a diaper, weigh a dry diaper, then weigh the wet diaper and subtract the weight of the dry diaper; the difference is the amount to record as the output.

Enteral Nutrition

Sometimes infants or children who have had surgery or have a chronic or serious condition are unable to take adequate food and fluid by mouth. The nutritional needs of these children are met by means **of an enteral tube feeding**.

Gavage Feeding

Gavage feeding provides nutrition through a tube passed directly into the stomach through the nose (nasogastric) (Fig. 30-6) (Nursing Procedure 30-1) or mouth (orogastric). This procedure is particularly appropriate in infants but may also be used in the older child. These feedings may be given intermittently as a **bolus feeding** where a specific amount of feeding is given over a short period of time, usually 15 to 30

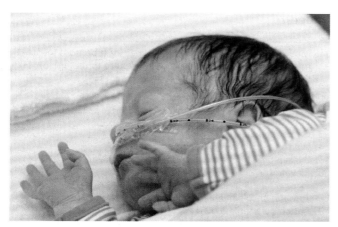

FIGURE 30-6 The infant receives nutrition via an enteral feeding tube (nasogastric) and oxygen via a nasal cannula.

signs such as gagging, vomiting, coughing, or respiratory distress which might indicate the tube is incorrectly placed.

As well as verifying tube placement, the **gastric residual**, the amount remaining in the stomach, which indicates absorption of feedings and gastric emptying, is aspirated, measured, recorded, and observed, and the characteristics of the aspirate are documented. The gastric aspirate is returned to the stomach through the tube unless the amount is larger than the health care provider has specified.

If enteral feedings are not well tolerated, stop the feeding, report observations, and await alternate orders from the health care provider.

> **Warning!**
> Verifying positioning of a gavage feeding tube by inserting air (using an Asepto syringe) and listening with a stethoscope for sounds in the stomach is considered an *unreliable* method of checking for tube placement and is not recommended.

Gastrostomy Feeding

If feedings will be given continuously or are required over a longer period of time, then a gastrostomy tube is often placed. Whereas a gavage feeding tube is inserted into the stomach through the nose or mouth, a **gastrostomy tube** is inserted through the abdominal wall into the stomach (Fig. 30-7A). The gastrostomy tube is usually inserted surgically with the child under general anesthesia. Following placement, the site must be kept clean and dry and be monitored for signs of infection and irritation. The child may need to be restrained to prevent pulling on the tube, which may cause leakage of caustic gastric juices. Gastrostomy tubes are often used in children who have conditions that interfere with their ability to eat or

minutes, and then feedings are given at specific time intervals. The feedings may be given continuously at a slower rate over a longer period of time. If given as a continuous feeding, an enteral feeding pump is used to regulate and monitor the infusion flow rate of the feeding. Many times, continuous feedings are given through the night to allow the child to be disconnected from the feeding during the day. This allows the child to be less restricted in daytime activities.

Prior to giving an enteral feeding checking for tube placement is a priority. Methods of verifying tube placement include radiographic confirmation, appearance and pH of gastric aspirate, and measuring the external length of the tube from the exit mark to the end of the tube. Following institution policies and procedures and using more than one method of checking for placement is important. Monitor for

NURSING PROCEDURE 30-1 Gavage Feeding

EQUIPMENT
Enteral feeding tube
Nonsterile gloves
Water-soluble lubricant
Tape or marking pen
Catheter-tip syringe (Asepto syringe)
pH tape
Feeding solution

PROCEDURE
Inserting an enteral feeding tube
1. Explain procedure to the child and family caregiver.
2. Wash hands.
3. Position the infant in a supine position with a towel or pillow under the shoulders to elevate the head. Position the child in a sitting position, if possible.
4. Use a swaddle restraint or have a second person securely hold the infant or child.
5. Determine the length of tubing to use by measuring from the tip of the child's nose to the earlobe, and from the earlobe down to the tip of the sternum (Fig. A).

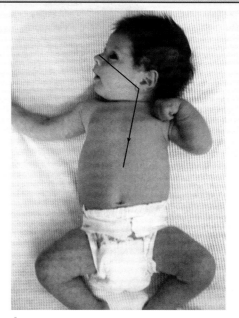

A

(Continued)

NURSING PROCEDURE 30-1 Gavage Feeding (Continued)

6. Mark this length on the tube with tape or a marking pen.
7. Put on nonsterile gloves.
8. Lubricate the end of the tube to be inserted with water-soluble lubricant (never an oily substance because of the danger of oil aspiration into the lungs).
9. Insert tube nasally (nasogastric) or orally (orogastric). Pass tube until the insertion mark is at the opening of the nose.
10. Temporarily secure tube until placement is verified.
11. Confirm placement by radiologic confirmation, the most accurate method of verifying tube placement and position. Because of the risks of repeated radiation exposure, this procedure cannot be used before each feeding (see the procedure for checking placement before feeding below).
12. Secure tubing to the child's nose using adhesive tape (Fig. B).

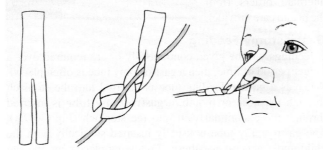

B

13. Further secure tubing for the child's comfort by gently placing tubing behind the ear and securing to the child's cheek (Fig. C).

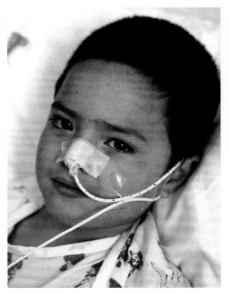

C

14. Measure the length of the external part of tube from the marking on the tube (at the nose or mouth) to the end of the tube, and document this measurement.

Administering gavage feeding

1. Verify order for gavage feeding.
2. Wash hands.
3. Gather supplies
4. Warm feeding to room temperature.
5. Explain procedure to child and family caregiver.
6. Elevate the child's head and shoulders.
7. Place a rolled-up towel behind the neck.
8. Turn the child's head and align the body to the right.
9. Put on nonsterile gloves.
10. Insert the feeding syringe (bulb or Asepto syringe) into feeding tube.
11. Verify placement of tube to ensure that the tube is in the stomach:
    a. Measure length of the external part of tube (from the marking on the tube at the nose or mouth to the end of tube) and compare measurement to the documented measurement.
    b. Aspirate stomach contents. Check the pH of the fluids aspirated. The pH of gastric contents is acidic, rather than alkaline, which would be noted if the fluids were respiratory in nature.
12. Measure and replace stomach contents that have been aspirated.
13. Remove plunger from catheter-tip syringe, attach syringe to end of tubing, pour feeding into syringe.
14. Slowly administer feeding over 15 to 30 minutes, letting it flow by gravity.
15. Observe for signs of distress, such as gasping, coughing, or cyanosis, which might indicate tube is incorrectly placed. Stop the feeding and withdraw the tube if any of these signs are noted.
16. Flush the tube with water after the feeding to maintain the patency of the tube.
17. Burp the infant.
18. Position the infant or child on the right side for at least 1 hour to prevent regurgitation and aspiration.
19. Discard any leftover feeding at the completion of the procedure.
20. Document the following:
    a. Date and time of feeding
    b. Type and size of tubing used
    c. Method of placement and tube patency
    d. Type and amount of contents aspirated, pH of residual
    e. Type and amount of feeding given
    f. Child's response to and tolerance of procedure
    g. Positioning of child following feeding

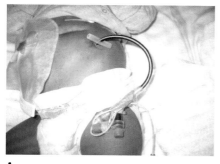

A

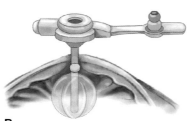

B

FIGURE 30-7 **(A)** A gastrostomy tube or **(B)** gastrostomy button is placed when long-term enteral feedings will be needed.

drink; surgical repairs in the mouth; swallowing, throat, or esophageal concerns; severe gastroesophageal reflux disease (GERD); respiratory distress; or who are respirator-dependent.

For long-term gastrostomy feedings, a gastrostomy button may be inserted (Fig. 30-7B). Some advantages of buttons are that they are more desirable cosmetically, are simple to care for, and cause less skin irritation. When regular oral feedings are resumed, the gastrostomy tube or button is surgically removed, and the opening usually closes spontaneously.

Procedures for positioning and feeding the child with a gavage feeding tube or a gastrostomy tube are similar. Elevate the child's head and shoulders during feeding. Before administering a gastrostomy feeding, observe the tube for placement and, as with a gavage feeding, check the **gastric residual**. Following any feeding, flush the tube with water to clear the tubing and prevent the feeding solution from occluding the tube. After each feeding, place the child on the right side with the head slightly elevated.

Take Note

Both gavage and gastrostomy tubes can also be used to administer liquid or dissolved forms of oral medications (see Chapter 31). Following medication administration, always flush the tube adequately with water to prevent the tube from being occluded.

Remember **Reyna** from the beginning of the chapter? Why do you think Reyna is getting enteral feedings? What is the process you will follow to administer Reyna's nasogastric feedings? Write the steps of the procedure.

TEST YOURSELF

✔ When might a cooling device be used?

✔ Why is it important to monitor and document a child's intake?

✔ When are enteral feedings used?

✔ What is the difference between a gavage tube and a gastrostomy tube?

PERFORMING PROCEDURES RELATED TO RESPIRATION

Oxygen administration, nasal and oral suctioning, and caring for the child with a tracheostomy are procedures you might be called on to perform for the child with a respiratory condition. Monitoring and maintaining adequate oxygenation are nursing responsibilities.

Oxygen Administration

Oxygen is administered to treat symptoms of respiratory distress or when the oxygen saturation level in the blood is below normal (see Chapter 28 for measurement of oxygen saturation). Depending on the child's age and oxygen needs, many different methods are used to deliver oxygen (Table 30-1). Infants, as well as older children, might have oxygen administered by nasal cannula (see Fig. 30-6) or prongs, mask (Fig. 30-8), or an oxygen hood (Fig. 30-9). Oxygen tents are used infrequently because the oxygen concentration is more difficult to maintain.

Whatever equipment is used to administer oxygen, explain the procedure and equipment to the child and the family caregiver. Letting the child hold and feel the equipment and flow of oxygen through the device helps decrease the child's fear and anxiety about the procedure. Most devices warm and humidify oxygen to prevent the recipient's nasal passages from becoming dry. Closely monitor children receiving oxygen therapy; when oxygen is to be discontinued, it is done gradually. Check equipment frequently to ensure proper functioning, cleanliness, and correct oxygen flow rate. Exposure to high concentrations of oxygen can be dangerous to small infants and children with respiratory diseases.

Safety First

Use only water-based products for lubrication for dry nasal passages for the child who is receiving oxygen. Always *avoid* petroleum-based lotions or creams, like Vaseline, on the child's face and chest. These products are highly flammable and should not be used in the presence of oxygen.

TIPS FOR REINFORCING FAMILY TEACHING

Oxygen Safety

- Keep equipment clean. Dirty equipment can be a source of bacteria.
- Use signs noting that oxygen is in use.
- Give good mouth care. Use swabs and mouthwash.
- Offer fluids frequently.

- Keep nose clean.
- Do not use electric or battery-powered toys.
- Do not allow smoking, matches, or lighters nearby.
- Do not keep flammable solutions in the room.
- Do not use wool or synthetic blankets.

TABLE 30-1 Methods of Oxygen Administration

METHOD	AGE OR REASON TO USE	NURSING CONCERNS WHEN USING
Nasal prongs/ cannula	Many sizes available Nasal prongs fit into child's nose	Not always humidified; causes dryness Keep nasal prongs clean and clear of secretions Monitor nostrils for irritation Toddlers may pull out of nose; other methods better
Mask	Various sizes available Covers mouth and nose, not eyes Humidified, decreases dryness	Not used in comatose children
Hood	Fits over head and neck of child Clear so child can be seen	May be frightening for child
Oxygen tent	Equipment does not come in contact with face Allows for movement inside tent	Difficult to see child in tent Difficult for child to see out Child feels isolated Change clothing and linen often Keep side rails up
Tracheostomy	Used in emergencies or when long-term oxygen is needed	Must be kept clean with airway patent Suction when needed

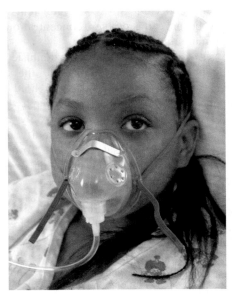

FIGURE 30-8 The child receives oxygen via a facemask.

Many times children are cared for in a home setting while receiving oxygen. Reinforce with the family caregiver information regarding oxygen administration, equipment, and safety measures (see Tips for Reinforcing Family Teaching: Oxygen Safety).

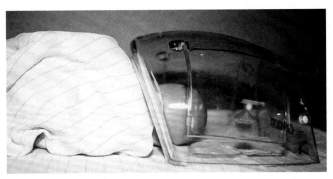

FIGURE 30-9 Oxygen hood used for an infant. (Reprinted with permission from Rosdahl C. B., & Kowalski M. T. (2017). *Textbook of basic nursing* (11th ed., p. 1179, Fig. 71.7). Wolters Kluwer.)

Nasal/Oral Suctioning

Excess secretions in the nose or mouth can obstruct the infant's or child's airway and decrease respiratory function. Coughing often clears the airway, but when the infant or child is unable to remove secretions, they are removed by suctioning. Use a bulb syringe to remove secretions from the nose and mouth (Fig. 30-10). Sterile normal saline drops may be used to loosen dried nasal secretions. Nasotracheal suctioning with a sterile suction catheter may be needed if secretions cannot be removed by other methods.

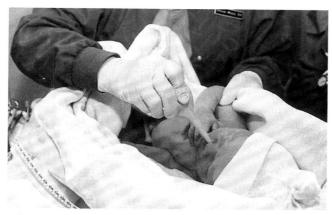

FIGURE 30-10 A bulb syringe is used to remove secretions from the nose and mouth.

Tracheostomy Care

A **tracheostomy** is a surgical procedure in which an opening is made into the trachea and a tube is put in place to give the child a patent airway. A tracheostomy is performed in emergency situations or in conditions in which an infant or child has an obstructed airway. The tracheostomy may be temporary or permanent. Mechanical ventilation and oxygen can be supplied using a ventilator, when needed.

Children with tracheostomies are cared for initially in the hospital setting; children with long-term conditions are often cared for at home or in long-term care facilities. The tracheostomy tube is suctioned to remove mucus and secretions and to keep the airway patent. With a new tracheostomy, sterile technique is used. Depending on the respiratory status, the child may be preventilated prior to being suctioned and ventilated again following the procedure, using a manual ventilation bag. The plastic or metal tracheostomy tube must be cleaned often to decrease the possibility of infection. When doing tracheostomy care, a second person helps to hold or secure the tracheostomy while the ties or self-fastening securing devices are being changed to prevent accidental dislodgement. Care of the skin around the site will prevent breakdown. A dressing may be placed around the stoma if there are excessive secretions. If ties are used to secure the tracheostomy, they should be tied on the side of the neck to decrease skin breakdown. A tracheostomy collar or ventilator provides moisture and humidity. The tracheostomy prevents the child from being able to cry or speak, so monitor closely, leave the call bell within reach, and find alternative methods of communicating with the child. In case of an accidental dislodgement, a spare tracheostomy and a second one a size smaller are kept at the bedside.

PERFORMING PROCEDURES RELATED TO CIRCULATION

Heat or cold therapy may be used to treat problems associated with circulation. After a health care provider has written an order for heat or cold therapy, you may be responsible for applying the treatment, closely monitoring the effects of the treatment, and documenting those observations.

Heat Therapy

The local application of heat increases circulation by vasodilatation and promotes muscle relaxation, thereby relieving pain and congestion. It also speeds the formation and drainage of superficial abscesses.

Artificial heat should never be applied to the child's skin without a specific order from the health care provider. Tissue damage can occur, particularly in fair-skinned people or in those who have experienced sensory loss or impaired circulation. Children require close monitoring, and none should receive heat treatments longer than 20 minutes at a time, unless specifically ordered by the health care provider.

Moist heat produces faster results than does dry heat and is usually applied in the form of a warm compress or soak.

> **Be Alert for Client Safety!**
> If towels are used to provide moist heat, they should not be warmed in the microwave because the microwave may unevenly heat the towels, which in turn may burn the child.

Dry heat may be applied by means of an electric heating pad or a K-pad (a unit that circulates warm water through plastic-enclosed tubing). Many children have been burned because of the improper use of hot water bottles; therefore, these devices are not recommended. Electric heating pads and K-pads should be covered with pillowcases, towels, or stockinettes. Document the application type, start time, therapy duration, and the skin's condition before and after the application.

Cold Therapy

As with heat, a health care provider must order the use of cold applications. In addition to reducing body temperature (see the section on Cooling Devices), the local application of cold may also help prevent swelling, control hemorrhage, and provide an anesthetic effect. Intervals of about 20 minutes are recommended for both dry cold (ice bag and commercial instant-cold preparation) and moist cold (compress, soak, and bath) treatments. Lightly cover dry cold applications to protect the child's skin from direct contact. Because cold decreases circulation, prolonged chilling may result in frostbite and gangrene.

Inspect the child's skin before and after the cold application to detect skin redness or irritation. Document the application type, start time, therapy duration, and the skin's condition before and after the application.

Detailed instructions for the therapeutic application of cold and heat may be obtained in the procedures manual of each facility and from manufacturers of commercial devices.

> ## TEST YOURSELF
> ✔ What are some methods used to administer oxygen to children?
> ✔ What is a tracheostomy, and when would one be used?
> ✔ For what reasons might heat therapy be used?
> ✔ For what reasons might cold therapy be used?

PERFORMING PROCEDURES RELATED TO ELIMINATION

As the nurse in the pediatric setting, you may be responsible for performing procedures related to elimination. You might administer an enema to a child as a treatment or as a preoperative procedure. When a child has a colostomy, ileostomy, or urostomy, you may care for the ostomy site and document the output from the ostomy.

Enema Administration

An enema may be used in an infant or child as treatment for some disorders or before a diagnostic or surgical procedure. Administering the enema can be uncomfortable and threatening, so it is important to discuss the procedure with the child before giving the enema. The type, amount of fluid, and the distance the rectal tube is inserted vary according to age. Lubricate the tube with a water-soluble jelly before insertion. Never force the rectal tube; if there is resistance, remove the tube. Because the infant or younger child cannot retain the solution, hold the buttocks for a short time to prevent the fluid from being expelled. With an explanation before the procedure, the older child can usually hold the solution. A diaper or bedpan is used, and the child's back and head are supported by a pillow. Make sure a bedpan or bathroom is available before starting the enema.

Ostomy Care

Infants and children may have an ostomy (also called a stoma) surgically created for various disorders and conditions that prevent the child from having normal bowel or bladder elimination. A **colostomy** is made by bringing a part of the colon through the abdominal wall to create an outlet for fecal material elimination. Colostomies can be temporary or permanent. A new colostomy may be left to open air or a bag, pouch, or appliance may be used to collect the stool. An **ileostomy** is a similar opening in the small intestine. The drainage from the ileostomy contains digestive enzymes, so the stoma must be fitted with a collection device to prevent skin irritation and breakdown. It is important to reinforce teaching with the child or family caregiver about how to care for the stoma and skin with any ostomy. Preventing skin breakdown is a priority. A **urostomy** may be created to help in the elimination of urine.

Check ostomy bags for leakage, empty them frequently, and change the bags when needed. A variety of collection bags, devices, and products are available to be used with ostomies. Review and follow institution procedures regarding the products used and the procedure for changing the bags or appliances. The output from any ostomy must be recorded accurately.

PERFORMING PROCEDURES FOR SPECIMEN COLLECTION

Collecting or assisting in the collection of specimens is often a nursing responsibility. Standard precautions (see Appendix A) are followed in collecting and transporting specimens, no matter the source of the specimen.

Nose and Throat Specimens

Specimens from the nose and throat are used to help diagnose infection. To diagnose respiratory syncytial virus (Chapter 36), a nasal washing may be done. A small amount of saline is instilled into the nose; then the fluid is aspirated and placed into a sterile specimen container.

To collect a nasal or throat specimen, swab the nose or the back of the throat and tonsils with a special collection swab. The swab is placed directly into a culture tube and taken to the laboratory for analysis. If epiglottitis (Chapter 36) is suspected, a throat culture should not be done because of possible trauma and airway occlusion.

Urine Specimens

Urine is collected for a variety of reasons, including output measurement. To monitor the output, all urine is collected and measured, whether voided into a diaper, urinal, bedpan, or toilet collection device (see Intake and Output Measurement). Several methods and collection devices can be used to obtain urine specimens for diagnostic purposes such as urinalysis; urine cultures; specific gravity; and dip sticking urine for glucose, protein, and pH. In the infant, after cleaning the perineal area, cotton balls can be placed near the urethra and the diaper replaced. When the infant voids, the urine squeezed from the cotton ball can be collected and used for many urine tests. Because toddlers and young children cannot usually void on command, offer them fluids 15 to 20 minutes before the urine specimen is needed. Offering privacy to the older child and adolescent is important when obtaining a urine specimen.

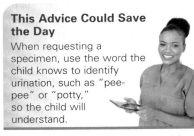

This Advice Could Save the Day

When requesting a specimen, use the word the child knows to identify urination, such as "pee-pee" or "potty," so the child will understand.

In preparation for collecting a urine specimen, position the infant or child so that the genitalia are exposed and the area can be cleansed. On a client who is a boy, wipe the tip of the penis with a soapy cotton ball, followed by a rinse with a cotton ball saturated with sterile water. In a client who is a girl, clean the labia majora front to back using one cotton pad for each wipe. Then expose and clean the labia minora in the same fashion (Fig. 30-11). Rinse the area with a cotton ball saturated with sterile water. Allow the male or female genitalia to air-dry before collection methods are followed (see later discussion).

After the collection, the specimen may be sent to the laboratory in the plastic collection container or in a specimen container preferred by the laboratory. All specimens must be labeled with the client's identifying information. Appropriate documentation includes the time of specimen collection, the amount and color of the urine, the test to be performed, and the condition of the perineal area.

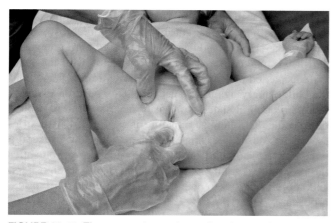

FIGURE 30-11 The nurse cleans the perineal area of the girl from front to back.

Collection Bag

To collect a urine specimen from infants and toddlers who are not toilet trained, use a pediatric urine collection bag (Fig. 30-12A). For the collection bag to stay in place, the skin must be clean, dry, and free of lotions, oils, and powder. The device is a small plastic bag with a self-adhesive material to apply it to the child's skin. Remove the paper backing from the urine collection container, and for a boy, place the penis and scrotum into the bag opening and apply the adhesive surface to the perineum. For a girl apply the bag over the lower perineum, the press the upper part of the bag over the vulva. Replace the child's diaper. Usually within a short period of time, the child will void and the specimen can be obtained. Remove the collection device as soon as the child voids (Fig. 30-12B).

Clean Catch

If an uncontaminated urine specimen is needed for a culture, the older child may be able to cooperate in the collection of a midstream specimen. Instruct the child as to the procedure so they understand what to do. The genital area is cleaned (as described earlier), the child urinates a small amount, stops the flow, then continues to void into a specimen container.

Catheterization

Occasionally, children must be catheterized to obtain a specimen, particularly if a sterile specimen is required. If the catheter is only needed to get a specimen, often a small sterile feeding tube is used. If an indwelling catheter is needed after catheterization, the catheter is left in place, the balloon inflated, and a collection bag attached.

24-Hour Urine Collection

Timed urine collections are sometimes done for a period of as long as 24 hours. The family caregiver can often assist and should be instructed in the procedure. The child should void and empty the bladder, that specimen is discarded, and then the 24-hour collection begins. The urine is kept on ice in a special bag or container during the collection time period. At the end of the timed collection, the entire specimen is sent to the laboratory. If any urine is accidently discarded after collection begins, the collection must be started again.

Stool Specimens

Stool specimens are tested for various reasons, including the presence of occult blood, ova and parasites, bacteria, glucose, or excess fat. Put on gloves and use a tongue blade to collect these specimens from a diaper or bedpan. Place the specimens in clean specimen containers. Stool specimens must not be contaminated with urine, and they must be labeled and delivered to the laboratory promptly. Document the time of specimen collection; stool color, amount, consistency, and odor; the test to be performed; and the skin condition.

ASSISTING WITH PROCEDURES RELATED TO COLLECTION OF BLOOD AND SPINAL FLUID

As a pediatric nurse, one of your roles is to assist with procedures performed on children. You might assist with the collection of blood samples or in holding and supporting a child during a lumbar puncture.

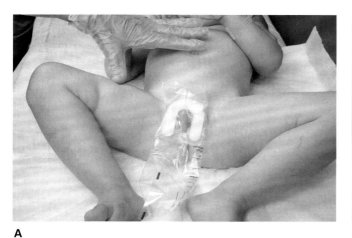

A

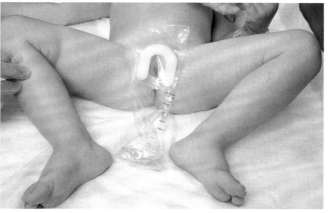

B

FIGURE 30-12 A. The skin must be clean and dry in order for the urine collection bag to adhere to the child's skin. **B.** The urine collection bag should be removed as soon as the child voids.

Blood Collection

Blood tests are part of almost every hospitalization experience and many times must be done in other settings to help with diagnosis. Although laboratory personnel or a health care provider usually obtains the specimens, you must be familiar with the general procedure to explain it to the child. You may be asked to help hold or restrain the child during the procedure. Blood specimens are obtained either by pricking the heel, great toe, earlobe, or finger or by venipuncture. In infants, the jugular or scalp veins are most commonly used; sometimes the femoral vein is used (Fig. 30-13). In older children, the veins in the arm are used.

A Personal Glimpse

I have been sick so many times that I don't know which one to write about. When I had hepatitis, I was very sick for a very long time. I missed a lot of school. I had to get blood tests, urine tests, and medications all the time, and I slept a lot because I felt tired all the time. Every time I had to get a blood test, I would cry because I didn't want to go. After a very long time, I got well enough to go back to school, but I couldn't play any gym games or activities because I couldn't get hit in my belly.

Justin, age 9 years

Learning Opportunity: What approach would be appropriate for the nurse to take with this client if he were to become ill again and need medical care? What would you say to him before any treatment or procedure was done?

Lumbar Puncture

When analysis of cerebrospinal fluid is necessary, a lumbar puncture is performed. Children undergoing this procedure may be too young to understand its explanation. Tell the child, however, that it is important to hold still and that they will have help to do this. During the procedure, restrain the child in the position shown in Figure 30-14 until the procedure is completed. Grasp the child's hands with the hand that has passed under the child's lower extremities and hold the child snugly against your chest. This position enlarges the intervertebral spaces for easier access with the aspiration needle. The lumbar puncture is performed with strict asepsis. A sterile dressing is applied when the procedure is complete. The child must remain quiet for 1 hour after the procedure. Monitor vital signs, level of consciousness, and motor activity frequently for several hours after the procedure.

ASSISTING WITH PROCEDURES RELATED TO DIAGNOSTIC TESTS AND STUDIES

A variety of healthcare personnel in the radiology, nuclear imaging, and other departments of the healthcare setting perform many diagnostic tests and procedures. These diagnostic studies include radiography, arteriograms, computed tomography scans, intravenous pyelograms, bone or brain scans, electrocardiograms, electroencephalograms, magnetic resonance imaging scans, and cardiac catheterizations.

As the nurse, your role for these tests is often to reinforce teaching and prepare the child and the family caregiver for the procedures. After the health care provider has written orders, request and schedule the tests or studies to be done. See that the required paperwork is completed and informed consents are signed. If the child must receive nothing by mouth (NPO) before the study, ensure that the NPO status is maintained. Clarify and document any allergies on the consent and requisition forms. During the procedure, you might be called on to support and comfort or restrain the child. After the procedure, perform and document the care needed.

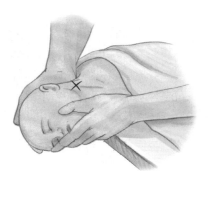

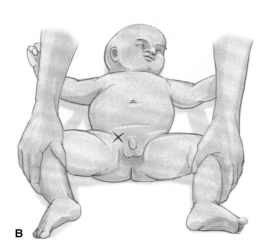

A　　　　　　**B**

FIGURE 30-13 A. Position of infant for jugular venipuncture. **B.** Position of infant for femoral venipuncture.

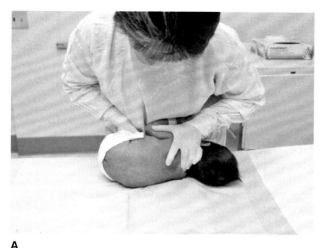

A

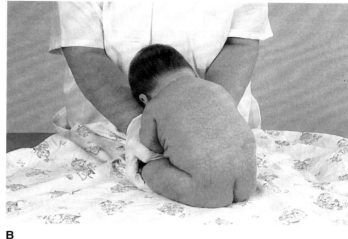

B

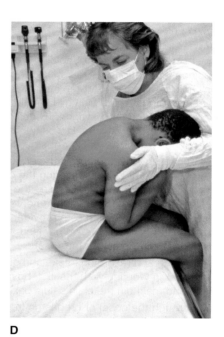

C

D

FIGURE 30-14 Positions of infant or child for lumbar puncture: **(A)** infant side-lying; **(B)** infant sitting; **(C)** child side-lying; **(D)** child sitting.

TEST YOURSELF

✔ How do a colostomy, an ileostomy, and a urostomy differ?

✔ How are nose and throat specimens obtained?

✔ Describe various methods for obtaining urine specimens in children.

✔ What are the reasons a stool specimen might be obtained?

For what reasons might restraints be used in caring for **Reyna**? What types of restraints might be used to keep her safe? What will you reinforce with her parents about ways to keep Reyna safe? What will you be monitoring related to the oxygen Reyna is receiving?

KEY POINTS

- When preparing for a procedure, nursing responsibilities include supporting and reinforcing teaching with the child and family to decrease their anxiety. Follow guidelines and policies of the healthcare setting, such as verifying the child's identity and ensuring signed informed consent is obtained.

- After any procedure or treatment, nursing responsibilities include ensuring the child is in a safe position, comforting and reassuring the child, answering questions, and following documentation and procedure policies of the healthcare setting.

- Types of restraints used for children include mummy restraints, papoose boards, clove hitch, elbow, jacket, and crib top restraints. Children in restraints require regular, careful observation, including monitoring circulation and neurovascular status, to prevent injury or complications. Family caregivers need explanations about the need for restraints.

- The three most common methods of holding a child are the cradle position, upright or over the shoulder position, or the football hold. Always support the infant's head and back. When transporting a child, the child should be held or placed in a crib, bassinet, bed, wagon, wheelchair, or stroller; use seat belts or safety straps. Position infants on their backs or supported on their sides for sleeping.

- Methods of reducing an elevated body temperature include not overdressing or heavily covering the child, encouraging the child to drink fluids, keeping the room environment cool, and using acetaminophen or other antipyretics according to the health care provider's instructions. A cooling device may also be used. With any method, closely monitor the child's temperature.

- Accurately measuring and recording intake and output are especially important in working with the ill or hospitalized child to monitor and maintain the child's fluid balance.

- A nasogastric (through the nose) or orogastric (through the mouth) tube is used to administer gavage feedings directly into the stomach for a child who is unable to get adequate food and fluid by mouth. Refer to Nursing Procedure 30-1.

- If enteral feedings are needed for a long period of time, a gastrostomy tube may be surgically inserted into the stomach through the abdominal wall. After the incision is made, a catheter is inserted and used as the feeding tube.

- The infant often receives oxygen while in an isolette or incubator. Other methods of oxygen administration include nasal cannula or prongs, mask, oxygen hood, or oxygen tent. High concentrations of oxygen can be dangerous to children, so close monitoring is needed.

- Oxygen safety measures are taught to family caregivers and followed by healthcare personnel.

- Oral and nasal secretions can obstruct the airway and are removed by coughing or suctioning.

- In emergency situations, a tracheostomy is surgically performed to create an opening in the trachea and a tube is put in place to give the child a patent airway. The tracheostomy must be monitored closely, suctioned, and kept clean to decrease possibilities of infection. The tracheostomy prevents the child from being able to cry or speak. Close observation and finding ways to communicate with the child are important.

- Local application of heat increases circulation by vasodilatation and promotes muscle relaxation, thereby relieving pain and congestion. It also speeds the formation and drainage of superficial abscesses. The local application of cold may help prevent swelling, control hemorrhage, and provide an anesthetic effect.

- A colostomy is created as an outlet for fecal material elimination. An ileostomy is a similar opening in the small intestine, and the drainage contains digestive enzymes. A urostomy may be created to help in the elimination of urine.

- Nasal washings and specimens taken from the nose or throat may be used to diagnose infection.

- To collect a urine specimen from an infant, cotton balls can be placed near the urethra in the diaper. When the infant voids, the urine is squeezed from the cotton ball into a collection container and used for urine tests. Other urine collection methods include using a pediatric urine collection bag, or collecting a midstream specimen (clean catch), catheterization, and 24-hour collection.

- Wear gloves and use a tongue blade to collect a stool specimen from the diaper or bedpan.

- For blood collection or lumbar puncture, explain the procedure to the child and family and help hold the child still. For diagnostic tests and studies, assist by supporting and reinforcing teaching with the child and family caregiver, preparing the child for the procedure, completing required paperwork, verifying informed consents are signed, maintaining NPO status, clarifying allergies, and documenting what has been done.

INTERNET RESOURCES

Tracheostomy
www.tracheostomy.com

International Foundation for Functional Gastrointestinal Disorders
www.aboutkidsgi.org

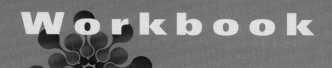

NCLEX-STYLE REVIEW QUESTIONS

1. When the nurse is performing or assisting the health care provider with a procedure, which of the following actions by the nurse would be the highest priority?
   a. Explain the procedure to the child.
   b. Gather the needed supplies.
   c. Identify the child before beginning the procedure.
   d. Document the procedure immediately after completion.

2. The nurse is inserting a nasogastric tube on a toddler. Which of the following restraints would be the most appropriate for the nurse to use with this child during this procedure?
   a. Mummy restraint
   b. Clove hitch restraint
   c. Elbow restraint
   d. Jacket restraint

3. When reviewing instructions with the child's family caregiver regarding methods used to reduce an elevated temperature, the caregiver makes the following statements. Which statement would require follow-up by the nurse?
   a. "The last time my child had immunizations, I gave her Tylenol."
   b. "When my older child had a fever, I always gave him a cold bath."
   c. "I have had trouble getting my child to drink juice."
   d. "My child likes only a small blanket over her."

4. When caring for a 3½-year-old child who is receiving oxygen in an oxygen tent, which of the following toys or activities would be best to offer this child?
   a. A radio playing soothing music
   b. Age-appropriate books
   c. A favorite blanket belonging to the child
   d. Board games the child can play alone

5. The practical nurse is participating in the development of a plan of care for a child who has a new ileostomy. Of the following nursing care focuses, which would be the highest priority for this child?
   a. Risk for altered development
   b. Family coping impairment
   c. Bowel incontinence
   d. Altered skin integrity risk

6. The nurse needs to calculate the intake and output during the 7 AM to 7 PM shift. The child is receiving supplemental gavage feedings in addition to oral intake. The child had a bowl of cereal with 2 oz of milk and a 3-oz glass of orange juice for breakfast. At 10 AM, the child voided 75 mL of urine. The child refused lunch and was given a gavage feeding of 120 mL of supplemental feeding. Early in the afternoon, the child had an emesis of 50 mL. Throughout the afternoon, the child sucked on 4 oz of ice chips. At 3 PM, the child had 25 mL of apple juice and several crackers. At 4 PM, the child voided 45 mL of urine and had a small-formed stool. The child again refused to eat any supper and was given a 120-mL gavage feeding. Calculate the child's 12-hour intake and output. Express your answer in milliliters (mL).

STUDY ACTIVITIES

1. Using the table below, list the types of restraints, describe each restraint, and explain the purpose of using this type of restraint in the pediatric client.

Type of Restraint	Description	Purpose

2. Develop a teaching plan to be used in reinforcing teaching with a group of family caregivers about caring for a child who has a fever. Include in your plan when and how to take a temperature, what to do to reduce the fever, and when it would be important for the family caregiver to call the health care provider.

3. Do an Internet search using the key term "fever management." Find sites that would be helpful for the pediatric nurse. Answer the questions below, and discuss what you found with your peers.
   a. At what body temperature is it considered that a child has an elevated temperature?
   b. What are some ways to treat a fever without using medications?

CRITICAL THINKING: WHAT WOULD YOU DO?

1. Three-year-old Denise has an elevated temperature of 104.4°F (40.2°C).
   a. What specific steps would you follow in caring for this child?
   b. What explanations would you give this child and family caregiver about what you are doing?
   c. What would be your highest priority for this child?
   d. What complication would you be most concerned about for this child?

2. The family caregiver of a 2-year-old child seems upset when you enter the client's room. The child has an enteral feeding tube in place, as well as an intravenous line. The caregiver says, "My child does not like to have her hands tied down. Why don't you just untie her?"

    a. What explanation would you give to the family caregiver?

    b. What could you do to help reassure this caregiver?

    c. What could you do to support this child?

3. You are the nurse on the pediatric unit leading a discussion with a group of your peers about caring for children receiving oxygen.

    a. What are some reasons a child might be receiving oxygen?

    b. What are the methods of oxygen delivery that might be used for children of different ages?

    c. What safety factors are important to follow when caring for the child receiving oxygen?

    d. Why must these factors be considered?

31

Medication Administration and Intravenous Therapy

Key Terms

acid–base balance
acidosis
alkalosis
azotemia
body surface area (BSA) method
body weight method
electrolytes
extracellular fluid
extravasation
homeostasis
induration
infiltration
intermittent infusion device
interstitial fluid
intracellular fluid
intravascular fluid
total parenteral nutrition (TPN)
West nomogram

Learning Objectives

At the conclusion of this chapter, you will:

1. Discuss the "rights" of medication administration.
2. Describe developmental behaviors and nursing actions to consider when giving medications to children.
3. Explain the body weight method of calculating pediatric drug dosages.
4. Calculate low and high safe dosages of medications for children using body weight.
5. Explain the body surface area method of calculating pediatric drug dosages.
6. Discuss various routes of medication administration used in children.
7. Identify the muscle preferred for intramuscular (IM) injections in the infant and explain the process of administering the IM injection in that muscle.
8. Identify the reasons children might receive intravenous (IV) therapy.
9. Discuss the importance of maintaining a fluid and electrolyte balance in children.
10. Differentiate between intracellular fluid and extracellular fluid.
11. Discuss what needs to be observed for and monitored in the child receiving IV therapy.
12. State the reason infusion control devices, volume control chambers, and syringe pumps are used in pediatric IV infusions and medication administration.

As the nurse in the pediatric clinic, you are administering medications. **Cora Chan**, age 4, needs an oral antibiotic administered. **Jaylor Mason**, age 10, needs to have eye drops administered. In addition, he will be taking eye drops at home, and his mother Sandra needs reinforcement of teaching on how to administer this medication. **Amin Das**, age 15 months, needs immunizations. One is to be given by the IM route and one is a subcutaneous immunization. Review characteristics of normal growth and development (Chapters 22–27). As you read this chapter, consider how you will administer each of these medications to these children.

MEDICATION ADMINISTRATION

Caring for children who are ill challenges every nurse to function at the highest level of professional competence. Giving medications is one of the most important nursing responsibilities. Medication administration calls for accuracy, precision, and considerable psychological skill. Before

649

administering any medication, always know the use, in particular the reason this client is receiving this medication, action, contraindications, side effects, and any nursing considerations.

Rights and Guidelines

Basic to administering medications to a person of any age are the following "rights" of medication administration:

- *The right patient.* Two identifiers are used to confirm identification of the client. Check the identification bracelet each time that a medication is given and always verify the child's name and birthdate with the child and family caregiver. Use technology such as a bar code system when available.
- *The right medication.* Check the drug label to confirm that it is the correct drug. Verify it is the drug and form ordered. Do not use a drug that is not clearly labeled. Check the expiration date of the drug.
- *The right dose.* Always double-check the dose by calculating the dosage according to the child's weight. Question the order if it is unclear. Have another qualified person double-check dosage calculations and any drugs governed by the facility's policy, such as insulin and digoxin. Use drug references or check with the health care provider or pharmacist for the appropriateness of the dose. Orders must be questioned before the drug is given.
- *The right route.* Give the drug only by the route ordered. Question the order if it is unclear or confusing. If a child is vomiting or a drug needs to be given by an alternate route, always get an order from the health care provider before administration.
- *The right time.* Administering a drug at the correct time and frequency helps to maintain the desired blood level of the drug. Some medications are given before meals, others with food. When giving an as-needed medication (PRN), always check the last time it was given, and clarify how much has been given during the past 24 hours.
- *The right reason.* Verify the rationale for why the drug is ordered and that the drug is appropriate to treat the client's condition.
- *The right documentation.* AFTER the medication is administered record that it was given and any pertinent information (site of administration, vital signs, laboratory values). Recording the administration of the medication, especially as-needed medications (PRN), is critical to avoiding potential errors in medication administration.
- *The right response.* Monitor and document the client's response to the drug administered, and verify the client had the desired effect from the drug.

Use What You Know

The right approach. Use your knowledge of the child's stage of growth and development to determine the best positive, age-appropriate approach when giving medications.

Administering medications to children is much more complex than these guidelines indicate. Accurate administration of medications is especially critical because of the variable responses to drugs that children

have as a result of immature body systems. It is important to understand the factors that influence or alter how the child absorbs, metabolizes, and excretes the medication and any allergies the child has. You may be responsible for administration of medications as well as for reinforcing teaching and giving information to the client and family caregivers about the purpose, effects, and possible side effects of medications given.

Ten rules to guide medication administration are presented in Box 31-1. Evaluate each child from a developmental point of view to administer medications successfully. Understanding, planning, and implementing nursing care that considers the child's developmental level and coping mechanisms helps minimize trauma for the child receiving medication (Table 31-1).

Medication errors can occur because nurses are human and not perfect. To admit an error is often difficult, especially if there has been carelessness concerning the rules. A person may be strongly tempted to adopt a "wait and see" attitude, which is the gravest error of all. It is important to accept responsibility for your actions. Serious consequences for the child may be avoided if a mistake is disclosed promptly.

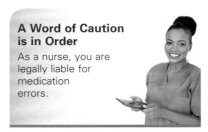

A Word of Caution is in Order

As a nurse, you are legally liable for medication errors.

TEST YOURSELF

✔ What are the "rights" of medication administration?

✔ Why are the "rights" especially important when administering medication to children?

✔ Why is it necessary for the nurse to always calculate and have another nurse double-check medication dosages for children?

Pediatric Dosage Calculation

Administering the correct dose of medication is vital, and especially in children the correct dosage needs to be calculated. Two methods of computing dosages are used to determine accurate pediatric medication dosages. As the nurse, you must use these methods to verify that the dosages ordered are appropriate and accurate. The first method uses the child's weight in kilograms to determine dosage. The second method uses the child's body surface area (BSA).

Body Weight Method

The **body weight method** uses the child's weight as a basis for computing the medication dosage. You must first convert the child's weight to kilograms if it is recorded in pounds. Often a drug reference provides a dosage range of

- Never give a child a choice of whether or not to receive medicine. The medication is ordered and is necessary for recovery; therefore, there is no choice to be made.
- Do give choices that allow the child some control over the situation, such as the kind of juice or the number of bandages.
- Never lie. Do not tell a child that an injection will not hurt.
- Keep explanations simple and brief. Use words that the child will understand.
- Assure the child that it is all right to be afraid and that it is OK to cry.
- Do not talk in front of the child as though they were not there. Include the child in the conversation when talking to family caregivers.
- Be positive in approaching the child. Be firm and assertive when explaining to the child what will happen.
- Keep the time between explanation and execution to a minimum. The younger the child, the shorter the time should be.
- Preparations, such as setting up an injection, solutions, or instrument trays, should be done out of the child's sight.
- Obtain cooperation from family caregivers. They may be able to calm a frightened child, persuade the child to take the medication, and achieve cooperation for care.

milligrams of a medication to number of kilograms the child weighs. To calculate a safe dose range for a child, use the child's weight in kilograms and the dosage range provided by the drug manufacturer.

Converting Pounds to Kilograms

To use the body weight method of dosage calculation, you must first convert a child's weight into kilograms if the weight has been recorded in pounds. To do this, set up a proportion using the number of pounds in a kilogram in one fraction and the known weight in pounds and the unknown weight in kilograms in the other fraction. For a child weighing 42 lb, set up the conversion as follows:

$$2.2 \, \text{lb}/1 \, \text{kg} = 42 \, \text{lb}/X \, \text{kg}$$

Then cross-multiply the fractions:

$$2.2 \, \text{lb} \times X \, \text{kg} = 1 \, \text{kg} \times 42 \, \text{lb}$$

Solve the problem for X. Divide each side by 2.2, and cancel the units that are in both the numerator and the denominator.

$$(2.2 \, \text{lb} \times X \, \text{kg})/2.2 \, \text{lb} = (1 \, \text{kg} \times 42 \, \text{lb})/2.2 \, \text{lb}$$
$$X = 42/2.2$$
$$X = 19 \, \text{kg}$$

The child who weighs 42 lb weighs 19 kg.

Calculating Dosage Using Body Weight Method

After converting the child's weight into kilograms, calculate a safe dose range for that child. For example, if a dosage range of 10 to 30 mg/kg of body weight is a safe dosage range and a child weighs 20 kg, calculate the low safe dose using the following:

$$10 \, \text{mg}/1 \, \text{kg} = X \, \text{mg}/20 \, \text{kg}$$

Cross-multiply the fractions:

$$10 \, \text{mg} \times 20 \, \text{kg} = 1 \, \text{kg}/X \, \text{mg}$$

Solve for X by dividing each side of the equation by 1 (canceling the units that are in both the numerator and the denominator):

$$(10 \, \text{mg} \times 20 \, \text{kg})/1 \, \text{kg} = (1 \, \text{kg} \times X \, \text{mg})/1 \, \text{kg}$$
$$200 \times 1 = 1X$$
$$200 = X$$

The low safe dose range of this medication for the child who weighs 20 kg is 200 mg.

To calculate the high safe dose for this child, use the following:

$$30 \, \text{mg}/1 \, \text{kg} = X \, \text{mg}/20 \, \text{kg}$$

Cross multiply the fractions:

$$30 \, \text{mg} \times 20 \, \text{kg} = 1 \, \text{kg} \times X \, \text{mg}$$

Solve for X by dividing each side of the equation by 1 (canceling the units that are in both the numerator and the denominator):

$$30 \, \text{mg} \times 20 \, \text{kg} = 1 \, \text{kg} \times X \, \text{mg}/1 \, \text{kg}$$
$$600 \times 1 = 1X$$
$$600 = X$$

The high safe dose range of this medication for the child who weighs 20 kg is 600 mg. The safe dose range for this medication for the child who weighs 20 kg is 200 to 600 mg.

Body Surface Area Method

The second formula used to calculate dosages is the **body surface area (BSA) method**. The **West nomogram**, commonly used to calculate BSA, is a graph with several scales arranged so that when two values are known, the third can be plotted by drawing a line with a straight edge (Fig. 31-1). Mark the child's weight on the right scale, and mark the height on the left scale. Use a straight edge to draw a line between the two marks. The point where the lines cross the

TABLE 31-1 Developmental Considerations in Medication Administration

AGE	BEHAVIORS	NURSING ACTIONS
Birth–3 months	Reaches randomly toward mouth and has a strong reflex to grasp objects	The infant's hands must be held to prevent spilling of medications
	Poor head control	The infant's head must be supported while medications are given
	Tongue movement may force medication out of mouth	A syringe or dropper should be placed along the side of the mouth
	Sucks as a reflex with stimulation	Use this natural sucking desire by placing oral medications into a nipple and administering in that manner
	Stops sucking when full	Administer medications before feeding when infant is hungry. Be aware that some medications' absorption is affected by food
	Responds to tactile stimulations	The likelihood that the medication is taken will increase if the infant is held in a feeding position
3–12 months	Begins to develop fine muscle control and advances from sitting to crawling	Medication must be kept out of reach to avoid accidental ingestion
	Tongue may protrude when swallowing	Administer medication with a syringe
	Responds to tactile stimuli	Physical comfort (holding) given after a medication is helpful
12–30 months	Advances from independent walking to running without falling	Allow the toddler to choose position for taking medication
	Advances from messy self-feeding to proficient feeding with minimal spilling	Allow the toddler to take medicine from a cup or spoon
	Has voluntary tongue control; begins to drink from a cup	Disguise medication in a small amount of nonessential food such as applesauce (clarify medication compatibility with pharmacist) to decrease incidence of spitting out medication
	Develops second molars	Chewable tablets may be an alternative
	Exhibits independence and self-assertiveness	Allow as much freedom as possible. Use games to gain confidence. Use a consistent, firm approach. Give immediate praise for cooperation
	Responds to sense of time and simple direction	Give direction to "drink this now" and "open your mouth"
	Responds to and participates in routines of daily living	Involve the family caregivers and include the toddler in medicine routines
	Expresses feelings easily	Allow for expression through play
30 months–6 years	Knows full name	Ask the child their name before giving medicine
	Is easily influenced by others when responding to new foods or tastes	Approach the child in a calm, positive manner when giving medications
	Has a good sense of time and a tolerance for frustration	Use correct immediate rewards for the young child and delayed gratification for the older child
	Enjoys making decisions	Give choices when possible
	Has many fantasies; has fear of mutilation	Give simple explanations. Stress that the medication is not being given as punishment
	Is more coordinated	Child can hold cup and may be able to master pill-taking
	Begins to lose teeth	Chewable tablets may be inappropriate because of loose teeth
6–12 years	Strives for independence	Give acceptable choices. Respect the need for regression during hospitalization
	Has concern for bodily mutilation	Give reassurance that medication, especially injectables, will not cause harm. Reinforce that medications should be taken only when given by nurse or family caregiver

AGE	BEHAVIORS	NURSING ACTIONS
	Can tell time	Include the child in daily schedule of medication. Make the child a poster of medications and time due so they can be involved in care
	Is concerned with body image and privacy	Provide private area for administration of medication, especially injections
	Peer support and interaction are important	Allow child to share experiences with others
12+ years	Strives for independence	Write a contract with the adolescent, spelling out expectations for self-medication
	Can understand abstract theories	Explain why medications are given and how they work
	Decisions are influenced by peers	Encourage teens to talk with their peers in a support group. Work with teens to plan medication schedule around their activities. Differentiate medication use from substance abuse
	Questions authority figures	Be honest and provide medication information in writing
	Is concerned with sex and sexuality	Explain relationships among illness, medications, and sexuality. For example, emphasize, "This medication will not react with your birth control pills"

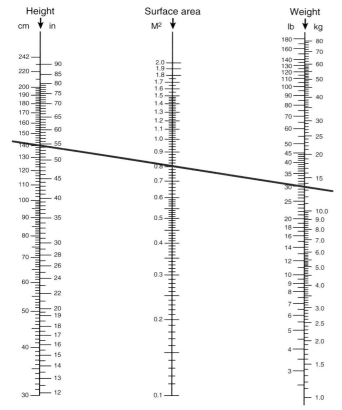

FIGURE 31-1 West nomogram for estimating body surface area of infants and young children. To determine the body surface area, draw a straight line between the point representing the child's height on the left scale to the child's weight on the right scale. The point at which this line intersects the middle scale is the child's body surface area in square meters.

column labeled SA (surface area) is the BSA, expressed in square meters (m²). The average adult BSA is 1.7 m²; thus, the formula to calculate the appropriate dosage for a child is as follows:

$$\text{Estimated child's dose} = \text{child's BSA}\,(m^2)/1.7\ m^2$$
$$(\text{adult BSA}) \times \text{usual adult dose}$$

For example, a child is 37 inches (95 cm) tall and weighs 34 lb (15.5 kg). The usual adult dose of the medication is 500 mg. Place and hold one end of a straight edge on the first column at 37 inches and move it so that it lines up with 34 lb in the far right column. On the SA column, the straight edge falls across 0.64 (m²). You are ready to do the calculation.

$$\text{Estimated child's dose} = 0.64 m^2/1.7\ m^2 \times 500\ mg$$
$$= 0.38 \times 500\ mg$$
$$= 190\ mg$$

Dividing the child's BSA by the average adult BSA tells you that this child's BSA is 0.38 times that of the average adult. Multiplying 0.38 times 500 mg (the usual adult dose) gives you the child's dose. The child's dose is 190 mg.

After computing any dosage, always have the computation checked by another staff person qualified to give medication or by someone in the department who is delegated for this purpose. Errors are easy to make and easy to overlook. A second person should do the computation separately; then both results should be compared.

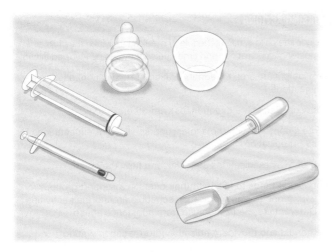

FIGURE 31-2 Examples of devices used to administer oral medications to children.

Oral Administration

Oral medications come in liquids, powders, capsules, and tablets. The age of the child and the type of medication helps determine the form in which it is given. For example, small babies who are hungry may suck almost anything liquid, including liquid medicines, through a nipple unless the medicine is bitter. Medications that are available in syrup or fruit-flavored suspensions are easily administered this way. Many calibrated devices are used to give liquid oral medications to children (Fig. 31-2). One method of administering oral medications is to drop them slowly into the child's mouth with a plastic medicine dropper or an oral syringe which has a

This is Important

Always use calibrated devices or medication cups to administer liquid oral medications. Using a household measuring device may deliver an incorrect dosage.

smooth tip rather than a luer-lock (preventing a needle from being attached and the medication being inadvertently administered by injection). When using an oral syringe, place it on the side of the tongue and slowly drip small amounts of the medication into the infant or child's mouth (Fig. 31-3). Allow the child to swallow between amounts. To avoid aspiration, keep the infant or child in an upright position while giving oral medications. Medication cups and spoons can be used to administer liquid medications to the older child.

Liquid medications may be in the form of elixirs, syrups, or suspensions. Elixirs contain alcohol and may cause choking unless they are diluted. Syrups and suspensions are thick and may need dilution to ensure that the child gets the full dose. Always check with the pharmacist before diluting any medication. To ensure the liquid medication is evenly distributed, some medications, especially suspensions, must be shaken well before the dose is given.

When a child is old enough to swallow a capsule or tablet, make sure that the pill is actually swallowed. When asked to open their mouths, children usually cooperate so well and open so wide that their tonsils can be inspected. While the mouth is open, look under the tongue to be sure the medication is not hidden.

It is usually best to give medicine in solution form to a small child. Some tablets can be crushed and some capsules can be opened and dissolved in a small amount of water or liquid. Consult the pharmacist before crushing a tablet or opening a capsule to be sure it is safe to administer the medication this way. Enteric-coated and time-release forms of medications can deliver an incorrect and even dangerous dosage of medication if crushed or opened and, thus, should *never* be crushed or opened to administer. Do not use orange juice for a solvent unless specifically ordered to do so; the child may always associate the taste of orange juice with the unpleasant medicine. If the medicine is bitter, corn syrup may disguise the taste. The child may develop a dislike for corn syrup, but that is not as problematic as a lifelong dislike of orange juice.

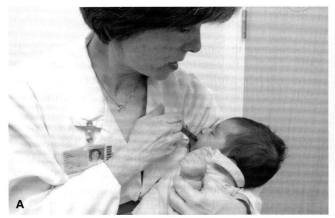
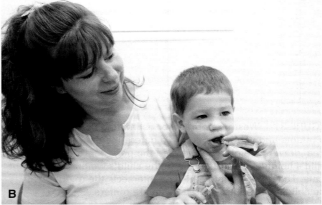

FIGURE 31-3 An oral syringe may be used to administer an oral medication. **A.** The nurse tucks the arm of the infant under hers and supports the infant's head as the medication is administered by placing the syringe on the side of the tongue. **B.** The medication is given to the young child by placing the syringe at the side of the tongue.

TIPS FOR REINFORCING FAMILY TEACHING

Giving Oral Medications

Before giving the medication, know:

- the name of the medication,
- what the drug is and what it is used for,
- how the medication will help your child,
- how often and for how long your child will need to take it,
- if it should be taken with meals or on an empty stomach,
- what the correct dose is and how to measure it in the calibrated device,
- the correct way to give the medication,
- how soon the medication will start working,
- what the possible side effects are and when the health care provider should be called,
- what to do if a dose is missed, spit up, or vomited, and
- if there are any concerns about your child taking this medication and other medications at the same time.

When giving the medication:

- Read the entire label and instructions each time it is given.
- Check the medicine's expiration date.
- Give the right dose at the right time interval.
- Use a calibrated dosing instrument that will administer an exact dose such as the following:
  - Plastic medication cup
  - Oral syringe with smooth tip
  - Medication dropper
  - Cylindrical dosing spoon
- Measure the medication carefully and read at eye level.

- ALWAYS remove the cap on the syringe before giving the medication.
- Throw the cap away or place it out of the reach of children.
- Slowly drip medication along the side of the tongue (a little at a time).
- Blowing gently on your child's face after giving the medication will cause them to swallow, if they are reluctant.
- Make the medication more palatable by mixing it with a small amount of liquid or soft food (such as applesauce); use only a small amount of food, and make sure your child eats the entire portion. (*Always* check with your child's pharmacist before doing so, however, because the effectiveness of some drugs may be compromised.)
- *Never* tell your child the medication is candy to get the child to take it.

After the medication is given:

- *If the child is wheezing, has trouble breathing, or has severe pain after taking a medication, seek emergency help by calling 911 or going to the emergency department immediately.*
- Watch closely for side effects or allergic reactions.
- ALWAYS use child-resistant caps and store all medications in a safe place, out of reach of children and pets.
- Refrigerate the medication if required to do so.
- Do not give medication prescribed for one child to another child.
- Keep a chart, and mark it each time your child takes the medication.

As a general rule, medications should not be given in food because if the child does not consume the entire amount of food, the dosage of medication will not be accurate. In addition, if given with food, the child may eventually associate the bad taste of the medication with food and may refuse to eat that food. If a medication is ever given with food, it should be only a small amount of a nonessential food (such as applesauce), and the entire amount needs to be eaten.

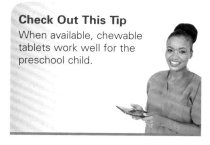

Check Out This Tip

When available, chewable tablets work well for the preschool child.

Do not restrain or force a child to take medication. The danger of aspiration is real. A child's sense of dignity must be respected, and finding alternative methods of encouraging the child to take the medication is important. Refer to Table 31-1 to review the developmental characteristics to consider at each age. For guidelines to help family caregivers administering oral medications at home, see Tips for Reinforcing Family Teaching: Giving Oral Medications.

Ophthalmic, Otic, Nasal, and Rectal Administration

Medications are also commonly administered through the ophthalmic (eye), otic (ear), nasal (nose), or rectal (rectum) routes. With few variations, the principles of administering medications by these routes are much the same as those for adults. Eye, ear, and nose drops should be warmed to room temperature before being administered. The infant or young child may need to be restrained for safe administration. This restraint may be accomplished with a mummy restraint or the assistance of a second person. It is important to realize that these are invasive procedures and that the young child may be resistant. Approaching the child with patience, explanations, and praise for cooperation helps gain the child's cooperation. Documentation must be completed after the administration of any medication.

Ophthalmic

To administer eye drops or ointment, place the child in a supine position. To instill drops, pull the lower lid down to form a pocket, and drop the solution into the pocket. Be careful not to touch the eye with the dropper to prevent contamination of the dropper or medication. Have the child

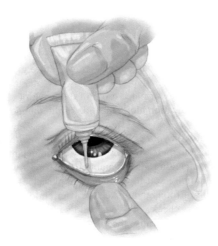

FIGURE 31-4 Administering eye ointment. Gently pull the lower lid down to form a pocket, and apply the ointment from the inner to the outer canthus with care not to touch the eye with the tip of the dropper or tube.

hold the eye shut briefly, if possible, to help distribute the medication to the conjunctiva. Apply gentle pressure to the inner canthus to decrease systemic absorption. Ointment is applied from the inner to the outer canthus, with care not to touch the eye with the tip of the dropper or tube (Fig. 31-4). Have the child keep the eye closed for 1 minute after ointment has been administered.

How will you approach **Cora Chan**, age 4, who needs an oral antibiotic administered? What steps will you follow to administer her medication? What aspects of normal growth and development did you review that will help you administer eye drops to **Jaylor Mason**, age 10? What teaching will you reinforce with Sandra, Jaylor's mother, about giving him his medications at home?

Otic

To administer ear drops, place the infant or young child in a side-lying position with the affected ear up. In an infant or toddler, pull the pinna (the outer part of the ear) down and back to straighten the ear canal. In a child older than 3 years, pull the pinna up and back, as with adults, to straighten the canal (Fig. 31-5).

After instilling the drops, gently massage the area in front of the ear. Keep the child in a position with the affected ear up for 5 to 10 minutes. A cotton ball may be loosely inserted into the ear to prevent leakage of medication.

Nasal

Before nose drops are instilled, the child should blow their nose or the nostrils should be suctioned with a bulb syringe to clear any mucus or secretions. For instillation, hold an infant with their head hyperextended over your arm. For a toddler or older child, place the head over a pillow while the child is lying flat. The infant or child should maintain the hyperextended position for at least a minute to ensure distribution of the medication. To administer a nasal spray, have the child sit upright with their head slightly tilted back. As the spray is being instilled have the child draw a breath through the nostril. Do one nostril at a time while holding the other nostril closed.

Rectal

Administration of medications by the rectal route is invasive and can be upsetting and embarrassing to the child. As well, rectal absorption is unpredictable, so other routes are preferable. If a child is vomiting or NPO and the rectal route must be used, age-appropriate explanations and support are necessary. To administer rectal medications, place the child in a left lateral side-lying position, and wear gloves or a finger cot. Lubricate the suppository with a water-soluble lubricant and then insert it into the rectum, followed by a finger, up to the first knuckle joint. The little finger should be used for insertion in infants. After the insertion of the suppository, hold the buttocks tightly together for 1 or 2 minutes until the child's urge to expel the suppository passes.

Intramuscular Administration

Medications administered by any injectable route can be uncomfortable and may be frightening, especially for children. Other routes of administration are used when possible, but medications such as immunizations are given into the muscle by intramuscular administration. When giving intramuscular (IM) or other injections, a swift, sure thrust with insertion is the best way to minimize pain, but it is important to stay calm and sure and be prepared for the child's squirming. Have a second nurse help hold the child, especially a young child or if this is the child's first injection.

Using nonpharmacologic interventions such as distraction and positioning may decrease anxiety, help relax the muscle, and make the injection process less traumatic. Have an adhesive bandage ready to cover the injection site. This technique prevents young children from worrying that they might "leak out" of the hole. A bandage, sticker, or small reward serves as a badge of courage or bravery and may provide comfort.

> **Something to Always Remember**
>
> Whenever possible, give injections and do treatments in the treatment room. Keep the bed and playroom as "safe" places for the child.

Table 31-2 describes IM injection sites, how to locate them, the suggested needle size, and the amount of medication to inject.

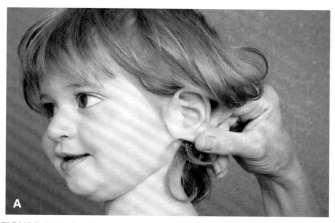
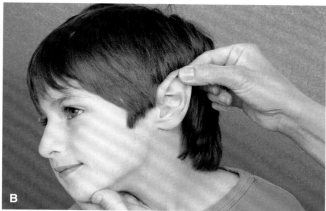

FIGURE 31-5 Positioning for administering ear drops. **A.** In the child younger than 3 years, the pinna is pulled down and back. **B.** In the child older than 3 years, pull the pinna up and back.

 A Personal Glimpse

When I was 5 years old, I went to the doctor's office. I had to get shots my mom said were for school. I don't know what they were for. I felt scared before I went. My mom told me ideas to think about when I got the shots so I wouldn't think about it hurting. She told me to think about my puppy dog and flowers and sailing ships. The nurse told me it would hurt a little. It hurt when the nurse stuck a needle in my leg. It didn't hurt as much as I thought it would. The nurse was nice and told me I was a brave girl. I am glad I thought about my dog Cheeto. I was happy to go to kindergarten.

Adriel, age 6 years

Learning Opportunity: *Why is it important to prepare children for medication administration? What would be important for the nurse to talk about with the child before giving IM injections?*

TABLE 31-2   Intramuscular Injection Sites

MUSCLE SITE	NEEDLE SIZE	MAXIMUM AMOUNT	PROCEDURES
Vastus lateralis Greater trochanter Site of injection (vastus lateralis) Knee joint	Infant: 25 gauge, 5⁄8 inch or 23 gauge, 1 inch Older: 22 gauge, 1 inch–1.5 inches	1.0 mL 2.0 mL	This main thigh muscle is used almost exclusively in infants for IM injections but is used frequently in children of all ages. Locate the trochanter (hip joint) and knee as landmarks. Divide the area between landmarks into thirds. Inject into the middle third section, using the lateral aspect. Inject at a 90-degree angle
Ventrogluteal Iliac crest Anterior superior iliac spine Site of injection Palm over greater trochanter	Assess child's muscle mass. 22–25 gauge, 5⁄8 inch–1 inch Infant: Toddler: School age and older:	 0.5–0.75 mL 1.0 mL 1.5–2.0 mL	With thumb facing the front of the child, place forefinger on the anterior superior iliac spine with middle finger on the iliac crest and the palm centered over the greater trochanter. Inject at a 90-degree angle below the iliac crest within the triangle defined. No important nerves are in this area

(Continued)

TABLE 31-2 Intramuscular Injection Sites (continued)

MUSCLE SITE	NEEDLE SIZE	MAXIMUM AMOUNT	PROCEDURES
Deltoid	Not recommended for infants Older: 22–25 gauge, 0.5 inch–1 inch	Small muscle limits amount to 0.5–1.0 mL	Expose entire arm. Locate the acromion process at the top of the arm. Give the injection in the densest part of the muscle below the acromion process and above the armpit. Not recommended for repeated injections. Can be used for one-time immunizations. Angle needle slightly toward the shoulder
Dorsogluteal	This site is not recommended in children who have not been walking for at least 1 or 2 years Not recommended for infant or toddler School age and older: 20–25 gauge, 0.5 inch–1.5 inch	1.5–2.0 mL	Because of the location of the sciatic nerve, use of this site is discouraged in younger children. Place child on abdomen with toes pointing in; this relaxes the gluteus. Locate the posterior superior iliac crest and the greater trochanter of the femur. Draw an imaginary line between the two. Give the injection above and to the outside of this line. The needle should be inserted at a 90-degree angle. The accompanying figure shows (A) how to locate the dorsogluteal IM injection site and (B) a child in position for a dorsogluteal injection. The site is marked by an X

Subcutaneous and Intradermal Administration

Subcutaneous injections are often used to administer insulin, allergy shots, and some immunizations. The medication is injected into the fatty tissue between the skin and the muscle. Sites most frequently used are the upper arm, abdomen, and the anterior thigh. The needles used for subcutaneous injections are small in gauge (26 to 30 gauge) and short in length (3/8 to 5/8 inches). The angle of administration is either 45 or 90 degrees, depending on the size of the needle and the size of the child.

Intradermal injections may be used for tuberculosis screening and allergy testing. The forearm is the site most often used. The needle is inserted just under the skin, and a small amount of solution is administered. A short and small-gauged needle is used.

Intravenous Administration

Medications are often administered intravenously to pediatric clients by registered nurses. Some drugs must be administered intravenously to be effective; in some clients, the quick response gained from IV administration is important. Delivering medications intravenously is actually less traumatic than administering multiple IM injections. Extra caution is necessary to observe for irritation of small pediatric veins from irritating medications. Syringe pumps and volume control devices are commonly used to administer IV medications (see discussion later in chapter). Double-checking the medication label before hanging the IV fluid bottle is important to ensure that the medication is correct for the correct patient, that it is being administered at the correct time, and that it is not outdated. IV devices and sites are covered in the discussion of IV therapy that follows.

INTRAVENOUS THERAPY

As with IV administration of medications, the registered nurse initiates and administers IV fluids in the pediatric client. In some states, depending on the Nurse Practice Act and scope of practice for that state, the practical nurse administers IV fluids.

Know the Rules and Regulations

If the scope of practice in a state allows the practical nurse to perform IV therapy, the nurse must follow the laws and statutes of the state. The nurse must have the knowledge and skills (attained through formal education and training), demonstrate clinical competence, and follow the policies and procedures of the institution.

IV therapy is commonly administered in the pediatric client for the following reasons:

- To administer fluids to maintain fluid and electrolyte balance
- To administer medications, especially antibiotics, pain medication, and chemotherapeutic agents
- To administer blood or blood products
- To administer nutrients

Candidates for IV therapy include children who have poor gastrointestinal absorption caused by diarrhea, vomiting, and dehydration; those who need a high serum concentration of a drug; those who have resistant infections that require IV medications; those with emergency problems; and those who need continuous pain relief.

Planning nursing care for the child receiving IV therapy requires knowledge of the physiology of fluids and electrolytes. It also requires understanding of the child's developmental level and the emotional aspects of IV therapy for children.

Fundamentals of Fluid and Electrolyte Balance

Maintenance of fluid balance in the body tissues is essential to health. Uncorrected, severe imbalance causes death, as in clients with serious dehydration resulting from severe diarrhea, vomiting, or loss of fluids in extensive burns. The fundamental concepts of fluid and electrolyte balance in body tissue are reviewed briefly to illustrate the importance of adequate fluid therapy for the sick child.

Water

A continuous supply of water is necessary for life. At birth, water accounts for about 77% of body weight. Between ages 1 and 2 years, this proportion decreases to the adult level of about 60%.

In health, the body's water requirement is met through the normal intake of fluids and foods. Intake is regulated by the person's thirst and hunger. Normal body losses of fluid occur through the lungs (breathing) and the skin (sweating) and in the urine and feces. In the normal state of health, intake and output amounts balance each other, and the body is said to be in a state of **homeostasis** (a uniform state). Homeostasis biologically signifies the dynamic equilibrium of the healthy organism. This balance is achieved by appropriate shifts in fluid and electrolytes across the cellular membrane and by elimination of the end products of metabolism and excess electrolytes.

Body water, which contains electrolytes, is situated within the cells, in the spaces between the cells, and in the plasma and blood. Imbalance (failure to maintain homeostasis) may be the result of some pathologic process in the body. Some of the disorders associated with imbalance are pyloric stenosis, high fever, persistent or severe diarrhea and vomiting, and extensive burns. Retention of fluid may occur through impaired kidney action or altered metabolism.

Intracellular Fluid

Intracellular fluid is contained within the body cells. Nearly half the volume of body water in the infant is intracellular. Intracellular fluid accounts for about 40% of body weight in both infants and adults. Each cell must be supplied with oxygen and nutrients to keep the body healthy. In addition, the body's water and sodium levels must be kept constant within narrow parameters.

A semipermeable membrane that retains protein and other large constituents within the cell surrounds cells. Water, certain salts and minerals, nutrients, and oxygen enter the cell through this membrane. Waste products and useful substances produced within the cell are excreted or secreted into the surrounding spaces.

Extracellular Fluid

Extracellular fluid is situated outside the cells. It may be **interstitial fluid** (situated within the spaces or gaps of body tissue) or **intravascular fluid** (situated within the blood vessels or blood plasma). Blood plasma contains protein within the walls of the blood vessels and water and mineral salts that flow freely from the vascular system into the surrounding tissues.

Interstitial fluid (also called intercellular or tissue fluid) has a composition similar to plasma, except that it contains almost no protein. In the infant, about 25% to 35% of body weight is attributable to interstitial fluid. In the adult, interstitial fluid accounts for only about 15% of body weight (Fig. 31-6).

This reservoir of fluid outside the body cells decreases or increases easily in response to disease. An increase in interstitial fluid results in edema. Dehydration depletes this fluid before the intracellular and plasma supplies are affected.

Infants and children can become dehydrated in a short amount of time. In part, this dehydration occurs because of a greater fluid exchange caused by the rapid metabolic

activity associated with infants' growth. It also occurs because of the increased body surface area (BSA) relative to the body fluid volume; the ratio is two or three times that in adults. Because of this, larger quantities of fluid are lost through the skin in the infant.

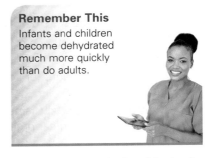

Because of these factors, the infant who is taking in no fluid loses an amount of body fluid equal to the extracellular volume in about 5 days, or twice as rapidly as does an adult. The infant's relatively larger volume of extracellular fluid may be designed to compensate partially for this greater loss.

TEST YOURSELF

✔ What are the different reasons children might receive IV therapy?

✔ What are some disorders that might cause an imbalance of water in children?

✔ What is the difference between intracellular and extracellular fluid?

Electrolytes

Electrolytes are chemical compounds (minerals) that break down into ions when placed in water. An ion is an atom with a positive or a negative electrical charge. Important electrolytes in body fluids are sodium (Na^+), potassium (K^+), magnesium (Mg^{2+}), calcium (Ca^{2+}), chloride (Cl^-), phosphate (PO_4^-), and bicarbonate (HCO_3^-). Electrolytes have the important function of maintaining acid–base balance. Each water compartment of the body has its own normal electrolyte composition.

Acid–Base Balance

Acid–base balance is a state of equilibrium between the acidity and the alkalinity of body fluids. The acidity of a solution is determined by the concentration of hydrogen (H^+) ions. Acidity is expressed by the symbol pH. Neutral fluids have a pH of 7, acid fluids lower than 7, and alkaline fluids higher than 7. Normally, body fluids are slightly alkaline. Internal body fluids have a pH of 7.35 to 7.45. Body excretions, however, are products of metabolism and become acid; the normal pH of urine, for example, is 5.5 to 6.5.

Defects in the acid–base balance result either in **acidosis** (excessive acidity of body fluids) or **alkalosis** (excessive alkalinity of body fluids). Acidosis may occur in conditions such as diabetes, kidney failure, and diarrhea. Hyperventilation is a frequent cause of alkalosis.

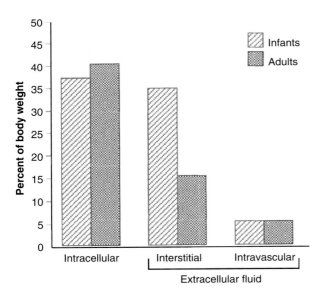

FIGURE 31-6 Distribution of fluid in body compartments. Comparison between the infant and adult fluid distribution in body compartments shows that the adult total is about 60% of body weight, whereas the infant total is more than 70% of body weight.

Regulation of Fluids and Electrolytes

In normal health, the fluid and electrolyte balance is maintained through the intake of a well-balanced diet. The kidneys play an important part in regulating concentrations of electrolytes in the various fluid compartments. In illness, the balance may be disturbed because of excessive losses of certain electrolytes. Replacement of these minerals is necessary to restore health and maintain life. When the infant or child can take sufficient fluids orally, that is the preferred route; often though, it is necessary to administer IV fluids.

IV Therapy Administration

IV fluids are administered to provide water, electrolytes, and nutrients that the child needs. As stated earlier, blood products, medications, and parenteral nutrition (see discussion that follows) are also administered intravenously. The type and purpose of IV therapy influence the equipment and site used.

Peripheral Intravenous Access

IV infusions may be administered through a peripheral vein. Over-the-needle catheters or winged-infusion needles, sometimes called "butterflies" or scalp vein needles, are used. Site selection in the pediatric client varies with the child's age. The best choice of sites is the one that least restricts the child's movements. Sites used include the hand, wrist, forearm, foot, and ankle. The antecubital fossa, which restricts movement, is sometimes used only if other sites are not available. The scalp vein has an abundant supply of superficial veins in infants and toddlers and may be used if no other site can be accessed. Using the scalp vein site may be upsetting to the family caregivers and the child's hair may need to be shaved in a small area. Explain the procedure and reason for using the scalp vein site to help alleviate the family's concerns.

Older children may be permitted some choice of site, if possible. The child should be involved in all aspects of the procedure within age-appropriate capabilities. The preschool child can often cooperate if given adequate explanation. Play therapy in preparation for IV therapy may be helpful. Honesty is essential with children of any age. The older school-aged child and adolescent may have many questions that should be answered at their level of understanding. Family caregivers also need explanations and should be included in the preparation for the procedure. By their presence and reassurance, family caregivers may provide the emotional support the child needs and may help the child remain calm throughout the procedure.

In preparation for starting a peripheral IV line, all the equipment that may be needed should be collected. A site is selected and a plastic cannula or winged small-vein needle, usually between 22 and 25 gauge (depending on the child's size), is inserted. To protect and allow for observation of the IV site, a transparent dressing is often applied. An IV house may be placed to prevent movement of the IV catheter and decrease the risk of the IV becoming dislodged (Fig. 31-7A,B). For the scalp vein insertion, the needle is stabilized with U-shaped taping, and a loop of the tubing is taped so that if the child pulls on the tubing, the loop will absorb the pull and the site will remain intact (Fig. 31-7C). With the use of soft, pliable IV catheters rather than metal needles, the need for padded boards and splints to restrain and immobilize the IV site is rarely necessary.

If the child does not require continuous IV fluid infusion but may still require IV fluids or medications intermittently, an **intermittent infusion device**, sometimes referred to as a saline or heparin lock, may be used. This method frees the child from IV tubing between medication administrations. The veins on the back of the hand are often used for saline lock insertion (Fig. 31-8). Medication is administered

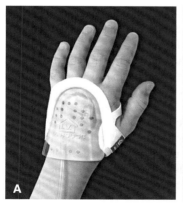
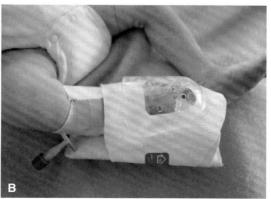
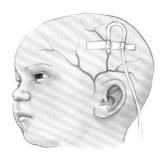

FIGURE 31-7 Protection of the IV site: **A.** IV house over the site on the child's hand; **B.** IV house over the site on an infant's foot; **C.** scalp vein IV site with U-shaped tubing taped so that if the child pulls on the tubing, the loop will absorb the pull and the site will remain intact.

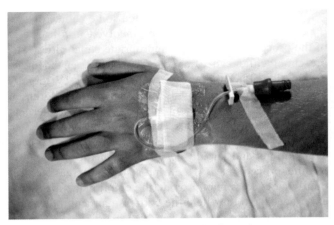

FIGURE 31-8 The saline or heparin lock allows for more freedom of movement between uses.

through the lock; when the administration is completed, the needle and tubing are removed, and the saline lock is flushed. A self-healing rubber stopper closes the saline lock so that it does not leak between administrations. This method may also be used for a child who must have frequent blood samples drawn. The saline lock is flushed every 4 to 8 hours with saline or heparin, according to the facility's procedure.

It is sometimes difficult to gain access to children's small veins, and they may easily be "blown." Only nurses skilled in the procedure should start an IV infusion in children. You may serve as the child's advocate when the IV is being started. especially if you have cared for the child and have the child's trust and confidence.

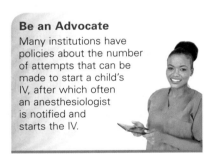

Be an Advocate

Many institutions have policies about the number of attempts that can be made to start a child's IV, after which often an anesthesiologist is notified and starts the IV.

Central Venous Access

Some solutions are administered through a central venous access line. Some of these catheters are peripherally inserted central catheters (PICC) and are threaded into the superior vena cava. Most central venous infusions are administered through a large vein such as the jugular or subclavian vein. The line is inserted by surgical technique and is sutured into place. These catheters may exit through a tunnel in the subcutaneous tissue on the chest. Some brand names of central venous lines are Hickman, Broviac, or Groshong catheters. Caring for a child with a central venous line calls for skilled nursing care because of the danger of complications, such as contamination, infection, thrombosis, dislodging of the catheter, and **extravasation** (fluid escaping into surrounding

tissue). The infant or child must be closely monitored for hyperglycemia, dehydration, or **azotemia** (nitrogen-containing compounds in the blood).

Another type of central venous access is a vascular access port. A small stainless steel port with a catheter attached is implanted under the skin and used for medication administration or for long-term fluid administration. Examples are brands such as Port-A-Cath and Infuse-A-Port. Special needles are used to access these ports. The advantages of vascular access ports are that they are low risk for infection, blood samples can be removed through the port, they are not visible, and they do not need a dressing over them.

When assisting with the insertion of a central venous line, gather the equipment required for the procedure. Your role will be to support the child during the procedure and to be available to assist in the procedure. Dressing changes are routinely performed on the external site of a central venous device. The institution's policies must always be clarified and followed; practical nurses often assist with this dressing change. This is a sterile procedure, so sterile gloves and forceps are used. After the dressing change, the procedure is documented, as is skin condition, including any redness, swelling, drainage, or irritation.

Infusion Control

A variety of IV infusion control devices are suitable for pediatric use. These electronic devices monitor the rate and flow of intravenous infusions and have alarms which indicate any concern with the infusion. The rate of infusion for infants and children must be carefully monitored, and an infusion control device must be used (Fig. 31-9A). To avoid overloading the circulation and inducing cardiac failure, the IV drip rate must be slow, especially for the small child. The tubing used with some infusion control devices is made to decrease the size of the drop to a "mini" or "micro" drop of 1/50 mL or 1/60 mL, thus delivering 50 or 60 minidrops or microdrops per milliliter, rather than the 15 drops per milliliter of most regular sets. A control chamber may be used which holds 100 to 150 mL of fluid and is designed to deliver controlled volumes of fluid to avoid the accidental entrance of too great a fluid volume into the child's system (Fig. 31-9B).

A syringe pump that can be programmed to deliver a small amount of fluid over a period of time may be used to deliver IV fluids or for IV medication administration (Fig. 31-10).

Regardless of the control systems and safeguards, the child and the IV infusion require monitoring as frequently as every hour. Check the IV site to see that it is intact and that the IV is infusing at the set flow rate. If the IV catheter becomes dislodged, **infiltration**, or fluid leaking into the surrounding tissues, can occur. Signs that might indicate infiltration include cool, blanched, or swollen skin. Observe for signs of inflammation including warmth,

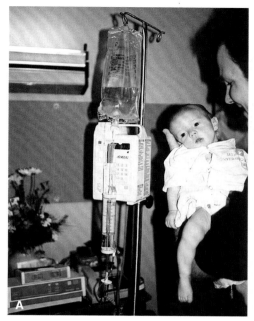
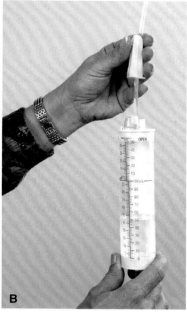

FIGURE 31-9 A. An infant with an infusion control device and a volume control chamber. **B.** The volume control chamber holds a small amount of IV fluid and has a "mini" dropper to reduce the size of the drops.

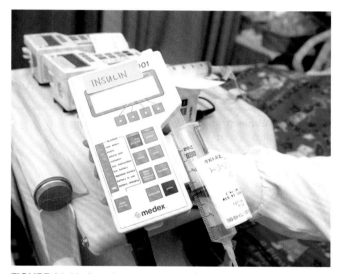

FIGURE 31-10 A syringe pump may be used to administer IV fluids or medications over a period of time.

Peripheral vein parenteral nutrition may occasionally be used on a short-term basis. Extra care must be taken to avoid infiltration because tissue injury and sloughing may be severe.

For long-term administration of TPN, a central venous access device may be inserted (see discussion of central venous access earlier in the chapter). Children can be discharged from the hospital on TPN therapy after family caregivers have been instructed in the care of the device, thus reducing hospital time and expense.

Check the Levels

When a child is on TPN, the blood glucose levels are checked frequently. Insulin may need to be given to treat hyperglycemia.

swelling, redness, burning, pain, or **induration** (hardness) of the area. Documentation is sometimes done on an IV flow sheet that lists the flow rate, the amount in the bottle, the amount in the control chamber, the amount infused, and the condition of the site.

Monitor Closely

It is critical to monitor the child receiving IV therapy. Monitor the IV flow rate and infusion control device. Monitor the site for any signs of infiltration, inflammation, pain, leakage, or infection. Accurate documentation is vital.

TEST YOURSELF

✔ What is the difference between peripheral and central IV access?

✔ What sites might be used for peripheral IV therapy in children?

✔ Why is it important to use an infusion control device for IV therapy in children?

Amin Das, age 15 months, needs immunizations. One is to be given by the IM route and one is a subcutaneous immunization. How will you determine what sites and techniques you will use to locate the sites? What steps will you follow to administer the medications? What specific aspects of this child's growth and development will you consider as you administer the medications?

Parenteral Nutrition Administration

Total parenteral nutrition (TPN) is the administration of dextrose, lipids, amino acids, electrolytes, vitamins, minerals, and trace elements into the circulatory system to meet the nutritional needs of a child whose needs cannot be met through the gastrointestinal tract.

KEY POINTS

- The "rights" of medication administration include the right patient, medication, dose, route, time, reason, documentation, and response. Using the right approach takes into consideration the child's stage of growth and development.

- Administering medications to children is complex because of their immature body systems and varying sizes. Age-related behaviors and developmental considerations should be kept in mind, and age-appropriate nursing actions should be used when administering medications to children.

- To use the body weight method of pediatric dosage calculation, always calculate the child's weight in kilograms if the medication is ordered as a dose per kilogram. Then calculate the safe low and high doses by using the child's body weight. Always have another person check computations of drug dosage before administering medications to children.

- The body surface area (BSA) method can also be used to calculate pediatric dosages. A West nomogram is used to determine the child's BSA based on their height and weight. Then use the BSA and usual adult dosage of the medication to calculate the child's dose.

- Routes of pediatric medication administration are oral, ophthalmic, otic, nasal, rectal, IM, subcutaneous, intradermal, and IV. Oral is the most common route.

- The muscle preferred for intramuscular (IM) injections in the infant is the vastus lateralis. To use the vastus lateralis muscle for an IM injection, locate the trochanter (hip joint) and knee as landmarks. Divide the area between landmarks into thirds. Using the middle section of the three sections, follow correct procedure for drawing up the medication and inject the needle into the lateral aspect of the leg at a 90-degree angle.

- Maintaining fluid balance in the body tissues is essential to health. Severe imbalance can occur rapidly in children because they dehydrate much faster than do adults. Serious dehydration can result from diarrhea, vomiting, or loss of fluids in extensive burns. Electrolytes help maintain the acid–base balance in the body, so the electrolyte balance in the body is also essential.

- Intracellular fluid is contained within the body cells and makes up 40% of body weight in children and adults. Extracellular fluid is situated outside the cells and is either interstitial fluid (situated within the spaces or gaps of body tissue) or intravascular fluid (situated within the blood vessels or blood plasma).

- IV therapy might be administered to children to provide water, electrolytes, blood products, medications, or nutrients (total parenteral nutrition [TPN]) the child needs.

- IV fluid administration requires careful observation of the child's appearance, vital signs, intake and output, and the fluid's flow rate.

- IV flow rate is regulated by the use of an infusion control device in order to closely monitor the rate of infusion. A control chamber is used to deliver a controlled volume of fluid. IV infusion sites must be monitored to avoid infiltration and tissue damage.

INTERNET RESOURCES

Medication Administration
www.childhealthonline.org
www.pediatriccareonline.org

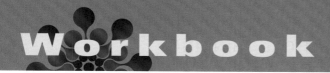
NCLEX-STYLE REVIEW QUESTIONS

1. The pediatric nurse is administering oral liquid medications to a 4-year-old child. Which statement by the nurse indicates an understanding of the child's developmental level?
   a. "Your mom will help me hold your hands."
   b. "Would you like orange or apple juice to drink after you take your medicine?"
   c. "You can make a poster of the schedule for all your medications."
   d. "This booklet tells all about how this medicine works."

2. The nurse is calculating a medication dosage for an infant who weighs 16 lb. How many kilograms does the child weigh?
   a. 0.72 kg
   b. 1.7 kg
   c. 7.3 kg
   d. 9 kg

3. The dosage range of meperidine for a school-aged child is 1.1 to 1.8 mg/kg. Which dosage would be appropriate to give a school-aged child who weighs 76 lb?
   a. 24.4 mg
   b. 30 mg
   c. 60 mg
   d. 110 mg

4. When administering an IM injection to a 4-month-old infant, the best injection site to use would be the:
   a. vastus lateralis
   b. ventrogluteal
   c. deltoid
   d. dorsogluteal

5. Infusion pumps and volume control devices are used when children are given IV fluids. The most important reason these devices are used is to:
   a. regulate the rate of the infusion
   b. decrease the size of the drops delivered
   c. reduce the chance of infiltration
   d. administer medications

6. The nurse is administering an IM injection using the vastus lateralis muscle. Mark an X on the location of the vastus lateralis muscle in this child's right leg.

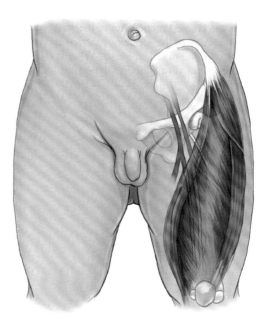

STUDY ACTIVITIES

1. Caitlin weighs 28.5 lb (13 kg) and measures 35.5 inches (90 cm). Find her BSA using the West nomogram. Calculate the dose of a medication for her if the adult dosage is 750 mg.

2. Describe how you would approach each of the following children when giving oral medications and IM medications.

	Oral Medications	Intramuscular Medications
6-month-old Kristi		
18-month-old Jared		
3-year-old Sarah		
4.5-year-old Miguel		
8-year-old Danika		
16-year-old Jon		

2. Identify each of the IM injection sites, state how to locate each of the sites, and name the landmarks used.

3. Do an internet search on "preventing medication errors in children."
   a. List some of the sites you found for this topic.
   b. What are some recommendations for ways to prevent medication errors in children?
   c. What recommendations did you find that you would share with your nursing peers?

4. Research the Nurse Practice Act in the state you live. What is included in the scope of practice and rules and regulations for the practical nurse? What is the role of the practical nurse in your state in relationship to IV therapy?

CRITICAL THINKING: WHAT WOULD YOU DO?

1. You have been asked to lead a discussion with a group of your peers about medicating children.
   a. What is the importance of following the "rights" of medication administration?
   b. What do you think are the most important responsibilities of the nurse when medicating children?
   c. How does medicating children differ from medicating adults?
   d. What steps would you take if you discovered that you had made a medication error?
   e. What are your legal responsibilities related to medication errors?

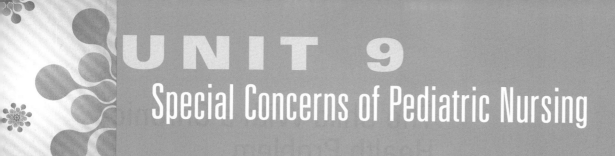

UNIT 9
Special Concerns of Pediatric Nursing

The Child With a Chronic Health Problem

32

Key Terms

chronic condition
denial
gradual acceptance
overprotection
rejection
respite care
stigma

Learning Objectives

At the conclusion of this chapter, you will:

1. Identify 14 chronic conditions that may be seen in children.
2. Explain 10 concerns common to many families of children with chronic conditions.
3. Discuss the effects chronic conditions may have on the child's parents and family caregivers.
4. Discuss the effects chronic conditions may have on the child's growth and development.
5. Describe the effects the child's chronic condition may have on siblings in the family, including positive and negative sibling responses.
6. Identify ways the nurse may encourage growth and development, self-care, and socialization in the child with a chronic condition.
7. Describe how the nurse can help the family adjust to the child's chronic condition.
8. Discuss general guidelines for preparing the family for home care of the child with a chronic condition.

Gauge Watson is 3 years old and is diagnosed with muscular dystrophy. Gauge has a 7-year-old sister and an 11-year-old brother. As you read this chapter, think about how having a child with a chronic condition such as muscular dystrophy might affect the family and the child's siblings.

A chronic condition is one of long duration or one that progresses slowly, shows little change, and often interferes with daily functioning. Chronic conditions during childhood may affect a child's physical, psychosocial, and cognitive development. The condition also affects the entire family. As a nurse, you may be involved in caring for these children and their families at the stage of diagnosis and as they continue to experience ongoing and long-term needs over many years. Therefore, you can play a vital role in helping the family adjust to the condition.

CAUSES OF CHRONIC CONDITIONS IN CHILDREN

Chronic conditions are a leading health problem in the United States. The number of children with chronic conditions is growing as more infants and children survive prematurity, difficult births, congenital anomalies, accidents, and illnesses that were once fatal. Most children

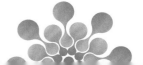

experience only brief, acute episodes of illness; however, a significant number are affected by chronic health problems.

Conditions considered chronic in children include congenital heart disease, Down syndrome, spina bifida, blindness, cerebral palsy, asthma, cystic fibrosis, sickle cell disease, hemophilia, diabetes, muscular dystrophy, juvenile rheumatoid arthritis, cancer, and acquired immunodeficiency syndrome. These specific chronic health problems of children are discussed in chapters throughout this text. Each requires individualized management based on the disease process and the abilities of the client and family to understand and comply with the treatment regimen.

EFFECTS OF CHRONIC CONDITIONS ON THE FAMILY

The diagnosis of a chronic health problem causes a crisis in the family, whether it happens during the first few hours or days of the child's life or even much later in life. Although the specific disorders that cause chronic conditions are varied, all chronic health problems create some common challenges for clients and families. Some of these concerns include:

- financial concerns such as payment for treatment, living expenses at a distant healthcare facility, or caregiver's job loss because of time not at work
- administration of treatments and medications at home
- disruption of family life such as vacations, family goals, and careers
- educational opportunities for the child
- social isolation because of the child's condition
- family adjustments because of the disease's changing course
- reactions of siblings
- stress among family caregivers
- guilt about and acceptance of the chronic condition
- care of the child when family caregivers can no longer provide care

The effects of these challenges on the family depend, in part, on family member coping abilities. How families cope with chronic conditions varies greatly from one family to another. Families who have strong support systems are usually better able to meet these challenges.

Parents and Chronic Conditions

When family caregivers learn of the child's diagnosis, their first reactions may be shock, disbelief, and denial. These reactions may last for a varied amount of time, from days to months. The initial response may be one of mourning for the "perfect" child they lost combined with guilt, blame, and rationalization. The caregivers may seek advice from other professionals and actually may go "shopping" for another health care provider in the hopes that they may find the diagnosis is incorrect or not as serious as they have been told. They may refuse to accept the diagnosis or talk about it, or they may delay seeking or agreeing to treatment. However, they gradually adjust to the diagnosis. They may

enter a period of chronic sorrow when they adapt to the child's chronic condition but do not necessarily accept it. They often waver between the stages, and they experience emotional highs and lows as they care for the child and meet the challenges of daily life.

Several typical caregiver responses have been identified: overprotection, rejection, denial, and gradual acceptance. Caregivers responding with **overprotection** try to protect the child at all costs. They may hover, which prevents the child from learning new skills. They may fail to use discipline. They may use any means to prevent the child from experiencing any frustration. Caregivers in **rejection** emotionally distance themselves from the child. Although they provide physical care, they tend to scold and correct the child continuously. Caregivers in **denial** behave as though the condition does not exist, and they encourage the child to overcompensate for any disabilities. Caregivers who respond with **gradual acceptance** take a commonsense approach to the child's condition; they help the child set realistic goals for self-care and independence and encourage the child to achieve social and physical skills within their capability (Fig. 32-1).

Economic pressures can become overwhelming to the families of children with chronic conditions. If the family does not have adequate health insurance, the costs of treatment may be enormous. Away-from-home living costs may become a problem if the child must go to a distant hospital for further diagnosis or treatment. To keep health insurance benefits, a family caregiver may feel tied to a job, which creates additional stress. The time required to take the child to medical appointments can be excessive and may threaten job security because of the time lost from the job.

Families must make many adjustments to care for the child with a chronic condition. The family caregivers may have to learn to perform treatments and give medications. Family life is often disrupted. Vacations may be nonexistent, and the family may be limited in how they can spend their leisure time. Families may have difficulty finding babysitters and have little opportunity for a break from the routine. Some families become isolated from customary

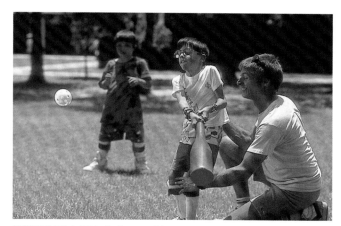

FIGURE 32-1 This father and brother encourage a child with a disability to participate in outdoor activities.

social activities because of the responsibilities of caring for the child. **Respite care** (care of the child so that the caregivers can have a period of rest and refreshment) is often desperately needed but is not readily available in many communities. Families in which both parents work may have to forgo a second income so that one adult can stay home with the child.

As the child grows, concerns about education may become foremost among caregiver worries. These concerns include the availability of appropriate education, early learning opportunities, physical accessibility of the facilities, acceptance of the child by school personnel and classmates, inclusive versus segregated classes, availability and quality of homebound teaching, and general flexibility of school teachers and administrators. Few schools are prepared to accommodate treatments at school that would otherwise require the child to leave during the school day. Family caregivers often must become the child's advocate to preserve as much normalcy as possible in the child's educational experience.

As the child's condition changes, the family must make additional changes. All of these stressors may strain a marriage, and couples may have little time left for each other when caring for a child with a chronic condition. Sometimes partners in relationships blame each other for the child's problems, which further strains the relationship. Single-parent families have significant needs to which healthcare personnel must be especially sensitive.

The Child and Chronic Conditions

The child with a chronic condition may face many problems that interfere with normal growth and development. These problems vary with the diagnosis and condition. For example, some conditions require the child to be immobilized. If this occurs for a school-aged child during the stage of industry and inferiority, the child cannot complete tasks of industry, such as helping with household chores or working on and completing special projects with siblings or peers. The child's attitude toward the condition is a critical element in its long-term management and the family's adjustment.

 A Personal Glimpse

I am 16 years old, and I was diagnosed with cystic fibrosis at birth. Every morning, I wake up and have many things that I have to accomplish; taking a breathing treatment, having percussion done, and taking many pills. I guess it isn't so bad if you are used to doing it every day, but it is a bit annoying having the same routine all the time. I have been doing all of this for 16 years. I sometimes feel that I am very different from other people. My friends don't feel it is weird having me as a friend, but they know that I have this disease, and they are afraid of what can happen to me. My friends don't treat me any differently. I think that is the most important thing. It is good that I have friends who can care so much that they don't let it bother them.

I don't like it when I have to cough all the time; everyone stares at me. When I am in school, at lunch I have to take pills before I eat. Everyone is always asking me why I am taking the pills. Even when I go to a friend's house, I have to take my medication and get my percussions done. My friends usually help out with the percussions.

A lot of times, I feel very lonely because I am the only one in my family who has this disease. No one knows what I am feeling, and that sometimes makes me very lonely and afraid. I have a twin brother who really cares for me a lot. When anyone asks about my illness, he is usually the person to explain it to them. He has always been there for me when I needed him. When I have to go in the hospital, he gets my school work for me. We are very close. I am glad to have a brother like him.

I am very lucky to have a family that cares for me and loves me like they do. They are always helping me when I need percussions done, and they are very supportive. I don't know what I would do without their help. They all took care of me when I couldn't. They still do now. I owe them a lot of credit. I love them very much and always will.

Gretchen, age 16 years

Learning Opportunity: *Do you think this adolescent has accepted her disease? What are the things she shared that show that she has or has not accepted her condition? What are your thoughts about her family and friends?*

The child's response to the chronic condition is influenced by the response of family caregivers. Whether caregivers respond with overprotection, rejection, denial, or gradual acceptance, as discussed earlier, may greatly affect the child's attitude and motivation to participate in self-care activities.

As with any illness, children may perceive a chronic condition as punishment for a bad thought or action, depending on the child's developmental stage at the time of diagnosis. This perception is also influenced by the attitudes of parents and peers. Rejection by caregivers, for example, may further convince the child that the condition is a punishment. The child's perception is also shaped by whether the dysfunctional body part is visible. Problems such as asthma, allergies, and epilepsy are difficult for young children to understand because "what's wrong" is inside, not outside.

The child's family, peers, and school personnel comprise the support system that can affect the child's adaptation. Sometimes the efforts necessary to meet the child's physical needs are so great that finding time and energy to meet the child's emotional needs can be difficult for members of the support team. The older child with a chronic condition also has developing sexual needs that should not be ignored but must be acknowledged and respected.

Disease progression can add additional stresses over time. For instance, Hodgkin disease can be successfully treated for a time with chemotherapy and radiation therapy, but this adds the side effects of treatment (steroid-induced acne, edema, and alopecia) to the disease manifestations of night sweats, chronic fatigue, pruritus, and gastrointestinal bleeding. The child with Duchenne muscular dystrophy gradually weakens so that in adolescence they may be wheelchair-bound during a time when their peers are actively involved in sports and exploring sexual relationships. These stresses can add up and become difficult for the young person to cope and deal with.

Discrimination continues to be present in the life of the child with a chronic condition and the family. Discrimination can occur in relationships among children, and social exclusion of the child is common. Physical barriers may present problems that families must struggle with to help their child overcome. Sometimes hurtful discrimination is as simple as being stared at in public places.

Siblings and Chronic Conditions

Some degree of sibling rivalry can be found in most families with healthy children, so it is not surprising that a child with a chronic health problem can seriously disrupt the lives of brothers and sisters. Much of the family caregiver's time, attention, and money is directed toward management of the child's chronic problem. This can cause anger, resentment, and jealousy in the siblings. The caregiver's failure to set limits for the child's behavior while maintaining discipline for the siblings can cause further resentment. Some family caregivers unknowingly create feelings of guilt in the other children by overemphasizing the needs of the child with the chronic condition.

Siblings may feel that having a brother or sister with a chronic condition is a **stigma**, a mark of embarrassment, or shame, especially if the child has a physical disfigurement or apparent cognitive deficit. Siblings may choose not to tell others about them or may be selective in whom they tell, choosing to tell only people they can trust. An older sibling is more likely to tell others than a younger one, perhaps because the older child tends to understand more about the condition and its effect.

Siblings of a child with a chronic condition may display both positive and negative behaviors. Some siblings may react with anger, hostility, jealousy, increased competition for attention, social withdrawal, or poor school performance. On the other hand, many siblings demonstrate positive behaviors such as caring and concern for the child, cooperating with family caregivers in helping care for the child, protecting the child from negative reactions of others, and including the child in activities with peers (Fig. 32-2).

How siblings react to a sibling with a chronic condition may ultimately depend on how the family copes with stress and how its members feel about one another. This delicate balance is challenging and takes great effort and caring for a family to sustain, but the results are well worth it. (See Tips for Reinforcing Family Teaching: Helping Siblings Cope With a Chronic Condition for additional information.)

TIPS FOR REINFORCING FAMILY TEACHING

Helping Siblings Cope With a Chronic Condition

- Find time for special activities with healthy children.
- Explain the child's chronic condition as simply as possible.
- Depending on the developmental ability of the healthy siblings, involve them in the care of the child.
- Set behavioral limits for all children in the family.

Gauge Watson has a chronic condition. He has a 7-year-old sister and an 11-year-old brother. What are some ways Gauge's diagnosis might affect his siblings? What are some of the feelings Gauge's siblings might have and what are some ways they might respond to their feelings?

TEST YOURSELF

✔ What effect does a chronic condition have on the parents of the child with a chronic condition?

✔ What problems might the child with a chronic condition face?

✔ What effect do chronic conditions have on the siblings of the child with a chronic condition?

THE ROLE OF THE NURSE

As the nurse, you play an important role in providing care for the child with a chronic condition and in helping the child and family learn to cope. Be aware of individual needs and abilities to cope with the condition. Encourage the child and family to share their feelings and reactions to the situation. Support by listening and providing appropriate interventions.

Nursing Process and Care Plan *for the Family and the Child With a Chronic Condition*

Assessment (Data Collection)

The assessment of the family and the child with a disability or chronic condition is an ongoing process by the healthcare team. The information and data collected are reviewed and updated with each visit the child makes to the healthcare facility. Include the child in the admission and ongoing interview processes if they are old enough and

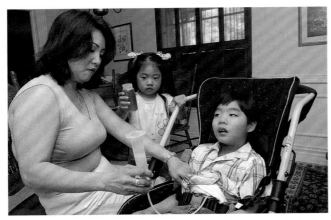

FIGURE 32-2 This sibling demonstrates caring, concern, and helping with the child who has a chronic condition.

able to participate. Unless the child is newly diagnosed, the family caregivers may have a good understanding of the condition. Observe for evidence of the family's knowledge and understanding so that plans can be made to supplement it as needed.

During any interview with the child or family caregivers, determine how the family is coping with the child's condition and observe for the family's strengths, weaknesses, and acceptance of the diagnosis. Identify the needs that change with the child's condition and include them in planning care. Also, consider needs that change with the child's growth and development.

Adjust the physical examination to correspond with the child's current condition. Make every effort to gain the child's cooperation and explain what is being done in terms the child can understand throughout the physical examination. Praise the child for cooperation throughout the process to gain the child's (and the family caregivers') goodwill.

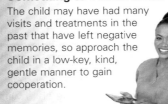

Something to Think About!

The child may have had many visits and treatments in the past that have left negative memories, so approach the child in a low-key, kind, gentle manner to gain cooperation.

Nursing Care Focus

When selecting nursing care focuses for the family and the child with a chronic condition, the possibility of the child being behind anticipated stages of normal growth and development, self-care deficits and anxiety are considerations. The child and family may be socially isolated and have feelings of grief and loss. Those feelings and other changes in family life may arise related to the care of the child in the home and must be considered in caring for the child and family.

Outcome Identification and Planning

Major goals for the child with a chronic condition are to accomplish growth and development milestones, perform self-care tasks, decrease anxiety, and experience more social interaction. Goals for the caregiver or family are to increase their social interaction; decrease their feelings of grief, anger, and guilt; increase their adjustment to living with a child with a chronic condition; and reinforce teaching with them about caring for the child.

Nursing Care Focus

- Growth and development concerns related to decreased ability to achieve developmental tasks or family caregiver reactions to the child's condition

Goal

- The child will achieve the highest level of growth and development within constraints of their chronic condition, and the family caregivers will acknowledge appropriate growth and development expectations.

Implementations for Encouraging Optimal Growth and Development

The family caregivers may become overprotective and prevent the child from attempting developmental challenges appropriate for their age and disability. Help the caregivers recognize the child's potential and set realistic growth and development goals. Consistent care by the same staff helps provide a sense of routine in which the child can be encouraged to have some control and perform age-appropriate tasks within the limitations of the disability. Set age-appropriate limits and enforce appropriate discipline. Accomplish this gradually by displaying a kind and caring attitude. Give the child choices within the limits of treatments and other aspects of required care. Encourage the child to wear regular clothes rather than stay in pajamas to reduce feelings of being an invalid. Encourage the child to learn about the condition. Introducing the child to other children with the same or a similar condition can help dispel feelings that they are the only person with such a condition.

An older child or adolescent benefits from social interaction with peers with and without disabilities (Fig. 32-3). Encourage family caregivers to help the adolescent join in age-appropriate activities. The adolescent may also need some help dressing or styling their look. This help with personal appearance from a caregiver will aid in minimizing any physical disability.

Evaluation of Goal/Desired Outcome

- The child attains growth and development milestones within their capabilities.
- The family caregivers acknowledge the child's capabilities, encourage the child, and set realistic goals for the child.

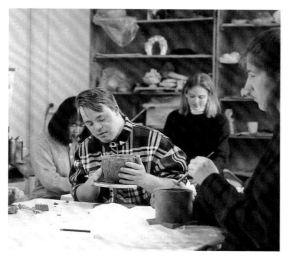

FIGURE 32-3 The adolescent with disabilities benefits from social interaction.

Nursing Care Focus

- Activities of daily living deficit related to self-care

Goal

- The child will become involved in self-care activities.

Implementations for Promoting Self-Care

To encourage the child to assist in self-care, devise aids to ease tasks. Creative problem-solving can equip the child with skills that they can use in the future. When appropriate, integrate play and toys into the care to help encourage cooperation. Do not expect the child to perform tasks beyond their capabilities. Make certain that the child is well rested before they attempt any energy-taxing tasks. Remember, these tasks are often hard work for the child.

Praise and reward the child genuinely and generously for tasks attempted, even if they are not totally completed. Positive reinforcement increases self-confidence, promotes pride in accomplishments, and encourages the child to try new things.

> **Try This!**
> Use a chart or other visual aid with listed tasks as a tool to help the child reach a desired goal. Stickers can record the child's progress. School-aged children often respond well to contracts. For instance, a special privilege or other incentive is awarded when a set number of stickers are earned.

Evaluation of Goal/Desired Outcome

- The child participates in self-care as appropriate for their age and capabilities, and they use creative problem-solving techniques.
- The child demonstrates a positive outlook about their achievements.

Nursing Care Focus

- Acute anxiety related to procedures and treatments

Goal

- The child's anxiety will be decreased.

Implementations for Reducing Anxiety About Procedures and Treatments

Periodically, the child may need to undergo procedures, tests, and treatments. The child may also be hospitalized frequently. Many of the procedures may be painful or at least uncomfortable. Explain the tests, treatments, and procedures ahead of time, and encourage the child to ask questions. Acknowledge when a particular procedure is painful, and help them plan ways to cope with the pain. Advise family caregivers that they should also help the child prepare for hospitalization ahead of time whenever possible.

Evaluation of Goal/Desired Outcome

- The child's anxiety is minimized as evidenced by cooperation with care and treatments.

Nursing Care Focus

- Psychosocial needs related to social isolation

Goal

- The child and family will actively socialize with others.

Implementations for Preventing Social Isolation

The child with a chronic condition may feel isolated from peers. When the child is hospitalized, consider arranging for contact with peers by phone, technology devices, in writing, or through visits. Many pediatric units have special programs that help children deal with chronic conditions and hospitalizations. Encourage regular school attendance as soon as the child is physically able. If the child is a member of an inclusive classroom, suggest that the caregiver make arrangements with the school for rest periods, as needed. Ask the child about their interests. There might be suitable after-school activities that the child can participate in and will increase their interactions with peers. Make suggestions and confer with family caregivers to ensure that proposed plans are carried out.

> **Listen Carefully!**
> The child's discussions about social activities can help you gain insight into their feelings about socialization.

Family caregivers may also be at risk for social isolation. Having a child who requires constant or frequent attention often can be exhausting. The care requirements and exhaustion may leave little time for the caregivers to socialize. The family lacking close extended family and few close friends may find getting away for rest and relaxation, even for an evening, almost impossible. Help the family caregivers find resources for respite care. Any caregiver, no matter how devoted, needs to have a break from everyday cares and concerns. Refer the family to social services where they can get help. Sometimes a caregiver may feel that another person cannot care for the child adequately. Encourage this caregiver to express fears and anxieties about leaving the child. This helps the family caregiver work through some of these anxieties and feel more confident about getting away for a period of rest.

Evaluation of Goal/Desired Outcome

The child and family use opportunities to socialize with others.
The family seeks and finds adequate respite care for the child.

Nursing Care Focus

● Psychosocial needs of caregivers related to acceptance of the child's condition

Goal

● The family will deal with their feelings of anger, grief, guilt, and loss.

Implementations for Aiding Caregiver Acceptance of the Condition

A grief reaction occurs whenever anyone suffers a serious loss. This is true of family caregivers when they first learn that their child has a chronic condition. Encourage family caregivers to express these feelings to help them understand that this reaction is common and acceptable.

Denial is usually the first reaction that family caregivers have to the diagnosis. This is a time when they say, "How could this be?" or "Why my child?" Let them express their emotions and respond in a nonjudgmental way. Staying with them and offering quiet, accepting support may be helpful. Statements such as "it will seem better in time" are inappropriate. Acknowledge the caregiver feelings as acceptable and reasonable.

Guilt is the next stage. During this stage, listen to the caregivers express their feelings of guilt and remorse. Again, acknowledging their feelings is useful. Accept family caregiver expressions of anger without viewing them as personal attacks. Use active listening techniques that reflect the caregiver feelings, such as "you sound upset"; this is a helpful method of handling these emotions.

Grief reactions may also occur when the family caregivers are informed that the child is deteriorating or has experienced a setback. Caregivers usually cycle through these reactions much more quickly as they experience them again; regardless the same methods are useful.

Evaluation of Goal/Desired Outcome

The family caregivers:

● express their feelings of guilt, fear, and anxiety.
● receive support while working toward accepting the child's condition.

Nursing Care Focus

● Altered health maintenance related to the child's chronic health condition

Goal

● The family caregivers will adjust to the requirements of caring for the child with chronic condition or disability.

Implementations for Helping the Family Adjust to the Child's Condition

The family's adjustment to the condition is considered during initial and ongoing interviews. Adjustment may depend on how recently the child has been diagnosed or on the current status of the child's condition. After determining the family's needs, provide an opportunity for the family members to express their feelings and anxieties. Help them explore any feelings of guilt or blame about the child's condition. Encourage them to express doubts they may have about their ability to cope with the child's future. Help the caregivers look realistically at their resources, and give them suggestions about ways to cope. Serve as a role model when caring for the child, and express a positive attitude toward the child's condition.

Question the family to determine the resources and support systems available to them. Remind them that these support systems may include immediate family members, extended family, friends, community services, and health care providers.

Encourage the caregivers to discuss sibling needs and their adjustments to the child's condition. Help the family meet sibling needs, and help the siblings feel comfortable with the problems and needs of the child with the chronic condition. Assist the family in setting reasonable expectations for all their children.

Evaluation of Goal/Desired Outcome

The family caregivers:

● express ways they can cope with their child's condition.
● list the resources and support systems available to them.

Nursing Care Focus

● Discharge planning related to home care for the child

Goal

● The family caregivers will actively participate in the child's home care.

Implementations for Planning for Home Care

Home care planning begins when the child is admitted to the healthcare facility and continues until discharge. Focus plans for care at home on the continuing care, medications, and treatments the child will need. During a healthcare visit or hospitalization, include family caregivers when caring for the child so that they become comfortable with the care. Demonstrate the use of special equipment and treatments, and give the family caregivers a chance to perform the treatments under guidance and supervision. A discussion of the home's facilities may be appropriate to help the family accommodate the child's special needs. Give the caregivers a list of community services and organizations that they can turn to for help and support, including appropriate disease or disability-specific organizations.

Reinforce teaching with the caregivers about growth and development guidelines so that they have a realistic concept of what to expect as the child develops. Throughout the child's hospital stay, encourage caregivers to express their concerns to help solve whatever problems the family anticipates having while caring for the child at home. Give the family the name and telephone number of a contact person they can call for support.

You Can Make a Difference!

Families face many hurdles while caring for a child with a chronic condition, but they are more likely to feel that they can competently face the future with the reassurance that help is just a telephone call away.

Caring for a child with a chronic condition can be an overwhelming task that requires cooperation from all involved with the child and family. Family caregivers deserve all the help they can get.

Evaluation of Goal/Desired Outcome

The family caregivers:

- ask pertinent questions.
- contact support groups and community agencies for help.
- demonstrate their ability to perform care and treatments.

TEST YOURSELF

✔ How might a chronic condition affect a child's growth and development?

✔ What can you do to help decrease the social isolation of the child with a chronic condition?

✔ Why is it important for you to try to determine how the family and child are coping with a chronic condition?

Remember **Gauge Watson** from the beginning of the chapter. He was diagnosed with muscular dystrophy. What challenges do you think his parents will have to face related to his diagnosis? As the nurse working with this family, what can you do to support Gauge, his parents, and his brother and sister?

KEY POINTS

- Chronic conditions seen in children include congenital heart disease, Down syndrome, spina bifida, blindness, cerebral palsy, asthma, cystic fibrosis, sickle cell disease, hemophilia, diabetes, muscular dystrophy, juvenile rheumatoid arthritis, cancer, and acquired immunodeficiency syndrome. Concerns common to many families of children with chronic conditions include financial, administration of treatments and medications at home, disruption of family life, educational opportunities for the child, social isolation, family adjustments, reaction of siblings, stress among caregivers, guilt about and acceptance of the chronic condition, and care of the child when family caregivers can no longer provide care.

- Economic pressures, such as adequate health insurance, away-from-home living costs, the stress of having to keep a job (especially when the child needs the caregiver's time and attention), and the threat to job security because of time away from the job, can become overwhelming to the families of children with chronic conditions.

- Respite care is important so that family caregivers can have time away from the child with a chronic condition and a break in the routine. Time away will help keep the caregivers from becoming isolated and enable them to participate in normal social activities.

- Caregivers of a child with a chronic condition may respond by overprotecting the child, which may prevent the child from learning new skills. Sometimes caregivers distance themselves emotionally (rejection) or are in denial and behave as though the condition does not exist. Caregivers with acceptance are able to help the child set realistic goals.

- A chronic condition may interfere with normal growth and development depending on the diagnosis, age of the child when diagnosed, and the overall condition, severity, and long-term disability the condition may cause.

- Siblings may respond negatively to the child's chronic condition by showing anger, hostility, jealousy, increased competition for attention, social withdrawal, or poor school performance. Many siblings demonstrate positive responses to the child including helping to care for the child, protecting the child from negative reactions of others, and including the child in activities with peers.

- To help promote normal growth and development, encourage the child to participate in age-appropriate activities and to do tasks within the limitations of the child's disability. Encourage self-care by the child by devising aids to ease tasks, integrating play and toys into the care, praising the child for tasks attempted, being sure the child is well rested before attempting tasks, and by using charts, visual aids, and stickers as ways to reward the child.

- Help the family adjust to the child's condition by encouraging the family caregivers to express their feelings of anger, guilt, fear, and remorse by responding in a nonjudgmental way. Encourage the family to express doubts they may have about their ability to cope with the child's future and to look realistically at their resources. Offer suggestions about ways to cope, be a role model when caring for the child, and have a positive attitude.

- Preparing the family for home care of the child may include having the family caregivers observe the nurse when caring for the child so that they become comfortable performing continuing care, using equipment, giving medications, and doing treatments when the child goes home.

INTERNET RESOURCES

Make a Wish Foundation
www.wish.org

Fathers Network
www.fathersnetwork.org

CoachArt
www.coachart.org

Dream Factory of Greater Kansas City
www.kcdream.org

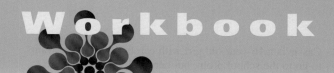

NCLEX-STYLE REVIEW QUESTIONS

1. In planning nursing care for a child with a chronic condition, which goal would *most likely* be part of this child's plan of care?
   a. The child will achieve the highest levels of growth and development.
   b. The child will participate in age-appropriate activities.
   c. The child will eat at least 75% of each meal.
   d. The child will share feelings about changes in body image.

2. The nurse is working with the family caregivers of a child who has a chronic condition. Which statement made by the child's caregivers is an example of the common response called overprotection?
   a. "My child was born with this, and it will always be part of our lives."
   b. "She should be punished when she breaks things because she knows better."
   c. "I know I should let her try new activities, but she just gets frustrated."
   d. "My child just isn't what I expected when I decided to become a parent."

3. The nurse is working with the caregivers of a child who has a chronic condition. Which statement made by the child's caregivers is an example of the common response called acceptance?
   a. "My child was born with this, and it will always be part of our lives."
   b. "She should be punished when she breaks things because she knows better."
   c. "I know I should let her try new activities, but she just gets frustrated."
   d. "My child just isn't what I expected when I decided to become a parent."

4. In working with families of children who have chronic conditions, what is important for the nurse to encourage family members to do?
   a. Refrain from talking about the condition.
   b. Openly express their feelings.
   c. Prevent the child from overhearing conversations.
   d. Tell stories about themselves.

5. In working with siblings of children who have chronic conditions, it is important for the nurse to recognize which statement may be true about the siblings in many cases?
   a. Siblings may feel embarrassed about their brother's or sister's condition.
   b. Siblings are the primary caregiver for the sick child.
   c. Siblings excel in school in an effort to decrease the family stress.
   d. Siblings get jobs at a young age to help support the family.

6. When working with the family caregivers of a child with a chronic condition, the nurse may note the family experiences a grief reaction before coming to an acceptance of the child's condition. Which of the following behaviors by the nurse would be helpful in working with these family caregivers? Select all that apply.
   a. Encouraging the family to express their feelings.
   b. Responding in a nonjudgmental way.
   c. Stating, "It won't be so hard as time goes on."
   d. Reminding the family that anger is inappropriate.
   e. Staying quietly with the family.

STUDY ACTIVITIES

1. Lena and Josh are the young parents of Nina, a 12-month-old girl with meningomyelocele (spina bifida). Nina must be catheterized at least four times a day and also has mobility problems. Describe some of the economic and other stresses that this young couple faces.

2. Do a search online (or use your local telephone book) to make a list of agencies to which you could refer families for assistance and support in the care of a child with a chronic condition.

3. Eight-year-old Jason, a client in your pediatric unit, is undergoing chemotherapy. He seems very lonely and sad, although his family visits him regularly. You decide he may need contact with children his own age. Describe plans that you will make to provide contact with peers.

4. Go to the following website: www.lehman.cuny.edu/faculty/jfleitas/bandaides/. See "Bandaides and Blackboards." Click on "Kids." Click on the star next to the section "To tell or not to tell," and read this section.
   a. List five reasons kids choose *not* to tell others that they have a chronic health condition.
   b. List five reasons kids choose to tell others that they have a chronic health condition.

CRITICAL THINKING: WHAT WOULD YOU DO?

1. You are caring for 5-year-old Abby, who has cystic fibrosis. Her mother, Mattie, has been overprotective and has always done everything for her.
   a. What will you do to involve Abby in caring for herself?
   b. What will you say or do to help and encourage Mattie to encourage Abby to do more of her own care?
   c. What are the reasons you think Mattie is overprotective of her child?

2. Nine-year-old Tyson is angry. He tells you that he hates his 6-year-old brother, Josh, who has Down syndrome.
   a. What would you say to Tyson to begin a discussion with him about his feelings?
   b. What are some of the factors you think might be causing Tyson to be angry?
   c. What would you say or suggest if you had the opportunity to talk to Tyson and Josh's family caregiver?

3. Cassie is a 16-year-old girl with cerebral palsy. She wants to go to the school prom, but her family caregivers are resistant to the idea. Cassie pleads with you to talk to them.
   a. How will you approach this problem?
   b. What are your responses to Cassie and to her caregivers?

Abuse in the Family and Community

Key Terms
child abuse
child maltreatment
child neglect
codependent parent
dysfunctional family
human trafficking
incest
sexual abuse
sexual assault

Learning Objectives

At the conclusion of this chapter, you will:

1. Discuss factors that may lead to child maltreatment.
2. Identify the circumstances under which physical punishment can be classified as abusive.
3. Describe the differences between bruises that occur accidentally to a child and those that result from physical abuse.
4. Explain the injuries that occur as a result of abusive head trauma (shaken baby syndrome).
5. Describe Munchausen syndrome by proxy.
6. Discuss how a child may be emotionally abused.
7. Explain child neglect.
8. Discuss sexual abuse and the effects on the child.
9. Describe the nursing responsibilities for the child who has been abused.
10. Discuss concerns related to human trafficking.
11. Discuss bullying and the effects on the child.
12. Describe the unpredictable behavior of a parent with substance addiction and its effect on the child.
13. Identify behaviors that suggest there is an addiction problem in the child's family.

Shantell Williams is brought to the clinic by her mother. In collecting data, you find that Shantell is almost 2 years old and lives with her mother and her mother's boyfriend who is not Shantell's father. You note that Shantell has an unusual mark on her upper thigh, and you suspect she might be abused. As you read this chapter, think about the questions you will ask Shantell's mother.

Every family faces many types of stress at one time or another. Events that create stress for a family include illness, job loss, economic crisis or poverty, relocation, birth, death, and trauma. How the family handles these stresses greatly affects the emotional, social, and physical health of each member of the family. A **dysfunctional family** is one that cannot resolve these stresses and work through them in a positive, socially acceptable manner. Families often face multiple pressures at the same time; this dynamic creates additional stress and adds to the risk of dysfunctional coping. The atmosphere in a dysfunctional family creates additional stress for all family members. Because of the lack of support within the dysfunctional family for individual members, these members respond negatively to real or perceived problems. This family climate may set the stage for abuse and other unhealthy coping behaviors.

Abuse in the family can take various forms. Parents or caregivers may abuse the child, spouses, other family members, or substances. Bullying, a form of peer abuse often occurs in the community. Child abuse can have a significant negative impact on the child's growth and development and physical and emotional health. Likewise, the family problems of domestic violence or parental substance abuse negatively affect the child. In some cases, domestic violence or parental substance abuse may lead to child abuse, but this is not always the case. As the nurse, you must be alert to signs of abuse in the family and be aware of the potential effects on the child.

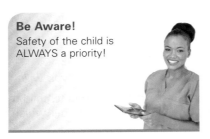

Be Aware!
Safety of the child is ALWAYS a priority!

CHILD MALTREATMENT

Today, in the United States, any sort of mistreatment and abuse of children is regarded as unacceptable. The term **child maltreatment** is a broad term used to define all types of child abuse including physical, sexual, emotional, and any acts of negligence. Child maltreatment is usually committed by a person responsible for the care of the child. The term **child abuse** is used to describe acts of commission which may result in harm or a threat of harm to the child. **Child neglect** is used to describe acts of omission in which there is a failure to provide for the child's needs or to protect the child from harm.

Each year, increasing numbers of child maltreatment cases are brought to the attention of authorities. Estimates of the number of children treated in emergency departments after an episode of abuse range from 700,000 to 1.25 million annually. However, the actual number of abused children may be much higher because many more cases may go undetected.

Child maltreatment is not limited to one age group and can be detected at any age. The courts have even viewed fetal exposure to drugs and alcohol as child abuse. The age group of children from birth to 4 years has the highest number of victims of child abuse (Boos, 2021). Abusive parents can be found at all socioeconomic levels, but families with greater financial means may be able to evade detection more easily. Low-income families show greater evidence of violence, neglect, and sexual abuse according to some studies. Commonly, abusive parents have inadequate parenting skills; if they have unrealistic expectations of the child, they may not respond appropriately to the child's behavior.

State laws require healthcare personnel to report suspected child abuse. This requirement overrides the concern for confidentiality. Laws have been enacted that protect the nurse who reports suspected child abuse from reprisal by a family caregiver (e.g., being sued for slander), even if it is found that the child's situation is not a result of abuse. If you do not report suspected child abuse, the penalty can be loss of your nursing license.

If abuse is suspected, the healthcare facility can hold the child for a certain period of time, and then a court holds a hearing to determine if the charges are true and to decide where the child should be placed.

This is Critical to Remember!
Suspected child abuse must be reported. A healthcare facility can usually hold a child for 72 hours after suspected abuse has been reported so that a caseworker can investigate the charge.

Types of Child Maltreatment
Physical Abuse

Physical abuse may occur when the family caregiver is unfamiliar with normal child behavior. Inexperienced caregivers may not know what normal behavior is for a child and become frustrated when the child does not respond in the way they expect. If inexperience is coupled with dysfunctional coping, the caregiver may physically abuse the child. Some young women become pregnant to have a child to love, and they expect that love to be returned in full measure. When the child resists the caregiver's control or seems to do the opposite of what is expected, the caregiver may take it as a personal affront and become angry, possibly responding with physical punishment. Some cultures support physical punishment for children, citing the principle "spare the rod, spoil the child." Despite evidence that physical punishment often results in negative behavior and that other forms of punishment are more effective, corporal punishment continues to be approved occasionally, even in some schools. However, physical punishment that leaves marks, causes injury, or threatens the child's physical or emotional well-being is considered abusive.

When a child's physical injury requires medical attention, family caregivers may attribute the injury to some action of the child's that is not in keeping with the child's age or level of development. For example, the caregiver may attribute an injury to the child's playing in a competitive sport that the child is too young to play. The caregiver may also attribute the injury to an action of a sibling. When the child's symptoms do not match the injury the caregiver describes, be alert for possible abuse. However, do not accuse the caregiver before a complete investigation takes place.

Pay Attention to What You See!
An important role of the healthcare team is to identify abusive or potentially abusive situations as early as possible.

Young, active children often have a number of bruises that occur from their usual activities. Most of these bruises occur over bony areas such as the knees, elbows, shins, and forehead. Bruises that occur in areas of soft tissue, such as the buttocks, genitalia, thighs, back of the knees, upper back, and nose and eyes, may be suspect (Fig. 33-1).

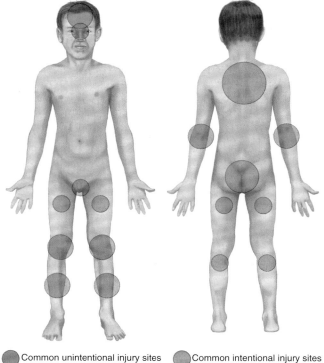

Common unintentional injury sites Common intentional injury sites

A

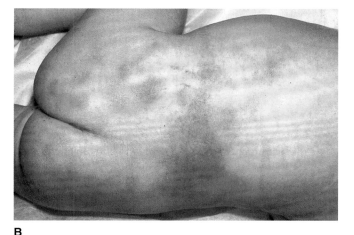

B

Figure 33-1 A. Common unintentional injury sites and common intentional injury sites, suspicious for physical abuse. **B.** Example of suspicious bruises.

Bruises in the inner aspect of the upper arms may indicate that the child raised the arms to protect the face and head from blows.

Bruises may be distinctive in outline, clearly indicating the instrument that was used. Cigarettes, hangers, belt buckles, electrical cords, handprints, teeth (from biting), and sticks leave identifiable marks (Fig. 33-2). The injuries may be in varying stages of healing, indicating that not all the injuries occurred during one episode.

Signs or possible evidence of child abuse can be further evaluated by the use of technology. On an x-ray, bone fractures in various stages of healing may be noted. Spiral

fractures of the long bones of a young child are not common, and their presence might indicate possible abuse. Children who have been harshly shaken may not show a clear picture of abuse, but computed tomography may demonstrate cerebral edema or cerebral hemorrhage.

Burns are another common type of injury seen in the abused child (Fig. 33-3). Although burns may be accidental in young children, certain types of burns are highly suspicious. Cigarette burns, for example, are common abuse injuries. Burns from immersion of a hand in hot liquid, a hot register (as evidenced by the grid pattern), a steam iron, or a curling iron are other common abuse injuries. Caregivers may immerse the buttocks of a child in hot water if they thought the child was uncooperative in toilet training. Caregivers are often unaware of how quickly a child can be seriously burned. A burn that is neglected or not immediately reported must be considered suspicious until all the facts can be gathered and examined.

After observing the unusual mark on **Shantell Williams**, what other things will you observe for and what information will you document regarding your findings?

Abusive Head Trauma (Shaken Baby Syndrome)

Shaken baby syndrome is one form of abusive head trauma and occurs when a small child is shaken by the arms or shoulders in a repetitive, violent manner. Shaking causes a whiplash-type injury to the child's neck. In addition, the child may have edema to the brain stem and retinal or brain hemorrhages. Loss of vision, cognitive impairment, or even death may occur in these children. Clinical manifestations may include lethargy, irritability, poor feeding, vomiting, and seizures, but often the signs of this form of child abuse are not easily observed and may be missed during physical examination. Internal symptoms are detected by the use of computed tomography and magnetic resonance imaging.

Munchausen Syndrome by Proxy

In Munchausen synby proxy (may be referred to as caregiver-fabricated illness or medical child abuse), one person either fabricates or induces illness in another to get attention. When a caregiver has this syndrome, they frequently bring the child to a healthcare facility and report symptoms of illness when the child is actually well. The child's mother is most often the person who has the syndrome. Often the mother injures the child to get the attention of medical personnel. She may slowly poison the child with prescription drugs, alcohol, or other drugs, or she may suffocate the child to cause apnea. Many times, the symptoms, such as seizures or abdominal pain, are not easy to find on physical examination but are reported as history. The mother appears very attentive to the child and is often familiar with medical terminology. This situation is frustrating for healthcare personnel because it is difficult to catch the suspect in the act of endangering the child. Close observation

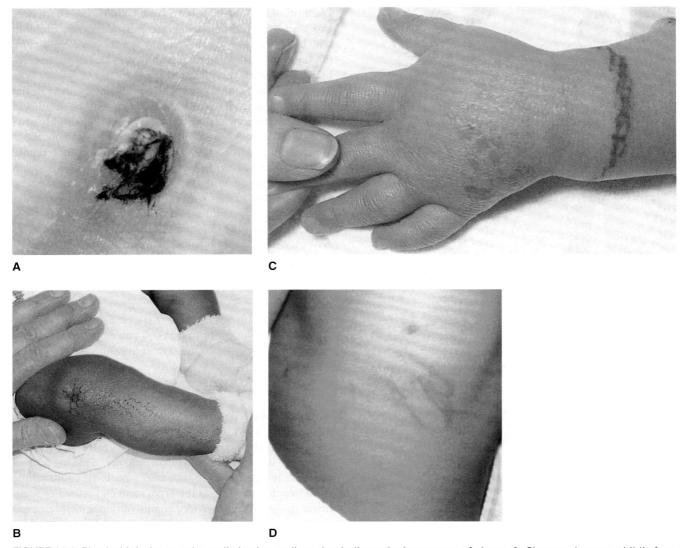

FIGURE 33-2 Physical injuries may have distinctive outlines that indicate the instrument of abuse. **A.** Cigarette burn on child's foot. **B.** Imprint from a radiator cover. **C.** Rope burn from being tied to crib rail. **D.** Imprint from a looped electrical cord.

of the caregiver's interactions with the child is necessary. For instance, if episodes of apnea occur only in the presence of the caregiver, be alert for this syndrome. The caregiver who suffers from this syndrome must receive psychiatric help.

Emotional Abuse

Injury from emotional abuse can be just as serious and lasting as that from physical abuse, but it is much more difficult to identify. Several types of emotional abuse can occur, including the following:

- Verbal abuse such as humiliation, scapegoating, unrealistic expectations with belittling, and erratic discipline
- Emotional unavailability when caregivers are absorbed in their own problems
- Insufficient or poor nurturing, or threatening to leave the child or otherwise end the relationship
- Role reversal in which the child must take on the role of parenting the parent and is blamed for the parent's problems

Children may show evidence of emotional abuse by appearing worried or fearful or having vague complaints of illness or nightmares. Family caregivers may display signs of inappropriate expectations of the child when in the healthcare facility by sometimes mocking or belittling the child for age-appropriate behavior. In young children, failure to thrive may be a sign of emotional abuse. In the older child, poor school performance and attendance, poor self-esteem, and poor peer relationships may be clues.

Neglect

Child neglect is failure to provide adequate hygiene, healthcare, education, nutrition, love, nurturing, and supervision needed for growth and development. If a child is not given adequate care for a serious medical condition, the caregivers are considered neglectful. For example, if a child is seriously burned, even accidentally, and the caregivers do not take the child for evaluation and treatment until several days later, they may be judged to be neglectful. Often, the

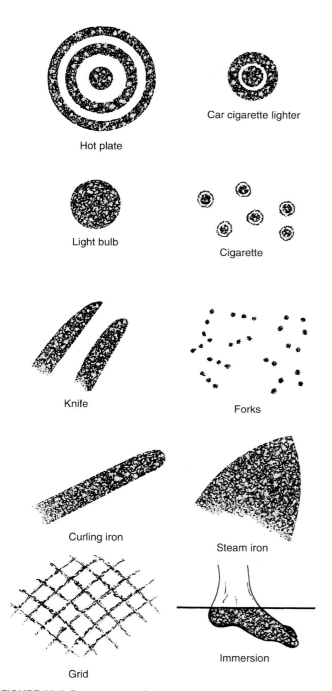

FIGURE 33-3 Burn patterns from objects used for inflicting burns in child abuse.

child with failure to thrive as a result of being underfed, deprived of love, or constantly criticized can be classified as neglected; however, be careful not to make an unsubstantiated accusation of neglect.

Sexual Abuse

The Federal Child Abuse Prevention and Treatment Act defines **sexual abuse** as "the employment, use, persuasion, inducement, enticement, or coercion of any child to engage in, or assist any other person to engage in, any sexually

explicit conduct or simulation of such conduct for the purpose of producing a visual depiction of such conduct; or the rape, and in cases of caretaker or interfamilial relationships, statutory rape, molestation, prostitution, or other form of sexual exploitation of children, or incest with children" (*Child Abuse Prevention and Treatment Act as Amended by the CAPTA Reauthorization Act of 2010*).

Sexual abuse of children has existed in all ages and cultures, but it has seldom been admitted when perpetrated by parents or other relatives in the home. The abuser is often a trusted adult man and **incest** (sexually arousing physical contact between family members not married to each other) is common in sexual abuse cases. As with other types of child abuse, sexual abuse knows no socioeconomic, racial, religious, or ethnic boundaries. However, substance abuse, job loss, and poverty are contributing factors. Like other forms of child abuse, sexual abuse is being recognized and reported more often.

Several terms are commonly used when sexual abuse is discussed. *Sexual contact* includes fondling of breasts or genitalia, intercourse (vaginal or anal), oral–genital contact, exhibitionism, and voyeurism. From a legal viewpoint, sexual contact between a child and another person in a caregiving position, such as a parent, babysitter, or teacher, is classified as sexual abuse. A sexual contact made by someone who is not functioning in a caregiver role is classified as **sexual assault**. When a person has power or control over a child, that person, even if a child as well, can be a sexual abuser.

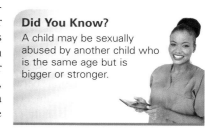

Did You Know?

A child may be sexually abused by another child who is the same age but is bigger or stronger.

When a child is sexually assaulted by a stranger, the family caregivers usually become aware of the incident, promptly report it, and take the child for a physical examination. However, in the case of incest, the child rarely tells another person what is happening; the family member committing the acts often intimidates the child with threats, appeals to the child's desire to be loved and to please, and convinces the child of the importance of keeping the act secret. The child may exhibit physical complaints such as various aches and pains, gastrointestinal upsets, changes in bowel and bladder habits (including enuresis), nightmares, and acts of aggression or hostility. Some of these complaints or behaviors may be the presenting problem when a health care provider sees the child.

Regardless of the relationship of the perpetrator to the child, the outcome of the abuse is devastating. Sexual abuse by a person the child trusts seems to be the most damaging type.

Effects on the Child and Family

Child maltreatment has long-term as well as immediate effects. The abused child may be hyperactive; may exhibit angry, antisocial behavior; or may be especially withdrawn.

When child abuse is suspected or confirmed, the child may be removed from the home or separated from the family for protection. Abusive parents were often abused themselves as children; thus, the problem of child abuse continues in a cyclical fashion from generation to generation.

TEST YOURSELF

✔ What are the different types of child maltreatment often seen?

✔ What differentiates punishment for inappropriate behavior from child abuse?

✔ Who is the person who usually has the disease in Munchausen syndrome by proxy?

Nursing Process and Care Plan *for the Child Who is Abused*

Assessment (Data Collection)

When collecting data on a child who may have been abused or neglected, it is important to observe and document thoroughly and completely. The child should have a complete physical examination; carefully describe and accurately document all bruises, blemishes, lacerations, areas of redness and irritation, and marks of any kind on the child's body. It may be necessary to request that photographs be taken.

Observe the interaction between the child and the caregiver, and carefully document your observations using nonjudgmental terms. The child's body language may be revealing, so be alert for significant information. For example, if the child shrinks away from contact by the caregiver or health care provider or, on the other hand, is overly clingy or obedient to the caregiver, watch for other signs of inappropriate behavior. These assessments vary with the child's age (Table 33-1).

Perhaps the most difficult part may be to maintain a nonjudgmental attitude throughout the interview and examination. Be calm and reassuring with the child; let the child lead the way when possible.

Nursing Care Focus

When developing evidence-based nursing care focuses for the child and family who may be or have been in an abusive situation, anxiety and fear are concerns. Safety of the child is of utmost importance. Dysfunctional family patterns and coping skills among members of the family must be addressed.

Outcome Identification and Planning

Major goals for the abused child include caring for any injuries the child has sustained as well as relieving anxiety and fear and reducing the risk for injury. An important family goal is to improve parenting and coping skills of the caregiver or family.

Nursing Care Focus

● Anxiety, fear by child related to history of abuse, and fear of abuse from others

Goal

● The child will exhibit decreased signs of anxiety and fear.

Implementations for Relieving the Child's Anxiety and Fear

Observe the child for behavior that indicates anxiety or fear such as withdrawal, ducking or shying away from the nurse or caregivers, and avoiding eye contact. One nurse should be assigned to care for the child so that the child can relate to one person consistently. Provide physical contact, such as hugging, rocking, and caressing, only if the child accepts it. Identify nursing actions that seem to comfort the child, and use them consistently. Use a calm, reassuring, and kind manner, and provide a safe atmosphere in which the child has an opportunity to express feelings and fears. Use play to help the child express some of these emotions. Be careful not to do anything that might alarm or upset the child. Psychological support is provided through social services or an abuse team.

Evaluation of Goal/Desired Outcome

The child:

● demonstrates relaxed play, facial expressions, and posture.
● displays no withdrawal or guarding during contacts with the nursing staff.

Nursing Care Focus

● Injury risk for the child related to caregiver situational stressors or poor coping skills

Goal

● The child will remain free from injury and the family caregiver will exhibit positive interaction with the child.

Implementations for Observing Interaction Between the Caregiver and Child

While caring for the abused child when the family caregiver is present, take the opportunity to observe how the caregiver relates to the child and how the child reacts to the caregiver. Give the caregiver the same courtesy extended to all caregivers. Offer a compliment when the caregiver does something well in caring for the child. Give the caregiver an opportunity to discuss in private any concerns; during this time, you may be able to gain their confidence.

TABLE 33-1 Signs of Maltreatment in Children

PHYSICAL SIGNS	BEHAVIORAL SIGNS
Physical Abuse	
Bruises and welts: may be on multiple body surfaces or soft tissue; may form regular pattern (e.g., belt buckle)	Less compliant than average
	Signs of negativism, unhappiness
Burns: cigar or cigarette, immersion (stocking/glovelike on extremities or doughnut-shaped on buttocks or genitals), or patterned as an electrical appliance (e.g., iron)	Anger, isolation
	Destructive
	Abusive toward others
Fractures: single or multiple; may be in various stages of healing	Difficulty developing relationships
Lacerations or abrasions: rope burns; tears in and around mouth, eyes, ears, genitalia	Either excessive or absent separation anxiety
	Inappropriate caregiving concern for parent
Abdominal injuries: ruptured or injured internal organs	Constantly in search of attention, favors, food, etc.
Central nervous system injuries: subdural hematoma, retinal or subarachnoid hemorrhage	Various developmental delays (cognitive, language, motor)
Emotional Abuse	
Delays in physical development	Delayed, immature emotional development
Failure to thrive	Deteriorating conduct
	Increased anxiety, fear
	Apathy or depression
	Developmental lags
Neglect	
Malnutrition	Lack of appropriate adult supervision
Repeated episodes of pica	Repeated ingestions of harmful substances
Constant fatigue or listlessness	Poor school attendance
Poor hygiene	Exploitation (forced to beg or steal; excessive household work)
Inadequate clothing for circumstances	Role reversal with parent
Inadequate medical or dental care	Drug or alcohol use
Sexual Abuse	
Difficulty walking or sitting	Direct or indirect disclosure to relative, friend, or teacher
Thickening or hyperpigmentation of labial skin	Withdrawal with excessive dependency
Vaginal opening measures greater than 4 mm horizontally in preadolescence	Poor peer relationships
	Poor self-esteem
Torn, stained, or bloody underclothing	Frightened or phobic of adults
Bruises or bleeding of genitalia or perianal area	Sudden decline in academic performance
Lax rectal tone	Pseudomature personality development
Vaginal discharge	Suicide attempts
Recurrent urinary tract infections	Regressive behavior
Nonspecific vaginitis	Enuresis or encopresis
Venereal disease	Excessive masturbation
Sperm or acid phosphatase on body or clothes	Highly sexualized play
Pregnancy	Sexual promiscuity

Evaluation of Goal/Desired Outcome

The child:

- remains free from injury from the caregiver.

The family caregiver:

- talks with the child and is sensitive to their needs.
- refrains from making unreasonable demands on the child.

Nursing Care Focus

- Family coping impairment related to unrealistic expectations of the child by the family caregiver

Goal

- The family caregiver will be involved in the child's care and will verbalize examples of normal growth and development and ways to handle the child's misbehavior.

Implementations for Promoting Parenting Skills and Coping

Maltreatment often occurs when a family caregiver is unfamiliar with normal growth and development and the behaviors common to a particular stage of development. Help the caregiver develop realistic expectations of the child. To help accomplish this goal, when helping design a teaching plan include the caregiver in caring for the child. Discuss with the caregiver the child's expected responses and help them learn about normal development. Praise the caregiver for displaying positive behaviors. Point out specific behaviors of the child and explain them to the caregiver. Discuss specific behaviors of the child that are upsetting to the caregiver and explain that these are common for the child's age. Explore the reasons for the caregiver's absence when they do not visit regularly.

The family caregiver may be facing temporary or permanent placement of the child in another home. Help the caregiver and the child accept this change. Emotions that a caregiver has had for a long period cannot be easily eliminated and must be recognized and acknowledged. The assistance of social services and a child life specialist is beneficial in these situations. Act as a member of the team to aid in the transition. The foster parents may need support from the nursing staff to help ease the child's transition to the new home. Abused children must be followed up carefully after discharge from the healthcare facility to ensure that their well-being is protected.

Evaluation of Goal/Desired Outcome

The family caregiver:

- states age-appropriate behavior for the child.
- discusses ways to handle the child's irritating behavior.
- is involved in counseling and discharge plans.

Nursing Care Focus

- Coping impairment by the nonabusive caregiver related to fear of violence from abusive partner or feelings of powerlessness

Goal

- The nonabusive caregiver will begin to cope with fears and feelings of powerlessness.

Implementations for Supporting the Nonabusive Caregiver

In some cases, one caregiver in the family may be an abuser and the other is not. The nonabusive caregiver is a victim, as is the child. Give the nonabusive caregiver an opportunity to express fears and anxieties. They may feel powerless in the situation. Support the nonabusive caregiver in deciding whether to continue or leave the relationship with the abuser. Try to preserve the caregiver's self-esteem because this is not an easy decision to make. Remember that building trust is essential when discussing the problems and issues of the situation.

Evaluation of Goal/Desired Outcome

The nonabusive caregiver:

- expresses fears and concerns.
- makes plans to resolve problems.

HUMAN TRAFFICKING

Human trafficking is a modern form of slavery in which people are deceived and misled and end up in a situation where one person exerts control over another person for the purpose of exploitation in some form. There are different forms of human trafficking including sex trade, forced labor, or begging. Many times individuals are trapped through coercion and false promises.

Women and children are the most frequent victims of human trafficking. Often poverty and lack of economic opportunities cause vulnerability and allow these individuals to be tricked and to become stuck in trafficking situations. Other risk factors that may lead to human trafficking include being a young girl (ages 12 to 16 years old are at greatest risk), rural location, lack of education, disability, inadequate family support and protection, runaway or throwaway youth, migrant workers, and a history of childhood abuse. Trafficking can happen in any community and individuals of any age, race, gender, or nationality may be victims.

Victims of human trafficking may present to the healthcare setting with concerns related to sexually transmitted infections (STIs), physical injuries, burns, malnutrition, depression, pregnancy care, and HIV/AIDS. Nurses and health care providers may be one of the few contacts the victim has outside of the abusive situation. Rarely do the victims of human trafficking report what is happening to them. Often they have been threatened and are afraid for themselves and their families. The healthcare team is in a unique position to recognize and get help for these victims and must be aware of the potential "red flags" and how to best support the client. See Box 33-1 Guidelines for Caring for Victims of Human Trafficking.

The United States National Human Trafficking Hotline (telephone 1-888-373-7888) can be used by health care providers or clients to report human trafficking (even if suspected but not disclosed).

DOMESTIC VIOLENCE IN THE FAMILY

Millions of children are exposed to domestic violence each year (Franchek-Roa, 2021). Sometimes referred to as family violence, domestic violence is a serious concern seen in families of all races, socioeconomic groups, and educational backgrounds. In cases of domestic violence, a person uses power and control over a person who is a partner or family member. Physical violence, threats, emotional abuse, harassment, and stalking are forms of violence often seen. Children who are exposed to or witness domestic violence are greatly impacted.

Effects on the Child and Family

The impact of domestic violence on the family is great. Even if all family members are not victims of the violence, each family member is affected. The child may witness domestic violence, overhear it from another room, or see physical evidence, such as bruises or broken bones on the victimized parent. The child may even be injured during an

Warning signs that may indicate the person is a victim:
- Delay in seeking medical treatment
- Accompanied by a person who will not let the client speak for themselves
- Hesitant to answer questions about injury or illness
- Clinical presentation does not match the stated history
- Does not know facts such as their address, the date, the time, where they are
- Appears nervous, fearful, avoids eye contact
- Evidence of markings or tattoos that might indicate "branding," such as "property of" and "for sale"
- Inappropriate clothes for the setting or the weather

Supportive measures for the potential victim:
- Give the client privacy for interviewing and maintain confidentiality.
- Be observant for verbal and nonverbal clues that offer openings for further inquiries about the client's situation.
- Listen, use eye contact, show concern with a supportive approach.
- Use a professional interpreter if language is a barrier.
- Recognize that client's safety is of paramount concern and they must build trust which may take time to develop.

episode of violence. In most cases, the victim of domestic violence is the mother, but not always. The older child, especially adolescent boys, may feel a need to intervene to protect the mother. The person who is violent toward a spouse will often abuse their children as well.

Clinical Manifestations in the Child

Children affected by domestic violence may show signs and symptoms that result from the violent situation. These symptoms may be referred to as symptoms of posttraumatic stress disorder and may include inability to sleep, bedwetting, temper tantrums, withdrawal, and feelings of guilt for not being able to protect the victim. The school-aged child may have academic problems, frequent absences, behavior issues, self-isolation, or physical complaints such as headaches and stomachaches. The older child will often use drugs or alcohol; get into legal trouble, many times by committing a crime against another person; or suffer from depression and attempt or commit suicide. Children who witness domestic violence in their homes may become victims or perpetrators as they grow into adulthood.

As a nurse, you must be aware of the signs and symptoms that families affected by domestic violence might exhibit. Shame and embarrassment may prevent children from talking about the violent behavior they have witnessed. Sometimes the abuser has threatened further violence if anyone in the family tells others about the situation. Asking direct and specific questions when domestic violence is suspected will encourage the child or family member to be honest about the situation.

Members of the family may have to seek emergency help from relatives, friends, or community shelters in order to be safe. Shelters for battered women and their children are available in many communities. The National Domestic Violence Hotline (1-800-799-SAFE [7233]) is available for families and victims. The child needs support to deal with the fear and disruption these events cause. In cases in which the child becomes a victim of the domestic violence, the child may even be removed from the home, causing even further trauma.

BULLYING

Bullying, sometimes called peer abuse, is a form of aggressive behavior which is deliberate and repeated, usually toward a person who is physically weaker, shy, or less able to defend themselves from the abuser. The abuse can be physical (hitting, kicking, taking belongings); verbal (teasing, name calling, insulting); psychological (spreading rumors, exclusion); or cyber (text messaging, e-mail, social networking) in nature. In discussing bullying, one person is the victim of the bully, and another person or group of people acts as the bully. This section discusses the child who is the victim of bullying. For discussion of the child who acts as the bully, see Chapter 42.

Effects on the Child
Being the victim of a bully can have long-lasting psychological effects on the child.

The child who is a victim of bullying is singled out because they are somehow different (size, clothing, intelligence, religion, sexual orientation). The victim may have some physical disability or defect or have a socioeconomic status that prevents the child from being "like" other children. For example, a child from a family who has a limited income may not be able to dress like or have the same amounts of spending money that other children may have. The child may feel self-conscious or may be shy, thus becoming a potential target for the bully.

Clinical Manifestations in the Child
The child who is being bullied may have injuries and bruises, but symptoms are often difficult to differentiate from other concerns. They may have physical signs such as headaches, stomachaches, eating and sleeping issues, or more subtle signs such as anxiety, changes in mood, decreasing school performance, or avoidance of certain situations. The child may try to avoid doing certain things such as taking the school bus or playing on the school playground because that is where the bullying is occurring. Parents, teachers, and nurses need to be observant for these behaviors and be a trusted resource for the child who is the victim of bullying (see Tips for Reinforcing Family Teaching: Bullying).

PARENTAL SUBSTANCE ABUSE

The problem of substance abuse has grown to alarming proportions. More than 10% of children come from a home affected by the alcoholism of one or both parents. Alcoholism exacts a terrible toll on the functioning of the

TIPS FOR REINFORCING FAMILY TEACHING

Bullying

- Watch for signs that might indicate your child is the victim of a bully.
- If you think your child may be being bullied but is hesitant to tell you, have a conversation with your child using an indirect approach. For instance, after seeing a situation on TV related to some type of bullying behavior, ask your child, "Have you ever seen anything like this happen?" "Has anyone ever treated you like that?" "What do you think that child should do?"
- Encourage your child to talk to you, a teacher, counselor, or school nurse if they are being bullied or sees someone else being bullied.
- Discuss ways the child might deal with a bullying situation:

- Avoid the bully or the situation (e.g., use a different bathroom; go to your locker at a time other than when the bully is present)
- Have or be a "buddy" in places where the bully might be present (e.g., on the school bus, on the playground, in the school lunchroom)
- Rather than react to the bully, tell the bully to stop, then walk away and ignore the bully and behavior
- Remove the motive; for example, if the bully is trying to take lunch money, bring your lunch to school
- Encourage your child to develop self-confidence. Developing a skill such as music, art, sports, martial arts, or proficiency with computers may help the child develop new friendships and feel better about themselves.

family. Children of alcoholics have an increased risk of becoming alcoholics themselves. When other substances are included, the number of affected homes increases substantially. Adverse childhood experiences, such as physical, emotional, or sexual abuse, have a strong influence on alcohol and drug abuse as adults.

Effects on the Child and Family

Substance abuse is a family problem. If one member of the family abuses alcohol and/or drugs, every member of that family is affected. Children who have at least one parent who is a substance abuser are at risk for a variety of problems that researchers relate to substance abuse in the family. For example, developmental delays occur in young children of substance abusers, and infants of cocaine abusers avoid the caregiver's gaze, which contributes further to bonding delays.

The parent who is addicted may be so involved in procuring the drug that they forget any parenting responsibilities. Caught in the ups and downs of addiction, the parent is not dependable and cannot provide any stability for the child. The parent may waver between overindulgence—smothering the child with attention, leniency, and gifts—and the opposite behavior of irritability, unreasonable accusations, threats, and anger. This unpredictable behavior has a severely negative impact on relationships in the family.

Children of substance-abusing parents often become loners and avoid relationships with others for fear that the substance-abusing parent might do or say something to embarrass them in front of their peers. As the parent's substance abuse worsens, the family's dysfunction and social isolation increase. The **codependent parent** directly or indirectly supports the addictive behavior of the other parent. This behavior usually involves making excuses for the addict's actions and expecting others (i.e., the children) to overlook the parent's moodiness, erratic behavior, and consumption of alcohol or drugs. Codependency adds to the dilemma of children living with an addicted parent.

Clinical Manifestations in the Child

Children react to parental substance addiction in a variety of ways. Children rarely talk about the parent's problem even to the other parent. These children often experience guilt, anxiety, confusion, anger, depression, and addictive behavior. An older child, often a girl, may take on the responsibility of running the household, taking care of the younger children, making meals, and performing the tasks that the parent normally should do. These children may become overachievers in school but remain emotionally isolated from their peers and teachers. This child does not usually bring negative attention to the family, and substance abuse in the family is not often suspected based on the behavior of this child. Another child in the family may try to deflect the embarrassment and anger of the other siblings by trying to make everyone feel good. As these children become adolescents or young adults, they may have problems such as their own substance abuse or eating disorders. The child in the family who "acts out" and engages in delinquent behavior is most likely to come to the attention of social services and be identified as a child who needs help.

 A Personal Glimpse

When I was little, we had such happy times. We used to go places together and even when we stayed home, we laughed and had fun. My brother was born when I was 3 and then my little sister was born when I was 8. Sometimes after she was born, I could hear my parents arguing and shouting downstairs when they thought I was asleep. I couldn't usually hear the words they were saying, but it scared me to hear them. The next day they would act like nothing had happened and things were fine. I thought the way they argued was just what parents did. I worked hard in school, got good grades, and never got into trouble. I helped take care of my little brother and sister. I kept my room clean and helped with cooking and laundry. I noticed my mom always had a glass in her hand; I thought it was soda when I was little. As I got older, I realized that my mom was drinking. Sometimes when my parents were arguing it was so loud, I tried to cover my ears and my brother's and sister's ears so they wouldn't hear. Words like "alcoholic," "drunk," and "drinking," were always part of the screaming. If I ever asked my dad about my mom, he would always excuse her behavior or apologize to me and tell me he would talk to her, and things would be better.

By the time I was in eighth grade, I was used to walking home from school because my mother forgot to pick me up. When I would get home, she would be passed out on the couch. I made excuses to my friends why they couldn't come to my house. I was so afraid my mom would show up at a school meeting drunk that I didn't even tell her about the meetings. She would get mad and blame me for things I didn't do and then turn around and promise me she would take me places or do things with me. I would get excited and think finally things with my mom would be better. Over and over, she would forget her promises, and I would feel hurt again.

By the time I was in high school, I just couldn't wait to get away from home. I was so embarrassed, I never told anyone my mom drank or what really happened at my house. I worked so hard to keep our secret. My brother was always in trouble, and one day the school counselor called me in to her office. She asked me how things were at my house and finally I couldn't keep the pain inside anymore. I am thankful she listened. We started to go to counseling, and my dad started going to Al-Anon. I wish I could say my mom stopped drinking. My parents got a divorce, and we live with my dad. I hope someday my mom will get help.

Caitlyn, age 17 years

Learning Opportunity: *What are some of the things this father did that enabled the addictive behavior of this mother? What are some ways that children deal with a parent's substance abuse?*

Behaviors that may alert nurses and other healthcare personnel to an addiction problem in the family include the following:

• The loner child who avoids interaction with classmates
• The child who is failing in school or has numerous episodes of unexcused absences or truancy
• The child with frequent minor physical complaints, such as headaches or stomachaches
• The child who steals or commits acts of violence
• The aggressive child
• The child who abuses drugs or alcohol

Nurses and others who work with children must be alert to these signals for help. Children can benefit from programs that support them and help them understand what is happening at home. Such a program may include group therapy sessions at school in which the child learns that others have the same problems; this reduces their feelings of isolation. Other programs may include the whole family, perhaps as part of the program for the addicted parent who is

trying to break the addiction. Professional help is necessary to prevent the child from developing more serious problems. The earlier the child can be identified and treatment begun, the better the prognosis. Tips for Reinforcing Family Teaching: Resources for Information and Help with Drug and Alcohol Problems in Chapter 42 provides a list of resources for information and help with drug and alcohol problems.

Don't be Afraid to Speak Up!

There is help for the child in a home where substance abuse is an issue. You can provide referrals and support that benefit the child and family.

TEST YOURSELF

✔ What are some examples of the forms of domestic violence often seen?

✔ The signs and symptoms seen in children as a result of a violent situation may be referred to as symptoms of what?

✔ What term is used to describe the parent who supports, directly or indirectly, the addictive behavior of the other parent?

As **Shantell Williams's** nurse, after observing and documenting your findings, what types of maltreatment or abuse might she possibly be the victim? What are your responsibilities in caring for Shantell and her mother?

KEY POINTS

• Family stressors and how the family handles these stresses may lead to child maltreatment. Poor parenting skills may lead to child abuse if the parent has unrealistic expectations of the child or dysfunctional coping skills.

• Physical punishment can be classified as abusive if it leaves marks, causes injury, or threatens the child's physical or emotional well-being.

• Bruises that occur accidentally to a child usually appear over bony areas such as the knees, elbows, shin, and forehead. Those that have been inflicted in an abusive manner may be found in soft tissue such as the buttocks, genitalia, thighs, back of the knees, upper back, and nose and eyes.

• Abusive head trauma (shaken baby syndrome) causes a whiplash-type injury in the neck. In addition, the child may have edema to the brain stem, brain hemorrhages, loss of vision, cognitive impairment, or even death. The child might have clinical manifestations of lethargy, irritability, poor feeding, vomiting, and seizures or have no easily noted symptoms.

- Munchausen syndrome by proxy (may be referred to as caregiver-fabricated illness or medical child abuse) occurs when one person, commonly the mother, either fabricates or induces illness in another (usually the child) to get attention.
- A child may be emotionally abused verbally or by emotional unavailability of the family caregiver, poor nurturing, threats involving leaving the child, or role reversal, in which the child must take on the role of parenting or is blamed for the parent's problems.
- Child neglect is failure to provide adequate hygiene, healthcare, nutrition, love, nurturing, and supervision.
- Sexual abuse can be incest, sexual contact, or sexual assault and occurs in all socioeconomic, racial, religious, and ethnic groups. Substance abuse, job loss, and poverty are often contributing factors.
- Nursing care goals for the child who has been abused focus on caring for any injuries the child has sustained as well as relieving anxiety and fear and reducing the child's risk for injury. Nursing care that promotes parenting skills and coping benefits the child as well.
- Human trafficking is a modern form of slavery in which people end up in a situation where one person exerts control over another person for the purpose of exploitation in some form. Poverty, lack of economic opportunities, being a young girl, living in a rural location, lack of education, disability, inadequate family support and protection, runaway or throwaway youth, migrant workers, and a history of childhood abuse are risk factors. When victims are seen in a healthcare setting, nurses and health care providers are in a unique position to identify and support these victims.
- In cases of domestic violence, the child may have witnessed, heard, or seen evidence of the violence. The child may be injured or have symptoms such as inability to sleep, bed-wetting, temper tantrums, withdrawal, and feelings of guilt. They may have academic problems, frequent absences, behavior issues, isolate themselves from others, or have physical complaints such as headaches and stomachaches. The older child may use drugs or alcohol, commit crimes, suffer from depression, and attempt or commit suicide. These children may become victims or perpetrators of domestic violence as adults.
- The child being bullied may be the victim of physical, verbal, psychological, or cyber abuse. Often the victim is perceived as somehow being different from others and thus "weaker." Symptoms may be physical or less obvious such as anxiety, changes in mood, decreasing school performance, or avoidance of certain situations. Support from trusted adults may help the child develop self-confidence and be more able to cope with the bullying situation.
- The parent with substance addiction is not dependable and cannot provide stability for the child. The parent may waver between overindulgence and the opposite—unreasonable and unpredictable behavior toward the child.
- Behaviors seen in children who have an addicted parent include avoidance of interaction with classmates, failing in school, unexcused absences or truancy, frequent minor physical complaints, stealing or committing acts of violence, aggressive behavior, and abuse of drugs or alcohol. Sometimes children behave in a positive manner to prevent attention being drawn to the family. These children may take on the responsibilities the adult would normally take on, may become overachievers in school, or they may attempt to deflect the behaviors of their siblings by trying to make everyone feel good.

INTERNET RESOURCES

Child Welfare Information Gateway
www.childwelfare.gov

Prevent Child Abuse America
www.preventchildabuse.org

Tennyson Center for Children at Colorado Christian Home
www.childabuse.org

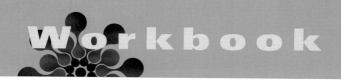

NCLEX-STYLE REVIEW QUESTIONS

1. The nurse is assisting with a physical examination on a child who has been admitted with a diagnosis of possible child abuse. Which finding might alert the nurse to the possibility that the child has been abused?
   a. A fractured bone
   b. Bruises on the knees and elbows
   c. Hyperactive and angry behavior
   d. A burn that has not been treated

2. The nurse is interviewing the family caregiver of a 5-year-old child who has been admitted with bruises on the abdomen and thighs as well as additional bruises in various stages of healing. Which statement made by the family caregiver might alert the healthcare team to the possibility of child abuse?
   a. "His brother just plays too rough with him."
   b. "My child goes to the day care after school."
   c. "He just learned to ride his bicycle."
   d. "When he is in trouble, I make him go to his room."

3. In caring for a child who has been admitted after being sexually abused, which intervention would be included in the child's plan of care?
   a. Observe for signs of anxiety.
   b. Weigh on the same scale each day.
   c. Encourage frequent family visits.
   d. Test the urine for glucose upon admission.

4. The nurse is discussing the topic of bullying with a group of parents of school-age children. Which statements made by parents in the group would indicate an understanding of the topic? Select all that apply.
   a. "I am concerned my child is being bullied; his grades keep dropping."
   b. "The little girl next door is timid and shy, and she just had braces put on. She is a target for bullying."
   c. "It is not considered bullying if children write unkind messages on social networking sites."
   d. "Bullying usually occurs among family members, rather than among school peers."
   e. "It is good for the child to tell the bully to leave them alone and then walk away from the situation."

STUDY ACTIVITIES

1. You are on duty in the emergency department when an infant is admitted with injuries that cause you to suspect abuse. The mother says her boyfriend was babysitting for her. State how you feel about this. Describe the observations that you will make when collecting data on the infant. What are your plans to approach the mother? Write out an effective communication you might have with the mother.

2. Children react differently to living with a family caregiver who is addicted. Make a list of the behaviors you might see that would cause you to be alert to a child with such a family problem. Research your community for resources available to children from families in which addiction is a problem. Share the information you find with your classmates.

3. Research the internet to find at least three reliable websites that give information regarding substance abuse in parents and how a child is affected by a parent's use of substances.

CRITICAL THINKING: WHAT WOULD YOU DO?

1. Your neighbor, 17-year-old Holly, has an active 18-month-old toddler named Jason. You overhear Holly screaming at him and saying, "I'm going to beat you if you don't listen to me!"
   a. Describe your feelings about the comment the mother made.
   b. What might be some factors that contributed to this situation?
   c. What would you say and do regarding this situation?

2. At a well-child visit, a mother confides in you that her husband's drinking is a concern to her. She tells you she has tried to get him to stop drinking because she thinks his drinking is affecting the children.
   a. Explain how the codependent parent supports, either directly or indirectly, the addictive behavior of the other parent.
   b. What are some behaviors that might be seen in the children in this family?
   c. What would you say to this mother?

34

The Dying Child

Key Terms
anticipatory grief
hospice
thanatologist
unfinished business

Learning Objectives

At the conclusion of this chapter, you will:

1. Discuss reasons why nurses may have difficulty working effectively with dying children.
2. Discuss how a nurse can personally prepare to care for a dying child.
3. Explain factors that affect the child's understanding of death.
4. Describe how a child's understanding of death changes at each developmental level.
5. Describe the role of anticipatory grief in the grieving process.
6. Describe the reactions of family caregivers when a child has a terminal illness.
7. Explain why a family may suffer excessive grief and guilt when a child dies suddenly.
8. Describe possible reactions in a child when a sibling dies.
9. Identify settings for caring for the dying child and the advantages and disadvantages of each.
10. Discuss the role of the nurse in caring for the dying child and the child's family.

After many months of intense treatment for leukemia, **Lee Anderson**, age 6, is in the terminal stage of the disease. Lee lives with his parents and his 4-year-old sister and 12-year-old brother. The health care provider has talked to Lee's parents and has told them that most likely Lee has less than a month to live. As you read this chapter, think about Lee and his family and what responses you might see in each family member when they are told about Lee's condition.

Death is a tragic reality for thousands of children each year. Accidents are the leading cause of death in children between the ages of 1 and 14 years; cancer is the number one fatal disease in this age group (American Childhood Cancer Organization, 2021). Nearly all these children leave behind at least one grieving family caregiver and perhaps brothers, sisters, and grandparents. As a nurse caring for children and families, you must be prepared for encounters with the dying and the bereaved.

Death of a child is the most difficult death to accept. We may more easily accept that senior clients have lived a full life and that life must end, but the life of a child still holds the hopes, dreams, and promises of the future. When a child's life ends early, whether abruptly, such as the result of an accident, or after a prolonged illness, we ask ourselves, "Why? What's the justice of this?"

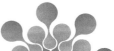

Caring for a family facing the death of their child calls on all your personal and professional skills as a nurse. It means offering sensitive, gentle, and physical care and comfort measures for the child and continuing emotional support for the child, the family caregivers, and the siblings. This kind of caring demands an understanding of your own feelings about death and dying, knowledge of the grieving process that clients and their families experience during a terminal illness or when facing an unexpected death, and a willingness to become involved.

Like chronic conditions, terminal illness creates a family crisis that can either destroy or strengthen the family as a unit and as individuals. Nurses and other health professionals who can offer knowledgeable, sensitive care to these families help make the remainder of the child's life more meaningful and the family's mourning experience more healing. Helping a family struggle through this crisis and emerge stronger and closer can yield deep satisfaction.

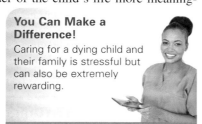

You Can Make a Difference!

Caring for a dying child and their family is stressful but can also be extremely rewarding.

THE NURSE'S REACTION TO DEATH AND DYING

Healthcare workers are often uncomfortable with dying clients, so they avoid them and are afraid that the clients will ask questions they cannot or should not answer. These caregivers signal by their behavior that the client should avoid the fact of their impending death and should keep up a show of bravery. In effect, they are asking the client to meet their needs, instead of trying to meet the client's needs.

 A Personal Glimpse

I am a student nurse. I am dying. I write this to you who are and will become nurses in the hope that by sharing my feelings with you, you may someday be better able to help those who share my experience... You slip in and out of my room, give me medications, and check my blood pressure. Is it because I am a student nurse myself, or just a human being, that I sense your fright? And your fears enhance mine. Why are you afraid? I am the one who is dying!

I know you feel insecure, don't know what to say, don't know what to do. But please believe me, if you care, you can't go wrong. Just admit that you care.... Don't run away— wait—all I want to know is that there will be someone to hold my hand when I need it.... If only we could be honest, both admit our fears, touch one another. If you really care, would you lose so much of your valuable professionalism if you even cried with me? Just person to person? Then it might not be so hard to die in a hospital—with friends close by.

(American Journal of Nursing, 1970)

Learning Opportunity: *Describe your feelings about the student nurse's story. How might this person's experience influence your approach to caring for the dying client?*

Death reminds us of our own mortality, a thought with which many of us are uncomfortable. The thought that someone even younger than us is about to die makes us feel more vulnerable.

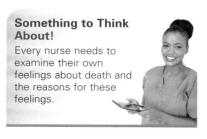

Something to Think About!

Every nurse needs to examine their own feelings about death and the reasons for these feelings.

How have you reacted to the death of a friend or a family member? When growing up, was talking and thinking about death avoided because of your family's attitudes? Admitting that death is a part of life and that clients should be helped to live each day to the fullest until death are steps toward understanding and being able to communicate with those who are dying. Attending a workshop, conference, or seminar in which you can explore your own feelings about life and death is useful in preparing you to provide nursing care for the dying child and family (Box 34-1).

Learning to care for the dying client requires talking with other professionals, sharing concerns, and comforting each other in stressful times. It calls for reading studies about death to discover how dying clients feel about their care, their illness, and their families and how they want to spend the rest of their lives. It also requires being a sensitive, empathic, nonjudgmental listener to clients and families who need to express their feelings, even if they may not be able to express them to each other. Caring for the dying is usually a team effort that may involve a nurse, a health care provider, a religious leader, a social worker, a psychiatrist, a hospice nurse, or a **thanatologist** (a person, sometimes a nurse, trained especially to work with the dying and their families), but the nurse is often the person who coordinates the care.

THE CHILD'S UNDERSTANDING OF DEATH

Stage of development, cognitive ability, and experiences all influence children's understanding of death. The child's first experience with death may be the death of a pet or a family member. How the family deals with the experience has a great impact on the child's understanding of death, but children usually do not have a realistic comprehension of the finality of death until they near preadolescence. Although the dying child may be unable to understand death, the emotions of family caregivers and others alert the child that something is threatening their secure world. Dealing with the child's anxieties with openness and honesty restores the child's trust and comfort.

Developmental Stage
Infants and Toddlers
Infants and toddlers have little if any understanding of death. The toddler may fear separation from beloved family caregivers but have no recognition of the fact that death is nearing and irreversible. A toddler may say,

The following questions can be used in a group with a hospice or other facilitator. They can be used to help heighten your awareness of yourself: Who are you? How you have gotten to where you are today? What you are doing with your life and why? How you would change the way you live? What are your feelings about death in general in relation to your friends and family and in regard to your own death?

Some Considerations in the Resolution of Death and Dying

- What was your first conscious memory of death? What were your feelings and reactions?
- What is your most recent memory of death? How was it the same or different from your first memory?
- What experience of death had the most effect on you? Why?

Get Comfortable and Imagine Now

- You have just been told you have 6 months to live. What is your first reaction to that news?
- *Three months later:* What relationships might require you to tie up loose ends? What unfinished business do you have to deal with? You and your significant other are trying to cope with the news, what changes occur in your relationship?
- *One month remains:* What do you need to have happen in the remaining time? What hopes, dreams, and plans can or need to be fulfilled?
- *One week remains:* You are very weak and barely have enough energy to talk. You don't even want to look at yourself. Nausea and vomiting are constant companions. Write a letter to the one person you feel would be the most affected by your dying.
- *Twenty-four hours remain:* You are dying. Breathing is difficult, you feel very hot inside, and overwhelming fatigue is ever present. How would you like to spend this last day?

"Gramma's gone bye-bye to be with God" or "Grampy went to heaven" and a few moments later ask to go visit the deceased person. This is an opportunity to explain to the child that Gramma or Grampy is in a special place and cannot be visited, but the family has many memories of them that they will always treasure. The child should not be scolded for not understanding. Questions are best answered simply and honestly.

If the infant's or toddler's own death is approaching, family caregivers can be encouraged to stay with the child to provide comfort, love, and security. Maintaining routines as much as possible helps give the toddler a greater sense of security.

Preschool Children

The egocentric thinking of preschool children contributes to the belief that they may have caused a person or pet to die by thinking angry thoughts. Magical thinking also plays an important part in the preschool-aged child's beliefs about death. It is not unusual for a preschool child to insist on burying a dead pet or bird, then in a few hours or a day or two dig up the corpse to see if it is still there. This may be especially true if the child has been told that it will "go to heaven." Many preschool-aged children think of death as a kind of sleep; they do not understand that the dead person will not wake up. They may fear going to sleep after the death of a close family member because they fear that they may not wake up. Family caregivers must watch for this kind of reaction and encourage children to talk about their fears while reassuring them that they need not fear dying while sleeping. The child's feelings must be acknowledged as real, and the child must be helped to resolve them. The feelings must never be ridiculed.

A preschool child may view personal illness as punishment for thoughts or actions. Because preschool-aged children do not have an accurate concept of death, they fear separation from family caregivers. Caregivers can provide security and comfort by staying with the child as much as possible.

TEST YOURSELF

✔ Why is it important for the nurse to examine their own feelings about death?

✔ What does the toddler fear in relationship to death and dying?

✔ How does magical thinking in preschool children relate to their understanding of death?

School-Aged Children

The child who is 6 or 7 years old is still in the magical-thinking stage and continues to think of death in the same way as the preschool child does. At about 8 or 9 years of age, children gain the concept that death is universal and irreversible. Around this age, death is personified—that is, it is given characteristics of a person and may be called the devil, God, a monster, or the bogeyman. Children of this age often believe they can protect themselves from death by running past a cemetery while holding their breath, keeping doors locked, staying out of dark rooms, staying away from funeral homes and dead people, or avoiding stepping on cracks in the sidewalk.

When faced with the prospect of their own deaths, school-aged children are usually sad that they will be leaving their family and the people they love (Fig. 34-1). They may be apprehensive about how they will manage when they no longer have their parents around to help them. They often view death as another new experience, like going to school, leaving for camp, or flying in an airplane for the first time. They may fear the loss of control that death represents to them and express this fear through vocal aggression. Family caregivers and nurses must recognize this as an expression of fear and avoid scolding or disciplining them for this behavior. This is

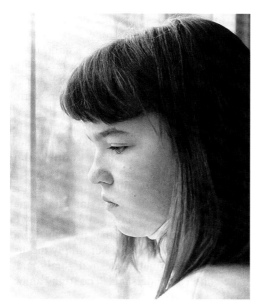

FIGURE 34-1 School-aged children are often sad when faced with their own death and leaving their family.

a time when the people close to the child can help them voice anxieties about the future and provide an outlet for these aggressive feelings. The presence of family members and maintenance of relatively normal routines help give the child a sense of security. Tips for Reinforcing Family Teaching: Talking to Children About Death provides help for caregivers in talking with their children about death.

Adolescents

Adolescents have an adult understanding of death but feel that they are immortal—that is, death will happen to others but not to them. This belief contributes to adolescent behavior that is sometimes dangerous or life-threatening. This denial may also contribute to an adolescent's delay in reporting symptoms or seeking help.

Diagnosis of a life-threatening or terminal illness creates a crisis for the adolescent. To cope with the illness, the adolescent must draw on cognitive functioning, past experiences, family support, and problem-solving ability.

The adolescent with a terminal illness may express helplessness, anger, fear of pain, hopelessness, and depression. Adolescents often try to live the fullest lives they can in the time they have.

Adolescents may be upset by the results of treatments that make them feel weak and alter their appearance such as alopecia, edema resulting from steroid therapy, and pallor. They may need assistance in presenting themselves as attractively as possible to their peers. Adolescents need opportunities to acknowledge their impending death and can be encouraged to express fears and anxieties and ask questions about death. Participating in their usual activities helps adolescents feel in control.

> **This is Important to Remember!**
>
> A child's understanding of death and dying is affected by the child's stage of growth and development, so it is important for you to be aware of what the child may understand and think.

> **TEST YOURSELF**
>
> ✔ At what age does the child understand the concept that death is universal and irreversible?
>
> ✔ What belief do adolescents have regarding dying that allows them to sometimes participate in dangerous, life-threatening behaviors?

Experience With Death and Loss

Every death that touches the life of a child makes an impression that affects the way the child thinks about every other death, including their own. Attitudes of family members are powerful influences. Family caregivers must be able to discuss death with children when a grandparent or other family member dies, even though the discussion may be painful. Otherwise, the child thinks that death is a forbidden topic; avoiding the subject leaves room for fantasy and distortion in the child's imagination.

Many books are available to help a child deal with loss and death. Reading a story to a child provides the adult with

---

TIPS FOR REINFORCING FAMILY TEACHING

Talking to Children About Death

- Encourage children to talk about the topic of death.
- Talk about the subject when the child wants to talk.
- Share information at the child's level of understanding.
- Listen to what the child is saying and asking.
- Accept the child's feelings.
- Be open and honest, and give simple, brief answers, especially when talking with the younger child.

- Answer the question each time the child asks; sometimes children need to ask the same question more than once.
- Say "I don't know" to questions you don't have answers for.
- Use the words "death," "died," and "dying."
- Talk about death when less emotion is involved, such as dead flowers, trees, insects, and birds.
- Explain death in terms of the absence of things that occur in everyday life, such as when people die they don't breathe, eat, talk, think, or feel.

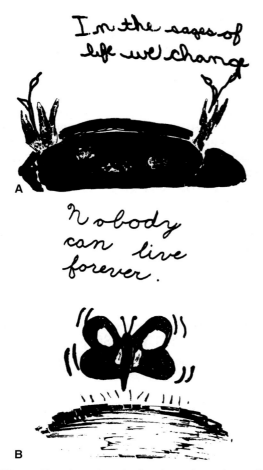

FIGURE 34-2 Drawings done by fourth-grade students after a presentation about death that included a reading of *Water Bugs and Dragonflies*. **A.** In the s[t]ages of life, we change. At the center of the drawing is a pond with three lily pads. The stems at the end represent plants that water bugs crawl up on before turning into dragonflies. **B.** Nobody lives forever. (Courtesy of Ruth Anne Sieber.)

the perfect opening to discuss loss. A small booklet that is excellent to use with any age group is *Water Bugs and Dragonflies*. This story approaches life and death as stages of existence by illustrating that after a water bug turns into a dragonfly, he can no longer go back and tell the other curious water bugs what life is like in this beautiful new world to which he has gone. This story can serve as the foundation for further discussion about death (Fig. 34-2).

Available books on death vary in their approaches. A number of books focus on the death of an animal or a pet. Many stories deal with death as a result of old age. Several books have an accident as the cause of death. Most of the books are fiction, but several nonfiction books are available for older children (Table 34-1). There is no discussion of one's own death in these books, which is consistent with the Western philosophy of handling death as something that happens to others but not to oneself.

Awareness of Impending Death

Children know when they are dying. They sense and fear what is going to happen, even if they cannot identify it by name. Their play activities, artwork, dreams, and symbolic language demonstrate this knowledge.

Family caregivers who insist that a child not learn the truth about their illness place healthcare professionals at a disadvantage because they are not free to help the child deal with fears and concerns. If family caregivers permit openness and honesty in communication with a dying child, the healthcare staff can meet the child's needs more effectively, dispel misunderstandings, and see that the child and the family are able to resolve any problems or **unfinished business**. Completing unfinished business may mean spending more time with the child, helping siblings understand the child's illness and impending death, and giving family members a chance to share their love with the child. Allowing openness does not mean that nurses and other personnel offer information not requested by the child but simply means that the child be given the information desired gently and directly in words the child can understand. The truth can be kind as well as cruel.

 Cultural Snapshot

Death and dying are not discussed openly in many cultures. In some cultures, the fact that a person is dying is discussed only in very private settings and often not with the dying individual. In front of the dying child for instance, the atmosphere might be jovial, with eating, joking, playing games, and singing.

Adolescents are usually sensitive to what is happening to them and may need you to be an advocate for them if they have wishes they want to fulfill before dying. An adolescent who senses your willingness and ability may discuss feelings that they are uncomfortable discussing with family members. You can talk with the adolescent and work with the family to help them understand the adolescent's desires and needs. You can call on hospice workers, social or psychiatric services, or a member of the clergy to help the family express and resolve their concerns and recognize the adolescent's needs.

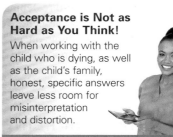

Acceptance is Not as Hard as You Think!

When working with the child who is dying, as well as the child's family, honest, specific answers leave less room for misinterpretation and distortion.

THE FAMILY'S REACTION TO DYING AND DEATH

The death of a child sends feelings of shock, disbelief, and guilt through every family member. Family members typically go through the stages of the grieving process: denial and isolation, anger, bargaining, depression and acute grief, and finally acceptance. Not every child or family will complete the process because each family, as well as each death, is personal and unique.

TABLE 34-1 Books About Death for Children

AUTHOR	BOOK	PUBLISHER	WHO DIES	AGE APPROPRIATE
Blume, J.	*Tiger Eyes*	Scarsdale, NY: Bradbury Press	Father	11–15
Bunting, E.	*The Happy Funeral*	New York, NY: Harper & Row	Grandfather	3–7
Buscaglia, L.	*The Fall of Freddie the Leaf*	San Francisco, CA SLACK, Inc.		All ages
Carrick, C.	*The Accident*	New York, NY: Houghton Mifflin, Clarion Books	Dog	6–11
Claudy, A. F.	*Dusty Was My Friend*	New York, NY: Human Sciences Press	Friend	6–11
dePaola, T.	*Nana Upstairs & Nana Downstairs*	New York, NY: G.P. Putnam's Sons	Grandmother	4–9
Edleman, H.	*Motherless Daughters*	New York, NY: Dell Publishing Company	Mother	14 and up
Geithner, C.	*If Only*	New York, NY: Scholastic Press	Mother	10–15
Graeber, C.	*Mustard*	New York, NY: MacMillan Publishing Co.	Cat	6–10
Hemery, K.	*The Brightest Star*	Omaha, NE: Centering Corporation	Mother	4–8
Henkes, K.	*Sun & Spoon*	New York, NY: Greenwillow Books	Grandmother	9–13
Hermes, P.	*You Shouldn't Have to Say Goodbye*	New York, NY: Harcourt Brace Jovanovich	Mother	9–13
Hesse, K.	*Poppy's Chair*	New York, NY: MacMillan Publishing Co.	Grandfather	6–11
Hickman, M. W.	*Last Week My Brother Anthony Died*	Nashville, TN: Abington Press	Brother	3–7
Holmes, M. and Mudlaff, S.	*Molly's Mom Died*	Omaha, NE: Centering Corporation	Mother	5–9
Karst, P.	*The Invisible String*	Camarillo, CA: Devorss & Co.		3 and up
Lorenzen, K.	*Lanky Longlegs*	New York, NY: Atheneum. A Margaret K. McElderry Book	Brother	9–13
Mellonie, B.	*Lifetimes: The Beautiful Way to Explain Death to Children*	New York, NY: Bantam Books	Plants Animals People	All ages
Schotter, R.	*A Matter of Time*	New York, NY: Collins Press	Mother	14 and up
Schwiebert, P.	*Tear Soup*	Portland, OR: Grief Watch		8 and up
Scrivani, M.	*I Heard Your Mommy Died*	Omaha, NE: Centering Corporation	Mother	3–7
Scrivani, M.	*I Heard Your Daddy Died*	Omaha, NE: Centering Corporation	Father	3–7
Scrivani, M.	*When Death Walks In: For Teens Facing Grief*	Omaha, NE: Centering Corporation		13 and up
Shook-Hazen, B.	*Why Did Grandpa Die?*	Racine, WI: Western Publishing Co.	Grandfather	3–7
Smith, D. B.	*A Taste of Blackberries*	Boston, MA: Thomas Crowell Company	Friend	6–11
Thomas, J. R.	*Saying Goodbye to Grandma*	New York, NY: Clarion Books	Grandmother	6–11
Thomas, P.	*I Miss You*	Hayppauge, NY: Barron's Educational Series		4 and up
Tiffault, B.	*A Quilt for Elizabeth*	Omaha, NE: Centering Corporation	Father	4–8
Vigna, J.	*Saying Goodbye to Daddy*	Morton Grove, IL: Albert Whitman & Co.	Father	6–9
Viorst, J.	*The Tenth Good Thing About Barney*	New York, NY: Simon and Schuster	Cat	6–9

When death is expected, as in a terminal illness, the family begins to mourn in anticipation of the death, a phenomenon called **anticipatory grief**. For some people, this shortens the period of acute grief and loss after the child's death. Anticipatory grief begins when a potentially fatal disease (such as acquired immunodeficiency syndrome, leukemia, or other cancer) is diagnosed and continues until remission or death. When the disease rapidly advances, anticipatory grief may be short-lived as the child's death nears. In cases of accidental or sudden death, the family has no time to anticipate or begin grieving the loss of the child. Their grief may last longer and be more difficult to resolve.

Grief for the death of a child is not limited in time but may continue for years. Sometimes professional counseling is necessary to help family members work through grief. The support of others who have experienced the same sort of loss can be helpful. Two national organizations founded to offer support are the American Childhood Cancer Organization and The Compassionate Friends (see Internet Resources). These organizations have many local chapters.

Family Caregiver Reactions

Family caregivers may grieve the death of a child that follows a terminal illness or that is sudden and unexpected.

Terminal Illness

The family caregivers of children in the final stages of a terminal illness may have had to cope with many hospital admissions between periods at home. During this time, the family may face decisions about the child's physical care, as well as learning to live with a dying child. As the child's condition deteriorates, you can encourage the family to talk to their child about dying. This is a task they may find very difficult. Support from a religious counselor, hospice nurse, or social service or psychiatric worker can help them through this difficult task. Family caregivers can be encouraged to provide as much normalcy as possible in the child's schedule. School attendance and special trips can be encouraged within the child's capabilities and desires.

During this time, family caregivers may go through a grieving process of anger, depression, ambivalence, and bargaining over and over again. The caregivers may direct anger at the hospital staff, themselves (because of guilt), each other, or the child. Reassure the caregivers that these are normal reactions, but avoid taking sides.

If the child improves enough to go home again, parents may find themselves overprotecting the child. As in chronic conditions, this overprotective attitude reinforces the child's sick behavior and dependency and is usually accompanied by a lack of discipline. Failure to set limits accentuates the child's feelings of being different and creates problems with siblings. The child learns to manipulate family members, only to find that this kind of behavior does not bring positive results when attempted with peers or healthcare personnel.

When the child has to return to the hospital because of increasing symptoms, family caregivers may once again

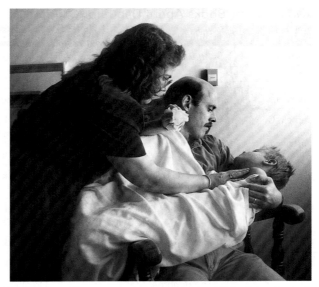

FIGURE 34-3 The parents hold the dying child, giving both the child and parents comfort.

experience all stages of the grieving process. The family members dread the child's approaching death and fear that the child will be in great pain or may die when they are not present. You can help relieve these fears by keeping the family informed about the child's condition, making the child as comfortable as possible, and reassuring the family members that they will be summoned if death appears to be near.

When death comes, it is perfectly appropriate to share the family's grief, crying with them, then giving them privacy to express their sorrow. You can stay with the family for a while, remaining quietly supportive with an attitude of a comforting listener. An appropriate comment may be, "I am so sorry" or "This is a very sad time." Keep the focus on the family's grief and what you can do to support them.

The family may want to hold the child to say a final goodbye, and you can encourage and assist them in this. Intravenous lines and other equipment can be removed to make holding the child easier. The family may be left alone during this time if they desire. Be sensitive to the family's needs and desires to provide them with comfort (Fig. 34-3).

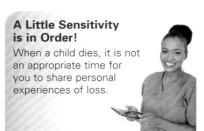

A Little Sensitivity is in Order!

When a child dies, it is not an appropriate time for you to share personal experiences of loss.

TEST YOURSELF

✔ What does the term *anticipatory grief* mean?

✔ How is anticipatory grief helpful to the family who has lost a child by death?

✔ Why is it important for family caregivers to refrain from being overprotective with the dying child?

Sudden or Unexpected Death

When a child dies suddenly and unexpectedly, the family is not able to prepare for the death as they could with a terminal illness. They do not have the opportunity to complete unfinished business or go through anticipatory grief. Such a family may have excessive guilt and remorse for something they felt they left unsaid or undone. Even if a child has had a traumatic death with disfigurement, the family must be given the opportunity to be with, see, and hold the child to help with closure of the child's life. You can prepare the family for seeing the child, explaining why parts of the body may be covered. Viewing the child, even if the body is severely mutilated, helps the family have a realistic view of the child and aids in the grief process.

The family may face a number of decisions that must be made rather quickly, especially when the child's death is unexpected. Families of terminally ill children have usually made some plans for the child's death and may know exactly what they want done. However, when the child dies unexpectedly, decisions may be necessary concerning organ donation, funeral arrangements, and an autopsy. If the death has been the result of violence or is unexplained, law requires an autopsy, but there may be other reasons that an autopsy is desired. An autopsy might be helpful in finding causes and treatments for other children diagnosed with the same disease, especially if it is a diagnosis about which little research is available. Organ donation can be discussed with the family by the hospital's organ donor coordinator or other designated person. The family needs to be well informed and must be supported throughout these difficult decisions.

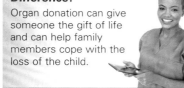

This Could Make a Difference!

Organ donation can give someone the gift of life and can help family members cope with the loss of the child.

A Personal Glimpse

As I sit here each morning after losing my little girl, I know I'll make it through another day. I know this because I told her every day how happy I was that she was my child. As she was developing into a young woman, I never forgot to say how gorgeous she looked. I also know in my heart I can sleep each night hereafter, because from the day I gave birth to her I told her to always come back to me. Don't get me wrong! I always worried endlessly, but I felt it was important for her not to know these fears. As parents, we hope our kids will always do the right thing. I wanted my children, and still do Michael, to know that whatever they did or do I would stand behind them, beside them, and always in my heart near them. I spent every waking day with Nicole and Michael as they were growing. I enjoyed all their developmental years. I reveled in their games, ideas, and thoughts. I know now that I was growing vicariously through them. Not a day went by that I didn't want them with me. Maybe because of this I was not as good a wife as I should have been, but I can sleep at night knowing that I was and am a great mother to my children.

You are all saying how strong I am. This is not strength. This is the power of knowing I tried through it all to be supportive and share with them what little knowledge I had. I understood that these little bodies were given to me to mold and build into productive, loving, caring human beings, and with that, I held the future so that my grandchildren would be better people. Nicole would have definitely gone on to bigger and better things. I know her part in society would have made a difference. Her impact on the future would have changed things for the better. Cry? I really can't cry, for I know my Nikki will never leave me. I'll always see her smile. I'll always remember her voice. I'll always remember all the little things she needed to cultivate to become the adult that she would have become.

Sunday night the skies were in such turmoil. I found deep solace in that for I knew that they were letting her in. She was probably fighting with others and found her way to the front of the line. I know in my heart that once she got there she began checking the situation carefully and assessing what needed to be done and the tasks that she wanted to take on to make a difference up there. How do I know this? The skies were rumbling, the lightning was crashing, and then a heavy downpour began. I knew the angels were crying—so happy and confused as to why someone with so much to give on Earth would be up in Heaven so early. This went on for a good 10 min. It was pouring like crazy and then in my Nikki's infinite wisdom she spoke to them, explained the stupidity of that night, and everyone settled down. I also found great comfort, for at this time, the sun, which hadn't appeared all day, broke through the clouds and shined on me. I was sitting where she knows I always sit when I need quiet time, and through an opening in these clouds, she spoke directly to me and said, "Ma, I'm here. It's OK. I tried to get home. I would have told you some of the things of how my night was. But, Ma, I screwed up, and I'll be waiting here for all of you!" This, my friend, is what has given me comfort. To love has many different meanings, but I am by far a better person for having her in memories with me always. Thanks Nikki. I will always love you.

Marie (after losing her 16-year-old daughter Nicole in a car accident)

Learning Opportunity: What are some of the experiences this mother shared that gave her strength in dealing with her daughter's death? What are your feelings about the death of a child or an adolescent?

The Child's Reaction

The child who has a terminal illness also experiences anticipatory grief. Even young children are aware of the seriousness of their illness because of the actions and emotions of the people around them. The child realizes that they are going to die and that there is no cure for them. Sadness and depression are common. The child may have fears about dying as well as concerns for the family members who will be left behind. It is important for the child to have the opportunity to talk about fears, anger, and concerns, as well as to be able to express feelings about the joys and happiness in their life. When the child is ready to talk about these things, encourage them to do so. The child needs support, honesty, and answers to questions regarding the illness, treatment, and prognosis. Children should be encouraged to express their feelings through crying, playing, acting out, or drawing. The child may fear that pain is a part of death and should be reassured that medications can be used to control pain and keep the child comfortable. Religious and spiritual beliefs can help the child deal with feelings regarding separation from family. Reassure the child that they will not be alone at the time of death.

The dying child may have a decreased level of consciousness, although hearing remains intact. Family members at the bedside and healthcare personnel may need to be reminded to avoid saying anything that would not be said if the child were fully conscious. Gentle touching and caressing may provide comfort to the child.

Excellent nursing care is required. Medications for pain are given intravenously because they are poorly absorbed from muscle caused by poor circulation. Keep mucous membranes clean, and apply petroleum jelly (Vaseline) to the lips to prevent drying and cracking. Moisten the conjunctiva of the eyes with normal saline eye drops, such as artificial tears, if drying occurs. Keep the skin clean and dry, and turn and position the child regularly to provide comfort and to prevent skin breakdown. While caring for the child, talk to them and explain everything that is being done.

As death approaches, the internal body temperature increases; thus, dying clients seem to be unaware of cold even though their skin feels cool. Explain this to family members so they do not think the child needs additional covering. Just before death, the child who has remained conscious may become restless, followed by a time of peace and calm. Be aware of these reactions, and know that death is near; keep family members informed as well.

TEST YOURSELF

✔ What feelings might the family of a child who dies suddenly and unexpectedly have?

✔ For what reason should caregivers and families never say anything in the presence of a comatose child that they would not say if the child were alert?

Sibling Reactions

The siblings of a child who is dying of a terminal illness have an opportunity to themselves go through a period of anticipatory grieving. If a sibling dies suddenly, the sibling begins the process of grief at the time of the death. Siblings may feel confused, lonely, and frightened about the sudden loss of their brother or sister. The unexpected change in the atmosphere of the household can be upsetting.

Just as in the case of chronic conditions, siblings resent the attention given to the ill child and are angry about the disruption in the family. Reaction varies according to the sibling's developmental age and parental attitudes and actions. Younger children find it almost impossible to understand what is happening; it is difficult even for older children to grasp. Reaction to the illness and its accompanying stresses can cause classroom problems for school-aged siblings; these may be incorrectly labeled as learning disabilities or behavioral disorders unless school personnel are aware of the family situation.

When the child dies, young siblings who are still prone to magical thinking may feel guilty, particularly if a strong degree of rivalry existed before the illness. These children need continued reassurance that they did not cause or help cause the sibling's death.

The decision of whether or not a sibling should attend funeral services for the child may be difficult. Although there has been little research, the current thinking among many health professionals supports the presence of the sibling. The sibling may be encouraged to leave a token of love and goodbye with the child—a drawing, note, toy, or another special memento. Siblings can visit the dead child in privacy with few other mourners present. Dealing with the realities of the brother's or sister's death openly is likely to be more beneficial than avoiding the issue and allowing the sibling to use their imagination about death (Box 34-2).

Remember **Lee Anderson** and his family from the beginning of the chapter. What would you anticipate would be the reactions of Lee's parents, his brother, and his sister when they are told that Lee has little time left to live? What would you anticipate about Lee's response to this news?

SETTINGS FOR CARE OF THE DYING CHILD

Where the child dies can greatly influence the family's response to and acceptance of a child's death. In a hospital, the child may receive the most professional care and the most technologically advanced treatment. However, having a child in the hospital can contribute to family separation, a feeling of loss of control, and a sense of isolation. An increasing number of families are choosing to keep the child at home to die.

Hospice Care

In medieval times, a **hospice** was a refuge for various travelers—not only those traveling through the countryside, but also the terminally ill who were leaving this life for another. Hospices often were operated by religious orders and became havens for the dying. The current hospice movement in healthcare began in England, when Dr. Cicely Saunders founded St. Christopher's Hospice in London in 1967. This institution has become the model for others in the United States and Canada, with an emphasis on sensitive, humane care for the dying. Hospice principles of care include relief of pain, attention to the needs of the total person, and absence of heroic life-saving measures.

The first hospice in the United States was the New Haven Hospice in Connecticut. Many communities now have hospice programs that may or may not be affiliated

BOX 34-2 Guidelines for Helping the Children Cope With Death

Do
- Know your own beliefs
- Begin where the child is
- Be there
- Confront reality
- Encourage expression of feelings
- Be truthful
- Include the child in family rituals
- Encourage remembrance
- Admit when you don't know the answer
- Use touch to communicate
- Start death education early and simply, using naturally occurring events
- Recognize symptoms of grief, and deal with the grief
- Accept differing reactions to death

Don't
- Praise stoicism (detached, unemotional behavior)
- Use euphemisms (mild expressions substituted for the ones that might be offensive)
- Be nonchalant
- Glamorize death
- Tell fairy tales or half-truths
- Close the door to questions
- Be judgmental of feelings and behaviors
- Protect the child from exposure to experiences with death
- Encourage forgetting the deceased
- Encourage the child to be like the deceased

with a hospital. Some programs offer a hospice setting to which clients go in terminal stages of illness; others provide support and guidance for the client and family whereas the client remains in the hospital or is cared for at home. Most of these hospice programs are established primarily for adults, but some programs also accept children as clients.

Children's Hospice International, founded in 1983, is an organization dedicated to hospice support of children. Through an individualized plan of care, Children's Hospice addresses the physical, developmental, psychological, social, and spiritual needs of children and families in a comprehensive and consistent way. It serves as a resource and advocacy center, providing education for family caregivers and professionals. The organization conducts seminars and conferences and publishes training manuals. Its website (www.chionline.org) provides information for adults, as well as games, books, and an excellent list of websites for children.

Home Care

Caring for the young or old dying client at home has become increasingly common in recent years. More families are choosing to keep the child at home during the terminal stage of illness. Factors that contribute to the decision to care for a child at home include the following:

- Concerns about costs for hospitalization and nonmedical expenses such as the family's travel, housing, and food

- Stress from repeated family separations
- Loss of control over the care of the child and the family life

Families feel that the more loving, caring environment of the home draws the family closer and helps reduce the guilt that is often a part of bereavement. All family members can be involved to some extent in the child's care and in this way gain a feeling of usefulness. Family caregivers feel that they remain in control.

There are disadvantages of home care, however. Costs that would have been covered by health insurance if the child was hospitalized may not be covered if the child is cared for at home. Caring for a dying child can be extremely difficult emotionally and physically. Not every family has someone who can carry out the procedures that may need to be performed regularly. In some instances, home nursing assistance is available, but this varies from community to community. Usually the home care nurse visits several days a week and may be on call the rest of the time. In some communities, hospice nurses may provide the teaching and support that families need.

Deciding whether or not to care for a dying child at home is an extremely difficult decision for a family. Family members need support and guidance from healthcare personnel when they are trying to make the decision, after the decision is made, and even after the child dies.

Hospital Care

Dying in a hospital has both limitations and advantages. The child and the family may find support from others in the same situation. Family members may not have the physical or emotional strength to cope with total care of the child at home, but they can participate in care supported by the hospital staff (Fig. 34-4).

Hospital care is much more expensive, but this may not be important to some families, especially those with health insurance. The hospital is still the culturally accepted place to die, and this is important to some people. Clients and families who choose hospital care need to know that they have rights and can exert some control over what happens to them.

TEST YOURSELF
✔ What are the principles of hospice care for the dying child?
✔ What factors contribute to the decision to care for a dying child at home?
✔ What might be helpful for the family of a dying child if the child is hospitalized?

THE ROLE OF THE NURSE

As the nurse, you play an important role in providing both physical care for the child who is dying and emotional care for both the child and family. Provide information

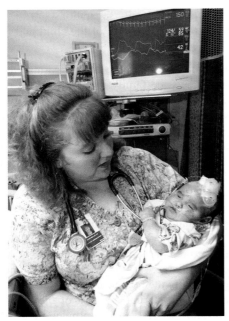

FIGURE 34-4 The nurse helps support the dying child in the hospital setting.

as clearly and simply as possible. Open, honest communication is important. Encourage the child and family to share their feelings and reactions to the situation and to ask questions. Support by listening and providing appropriate interventions.

Nursing Process and Care Plan *for the Dying Child*

Assessment (Data Collection)

The assessment of the terminally ill child and family is an ongoing process over a period of time by the healthcare team. The healthcare team's assessment covers the child's developmental level, the influence of cultural and spiritual concerns, the family's support system, present indications of grieving (e.g., anticipatory grief), interactions among family members, and unfinished business. To understand the child's view of death, consider the child's previous experiences, developmental level, and cognitive ability.

Nursing Care Focus

Nursing care focuses for the dying child include those appropriate for the child's illness and managing the child's pain. Other nursing care focuses are specific to the dying process, such as social isolation and anxiety. In caring for the family coping skills and the powerlessness the family experiences are important.

Outcome Identification and Planning

Goals and plans of care depend on the stage of the illness, the child's and the family's acceptance of the illness, and their attitudes and beliefs about death and dying. Major goals for the child include minimizing pain, diminishing feelings of abandonment by peers and friends, and relieving anxiety about the future. Goals for the family include helping cope with the impending death and identifying feelings of powerlessness.

Nursing Care Focus

- Acute pain related to illness and weakened condition

Goal

- The child will have minimal pain.

Implementations for Relieving Pain and Discomfort

The child may be in pain for many reasons such as chemotherapy; nausea, vomiting, and gastrointestinal cramping; pressure caused by positioning; or constipation. Until the child is comfortable and relatively pain-free, all other nursing interventions are fruitless; pain becomes the child's primary focus until relief is provided. Nursing measures to relieve pain may include positioning, using pillows as needed; changing linens; providing conscientious skin and mouth care; protecting skin surfaces from rubbing together; offering back rubs and massages; and administering antiemetics, analgesics, and stool softeners as appropriate. Some measures may relieve pain in one situation but not in another, so a variety of measures may be needed to relieve the child's pain.

Evaluation of Goal/Desired Outcome

The child:

- has uninterrupted periods of quiet rest.
- indicates minimal or no pain, or relief from pain when using a pain scale.

Nursing Care Focus

- Psychosocial needs related to isolation and terminal illness

Goal

- The child will have social interaction with others.

Interventions for Providing Appropriate Social Interactions

Encourage the child's siblings and friends to maintain contact. Provide opportunities for peers to visit, write, or telephone, as the child is able. Read to the child, and engage in other activities that they find interesting and physically tolerable. When possible, encourage the child to make decisions to foster a feeling of control. Explain all procedures and how they will affect the child. Provide the child with privacy, but do not neglect them. Provide ample periods of rest. Continue to talk to and tell the child what you are doing, even though the child may seem unresponsive. Hearing is often the last sense to shut down, the child will feel reassured by your voice and presence.

Evaluation of Goal/Desired Outcome

● Within physical capabilities, the child engages in activities with peers, family, and others.

Nursing Care Focus

● Death anxiety related to condition and prognosis

Goal

● The child will express feelings of anxiety and use available supports to cope with anxiety.

Implementations for Easing the Child's Anxiety

Ask family caregivers about the child's understanding of death and previous experiences with death. Observe how the child exhibits fear, and ask family caregivers for any additional information. Encourage the child to use a doll, a pillow, or another special "warm fuzzy" for comfort. Use words such as "dead" or "dying," if appropriate, in conversation because this may give the child an opening to talk about death. Nighttime is especially frightening for children because they often think they will die at night. Provide company and comfort, and be alert for periods of wakefulness when the child may need someone with whom to talk. A night light provides a sense of security. Be honest and straightforward, and avoid injecting your beliefs into the conversation. If appropriate, read a book about death to the child to initiate conversation (although ideally this would have been done much earlier in the child's care).

Evaluation of Goal/Desired Outcome

● The child keeps a "warm fuzzy" close by for comfort and talks about death to the nurse or the family.
● When awake at night, the child is comforted by the presence of someone with whom to talk.

Nursing Care Focus

● Family coping impairment related to approaching death.

Goal

● The family members will develop ways to cope with the child's approaching death.

Implementations for Helping the Family Cope

Family caregivers may need encouragement to discuss their feelings about the child. They may feel they need to "keep up a brave front" for the child and siblings. Acknowledge emotions and fears, and reassure caregivers that their reactions are normal. The support of a member of the clergy may be helpful during this time. Help family members contact their own spiritual counselors, or offer to contact the hospital chaplain if the family desires. Encourage family caregivers to eat and rest properly so they will not become ill or exhausted

themselves. Explain the child's condition to the family, and answer any questions. Reassure the family that everything is being done to keep the child as comfortable and pain-free as possible. Interpret signs of approaching death for the family.

If appropriate, ask the family about the siblings: what they know, how much they understand, and whether the family has discussed the approaching death. Offer to help the family caregivers talk with siblings.

Evaluation of Goal/Desired Outcome

● The family members express their feelings, identify signs that indicate approaching death, and use available support systems and people.
● The siblings visit and talk about their feelings regarding the approaching death of their sister or brother.

Nursing Care Focus

● Psychosocial needs of family caregivers related to inability to control child's condition

Goal

● The family members will be involved in the child's care to decrease feelings of powerlessness.

Implementations for Helping the Family Feel Involved in the Child's Care

Respond to the family's need to feel some control over the situation by suggesting specific measures they can perform to provide comfort for the child such as positioning, moistening lips, and reading or telling a favorite story. Encourage the caregivers to talk to the child even if the child does not respond. Discourage whispered conversations in the room. Encourage and help the family carry out cultural customs if they wish. Help the family complete any unfinished business on the agenda; this may include the need for the child to go home to die. Help family contact support people such as hospice workers or social services.

Evaluation of Goal/Desired Outcome

The family members:

● provide comfort measures for the child and talk to the child.
● complete unfinished business with the child.

Lee Anderson has been placed in Hospice Care and the family is caring for Lee in their home. As Lee's nurse, what are your responsibilities for both Lee and his family? What concerns do you think the family may have during this time? What are some of the things you will encourage the family to do when caring for Lee?

KEY POINTS

- Anticipatory grief shortens the period of acute grief and loss after the child's death.

- Nurses and other healthcare workers are often uncomfortable with dying clients because they are afraid that the clients will ask questions they cannot or should not answer. In addition, death reminds us of our own mortality, a thought with which many of us are uncomfortable. It is important to examine your own feelings about death and the reasons for these feelings.

- You can personally prepare to care for dying children by exploring your own feelings about life and death. Attending a workshop, conference, or seminar in which one's own feelings about death are explored can be helpful. Talking with other professionals, sharing concerns, comforting each other in stressful times, and reading studies about death to discover how dying clients feel about the situation can also be helpful in preparing to work with dying clients.

- Factors that affect the child's understanding of death include their stage of development, cognitive ability, experiences, and how the family deals with death. Most children do not understand the finality of death until they near preadolescence.

- Infants and toddlers have little understanding of death; the toddler may fear separation but has no recognition of the fact that death is nearing and irreversible. The preschool child may believe that death happens because of angry thoughts. Magical thinking about death and thinking of death as a kind of sleep are seen in preschool-aged children until about 8 or 9 years of age. After age 9, children gain the concept that death is universal and irreversible. Adolescents have an adult understanding of death, but feel that they are immortal—that is, death will happen to others but not to them.

- When a child has a terminal illness, family caregivers go through anticipatory grieving. Families have the opportunity to complete unfinished business by spending time with the dying child, helping siblings understand the child's illness and impending death, and giving family members a chance to share their love with the child.

- When a child dies suddenly, a family may suffer excessive grief and guilt for something they felt they left unsaid or undone.

- When a sibling dies, possible reactions seen in children depend on the stage of development of that sibling. Young siblings find death impossible to understand. School-aged siblings may have classroom problems, behavioral issues, and feelings of guilt about the death of their sibling. Dealing with the realities of the brother's or sister's death openly is likely to be more beneficial than avoiding the issue.

- Settings for caring for the dying child include the home, hospice, and hospital settings. The home provides a loving, caring environment and may decrease costs and family separations. Home settings may prevent some expenses from being covered and may be difficult emotionally and physically for the family. Hospice principles of care include relief of pain, attention to the needs of the total person, and absence of heroic life-saving measures. In the hospital setting, the child and the family may find support from others in the same situation, support from the hospital staff, and technologically advanced treatment. Hospital care is much more expensive, but this may not be important to some families. The hospital is still the culturally accepted place to die, but having a child in the hospital can contribute to family separation, a feeling of loss of control, and a sense of isolation.

- Nursing care for the dying child focuses on minimizing pain, diminishing feelings of abandonment by the child's peers and friends, and relieving anxiety about the future. Care also aims to help the family find ways to cope with the impending death and to identify feelings of powerlessness.

INTERNET RESOURCES

American Childhood Cancer Organization
www.acco.org

Children's Hospice International
www.chionline.org

The Compassionate Friends
www.compassionatefriends.org

Hospice Foundation of America
www.hospicefoundation.org

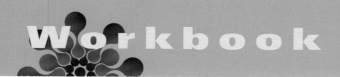

NCLEX-STYLE REVIEW QUESTIONS

1. While the nurse is working with the family of a child who is terminally ill, the child's sibling makes the following statement to the nurse. Which statement is an example of the stage of grief referred to as bargaining?
   a. "I will share my toys if he can just come to my birthday party next month."
   b. "It makes me mad that they said my brother is going to die."
   c. "I think he will get well now that he has a new medicine."
   d. "When he dies, at least he won't have any more pain."

2. When working with the family of a child who is terminally ill, the child's sibling makes the following statement to the nurse. Which statement is an example of the stage of grief referred to as denial?
   a. "I will share my toys if he can just come to my birthday party next month."
   b. "It makes me mad that they said my brother is going to die."
   c. "I think he will get well now that he has a new medicine."
   d. "When he dies, at least he won't have any more pain."

3. The nurse is working with a group of 4- and 5-year-old children who are talking about death and dying. One child in the group recently experienced the death of the family pet. Which statement would the nurse expect a 5-year-old child to say about the death of the pet?
   a. "I think he was sad to leave us."
   b. "He's only a little dead."
   c. "A monster came and took him during the night."
   d. "I will be real good so I won't die."

4. The nurse is discussing the subject of death and dying with a group of adolescents. Which statement would be expected considering the adolescent stage of growth and development?
   a. "I always hold my breath and run past the cemetery to protect myself."
   b. "It would be sad to die because my girlfriend would really miss me."
   c. "Others die in car wrecks, but even if I had a wreck, I wouldn't be killed."
   d. "It makes me nervous to go to sleep. I am afraid I won't wake up."

5. The nurse is with a family whose terminally ill child has just died. Which statement made by the nurse would be the *most* therapeutic statement?
   a. "It will not hurt as much as time passes."
   b. "My sister died when I was a teenager. I know how you feel."
   c. "I will leave the call light here. Call me if you need me."
   d. "This is a really sad and difficult time."

6. The family of a child with a terminal illness might go through a process known as anticipatory grief. Which of the following might occur for the family during this process? Select all that apply.
   a. Having an opportunity to complete unfinished business
   b. Preparing for the eventual death of the child
   c. Having no feelings of guilt or remorse
   d. Beginning the process of preparing for the funeral
   e. Helping the child's siblings deal with the coming death

STUDY ACTIVITIES

1. List and compare thoughts and ideas a child of each of the following ages would most likely have regarding death and dying.

Toddler	Preschool	School-Aged	Adolescent

2. Research your community to find the procedure for organ donation. Make arrangements for a speaker from the organization to discuss organ donation with your class. If such a person is not available, research organ donation on the internet and share your findings with your class.

3. Survey your community to see if there is a hospice available. Describe how it functions. Find out if it accepts children as clients and if there are any restrictions concerning children. Discuss your findings with your peers.

4. Do an internet search on "sibling loss." Find a site dealing with ways to help children deal with the loss of a sibling.

CRITICAL THINKING: WHAT WOULD YOU DO?

1. The Andrews family has an 8-year-old daughter with a terminal illness.
   a. What factors do you think the family needs to consider when deciding if they will care for the child at home?
   b. With what feelings do you think the family might be dealing?

2. The Andrews family decides they cannot care for the child at home.
   a. What are your feelings about this decision?
   b. What would you say to this family to support them in their decision?

UNIT 10
The Child with a Health Disorder

35

The Child With a Sensory/Neurologic Disorder

Key Terms

amblyopia
astigmatism
ataxia
aura
binocular vision
cataract
clonus
conjunctivitis
diplopia
dysarthria
esotropia
exotropia
febrile seizures
focal (partial) seizures
generalized seizures
goniotomy
hordeolum
hyperopia
lacrimation
myopia
myringotomy
nuchal rigidity
nystagmus
opisthotonos
orthoptics
papilledema
photophobia
purpuric rash
refraction
strabismus
traumatic brain injury (TBI)

Learning Objectives

At the conclusion of this chapter, you will:

1. Discuss ways an infant's and child's eyes, ears, and nervous system differ from an adult's.
2. Compare different types of vision impairment.
3. Describe eye conditions and treatment for these conditions.
4. Differentiate types of hearing impairment, and explain the difference between a child who is hard of hearing and one who is deaf.
5. Explain otitis media, including the behaviors seen in the child with acute otitis media.
6. Discuss the symptoms, diagnosis, and treatment of Reye syndrome.
7. Discuss the causes of acute or nonrecurrent seizures.
8. Discuss seizure disorders and the nursing care specific to a child at high risk for seizures.
9. Describe (a) focal onset aware seizures, (b) focal onset impaired awareness seizures, and (c) generalized onset seizures.
10. Describe (a) tonic–clonic seizures, (b) absence seizures, (c) atonic seizures, (d) myoclonic seizures, and (e) infantile spasms.
11. Explain status epilepticus and the treatment for this disorder.
12. Discuss the causes, symptoms, treatment and potential complications of meningitis.
13. Describe cerebral palsy and its causes.
14. Differentiate between types of cerebral palsy.
15. Identify the healthcare professionals involved in the care of the child with cerebral palsy.
16. List the possible causes of intellectual disability.
17. Discuss the nursing care of the child with cognitive impairment.
18. Discuss clinical manifestations seen in children with brain tumors.
19. Describe head trauma and head injuries seen in children.
20. Discuss drowning in children and the immediate care of a drowning victim.

Chesa Andres, 5 years old, comes to the clinic for her prekindergarten well-child checkup. The family caregivers report that Chesa has been diagnosed with a seizure disorder following a serious automobile accident in which Chesa had a head injury. As you read this chapter, think about Chesa's diagnosis and what might be some concerns for Chesa and her family.

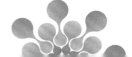

Neurologic disorders can be caused by many different factors. Nerve cells do not regenerate, and complications from these disorders can be serious and permanent. If neurologic damage has occurred, your role as the nurse is often one of support and guidance to the child and family dealing with the neurologic disorder.

Children learn about the world they live in through their senses. Any disorder related to the eyes and ears can have significant impact on the normal growth and development of the child.

GROWTH AND DEVELOPMENT OF THE EYES, EARS, AND NERVOUS SYSTEM

The Nervous System

The nervous system is the communication network of the body. The central nervous system is made up of the brain and spinal cord. The peripheral nervous system is made up of the nerves throughout the body. A fluid known as cerebrospinal fluid flows through the chambers of the brain and through the spinal cord, serving as a cushion and protective mechanism for nerve cells.

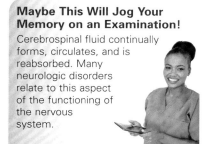

Maybe This Will Jog Your Memory on an Examination!
Cerebrospinal fluid continually forms, circulates, and is reabsorbed. Many neurologic disorders relate to this aspect of the functioning of the nervous system.

Nerves go from the brain and spinal cord to all parts of the body. These nerves quickly transmit information from the central nervous system. Stimuli of all types cause signals called nerve impulses to occur. These nerve impulses activate, coordinate, integrate, and control all of the body functions.

A part of the peripheral nervous system, the autonomic nervous system, regulates the involuntary functions of the body, such as the heart rate. At birth, the nervous system is immature. As the child grows, the quality of the nerve impulses sent through the nervous system develops and matures. As these nerve impulses become more mature, the child's gross and fine motor skills increase in complexity. The child becomes more coordinated and able to develop motor skills.

Sensory Organs

The eyes and ears are specialized organs of the nervous system. These organs transmit impulses to the central nervous system.

Eyes

The eye is a sensory organ that detects light, the stimuli, from the environment. Parts of the eye respond to the light and produce and transmit a nerve impulse to the brain. That information and image is interpreted in the brain, and thus the person "sees" the object.

Newborns do not focus clearly, but will stare at a human face directly in front of them. By 2 months of age, the infant can focus and follow an object with the eyes (Fig. 35-1). By 7 months of age, depth perception has matured enough so that the infant can transfer objects back and forth between their hands. Visual acuity of children gradually increases from birth, when the visual acuity is usually between 20/100 and 20/400 until about 5 years of age, when most children have 20/20 vision (Coats, 2021).

Ears

Ears function as the sensory organ of hearing as well as the organ responsible in part for equilibrium and balance. Sound waves, vibrations, and fluid movements create nerve impulses that the brain ultimately distinguishes as sounds.

The ear is made up of the external, middle, and inner ear. The eardrum or tympanic membrane is in the external ear. In the middle ear, the eustachian tube connects the throat with the middle ear. In infants and young children, this tube is straighter, shorter, and wider than in the older child and adult (Fig. 35-2). Initial hearing screening is done before the newborn is discharged (see Chapter 14). Hearing in children is acute, and the infant will respond to sounds within the first month of life.

VISION IMPAIRMENT

Good vision is essential to a child's normal development. How well a child sees affects their learning process, social development, coordination, and safety. One in 1,000 children of school age has serious vision impairment. The sooner these impairments are corrected, the better a child's chances are for normal or nearly normal development.

Children with vision impairments are classified as sighted with eye problems, partially sighted, or legally blind.

Types of Vision Impairment

Refractive Errors

Among sighted children with eye problems, errors of **refraction** (the way light rays bend as they pass through the lens to the retina) are the most common. About 10% of school-aged children have **myopia** (nearsightedness), which means that the child can see objects clearly at close range but not at a distance. When proper lenses are fitted, vision is corrected to normal. If uncorrected, this defect may cause a child to be labeled inattentive or intellectually disabled. Myopia tends to be seen in families; it often progresses into adolescence and then levels off.

Hyperopia (farsightedness) is a refractive condition in which the person can see objects better at a distance than close up. It is common in young children and often persists into the first grade or even later. The ocular specialist examining the child must decide whether corrective lenses are needed on an individual basis. Usually correction is not needed in a preschool-aged child. Teachers and family caregivers should be aware that considerable eye fatigue might result from efforts at accommodation for close work.

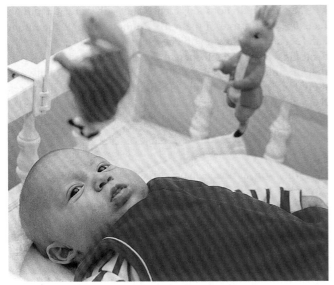

FIGURE 35-1 A 2-month-old focusing on a simple mobile.

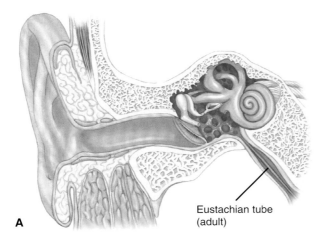

A

Eustachian tube
(adult)

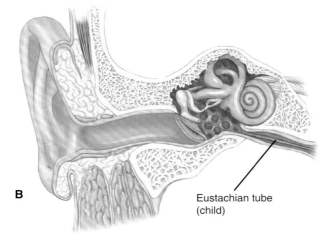

B

Eustachian tube
(child)

FIGURE 35-2 Comparison of the eustachian tube **(A)** in the adult and **(B)** in the infant or young child. Note the child's shorter, wider, and more horizontal eustachian tube.

Astigmatism, which may occur with or without myopia or hyperopia, is caused by unequal curvatures in the cornea that bend the light rays in different directions; this produces a blurred image. Slight astigmatism often does not require correction, moderate degrees usually require glasses for reading and watching television and movies, and severe astigmatism requires glasses at all times.

Partial Sight

Children with partial sight have a visual acuity between 20/20 and 20/200 in the better eye after all necessary medical or surgical correction. These children also have a high incidence of refractive errors, particularly myopia. Eye injuries also cause loss of vision, as do conditions such as cataracts, which can be improved by treatment but result in diminished sight.

Blindness

Blindness is legally defined as a corrected vision of 20/200 or less, or peripheral vision of less than 20 degrees in the better eye. Many causes of blindness, such as retinopathy of prematurity (ROP) (caused by excessive oxygen concentrations in newborns) (see Chapter 20) and trachoma, a viral infection, have been reduced or eliminated. Maternal infections are still a common cause of blindness.

Good News!
The incidence of maternal rubella causing blindness in infants has decreased significantly since immunizations for measles, mumps, and rubella are now being given routinely.

Between the ages of 5 and 7 years, children begin to form and retain visual images; they have memory with pictures. Children who become blind before 5 years of age are missing this crucial element in their development.

Blindness can seriously hamper the child's ability to form human attachments; learn coordination, balance, and locomotion; distinguish fantasy from reality; and interpret the surrounding world. How well the blind child learns to cope depends on the family's ability to communicate, teach, and foster a sense of independence in the child.

Clinical Manifestations and Diagnosis

Squinting and frowning while trying to read a blackboard or other material at a distance, tearing, red-rimmed eyes, holding work too close to the eyes while reading or writing, and rubbing the eyes are all signs of possible vision impairment. Although blindness is likely to be detected in early infancy, partial sightedness or correctable vision problems may go unrecognized until a child enters school unless vision screening is part of routine health maintenance (Fig. 35-3).

The Snellen eye chart is a familiar test in which the letters on each line are smaller than those on the line above. If the child can read the 20-ft line standing 20 ft away from the chart, visual acuity is stated as 20/20. If the child can read only the line marked 100, acuity is stated as 20/100. Picture

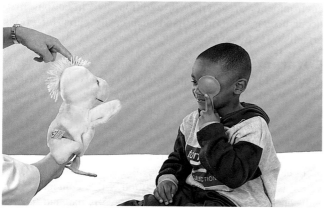

FIGURE 35-3 Vision screening on a preschool child as part of a routine examination.

charts for identification are also used but are not considered as accurate. A child can memorize the pictures and guess from the general shape without being able to see distinctly. A simple eye test chart for young children is available for home use by family caregivers or visiting nurses (see Tips for Reinforcing Family Teaching: Home Eye Test for Children).

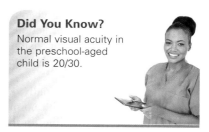

Did You Know?

Normal visual acuity in the preschool-aged child is 20/30.

TIPS FOR REINFORCING FAMILY TEACHING

Home Eye Test for Children

The chart used to do a home eye test for children is an adaptation of the Snellen E chart used for testing children who have not learned to read. To use the E chart, the child covers one eye and then points the fingers in the same direction as the "fingers" on each E, beginning with the largest. Some examiners refer to these as "legs on a table."

Line	20/	Distance	#
	20/200	200 FT / 61 M	1
	20/100	100 FT / 30.5 M	2
	20/70	70 FT / 21.7 M	3
	20/50	50 FT / 15.2 M	4
	20/30	30 FT / 9.1 M	5
	20/20	20 FT / 6.1 M	6
	20/15	15 FT / 4.6 M	7
	20/10	10 FT / 3.05 M	8

Supplies Needed

- Printed copy of the "Children's Home Eye Test" chart from https://www.aao.org/eye-health/tips-prevention/home-eye-test-children-adults
- Eye cover (paper cup, facial tissue)
- Tape or tack to attach chart to wall
- Yardstick or tape measure to measure distance to wall
- Flashlight
- Pencil or pen to record results

Prepare Test Area

- Measure 10 ft from bare wall with no windows
- Place chair at 10 foot mark
- Tape or tack chart to wall at eye level of child when seated on chair

Testing Child's Vision (Age 3 or Older)

- Use a practice "E" card and explain to child how to point in the same direction that the E is "pointing." Turn the practice E card up, down, right, left and have child point in the four different directions according to how the "E" is pointing.
- Practice with child until they can point in the four directions without help.
- Seat child in chair (10 ft from chart).
- Have child gently cover one eye (no peeking).
- Shine flashlight on letters if chart is too dark.
- Point at each E starting with the largest, have child point in the direction the E is pointing.
- Write down the number of the smallest line the child can correctly see (more than half of the E's correctly identified).
- Repeat the test with the other eye.

Results

The home eye test can help discover a concern or problem with the child's vision, but is not as accurate as an examination done by a vision health care provider. The home test should not be substituted for a complete medical eye examination.

Treatment and Education

Significant medical and surgical advances have occurred in the treatment of cataracts, strabismus, and amblyopia, discussed shortly. The earlier the child is treated, the better the child's chances of adequate vision for normal development and function. Errors of refraction are usually correctable. Corrective lenses for minor vision impairments should be prescribed early and checked regularly to be sure they still provide adequate correction.

Children who are partially sighted or totally blind benefit from association with normally sighted children. In most communities, education for these children is provided within the regular school or in classrooms that offer the child more specialized equipment and instruction.

Specialized equipment includes printed material with large print, pencils with large leads for darker lines, voice recordings, magnifying glasses, and keyboards. For a child with a serious impairment that sharply curtails participation in regular activities, talking books, raised maps, and Braille equipment are needed as well. These devices prevent isolation of the visually impaired child and minimize any differences from the other children.

Nursing Care

Children with visual impairments have the same needs as other children, and these should not be overlooked. The child who is blind needs emotional comfort and sensory stimulation, most of which must be communicated by touch, sound, and smell. Explain sounds and other sensations that are new to the child, and let them touch the equipment that will be used in procedures. A tactile tour of the room helps orient the child to the location of furniture and other facilities.

Identify yourself when you enter the room, and tell the child when you leave. Explanations of what is going to happen reduce the child's fear, anxiety, and the possibility of being startled by an unexpected touch. The child with a visual impairment should be involved with as many peers and their activities as possible. The child should also be encouraged to be as independent as possible. One step is to provide the child with finger foods and encourage self-feeding after orienting the child to the plate. A small bowl, instead of a plate, is useful so that food can be scooped against the side to get it on the spoon. Eating can be a time-consuming and messy affair, but having the opportunity to learn to feed themselves is essential to the growth of independence in all children.

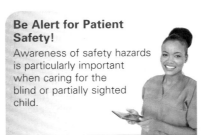

Be Alert for Patient Safety!

Awareness of safety hazards is particularly important when caring for the blind or partially sighted child.

EYE CONDITIONS

Vision screening is part of routine health maintenance. Cataracts, glaucoma, and strabismus are disease conditions that may need to be dealt with during childhood. Eye injuries can occur when children are exploring their environments or playing. In addition, eye infections may occur because exploring hands can easily carry infectious organisms to the eyes.

Cataracts

A **cataract** is a development of opacity in the crystalline lens that prevents light rays from entering the eye. Congenital cataracts may be hereditary, or cataracts may develop from eye injury, metabolic disturbances, such as galactosemia and diabetes, or long-term use of systemic corticosteroids.

Surgical extraction of the cataracts can be performed at an early age. With early removal, the prognosis for good vision is improved. The child is fitted with a contact lens. If only one eye is affected, the "good" eye is patched to prevent amblyopia (see discussion in the "Strabismus" section). As the child gets older, numerous lens changes are needed to modify the strength of the lens.

Glaucoma

There are three types of glaucoma in children. The congenital infantile type occurs in children younger than 3 years of age; the juvenile type shows clinical manifestations after 3 years; and the secondary type results from injury or disease. Increased intraocular pressure caused by overproduction of aqueous fluid causes the eyeball to enlarge and the cornea to become large, thin, and sometimes cloudy. Untreated, the disease slowly progresses to blindness. Pain may be present.

Goniotomy (surgical opening into Schlemm canal) provides drainage of the aqueous humor and is often effective in relieving intraocular pressure. Goniotomy may need to be performed multiple times to control intraocular pressure. Surgery is performed as early as possible to prevent permanent damage.

Strabismus

Strabismus is the failure of the two eyes to direct their gaze at the same object simultaneously. This condition is commonly called "squint" or "crossed eyes" (Fig. 35-4).

Normally, **binocular** (normal) **vision** is maintained through the muscular coordination of eye movements so that a single vision results. In strabismus, the visual axes are not parallel, and **diplopia** (double vision) results. In an effort to avoid seeing two images, the child's central nervous system suppresses vision in the deviant eye, causing **amblyopia** (dimness of vision from disuse of the eye), which is sometimes called "lazy eye."

A wide variation in the manifestation of strabismus exists. There may be monocular strabismus, in which one eye deviates while the other eye is used, or alternating strabismus, in which deviation alternates from one eye to the other. The term **esotropia** is used when the eye deviates toward the other eye; **exotropia** denotes a turning away from the other eye (Fig. 35-5).

Treatment depends on the type of strabismus present. In monocular strabismus, occlusion of the better eye by patching to force the use of the deviating eye should be initiated at an early age. Patching is continued for weeks or months. The younger the child is, the more rapid the

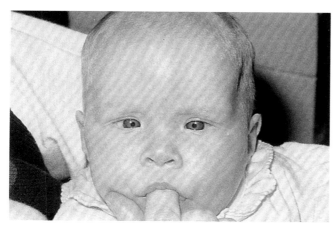

FIGURE 35-4 Strabismus in an infant.

improvement. The patching may be done for set periods of time or be continuous, depending on the child's age. For example, an older child usually needs continuous periods of patching, whereas a younger one may respond quickly to short periods of patching.

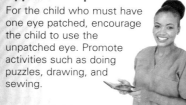

Some Nurses Find This Approach Helpful!
For the child who must have one eye patched, encourage the child to use the unpatched eye. Promote activities such as doing puzzles, drawing, and sewing.

Glasses can correct a refractive error if amblyopia is not present. **Orthoptics** (therapeutic ocular muscle exercises) to improve the quality of vision may be prescribed to supplement the use of glasses or surgery.

Early detection and treatment of strabismus are essential for a successful outcome. Surgery on the eye muscle to correct the defect is necessary for children who do not respond to glasses and exercises. Many children need surgery after amblyopia has been corrected. The surgical correction is believed to be necessary before the child reaches age 6 or the visual damage may be permanent. However, some authorities believe that correction can be successful up to age 10.

Eye Injury and Foreign Objects in the Eye

Eye injuries are fairly common, particularly in older children. Ecchymosis of the eye (black eye) is of no great importance unless the eyeball is involved. A penetrating wound of the eyeball is potentially serious—BB shots in particular are dangerous—and requires the ophthalmologist's attention.

With any history of an injury, a thorough examination of the entire eye is necessary.

Sympathetic ophthalmia, an inflammatory reaction of the uninjured eye, may follow perforation wounds of the globe, even if the perforations are small. Sympathetic ophthalmia often includes **photophobia** (intolerance to light), **lacrimation** (secretion of tears), pain, and some dimness of vision. The retina may become detached, and atrophy of the eyeball may occur. Prompt and skillful treatment at the time of the injury is essential to avoid involvement of the other eye.

Small foreign objects, such as specks of dust that have lodged inside the eyelid, may be removed by rolling the lid back and exposing the object. If the object cannot be easily removed with a small piece of moistened cotton or soft clean cloth or flushed out with saline solution, the child should be seen by a health care provider.

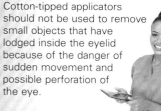

A Word of Caution is in Order!
Cotton-tipped applicators should not be used to remove small objects that have lodged inside the eyelid because of the danger of sudden movement and possible perforation of the eye.

Eye Infections

Hordeolum, known commonly as a stye, is a purulent infection of the follicle of an eyelash, generally caused by *Staphylococcus aureus*. Localized swelling, tenderness, pain, and a reddened lid edge are present. The maximal tenderness is over the infected site. The lesion progresses to suppuration, with eventual discharge of the purulent material. Warm saline compresses applied for about 15 minutes three or four times daily give some relief and hasten resolution, but recurrence is common. The stye should never be squeezed. Ophthalmic antibiotic ointment may help prevent accompanying conjunctivitis and recurrence.

Conjunctivitis is an acute inflammation of the conjunctiva. In children, a virus, bacteria, allergy, or foreign body may be the cause. Most commonly, conjunctivitis is caused by bacteria. The purulent drainage, a common characteristic, can be cultured to determine the causative organism. Because of the danger of spreading infection, bacterial conjunctivitis is treated with ophthalmic antibacterial agents.

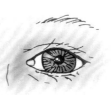

Here's a Pharmacology Fact!
Ophthalmic preparations of erythromycin, bacitracin, sulfacetamide, and polymyxin are often used to treat bacterial eye infections. Always clarify the preparation is ophthalmic.

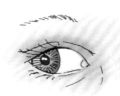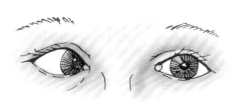

A   **B**

FIGURE 35-5 Types of strabismus. **A.** Esotropia. **B.** Exotropia.

Because ointments blur vision, eye drops are used during the day and ointments are used at night. Before medication is applied, warm moist compresses can be used to remove the crusts that form on the eyes. The child who has bacterial conjunctivitis should be kept separate from other children until the condition has been treated. The use of separate washcloths, towels, and disposable tissues is important in preventing the spread of infection among family members.

Nursing Care for the Child Undergoing Eye Surgery

When a child undergoes eye surgery, sensory deprivation is possible. Anyone experiencing sensory deprivation finds it difficult to stay in touch with reality.

A child who wakens from surgery to total darkness may go into a state of panic and anxiety evidenced by trembling and nervousness. The child needs a family caregiver or loved one to stay during the time when vision is restricted.

> **Think About This!**
> A child whose eyes are covered is particularly vulnerable to sensory deprivation. Nurses who have not experienced this deprivation do not always appreciate the implications of not being able to see. To better understand, cover one eye for a period of time and note the effects of this experience!

The child needs to be as well prepared for the event as possible. However, the small child has no experience to help in understanding what is actually going to happen. The darkness, pain, and total strangeness of the situation can be overwhelming. Using play can be helpful. For example, one preoperative preparation might be to play a game with a blindfold to help the child become accustomed to having their eyes covered (Fig. 35-6).

Restraints should not be used indiscriminately. However, most small children need some reminder to keep their hands away from the affected eye, unless someone is beside them to prevent them from rubbing it or from removing eye dressings. Elbow restraints are useful, although they do not prevent rubbing the eye with the arm. Soft, padded strips applied to the wrists in clove-hitch fashion can be tied to the bedsides in such a manner as to allow freedom of arm movement but to prevent the child from causing damage to the operative site.

Speak to the child to alert them as you approach. The child needs tactile stimulation; therefore, after speaking, you may stroke or pat the child. If permitted, hold the child for additional reassurance.

HEARING IMPAIRMENT

Hearing loss is one of the most common disabilities in the United States. About 1 to 2 of every 1,000 children are born with hearing impairments (Smith & Gooi, 2021). Depending on the degree of hearing loss and the age at detection,

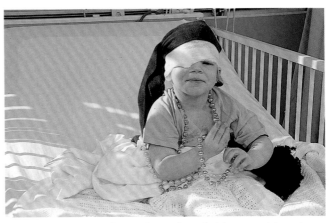

FIGURE 35-6 Pretending to be a pirate (with supervision close by) enables this toddler to prepare for having an eye patch after surgery.

a child's development can be moderately to severely impaired. Development of speech, human relationships, and understanding of the environment all depend on the ability to hear.

Hearing loss ranges from mild (hard of hearing) to profound (deaf). A child who is hard of hearing has a loss of hearing acuity but can learn speech and language by imitating sounds. A deaf child has no hearing ability.

Types of Hearing Impairment

There are four types of hearing loss: conductive, sensorineural, mixed, and central.

Conductive Hearing Loss

In conductive hearing loss, middle ear structures fail to carry sound waves to the inner ear. This type of impairment most often results from chronic serous otitis media or other infection and can make hearing levels fluctuate. Chronic middle ear infection can destroy part of the eardrum or the ossicles, which leads to conductive deafness. This type of deafness is seldom complete and responds well to treatment.

Sensorineural Hearing Loss

Sensorineural hearing loss may result from damage, disease, or disorders affecting the inner ear, in particular the nerve endings in the cochlea or the nerve pathways leading to the brain. Hereditary or congenital factors and toxic reactions to certain drugs may cause sensorineural hearing loss. It is generally severe and unresponsive to medical treatment.

Mixed Hearing Loss

Mixed hearing loss combines both conductive and sensorineural hearing impairments. In these instances, the conduction level determines how well the child can hear.

Central Auditory Processing Disorder

Although the child with central auditory processing disorder may have normal hearing, damage to or faulty development of the proper brain centers makes this child unable to use the auditory information received.

Clinical Manifestations

Children with hearing loss may have difficulty with normal conversation, especially if not facing the person speaking. Mild to moderate hearing loss often remains undetected until the child moves outside the family circle into preschool or kindergarten. The hearing loss may have been gradual, and the child may have become such a skilled lip reader that neither the child nor the family is aware of the partial deafness.

Certain reactions and mannerisms characterize a child with hearing loss. Observe the child for an apparent inability to locate a sound and a turning of the head to one side when listening. The child who fails to comprehend when spoken to, who gives inappropriate answers to questions, who consistently turns up the volume on the television or radio, or who cannot whisper or talk softly may have hearing loss.

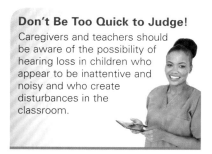

Don't Be Too Quick to Judge!
Caregivers and teachers should be aware of the possibility of hearing loss in children who appear to be inattentive and noisy and who create disturbances in the classroom.

Diagnosis

Children who are profoundly deaf are more likely to be diagnosed before 1 year of age than are children with mild to moderate hearing losses. The child who is suspected of having hearing loss should be referred for a complete audiologic assessment. Children with sensorineural impairment generally have a greater loss of hearing acuity, which may vary from slight to complete in the high-pitched tones. Children with a conductive loss are more likely to have equal losses over a wide range of frequencies.

A child's hearing should be tested in a soundproof room. Speech reception and speech discrimination tests measure the amount of hearing impairment for both speech and communication. Accurate measurements can usually be made in children as young as 3 years of age, especially if the test is introduced as a game.

Infants and very young children must be tested in different ways. An infant with normal hearing should be able to locate a sound at 28 weeks, imitate sounds at 36 weeks, and associate sounds with people or objects at 1 year of age. A commonly used screening test for very young children uses noisemakers of varying intensity and pitch. The examiner stands beside or behind the child who has been given a toy. As the examiner produces sounds with a rattle, buzzer, bell, or other noisemaker, a hearing child is distracted and turns to the source of the new sound, whereas a deaf child does not react in a particular way.

Deafness, intellectual disability, and autism are sometimes incorrectly diagnosed because the symptoms can be similar. Deaf children may fail to respond to sound or develop speech because they cannot hear. Children with intellectual disability or autism may show the same lack of response and development, even though they do not have a hearing loss.

Treatment and Education

When the type and degree of hearing loss have been established, the first step is to treat the underlying cause if possible. Some conditions can be treated with surgery. The child, or even the infant, may be fitted with a hearing aid. Hearing aids are helpful in conductive hearing loss. These devices only amplify sound; they do not restore the hearing to normal. Many models, styles, and electronic features are available. Bone conduction hearing devices transmit sound through the skull and often provide better sound for the child. Cochlear implants are surgically implanted and stimulate the cochlear nerve, which provides hearing.

Deaf children can best be taught to communicate by a combination of lip reading, sign language, and oral speech (Fig. 35-7).

The family members are the child's first teachers; they must be aware of all phases of development—physical, emotional, social, intellectual, and language—and seek to aid this development.

A deaf child depends on sight to interpret the environment and to communicate. Thus, it is important to be sure that the child's vision is normal and if it is not, to correct that problem. The child with hearing loss is likely to also have some vision impairment. Training in the use of all the other senses—sight, smell, taste, and touch—makes the deaf child better able to use any available hearing.

Preschool classes for deaf children exist in many communities. These classes attempt to create environments in which deaf children can have the same experiences and activities that hearing preschool-aged children have. Children are generally enrolled at age 2.5 years.

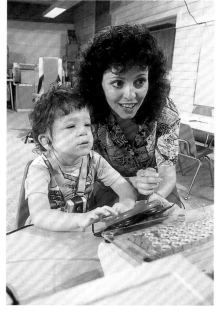

FIGURE 35-7 A young deaf girl learns to use the computer with the help of a speech therapist.

The John Tracy Clinic in Los Angeles, founded in 1943, is dedicated to children born with severe hearing loss or those who have lost hearing through illness before acquiring speech and language. The clinic provides services, support, and encouragement for children with hearing loss as well as their families. Their philosophy is that with early diagnosis and intervention, hearing-impaired children can develop speech, language, and listening skills they need to thrive in the hearing world. Their services include diagnostic testing, education, resources, training, and counseling. Information about the clinic can be obtained at www.jtc.org.

Federal law requires free and appropriate education for all disabled children. Children with hearing loss who cannot successfully function in regular classrooms are provided with supplementary services (speech therapist, speech interpreter, and signer) in special classrooms or in residential schools.

Nursing Care

When the deaf child is in a healthcare facility, the child's primary caregiver is encouraged to be present during the stay to help the child communicate needs and feelings. The deaf child's anxiety about unfamiliar situations and procedures can be greater than that of the child with normal hearing. When speaking to the deaf child, stand or sit face-to-face on the child's level. Be certain that a deaf child can see you before you touch them. Demonstrate each procedure before it is performed, showing the child the equipment or pictures of the equipment to be used. Follow demonstrations with explanations to be sure the child understands. Keep a night light in the child's room because sight is a critical sense to the deaf child.

> **A Little Sensitivity is in Order!**
> To understand the deaf child's helpless feeling, imagine being in a soundless, dark room. Be sure the child's room is well lit.

Hearing aids are expensive, so learning how to take care of and maintain them is important. Put the aid in a safe place when the child is not wearing it. Check linens before putting them into the laundry so as not to discard a hearing aid along with the dirty linens.

Use family members as important resources to learn about the child's habits and communication patterns. In many communities, signing classes are available for those working with hearing-impaired children and adults.

TEST YOURSELF

✔ What are the five types of vision impairment?

✔ What term is commonly used to describe strabismus?

✔ What are the four types of hearing loss?

✔ What are four examples of nursing interventions used when working with deaf children?

OTITIS MEDIA

Otitis media is one of the most common infectious diseases of childhood and frequently the reason infants are seen by health care providers, especially during their first year of life. Because the eustachian tube in an infant is shorter, wider, and straighter than that of the older child or adult (Fig. 35-2), nasopharyngeal secretions are able to enter the middle ear more easily. *Haemophilus influenzae* and *Streptococcus pneumoniae* are common causative agents of otitis media in infants and children. Infant immunizations have decreased the incidence of otitis media.

Clinical Manifestations

A restless infant who repeatedly shakes the head and rubs or pulls at one ear should be checked for an ear infection. These behaviors often indicate that the infant is having pain in the ears. Older children can express and describe the pain they are experiencing. In addition to pain, symptoms may include fever, irritability, decreased activity, lack of appetite, and hearing impairment. Vomiting or diarrhea may occur.

Diagnosis

The infant's ear is examined with an otoscope by pulling the ear down and back to straighten the ear canal. In the older child, the ear is pulled up and back. The examination reveals a bright red, bulging eardrum in otitis media. Spontaneous rupture of the eardrum may occur, in which case there will be purulent drainage, and the pain caused by the pressure buildup in the ear will be relieved. If present, purulent drainage is cultured to determine the causative organism and appropriate antibiotic antibiotic to be administered.

Treatment and Nursing Care

Antibiotics may be used during the period of infection and for several days after to prevent mastoiditis or chronic infection. A 10-day course of amoxicillin is a common treatment. Most children respond well to antibiotics. The health care provider considers the child's age, severity of symptoms, and improvement of symptoms to determine if antibiotic treatment should be used. Analgesics and antipyretics are used to control pain, discomfort, and fever. Some children have repeated episodes of otitis media. Children with chronic otitis media may be put on a prophylactic course of an antibiotic. **Myringotomy** (incision of the eardrum) may be performed to establish drainage and to insert tiny tubes into the tympanic membrane to facilitate drainage. In most cases, the tubes eventually fall out spontaneously. Attention to chronic otitis media is essential because permanent hearing loss can result from frequent occurrences.

Mastoiditis, infection of the mastoid sinus, is a possible complication of untreated acute otitis media, an untreated ruptured eardrum, or inadequate treatment of an acute episode.

Most infants and children with otitis media are cared for at home; therefore, your primary nursing responsibility is to reinforce teaching with the family caregivers about prevention and the care of the child (see Tips for Reinforcing Family Teaching: Otitis Media).

TIPS FOR REINFORCING FAMILY TEACHING

Otitis Media

The eustachian tube is a connection between the nasal passages and the middle ear. The eustachian tube is wider, shorter, and straighter in the infant, allowing organisms from respiratory infections to travel into the middle ear to cause infection (otitis media).

Prevention

- Hold infant in an upright position or with head slightly elevated while feeding to prevent formula from draining into the middle ear through the wide eustachian tube.
- Never prop a bottle.
- Do not give infant a bottle in bed. This allows fluid to pool in the middle ear, encouraging organisms to grow.
- Protect child from exposure to others with upper respiratory infections.
- Protect child from passive smoke (including wood smoke); do not permit smoking in child's presence.
- Remove sources of allergies from the home.
- Observe for clues to ear infection: shaking head, rubbing or pulling at ears, and fever combined with restlessness or screaming and crying.

- Be alert to signs of hearing difficulty in toddlers and preschool-aged children. This may be the first sign of an ear infection.
- Teach toddler or preschool-aged child gentle nose blowing.

Care of the Child With Otitis Media

- Have child with upper respiratory infection who shows symptoms of ear discomfort checked by a health care provider.
- Complete the entire amount of antibiotic medication prescribed, even if the child seems better before the prescription is complete.
- Use heat (such as a heating pad on low setting) to provide comfort; an adult must stay with the child.
- Soothe, rock, and comfort the child to help relieve discomfort. The child is more comfortable sleeping on side of infected ear.
- Give pain medications (such as acetaminophen or ibuprofen) as directed. Never give aspirin.
- Give medications such as acetaminophen or ibuprofen (to the child older than 6 months) to control fever.
- Provide liquid or soft foods; chewing causes pain.
- Know that hearing loss may last up to 6 months after infection.
- Schedule follow-up with hearing test as advised.

INSERTION OF FOREIGN BODIES INTO THE EAR OR NOSE

Children, especially toddlers and preschool-aged children, may insert small objects into their ears or noses. Irrigation of the ear may remove small objects, except paper, which becomes impacted as it absorbs moisture. The health care provider generally uses small forceps to remove objects not dislodged by irrigation.

The child may have placed a foreign body in the nose just inside the nares, but manipulation may push it in further. If the object remains in the nose for any length of time, infection may occur. When the object is discovered, a health care provider should inspect with a speculum and remove the object.

This is Important and Can Be Dangerous!

Children often put small objects, such as peas or beans, crumpled paper, beads, "button" batteries, and small toys, into their ears or noses.

REYE SYNDROME

Reye syndrome (rhymes with "eye") is characterized by acute encephalopathy and fatty degeneration of the liver and other abdominal organs. It occurs in children of all ages but is seen more frequently in young school-aged children than in any other age group. Reye syndrome usually occurs after a viral illness, particularly after an upper respiratory infection or varicella (chickenpox). Administration of aspirin during the viral illness has been implicated as a contributing factor. As a result, the American Academy of Pediatrics recommends that aspirin or aspirin compounds not be given to children with viral infections.

Clinical Manifestations

The symptoms appear within 3 to 5 days after the initial illness. The child recuperates unremarkably when symptoms of severe vomiting, irritability, lethargy, confusion, and disorientation occur. Immediate intervention is needed to prevent cerebral edema with increased intracranial pressure (IICP) and the possibility of seizures, coma, and respiratory arrest.

Diagnosis

The history of a viral illness is an immediate clue. Liver function tests show elevations because of poor liver function. Other diagnostics include liver biopsy, lumbar puncture, coagulation studies, blood glucose and ammonia levels. The child is often hypoglycemic and has delayed prothrombin time.

Treatment

The child with Reye syndrome is often cared for in the intensive care unit because the disease may progress rapidly. Medical management focuses on supportive measures—improving respiratory function, reducing cerebral edema, and controlling hypoglycemia. Osmotic diuretic drugs (e.g., mannitol) may be administered to reduce cerebral edema.

Nursing Care

Carefully observe the child for overall physical status and any change in neurologic status. This observation is essential in evaluating the progression of the illness. Accurate intake and output determinations are necessary to determine when fluids need to be adjusted to control cerebral edema and prevent dehydration. Monitor the blood glucose level and bleeding time. Low blood glucose levels can lead to seizures quickly in young children, and a prolonged bleeding time can indicate coagulation problems as a result of liver dysfunction.

This hospitalization period is a traumatic time for family members, so give them opportunities to deal with their feelings. In addition, keep the family caregivers well informed about the child's care. Having a child in intensive care is a frightening experience for the family, so make every effort to reassure them with sincerity and honesty.

Since the American Academy of Pediatrics made its recommendation to avoid giving aspirin to children, especially during viral illnesses, the number of cases of Reye syndrome has steadily decreased. The prognosis for children with Reye syndrome is greatly improved with early diagnosis and vigorous treatment. Reinforce teaching with family caregivers to avoid the use of aspirin in children.

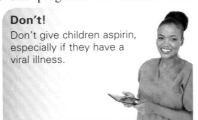

Don't!
Don't give children aspirin, especially if they have a viral illness.

TEST YOURSELF

✔ What is the physiologic reason otitis media occurs more often in young children than in older children and adults?

✔ What has greatly decreased the incidence of Reye syndrome?

ACUTE OR NONRECURRENT SEIZURES

A seizure (convulsion) may be a symptom of a wide variety of disorders. In children between the age of 6 months and 5 years (most occurring between 12 and 18 months of age), **febrile seizures** (seizures resulting from fever) are the most common. Febrile seizures usually occur in the form of a generalized seizure early in the course of a fever. Although commonly associated with high fever (102°F to 106°F [38.9°C to 41.1°C]), some children appear to have a low seizure threshold and convulse when a fever of 100°F to 102°F (37.8°C to 38.9°C) is present. These seizures are often one of the initial symptoms of an acute infection somewhere in the body.

Less common causes of seizures are intracranial infections, such as meningitis; toxic reactions to certain drugs or minerals such as lead; metabolic disorders; head trauma; and various brain disorders.

Clinical Manifestations and Diagnosis

A seizure may occur suddenly without warning; however, restlessness and irritability may precede an episode. The body stiffens, and the child loses consciousness. In a few seconds, clonic movements occur. These movements are quick, jerking movements of the arms, legs, and facial muscles. Breathing is irregular and the child cannot swallow saliva. These symptoms require prompt immediate action; further evaluation is made after the urgency of the seizure has passed.

Treatment

Protecting the child during the seizure is the primary concern (see Nursing Process and Care Plan for the Child at Risk for Seizures). If the seizure activity continues, diazepam or lorazepam may be administered IV to control the seizure. Acetaminophen may be administered to reduce the temperature.

SEIZURE DISORDERS

Seizure disorders, also referred to as convulsive disorders, are common in children and may result from a variety of causes. Unlike the acute febrile seizure that occurs with fevers and acute infections, epilepsy is a recurrent and chronic seizure disorder. Epilepsy can be classified as primary (idiopathic) with no known cause, or secondary, resulting from infection, head trauma, hemorrhage, tumor, or other organic or degenerative factors. Primary epilepsy is the most common.

Clinical Manifestations

Seizures are the characteristic clinical manifestation of both types of epilepsy and may be either focal (partial) onset, generalized onset, or of unknown onset. **Focal (partial) seizures** begin in a particular area of one side or hemisphere of the brain. Partial is a term used to describe seizures that are on one side of the brain, but the term focal is used to more accurately describe where the seizure began. **Generalized seizures** involve both hemispheres of the brain. Unknown onset seizures describe a seizure in which the beginning of the seizure is not known. The International League Against Epilepsy (ILAE) has used new terms to describe and classify seizures to more clearly describe the different types of seizures (Wilfong, 2021).

Focal (Partial) Onset Seizures

Manifestations of focal seizures vary depending on the area of the brain from which they arise. Focal seizures are classified as focal onset aware seizures or focal onset impaired awareness seizures. Depending on movement involved during the seizure, they are further classified as motor or nonmotor.

Focal Onset Aware Seizures (Formerly Called Simple Partial Seizure)

With the focal onset aware seizure, the child is awake and aware during the seizure.

• A focal onset motor seizure causes a localized motor activity such as jerking, shaking, or twitching of an arm, leg, or other part of the body. These may be limited to one side of the body or may spread to other parts.

- A focal onset sensory seizure may include sensory symptoms called an **aura** (a sensation that signals an impending attack) involving sight, sound, taste, smell, touch, or emotions (e.g., a feeling of fear). The child may also have numbness, tingling, paresthesia, or pain.

Focal Onset Impaired Awareness Seizures (Formerly Called Complex Partial Seizure)

With the focal onset impaired awareness seizure, the child is confused or their awareness is affected during the seizure. The child with impaired awareness is unable to respond normally to external stimuli. The seizure begins in a small area of the brain and changes or alters consciousness. These seizures can have motor and nonmotor symptoms. Nonpurposeful movements, such as hand rubbing, lip smacking, chewing, swallowing, and sucking, may occur. Older children may have repetitive actions such as flailing of the arms, jumping, running, screaming, spinning, kicking, or laughing without apparent reason. After the seizure, the child may be confused for a few minutes or may sleep for a period of time. The child is often unaware of the seizure.

 Concept Mastery Alert

Focal onset impaired awareness seizures cause confusion and lack of awareness during and after the seizure. Nonpurposeful movements may be involved (such as hand rubbing, lip smacking, and chewing). Repetitive actions such as flailing of the arms, running, screaming, and kicking may occur in the older child.

Generalized Onset Seizures

With the generalized onset seizure, both sides or hemispheres of the brain are affected at the same time. Types of generalized onset seizures include tonic–clonic, absence, atonic, myoclonic, and infantile spasms.

Tonic–Clonic Seizures

Tonic–clonic seizures consist of four stages: the prodromal period, which can last for days or hours; the aura, which is a warning immediately before the seizure; the tonic–clonic movements; and the postictal stage. Not all these stages occur with every seizure; the seizure may just begin with a sudden loss of consciousness. During the prodromal period, the child might be drowsy, dizzy, or have a lack of coordination. If the seizure is preceded by an aura, it is identified as a generalized onset seizure secondary to a focal seizure. The aura may reflect in which part of the brain the seizure originates. Young children may have difficulty describing an aura but may cry out in response to it. In the tonic phase, the child's muscles contract, the child may fall, and the child's extremities may stiffen. The contraction of respiratory muscles during the tonic phase may cause the child to become cyanotic and appear briefly to have respiratory arrest. The eyes roll upward, and the child might utter a guttural cry. The initial rigidity of the tonic phase changes rapidly to generalized jerking muscle movements in the clonic phase. The child may bite the tongue or lose control of bladder and

bowel functions. The jerking movements gradually diminish and then disappear, and the child relaxes. The seizure is usually brief, lasting less than 1 minute, but can be protracted, lasting 30 minutes or longer. The period after the tonic–clonic phase is called the postictal period. The child may sleep soundly for several hours during this stage or return rapidly to an alert state. Many children have a period of confusion, and others experience a prolonged period of stupor.

Absence Seizures

Absence seizures rarely last longer than 20 seconds. The seizure often interrupts conversation or physical activity such as eating or playing. The child loses awareness and stares straight ahead, but does not fall. The child may have blinking or twitching of the mouth or an extremity along with the staring. Immediately after the seizure, the child is alert and continues conversation but does not know what was said or done during the episode. Absence seizures can recur frequently, sometimes as often as 50 to 100 a day. If seizures are not fully controlled, the family caregiver needs to be especially aware of dangerous situations that might occur in the child's day, such as crossing a street on the way to school. These seizures often decrease significantly or stop entirely at adolescence.

Atonic Seizures

Atonic seizures cause a sudden momentary loss of consciousness, muscle tone, and postural control and can cause the child to fall. They can result in serious facial, head, or shoulder injuries. They may recur frequently, particularly in the morning. After the seizure, the child can stand and walk as normal.

Myoclonic Seizures

Myoclonic seizures are characterized by a sudden jerking of a muscle or group of muscles, often in the arms or legs, without loss of consciousness. Myoclonus occurs during the early stages of falling asleep in people who do not have epilepsy.

Infantile Spasms

Infantile spasms are most common in children younger than 2 years of age. They are characterized by flexion or extension of the arm, leg, or head. These seizures are often preceded or followed by a cry. Muscle contractions are sudden, brief, symmetrical, and accompanied by rolling eyes. Loss of consciousness does not always occur. They almost always indicate a cerebral defect and have a poor prognosis despite treatment.

Status Epilepticus

Status epilepticus is the term used to describe a seizure that lasts longer than 30 minutes or a series of seizures in which the child does not return to their previous normal level of consciousness. Immediate treatment decreases the likelihood of permanent brain injury, respiratory failure, or even death.

Take Note!

Status epilepticus is an emergency situation and requires immediate treatment. The drugs diazepam and lorazepam, given rectally or intravenously (IV), are used to treat the condition.

Diagnosis

The types of seizures can be differentiated through the use of electroencephalography, video and ambulatory electroencephalography, skull radiography, computed tomography, magnetic resonance imaging, brain scan, and physical and neurologic assessments. The child's seizure history is an important part of determining the diagnosis.

Treatment

The main goal of treatment, complete control of seizures, can be achieved for most people through the use of anticonvulsant drug therapy. A number of anticonvulsant drugs are available (Table 35-1). The drug is chosen based on its effectiveness in controlling seizures, side effects, and its degree of toxicity.

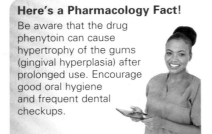

Here's a Pharmacology Fact!

Be aware that the drug phenytoin can cause hypertrophy of the gums (gingival hyperplasia) after prolonged use. Encourage good oral hygiene and frequent dental checkups.

Chewable or tablet forms of the medications are often used because suspensions separate and sometimes are not shaken well, causing the possibility of inaccurate dosage.

A few children may be candidates for surgical intervention when the focal point of the seizures is in an area of the brain that is accessible surgically and not critical to functioning. If the cause of the seizures is a tumor or other lesion, surgical removal may be possible. Vagus nerve stimulation (VNS) therapy is sometimes used to treat certain types of seizure disorders in older children and adolescents.

Ketogenic diets (high in fat, low in carbohydrates, and moderate in amounts of protein) cause the child to have high levels of ketones, which help to reduce seizure activity. These diets are prescribed, but long-term maintenance is challenging because the diets are difficult to follow and may be unappealing to the child.

Remember **Chesa Andres**. What types of seizures might Chesa have? How do you think Chesa is likely being treated for her seizure disorder? What medications do you think Chesa has been taking since her diagnosis to prevent seizures? List some nursing concerns you will take into consideration as you work with Chesa and her family caregivers.

Nursing Care

In the hospital or home setting, keeping the child safe during a seizure is the highest priority. In the hospital setting, the nurse must as well document information related to seizure activity (see Nursing Process and Care Plan for the Child at Risk for Seizures). Reinforce teaching with the family caregiver of a child who has a seizure disorder about how to prevent injury if the child has a seizure (see Tips for Reinforcing Family Teaching: Precautions Before and During Seizures).

The child and family caregivers need complete and accurate information about the disorder and the results that can be realistically expected from treatment. Epilepsy does not inevitably lead to intellectual disability, but continued and uncontrolled seizures do increase its possibility. Thus, early diagnosis and control of seizures are very important.

Although the outlook for a normal, well-adjusted life is favorable, inform the child and family about restrictions they may encounter. Children with epilepsy should be encouraged to participate in physical activities but should not participate in sports in which a fall could cause serious injury. In many states, a person with uncontrolled epilepsy is legally forbidden to drive a motor vehicle; this could limit choice of vocation and lifestyle. Despite attempts to educate the general public about epilepsy, many people remain prejudiced about this disorder, and this can limit the epileptic person's social and vocational acceptance.

TIPS FOR REINFORCING FAMILY TEACHING

Precautions Before and During Seizures

Before

- Have the child swim with a companion.
- Have the child use protective helmet and padding for bicycle riding and skateboarding.
- Supervise when using power equipment.
- Carry or wear medical identification bracelet.
- Discuss the child's condition with teachers and school nurse.
- Know factors that trigger seizure activity.

During

- Stay calm.
- Move furniture or objects that could cause injury.
- Turn the child on side with head turned to one side.
- Remove glasses.
- Protect the child's head.
- Do not restrain the child.
- Do not try to put anything between the child's teeth.
- Keep people from crowding around the child.
- After seizure, notify health care provider for follow-up.
- If seizures continue without stopping, call for emergency help.

TABLE 35-1 Antiepileptic–Anticonvulsive Therapeutic Agents

DRUG	INDICATION	SIDE EFFECTS	NURSING IMPLICATIONS
Carbamazepine	Generalized tonic–clonic, focal	Drowsiness, dry mouth, vomiting, double vision, leukopenia, gastrointestinal upset, thrombocytopenia	There may be dizziness and drowsiness with initial doses. This should subside within 3–4 days.
Ethosuximide	Absence seizures, myoclonic	Dry mouth, anorexia, dizziness, headache, nausea, vomiting, gastrointestinal upset, lethargy, bone marrow depression	Use with caution in hepatic or renal disease.
Phenobarbital	Generalized tonic–clonic, myoclonic, focal	Drowsiness, alteration in sleep patterns, irritability, respiratory and cardiac depression, restlessness, headache	Alcohol can enhance the effects of phenobarbital. Monitor blood levels of drug. Liver function studies are necessary with prolonged use.
Phenytoin	Generalized tonic–clonic, focal	Double vision, blurred vision, slurred speech, nystagmus, ataxia, gingival hyperplasia, hirsutism, cardiac arrhythmias, bone marrow depression	Alcohol, antacids, and folic acid decrease the effect of phenytoin. Instruct the child or caregiver to notify the dentist that they are taking phenytoin to monitor hyperplasia of the gums.
Valproic acid	Absence, Generalized tonic–clonic, myoclonic, focal	Nausea, vomiting, or increased appetite, tremors, elevated liver enzymes, constipation, headaches, depression, lymphocytosis, leukopenia, increased prothrombin time	Physical dependency may result when used for prolonged period. Tablets and capsules should be taken whole. Elixir should be taken alone, not mixed with carbonated beverages. Increased toxicity may occur with administration of salicylates (aspirin).

General Nursing Considerations With Anticonvulsant Therapy
General nursing considerations with anticonvulsant therapy that apply to all or most of drugs given to children include the following:
1. Warn the client and family that clients should avoid activities that require alertness and complex psychomotor coordination (e.g., climbing).
2. Medication can be given with meals to minimize gastric irritation.
3. The anticonvulsant medications should not be discontinued abruptly, as this can precipitate status epilepticus.
4. Anticonvulsant medications generally have a cumulative effect, both therapeutically and adversely.
5. Alcohol ingestion increases the effects of anticonvulsant drugs, exaggerating central nervous system depression.
6. Many of the drugs can cause bone marrow depression (leukopenia, thrombocytopenia, neutropenia, megaloblastic anemia). Regular complete blood cell counts, including white blood cells, red blood cells, and platelets, are necessary to evaluate bone marrow production.
7. The child should receive periodic blood tests to monitor therapeutic levels as opposed to toxic levels.

Nursing Process and Care Plan *for the Child at Risk for Seizures*

Assessment (Data Collection)

During the family caregiver interview, ask about any history of a seizure disorder or any seizure activity before this admission. Have the caregivers describe any previous episodes, including if the child had an elevated temperature, how the child behaved immediately before the seizure, movements during the seizure, and any other information they believe to be relevant. Ask about the presence of any fever during the present illness. Promptly institute seizure precautions. A child whose fever, history, or other symptoms indicate that a seizure may be anticipated should be placed under constant observation.

When collecting data, obtain a baseline temperature measurement. Using a neurologic tool, observe and record the child's neurologic status, and make other observations appropriate for the present illness.

Nursing Care Focus

When determining nursing care focuses applicable to the child at risk for seizures, include the risk for aspiration and ineffective airway clearance and preventing injury during a seizure. The anxiety of family caregivers needs to be considered as well as the needs they have for reinforcement of teaching related to seizure prevention and precautions.

Outcome Identification and Planning

The immediate goals for the child during a seizure are preventing aspiration, maintaining an open airway, and preventing injury. Goals for the family include decreasing anxiety and reinforcing teaching to increase knowledge about seizures. With safety in mind, help develop the nursing plan of care according to these goals.

Nursing Care Focus

- Aspiration, ineffective airway clearance risk during seizure related to decreased level of consciousness

Goal

- The child's airway will remain patent throughout the seizure.

Implementations for Preventing Aspiration and Maintaining Airway

When a seizure starts, position the child to one side to prevent aspiration of saliva or vomitus. Loosen any tight clothing, especially around the neck and remove blankets, pillows, or other items that may block the child's airway. Have oxygen and suction equipment readily available for emergency use.

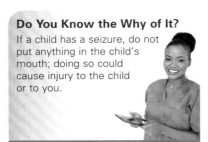

Do You Know the Why of It?

If a child has a seizure, do not put anything in the child's mouth; doing so could cause injury to the child or to you.

Evaluation of Goal/Desired Outcome

- The child's airway is patent with no aspiration of saliva or vomitus.

Nursing Care Focus

- Injury risk related to uncontrolled muscular activity during seizure

Goal

- The child will remain free from injury during the seizure.
- The child's seizure activity is accurately documented.

Implementations for Promoting Safety

Keep the child who has a history of seizures under close observation. The side rails are padded, objects that could cause harm are kept away from the bed, oxygen and suction are kept at the bedside, the side rails are in the raised position, and the bed lowered when the child is sleeping or resting. Do not, however, completely hide the view of the surroundings outside the crib because this could make the child feel isolated.

If the child begins to have a seizure, place the child on their side with the head turned toward one side. Stay calm, remain with the child to protect, but not restrain them. Remove any objects from around the child and protect the

child's head. If the child is not in bed when the seizure starts, move them to a flat surface.

During the seizure, note the following.

- time the seizure started
- what the child was doing when the seizure began
- any factor present just before the seizure (bright light, noise, smell)
- part of the body where seizure activity began
- movement and parts of the body involved
- any cyanosis
- eye position and movement
- incontinence of urine or stool
- time seizure ended
- child's activity after the seizure

When the seizure ends, monitor the child, paying close attention to their level of consciousness, motor functions, and behavior.

Document the seizure completely after the episode, including:

- type of movements (rigidity, jerking, and twitching)
- body parts involved
- duration of seizure
- pulse and respirations
- child's color
- deviant eye movements or other notable signs
- child's description of the aura

Be Sure to Ask!

The child may be able to describe the aura or sensation that occurred just before a seizure.

Evaluation of Goal/Desired Outcome

- The child is free from bruises, abrasions, concussions, or fractures after the seizure.
- The child's seizure activity is appropriately documented.

Nursing Care Focus

- Family caregiver anxiety related to the child's seizure activity

Goal

- The family caregiver anxiety will be reduced.

Implementations for Reducing Family Caregiver Anxiety

A seizure is very frightening to family caregivers. With a calm, confident attitude, reassure family caregivers. Explain that febrile seizures are not uncommon in small children. Reassure caregivers that the health care provider will evaluate the child to determine if the cause of the seizure was nervous system irritation resulting from the high fever or some other possible cause.

Evaluation of Goal/Desired Outcome

The family caregivers:

- verbalize their concerns and relate an understanding of seizures.
- have decreased anxiety.

Nursing Care Focus

- Knowledge deficiency of family caregivers related to seizure prevention and precautions during seizures

Goal

- The family caregivers will verbalize an understanding of seizure prevention and precautions.

Implementations for Reinforcing Family Teaching

Reinforce teaching with family caregivers about seizure precautions so they can handle a seizure that occurs at home. Clarify with them what observations to make during a seizure so they can report these to the health care provider to help in evaluating the child. Explain methods to control fever, cautioning caregivers to avoid using aspirin for fever reduction. Refer to Tips for Reinforcing Family Teaching: Reducing Fever, in Chapter 30, when reinforcing teaching with caregivers.

Evaluation of Goal/Desired Outcome

- The family caregivers state methods to prevent seizures and handle seizures at home.

MENINGITIS

Meningitis is an infection and inflammation of the meninges, which are the protective membranes surrounding the brain and spinal cord. A bacterium or virus causes the infection. Meningitis caused by a virus may be referred to as aseptic meningitis. The symptoms of viral meningitis are similar to those of bacterial meningitis, but usually less severe. Many different viruses can cause the infection, but often the virus enters the body through an infection in the nose or mouth of the child. *Enteroviruses* (EVs) are the most common cause of viral meningitis.

Bacterial meningitis in infancy and childhood is caused by a variety of agents, including *S. pneumoniae* (pneumococcal), group B *Streptococcus, Neisseria meningitides* (meningococcal), and *H. influenzae.* Transmission of the infection varies. For example, meningococcal and *H. influenzae* meningitis are spread by means of droplet infection from an infected person; other forms are contracted by invasion of the meninges via the bloodstream from an infection elsewhere. In addition to standard precautions, droplet transmission precautions should be observed for 24 hours after the start of antimicrobial therapy or until pathogens can no longer be cultured from nasopharyngeal secretions. Since the introduction of the *H. influenzae* type b (Hib) and pneumococcal conjugate vaccines, the incidence of bacterial meningitis has declined in children. Administration of the meningococcal vaccine has decreased the incidence of meningococcal meningitis in adolescents and young adults.

Clinical Manifestations

The onset may be either gradual or abrupt after an upper respiratory or ear infection. Infants with meningitis may have a fever, bulging fontanel (fontanelle), poor sucking and feeding, lethargy, and irritability. Other symptoms seen in children include headache, **nuchal rigidity** (stiff neck), which may progress to **opisthotonos** (arching of the back), positive Kernig and Brudzinski signs (see Fig. 35-8), photophobia, nausea/vomiting, and confusion. Generalized seizures are common in children. Coma may occur early, particularly in the older child. Meningococcal meningitis produces petechiae and a **purpuric rash** (caused by bleeding under the skin), in addition to the other symptoms.

Diagnosis

Early diagnosis and treatment are essential for uncomplicated recovery. A lumbar puncture (spinal tap) is performed promptly whenever symptoms raise a suspicion of meningitis. For accurate results, the procedure is done before antibiotics are administered. Assist by holding the child in the proper position (see Fig. 30-14 in Chapter 30). The spinal fluid pressure is measured to check for increased pressure, and laboratory examination of the fluid reveals increased white blood cells (WBCs) and protein and decreased glucose content. Early in the disease, the spinal fluid may be clear, but it rapidly becomes purulent. The causative organism can usually be determined from a Gram stain of the spinal fluid, enabling specific medication to be started early without waiting for growth of organisms on culture media.

Treatment

The child is initially placed on appropriate transmission-based precautions, and treatment is started using IV administration of antibiotics. Several antibiotics may be used in combination and are chosen for treatment depending on culture and sensitivity studies. The administration of IV steroids is started early in the course of the disease to prevent neurologic complications. Antipyretics are administered to reduce fever and as a comfort measure. If seizures occur, anticonvulsants are given. Later in the disease, medications may be given orally. Treatment continues as long as there is fever or signs of subdural effusion or otitis media.

Subdural effusion may complicate the condition in children during the course of the disease. Fluid accumulates in the subdural space between the dura and the brain. Needle aspiration through the open suture lines in the infant or burr holes in the skull of the older child are used to remove the fluid. Repeated aspirations may be required.

Complications of meningitis with long-term implications are deafness, intellectual disability, seizure disorders, hydrocephalus, and paralysis. The risk of complications is lessened when appropriate treatment is started early in the disease.

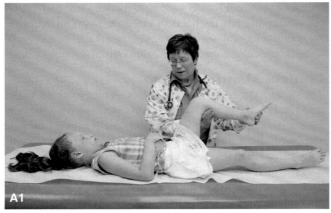
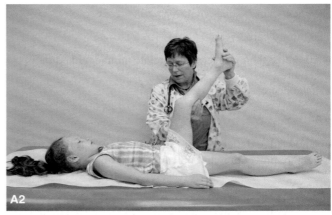
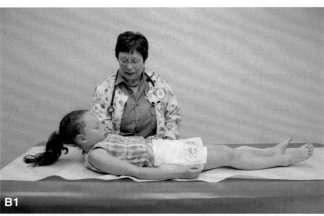
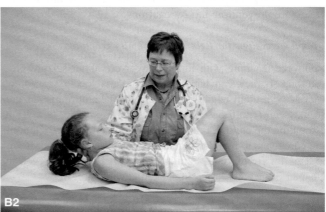

FIGURE 35-8 Kernig and Brudzinski signs indicate irritation of the meninges in a child with meningitis. **A.** Kernig sign is tested by flexing legs at the hips and knee **(A1)**, then extending the knee **(A2)**. A positive report of pain along the vertebral column and/or inability to extend knee is a positive sign and indicates irritation of the meninges. **B.** Brudzinski sign is tested by the child lying supine with the neck flexed **(B1)**. A positive sign occurs if resistance or pain is met. The child may also passively flex hip and knees in reaction, indicating meningeal irritation **(B2)**. (Reprinted with permission from Ricci, S., Kyle T., & Carman, S. (2021). *Maternity and pediatric nursing* (4th ed., Figure 38.14, p. 1360). Wolters Kluwer.)

TEST YOURSELF

✔ What types of seizures are seen in children?

✔ What factors should the nurse document after a seizure?

✔ How can bacterial meningitis be prevented?

Nursing Process and Care Plan *for the Child With Meningitis*

Assessment (Data Collection)

The child with meningitis is extremely sick, and the anxiety level of the family caregivers is understandably high. Be patient and sensitive to their feelings when doing an interview. Obtain a complete history with particular emphasis on the present illness, including any recent upper respiratory infection or middle ear infection. Information on other children in the family and their ages is also important.

Collecting data on the child is usually done after the lumbar puncture is completed and IV fluids and antibiotics are initiated because those procedures take precedence over everything else. Data collection on the child includes obtaining temperature, pulse, and respirations. Use a neurologic evaluation tool to monitor neurologic status, including the child's level of consciousness (see the section on neurologic evaluation in Chapter 28). Examine the infant for a bulging fontanel, and measure the head circumference for a baseline.

Nursing Care Focus

When developing evidence-based nursing care focuses for the child with meningitis, include the risk for injury related to neurologic status and increased intracranial pressure (IICP) and seizure activity. Potential for aspiration, dehydration, and fluid volume excess are considered. Recognize the need for reinforcing family teaching as well as helping the family cope with the anxiety they have related to having an ill child.

Outcome Identification and Planning

The goals for the child with meningitis include monitoring for complications related to neurologic compromise, preventing aspiration, keeping the child safe from injury during a seizure, and monitoring fluid balance. The goals for the family include reinforcing teaching about ways of preventing the transmission of infection and promoting family coping. The nursing care plan includes interventions, such as eliminating the infection by administering antibiotics and observing for signs of IICP.

Nursing Care Focus

- Injury risk related to neurologic status and increased intracranial pressure (IICP)

Goal

- The child will have a normal neurologic status.

Implementations for Monitoring for Complications and Preventing Increased Intracranial Pressure

Closely monitor the child for signs of IICP, including increased head size; headache; bulging fontanel; decreased pulse; vomiting; seizures; increased blood pressure; change in eyes, level of consciousness, or pupil response; and irritability or other behavioral changes. Vital signs require close monitoring. A change in blood pressure, pulse, neurologic signs, or signs of respiratory distress must be reported at once. Measure the infant's head circumference at least every 4 hours to detect complications of subdural effusion or obstructive hydrocephalus. Keep the child's room quiet and darkened to decrease stimulation that may cause seizures. While in the room, speak softly, avoid sudden movements, move quietly, and raise and lower side rails carefully. The head of the bed can be elevated.

Evaluation of Goal/Desired Outcome

The child's:

- neurologic status is stable.
- vital signs are within normal limits.

Nursing Care Focus

- Aspiration, ineffective airway clearance risk related to decreased level of consciousness

Goal

- The child's airway will remain patent and clear.

Implementations for Preventing Aspiration and Keeping Airway Clear

Position the child in a side-lying position with the neck supported for comfort and the head elevated. Remove pillows, blankets, and soft toys that might obstruct the airway. Watch for and remove excessive mucus as much as possible. Use suction sparingly.

Evaluation of Goal/Desired Outcome

The child's:

- position is side-lying with neck supported and head elevated.
- airway remains patent with no aspiration of saliva or vomitus.

Nursing Care Focus

- Injury risk related to seizure activity

Goal

- The child will remain free from injury.

Implementations for Promoting Safety

Keep the child under close observation. Implement seizure precautions and observe the child for seizure activity (see Nursing Process and Care Plan for the Child at Risk for Seizures). At least every 2 hours, monitor vital signs and neurologic signs, and observe for changes in level of consciousness.

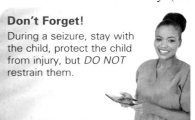

Don't Forget!
During a seizure, stay with the child, protect the child from injury, but *DO NOT* restrain them.

Evaluation of Goal/Desired Outcome

- The child is free from bruises, abrasions, concussions, or fractures during seizure activity.

Nursing Care Focus

- Dehydration risk related to vomiting, fever, and fluid restrictions

Goal

- The child will maintain normal fluid balance and skin turgor.

Implementations for Monitoring and Maintaining Fluid Balance

Fluid balance is an important aspect of this child's care. Strict intake and output measurements are critical. Observe the child's mucous membranes and skin turgor for signs of dehydration. To decrease concerns of dehydration caused by elevated temperature, methods of reducing fever may be used. The child may be kept NPO, especially if they have nausea and vomiting. Administer IV fluids while observing and monitoring the IV infusion site and following safety precautions to maintain the site.

Evaluation of Goal/Desired Outcome

The child's:

- intake and output are within normal limits.
- temperature is 98.6°F to 100°F (37°C to 37.8°C).
- skin turgor and mucous membranes are normal and show no signs of dehydration.

Nursing Care Focus

- Fluid overload risk related to syndrome of inappropriate antidiuretic hormone

Goal

- The child will maintain normal weight and have adequate urinary output.

Implementations for Prevention of Fluid Overload

The infectious process may increase secretion of the antidiuretic hormone produced by the posterior pituitary gland. As a result, the child may not excrete urine adequately, and body fluid volume excess will occur, further emphasizing the need for strict measurement of intake and output. Also, monitor daily weight and electrolyte levels. Signs that must be reported immediately are decreased urinary output, hyponatremia, increased weight, nausea, and irritability. The child is placed on fluid restrictions if these signs occur.

Evaluation of Goal/Desired Outcome

The child's:

- weight and electrolyte levels are within normal limits.
- hourly urine output is 0.5 to 1 mL/kg.

Nursing Care Focus

- Knowledge deficiency of family caregivers related to droplet transmission exposure to others

Goal

- The family caregivers will follow measures to prevent the transmission of bacteria to others.

Implementations for Reinforcing Family Teaching Regarding Spread of Infection

N. meningitides (meningococcal) and *H. influenza* are highly contagious organisms that may spread to other people by means of droplet transmission. Droplet transmission precautions must be maintained for the first 24 hours after antibiotic administration is started. Healthcare staff members and family caregivers must follow proper precautions, including standard transmission precautions. Meticulous handwashing is a key precaution. Other children in the family may need to be examined to determine if they should receive prophylactic antibiotics.

Evaluation of Goal/Desired Outcome

The family caregivers:

- identify measures for preventing the spread of bacteria.
- discuss the need for droplet transmission precautions to be followed.

Nursing Care Focus

- Family caregiver anxiety and coping impairment related to the child's condition and prognosis

Goal

- Family caregiver anxiety will decrease.

Implementations for Decreasing Family Caregiver Anxiety and Promoting Coping

Support family caregivers through every step of the process and encourage them to stay with their child if possible. Their anxiety about procedures, the child's seizures and condition, and the possible complications are all concerns. Family caregivers must be included and made to feel useful. If they are not too apprehensive, help them find small things they can do for their child. Keep them advised about the child's progress at all times.

Evaluation of Goal/Desired Outcome

The family caregivers:

- verbalize understanding of the disease process.
- relate the child's progress throughout the course of treatment.

CEREBRAL PALSY

Cerebral palsy (CP) is a group of disorders arising from a malfunction of motor centers and neural pathways in the brain. It is one of the most complex of the common permanent disabling conditions and often can be accompanied by seizures, intellectual disability, sensory defects, and behavior disorders. Research in this area is directed at adapting biomedical technology to help people with CP cope with the activities of daily living and achieve maximum function and independence.

Causes

Although the cause of CP cannot be identified in many cases, several causes are possible. It may be caused by damage to the parts of the brain that control movement; this damage generally occurs during the fetal or perinatal period, particularly in premature infants.

Common *prenatal* causes are the following:

- Any process that interferes with the oxygen supply to the brain such as separation of the placenta, compression of the cord, or bleeding
- Maternal infection (e.g., cytomegalovirus, toxoplasmosis, rubella)

- Nutritional deficiencies that may affect brain growth
- Acute bilirubin encephalopathy (kernicterus) resulting from Rh incompatibility
- Teratogenic factors, such as drugs and radiation

Common *perinatal* causes are the following:

- Prematurity because immature blood vessels predispose the neonate to cerebral hemorrhage
- Anoxia immediately before, during, and after birth
- Intracranial bleeding
- Asphyxia or interference with respiratory function
- Maternal analgesia (e.g., morphine) that depresses the sensitive neonate's respiratory center
- Birth trauma

About 10% to 20% of cases occur after birth. Common *postnatal* causes are the following:

- Head trauma (e.g., due to a fall, motor vehicle accident)
- Infection (e.g., encephalitis, meningitis)
- Neoplasms
- Cerebrovascular accident

Prevention

Because brain damage in CP is irreversible, prevention is the most important aspect of care. Prevention of CP focuses on the following:

- Prenatal care to improve nutrition, prevent infection, and decrease the incidence of prematurity
- Perinatal monitoring with appropriate interventions to decrease birth trauma
- Postnatal prevention of infection through breast-feeding, improved nutrition, and immunizations
- Protection from trauma of motor vehicle accidents, child abuse, and other childhood accidents

Clinical Manifestations and Types

Difficulty in controlling voluntary muscle movements is one manifestation of the central nervous system damage. Seizures, intellectual disability, hearing and vision impairments, and behavior disorders often accompany the major problem. Delayed gross motor development, abnormal motor performance (e.g., poor sucking and feeding behaviors), abnormal postures, and persistence of primitive reflexes are other signs of CP. Diagnosis of CP seldom occurs before 2 months of age and may be delayed until the second or third year, when the toddler attempts to walk and caregivers notice an obvious lag in motor development. Diagnosis is based on observations of delayed growth and development through a process that rules out other diagnoses.

Several major types of CP occur; each has distinctive clinical manifestations.

Spastic Type

Spastic CP is the most common type and is characterized by the following:

- A hyperactive stretch reflex in associated muscle groups.
- Increased activity of the deep tendon reflexes.

- **Clonus** (rapid involuntary muscle contraction and relaxation).
- Contractures affecting the extensor muscles, especially the heel cord.
- Scissoring caused by severe hip adduction.
- When scissoring is present, the child's legs are crossed and the toes are pointed down (Fig. 35-9).
- When standing, the child is on their toes. It is difficult for this child to walk on the heels or to run.

Athetoid Type (Dyskinetic)

Athetoid CP is marked by involuntary, uncoordinated motion with varying degrees of muscle tension. Children with this disorder are constantly in motion, and the whole body is in a state of slow, writhing muscle contractions whenever voluntary movement is attempted. Facial grimacing, poor swallowing, and tongue movements causing drooling and **dysarthria** (poor speech articulation) are also present. These children are likely to have average or above average intelligence, despite their abnormal appearance. Hearing loss is most common in this group.

Ataxic Type

Ataxia is essentially a lack of coordination caused by disturbances in the kinesthetic and balance senses. The least common type of CP, ataxic CP may not be diagnosed until the child starts to walk; the gait is awkward and wide-based.

Mixed Type

Children with signs of more than one type of CP, termed mixed type, are usually severely disabled. The disorder may have been caused by postnatal injury.

Diagnosis

The birth and family history may help in diagnosing the child with CP. Children with CP may not be diagnosed with certainty until they have difficulties when attempting to walk. They may show signs of intellectual disability, attention deficit disorder, or recurrent seizures. Developmental delays and screening also may give indications of CP. Magnetic resonance imaging (MRI) and a cranial ultrasound, for infants before closure of skull sutures, may be used to help determine the cause of CP.

Treatment and Special Aids

Treatment of CP focuses on helping the child make the best use of residual abilities and achieve maximum satisfaction and enrichment in life. A team of healthcare professionals—health care provider, surgeon, physical therapist, occupational therapist, speech therapist, and a social worker—works with the family to set realistic goals. Medications, such as baclofen, diazepam, and dantrolene, may be used to help relax the muscles and decrease spasticity.

Physical Therapy

Body control needed for purposeful physical activity is learned automatically by a normal child but must be consciously learned by a child who has problems with physical

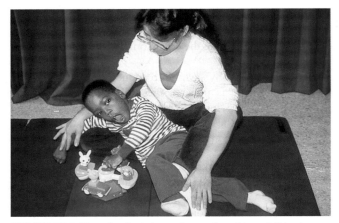

FIGURE 35-9 The physical therapist works with a child who has cerebral palsy. Note the scissoring of the legs.

mobility. Physical therapists attempt to teach activities of daily living that the child with CP has been unable to accomplish. Methods must be suited to the needs of each child, as well as to the general needs arising from the condition. These methods are based on principles of conditioning, relaxation, use of residual patterns, stimulation of contraction and relaxation of antagonistic muscles, and others. Various techniques are used. Because there are many variations in the disabilities caused by CP, each child must be considered individually and treated appropriately.

Orthopedic Management

Braces and other orthopedic devices are used as supportive and control measures to facilitate muscle training, to reinforce weak or paralyzed muscles, or to counteract the pull of antagonistic muscles. Various types are available; each is designed for a specific purpose (Fig. 35-10). Orthopedic surgery is sometimes used to improve function and to correct deformities, such as the release of contractures and the lengthening of tight heel cords.

Technologic Aids for Daily Living

Biomedical engineering, particularly in the field of electronics, has perfected a number of devices to help make the disabled person more functional and less dependent on others. The adaptive devices range from simple items, such as motorized wheelchairs, to completely electronic cottages furnished with voice-activated computer systems that facilitate independence in many areas of living.

A child who has difficulty maintaining balance while sitting may need a high-backed chair with sidepieces and a foot platform. Feeding may be a challenge, so family caregivers may need help finding a method that works for feeding the child. Sometimes controlling and stabilizing the jaw by hand will help with feeding. Feeding aids include spoons with enlarged handles for easy grasping or with bent handles that allow the spoon to be brought easily to the mouth. Plates with high rims and suction devices to prevent slipping enable a child to eat with little assistance. Covered cups set in holders with a hole in the lid to admit a straw help a child

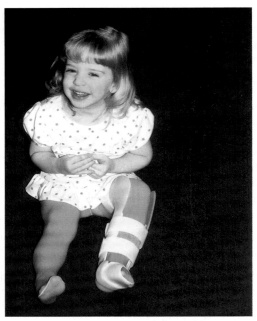

FIGURE 35-10 Ankle–foot braces are being used for this child with cerebral palsy to give support for walking.

who does not have hand control (Fig. 35-11). The severely disabled child may need a nasogastric or gastrostomy tube.

Manual skill can be aided by games that must be manipulated, such as pegboards and cards.

Computer programs have been designed to enable these children to communicate and improve their learning skills. Special keyboards, joysticks, and electronic devices help the child have fun and gain a sense of achievement while learning. Computers also have expanded the opportunities for future employment for these children.

Good News!

Keyboarding is an ego-boosting alternative for a child whose disability is too severe to permit legible writing.

Nursing Care

The child with CP may be seen in the healthcare setting at any age level. Interview and observe the child and the family to determine the child's needs, the level of development, and the stage of family acceptance and to set realistic long-range goals. The child and family facing a new diagnosis may need more guidance and support than the child and family who have been successfully dealing with CP for a long time.

When the child is hospitalized, communicate with the family to learn as much as possible about the child's activities at home. Encourage the child to maintain current self-care activities and set goals for attaining new ones. Positioning to prevent contractures, providing modified feeding utensils, and suggesting appropriate educational play activities are all important aspects of the child's care. If the child has been admitted for surgery, the child and family need appropriate preoperative and postoperative teaching,

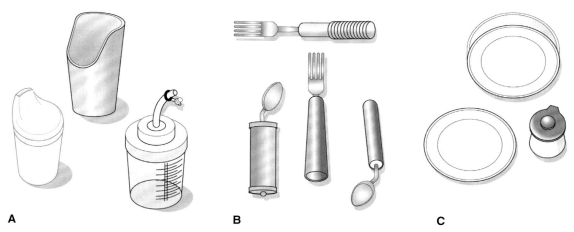

FIGURE 35-11 Feeding aids and devices: **(A)** cups, **(B)** utensils, and **(C)** dishes.

emotional support, and assistance in setting realistic expectations. The family may need help to explore educational opportunities for the child.

Like any chronic condition, CP can become a devastating drain on the family's emotional and financial resources. The child's future depends on many variables: family attitudes; economic and therapeutic resources; the child's intelligence; and the availability of competent, understanding healthcare professionals. Some children, when given the emotional and physical support they need, can achieve a satisfactory degree of independence. Some have been able to attend college and find fulfilling work. Vocational training is also available to an increasing number of these young people. Some people with CP will always need a significant amount of nursing care with the possibility of institutionalized care when their families can no longer care for them.

INTELLECTUAL DISABILITY

Intellectual disability is defined by the American Association on Intellectual and Development Disability (AAIDD) (2020) as a disorder with significant limitations in intellectual functioning (learning, reasoning, problem-solving)—an intelligence quotient (IQ) of 70 or lower, and concurrent deficits in adaptive behavior. Adaptive behavior refers to a person's conceptual skills (language, reading, writing, use of money, time, self-direction); social skills (social responsibility, interpersonal skills, ability to follow rules/obey laws); and practical skills (activities of daily living, occupational skills, healthcare, schedules, routines) expected for their age and cultural group (Pivalizza & Lalani, 2021). The onset occurs before the individual is 18 years of age. Intellectual disabilities often occur in combination with other physical disorders.

Causes

Many factors can cause intellectual disability.
Prenatal causes include the following:

- Inborn errors of metabolism such as phenylketonuria, galactosemia, or congenital hypothyroidism. Damage often can be prevented by early detection and treatment.

- Prenatal infection, such as toxoplasmosis or cytomegalovirus. Microcephaly, hydrocephalus, cerebral palsy (CP), and other brain damage can result from intrauterine infections.
- Teratogenic agents, such as drugs, radiation, and alcohol, can have devastating effects on the central nervous system of a developing fetus.
- Genetic factors—inborn variations of chromosomal patterns—result in a variety of deviations, the most common of which is Down syndrome.

Perinatal causes of intellectual disability include birth trauma, anoxia from various causes, prematurity, and difficult birth. In some instances, prenatal factors may have influenced the perinatal complications.
Postnatal causes include the following:

- Poisoning, such as lead poisoning. Children who develop encephalopathy from chronic lead poisoning usually have significant brain damage.
- Infections and trauma such as meningitis, seizure disorders, and hydrocephalus.
- Impoverished early environment, such as inadequate nutrition and a lack of sensory stimulation. Emotional rejection in early life may do irreparable damage to a child's ability to respond to the environment.

Clinical Manifestations and Diagnosis

A small percentage of children born in the United States have some level of cognitive impairment. About 15% of these are so severely impaired that diagnosis is made at birth or during the first year. Most of the other children are diagnosed when they begin school.

The most common classification of intellectual disability formerly was based on IQ, but IQ is no longer used to classify the severity of intellectual disability. The adaptive impairment and the level of support needed help identify the severity of the disorder. The severity is categorized as mild, moderate, severe, or profound.

The child with mild intellectual disability is a slow learner but can acquire basic skills. The child can learn to read, write, and do arithmetic to a fourth- or fifth-grade level but is slower than average in learning to walk, talk, and feed themselves. The disability may not be obvious to casual acquaintances. With support and guidance, this child usually can develop social and vocational skills adequate for self-maintenance. About 85% of children with intellectual disability are classified in this category.

The child with moderate intellectual disability has little, if any, ability to attain independence and academic skills and is referred to as trainable. Motor development and speech are noticeably delayed, but training in self-help activities is possible. This child may be able to learn repetitive skills in sheltered workshops. Some children may learn to travel alone, but few become capable of assuming complete self-maintenance. About 10% of cases of intellectual disability fall in the moderate category.

The development of the child who has severe intellectual disability is markedly delayed during the first year of life. The child cannot learn academic skills, but may be able to learn some self-care activities if sensorimotor stimulation is begun early. Eventually this child will probably learn to walk and develop some speech; however, a sheltered environment and careful supervision will always be required. About 3% to 4% of children with intellectual disability fall into the severe category.

The child with profound intellectual disability has minimal capacity for functioning and needs continuing care. Eventually the child may learn to walk and develop a primitive speech but will never be able to perform self-care activities. Only about 1% to 2% of children with intellectual disability are in this category.

Treatment and Education

Knowledge about teaching children with cognitive impairment has increased dramatically, and new teaching methods have been yielding encouraging results. People with mild and moderate intellectual disability are taught to perform tasks that enable them to achieve some degree of independence. More and better services are available for all cognitively impaired children and adults.

The child with cognitive impairment may not be identified until well into the preschool stage, because slow development can often be excused in one way or another. The family may be the best judge of the child's development, and healthcare personnel must listen carefully to any concerns or questions that family caregivers express.

When family members are faced with the fact that their child has an intellectual disability, they need to go through a grieving process, as do family members of any other child with a serious disorder. They need to mourn the loss of the normal child that was expected and resolve to give this child the best opportunities to develop their potential.

Early diagnosis and intervention are important. Tests done during infancy are difficult to administer, and the results are inaccurate, but they may provide the family with some idea about the child's potential. The family must be aware that these are only predictions based on unreliable test data.

The child is often kept at home in the supportive family environment where the child can relate closely to a few people whose role is to stimulate and encourage maximum development and learning. The individual attention, security, and sense of belonging to a family are important factors in every child's growth and development. In the United States, federal legislation supports services to provide early intervention and special education for children with intellectual disabilities. These programs focus on individual needs and abilities.

Nursing Process and Care Plan *for the Child With Intellectual Disability or Cognitive Impairment*

Assessment (Data Collection)

The child who has an intellectual disability or a cognitive impairment is seen in the healthcare setting for diagnosis, treatment, and follow-up, as well as the usual health maintenance visits. During these visits, communicating with the child may be a challenge. A thorough interview with the child's family caregiver can be helpful in learning about the child and family. Listen carefully to the caregiver, paying particular attention to any comments or concerns they have.

The process of data collection may be lengthy and detailed, depending partially on the circumstances of the child's primary need for healthcare. An unhurried atmosphere avoids placing undue stress on the child or the family. Aside from the data collection needed as dictated by the current healthcare needs, also collect information about the child's habits, routines, and personal terminology (such as nicknames and toileting terms). Be careful to communicate at the child's level of understanding, do not talk down to the child, and treat the child with respect. This approach helps gain cooperation from both the family and the child.

Nursing Care Focus

When determining the focus of nursing care for the child with intellectual disability or cognitive impairment, growth and development concerns, deficits related to activities of daily living, preventing injury, and impaired communication issues are addressed. The family may have concerns related to compromised coping skills and social isolation.

Outcome Identification and Planning

The major goals for the cognitively impaired child depend entirely on the child's abilities as determined during data collection and the interview. Common goals include promoting growth and development to reach the highest level of functioning (within the child's ability), promoting self-care (within the child's ability), fostering communication, and preventing injury. Goals for the family include promoting family coping and preventing social isolation.

Nursing Care Focus

- Growth and development concerns related to physical and intellectual disability

Goal

- The child will attain the milestones of their stage of growth and development according to mental age.
- The family caregivers verbalize an understanding of the child's level of development.

Implementations for Promoting Growth and Development

The child with cognitive impairment often has physical disabilities that affect growth and development. All but the most profoundly impaired children go through the sequence of normal development with delays at each stage; their abilities level off as the children reach the limits of their capabilities. A cognitively impaired child proceeds according to mental age, rather than chronologic age. Thus, an impaired 6-year-old child may be functioning on a mental level of 2 years, and the expected behavior must be essentially that of a 2-year-old child. Reinforce teaching with the family caregivers about the important landmarks of normal growth and development to help them understand the progressive nature of maturation and to improve planning for the child.

Environmental stimulation is essential for development in all children, but the cognitively impaired child needs much more environmental enrichment than does the average child. Suggested activities for providing this enrichment are summarized in Table 35-2.

Whether at home or in a healthcare facility, the child with cognitive impairment needs to know which behaviors are acceptable and which are unacceptable. Discipline is as important to this child as to any other. The limited ability of these children to adapt to varying circumstances makes consistent discipline essential, with instructions given in simple, direct, concise language. Using a positive approach with many examples and demonstrations achieves better results than a constant stream of "don't touch" or "stop that."

Obedience is an important part of discipline, especially for the child with decreased reasoning ability, but the objectives of discipline should be much broader than simply obedience. The child needs to know what to expect and finds security and support in routines and consistency. Use kindness, love, understanding, and physical comforting as a major part of discipline.

If discipline is needed, be certain it follows the misdeed immediately so that the cause-and-effect relationship is clear. Taking the child away from the group for a short time may help restore self-control. If the child is using misbehavior to get attention, praise and approval for good behavior may eliminate the need for wrongdoing.

Evaluation of Goal/Desired Outcome

- The child attains the highest level of functioning for their mental age.

- Family caregivers identify the child's developmental level and set realistic goals.

Nursing Care Focus

- Activities of daily living (ADL) deficit (bathing, dressing, feeding, and toileting) related to cognitive or neuromuscular impairment (or both)

Goal

- The child will develop skills to meet self-care needs within their ability.

Implementations for Promoting Self-Care

Instructing the child with intellectual disability can be time-consuming, frustrating, challenging, and rewarding. When the child is first seen in a healthcare setting, a teaching program that reflects their developmental level must be designed. Be certain that all personnel who care for the child and any involved family members are aware of the program. Break each element of care to be taught into small segments and repeat those steps over and over.

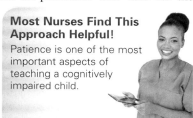

Most Nurses Find This Approach Helpful!

Patience is one of the most important aspects of teaching a cognitively impaired child.

Use praise generously, and give small material rewards as useful tools to aid in teaching. Challenge the child, but make the immediate small goals realistic and attainable. Brushing teeth, brushing or combing the hair, bathing, washing the hands and face, feeding oneself, dressing independently, and basic safety are all self-care areas in which the child needs instruction and positive reinforcement.

Instructing the cognitively impaired child requires the same principles used in teaching any child: Work at a level appropriate to the stage of the child's maturation, not the chronologic age. If the child has physical disabilities in addition to intellectual disability, the rate of physical development is also affected. One factor that makes the child with cognitive impairment different from the average child is the lack of ability to reason abstractly. This prevents transfer of learning or application of abstract principles to varied situations. Learning takes place by habit formation and emphasizing the "three R's": routine, repetition, and relaxation. Most cognitively impaired children increase in mental age, although slowly and to a limited level. Therefore, each child needs to be watched for evidence of readiness for a new skill.

Evaluation of Goal/Desired Outcome

- The child practices basic hygiene habits, as well as dressing/grooming, feeding, and toileting skills within their abilities with support and supervision.

TABLE 35-2 Examples of Developmental Stimulation and Sensorimotor Teaching for Infants and Young Children With Intellectual Disability

DEVELOPMENTAL SEQUENCE	POSSIBLE ACTIVITIES TO ENCOURAGE DEVELOPMENT
Sitting 1. Sit with support in caregiver's lap 2. Sit independently when propped 3. Sit with increasingly less support 4. Sit in chair without assistance 5. Sit without support	Hold child in sitting position on lap, supporting under armpits. Do several times a day, gradually lessening the support. Place child in sitting position against firm surface with pillow behind the back and on either side. Let the child sit this way several times a day. Allow child to sit on equipment that provides increasingly less support such as baby swing, feeder, walker, high chair. Place child in a chair with arms. Provide balance support at first, and then gradually withdraw. Leave for 10 minutes at a time. Place child on floor. Gradually withdraw assistance.
Self-Feeding 1. Sucking 2. Drink from a cup 3. Grasp piece of food and place in mouth 4. Transfer food from spoon to mouth 5. Scoop up food and transfer to mouth	Encourage child to suck by putting food on pacifier, putting a drop on tongue, and so forth. Put small amount of fluid in a baby cup. Raise cup to mouth by placing hands under the child's hand. Place bit of favorite food in child's hand. Guide hand and food to mouth. Gradually reduce support. Move spoon to child's mouth with hand supporting baby's mouth. Gradually reduce support. Have child hold spoon by handle, scoop up food, and transfer to mouth. Do not allow child to use fingers. Progress from bowl to flat plate.
Stimulation of Touch 1. Body sensation 2. Explore environment through touch 3. Explore environment through mouth 4. Explore tactile sensations 5. Explore with water	Hold, cuddle, rock child. Brush skin with objects of various textures (feathers, silk, sandpaper). Place objects of different textures near child. Move hand to object. Give child objects that can be chewed. Guide hand to mouth at first. Expose child to hard, soft, warm, and cold objects. Place hands or feet in water.

Nursing Care Focus

- Verbal communication impairment related to impaired receptive or expressive skills

Goal

- The child's communication skills will improve.

Implementations for Fostering Communication Skills

The child with cognitive impairment often has major problems with language skills. The child may have problems forming various speech sounds because of an enlarged tongue or other physical deviations, including hearing impairment. These problems can frustrate attempts at communication. In addition, the child may not be able to process the spoken word, which compounds communication problems. A speech therapist can evaluate the child and develop a program to help caregivers work with the child to improve both the child's understanding of what is said and the child's ability to use language.

Evaluation of Goal/Desired Outcome

- The child can communicate basic needs to healthcare staff and family caregivers.

Nursing Care Focus

- Injury risk related to physical or neurologic impairment (or both)

Goal

- The child will be free from injury and will learn basic safety rules.

Implementations for Preventing Injury

The child with cognitive impairment has faulty reasoning ability and a short attention span. As a result, the caregivers must be responsible for protecting the child. The healthcare facility and the home must be made safe. Teach elementary safety rules and reinforce them continuously.

Evaluation of Goal/Desired Outcome

- The child remains free from injury and cooperates with basic safety rules within their abilities.

Nursing Care Focus

- Family caregiver coping impairment related to emotional stress or grief

Goal

- The family caregiver will effectively cope with the child's diagnosis.

Implementations for Promoting Family Coping

Before effective treatment can begin, the family caregiver needs to acknowledge the reality of the child's situation and be willing to accept the difficult task of helping the child develop to their full potential. Diagnosis made at birth or during the first year affords the greatest hope of early acceptance and beginning education and training.

The family caregiver's first reaction to learning that the child may have cognitive impairment is grief because this is not the anticipated child of their dreams. A parent may feel shame, assuming that they cannot produce a perfect child. Some rejection of the child is almost inevitable, at least in the initial stages, but this must be worked through for the family to cope. Some family caregivers compensate for their early hostile feelings by overprotection or overconcern, making the child unnecessarily helpless and perhaps taking out their anger and frustration on the normal siblings. The family begins to function effectively only when the family caregivers accept the child as another family member to be helped, loved, and disciplined.

Evaluation of Goal/Desired Outcome

The family caregiver:

- verbalizes feelings and mourns the loss of the "perfect child."
- provides appropriate care to help the child reach optimum functioning.

Nursing Care Focus

- Psychosocial needs related to a risk of social isolation (family or child) associated with fear of and embarrassment about the child's behavior or appearance

Goal

- The family will interact with social groups and support networks.

Implementations for Preventing Social Isolation

Family members need to know that their feelings are normal. Talking with other families of impaired children can offer some of the best support and guidance, as family caregivers seek information to help them deal with the situation. One group that includes both families and healthcare professionals is the Arc (for people with intellectual and developmental disabilities), a volunteer organization with chapters in many communities (www.thearc.org). The National Down Syndrome Society is another excellent resource for the family of a child with Down syndrome (www.ndss.org). Participating in the Special Olympics is a good way for the child to begin to gain self-confidence.

 A Personal Glimpse

The mother of a developmentally delayed child knows her child has a problem before any doctor notices. Visually my son looked perfect. There were no outward signs of disability. He was a beautiful baby but he was often ill— severe croup, pneumonia, bronchitis, grand mal seizures because of fever, hospital stays, EEGs, spinal taps, tests and more tests—but he always bounced back, much better than his parents recovered.

Slowly, I started to notice that he was not the same as other kids of his age. His vocabulary was Mom and DaDa when other 3-year-olds were starting to put words together into little sentences. Everyone said he didn't talk because I spoiled him and got him everything he needed before he asked for it. I would try to believe people, including doctors, who would say, "Don't worry; you are just being an overprotective mother. Your son will be fine." You try to hide from the truth, but slowly you realize you have to get others to see what you see. You have to get help for your child—someone has to listen to you.

Finally, I forced my pediatrician to try some physical dexterity tests. My son failed these tests. I heard the doctor say the words that broke my heart: "I am sorry. I thought you were just another hysterical mother—but there is something wrong with your child. We must schedule him for more testing." Then I cried.

Patricia

Learning Opportunity: *What are some feelings parents of children diagnosed with intellectual disability might have? What are some ways that the nurse can support the mother and the child in the above situation?*

Evaluation of Goal/Desired Outcome

The family:

- freely voices feelings and concerns about the child and makes contact with support systems.
- establishes relationships with families of other cognitively impaired children.

TEST YOURSELF

- ✔ What is the difference between the five types of cerebral palsy (CP)?
- ✔ What is the most common way to classify intellectual disability?
- ✔ What is usually seen in the growth and development of a child with cognitive impairment?

BRAIN TUMORS

Brain tumors can be benign or malignant in nature. They are the second most common type of cancer seen in children and adolescents. The cause of most brain tumors is not known. Brain tumors, even if not malignant, can cause neurologic effects that can have long-term concerns. The prognosis for the child depends on the type, location, ability to remove the tumor, and the treatment that is done. Brain tumors can have signs and symptoms due to local invasion of tissues, compression of structures around the tumor, causing increased intracranial pressure (IICP), or by causing obstruction of the flow of cerebrospinal fluid. Tumors on the surface of the brain are easier to remove and treat than tumors that are deeper in the brain.

Clinical Manifestations and Diagnosis

The clinical manifestations of brain tumors may be subtle and nonspecific and vary with the child's age and the location of the tumor. In the infant or young child the cranial sutures are not fused and allow for increased pressure without necessarily showing neurologic changes which might indicate IICP. A large head, bulging fontanels, and irritability are symptoms often seen in the infant.

Nausea and vomiting are common in all ages. Other symptoms seen in older children include headache, impaired vision, visual disturbances such as diplopia (double vision), **nystagmus** (involuntary, rhythmic movements of the eyes), **papilledema** (swelling of the optic disc), abnormal gait, poor coordination, head tilting, and seizures. Changes in behavior or school performance, sleep disturbances, and growth impairment also may be indicative of brain tumors.

Magnetic resonance imaging (MRI) or computed tomography (CT) are used to identify brain tumors. To diagnose the type of tumor, tissue samples are taken and examined to identify cells that indicate certain tumor types. A lumbar puncture may be done to analyze the cerebrospinal fluid.

Treatment and Nursing Care

The tumor is removed and radiation, as well as chemotherapy, may be used as treatment. Radiation therapy is not usually done in children younger than 3 years. Chemotherapy is used depending on the type of tumor and the child's age. Anticonvulsant therapy is indicated for children who have tumors that cause the child to have seizures.

Nursing care prior to and after surgery to remove the tumor includes closely monitoring the child and preventing increased intracranial pressure (IICP). When the child undergoes chemotherapy treatment, it is important to offer support and encouragement while the child adjusts to the difficult course and effects of chemotherapy, such as hair loss, nausea, and vomiting. Reinforcing family teaching is ongoing throughout the entire process. Survival after diagnosis and treatment of a brain tumor varies considerably, depending on the age of the child and the type of tumor.

HEAD TRAUMA

Head trauma is a broad term used to describe head injuries that include any kind of distress to the scalp, skull, or brain, such as fractures, concussions, bleeding, or bruises. Serious injuries called **traumatic brain injury (TBI)** affect the brain. TBI can be mild, moderate, or severe in nature.

 TIPS FOR REINFORCING FAMILY TEACHING

Sports Concussion

Any sports injury can potentially cause a sports concussion. Preventing injuries is important, but should the child be hit on the head or any part of the body, the child should be monitored closely for the possibility of a sports concussion. Signs and symptoms need to be evaluated by a health care provider. The health care provider will determine when it is safe for the child to return to sports activities.

Prevention

- Wear good fitting, sport-appropriate headgear and safety equipment.
- Avoid dangerous play by using good technique, developing skills, and following rules.

If Child Is Hit or Head Is Injured

- The child should stop playing or participating in activity immediately.

- Remove the child from situation to avoid a second head injury.
- Monitor the child closely and provide medical care when needed.

Signs and Symptoms of Concussion (Can Happen Immediately or Hours, Days After Injury)

- Headache, vision changes, confusion
- Dizziness, trouble with balance or walking
- Nausea, vomiting
- Difficulty concentrating, thinking, memory loss
- Feeling sleepy, sleeping too much, unable to fall sleep
- Slurred speech, trouble talking, saying things that do not make sense
- Feeling anxious, irritable, behavior or mood changes
- Sensitive to noise or light

The Glasgow Coma Scale score (see Chapter 28) is used to classify the severity of a TBI. Head injuries are a significant cause of serious injury or death in children of all ages. The primary cause of a head injury varies with the child's age. Toddlers and young children may receive a head injury from a fall or child abuse; school-aged children usually experience such an injury as a result of a bicycling, inline skating, skiing, or motor vehicle accident. Adolescent injuries are often related to a motor vehicle accident or a sports-related head injury (sometimes referred to as a sports concussion). A sports concussion is a mild traumatic brain injury and occurs when an athlete has had a forceful contact to the face, neck, or another part of the body which jolts the head. Sports concussions are seen more frequently in athletes who play high impact sports such as football, hockey, soccer, and lacrosse (see Tips for Reinforcing Family Teaching: Sports Concussion).

Children, especially young children, seem to receive many head trauma injuries. Fortunately, most of them are not serious, but they are often frightening to the family caregiver. If a scalp laceration is involved, the caregiver may be quite alarmed by the amount of bleeding because of the large blood supply to the head and scalp. The caregiver can apply an ice pack and pressure until the bleeding is controlled. Applying ice cubes in a zip-closure sandwich bag wrapped in a washcloth works well at home. An open wound should be cleaned with soap and water and a sterile dressing applied. For an injury without a break in the skin, the caregiver can apply ice for an hour or so to decrease the amount of swelling.

The family caregiver should observe the child for at least 6 hours for vomiting or a change in the child's level of consciousness. If the child falls asleep, they should be awakened every 1 to 2 hours to determine that the level of consciousness has not changed. No analgesics or sedatives should be administered during this period of observation. The child's pupils are checked for reaction to light every 4 hours for 48 hours. The caregiver should notify the health care provider immediately if the child vomits more than three times, has pupillary changes, has double or blurred vision, has a change in level of consciousness, acts strange or confused, has trouble walking, or has a headache that becomes more severe or wakes them from sleep; these instructions should be provided in written form to the family caregiver.

Family caregivers are wise to take the child to a healthcare facility to have the injury evaluated if they have any doubt about its seriousness. Traumatic brain injury can occur with any head injury. Complications of head injuries can include hemorrhage, hypoxia, cerebral edema, and increased intracranial pressure (IICP). These conditions often require the child or adolescent to be cared for in a pediatric neurologic or intensive care unit.

The child is monitored closely for any signs of change in their neurologic status, using tools such as the Glasgow Coma Scale, so concerns can be detected and treated immediately.

Abusive head trauma is seen in children who are victims of child maltreatment and physical abuse. When head trauma is inflicted, injuries such as retinal hemorrhage and intracranial hemorrhage (subdural, subarachnoid, epidural) may lead to severe traumatic brain injury and even death of the child. One form of abusive head trauma is referred to as shaken baby syndrome, a form of abuse that can cause head injury without external signs of head trauma. Child maltreatment and abuse is discussed in Chapter 33.

DROWNING

Drowning is the second leading cause of accidental death in children. Toddlers and older adolescents have the highest actual rate of death from drowning. Drowning in children often occurs when the child has been left unattended in a body of water. Infants more commonly drown in a bathtub; toddlers and preschool-aged children drown in pools or small bodies of water. A pail of water may become something for the toddler to investigate, which could lead to accidental death. Many drowning deaths in this age group occur in home pools, including spas, hot tubs, and whirlpools. Drowning in older children often occurs because the child is playing or acting in an unsafe manner.

A responsible adult must continuously supervise all infants and young children when they are near any source of water. Older children and adolescents should not play alone around any body of water. Swimming in undesignated swimming areas, such as creeks, quarries, and rivers, is especially hazardous for older children and adolescents.

When a drowning victim of any age is discovered, cardiopulmonary resuscitation (CPR) should be started immediately and continued until the victim can be transported to a medical facility for additional care. Intensive care is carried out according to the client's needs. All adults who care for children in any capacity must learn CPR and be ready to perform it immediately (Table 35-3 and Fig. 35-12).

Think back to **Chesa Andres** from the beginning of the chapter. As Chesa's nurse, what will you do for her if she has a seizure? What will you observe for? What will you document? What teaching will you reinforce with her family caregivers?

TABLE 35-3 Summary of Basic Life Support Maneuvers in Infants and Children

MANEUVER	INFANT (<1 YEAR)	CHILD (1–8 YEARS)
Activate		
Emergency response system (lone rescuer)	For sudden, witnessed collapse, activate EMS after verifying that victim is unresponsive, obtain AED, begin CPR Unwitnessed, perform 2 minutes of CPR (five cycles), activate EMS, obtain AED	For sudden, witnessed collapse, activate EMS after verifying that victim is unresponsive, obtain AED, begin CPR Unwitnessed, perform 2 minutes of CPR, activate EMS, obtain AED
Circulation		
Pulse check (≤10 seconds)	Brachial	Carotid/femoral
Compression landmarks	Just below nipple line	Center of chest, between nipples
Compression method (push hard and fast; allow complete recoil)	One rescuer: Two fingers Two rescuers: Two thumb-encircling hands	Two hands: Heel of one hand with second on top or One hand: Heel of one hand only
Compression depth	Approximately 1/3 to 1/2 the depth of the chest	Approximately 1/3 to 1/2 the depth of the chest
Compression rate	Approximately 100/minute	Approximately 100/minute
Compression–ventilation ratio	30:2 (single rescuer) 15:2 (two rescuers)	30:2 (single rescuer) 15:2 (two rescuers)
Airway		
	Head tilt-chin lift (unless trauma present) Jaw thrust (if suspected trauma)	Head tilt-chin lift (unless trauma present) Jaw thrust (if suspected trauma)
Breaths		
Initial	Two effective breaths at 1 second/breath	Two effective breaths at 1 second/breath
Rescue breathing without chest compressions	12–20 breaths/minutes (approximately one breath every 3–5 seconds)	12–20 breaths/minutes (approximately one breath every 3–5 seconds)
Rescue breaths for CPR with advanced airway	8–10 breaths/minutes (approximately one breath every 6–8 seconds)	8–10 breaths/minutes (approximately one breath every 6–8 seconds)
Foreign-body airway obstruction	Back slaps and chest thrusts	Abdominal thrusts
Defibrillation		
AED	Manual defibrillator preferred If not available, use AED with a pediatric attenuator or standard AED	Use AED with a pediatric attenuator If not available use standard AED

AED, automated external defibrillator; CPR, cardiopulmonary resuscitation; EMS, emergency medical services.
Adapted from Ralston, M. E. (2021). *Pediatric basic life support for health care providers*. UpToDate. Retrieved May 2, 2021 from https://www.uptodate.com/contents/pediatric-basic-life-support-for-health-care-providers

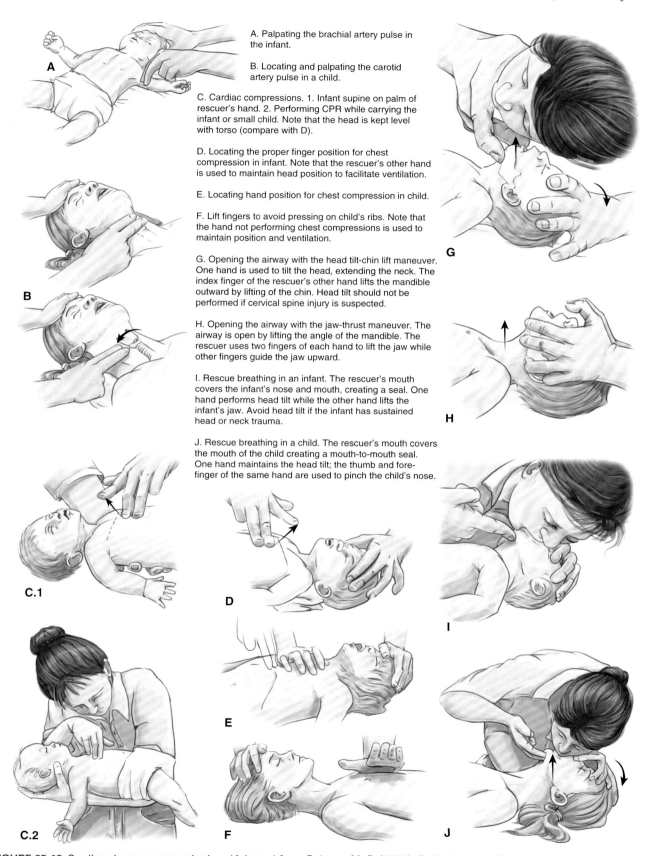

A. Palpating the brachial artery pulse in the infant.

B. Locating and palpating the carotid artery pulse in a child.

C. Cardiac compressions. 1. Infant supine on palm of rescuer's hand. 2. Performing CPR while carrying the infant or small child. Note that the head is kept level with torso (compare with D).

D. Locating the proper finger position for chest compression in infant. Note that the rescuer's other hand is used to maintain head position to facilitate ventilation.

E. Locating hand position for chest compression in child.

F. Lift fingers to avoid pressing on child's ribs. Note that the hand not performing chest compressions is used to maintain position and ventilation.

G. Opening the airway with the head tilt-chin lift maneuver. One hand is used to tilt the head, extending the neck. The index finger of the rescuer's other hand lifts the mandible outward by lifting of the chin. Head tilt should not be performed if cervical spine injury is suspected.

H. Opening the airway with the jaw-thrust maneuver. The airway is open by lifting the angle of the mandible. The rescuer uses two fingers of each hand to lift the jaw while other fingers guide the jaw upward.

I. Rescue breathing in an infant. The rescuer's mouth covers the infant's nose and mouth, creating a seal. One hand performs head tilt while the other hand lifts the infant's jaw. Avoid head tilt if the infant has sustained head or neck trauma.

J. Rescue breathing in a child. The rescuer's mouth covers the mouth of the child creating a mouth-to-mouth seal. One hand maintains the head tilt; the thumb and fore-finger of the same hand are used to pinch the child's nose.

FIGURE 35-12 Cardiopulmonary resuscitation. (Adapted from Ralston, M. E. (2021). *Pediatric basic life support for health care providers.* UpToDate. Retrieved May 2, 2021, from https://www.uptodate.com/contents/pediatric-basic-life-support-for-health-care-providers.)

KEY POINTS

- At birth, the nervous system is immature. As the child grows, the quality of the nerve impulses sent through the nervous system develops and matures, allowing for the development of gross and fine motor skills.

- Visual acuity of children gradually increases from birth until about 7 years of age, when most children have 20/20 vision. Hearing in children is acute, and the infant will respond to sounds within the first month of life.

- Vision impairment includes myopia (nearsightedness), hyperopia (farsightedness), astigmatism, partial sight, or blindness. Adequate vision and normal development are more likely with early treatment. Specialized equipment helps prevent isolation.

- Cataracts, glaucoma, and strabismus may be detected and treated, sometimes surgically, during childhood. Eye injuries and infections are common. Bacterial conjunctivitis is treated with ophthalmic antibacterial agents such as erythromycin, bacitracin, sulfacetamide, and polymyxin.

- Types of hearing loss and the treatment depend on the part of the ear or brain that is affected. A child who is hard of hearing has a loss of hearing but is able to learn speech and language. A child who is deaf has no hearing ability.

- The child with acute otitis media is usually restless, shakes the head, and rubs or pulls at the ear. The child may also have fever, irritability, decreased activity, lack of appetite, and hearing impairment. Antibiotics or a myringotomy, incision of the eardrum with tiny tubes placed in the tympanic membrane, is used to treat otitis media.

- Reye syndrome usually occurs after a viral infection. The child has severe vomiting, irritability, lethargy, confusion, and disorientation. The disease can progress rapidly. Supportive measures are used to treat the disease.

- Nursing care for the child at high risk for seizures includes monitoring for complications, such as signs of increased intracranial pressure (IICP), as well as preventing aspiration, keeping the child safe, monitoring intake and output, and supporting the child's family.

- A focal onset seizure begins on one side or hemisphere of the brain. Focal onset aware seizures (formerly called simple partial seizures) can either have motor or sensory symptoms. A focal onset motor seizure causes a localized motor activity such as shaking of an arm, leg, or other body part. A focal onset sensory seizure may include sensory symptoms called an aura, which signals an impending attack. Focal onset impaired awareness seizures (formerly called complex partial seizure) begin in a small area of the brain and cause confusion and a lack of awareness. The child is unable to respond normally to external stimuli. Nonpurposeful movements and repetitive actions without apparent reason are sometimes seen.

- In generalized onset seizures both sides or hemispheres of the brain are affected at the same time. Tonic–clonic seizures consist of four stages. In the prodromal period, the child may be drowsy or dizzy. An aura is a warning and occurs immediately before the seizure. During the tonic phase, the muscles contract and the extremities stiffen. The initial rigidity of the tonic phase changes to generalized jerking muscle movements in the clonic phase. The jerking movements gradually diminish and then disappear. Sleep usually occurs during the postictal stage.

- In absence seizures, there is loss of awareness, the child stares straight ahead, may have eye blinking or twitching, but does not fall. After the seizure, the child is alert and continues conversation. Atonic seizures cause a sudden momentary loss of consciousness, muscle tone, and postural control, and the child may fall. In myoclonic seizures, there is a sudden jerking of a muscle or group of muscles, often in the arms or legs. Infantile spasms usually indicate a cerebral defect and consist of muscle contractions and rolling of the eyes.

- Status epilepticus describes a seizure that lasts longer than 30 minutes or a series of seizures, in which the child does not return to a normal level of consciousness. Drug therapy is used to stop and control the seizure activity.

- Meningitis is an infection and inflammation of the meninges, the protective membranes surrounding the brain and spinal cord, caused by a bacterium or virus and spread by droplet transmission. Symptoms may include fever, bulging fontanel, poor sucking and feeding, lethargy, irritability, headache, nuchal rigidity, photophobia, nausea/vomiting, confusion, and seizures. Treatment includes administration of antibiotics and use of steroids to decrease the incidence of complications such as deafness, intellectual disability, seizure disorders, hydrocephalus, and paralysis.

- Cerebral palsy (CP) is a group of disorders arising from a malfunction of motor centers and neural pathways in the brain, often accompanied by seizures, intellectual disability, sensory defects, and behavior disorders.

- Prenatal causes of CP include oxygen deprivation, maternal infection, nutritional deficiencies, Rh incompatibility, and teratogenic agents, such as drugs and radiation. Perinatal causes include anoxia, intracranial bleeding, asphyxia, maternal analgesia, trauma, and prematurity. Postnatal head trauma, infection, neoplasms, or cerebrovascular accident can also cause CP.

- Spastic-type CP is characterized by a hyperactive stretch reflex in associated muscle groups; increased activity of the deep tendon reflexes; clonus; contractures of the extensor muscles, especially the heel cord; and scissoring caused by hip adduction. Athetoid (dyskinetic) type CP is marked by involuntary, uncoordinated motion with muscle tension; the child is in constant motion. Ataxic CP is a lack of coordination caused by disturbances in the kinesthetic and balance senses.

- Healthcare professionals involved in the care of the child with CP include a physical therapist, as well as individuals who specialize in orthopedic and technologic aids to help in activities of daily living.

- Prenatal causes of intellectual disability include inborn errors of metabolism; prenatal infection; teratogenic agents, such as drugs, radiation, and alcohol; and genetic factors. Birth trauma, anoxia, prematurity, and difficult birth are perinatal causes. Postnatal causes include poisoning, such as lead poisoning, infections, trauma, inadequate nutrition, and a lack of sensory stimulation.

- Promoting self-care, fostering communication, promoting growth and development to reach the highest level of functioning (within the child's ability), and preventing injury are the goals when working with cognitively impaired children.

- Brain tumors are a common type of cancer seen in children and adolescents. They can be benign or malignant. Clinical manifestations in infants may include a large head, bulging fontanels, and irritability. Other symptoms may be nausea, vomiting, headache, impaired vision, visual disturbances, abnormal gait, poor coordination, head tilting, and seizures. Changes in behavior or school performance, sleep disturbances, and growth impairment also may be indicative of brain tumors. Treatment is often removal of the tumor, as well as radiation and chemotherapy. Closely monitoring the child, preventing increased intracranial pressure (IICP), and reinforcing teaching are important nursing responsibilities. Prognosis depends largely on the age of the child and the type of tumor.

- Head trauma and head injuries are a significant cause of serious injury or death in children of all ages. Toddlers and young children may receive a head injury from a fall or child abuse; school-aged children usually experience such an injury as a result of a bicycling, inline skating, skiing, or motor vehicle accident. Adolescent injuries are often related to a motor vehicle accident or a sports-related head injury (sometimes referred to as a sports concussion). Serious injuries called traumatic brain injury (TBI) affect the brain. TBI can be mild, moderate, or severe in nature. The child with any head trauma is monitored closely and any change in the child is reported immediately.

- Drowning is the second leading cause of accidental death in children. Toddlers and older adolescents have the highest actual rate of death from drowning. Drowning in children often occurs when the child has been left unattended in a body of water. Cardiopulmonary resuscitation (CPR) should be started immediately when a drowning victim is discovered.

INTERNET RESOURCES

Epilepsy
www.efa.org

Febrile Seizures
https://www.ninds.nih.gov/Disorders/Patient-Caregiver-Education/
Fact-Sheets/Febrile-Seizures-Fact-Sheet

Hearing Loss
http://www.jtc.org/

Intellectual Disability
www.aamr.org

Otitis Media
www.nidcd.nih.gov/health/hearing

Reye Syndrome
www.reyessyndrome.org

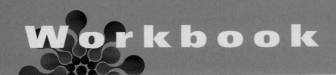

NCLEX-STYLE REVIEW QUESTIONS

1. If a child has a febrile seizure, what is the *highest* priority for the nurse?
   a. Document the child's behavior during the seizure.
   b. Instruct the caregivers about fever reduction methods.
   c. Protect the child during the seizure activity.
   d. Reassure the caregivers that seizures are common.

2. After discussing ways to lower a fever with the caregiver of an infant, the caregiver makes the following statements. Which statement requires further teaching?
   a. "I won't give my child baby aspirin when she has a fever."
   b. "I know I need to dress my baby lightly if she has a fever."
   c. "When my baby has a fever, I will sponge her in cool water for 20 minutes."
   d. "I need to recheck my baby's temperature until it is below 101."

3. The nurse admits a child with a diagnosis of meningitis. The child is being monitored for signs of increased intracranial pressure (IICP). Which would *most* likely be seen in the child with IICP?
   a. Headache, stiff neck
   b. Itching, swelling around eyes
   c. Weight gain or loss
   d. Decreased head size, sunken fontanel

4. The nurse has admitted a 6-year-old child who has received a diagnosis of a seizure disorder and has frequent tonic–clonic seizures. Which are characteristics of tonic–clonic seizures? Select all that apply.
   a. The seizure activity might be preceded by a sight, sound, taste, or smell.
   b. The seizure activity is usually limited to one side of the body.
   c. The seizure activity involves a phase in which the muscles are rigid.
   d. The seizure activity causes memory loss and staring.
   e. The seizure activity involves a phase in which there are jerking muscle movements.
   f. The seizure activity often is followed by a loss of control of bowel and bladder.

5. The nurse has admitted a 9-year-old child who is blind. Which actions would be important for the nurse to implement? Select all that apply.
   a. Identify self when entering the room.
   b. Quietly walk out of the room when they leave.
   c. Involve the child in activities with younger children.
   d. Encourage the child to be as independent as possible.
   e. Provide the child with only finger foods.
   f. Encourage self-feeding after orienting the child to the plate.

STUDY ACTIVITIES

1. Research your community for financial resources, supplies and equipment, and support groups available to children and families with the following disorders. Complete the following table and share the information with your peers.

Condition	Financial Resources	Supplies and Equipment	Support Groups
Vision impairment			
Hearing impairment			
Cerebral palsy			
Intellectual disability			

2. Create a poster or teaching aid to be used in instructing family caregivers of children who have seizure disorders. Include safety precautions, what to do when a child has a seizure and after the seizure, and medication considerations.

3. Perform a home eye test on a child you have contact with. Use the instructions on the website https://www.aao.org/eye-health/tips-prevention/home-eye-test-children-adults from the Tips for Reinforcing Family Teaching: Home Eye Test for Children in this chapter.
   a. Ask a family member, friend or neighborhood child for permission to perform the eye test.
   b. Gather the needed supplies and follow the steps outlined on how to do the test. Write down the results you get regarding the child's vision.
   c. What did you discover? Does this child appear to have any vision concerns? What suggestions might you give the family caregiver of this child?

CRITICAL THINKING: WHAT WOULD YOU DO?

1. Four-year-old Todd is blind. You are the nurse helping with his care. He is going to have surgery and will be hospitalized for 3 to 4 days.
   a. What will you do to orient him to the pediatric unit?
   b. What things will you talk to him about and do to prepare him for his hospital stay?
   c. What age-appropriate activities will you offer to him before and after surgery?

2. You are caring for 10-year-old Missy, who has a mild hearing impairment. She and her father have returned to the pediatric clinic for a follow-up visit.
   a. What information do you need to ask Missy's father that will help you in communicating with Missy?
   b. What will you do to adapt your nursing care to improve your communication with her?

3. You and your friend are working with a group of children with physical limitations. One of the children has cerebral palsy. Your friend asks you if cerebral palsy is inherited and if it can be prevented.
   a. What explanation will you give your friend regarding the causes of cerebral palsy?
   b. How will you answer the question regarding whether cerebral palsy can be prevented?
   c. What will you tell your friend about the types of cerebral palsy that children might have?

4. Dosage calculation: An infant with a diagnosis of otitis media is being treated with amoxicillin. The child weighs 13.2 lb. The usual dosage of this medication is 40 mg/kg per day in divided doses every 8 hours. Answer the following:
   a. How many kilograms does the child weigh?
   b. How much amoxicillin will be given in a 24-hour time period?
   c. How many milligrams per dose will be given?
   d. How many doses will the child receive in a day?

5. Dosage calculation: A school-aged child with a diagnosis of a seizure disorder is being treated with phenytoin. The child weighs 58 lb. The child is being given a dose of 6 mg/kg a day in three divided doses. Answer the following:
   a. How many kilograms does the child weigh?
   b. How many milligrams of phenytoin will the child receive in a 24-hour period of time?
   c. How many milligrams of phenytoin will the child receive in each dose?
   d. If the dose is increased by 20 mg a dose, how many milligrams will then be in each dose?
   e. How many milligrams will the child receive in a 24-hour period, after the dose has been increased?

36

The Child With a Respiratory Disorder

Key Terms

achylia
adenoids
circumoral
coryza
croup
dysphagia
hypochylia
metered-dose inhaler (MDI)
nebulizer
steatorrhea
stridor
teratogenicity
tonsils
wheezing

Learning Objectives

At the conclusion of this chapter, you will:

1. Discuss ways the infant's and child's respiratory system differs from the adult's system.
2. Name the most common complication of acute nasopharyngitis.
3. Discuss nursing care of the child with allergic rhinitis.
4. Discuss nursing care of the child with tonsillitis and adenoiditis.
5. Explain the most common complication of a tonsillectomy, and list the signs requiring observation.
6. Compare the croup syndrome disorders, including (a) spasmodic laryngitis, (b) acute laryngotracheobronchitis, and (c) epiglottitis.
7. Discuss the symptoms, diagnosis, and treatment of acute bronchiolitis/respiratory syncytial virus (RSV) infection.
8. Describe asthma, including (a) factors that can trigger an asthma attack, (b) the physiologic response that occurs in the respiratory tract during an asthma attack, (c) treatment, and (d) nursing care.
9. Explain the diagnosis of pneumonia including the treatment and nursing care.
10. Identify the basic defect and organs affected by cystic fibrosis, along with diagnostic procedures.
11. Name the most common type of complication in cystic fibrosis, and describe the dietary and pulmonary treatments of the disorder.
12. Discuss how tuberculosis is detected and treated.

Casey Wilson was diagnosed with asthma (reactive airway disease) when he was 4 years old. The asthma has been well controlled on medications. Casey's eighth birthday is next week, the day after Thanksgiving. Casey is now in the emergency department after awakening from his sleep having difficulty breathing; he is having an acute asthma attack.

Respiratory disorders in infants and children are common. They range from mild to serious, even life-threatening. They can be acute or chronic in nature. Sometimes these problems require hospitalization, which interrupts development of the child–family relationship and the child's patterns of sleeping, eating, and stimulation. Although

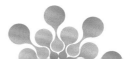

the illness might be acute, if recovery is rapid and the hospitalization brief, the child will probably experience few, if any, long-term effects. However, if the condition is chronic or so serious that it requires long-term care, both child and family may suffer serious consequences.

GROWTH AND DEVELOPMENT OF THE RESPIRATORY SYSTEM

The respiratory system is made up of the nose, pharynx, larynx, trachea, epiglottis, bronchi, bronchioles, and the lungs. These structures are involved in the exchange of oxygen and carbon dioxide and the distribution of the oxygen to the body cells. Tiny, thin-walled sacs called alveoli are responsible for distributing air into the bloodstream. It is also through the alveoli that carbon dioxide is removed from the bloodstream and exhaled through the respiratory system. The structures and organs found in the respiratory system cleanse, warm, and humidify the air that enters the body.

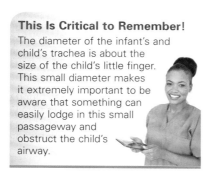

This Is Critical to Remember!
The diameter of the infant's and child's trachea is about the size of the child's little finger. This small diameter makes it extremely important to be aware that something can easily lodge in this small passageway and obstruct the child's airway.

Respiratory problems occur more often and with greater severity in infants and children than in adults because of their immature body defenses and small, undeveloped anatomic structures. The respiratory tract grows and changes until the child is about 12 years of age. During the first 5 years, the child's airway increases in length but not in diameter.

Infants and young children have larger tongues in proportion to their mouths, shorter necks, and narrower airways, and the structures are closer together. This leads to the possibility of respiratory obstruction, especially if there is edema, swelling, or increased mucus in the airways. The ability to breathe through the mouth when the nose is blocked is not automatic but develops as the child's neurologic development increases.

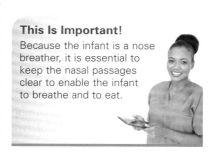

This Is Important!
Because the infant is a nose breather, it is essential to keep the nasal passages clear to enable the infant to breathe and to eat.

The tonsillar tissue is enlarged in the early school-age child, but the pharynx, which contains the tonsils, is still small, so the possibility of obstruction of the upper airway is more likely. In children older than 2 years, the right bronchus is shorter, wider, and more vertical than the left.

Infants use the diaphragm and abdominal muscles to breathe. Beginning at about age 2 to 3 years, the child starts using the thoracic muscles to breathe. The change from using abdominal to using thoracic muscles for respiration is

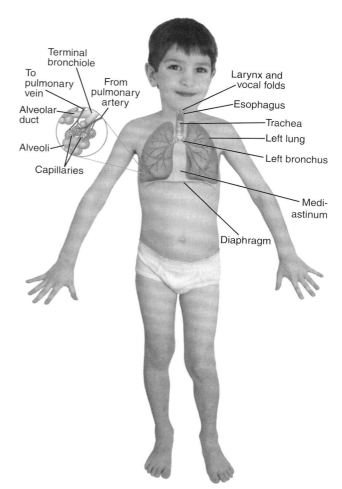

FIGURE 36-1 Anatomy of the child's respiratory tract.

completed by the age of 7 years. Because accessory muscle's are used for breathing, weakness of these muscles can cause respiratory failure (Fig. 36-1).

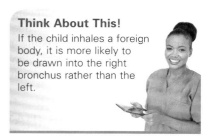

Think About This!
If the child inhales a foreign body, it is more likely to be drawn into the right bronchus rather than the left.

ACUTE NASOPHARYNGITIS (COMMON COLD)

The common cold is one of the most common infectious conditions of childhood. The young infant is as susceptible as the older child but generally is not exposed as frequently.

The illness is of viral origin such as rhinoviruses, coronaviruses, coxsackievirus, respiratory syncytial virus (RSV), influenza virus, parainfluenza virus, or adenovirus. Bacterial invasion of the tissues might cause complications such as ear, mastoid, and lung infections. The child appears to be more susceptible to complications than is an adult. The infant should be protected from people who have colds because complications in the infant can be serious.

Prevention of the common cold includes frequent hand-washing and not touching the mouth, nose, and eyes.

Clinical Manifestations

The infant usually develops fever early in the course of the infection, often as high as 102°F to 104°F (38.9°C to 40°C). The congested nasal passages can interfere with feeding, increasing the infant's irritability and fussiness. The older child has nasal congestion and discharge with sneezing and coughing. Because the older child can mouth breathe, nasal congestion is not as great a concern as in the infant. Fever is less common in the older child. Headache, decreased appetite, and difficulty sleeping may occur.

Diagnosis

This nasopharyngeal condition might appear as the first symptom of many childhood diseases and must be observed carefully. The common cold also needs to be differentiated from allergic rhinitis. Complications that may arise from the common cold include otitis media and sinusitis.

 Concept Mastery Alert

The nasal secretions associated with allergic rhinitis are clear and watery.

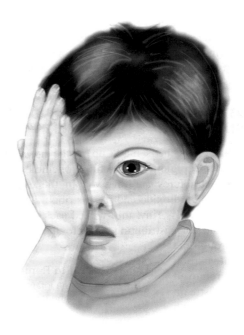

FIGURE 36-2 Back pressure to blood circulation around the eyes leads to dark areas under the eyes in the child with allergic rhinitis. The child pushes the nose upward in the "allergic salute" to relieve itching and open the airway.

Treatment and Nursing Care

The child with an uncomplicated cold may not need any treatment in addition to rest, increased fluids and adequate nutrition, normal saline nose drops, suction with a bulb syringe, and a cool-mist humidified environment. Acetaminophen or ibuprofen may be administered as an analgesic and antipyretic. Aspirin should not be used because of the concern of developing Reye syndrome (see Chapter 35 for discussion of Reye syndrome). If the nares or upper lip become irritated, cold cream or petrolatum (Vaseline) can be used. The child needs to be comforted by holding, rocking, and soothing. If the symptoms persist for several days, the child must be seen by a health care provider to rule out complications, such as otitis media.

ALLERGIC RHINITIS (HAY FEVER)

Allergic rhinitis in children is most often caused by sensitization to animal dander, house dust, pollens, and molds. Pollen allergy seldom appears before 4 or 5 years of age.

Clinical Manifestations

A watery nasal discharge, postnasal drip, sneezing, and allergic conjunctivitis are the usual symptoms of allergic rhinitis. Continued sniffing, itching of the nose and palate, and the "allergic salute," in which the child pushes their nose upward and backward to relieve itching and open the air passages in the nose, are common complaints. Because of congestion in the nose, there is backpressure to the blood circulation around the eyes, and dark circles are visible under the eyes (Fig. 36-2). Headaches are common in older children.

Treatment and Nursing Care

When possible, offending allergens are avoided or removed from the environment. Antihistamines and decongestants can be helpful for some children. Hyposensitization can be implemented, particularly if antihistamines are not helpful or are needed chronically. Reinforce teaching with the family caregivers about the importance of avoiding allergens and administering antihistamines to decrease symptoms.

TONSILLITIS AND ADENOIDITIS

Tonsillitis is a common illness in childhood resulting from pharyngitis. A brief description of the location and functions of the tonsils and adenoids serves as an introduction to the discussion of their infection and medical and surgical treatments.

A ring of lymphoid tissue encircles the pharynx, forming a protective barrier against upper respiratory infection. This ring consists of groups of lymphoid tonsils, including the faucial, the commonly known **tonsils**; pharyngeal, known as the **adenoids**; and lingual tonsils. Lymphoid tissue normally enlarges progressively in childhood between the ages of 2 and 10 years and shrinks during preadolescence. If the tissue itself becomes a site of acute or chronic infection, it may become hypertrophied and can interfere with breathing and swallowing, cause partial deafness, or become a source of infection in itself.

Clinical Manifestations and Diagnosis

The child with tonsillitis may have a fever of 101°F (38.4°C) or more; a sore throat, often with **dysphagia** (difficulty swallowing); hypertrophied tonsils; halitosis; and erythema of the soft palate. Exudate may be visible on the tonsils. The symptoms vary somewhat with the causative organism. Throat cultures are performed to diagnose tonsillitis and the causative organism. Frequently the cause of tonsillitis is viral, although β-hemolytic streptococcal infection may also be the cause.

Treatment and Nursing Care

Medical treatment of tonsillitis consists of administration of analgesics for pain, antipyretics for fever, and an antibiotic in the case of streptococcal infection.

Here's a Pharmacology Fact!

A standard 10-day course of antibiotics is often recommended for the treatment of tonsillitis. Stress the importance of completing the full prescription of antibiotic to ensure that the streptococcal infection is eliminated.

Reinforce with family caregivers that a soft or liquid diet is easier for the child to swallow, and to encourage the child to maintain good fluid intake. A cool-mist vaporizer may be used to ease respirations.

Tonsillectomies and adenoidectomies are controversial. One can be performed independent of the other, but they are often done together. No conclusive evidence has been found that a tonsillectomy in itself improves a child's health by reducing the number of respiratory infections, increasing the appetite, or improving general well-being. Currently, tonsillectomies are generally not performed unless other measures are ineffective or the tonsils are so hypertrophied that breathing and eating are difficult. If the child has obstructive sleep apnea, a tonsillectomy and adenoidectomy are often the treatment. Tonsillectomies are not performed while the tonsils are infected. The adenoids are more susceptible to chronic infection. An indication for adenoidectomy is hypertrophy of the tissue to the extent of impairing hearing or interfering with breathing. Performing only an adenoidectomy if the tonsil tissue appears to be healthy is an increasingly common practice. Tonsillectomy is postponed until after the age of 4 or 5 years, except in the rare instance when it appears it is urgently needed. Often when a child has reached the acceptable age, the apparent need for the tonsillectomy has disappeared.

Nursing Process and Care Plan *for the Child Having a Tonsillectomy*

Assessment (Data Collection)

Much of the preoperative preparation, such as complete blood count, bleeding and clotting time, and urinalysis, is done on a preadmission outpatient basis. In many facilities, the child is admitted on the day of surgery or the procedure is done in a day surgery setting. Psychological preparation is often accomplished through preadmission orientation.

Acting out the forthcoming experience, particularly in a group, with the use of puppets, dolls, and play-doctor or play-nurse material helps the child develop security. The amount and the timing of preparation before admission depend on the child's age. The child may become frightened about losing a body part. Telling the child that the troublesome tonsils are going to be "fixed" is a much better choice than saying that they are going to be "taken out." Include the child and the family caregiver in the admission interview. Ask about any bleeding tendencies because postoperative bleeding is a concern. Carefully explain all procedures to the child, and be sensitive to the child's apprehension. Take and record vital signs to establish a baseline for postoperative monitoring. The temperature is an important part of the data collection to determine that the child has no upper respiratory infection. Observe the child for loose teeth that could cause a problem during administration of anesthesia, and document findings.

Nursing Care Focus

When determining the focus of nursing care for the child having a tonsillectomy, consider that the child is at risk for aspiration, pain, and dehydration following the procedure. Recognize the need for reinforcing family caregiver teaching related to home care after discharge and signs and symptoms of complications.

Outcome Identification and Planning

The major postoperative goals for the child include preventing aspiration; relieving pain, especially while swallowing; and improving fluid intake. The major goal for the family is to increase knowledge and understanding of post discharge care and possible complications. Design the plan of care with these goals in mind.

Nursing Care Focus

- Aspiration risk related to impaired swallowing and bleeding at the operative site

Goal

- The child will not aspirate and the airway will remain clear after surgery.

Implementations for Preventing Postoperative Aspiration

Immediately after a tonsillectomy, place the child in a partially prone position with head turned to one side until the child is completely awake. This position can be accomplished by turning the child partially over and by flexing the knee where the child is not resting to help maintain the position. Keeping the head slightly lower than the chest helps facilitate drainage of secretions. Avoid placing pillows under the chest and abdomen, which may hamper respiration. Encourage the child to expectorate all secretions, and place an ample supply of tissues and a waste container near them. Discourage the child from coughing.

Check vital signs every 10 to 15 minutes until the child is fully awake, and then check every 30 minutes to an hour. Note the child's preoperative baseline vital signs to interpret the vital signs correctly. Hemorrhage is the most common complication of a tonsillectomy. Bleeding is most often a concern within the first 24 hours after surgery and the fifth to seventh postoperative day. During the 24 hours after surgery, observe, document, and report any unusual restlessness or anxiety, frequent swallowing, or rapid pulse that may indicate bleeding. Vomiting dark, old blood may be expected, but bright, red-flecked emesis or oozing indicates fresh bleeding. Observe the pharynx with a flashlight each time vital signs are checked. Bleeding can occur when the clots dissolve between the fifth and seventh postoperative days if new tissue is not yet present. Because the child is cared for at home by this time, give the family caregivers information concerning signs and symptoms for which to watch.

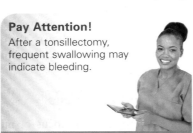

Pay Attention!
After a tonsillectomy, frequent swallowing may indicate bleeding.

Evaluation of Goal/Desired Outcome

The child:

- shows signs of an open and clear airway.
- expectorates saliva and drainage with no aspiration.

Nursing Care Focus

- Acute pain related to surgical procedure

Goal

- The child will show signs of being comfortable.

Implementations for Providing Comfort and Relieving Pain

Apply an ice collar postoperatively; however, remove the collar if the child is uncomfortable with it. Administer pain medication as ordered. Liquid acetaminophen is often prescribed. Rectal or intravenous analgesic medications may be given. Opioid analgesic medications may be used for pain unrelieved by other analgesic medications. Encourage the family caregiver to remain at the bedside to provide soothing reassurance. Crying irritates the raw throat and increases the child's discomfort; thus, it should be avoided if possible. Reinforce with the family caregiver what may be expected in drainage and signs that should be reported immediately to the nursing staff.

Evaluation of Goal/Desired Outcome

The child:

- rests quietly and does not cry.
- exhibits pulse rate that is regular and normal for their age.
- states that pain is lessened.

Nursing Care Focus

- Dehydration risk related to inadequate oral intake secondary to painful swallowing

Goal

- The child's fluid intake will be adequate for their age.

Implementations for Encouraging Fluid Intake

When the child is fully awake from surgery, give small amounts of clear fluids or ice chips. Decreasing discomfort by administering pain medications may encourage the child to increase fluid intake. Synthetic juices, carbonated beverages that are "flat," and frozen juice popsicles are good choices.

Avoid irritating liquids, such as orange juice and lemonade. Milk and ice cream products tend to cling to the surgical site and make swallowing more difficult; thus, they are poor choices, despite the old tradition of offering ice cream after a tonsillectomy. Continue administration of intravenous fluid and record intake and output until adequate oral intake is established.

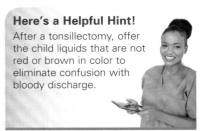

Here's a Helpful Hint!
After a tonsillectomy, offer the child liquids that are not red or brown in color to eliminate confusion with bloody discharge.

Evaluation of Goal/Desired Outcome

The child's:

- skin turgor is good.
- mucous membranes are moist.
- hourly urinary output is at least 0.5 to 1 mL/kg.
- parenteral fluids are maintained until oral fluid intake is adequate.

Nursing Care Focus

- Knowledge deficiency of family caregivers related to understanding of post discharge home care and signs and symptoms of complications

Goal

- Family caregivers will verbalize an understanding of post discharge care.

Implementations for Reinforcing Family Teaching

The child is typically discharged on the day of or the day after surgery if no complications are present. Instruct the family caregiver to keep the child relatively quiet for a few days after discharge. Recommend giving soft foods and nonirritating liquids for the first few days. Reinforce with family members that if at any time after the surgery they note any signs of hemorrhage (bright red bleeding, frequent swallowing, restlessness), they should notify the health care provider. Provide written instructions and telephone numbers before discharge. Advise the caregivers that a mild earache may be expected about the third day.

Evaluation of Goal/Desired Outcome

The family caregivers:

- give appropriate responses when questioned about care at home.
- verbalize signs and symptoms of complications.
- ask appropriate questions for clarification.

CROUP SYNDROMES

Croup is not a disease, but a group of disorders typically involving a barking cough, hoarseness, and inspiratory **stridor** (shrill, harsh respiratory sound). The disorders are named for the respiratory structures involved. Acute laryngotracheobronchitis, for instance, affects the larynx, the trachea, and the major bronchi.

Spasmodic Laryngitis

Spasmodic laryngitis occurs in children between ages 6 months and 3 years. The cause is undetermined; it may be of infectious or allergic origin, but certain children seem to develop severe laryngospasm with little, if any, apparent cause.

Clinical Manifestations and Diagnosis

The attack may be preceded by **coryza** (runny nose) and hoarseness or by no apparent signs of respiratory irregularity during the evening. The child awakens after a few hours of sleep with a barklike cough, increasing respiratory difficulty, and stridor. The child becomes anxious, restless, and markedly hoarse. A low-grade fever and mild upper respiratory infection may be present.

This condition is not serious but is frightening both to the child and to the family. The episode subsides after a few hours; little evidence remains the next day when an anxious family caregiver takes the child to the health care provider. Attacks frequently occur 2 or 3 nights in succession.

Treatment and Nursing Care

Humidified air is helpful in reducing laryngospasm. Cool-mist or humidifiers that produce mist at room temperature may be used in the child's bedroom to provide high humidity. Humidifiers must be cleaned regularly to prevent the growth of undesirable organisms. Sometimes the spasm is relieved by

Good News!

Although frightening to the child and the family, spasmodic laryngitis is not serious and can often be lessened quickly by taking the child into the bathroom, shutting the door, and turning on the hot water tap. This fills the room with steam or humidified air and relieves the child's symptoms.

exposure to cold air—when, for instance, the child is taken out into the night to go to the emergency department or to see the health care provider.

It is important to explain which symptoms can be treated at home (hoarseness, croupy cough, and inspiratory stridor) and which symptoms might indicate a more serious condition in which the child needs to be seen by the health care provider (continuous stridor, use of accessory muscles, labored breathing, lower-rib retractions, restlessness, pallor, and rapid respirations). The family must be aware that recurrence of these conditions may occur.

Acute Laryngotracheobronchitis

Laryngeal infections are common in small children, and they often involve tracheobronchial areas as well. Acute laryngotracheobronchitis (bacterial tracheitis or laryngotracheobronchitis) may progress rapidly and become a serious problem within a matter of hours. The toddler is the most frequently affected age group. This condition is usually of viral origin, but bacterial invasion, usually staphylococcal, may follow and cause a secondary infection. It generally occurs after an upper respiratory infection with fairly mild rhinitis and pharyngitis.

Clinical Manifestations and Diagnosis

The child develops hoarseness and a barking cough with a fever that may reach 102.2°F (39°C). As the disease progresses, marked laryngeal edema and inspiratory stridor occurs, and the child's breathing becomes difficult, the pulse is rapid, and cyanosis may appear. Acute respiratory distress can result.

Treatment and Nursing Care

The major goal of treatment for acute laryngotracheobronchitis is to maintain an airway and adequate air exchange. Corticosteroids are administered to decrease airway edema and inflammation. The child is placed in a humidified air atmosphere and oxygen may be administered to maintain oxygen saturation levels at 92% or above. To achieve bronchodilation, racemic or nebulized epinephrine may be administered, usually by a respiratory therapist. Nebulization often produces rapid relief because it causes vasoconstriction. However, the child requires careful observation for the reappearance of symptoms. If necessary, intubation with an endotracheal tube may be performed for a child with severe distress unrelieved by other measures. Antibiotic medications are administered if a secondary bacterial infection occurs.

Close and careful observation of the child is important. Observation includes checking the pulse, respirations, and color; listening for hoarseness and stridor; and noting any restlessness that may indicate an impending respiratory crisis. Pulse oximetry is used to determine the degree of hypoxia.

Epiglottitis

Epiglottitis is acute inflammation of the epiglottis (the cartilaginous flap that protects the opening of the larynx).

Previously the most common cause of epiglottitis was *Haemophilus influenzae* type B, but since the Hib conjugate vaccine is now given routinely, more often it is caused by other bacterium. The epiglottis becomes inflamed and swollen with edema. The edema decreases the ability of the epiglottis to move freely, which results in blockage of the airway and creates an emergency.

Clinical Manifestations and Diagnosis

The child may have been well or may have had a mild upper respiratory infection before the sudden onset of a severe sore throat, dysphagia (difficulty swallowing), and a high fever of 102.2°F to 104°F (39°C to 40°C). The dysphagia causes drooling which is a sign of significant concern. The child is very anxious, is restless, and prefers to breathe by sitting up and leaning forward with the mouth open and the tongue out. This is called the "tripod" position (Fig. 36-3). Immediate emergency attention is necessary.

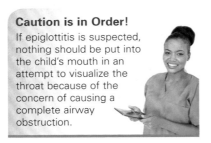

Caution is in Order!
If epiglottitis is suspected, nothing should be put into the child's mouth in an attempt to visualize the throat because of the concern of causing a complete airway obstruction.

Treatment and Nursing Care

Keep the child as calm as possible and avoid procedures likely to be upsetting or cause crying, which could lead to airway obstruction, until the child's airway is secure. Humidified oxygen is given if the airway is patent. The child may need endotracheal intubation or a tracheostomy if intubation cannot be performed because the epiglottis is swollen. Pulse oximetry is used to monitor oxygen

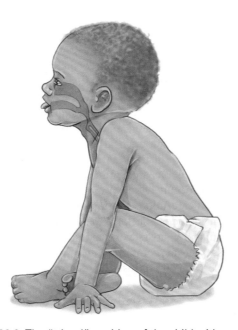

FIGURE 36-3 The "tripod" position of the child with epiglottitis.

saturation levels. Antibiotic medications are administered intravenously. Antibiotic therapy is usually continued for 10 days. This condition is not common and it is extremely frightening for the child and the family.

ACUTE BRONCHIOLITIS/RESPIRATORY SYNCYTIAL VIRUS INFECTION

Acute bronchiolitis (acute interstitial pneumonia) is most common during the first 6 months of life. Most cases occur in infants who have been in contact with older children or adults with upper respiratory viral infections. It usually occurs in the winter and early spring.

Acute bronchiolitis is caused by a viral infection. The causative agent in most cases has been shown to be respiratory syncytial virus (RSV). Other viruses associated with the disease are parainfluenza virus, adenoviruses, coronavirus, and other viruses not always identified.

The bronchi and bronchioles become plugged with thick, viscid mucus, causing air to be trapped in the lungs. The child can breathe air in but has difficulty expelling it. This hinders the exchange of gases, and cyanosis appears.

Clinical Manifestations

The onset of dyspnea is abrupt, sometimes preceded by a cough or nasal discharge. Manifestations include a persistent cough, respiratory distress including increased respiratory rate, nasal flaring, air hunger, and often marked cyanosis. Suprasternal and subcostal retractions are present. The chest becomes barrel-shaped from the trapped air. Respirations are 60 to 80 breaths per minute.

Fever is not extreme, seldom higher than 101°F to 102°F (38.3°C to 38.9°C). Dehydration may become a serious factor because of increased fluid needs and decreased oral intake. The infant appears apprehensive, irritable, and restless.

Diagnosis

Diagnosis is made from clinical findings and can be confirmed by laboratory testing of the mucus obtained by direct nasal aspiration or nasopharyngeal washing.

Treatment and Nursing Care

The child is usually hospitalized and treated with supportive care including nasal suctioning, rest, and increased fluids. Humidified oxygen may be administered via a nasal cannula, facemask, or an oxyhood (a clear plastic hood placed over the infant's head) if needed. Monitoring of oxygenation may be done by means of pulse oximetry or capillary blood gases. Antibiotics are not prescribed because the causative organism is a virus. Intravenous fluids are often administered to ensure an adequate intake and to permit the infant to rest. The hospitalized child is placed on contact and droplet transmission precautions to prevent the spread of infection.

Ribavirin is an antiviral drug that may be used to treat certain children with RSV. It is usually administered as an inhalant. The American Academy of Pediatrics states that the use of ribavirin must be limited to children who are immunocompromised and at high risk for severe or complicated RSV. Ribavirin is classified as a category X drug, signifying a high risk for **teratogenicity** (causing damage to a fetus). Healthcare personnel and others may inhale the mist that escapes into the room, so care must be taken when the drug is administered.

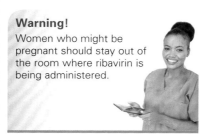

Warning!
Women who might be pregnant should stay out of the room where ribavirin is being administered.

TEST YOURSELF

✔ What is the most common complication after a tonsillectomy? During what two time periods is bleeding a concern after a tonsillectomy? Explain the reasons these time periods are a concern for bleeding.

✔ What is a fast and effective way to reduce laryngospasm for the child with croup?

✔ What is a complication often seen in the infant with a respiratory infection?

✔ What is the causative agent in many cases of bronchiolitis?

ASTHMA

Asthma is a spasm of the bronchial tubes caused by hypersensitivity of the airways in the bronchial system. When the child comes in contact with a trigger, inflammation occurs in the airways. Spasms of the smooth muscles cause the lumina of the bronchi and bronchioles to narrow. Edema of the mucous membranes lining these bronchial branches and increased production of thick mucus within them combine with the spasm to cause the airways to become narrowed and respiratory obstruction occurs (Fig. 36-4). Asthma is also sometimes referred to as reactive airway disease. This reversible obstructive airway disease affects millions of people in the United States, including 8.3% of all children in the United States.

Asthma attacks are often triggered by a hypersensitive response to allergens. In young children, asthma may be a response to certain foods including chocolate, milk, eggs, nuts, grains, or food additives. Asthma may be triggered by exercise, exposure to cold weather, irritants like wood-burning stoves, cigarette smoke, dust, pet dander, and fragrances or strong odors. Infections, such as bronchitis and upper respiratory infection, can provoke asthma attacks. In children with asthmatic tendencies, emotional stress or anxiety can trigger an attack. Some children with asthma may have no evidence of an immunologic cause for the symptoms.

Asthma can be either intermittent, with extended periods when the child has no symptoms and does not need medication, or chronic, with the need for frequent or continuous therapy. Chronic asthma affects the child's school attendance, academic performance, and general activities and may contribute to poor self-confidence and dependency.

Clinical Manifestations

The onset of an attack is usually slow over several days, but can occur suddenly with little warning. The attack is evidenced by a dry hacking cough, **wheezing** (a high-pitched sound of expired air being pushed through narrowed or obstructed airways), and difficulty breathing. Asthma attacks often occur at night and awaken the child from sleep. The child must sit up and is totally preoccupied with efforts to breathe. Attacks might last for only a short time, or might continue for several days. Thick, tenacious mucus might be coughed up or vomited after a coughing episode. In some asthmatic clients, coughing is the major symptom, and wheezing occurs rarely if at all. Many children no longer have symptoms after puberty, but this is not predictable. Other allergies may develop in adulthood.

Diagnosis

The history and physical examination are of primary importance in diagnosing asthma. When observing the child's breathing, dyspnea, use of accessory muscles, and labored

FIGURE 36-4 Note airway edema, mucus production, and bronchospasm occurring with asthma.

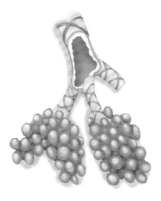

Normal airway

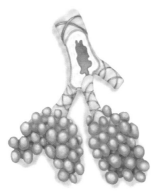

Airway with inflammation

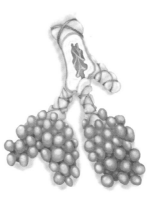

Airway with inflammation, bronchospasm, and mucus production

breathing may be noted, especially on expiration. When listening to the child's lung sounds (auscultation), the examiner hears wheezing, which is often generalized over all lung fields. Mucus production may be profuse. Pulmonary function tests and spirometry measurements are valuable diagnostic tools and indicate the amount of obstruction in the bronchial airways, especially in the smallest airways of the lungs. A definitive diagnosis of asthma is made when the obstruction in the airways is reversed with bronchodilators.

Treatment

Children and their families must be taught to recognize the symptoms that lead to an acute attack so they can be treated as early as possible. These symptoms include chest tightness, respiratory retractions, wheezing, shortness of breath, and an increased amount of coughing at night, in the early morning, or with activity. Use of a peak flow meter is an objective way to measure airway obstruction, and children as young as 4 or 5 years of age can be taught to use one (see Tips for Reinforcing Family Teaching: How to Use a Peak Flow Meter and Fig. 36-5).

A peak flow diary should be maintained and can also include symptoms, exacerbations, actions taken, and outcomes. Families must make every effort to eliminate any possible allergens from the home and to decrease or control asthma triggers for the child.

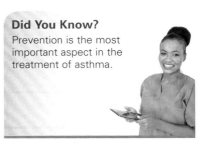

Did You Know?

Prevention is the most important aspect in the treatment of asthma.

TIPS FOR REINFORCING FAMILY TEACHING

How to Use a Peak Flow Meter

Your child cannot feel early changes in the airway. By the time the child feels tightness in the chest or starts to wheeze, they are already far into an asthma episode. The most reliable early sign of an asthma episode is a drop in the child's peak expiratory flow rate, or the ability to breathe out quickly, which can be measured by a peak flow meter. Almost every asthmatic child older than 4 years can and should learn to use a peak flow meter (Figs. A and B).

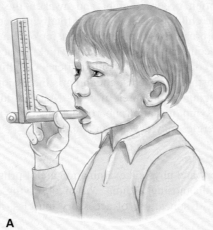

A

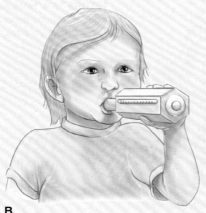

B

Steps to Accurate Measurements

1. Remove gum or food from the mouth.
2. Move the pointer on the meter to zero.
3. Stand up and hold the meter horizontally with fingers away from the vent holes and marker.
4. With mouth wide open, slowly breathe in as much air as possible.
5. Put the mouthpiece on the tongue and place lips around it.
6. Blow out as hard and fast as you can. Give a short, sharp blast, not a slow blow. The meter measures the fastest puff, not the longest.
7. Write down the result.
8. Repeat steps 1 to 7 three times. Wait at least 10 seconds between puffs. Move the pointer to zero after each puff.
9. Record the highest reading of the three.

Guidelines for Treatment

Each child has a unique pattern of asthma episodes. Most episodes begin gradually, and a drop in peak flow can alert you to start medications before the actual symptoms appear. This early treatment can prevent a flare-up from getting out of hand. One way to look at peak flow scores is to match the scores with three colors.

Green	Yellow	Red
80%–100% personal best	50%–80% personal best	Below 50% personal best
No symptoms	Mild-to-moderate symptoms	Serious distress
Full breathing reserve	Diminished reserve	Pulmonary function is significantly impaired
Mild trigger may not cause symptoms	A minor trigger produces noticeable symptoms	Any trigger may lead to severe distress
Continue current management	Augment present treatment regimen	Contact health care provider

Remember, treatment should be adjusted to fit the individual's needs. Your health care provider will develop a home management plan with you. When in doubt, consult your health care provider.

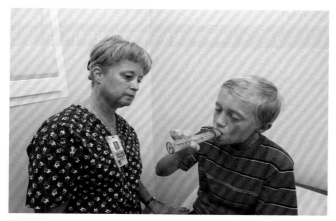

FIGURE 36-5 The child with asthma uses a peak flow meter and keeps track of readings on a daily basis.

The goals of asthma treatment include preventing symptoms, maintaining nearly normal lung function and activity levels, preventing recurring exacerbations and hospitalizations, and providing the best medication treatment with the fewest adverse effects. Depending on the frequency and severity of symptoms and exacerbations, a stepwise approach to the treatment of asthma is used to manage the disease. The steps are used to determine combinations of medications to be used (Table 36-1).

Medications used to treat asthma are divided into two categories: quick-relief medications for immediate treatment of symptoms and exacerbations and long-term control medications to achieve and maintain control of the symptoms. The classifications of drugs used to treat asthma include bronchodilators (sympathomimetics and xanthine derivatives). The sympathomimetics, also called β2-adrenergic agonists, can be used for quick relief of symptoms or for long-term control. The drugs are further described as short-acting β2-agonist (SABA) or long-acting β2-agonist (LABA). The xanthine derivatives (methylxanthines) are used for long-term control. Other antiasthmatic medications include systemic corticosteroids, inhaled corticosteroids (ICS), leukotriene modifiers (leukotriene receptor antagonists [LTRA]), and mast cell stabilizers. Inhaled corticosteroids and long acting β2-agonist (LABA) are sometimes given in combination for long-term control of symptoms. Table 36-2 lists some of the medications used to treat asthma.

Think About the "Why" of This!

A bronchodilator often is given to open up the airways just before the inhaled corticosteroid or the mast cell stabilizer is used.

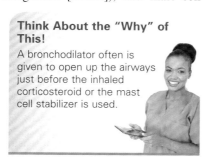

Many of these drugs can be given by either a **nebulizer** (medication administration device that turns liquid medication into a mist that can be more easily delivered into the lungs via an attached mouthpiece or face mask.); a **metered-dose inhaler (MDI)** (a handheld pressurized canister that delivers a premeasured dose of medication via an attached mouthpiece);

TABLE 36-1 Stepwise Approach to Treating Asthma

STEPS	SYMPTOMS
Step 1 Intermittent	Symptoms occur <2 times a week No symptoms between exacerbations Exacerbations brief Nighttime symptoms <2 times a month
Step 2 Mild persistent	Symptoms occur >2 times a week but <1 time a day Exacerbations may affect activity Nighttime symptoms >2 times a month
Step 3 Moderate persistent	Daily symptoms Daily use of inhaled short-acting β2 agonist Exacerbations affect activity Exacerbations >2 times a week, may last days Nighttime symptoms >1 time a week
Step 4 Severe persistent	Continual symptoms Limited physical activity Frequent exacerbations Frequent nighttime symptoms

or a dry powder inhaler (DPI). The MDI may have a spacer unit attached that makes it easier for the young child to use (Fig. 36-6).

Nursing Process and Care Plan *for the Child With Asthma*

Assessment (Data Collection)

Obtain information from the family caregiver about the asthma history, the medications the child takes, and the medications taken within the last 24 hours. Ask whether the child has vomited, because vomiting would prevent absorption of oral medications. Ask about any history of respiratory infections; possible allergens in the household such as pets; type of furniture and toys; if there is a damp basement (which could contain mold spores); any recent emotional stress or anxiety, and any history of breathing problems after exercise.

When collecting data, include vital signs; observe for diaphoresis and cyanosis, type of breathing and breathing position, alertness, chest movement, intercostal retractions, and breath sounds. Note any wheezing or coughing.

If the child is old enough and alert enough to cooperate, involve them in gathering the history, and encourage the child to add information. Ask questions that can be answered "yes" or "no" to minimize tiring the child, especially if they are having breathing issues.

TABLE 36-2 Medications Used in the Treatment of Asthma

GENERIC NAME	TRADE NAME	DOSE FORM	USES	ADVERSE REACTIONS/SIDE EFFECTS
Bronchodilators				
Action: Relax smooth muscles; open up the bronchi and narrowed airways which allows more air to enter lungs				
β2-Adrenergic Agonist (Sympathomimetic) *Short-Acting β2-Agonist (SABA)*				
Albuterol sulfate	Proventil, Ventolin	PO MDI Nebulizer DPI	Quick relief	Nervousness, anxiety, tachycardia, palpitations, insomnia, tremors
β2-Adrenergic Agonist (Sympathomimetic) *Long-Acting β2-Agonist (LABA)*				
Salmeterol	Serevent	MDI DPI	Long-term control	Headache, tremors, tachycardia
Formoterol	Foradil Symbicort	Nebulizer DPI	Long-term control	Headache, insomnia, tachycardia
Xanthine Derivative (Methylxanthines)				
Action: Stimulate the central nervous system to relax the smooth muscles and dilate the bronchioles				
Theophylline	Slo-Phyllin, Elixophyllin, Theo-Dur	PO Timed-release	Long-term control	Restlessness, headache, nervousness, irritability, tremors, tachycardia, insomnia, nausea, vomiting
Antiasthma Drugs				
Systemic Corticosteroids				
Action: Reduce inflammation and decrease obstruction in the airways				
Prednisone Prednisolone Methylprednisolone		PO IM IV	Quick relief	Adrenal suppression, nausea
Inhaled Corticosteroids (ICS)				
Action: Reduce inflammation; decrease the inflammatory process by being inhaled directly into the airways				
Beclomethasone	Beclovent	MDI Nebulizer	Long-term control	Throat irritation, cough, nausea, dizziness
Budesonide	Pulmicort	MDI Nebulizer	Long-term control	Throat irritation, headache, nausea
Flunisolide	AeroBid	MDI Nebulizer	Long-term control	Throat irritation, hoarseness, cough
Fluticasone	Flovent	MDI DPI	Long-term control	Restlessness, insomnia, nasal stuffiness
Triamcinolone	Azmacort	MDI	Long-term control	Throat irritation, cough, nausea, dizziness
Leukotriene Modifiers *Leukotriene Receptor Antagonists (LTRA)*				
Action: Inhibit leukotriene (substances released during the inflammatory process that cause bronchoconstriction) production; reduce inflammation and edema; cause bronchioles to dilate				
Montelukast	Singulair	PO	Long-term control	Headache, nausea, abdominal pain, diarrhea
Mast Cell Stabilizers				
Action: Stabilize the cell membrane by preventing mast cells from releasing the chemical mediators that cause bronchospasm and mucous membrane inflammation				
Cromolyn	Intal	Intranasal nebulizer	Long-term control	Few side effects, nasal and throat irritation, unpleasant taste, nausea

DPI, dry powder inhaler; MDI, metered-dose inhaler.

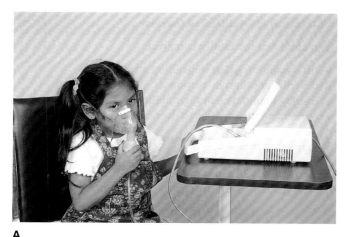

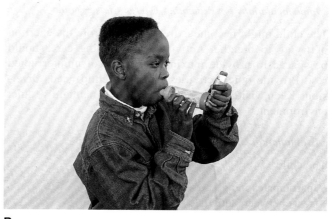

A

B

FIGURE 36-6 **A.** Child using a nebulizer with a mask. **B.** Child using a metered-dose inhaler with spacer.

Nursing Care Focus

Nursing care focuses for the child with asthma include concerns with maintaining an open airway and reducing the risk and monitoring for dehydration. Fatigue in the child and anxiety concerns of the child and family caregiver are addressed. Family caregiver teaching must be reinforced.

Outcome Identification and Planning

The initial major goals for the child include maintaining a clear airway, an adequate fluid intake, and relieving fatigue and anxiety. The family's goals include learning how to manage the child's life with asthma. Base the nursing plan of care on these goals.

Nursing Care Focus

- Ineffective airway clearance related to bronchospasm and increased pulmonary secretions

Goal

- The child's airway will remain open.

Implementations for Monitoring and Maintaining Respiratory Function

Continuously monitor the child while they are in acute distress from an asthma attack using pulse oximetry. Maintain oxygen saturation levels at 92% or higher. Take the child's respirations every 15 minutes during an acute attack and every 1 or 2 hours after the crisis is over. Listening to lung sounds should be done to further monitor the respiratory function. Observe for nasal flaring and chest retractions; observe the skin for color and diaphoresis.

Elevate the child's head. An older child may be more comfortable leaning forward on a pillow placed on an overbed table. Monitor the child for response to medications and their side effects such as restlessness, tremors, tachycardia, and gastrointestinal upset. Use humidified oxygen and suction as needed during periods of acute distress.

Evaluation of Goal/Desired Outcome

The child's:

- breath sounds are clear with no wheezing, retractions, or nasal flaring.
- skin color is good.

Nursing Care Focus

- Dehydration risk related to fluid loss from tachypnea, diaphoresis, and reduced oral intake

Goal

- The child's fluid intake will be adequate.

Implementations for Monitoring and Improving Fluid Intake

During an acute attack, the child may lose a great quantity of fluid through the respiratory tract and may have a poor oral intake because of coughing and vomiting. Monitor intake and output. Encourage oral fluids that the child likes. Intravenous (IV) fluids are administered as ordered. IV fluid intake is monitored and all precautions for parenteral administration are followed. Note the skin turgor and observe the mucous membranes at least every 8 hours. Weigh the child daily to help determine fluid losses.

Evaluation of Goal/Desired Outcome

The child's:

- hourly urine output is 0.5 to 1 mL/kg.
- skin turgor is good.
- mucous membranes are moist.
- weight remains stable.

Nursing Care Focus

- Fatigue related to dyspnea

Goal

- The child will have increased energy levels.

Implementations for Promoting Energy Conservation

The child might become extremely tired from the exertion of trying to breathe. Activities and nursing care should be spaced to provide maximum periods of uninterrupted rest. Provide quiet activities when the child needs diversion. Keep visitors to a minimum, and maintain a quiet environment.

Evaluation of Goal/Desired Outcome

The child:

- participates in age-appropriate activities.
- rests between activities.

Nursing Care Focus

- Acute anxiety related to sudden attacks of breathlessness

Goal

- Child and family caregiver anxiety and fear related to impending attacks will be minimized.

Implementations for Reducing Child and Family Caregiver Anxiety

The onset of an asthma attack can be frightening to the child and the family caregivers. Respond quickly when the child has an attack. Reassure the child and the family during an episode of dyspnea.

Reinforce teaching with the child and family caregiver about the symptoms of an impending attack and the immediate response needed to decrease the threat of an attack. This knowledge will help them to cope with impending attacks and plan how to handle the attacks. When they are prepared with information, the child and the family caregiver may be less fearful.

Following an asthma attack, reinforce teaching about breathing exercises to improve respiratory function and ways to control asthma attacks. These exercises teach children how to help control their own symptoms and

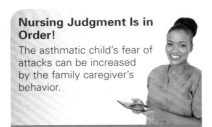

Nursing Judgment Is in Order!

The asthmatic child's fear of attacks can be increased by the family caregiver's behavior.

Check Out This Tip!

For the asthmatic child, if exercises can be taught as part of play activities, children are more likely to find them fun and to practice them more often.

thereby decrease anxiety and build self-confidence. Encourage the child and family caregiver to talk to others affected by asthma so they recognize they are not alone in this diagnosis.

Evaluation of Goal/Desired Outcome

The child and the family caregiver:

- list symptoms of an impending attack.
- describe appropriate responses.
- display confidence in their ability to handle an attack.
- participate in activities to decrease anxiety.

Nursing Care Focus

- Knowledge deficiency of the family caregiver related to disease process, treatment, home care, and control of disease

Goal

- The child and the family caregiver will gain knowledge of how to live with asthma.

Implementations for Reinforcing Family Teaching

Reinforcing child and family caregiver teaching is of primary importance in the care of the child with asthma. Family caregivers might overprotect the child because of the fear that an attack will occur when the child is with a babysitter, at school, or anywhere away from the caregiver. Asthma attacks can be prevented or decreased by prompt and adequate intervention. Reinforce teaching with the family caregiver and child, within the scope of the child's ability to understand, about the disease process, recognition of symptoms of an impending attack, environmental control, infection avoidance, exercise, and drug therapy.

Instruct the family caregiver and the child about how to use MDI medications and have them demonstrate correct usage (see Tips for Reinforcing Family Teaching: How to Use a Metered-Dose Inhaler). Give instructions on home use of a peak flow meter. Urge them to maintain a diary to record the peak flow as well as asthma symptoms, onset of attacks, action taken, and results. Include instructions about administering premedication before the child is exposed to situations in which an attack may occur.

Inform family caregivers of allergens that may be in the child's environment, and encourage them to eliminate or control the allergens as needed. Stress the importance of quick response when the child has a respiratory infection.

Reinforce with the family caregivers the importance of informing the child's classroom teacher, physical education teacher, school nurse, babysitter, and others who are responsible for the child about the child's condition. With a health care provider's order, including directions for use, the child should be permitted to bring medications to school and keep them so they can be used when needed.

Provide information on support groups available in the area. The American Lung Association has many materials available to families and can provide information about support groups, camps, and workshops (www.lung.org). The Asthma and Allergy Foundation of America (www.aafa.org) and the National Heart, Lung, and Blood Institute (www.nhlbi.nih.gov) are also resources.

Evaluation of Goal/Desired Outcome

The child and the family caregiver:

- verbalize an understanding of the disease process, treatment, and control.
- interact with healthcare personnel and ask and answer relevant questions.
- obtain information and make contact with support groups.

 A Personal Glimpse

The first time I put Bobbie in the hospital it was very scary. I knew the nurses, but I was still afraid for him. I felt like someone was punishing me. I couldn't leave him for a minute. I was afraid he wouldn't be alive when I came back. I was also afraid he would be frightened. He was so small; he needed me to protect him, but I couldn't help him. We were in the hospital every couple of weeks. He would get better then have another attack. It got to the point where I would call the doctor and say that Bobbie was having another attack, and they would just send us to admitting. After a few times, I got used to caring for him in the hospital. Finally I was able to go back to work during the day and care for him on my breaks and time off. It was very difficult each and every time, but we adjusted to hospital life. Although I was afraid for him, I knew he was a fighter, and I had to be too. I feel this experience made him a stronger person. He is now 8 years old and has had no severe attacks since he was about 2 years old. He has had a few mild attacks, but it doesn't affect him or myself.

Tracee

Learning Opportunity: *Give specific examples of what the nurse could do to support this mother and to help decrease the fear she had when her child was hospitalized.*

 TIPS FOR REINFORCING FAMILY TEACHING

How to Use a Metered-Dose Inhaler (MDI)

- When ready to use, shake the inhaler well with the cap still on.
- The child should stand, if possible.
- Remove the cap.
- Hold the inhaler with the mouthpiece down, facing the child.
- Be sure the child's mouth is empty.
- Hold the mouthpiece about 1 to 1.5 in. from the lips.[1]
- Breathe out normally. Open mouth wide and begin to breathe in.
- Press top of medication canister firmly while inhaling deeply. Hold breath as long as possible (at least 10 seconds—teach child to count slowly to 10).
- Breathe out *slowly* through nose or pursed lips.
- Relax 2 to 5 minutes, and repeat as directed by the health care provider.

[1]The mouthpiece can also be put between the lips, with the lips forming an airtight seal, or a spacer can be attached to the inhaler and the mouthpiece held between the lips.

Remember **Casey**? What do you think may have triggered the asthma attack for Casey? What signs and symptoms would you would expect to see in addition to his difficulty breathing? What treatments and medications do you think will be used to treat this acute attack? Describe the nursing care you would provide at this time.

TEST YOURSELF

✔ What is the most important aspect in the treatment of asthma?

✔ What are the two categories of medications used in the treatment of asthma?

✔ What are the routes of administration for many of the medications used to treat asthma?

PNEUMONIA

Pneumonia is an inflammation or infection in the lower respiratory tract of the child. It can be caused by a virus or a bacterium. A fungal infection can also cause pneumonia. Aspiration pneumonia occurs if foreign material gets into the lower respiratory tract.

The most common cause of pneumonia in children is a respiratory virus such as respiratory syncytial virus (RSV), influenza A and B, and coronaviruses. Good handwashing is the key to decreasing the spread of infection. Viruses are most often spread by the droplet method of transmission. If the pathogen is not known, the child may be placed on contact as well as droplet transmission precautions. Treatment of viral pneumonia is supportive care for symptoms.

Pneumococcal (*Streptococcus pneumoniae*) pneumonia is the most common form of bacterial pneumonia in infants and children. *H. influenzae* pneumonia also occurs in infants and young children. The incidence of each of these has decreased significantly since the introduction of the pneumococcal conjugate vaccine (PCV) and *H. influenzae* type B conjugate vaccine (HIB) as routine immunizations in early childhood. This disease occurs mainly during the late winter and early spring, principally in children younger than 4 years.

Children with chronic conditions such as asthma, cystic fibrosis, sickle cell disease, and congenital heart disease and children with exposure to cigarette or woodstove smoke are at higher risk of getting a community-acquired pneumonia. Potential complications of pneumonia include bacteremia, pleural effusion, lung abscess, pneumothorax, and empyema (pus in the lungs).

Clinical Manifestations

The onset of symptoms is usually abrupt, following a mild upper respiratory illness. Temperature increases rapidly to 103°F to 105°F (39.4°C to 40.6°C). Respiratory distress is marked with obvious air hunger, flaring of the nostrils, **circumoral** (around the mouth) cyanosis, and chest retractions. Tachycardia and tachypnea are present, with a pulse rate frequently as high as 140 to 180 beats per minute and respirations as high as 80 breaths per minute. Irritability, lethargy, poor feeding, nausea, and vomiting may also be noted. Cough may not be noticeable at the onset but may appear later. The child may have pain, especially with coughing and when taking deep breaths. Abdominal distention caused by swallowed air or paralytic ileus sometimes occurs.

Diagnosis

Diagnosis is based on clinical symptoms, chest radiography, and culture of the organism from secretions. The white blood cell count may be elevated, in particular with bacterial pneumonia.

Treatment

The use of anti-infectives early in the disease gives a prompt and favorable response. Amoxicillin has proved to be an effective treatment and is generally used unless the child has a hypersensitivity or allergy. Cephalosporin anti-infectives are also used. Antipyretics and analgesics may be used to control fever and alleviate discomfort. Oxygen started early in the disease process is important. An appropriate device for administering oxygen is used depending on the age and oxygen needs of the child (see Chapter 30, Table 30-1). Intravenous fluids are often necessary to supply the needed amount of fluids. Prognosis for recovery is excellent.

Nursing Process and Care Plan *for the Child With Pneumonia*

Assessment (Data Collection)

During the process of data collection, a thorough interview with the family caregiver is important. In addition to standard information, include specific data such as when the symptoms were first noticed, the course of the fever thus far, a description of respiratory difficulties, and the character of any cough. Collect data regarding how well the child has been taking nourishment and fluids. Ask about nausea, vomiting, urinary and bowel output, and history of exposure to other family members with respiratory infections.

When collecting data, include measurement of temperature, apical pulse, respirations (rate, respiratory effort, retractions [costal, intercostal, sternal, suprasternal, substernal], and flaring of nostrils) (see Chapter 28). Also note breath and lung sounds (crackles, wheezing), cough (dry, productive, hacking), irritability, restlessness, confusion, skin color (pallor, cyanosis), circumoral cyanosis, cyanotic nail beds, skin turgor, anterior fontanel (depressed or bulging), nasal passage congestion (color, consistency), mucous membranes (mouth dry, lips dry or cracked), and eyes (bright, glassy, sunken, moist, crusted). If the child is old enough to communicate verbally, ask questions to determine how the child feels.

Nursing Care Focus

When developing evidence-based nursing care focuses for the child with pneumonia, include the risk for ineffective airway clearance, impaired gas exchange, and altered breathing patterns. Potential for dehydration, hyperthermia, and further infection are also risks for the child with pneumonia. Anxiety, family coping impairment, and reinforcing family teaching are important aspects of caring for the child and the family.

Outcome Identification and Planning

The major goals for the child with pneumonia are maintaining respiratory function, preventing dehydration and fluid deficit, maintaining body temperature, preventing secondary infections such as otitis media, and relieving anxiety. Goals for the family include relieving anxiety, improving coping skills, and increasing family caregiver knowledge.

Nursing Care Focus

- Ineffective airway clearance related to obstruction associated with edema, mucus secretions, nasal and chest congestion

Goal

- The child's airway will remain clear and patent.

Implementations for Maintaining Airway Clearance

Elevate the head of the bed and use pillows to maintain the child's position to provide maximum ventilation and to keep airway open. Change positions at least every 2 hours. Observe frequently for slumping, which causes crowding of the diaphragm. Avoid use of constricting clothes and bedding. A humidified atmosphere is provided with a cool-mist humidifier or humidified oxygen. The moisturized air helps thin the mucus in the respiratory tract to ease respirations. Encourage intake of fluids; adequate hydration helps reduce thick mucus. Encourage older child to use incentive spirometer, cough, and expectorate secretions. Suction or clear secretions as needed to keep the nose and airway open.

Evaluation of Goal/Desired Outcome

The child's:

- airway is clear with no evidence of retractions, stridor, hoarseness, or cyanosis.
- mucus secretions are thin and scant; nasal passages are clear.

Nursing Care Focus

- Impaired gas exchange related to inflammatory process
- Altered breathing pattern related to increased respiratory rate

Goal

- The child's respiratory function will be within normal limits for age.

Implementations for Monitoring and Maintaining Adequate Respiratory Function

Be continuously alert for warning signs of airway obstruction. The need for immediate intubation is always a possibility; thus, vigilance is essential. Monitor the child at least every hour; uncover the child's chest, and observe the child's breathing efforts. Observe for tachypnea (rapid respirations), and note the amount of chest movement, shallow breathing, and retractions. Listen with a stethoscope for breath sounds, particularly noting the amount of stridor, which indicates difficult breathing. Oxygen saturation levels are monitored using pulse oximetry. Increasing hoarseness should be reported. In addition, observe for pallor, listlessness, circumoral cyanosis, cyanotic nail beds, and restlessness; these are indications of impaired oxygenation and should be reported at once. Cool, high humidity provides relief. Oxygen may be administered by an age-appropriate device. The child's energy must be conserved to reduce oxygen requirements; allow for sleep and rest.

Evaluation of Goal/Desired Outcome

- The child's respiratory rate is within normal range for child's age, respirations are regular, and breath sounds are clear.
- The infant no longer uses respiratory accessory muscles to aid in breathing.
- The child's oxygen saturation levels are within established limits.

Nursing Care Focus

- Dehydration risk related to respiratory fluid loss, fever, and difficulty swallowing

Goal

- The child's fluid intake will be adequate for age and weight.

Implementations for Promoting and Monitoring Adequate Fluid Intake

Blocked nasal passages may make eating food and drinking fluids difficult. It is important to clear the nasal passages immediately before feeding. For the infant, use a bulb syringe. Administer normal saline nose drops to thin secretions about 10 to 15 minutes before feedings and at bedtime. Feed the child slowly, allowing frequent stops with suctioning during feeding, as needed. Avoid overtiring the infant or child during feeding.

Maintaining adequate fluid intake may be a problem for children of any age because the child may be too ill to want to drink or eat. Offer warm, clear fluids to encourage oral intake. Between meals, offer juices and water appropriate for the infant or child's age. For infants, use a relatively small-holed nipple so they do not choke, but do not work too hard. Maintain accurate intake and output measurements.

Carefully observe for aspiration, especially in severe respiratory distress. The child may need to be kept NPO to prevent this threat. Parenteral fluids may be administered if the child is NPO or to replace fluids lost through respiratory loss, fever, and anorexia. Follow all safety measures for administration of parenteral fluids. Observe patency, placement, site integrity, and flow rate, at least hourly. Fluid needs are determined by the amount needed to maintain body weight with sufficient amounts added to replace the additional losses.

Monitor daily weights, at the same time each day, using the same scale and amount of clothing. Monitor serum electrolyte levels to ensure they are within normal limits. Observe and record the condition of mucous membranes, skin turgor, anterior fontanel (in infants), and urine output as these are good indicators of dehydration. For the infant, weigh diapers to determine the amount of urine output (1 mL urine weighs 1 gram).

Evaluation of Goal/Desired Outcome

The child:

- exhibits good skin turgor and moist, pink mucous membranes.
- has urine output of 0.5 to 1 mL/kg/hr.

Nursing Care Focus

- Hyperthermia related to infection process

Goal

- The child will maintain a temperature within normal limits.

Implementations for Monitoring and Maintaining Body Temperature

Monitor the child's temperature frequently, at least every 2 hours if it is higher than 101.3°F (38.6°C). If the child has a fever, remove excess clothing and covering. Encourage fluids as tolerated. Antipyretic medications may be ordered (see Chapter 30, Tips for Reinforcing Family Teaching: Reducing Fever).

Evaluation of Goal/Desired Outcome

- The child's temperature is 98.6°F to 100°F (37°C to 37.8°C).

Nursing Care Focus

- Infection risk related to possibility of transmitting organisms to others
- Secondary infection risk related to location and anatomic structure of the eustachian tubes

Goal

- The child will not spread infection to others and will have no signs of secondary infection (otitis media).

Implementations for Preventing Additional Infections

The child may need to be placed on transmission-based precautions, according to the policy of the healthcare facility, to prevent nosocomial spread of infection. Good handwashing and standard and transmission-based precautions must be followed by all healthcare personnel and visitors as well.

Turn the child from side to side every hour so that mucus is less likely to drain into the eustachian tubes, thereby reducing the risk for development of otitis media. An infant seat may help facilitate breathing and prevent the complication of otitis media in the younger child. Observe the child for irritability, shaking of the head, pulling at the ears, or complaints of ear pain. Do not give the infant a bottle while they are lying in bed. The best position for feeding is upright to avoid excessive drainage into the eustachian tubes.

Evaluation of Goal/Desired Outcome

The child:

- does not spread infection to others.
- shows no signs of ear pain such as irritability, shaking of the head, pulling on the ears.
- does not complain of ear pain.

Nursing Care Focus

- Acute anxiety related to dyspnea, invasive procedures, and separation from family caregiver

Goal

- The child will experience a reduction in anxiety.

Implementations for Reducing the Child's Anxiety

When frightened or upset and crying, the child with a respiratory condition may hyperventilate, which causes additional respiratory distress. For this reason, maintain a calm, soothing manner while caring for the child. When possible, the child should be cared for by a constant caregiver with whom a trusting relationship has been achieved. Offering support to the child during invasive procedures, such as when an IV is being started, will help decrease the child's anxiety.

The family can provide the child with a favorite blanket or toy. The family caregiver is encouraged to stay with the child if possible to provide reassurance and avoid separation anxiety in the child. Plan care to minimize interrupting the child's much-needed rest. Give the child age-appropriate explanations of treatment and procedures.

As the child's condition improves, provide age-appropriate diversional activities to help relieve anxiety and boredom. Make extra efforts to relieve the child's feelings of loneliness, especially when transmission-based precautions are being used.

Evaluation of Goal/Desired Outcome

The child:

- rests quietly with no evidence of hyperventilation.
- cooperates with care, cuddles a favorite toy for reassurance, smiles, and plays contentedly.

Nursing Care Focus

- Anxiety and coping impairment of family caregiver related to child's respiratory symptoms and child's illness

Goal

- The family caregiver's anxiety will be reduced.

Implementations for Decreasing Family Caregiver Anxiety and Promoting Coping

Watching a child with severe respiratory symptoms is frightening for the family caregiver. Family caregivers need reinforcement of teaching and reassurance. The family caregiver may feel helpless, and these feelings of anxiety and helplessness may be exhibited in a variety of ways. To alleviate these feelings, encourage the family caregiver to discuss them. Using easily understood terminology, explain equipment, procedures, treatments, the illness, and the prognosis to the caregiver. Include the family caregiver in the child's care as much as possible and encourage them to soothe and comfort the child. Actively listen to family caregivers and use communication skills to respond to their worries.

Evaluation of Goal/Desired Outcome

The family caregivers:

- cooperate with and participate in the child's care.
- appear more relaxed, verbalize their feelings, and soothe the child.

Nursing Care Focus

- Knowledge deficiency of the family caregiver related to child's condition and home care

Goal

- The family caregivers will verbalize an understanding of the child's condition and how to provide home care for the child.

Implementations for Reinforcing Family Teaching

Provide the family caregiver with thorough explanations of the condition's signs and symptoms. Reinforce teaching about the use of cool-mist humidifiers, including cleaning methods. Explain the effects, administration, dosage, and side effects of medications. To be certain the information was understood, have the family caregiver relate specific facts to you. Write the information down in a simple way so that it can be clearly understood, and determine that the family caregiver can read and understand the written material. When appropriate, observe the caregiver demonstrating care of equipment and any treatments to be done at home. See Tips for Reinforcing Family Teaching: Respiratory Infections.

Evaluation of Goal/Desired Outcome

The family caregivers:

- accurately describe facts about the child's condition.
- ask appropriate questions.
- relate signs and symptoms to observe in the child.
- state the effects, side effects, dosage, and describe the administration of medications.

TIPS FOR REINFORCING FAMILY TEACHING

Respiratory Infections

- Clear nasal passages with a bulb syringe for the infant.
- Allow the infant to bottle- or breast-feed without tiring.
- Frequently burp the infant to expel swallowed air.
- Feed the child slowly.
- Offer the child extra fluids.
- Soothe and comfort the child who is receiving oxygen via an oxygen device.
- Follow respiratory infection control precautions and good handwashing techniques.
- Discourage persons with infections from visiting the child.
- Use a cool mist humidifier at home after discharge.
- Clean humidifier properly and frequently.

CYSTIC FIBROSIS

Cystic fibrosis (CF) can affect many organs of the body because the gene mutation that occurs results in a dysfunction of all exocrine glands. The major organs affected are the lungs, pancreas, liver, and intestines. Because a large number of children with CF have pulmonary complications, this disorder is discussed here with other respiratory conditions.

CF is hereditary and transmitted as an autosomal recessive trait. Both parents must be carriers of the gene for CF to appear. With each pregnancy, the chance is one in four that the child will have the disease. In the United States, the incidence is about 1 in 3,200 children who are White, 1 in 10,000 children who are Hispanic, and 1 in 15,000 children who are Black.

The normal gene produces a protein, CF transmembrane conductance regulator (CFTR), which serves as a channel through which chloride enters and leaves cells. The mutated gene blocks chloride movement, which brings on the apparent signs of CF. The blocking of chloride transport results in a change in sodium transport; this in turn results in abnormal secretions of the exocrine (mucus-producing) glands that produce thick, tenacious mucus rather than the thin, free-flowing secretion normally produced. This abnormal mucus leads to obstruction of the secretory ducts of the pancreas, liver, and reproductive organs. Thick mucus obstructs the respiratory passages, causing trapped air and overinflation of the lungs. In addition, the sweat and salivary glands excrete excessive electrolytes, specifically sodium and chloride.

Newborn screening for CF has led to an increase in detecting CF in infants before symptoms are present. This early detection, before the onset of symptoms, has dramatically increased treatment options for these infants which leads to better lung function and outcomes.

Clinical Manifestations

Meconium ileus is the presenting symptom of CF in 10% to 20% of the newborns who later develop additional manifestations. Depletion or absence of pancreatic enzymes before birth results in impaired digestive activity and the meconium becomes viscid (thick) and mucilaginous (sticky). The thickened meconium fills the small intestine, causing complete obstruction. Clinical manifestations are bile-stained emesis, a distended abdomen, and an absence of stool. Intestinal perforation with symptoms of shock may occur. A symptom family caregivers sometimes note is that the skin of the newborn tastes salty when kissed because of the high sodium chloride concentration in their sweat.

If CF is not detected during a newborn screening, initial symptoms of CF may occur at varying ages during infancy, childhood, or adolescence. The symptoms depend on the severity of the disease and the organs affected. Respiratory symptoms, such as a persistent cough, tachypnea, and wheezing, may be the first sign. Later, frequent bronchial infections occur. Development of a barrel chest and clubbing of fingers (Fig. 36-7) indicate chronic lack of oxygen. Thickened secretions in the intestine block the ducts and cause a decrease in the flow of the normal fluids and enzymes which help digest food, causing gastrointestinal symptoms including abdominal distention and failure to thrive.

Pancreatic Involvement

Thick, tenacious mucus obstructs the pancreatic ducts, causing **hypochylia** (diminished flow of pancreatic enzymes) or **achylia** (absence of pancreatic enzymes). This achylia or hypochylia leads to intestinal malabsorption and severe malnutrition. Malabsorption of fats causes **steatorrhea** (fatty stools) with increased frequency of flatulence and large, bulky foul smelling stools. The incidence of diabetes is greater in these children than in the general population because of changes in the pancreas. The incidence of diabetes in clients with CF has increased as the life expectancy of individuals with CF has increased.

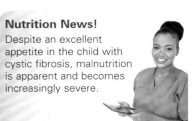

Nutrition News!
Despite an excellent appetite in the child with cystic fibrosis, malnutrition is apparent and becomes increasingly severe.

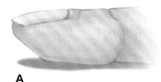 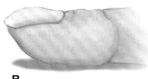 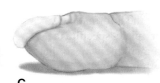

A **B** **C**

FIGURE 36-7 Clubbing of fingers indicates chronic lack of oxygen. **A.** Normal angle. **B.** Early clubbing—flattened angle. **C.** Advanced clubbing—the nail is rounded over the end of the finger.

Pulmonary Involvement

Respiratory complications pose the greatest threat to children with CF. The severity of pulmonary involvement differs in individual children, with a few showing only minor involvement. Abnormal amounts of thick, viscid mucus clog the bronchioles and provide an ideal medium for bacterial growth. *Staphylococcus aureus* can be cultured from the nasopharynx and sputum of most clients. *Pseudomonas aeruginosa* and *H. influenzae* also are frequently found. However, the basic infection appears most often to be caused by *S. aureus.*

Numerous complications arise from severe respiratory infections. Atelectasis and small lung abscesses are common early complications. Bronchiectasis and emphysema may develop with pulmonary fibrosis and pneumonitis; this eventually leads to severe respiratory insufficiency. In advanced disease, pneumothorax and pulmonary hypertension are complications which may cause respiratory failure.

Other Organ Involvement

The tears, saliva, and sweat of children with CF contain abnormally high concentrations of electrolytes. The loss of sodium, chloride, and fluid through sweating causes electrolyte imbalances. Additional fluid and salt should be given in the diet as a preventive measure, especially in hot weather. Males with CF will most likely be sterile because of the blockage or absence of the vas deferens. Females often have thick cervical secretions that prohibit the passage of sperm.

Diagnosis

Diagnosis is based on family history, newborn screening, clinical symptoms, elevated sodium chloride levels in the sweat chloride test, genetic tests to show CF gene mutation, a history of failure to thrive, chronic or recurrent respiratory infections, and radiologic findings of hyperinflation and bronchial wall thickening. In the event of a positive sodium chloride sweat test, at least one other criterion must be met to make a conclusive diagnosis.

The principal diagnostic test to confirm CF is a sweat chloride test using the pilocarpine iontophoresis method. This method induces sweating by using a small electric current that carries topically applied pilocarpine into a localized area of the skin. Elevations of 60 mEq/L or more are diagnostic. Although the test itself is fairly simple, conducting the test on an infant is difficult, and false-positive results do occur.

Treatment

In the newborn, meconium ileus is treated with hyperosmolar enemas administered gently. If this does not resolve the blockage of thick, gummy meconium, surgery is necessary. During surgery, a mucolytic drug, such as acetylcysteine, may be used to liquefy the meconium. If this procedure is successful, resection may not be necessary.

In the older child, treatment is aimed at correcting pancreatic deficiency, improving pulmonary function, and preventing respiratory infections. If bowel obstruction does occur (meconium ileus equivalent), the management includes an increase in fluids and administration of balanced electrolyte oral laxative solution. If needed hyperosmolar enemas are administered.

The overall treatment goals are to improve the child's quality of life and to provide for long-term survival. A healthcare team is needed, including a primary health care provider, a nurse, a respiratory therapist, a dietitian, and a social worker, to work together with the child and the family. Treatment centers with a staff of specialists are becoming more common, particularly in larger medical centers.

> **Good News!**
> With improved treatment, it is not unusual for a child with cystic fibrosis (CF) to live well into adulthood, with many adults with CF now living into their mid-40s and beyond.

Dietary Treatment

Commercially prepared pancreatic enzymes given during meals or with snacks aid digestion and absorption of fat and protein. Because pancreatic enzymes are inactivated in the acidic environment of the stomach, microencapsulated capsules are used to deliver the enzymes to the duodenum, where they are activated. These enzymes come in capsules that can be swallowed or opened and sprinkled on the child's food. A powdered preparation is used for infants.

The child's diet should be high in carbohydrates and protein, with no restriction of fats. The child may need one and a half to two times the normal caloric intake to promote growth. These children have large appetites unless they are acutely ill. However, even with their large appetites they can receive little nourishment without a pancreatic supplement. With proper diet and enzyme supplements, these children show evidence of improved nutrition, and their stools become relatively normal. Enteric-coated pancreatic enzymes essentially eliminate the need for dietary restriction of fat.

Because of the increased loss of sodium chloride, these children are allowed to use as much salt as they wish, even though onlookers may think it is too much. During hot weather, additional salt may be provided with pretzels, salted breadsticks, and saltine crackers.

Supplements of fat-soluble vitamins A, D, and E are necessary because of the poor digestion of fats. Vitamin K may be supplemented if the child has coagulation problems or is scheduled for surgery.

Pulmonary Treatment

The treatment goal is to prevent and treat respiratory infections. Respiratory drainage is provided by thinning the secretions and by mechanical means, such as postural drainage and clapping to loosen and drain secretions from the lungs. Antibacterial drugs for the treatment of infection are necessary as indicated. Some health care providers prescribe a prophylactic antibiotic regimen when the child receives the diagnosis of CF. Antibiotic medications may be administered orally or parenterally, even in the home. With home parenteral administration of antibiotic therapy, a central venous access device may be used. Immunization against childhood communicable diseases is extremely important for these children and immunizations should be kept up to date.

Physical activity is essential because it improves mucus secretion and helps the child feel good. The child can be encouraged to participate in any aerobic activity they enjoy. Physical activity should be limited only by the child's endurance.

Inhalation therapy can be preventive or therapeutic. A bronchodilators, such as a β-adrenergic agonist (metaproterenol, terbutaline, or albuterol), may be administered either orally or through nebulization. Recombinant human DNA breaks down DNA molecules in sputum, breaking up the thick mucus in the airways. A mucolytic, such as acetylcysteine, may be prescribed. Handheld nebulizers are easy to use and convenient for the ambulatory child.

Humidifiers provide a humidified atmosphere. In the summer, a room air conditioner can help provide comfort and controlled humidity.

Chest physiotherapy, a combination of postural drainage and chest percussion, is performed routinely at least every morning and evening, even if little drainage is apparent (Fig. 36-8). Performed correctly, chest percussion (clapping and vibrating of the affected areas) helps to loosen and move secretions out of the lungs. The physical therapist usually performs this procedure in the hospital and teaches it to the family. Mechanical devices may be used to help clear respiratory sections. The older child and adolescent may use some of these devices including a flutter-value device, a positive expiratory pressure (PEP) mask, or a high-frequency chest wall oscillation device (often called a percussion vest) (Fig. 36-9). As with chest physiotherapy, the purpose of any of these therapies is to mobilize secretions, clear airways, and improve pulmonary function. Chest physiotherapy, although time-consuming, is part of the ongoing, long-term treatment and should be continued at home.

Home Care

The home care for a child with CF places a tremendous burden on the family. This is not a one-time hospital treatment, and there is no prospect of cure to brighten the horizon.

Each day, much time is spent performing treatments. Family caregivers must learn to perform chest physiotherapy, how to operate respiratory equipment, and administer IV antibiotic medications when necessary. The child's diet must be planned with additional enzymes regulated according to need. Great care is needed to prevent exposure to infections.

Family caregivers must guard against overprotection and undue limitations of their child's physical activity. Caregivers must preserve a good family relationship, also giving time and attention to other members of the family.

Physical activity is an important adjunct to the child's well-being and is necessary to get rid of secretions. Capacity for exercise is soon learned, and the child can be trusted to become self-limiting as necessary, especially if given an opportunity to learn the nature of the disease.

> **A Little Fun Can be Good!**
> The younger child may find postural drainage fun when a caregiver raises the child's feet in the air and walks the child around "wheelbarrow" fashion. The older child with CF can learn to hang from a monkey bar by the knees, having fun and at the same time increasing postural drainage.

Providing as much normalcy as possible is always desirable. Hot-weather activity should be watched a little more closely with additional attention to increased salt and fluid intake during exercise.

Caring for a child with CF places great stress on a family's financial resources. The expense of daily medications, frequent clinic or office visits, and sometimes lengthy hospitalizations can be devastating to an ordinary family budget, even with medical insurance coverage. The Cystic Fibrosis Foundation (www.cff.org), with chapters throughout the United States, is helpful in providing education and services. Some assistance may be available through local agencies or community groups.

Nursing Process and Care Plan *for the Child With Cystic Fibrosis*

Assessment (Data Collection)

The collection of data on the child with CF varies, depending on the child's age and the circumstances of the admission. Conduct a complete parent interview that includes the standard information, as well as data concerning respiratory infections, the child's appetite and eating habits, stools, noticeable salty perspiration, history of bowel obstruction as an infant, and the family history for CF, if known. Also determine the family caregiver's knowledge of the condition.

When collecting data about vital signs, include observation of respirations, such as cough, breath sounds, and barrel chest; respiratory effort, such as retractions and nasal flaring; clubbing of the fingers; and signs of pancreatic involvement, such as failure to thrive and steatorrhea. Examine the skin around the rectum for irritation and breakdown from frequent foul stools. Involve the child in the interview process by asking age-appropriate questions, and determine the child's perception of the disease and this current illness.

Nursing Care Focus

When developing evidence-based nursing care focuses for the child with cystic fibrosis, concerns include the risk for ineffective airway and respiratory issues. Potential for infection and malnutrition are also risks for the child with cystic fibrosis. Anxiety, coping with a chronic condition, and reinforcing family teaching are important aspects of caring for the child and the family.

Outcome Identification and Planning

The goals for the child with CF depend on the reason for the specific admission. The child's age and ability for self-expression affect any goal-setting the child can do.

The major goals for the child include relieving immediate respiratory distress, maintaining adequate oxygenation, remaining free from infection, improving nutritional status, and relieving anxiety. The family caregivers' primary goal may include relieving problems related to this admission. However, other goals may include concerns about stress on the family related to the condition, as well as a need for additional information about the disease, treatment, and prevention of complications.

Nursing Care Focus

- Ineffective airway clearance related to thick, tenacious mucus production

Goal

- The child's airway will be clear.

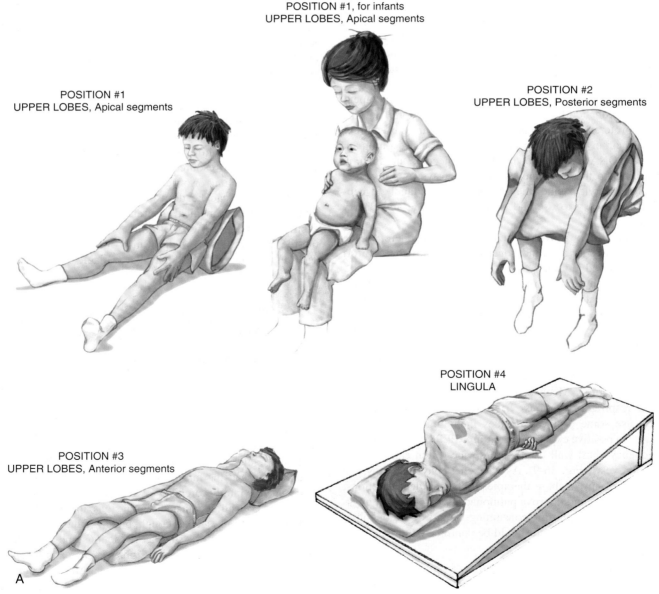

POSITION #1, for infants
UPPER LOBES, Apical segments

POSITION #1
UPPER LOBES, Apical segments

POSITION #2
UPPER LOBES, Posterior segments

POSITION #3
UPPER LOBES, Anterior segments

POSITION #4
LINGULA

A

FIGURE 36-8 Positions for postural drainage including segment of lung to be drained.

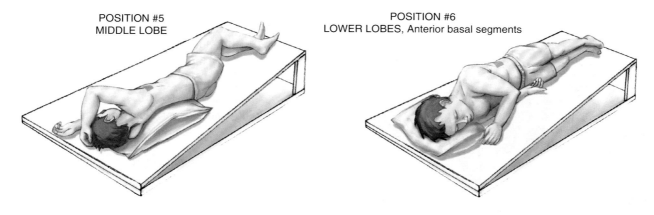

POSITION #5
MIDDLE LOBE

POSITION #6
LOWER LOBES, Anterior basal segments

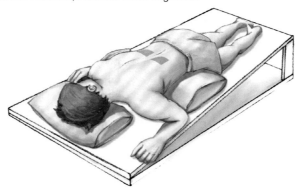

POSITION #7
LOWER LOBES, Posterior basal segments

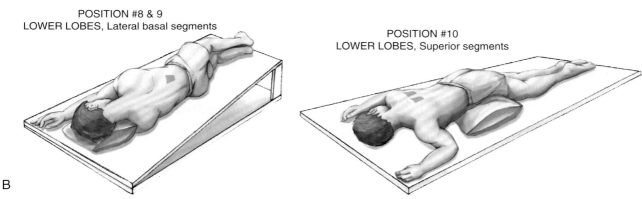

POSITION #8 & 9
LOWER LOBES, Lateral basal segments

POSITION #10
LOWER LOBES, Superior segments

B

FIGURE 36-8 Continued

Implementations for Improving Airway Clearance and Oxygen Exchange

Mucus obstructs the airways and diminishes gas exchange. Monitor the child for signs of respiratory distress, while observing for dyspnea, tachypnea, labored respirations with or without activity, retractions, nasal flaring, and color of nail beds. Administer medications to thin, loosen, and remove secretions. Encourage the child to cough effectively. Examine and document the mucus produced, noting the color, consistency, and odor. Send cultures to the laboratory, as appropriate. Increase fluid intake to help thin mucus secretions. Ask the child (or the family caregiver if the child is too young) what favorite drinks might be appealing. Intravenous fluids may be necessary. Provide humidified room air via a cool mist humidifier or humidified oxygen, as prescribed. Perform chest physiotherapy.

Evaluation of Goal/Desired Outcome

The child:

- effectively clears mucus from the airway and the airway remains patent.
- cooperates with chest physiotherapy.

Nursing Care Focus

- Altered breathing pattern related to tracheobronchial obstruction
- Impaired gas exchange related to decreased oxygenation

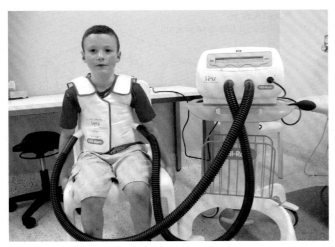

FIGURE 36-9 Child using a high frequency chest wall oscillation device (often called a percussion vest). (Reprinted with permission from Tagher C. G., & Knapp L. M. (2020). *Pediatric nursing: A case-based approach* (Fig. 20-20, p. 331). Wolters Kluwer.)

Goal

- The child will exhibit adequate respiratory function.

Implementations for Improving Respiratory Status

Maintain the child in a semi-Fowler position, with the upper half of the body elevated about 30°, or high Fowler position, with the upper half of the body elevated about 90°, to promote maximal lung expansion. Monitor oxygen saturation using pulse oximetry and maintain oxygen saturation higher than 90%. Administer oxygen as ordered if the oxygen saturation falls below this level. Administer mouth care every 2 to 4 hours, especially when oxygen is administered. Perform chest physiotherapy every 2 to 4 hours, as ordered. If respiratory therapy technicians or physical therapists do these treatments, observe the child after the treatment to determine effectiveness and if more frequent treatments may be needed. Supervise the child who can self-administer nebulizer treatments to ensure correct use.

Conserve the child's energy. Plan nursing and therapeutic activities so that maximal rest time is provided for the child. Note dyspnea and respiratory distress in relation to any activities. Plan quiet diversional activities as the child's physical condition warrants. Help the child and the family understand that activity is excellent for the child not in an acute situation. Remind them that exercise helps loosen the thick mucus and also improves the child's self-image.

Evaluation of Goal/Desired Outcome

The child:

- rests quietly with no dyspnea and the respiratory rate is even and appropriate for age.
- maintains oxygen saturation above 90%.

Nursing Care Focus

- Infection risk related to bacterial growth medium provided by pulmonary mucus and impaired body defenses

Goal

- The child will remain free of signs and symptoms of infection.

Implementations for Preventing Infection

The child with CF has low resistance, especially to respiratory infections. For this reason, take care to protect the child from any exposure to infectious organisms. Good handwashing techniques should be practiced by all; remind the child and the family about the importance of this first-line of defense. Practice and encourage other good hygiene habits. Carefully follow medical asepsis when caring for the child and the equipment. Monitor vital signs every 4 hours for any indication of an infectious process. Restrict people with an infection, such as staff, family members, other clients, and visitors, from contact with the child. Advise the family to keep the child's immunizations up-to-date. Administer antibiotic medications as prescribed, and clarify with the child or family caregiver home administration, as needed. Reinforce teaching with the family about the signs and symptoms of an impending infection so they can begin prophylactic measures at once.

Evaluation of Goal/Desired Outcome

- The child's vital signs are within normal limits for age.
- The child and the family follow infection-control practices.

Nursing Care Focus

- Malnutrition risk related to impaired absorption of nutrients

Goal

- The child's nutritional intake will be adequate to compensate for decreased absorption of nutrients and to provide for adequate growth and development.

Implementations for Maintaining Adequate Nutrition

Adequate nutrition helps the child resist infections. Increase the child's caloric intake to compensate for impaired absorption of nutrients and to provide adequate growth and development. In addition to increased caloric intake at meals, provide the child with high-calorie, high-protein snacks, such as peanut butter and cheese. Administer pancreatic enzymes with all meals and snacks. In addition, vitamins, especially fat-soluble vitamins, may be prescribed. Reinforce the need for these supplements to both the child and the family. The child also may require additional salt in the diet. Encourage the child to eat salty snacks. If the child has bouts of diarrhea or constipation, the dosage of enzymes may need to be adjusted. Report any change in bowel movements. Weigh and measure the child. Plot growth on a chart so that progress can easily be visualized.

Evaluation of Goal/Desired Outcome

The child:

- demonstrates weight gain appropriate for age.
- exhibits normal growth as indicated by growth chart.

Nursing Care Focus

- Acute anxiety related to hospitalization

Goal

- The child's anxiety will subside.

Implementations for Reducing the Child's Anxiety

Provide age-appropriate activities to help alleviate anxiety and the boredom that can result from hospitalization. Choose activities such as reading or arts and crafts according to age. Schoolwork may help ease some anxiety. Children may enjoy using electronic devices and participating in virtual games and activities, but watch the child for overexcitement. Encourage the family caregiver to stay with the child to help diminish some of the child's anxiety. Allow the child to have familiar toys or mementos from home. Stay with the child during acute episodes of coughing and dyspnea to reduce anxiety. Give the child age-appropriate information about CF. Talk with the child in a relaxed, friendly manner to help determine what the child knows and what information may be needed. Learning about CF can be turned into a game for some children, making it much more enjoyable.

Evaluation of Goal/Desired Outcome

- The child engages in age-appropriate activities and appears relaxed.

Nursing Care Focus

- Family coping impairment related to child's chronic condition and its demands on caregivers

Goal

- The family caregivers will verbalize feelings related to the child's chronic condition.

Implementations for Providing Family Support

The family with a child who has CF is faced with a long-term condition and may have already seen deterioration in the child's health. Give the family and the child opportunities to voice fears and anxieties. Respond with active listening techniques to help authenticate their feelings. Provide emotional support throughout the entire hospital stay. Demonstrate an interest and willingness to talk to the family; do not make family members feel as though they are intruding on time needed to do other things. As the nurse, you are the person who can best provide overall support.

Evaluation of Goal/Desired Outcome

- The family caregivers verbalize fears, anxieties, and other feelings related to the child's condition.

Nursing Care Focus

- Knowledge deficiency of the family caregiver related to diagnosis, treatment, and home care

Goal

- The family caregivers will verbalize an understanding of the child's condition and treatment.

Implementations for Reinforcing Family Teaching

Evaluate the family's knowledge about CF to determine their teaching needs. The family may need to have all the information repeated or may need clarification in just a few areas. Provide information for resources such as the Cystic Fibrosis Foundation, the American Lung Association (www.lung.org), and other local organizations. The family may have questions about genetic counseling and may need referrals for counseling.

Evaluation of Goal/Desired Outcome

The family caregivers:

- explain CF and describe treatments and possible complications.
- become involved in available support groups.

TEST YOURSELF

✔ What two immunizations have decreased the incidence of bacterial pneumonia in children?

✔ What major organs are affected by CF?

✔ What is the dietary treatment for CF?

✔ To what type of infection is the child with CF most susceptible?

PULMONARY TUBERCULOSIS

Tuberculosis (TB) is present in all parts of the world and is a concerning chronic infectious disease in terms of illness, death, and cost. The incidence of tuberculosis in children in the United States is low. Risk factors for children include being born or having a parent born in a foreign country or having lived outside of the United States, especially in a country where TB is widespread. Children are most likely to contract TB from an infected person in their household or in a crowded community setting such as a homeless shelter.

Cultural Snapshot

In some cultures, it is common for many people to live together in one home or in a close living arrangement. Respiratory illness is easily spread from person to person when people live in close contact with each other.

Tuberculosis is caused by *Mycobacterium tuberculosis*, a bacillus spread by droplets of infected mucus that become airborne when the infected person sneezes, coughs, talks, or laughs. The bacilli, when airborne, are inhaled into the respiratory tract of the unsuspecting person and become implanted in lung tissue. This process is the beginning of the formation of a primary lesion.

Clinical Manifestations

Primary tuberculosis is the original infection that goes through various stages and ends with calcification. Primary lesions in children are generally unrecognized and the child often has no symptoms. The most common site of a primary lesion is the alveoli of the respiratory tract. Most cases arrest with the calcification of the primary infection. However, in children with poor nutrition or health, the primary infection may invade other tissues of the body, including the bones, joints, kidneys, lymph nodes, and meninges. This is called miliary tuberculosis. In the small number of children with miliary tuberculosis, general symptoms of chronic infection, such as fatigue, loss of weight, and low-grade fever, may occur accompanied by cough and night sweats.

Secondary tuberculosis is a reactivation of a healed primary lesion. It often occurs in adults and contributes to the exposure of children to the organism. Although secondary lesions are more common in adults, they may occur in adolescents. Symptoms resemble those in an adult, including cough with expectoration, fever, weight loss, malaise, and night sweats.

Diagnosis

The tuberculin skin test is the primary means by which tuberculosis is detected. A skin test can be performed using an intradermal injection of 0.1 mL of purified protein derivative (PPD) on the inner aspect of the forearm. The site is marked and read at 48 to 72 hours after the test is administered. The site may have redness, but the measurement of the induration of the site is what indicates a positive reaction. Persons with a positive reaction are further examined by chest radiography, CT scan, and laboratory studies. Screening is recommended annually for children in high-risk situations or communities including children in whose family there is an active case. High-risk situations include children who recently immigrated from countries with high incidence of TB, children infected with human immunodeficiency virus, those who are homeless or live in overcrowded conditions, and those immunosuppressed for any reason.

Treatment

Drug therapy for tuberculosis includes administration of isoniazid (INH), often in combination with rifampin. Although INH has been known to cause peripheral neuropathy in children with poor nutrition, few problems occur in children whose diets are well-balanced. Rifampin is tolerated well by children but causes body fluids such as saliva, urine, sweat, tears, and feces to turn orange-red. A possible disadvantage for adolescents is that it may permanently stain contact lenses. In addition, rifampin can decrease the effect of hormonal birth control, so other forms of birth control should be used while taking the drug.

Drug therapy is continued for 9 to 12 months. After drug therapy has begun, the child or adolescent may return to school and normal activities unless clinical symptoms are evident. An annual chest x-ray is necessary from that time on.

Prevention

Prevention requires improvements in social conditions such as overcrowding, poverty, poor healthcare, contact tracing, and identification of individuals who have TB.

A vaccine called bacillus Calmette-Guérin (BCG) is used in countries with a high incidence of tuberculosis. It is given to tuberculin-negative persons, especially those who have a likelihood of being in contact with TB positive individuals. After administration of BCG vaccine, the skin test will be positive, so screening is no longer an effective tool.

Casey Wilson is now stabilized after his asthma attack. What treatments and medications would you expect will be used to manage Casey's asthma? What teaching would you reinforce with Casey and with his family?

KEY POINTS

- An infant or child's respiratory system, because of its small size and underdeveloped anatomic structures, is more prone to respiratory problems. Smaller structures lead to a greater chance of obstruction and respiratory distress. As the child grows, the use of the thoracic muscles takes the place of the use of the diaphragm and abdominal muscles for breathing.

- The most common complication of acute nasopharyngitis (common cold) is otitis media.

- Avoiding or removing allergens is the best way to prevent allergic rhinitis. Antihistamines and hyposensitization may be helpful for some clients.

- The child with tonsillitis may have a fever, sore throat, difficulty swallowing, hypertrophied tonsils, halitosis, and erythema of the soft palate. Exudate may be visible on the tonsils. Treatment of tonsillitis consists of analgesic, antipyretic, and antibiotic medications. Surgical removal of the tonsils and adenoids may be indicated.

- The most common complication of a tonsillectomy is hemorrhage or bleeding. The child must be observed, especially in the first 24 hours, after surgery and in the fifth to seventh postoperative days for unusual restlessness, anxiety, frequent swallowing, or rapid pulse. Vomiting bright, red-flecked emesis or bright red oozing or bleeding may indicate hemorrhage. If noted, these should be reported immediately.

- Spasmodic laryngitis may be of infectious or allergic origin. An attack is often preceded by a runny nose and hoarseness. The child awakens after a few hours of sleep with a barklike cough, respiratory difficulty, and stridor and may be anxious, restless, and hoarse. Humidified air is used to decrease the laryngospasm.

- Acute laryngotracheobronchitis is usually of viral origin, but bacterial invasion, usually staphylococcal, may follow and cause a secondary infection. The child may become hoarse and have a barking cough and elevated temperature. The child has laryngeal edema, inspiratory stridor, difficult breathing, and rapid pulse and cyanosis may occur. Corticosteroids are administered to decrease airway edema and inflammation. The child is placed in a humidified air atmosphere and oxygen administered. To achieve bronchodilation, racemic or nebulized epinephrine are given. Antibiotic medications are administered if a secondary bacterial infection occurs.

- Epiglottitis is an acute inflammation of the epiglottis and is not commonly seen. A mild upper respiratory infection often precedes the sudden onset of a severe sore throat, dysphagia (difficulty swallowing), high fever, and drooling which is a sign of significant concern. The child is better able to breathe in the "tripod" position.

- Bronchiolitis/RSV infection is caused by a viral infection. Dyspnea occurs as well as a persistent cough, respiratory distress including increased respiratory rate, nasal flaring, air hunger, and often marked cyanosis. Suprasternal and subcostal retractions are present with respirations as high as 60 to 80 breaths per minute. Diagnosis is made from clinical findings confirmed by laboratory testing of the respiratory secretions. The child is hospitalized, placed on contact and droplet transmission precautions, and treated with supportive care and humidified oxygen. Ribavirin, an antiviral drug, may be used.

- During an asthma attack, the combination of smooth muscle spasms, which cause the lumina of the bronchi and bronchioles to narrow, edema, and increased mucus production, cause respiratory obstruction.

- An asthma attack can be triggered by a hypersensitive response to allergens; foods such as chocolate, milk, eggs, nuts, grains, and food additives; exercise; or exposure to cold or irritants such as wood-burning stoves, cigarette smoke, dust, and pet dander. Infections, stress, or anxiety can also trigger an asthma attack.

- The goals of asthma treatment include preventing symptoms, maintaining nearly normal lung function and activity levels, preventing recurring exacerbations and hospitalizations, and providing the best medication treatment with the fewest adverse effects. Nursing care is focused on maintaining a clear airway, maintaining an adequate fluid intake, and relieving fatigue and anxiety.

- Pneumonia can be caused by a virus, bacterium, fungal infection, or aspiration of a foreign material. Pneumococcal (*Streptococcus pneumoniae*) pneumonia is the most common form of bacterial pneumonia. The onset is usually abrupt, following a mild upper respiratory illness. Symptoms may include a high temperature, respiratory distress with air hunger, flaring of the nostrils, circumoral cyanosis, and chest retractions. Tachycardia and tachypnea are present, with a pulse rate as high as 140 to 180 beats per minute and respirations as high as 80 breaths per minute. Irritability, lethargy, poor feeding, nausea, and vomiting may also be noted. Anti-infectives, such as amoxicillin have proved to be effective in the treatment. Cephalosporin anti-infectives are also used. Antipyretics and analgesics may be used to control fever and alleviate discomfort. Nursing care is focused on maintaining respiratory function, preventing fluid deficit, maintaining body temperature, preventing otitis media, conserving energy, and relieving anxiety.

- Cystic fibrosis (CF) causes the exocrine (mucus-producing) glands to produce thick, tenacious mucus, rather than thin, free-flowing secretions. These secretions obstruct the secretory ducts of the pancreas, liver, and reproductive organs.

- The sweat chloride test, which shows elevated sodium chloride levels in the sweat, is the principal diagnostic test used to confirm CF. Family history, newborn screening, clinical symptoms, genetic tests to show CF gene mutation, a history of failure to thrive, chronic or recurrent respiratory infections, and radiologic findings of hyperinflation and bronchial wall thickening help diagnose the disorder.

- The most common and serious complications of CF arise from respiratory infections, which may lead to severe respiratory concerns.

- Pancreatic enzymes given with meals and snacks are used in the dietary treatment of children with CF. The child's diet is high in protein and carbohydrates, and salt in large amounts is allowed. The use of chest physiotherapy, antibiotics, and inhalation therapy help in the prevention and treatment of respiratory infections.

- Tuberculosis can be detected by doing a tuberculin skin test using purified protein derivative. When a person has a positive reaction to the skin test, additional evaluation using radiography is done to confirm the disease. INH and rifampin are used to treat tuberculosis and are given for 9 to 12 months.

INTERNET RESOURCES

Cystic Fibrosis Foundation
www.cff.org

National Heart, Lung, and Blood Institute
www.nhlbi.nih.gov

Asthma and Allergy
www.aafa.org

American Lung Association
www.lung.org

American Academy of Allergy, Asthma and Immunology
www.aaaai.org

RSV
http://www.marchofdimes.org/complications/rsv.aspx

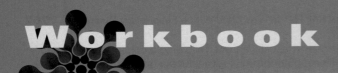
NCLEX-STYLE REVIEW QUESTIONS

1. The nurse is reinforcing teaching with the family caregivers of a child who has had a tonsillectomy the previous day and is being discharged. The nurse would reinforce that which reaction should be reported *immediately* to the child's health care provider?

   a. The child complains of a sore throat on the third post-operative day.

   b. The child refuses to leave the ice collar on for more than 10 minutes.

   c. The child vomits dark, old blood within 4 hours after being discharged.

   d. The child has frequent swallowing around the sixth day after surgery.

2. A toddler with a diagnosis of a respiratory disorder has a fever and decreased urinary output. When planning care for this child, what would be the *most* appropriate goal for this toddler?

   a. The child's anxiety will be reduced.

   b. The child's fluid intake will be increased.

   c. The child's caregivers will talk about their concerns.

   d. The child's caloric intake will be adequate for age.

3. The nurse is reinforcing teaching with a group of family caregivers of children who have asthma. The caregivers make the following statements. Which statement indicates a need for additional teaching?

   a. "We need to identify the things that trigger our child's attacks."

   b. "I always have him use his bronchodilator before he uses his steroid inhaler."

   c. "We will be sure our child does not exercise to prevent attacks."

   d. "She drinks lots of water, which I know helps to thin her secretions."

4. What intervention should be included in the plan of care for a child with cystic fibrosis?

   a. Maintain a flat-lying position when in bed.

   b. Provide low-protein snacks between meals.

   c. Perform postural drainage in the morning and evening.

   d. Reinforce isolation procedures when hospitalized.

5. After discussing the disease with the family caregiver of a child with cystic fibrosis, the caregiver makes the following statements. Which statement indicates a need for additional teaching?

   a. "It is good to know that my other children can't have the disease."

   b. "I will be sure to give my child the medication every time she eats."

   c. "It is important to let my child play with the other kids when she is at school."

   d. "When she exercises, I will feed her a salty snack."

6. The nurse is completing the intake and output record for a toddler who has a respiratory infection. The dry weight of the child's diaper is 38 grams. The child has had the following intake and output during the shift:

   Intake:
   3 oz of apple juice
   ½ serving of pancakes
   5 oz of milk
   4 saltine crackers
   ¼ cup of chicken soup
   2 oz of gelatin
   130 mL of IV fluid
   Output:
   Diaper with urine weighing 87 grams
   Diaper with stool only weighing 124 grams
   Diaper with urine weighing 138 grams
   Diaper with urine weighing 146 grams
   Diaper with urine weighing 95 grams

   a. How many milliliters should the nurse document as the child's total intake?

   b. How many milliliters should the nurse document as the child's urinary output?

STUDY ACTIVITIES

1. Draw a diagram to explain the heredity pattern of cystic fibrosis.

2. Research your community to find sources of help for families with children who have cystic fibrosis. What support groups and organizations are available that you might recommend to families of children with cystic fibrosis? Discuss with your peers what you found, and make a list of resources to share.

3. Do an internet search on "caring for children with asthma." Review several of the sites you find and do the following.

   a. Make a list of sites which you think would offer reliable information in caring for the child with asthma.

   b. List six areas you found on these sites that you think would be helpful to share with a family of a child with asthma.

   c. Discuss what you found on one of these sites that you think would be helpful for the nurse caring for the child with asthma.

CRITICAL THINKING: WHAT WOULD YOU DO?

1. Sandy calls the 24-hour pediatric health line at 10:30 PM about her 2.5-year-old child Jared. Jared had gone to bed at his usual bedtime of 8:00 PM after an uneventful evening. He had awakened with a barklike cough, respiratory difficulty, and a high-pitched harsh sound on inspiration.

   a. What questions would you ask this mother to further clarify Jared's situation?

   b. What would you suggest Sandy should do to decrease Jared's symptoms?

   c. What would you tell Sandy to watch for that might indicate Jared needs emergency attention?

2. Rachel, a 6-year-old girl, is brought to the clinic with a dry hacking cough, wheezing, and difficulty breathing. Rachel is coughing up thick mucus. Her parents are with her and are extremely anxious about Rachel's condition. The health care provider examines Rachel, and a diagnosis of an acute asthma attack is made.

   a. What other findings might have been noted during a physical examination of Rachel?

   b. What will most likely be done to treat Rachel's current condition?

   c. What medications might have been given?

   d. What would you discuss with Rachel's parents about prevention of additional attacks?

3. Dosage calculation: A toddler with a diagnosis of cystic fibrosis is being treated with the bronchodilator theophylline. The child weighs 32 lb. The usual dosage of this medication is 4 mg/kg/dose every 6 hours. Answer the following.

   a. How many kilograms does the child weigh?

   b. How many milligrams per dose will be given?

   c. How many doses will the child receive in a day?

   d. How much theophylline will be given in a 24-hour period?

37

The Child With a Cardiovascular/Hematologic Disorder

Key Terms

adenopathy
alopecia
arthralgia
bradycardia
carditis
chorea
congestive heart failure
digitalization
erythema marginatum
epistaxis
granulocytes
hemarthrosis
intrathecal administration
leukemia
lymphoblast
lymphocytes
monocytes
petechiae
polyarthritis
purpura

Learning Objectives

At the conclusion of this chapter, you will:

1. Describe the cardiovascular and hematologic systems and how they function.
2. Discuss ways the child's cardiovascular and hematologic systems differ from the adult's systems.
3. Discuss congestive heart failure (CHF), including care of the child with CHF.
4. Name the bacterium usually responsible for the infection that leads to the development of acute rheumatic fever.
5. List the major manifestations of acute rheumatic fever and describe the nursing care.
6. Explain Kawasaki disease and state the most serious concern for the child suffering from it.
7. Discuss iron-deficiency anemia and identify the common causes.
8. Explain how (a) sickle cell trait and (b) sickle cell disease are inherited.
9. Describe the shape of the red blood cell and the effect it has on the circulation in sickle cell disease.
10. Discuss the nursing care for the child with sickle cell disease.
11. Discuss the common complications and prognosis for the child with thalassemia.
12. Name the most common types of hemophilia and state how they are inherited.
13. Discuss the treatment and nursing care for the child with hemophilia.
14. Describe the symptoms noted in the child with immune thrombocytopenia (ITP).
15. Explain the diagnosis of leukemia, including the symptoms, treatment, and nursing care.

Amalia Romero is 9 years old. She comes to the clinic this afternoon with her father who tells you she is complaining of muscle, joint, and abdominal pain. Amalia is pale, has a low-grade fever, and appears fatigued. As you read this chapter, make a list of questions you will ask Amalia's father regarding her present symptoms.

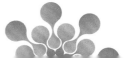

ardiovascular system disorders and hematologic disorders, which are disorders having to do with the blood and the blood-forming tissues, are usually serious and may be chronic or long-term conditions. Many of these conditions are hereditary and often present at birth. Congenital heart disorders are discussed in Chapter 21. The seriousness of disorders related to the cardiovascular system creates fear and concern in the child and family. An understanding of the cardiovascular system and how it functions can be helpful in decreasing the anxiety these families have.

GROWTH AND DEVELOPMENT OF THE CARDIOVASCULAR AND HEMATOLOGIC SYSTEMS

All systems of the body depend on the cardiovascular system. It works to carry the needed chemicals to and from the cells in the body so they can function properly. The major organ of the cardiovascular system is the heart, which is the pump that keeps the blood, containing oxygen and nutrients, circulating through the body. The hematologic system includes the blood and blood-forming tissues. The cardiovascular and hematologic systems work together to remove the waste products from the cells so they can be excreted from the body. The vessels, which carry the blood to and from the heart and through the body, include the arteries, veins, and capillaries. Arteries carry blood away from the heart to the body, and veins collect the blood and return it to the heart. Capillaries are the exchange vessels for the materials that flow through the body. Blood is a fluid composed of many elements, including plasma, red blood cells (RBCs), white blood cells (WBCs), and platelets. Each of these elements has a different function. These blood cells are formed in the bone marrow. The diseases and disorders of the circulatory system and the blood-forming tissues occur when the heart itself or the blood or blood-forming tissues are genetically altered, infection or damage has occurred, the organs or tissues are not shaped or functioning normally, or when the elements in the blood are increased or decreased in amount.

DIFFERENCES BETWEEN THE CHILD'S AND ADULT'S CARDIOVASCULAR AND HEMATOLOGIC SYSTEMS

Normal fetal circulation and the changes that occur in the cardiovascular system when the infant is born are covered in Chapter 21. Congenital heart disorders often occur in infants because the heart is not formed properly or the structures do not close at birth. At birth, both the right and left ventricles are about the same size, but by a few months of age, the left ventricle is about two times the size of the right. The infant's heart rate is higher than the older child's or adult's so that the infant's cardiac output can provide adequate oxygen to the body. If the infant has a fever, respiratory distress, or any increased need for oxygen, the pulse rate goes up to increase the cardiac output. Although the size is smaller, by the time the child is 5 years old the heart has matured, developed,

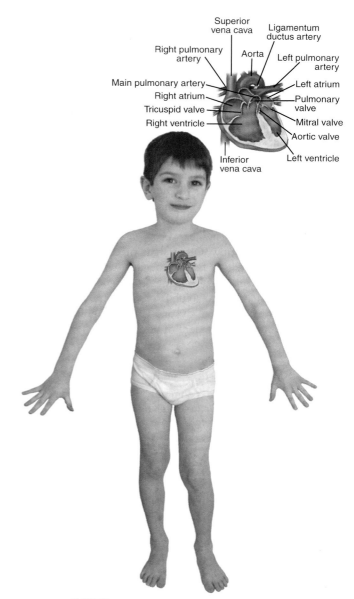

FIGURE 37-1 Anatomy of the normal heart.

and functions just as the adult's heart (Fig. 37-1). The blood volume in the body is proportionate to the body weight. The younger the child is, the higher the blood volume is per kilogram of body weight.

CONGESTIVE HEART FAILURE

Congestive heart failure (CHF) occurs when blood and fluids accumulate in the organs and body tissues. This accumulation happens because the heart is not able to pump and circulate enough blood to supply the oxygen and nutrient needs of the body cells. Manifestations of CHF may appear in children with conditions such as congenital heart disorders (see Chapter 21 for additional discussion), rheumatic fever, or Kawasaki disease. The condition places an increased workload on the ventricles of the heart.

Clinical Manifestations

The indications of CHF vary in children of different ages. Signs in the infant may be hard to detect because they are subtle. These include easy fatigability, which is manifested by feeding problems. The infant tires easily; breathes hard; and may have rapid respirations with an expiratory grunt, flaring of the nares, and sternal retractions. The infant may refuse the bottle after just 1 or 2 ounces, but soon becomes hungry again. During feeding, the infant may even become diaphoretic from the effort of feeding. Lying flat causes stress for the infant, who may appear more comfortable if held upright over an adult's shoulder. Periorbital edema may be present. A rapid weight gain may also indicate CHF.

In infants and older children, one of the first signs of CHF is tachycardia. The heart beats faster in an attempt to increase the blood flow. Other signs of CHF often seen in the older child include failure to gain weight, abdominal pain, nausea, vomiting, weakness, fatigue, restlessness, irritability, and a pale, mottled, or cyanotic color. Rapid respirations or tachypnea, dyspnea, and coughing are also seen. Edema and enlargement of the liver and heart may be present.

 Concept Mastery Alert

Failure to gain weight is a common finding in congestive heart failure. Congestive heart failure results in greater metabolic activity; therefore, the patient does not gain weight and muscle mass normally.

Diagnosis

The clinical symptoms are the primary basis for diagnosis of CHF. Chest x-rays reveal an enlarged heart; electrocardiography may indicate ventricular hypertrophy, and an echocardiogram may be done to note cardiac function.

Treatment

The underlying cause of the CHF is corrected when possible to reverse the heart failure. Treatment of CHF includes improving the cardiac function using cardiac glycosides, such as digoxin, removing excess fluids with the use of diuretic drugs, decreasing the workload on the heart by limiting physical activity, and improving tissue oxygenation. Digoxin is used to improve the cardiac efficiency by slowing the heart rate and strengthening the cardiac contractility. The use of large doses of digoxin, at the beginning of therapy, to build up the blood levels of the drug to a therapeutic level is known as **digitalization**. A maintenance dose is given, usually daily, after digitalization. Angiotensin-converting enzyme (ACE) inhibitors, such as captopril and enalapril, are given to increase vasodilatation. Beta blockers such as carvedilol or metoprolol may be used. The use of diuretic drugs, such as furosemide, thiazide diuretic drugs, or spironolactone, and fluid restriction in the acute stages of CHF help eliminate excess fluids. The child should be placed with the head elevated to allow for lung expansion. Oxygen is administered to increase oxygenation of tissues. Energy requirements should be minimized to ease the workload of the heart. Small, frequent feedings improve nutrition with minimal energy output.

Nursing Process and Care Plan *for the Child With Congestive Heart Failure*

Assessment (Data Collection)

An interview with the family caregiver of a child with CHF must include the gathering of information about the current illness and any previous episodes. Ask about any problems the child may have during feeding, episodes of rapid or difficult respirations, episodes of turning blue, and difficulty with lying flat. Determine if the child has been gaining weight.

The physical examination of the child includes a complete measurement of vital signs. Note the quality and rhythm of the apical pulse. Observe respiratory status, including any use of accessory muscles, retractions, breath sounds, rate, and type of cry. Examine the skin and extremities for color, skin temperature, and evidence of edema. Observe the child closely for signs of easy fatigability or an increase in symptoms on exertion.

Nursing Care Focus

When determining the focus of nursing care for the child with congestive heart failure, improving the cardiac output and monitoring for adequate tissue perfusion are important. In addition, concerns of sufficient oxygenation, nutrition, and activity intolerance must be addressed. Reinforcing family caregiver teaching related to the child's illness is included.

Outcome Identification and Planning

The major goals include improving cardiac output and oxygenation, relieving inadequate respirations, maintaining adequate hydration and nutritional intake, and conserving energy. The family's goals include increasing understanding of the condition and its prognosis.

Nursing Care Focus

- Altered cardiac tissue perfusion related to structural defects or decreased cardiac functioning

Goal

- The child's cardiac output will improve and be adequate to meet the child's needs.

Implementations for Monitoring Adequate Tissue Perfusion

Monitor vital signs regularly to detect symptoms of decreased cardiac output. Monitor pulse rates closely. Digoxin is frequently ordered for the child. Always check the dosage of digoxin with another nurse before administering it. Observe closely for any signs of digoxin toxicity, such as anorexia, nausea and vomiting, irregular pulse, or decreased pulse rate (**bradycardia**).

Regularly observe the child for evidence of periorbital or peripheral edema. Weigh the undressed child early in the morning before the first feeding of the day, using the same scale every time. Maintain careful intake and output measurements. If diuretic drugs are administered, monitor serum electrolyte levels, especially potassium levels.

Here's a Pharmacology Fact!
If digoxin is ordered, count the apical pulse for a full minute before administering digoxin. Withhold digoxin, and notify the health care provider if the apical rate is lower than the established norms for the child's age and baseline information (90 to 110 bpm for infants, 70 to 85 bpm for older children).

Evaluation of Goal/Desired Outcome

The child:

- has a heart rate within the normal limits for their age.
- is free from arrhythmias or evidence of edema.
- maintains adequate peripheral perfusion.

Nursing Care Focus

- Altered breathing pattern related to pulmonary congestion and anxiety

Goal

- The child's respiratory function will improve.

Implementations for Improving Respiratory Function

Elevate the head of the crib mattress so that it is at a 30-degree to 45-degree angle. Do not allow the child to shift down in the crib and become "scrunched up," which causes decreased expansion room for the chest and lungs. Avoid constricting clothing. Administer oxygen as ordered. Monitor respirations at least every 4 hours, paying close attention to breath sounds, dyspnea, tachypnea, and retractions. Observe the child for cyanosis, especially noting the color of the nail beds and around the mouth, lips, hands, and feet. Monitor oxygen saturation levels with pulse oximetry. Respiratory infections can be a concern for the child with CHF. The child has a decreased resistance to these infections, and exposure to people who have respiratory infections should be avoided. Monitor closely for any signs of infection and report any findings.

Evaluation of Goal/Desired Outcome

The child's:

- respirations are regular with no retractions.
- breath sounds are clear.
- oxygen saturation is within the acceptable range for the child's status.

Nursing Care Focus

- Malnutrition risk related to fatigue and dyspnea

Goal

- The child's caloric intake will be adequate to maintain nutritional needs for growth.

Implementations for Maintaining Adequate Nutrition

Give frequent feedings in small amounts to avoid overtiring the infant or child. Rest periods may be needed during feedings. For the infant, use a soft nipple with a large opening to ease the child's workload. If adequate nutrition cannot be taken during feedings, enteral feedings via a nasogastric tube may be necessary.

Evaluation of Goal/Desired Outcome

The child:

- consumes adequate amount of the feeding each time and feeds with minimal tiring.
- has appropriate weight gain for age.

Nursing Care Focus

- activity intolerance related to insufficient oxygenation

Goal

- The child will have increased levels of energy.

Implementations for Promoting Energy Conservation

Nursing care is planned so that the child has long periods of uninterrupted rest. While carrying out nursing procedures, talk to the child softly and soothingly, and handle them gently with care. Respond to the infant's cries quickly and plan simple age-appropriate activities to avoid tiring the child.

Evaluation of Goal/Desired Outcome

The child:

- rests quietly during uninterrupted periods of rest.
- does not become overly tired when awake.

Nursing Care Focus

- Knowledge deficiency of caregivers related to the child's illness

Goal

- The family caregivers are prepared for the child's home care.

Implementations for Reinforcing Family Teaching

The family of this child has reason to be apprehensive and anxious. It is important to be understanding, empathic, and nonjudgmental when communicating with them. Give them information about CHF in a way that they can understand. Repeat information about signs and symptoms, and offer explanations as many times as necessary. Reinforce teaching about medication, feeding and caring techniques, growth and development expectations, and future plans for correction of the defect, if known. Involve the family in the child's care as much as possible within the limitations of the child's condition.

Evaluation of Goal/Desired Outcome

The family:

- verbalizes anxieties.
- asks appropriate questions.
- participates in the child's care.
- discusses the child's condition.

ACUTE RHEUMATIC FEVER

Acute rheumatic fever (ARF) is a chronic disease of childhood, affecting the connective tissue of the heart, joints, and central nervous system. An autoimmune reaction to group A *Streptococcus* pharyngeal infection, rheumatic fever occurs throughout the world. The incidence of ARF in the United States is most commonly seen in children ages 5 to 15.

Rheumatic fever is precipitated by a streptococcal infection, such as strep throat, tonsillitis, scarlet fever, or pharyngitis, which may be undiagnosed or untreated. The resultant rheumatic fever manifestation may be the first indication of concern.

Clinical Manifestations

A latent period of 2 to 4 weeks follows the initial infection. The onset is often slow and subtle. The child may have a low-grade fever and complain of vague muscle, joint, or abdominal pain and fatigue. None of these is diagnostic by itself, but if such signs persist, the child should be seen by a health care provider.

The onset may be acute, rather than insidious, with severe carditis or arthritis as the presenting symptom. Major manifestations of acute rheumatic fever include carditis, polyarthritis, and Sydenham chorea. Sydenham chorea generally has an insidious onset. Other major manifestations include subcutaneous nodules that appear on a bony surface or tendon such as the elbows and **erythema marginatum** (a pink-red rash on the trunk).

The minor manifestations of acute rheumatic fever include **arthralgia** (joint pain), fever, elevated C-reactive protein (CRP) and erythrocyte sedimentation rate (ESR), and a prolonged PR interval on the electrocardiogram. Elevated CRP, elevated ESR, and leukocytosis indicate the presence of an inflammatory process.

Carditis

Carditis refers to inflammation of the heart. It is the major cause of permanent heart and heart valve damage, especially the mitral and aortic valves, and disability among children with rheumatic fever. Carditis may occur alone or as a complication of either arthritis or chorea. Presenting symptoms may be vague enough to be missed. The child may have a poor appetite, pallor, pain, or slight dyspnea on exertion. Physical examination reveals tachycardia and a murmur over the apex of the heart.

Polyarthritis

Polyarthritis, or migratory arthritis, moves from one major joint to another (ankles, knees, wrists, elbows). The joint becomes inflamed; painful to touch or with movement (arthralgia); and appears red, hot, and swollen. Body temperature is moderately elevated; the erythrocyte sedimentation rate (ESR) is increased. Although extremely painful, this type of arthritis does not lead to the disabling deformities that occur in rheumatoid arthritis.

Sydenham Chorea

Sydenham **chorea** is a disorder characterized by emotional instability, involuntary movements, and muscular weakness. The onset of chorea is gradual, often more evident on one side, stops during sleep, and is more commonly noted in females. Movements may be mild and remain so, or they may become increasingly severe. Active arthritis is rarely present when chorea is the major manifestation. Carditis occurs, although less commonly seen with chorea than when polyarthritis is the major condition.

Diagnosis

Acute rheumatic fever can be difficult to diagnose and differentiate from other diseases. The possible serious effects of the disease demand early and conscientious medical treatment.

The Jones criteria (Fig. 37-2) are used to diagnose and treat acute rheumatic fever. The criteria are divided into major and minor manifestations. The presence of two major or one major and two minor criteria indicates a high probability of rheumatic fever if supported by evidence of a preceding streptococcal infection. Additional manifestations can help confirm the diagnosis.

Remember Amalia from the beginning of the chapter? What do you think **Amalia Romero**'s diagnosis might be? If you determined that Amalia has rheumatic fever, you are correct. What would you anticipate regarding Amalia's history? What other symptoms might you note in Amalia? Think about what diagnostic tests might be done to collect data related to Amalia's condition.

Treatment

The treatment of acute rheumatic fever includes administering antibiotic medications such as penicillin to eliminate the group A streptococci. If the child is allergic to penicillin, erythromycin is used. Penicillin administration continues after the acute phase of the illness to prevent the recurrence of rheumatic fever. Anti-inflammatory drugs (NSAIDs) such as naproxen or ibuprofen help relieve the arthritis joint pain

The child with severe Sydenham chorea must be observed closely and protected from injury. Antiseizure drugs such as carbamazepine or valproic acid may be given.

Prevention

The overall approach to prevention is to promote health supervision and continuity of care for all children, especially school-aged children since the peak of onset of acute rheumatic fever occurs in this age group. Reinforcement of teaching includes informing the public about the need to have upper respiratory infections evaluated for group A streptococci and the need for treatment with penicillin if the throat culture is positive. Prophylactic antibiotic medications are sometimes given for a long period of time to prevent recurrence.

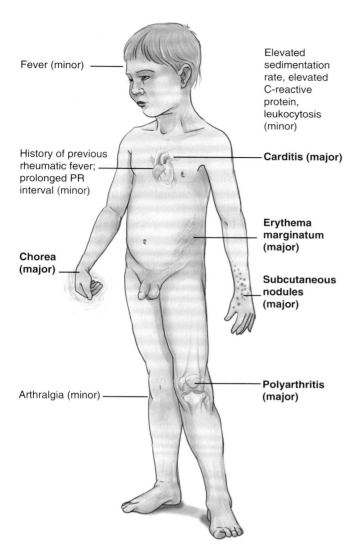

Fever (minor)

Elevated sedimentation rate, elevated C-reactive protein, leukocytosis (minor)

Carditis (major)

History of previous rheumatic fever; prolonged PR interval (minor)

Erythema marginatum (major)

Chorea (major)

Subcutaneous nodules (major)

Arthralgia (minor)

Polyarthritis (major)

FIGURE 37-2 Major and minor manifestations of rheumatic fever.

TEST YOURSELF

✔ What are the common symptoms and treatments for CHF?

✔ What type of infection would likely be found in the history of a child who has acute rheumatic fever?

✔ Explain the terms carditis, polyarthritis, and Sydenham chorea.

✔ What are the two important aspects in the prevention of acute rheumatic fever?

Nursing Process and Care Plan *for the Child With Acute Rheumatic Fever*

Assessment (Data Collection)

Conduct a thorough examination of the child. Begin with a careful review of all systems, and note the child's physical condition. Observe for any signs that may be classified as major or minor manifestations. In the physical examination, observe for elevated temperature and pulse, and carefully examine for erythema marginatum, subcutaneous nodules, swollen or painful joints, or signs of chorea. A throat culture determines whether there is an active infection. Obtain a complete up-to-date history from the child and the family caregiver. Ask about a recent sore throat or upper respiratory infection. Find out when the symptoms began, the extent of the illness, and what, if any, treatment was obtained. Include the school-aged child in the interview to help contribute to the history.

Nursing Care Focus

The nursing care focuses for the child with acute rheumatic fever include treating and managing joint pain. Helping the child cope with being on bed rest, having activities restricted, risk for injury, and adhering to prophylactic drug therapy are also concerns. Recognize the need for reinforcing family teaching about the condition, need for long-term therapy, and risk factors.

---

and are administered until those symptoms resolve.

A chief concern in caring for a child with rheumatic fever is the prevention and treatment of residual heart disease. Heart disease is treated in accordance with its severity and its type with cardiac medications, restricted activities, diuretic drugs, and a low-sodium diet as indicated. Corticosteroids may be given with severe carditis.

Here's a Pharmacology Fact!

Ensure that the child takes the complete prescription of penicillin (usually 10 days' supply). Even though the symptoms disappear and the child feels well, the infection can return if the entire course of antibiotics is not taken.

This Could Make a Difference!

As long as the rheumatic process is active, progressive heart damage is possible, so bed rest is essential for the child with acute rheumatic fever to reduce the heart's workload.

Outcome Identification and Planning

The goals are determined in cooperation with the child and the family caregiver. Goals for the child include reducing pain, providing diversional activities and sensory stimulation, conserving energy, and preventing injury. Goals for the family caregiver include complying with drug therapy and increasing knowledge about the long-term care of the child. Throughout planning and implementation, bear in mind the child's developmental stage.

Nursing Care Focus

- Acute pain related to joint pain when extremities are touched or moved

Goal

- The child's joint pain will be minimal.

Implementations for Providing Comfort Measures and Reducing Pain

Position the child to relieve joint pain. Large joints, including the knees, ankles, wrists, and elbows, are usually involved. Carefully handle the joints when moving the child to help minimize pain. Warm baths and gentle range-of-motion exercises help alleviate some joint discomfort. Use pain indicator scales with children so they are able to express the level of their pain (see Fig. 29-9).

Watch Out!
Even the weight of blankets may cause pain for the child with acute rheumatic fever. Be alert to this possibility and improvise covering as needed.

Anti-inflammatory drugs (NSAIDs) such as naproxen or ibuprofen are given to reduce fever and relieve joint inflammation and pain. Therapy is usually continued until laboratory findings are normal.

Evaluation of Goal/Desired Outcome

- The child verbalizes or indicates by using a pain scale to express degree of pain that the pain level is decreased.

Nursing Care Focus

- Coping impairment related to prescribed bed rest

Goal

- The child will become engaged in activities while on bed rest.

Implementations for Providing Diversional Activities and Sensory Stimulation

Children vary greatly in how poorly they feel during the acute phase of acute rheumatic fever. For those who do not feel very ill, being placed on bed rest can cause distress or resentment. Be creative in finding diversional activities that allow bed rest, but prevent restlessness and boredom. This may be a good time to choose a book that involves the child's imagination and has enough excitement to create ongoing interest. Quiet games can provide some entertainment. Television should be used minimally as a diversional activity. Use of a computer or electronic devices can be beneficial, because both entertaining and educational activities are available, and most children enjoy doing these. Simple needlework and model building are other appropriate diversional activities. Make efforts during the school year (or encourage the family caregiver) to provide the child with a tutor and work from school; this helps relieve boredom and also maintains contact with peers. Plan all activities with the child's developmental stage in mind. The pain of arthralgia may be so great that the child will not want to be involved in any kind of activity. Administer analgesic medications as ordered to help decrease the inflammation of the joints and decrease the pain so the child will want to participate in age-appropriate activities.

Evaluation of Goal/Desired Outcome

The child:

- displays interest in participating in activities.
- is actively involved in age-appropriate activities.

Nursing Care Focus

- Activity intolerance related to carditis or arthralgia

Goal

- The child will learn when and how to conserve energy.

Implementations for Promoting Energy Conservation

Provide rest periods between activities to help pace the child's energies and provide for maximum comfort. During times of increased cardiac involvement or exacerbations of joint pain, the child may want to rest and perhaps have someone read a story. Peers may be encouraged to visit, but these visits must be monitored so that the child is not overly tired. The child's classmates could be encouraged to write to the child to provide contact with everyday school activities and keep the child in touch. If the child has chorea, inform visitors that the child cannot control these movements, which may be as upsetting to others as they are to the child.

Evaluation of Goal/Desired Outcome

The child:

- rests quietly during rest periods.
- identifies when they need rest.
- engages in quiet diversional activities.

Nursing Care Focus

- Injury risk related to chorea

Goal

- The child will remain free of injury from chorea movements, and a safe environment is maintained.

Implementations for Preventing Injury

The child with chorea may be frustrated with their inability to control the movements. Provide an opportunity for the child to express feelings. Protect the child from injury by keeping the side rails up and padding them. Do not leave a child with chorea unattended in a wheelchair. Use all appropriate safety measures.

Evaluation of Goal/Desired Outcome

The child:

- has no evidence of injury.
- follows safety measures.

Nursing Care Focus

- Risk for nonadherence to prophylactic drug therapy related to financial or emotional burden of lifelong therapy

Goal

- The family caregivers will comply with follow-up drug therapy, and the child will take prophylactic medications.

Implementations for Promoting Compliance With Drug Therapy

A child does not become immune from future attacks of acute rheumatic fever after the first illness. Acute rheumatic fever can recur whenever the child has a group A streptococcal infection if the child is not properly treated. For this reason, often the child who has had acute rheumatic fever must be maintained on prophylactic doses of penicillin for 5 years or longer. Whenever the child is to have oral surgery, including dental work, extra prophylactic precautions should be taken, even in adulthood. Because of this long-term therapy, noncompliance for both financial and emotional reasons can become a problem. Oral penicillin is usually prescribed, but if compliance is poor, monthly injections of antibiotic medications such as penicillin G benzathine may be substituted. Encourage the family to contact the local chapter of the American Heart Association (www.americanheart.org) for help finding economical sources of medications. Become informed about other resources that may be available in your community. Emphasize to the child and the family the need to prevent recurrence of the disease because of the danger of heart damage. Follow-up care must be ongoing, even into adulthood.

Evaluation of Goal/Desired Outcome

The child and family caregivers:

- verbalize an understanding of the importance of prophylactic medication.
- identify means for obtaining medications.

Nursing Care Focus

- Knowledge deficiency of caregiver related to the condition, need for long-term therapy, and risk factors

Goal

- The family caregivers will verbalize an understanding of the child's condition, need for long-term therapy, and risk factors.

Implementations for Reinforcing Family Teaching

Reinforce with the family and the child the importance of having all upper respiratory infections checked by a health care provider to prevent another episode of a streptococcal infection. Be certain that they understand the child can have recurrences and that a future recurrence could have much more serious effects. If the child has had carditis and heart damage has occurred, reinforce with the family caregiver that the child must receive regular follow-up evaluations of the damage. The child may need to be maintained on cardiac medications. Reinforce teaching with the family about these medications. Mitral valve dysfunction is a common aftereffect of severe carditis. A female who has had mitral valve damage from cardiac involvement may have problems in adulthood during pregnancy. Reinforce with the family caregiver that heart failure for such a girl is a possibility during pregnancy and that she should be monitored closely to determine heart problems in the event that a mitral valve replacement is needed.

When talking with the child and family caregiver, take every opportunity to stress the importance of preventing rheumatic fever. Other children in the family may benefit if family caregivers are given this information.

Evaluation of Goal/Desired Outcome

The family caregivers:

- discuss the child's condition and need for follow-up care for the child.
- indicate how they will obtain follow-up care.

KAWASAKI DISEASE

Kawasaki disease (mucocutaneous lymph node syndrome) is an acute, febrile disease that is most often seen in boys younger than 5 years. The etiology is unknown, but the disease appears to be caused by an infectious agent. After an infection, an alteration in the immune system occurs. Genetic factors may also contribute to the cause of the disease. Most cases occur in the late winter or early spring. The major concern for the child is development of cardiac involvement.

Clinical Manifestations and Diagnosis

From the first day of the illness, the child presents with an elevated temperature (101.3°F to 104°F [38.5°C to 40°C]) which may continue 1 to 3 weeks. For Kawasaki disease to be diagnosed, the child must have had the elevated temperature for at least 5 days and in addition, four of the following symptoms:

- cervical lymphadenopathy
- conjunctivitis (bilateral)
- oral mucous membrane changes—red, cracked lips or strawberry-colored tongue
- extremity changes—edema, redness of hands and feet
- rash on trunk, extremities, perineal area

Other manifestations that may be seen include irritability, lethargy, cough, runny nose, diarrhea, and vomiting as well as joint and abdominal pain. Inflammation of the arteries, veins, and capillaries occurs, and this inflammation can lead to serious cardiac concerns, including aneurysms and thrombus. Electrocardiograms and echocardiograms may show cardiac involvement.

The white blood cell (WBC) count, eosinophil sedimentation rate (ESR), and C-reactive protein (CRP) are elevated. During the subacute stage, the platelet count increases, and this may lead to blood clotting and cardiac problems.

The disease occurs in three stages:

- Acute—high fever that does not respond to antibiotic or antipyretic medications; child is irritable, has symptoms as described above, and often has extreme tachycardia.
- Subacute—fever resolves, irritability continues; skin on the fingers and toes peels in layers; lack of appetite; greatest risk for aneurysms.
- Convalescent—symptoms are gone; phase continues until laboratory values are normal, and child's energy, appetite, and temperament have returned.

Treatment and Nursing Care

A high dose of intravenous immunoglobulin (IVIG) therapy is given to relieve the symptoms and prevent coronary artery abnormalities. Aspirin is used to control inflammation and fever and may be continued for as long as 1 year in lower doses as an antiplatelet medication.

> **Pay Attention!**
>
> Although not normally given to children, one of the few times aspirin is given is to the child with Kawasaki disease. The anti-inflammatory and antiplatelet effects help to decrease the concerns of coronary artery complications.

Nursing care for the child with Kawasaki disease focuses on management of the symptoms. It is important that you relieve pain and discomfort. Closely monitor temperature, cardiac status, intake and output, and daily weight. Offer extra fluids and soft foods, and provide mouth and lip care to help decrease the soreness. Encourage use of passive range-of-motion exercises that increase joint movement. Dealing with the irritability may be difficult for you as well as the child's family. Promote rest and a quiet environment to help decrease irritability. It is essential that you encourage the family caregivers to have times away from the child to help them cope with the stress of the illness. Reinforce teaching regarding the disease and symptoms, which may persist for a period of time, and follow-up treatments, visits, medication routines, and side effects. Most children recover without long-term effects, but the cardiac involvement may not be seen for a period of time after the child's recovery.

> **Do You Know the Why of It?**
>
> Immunizations, especially live vaccines, such as measles, mumps, and rubella (MMR), should not be given for 3 to 6 months to a child who has been treated with immunoglobulin (IVIG). The immunoglobulin prevents the body from building antibodies, so the vaccine will likely be ineffective in preventing the disease it is being given to prevent.

IRON-DEFICIENCY ANEMIA

Iron-deficiency anemia is a common nutritional deficiency in children. It is a hypochromic, microcytic anemia—in other words, the blood cells are deficient in production of hemoglobin and are smaller than normal—and is common between the ages of 9 and 24 months. The full-term newborn has a high hemoglobin level (needed during fetal life to provide adequate oxygenation) that decreases during the first 2 or 3 months of life. Considerable iron is reclaimed and stored, however, usually in sufficient quantity to last for 4 to 9 months of life.

A child needs to absorb 0.7 to 1.5 mg of iron per day. Because only 10% of dietary iron is absorbed, a diet containing 7 to 10 mg of iron is needed for good health. During the first years of life, obtaining this quantity of iron from food is often difficult for a child. If the diet is inadequate, anemia quickly results. In addition, some adolescents, females in particular, may have iron-deficiency anemia because of improper dieting to lose weight.

Babies with an inordinate fondness for milk can take in an astonishing amount and with their appetites satisfied, show little interest in solid foods. These babies are prime candidates for iron-deficiency anemia. They may have a history of consuming 2 or 3 quarts of milk daily while not accepting any other foods or, at best, only foods with a high carbohydrate content. Many family caregivers incorrectly believe that milk is a perfect food and that they should let the baby have all the milk desired. These children are commonly known as milk babies. They have pale, almost translucent (porcelain-like) skin and are chubby and susceptible to infections.

Many children with iron-deficiency anemia, however, are undernourished because of the family's economic situation. Along with the economic factor, a caregiver's

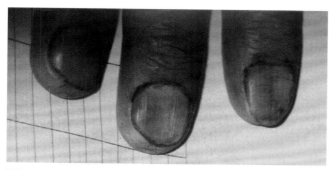

FIGURE 37-3 Concave or "spooning" of fingernails seen in iron-deficiency anemia.

knowledge deficit about nutrition is often present. The Women, Infants, and Children (WIC) program, discussed in Chapter 23, does much to alleviate this problem.

Clinical Manifestations and Diagnosis

The signs of iron-deficiency anemia include below-average body weight, pale mucous membranes, pallor, anorexia, delayed growth, fatigue, lethargy, and irritability, in addition to the characteristics of milk babies described earlier. Concave or "spooning" fingernails may be seen (Fig. 37-3).

In blood tests that measure hemoglobin, a level of less than 11 g/dL is highly suspect. Stool is tested for occult blood to rule out lower gastrointestinal bleeding as a cause for the depleted hemoglobin.

Treatment and Nursing Care

Treatment consists of improved nutrition, including iron-rich foods in the diet. Ferrous sulfate may be administered between meals with juice (preferably orange juice, because vitamin C aids in iron absorption). For best results, iron should not be given with meals. Tell the family

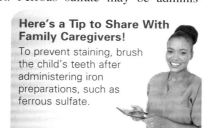

Here's a Tip to Share With Family Caregivers!
To prevent staining, brush the child's teeth after administering iron preparations, such as ferrous sulfate.

caregivers that ferrous sulfate can cause constipation or turn the child's stools black.

A few children have an intolerance to oral iron therapy, a hemoglobin level extremely low, or anorexia so acute that they need additional therapy. Iron sucrose or iron-dextran is given intravenously to these children. For children who are seriously ill, refer to Nursing Process and Care Plan for the Child With Malnutrition and Nutritional Problems in Chapter 38.

For most children with iron-deficiency anemia, diet and nutrition information is needed. When reinforcing teaching with caregivers, remember that attitudes and food choices are often influenced by cultural differences. See Tips for Reinforcing Family Teaching: Iron-Deficiency Anemia.

SICKLE CELL DISEASE

Sickle cell disease is a hereditary trait occurring most commonly in individuals of African descent. The sickling trait occurs in about 8% of people who are African Americans; the disease itself has an incidence of 1 out of every 365. The disease is characterized by the production of abnormal hemoglobin that causes the RBCs to assume a sickle shape. It appears as a trait without symptoms when the sickling trait is inherited from one parent alone (heterozygous state). There is a 50% probability that each child born to one parent carrying the sickle cell trait will inherit the trait from that parent. When the trait is inherited from both parents (homozygous state), the child has sickle cell disease, and anemia develops (Fig. 37-4). A rapid breakdown of RBCs carrying hemoglobin S, the abnormal hemoglobin, causes a severe hemolytic anemia. Persons who inherit the gene for the sickle cell trait from only one parent have no symptoms, normal hemoglobin levels, and normal RBC counts.

Clinical Manifestations

Clinical symptoms of the disease usually do not appear before the latter half of the first year of life because sufficient fetal hemoglobin is still present to prevent sickling. Sickle cell disease causes a chronic anemia with a

---

 TIPS FOR REINFORCING FAMILY TEACHING

Iron-deficiency Anemia

- One of the most important things you can do for your child and family is to learn about the foods that will help them stay healthy.
- Milk is good for your child, but no more than a quart a day (four 8-ounces bottles for the infant).
- Liquid iron preparations should be taken through a straw to prevent staining of teeth.

Foods Rich in Iron

- Baby cereals fortified with iron.
- For older children, fortified instant oatmeal and cream of wheat are good sources of iron.

- Some infant formulas are iron fortified.
- Egg yolks are rich in iron. Avoid egg whites for young children because of allergies.
- Green, leafy vegetables are good sources of iron.
- Dried beans, dried peas, canned refried beans, and peanut butter provide good iron sources for toddlers and older children.
- Fruits that are iron rich include peaches, prune juice, and raisins (do not give to a child younger than 3 years because of danger of choking).
- Read labels to check for iron content of processed foods.
- Organ meat, poultry, and fish are good iron sources.
- Orange juice helps the body absorb iron.

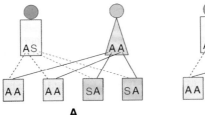
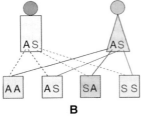

FIGURE 37-4 Inheritance patterns. **A.** Heterozygous type. One parent carries a hemoglobin S gene, and one does not. Two children will be free of the gene (AA), and two will be carriers (AS). **B.** Homozygous type. Each parent is carrying one hemoglobin A gene and one hemoglobin S gene. One child is free of the gene (AA), two are carriers (AS), and one has sickle cell disease (SS).

hemoglobin level of 6 to 9 g/dL (the normal level in an infant is 11 to 15 g/dL). The chronic anemia causes fatigue, a poor appetite, and pale mucous membranes.

Sickle cell crisis, vaso-occlusive crisis, is the most severe manifestation of the condition. Normal RBCs, which carry oxygen to the tissues, are disk-shaped and normally move through the blood vessels while bending and flexing to flow through smoothly. The smooth, uniform shape of the RBCs and the low viscosity (thickness) of the blood is such that these cells split relatively easily at Y-intersections and go single file through the capillaries with little or no clustering. The affected RBCs (hemoglobin S) do much the same thing until an episode causes sickling. An episode (a sickle cell crisis) can be precipitated by low oxygen levels, which can be caused by a respiratory infection or extremely strenuous exercise, dehydration, acidosis, or stress. When sickling occurs, the affected RBCs become crescent shaped and therefore do not slip through as easily as do the disk-shaped cells. The viscosity of the blood increases (becomes thicker), causing slowdown and sludging of the RBCs. The impaired circulation results in decreased oxygen to the tissues; and ischemia, occlusion, and infarction occur.

Vaso-occlusive crisis may be the first clinical manifestation of the disease and may recur frequently during early childhood. These acute painful episodes occur because of decreased circulation, causing decreased oxygenation, and present as a variety of symptoms, depending on the site of the occlusion. The pain can be in the abdomen, back, chest, joints, extremities, hands, and feet. Symptoms and complications from a vaso-occlusive crisis can occur in every system and organ of the body (Fig. 37-5). An occlusion in the brain can lead to cerebral ischemia or a stroke.

Diagnosis

Sickle cell disease is identified by newborn screening. Screening for the presence of hemoglobin S may be done with a test called Sickledex, a fingerstick screening test that gives rapid results. Definite diagnosis is made through hemoglobin electrophoresis. If the Sickledex screening results are positive, diagnosis can be done to determine if the child is carrying the trait or has sickle cell disease.

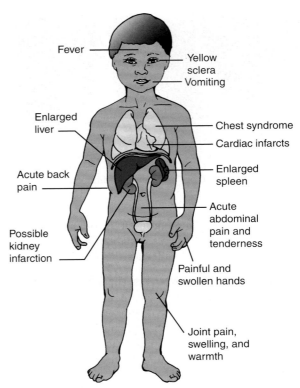

FIGURE 37-5 Sickle cell disease can affect many different areas of the child's body. (Reprinted with permission from Tagher, C. G., & Knapp, L. M. (2020). *Pediatric nursing: A case-based approach*, (Fig. 25-4, p. 499). Wolters Kluwer.)

Treatment

Prevention of crises is the goal between episodes. Hydroxyurea is used to decrease the incidence of vaso-occlusive pain episodes and strokes. Avoidance and early treatment of any type of infection is important. Adequate hydration is vital; fluid intake of 1,500 to 2,000 mL daily is desirable for a child weighing 20 kg and should be increased to 3,000 mL during the crisis. The child should avoid extremely strenuous activities that may cause oxygen depletion. Visiting areas of high altitude can increase oxygen needs, which could be a potential trigger for a crisis. Blood transfusions help bring the hemoglobin to a near-normal level and are used when needed.

Treatment for a crisis is supportive for each presenting symptom, and bed rest is indicated. Oxygen may be administered. Analgesic medications are given for pain. Dehydration and acidosis are vigorously treated.

Nursing Process and Care Plan *for the Child With a Sickle Cell Crisis*

Assessment (Data Collection)

The parents who have a child with sickle cell disease may experience a great deal of guilt for having passed the disease to their child. Take care not to increase this guilt, but help them cope with it. During the interview with the family

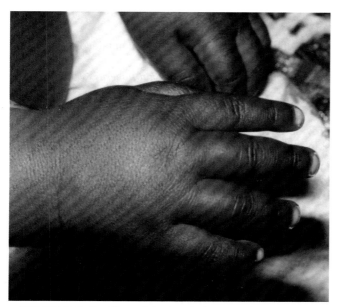

FIGURE 37-6 Swelling of the hands (dactylitis) in a toddler.

caregivers, ask about the activities or events that led to this crisis, obtain a history of the child's health and any previous episodes, and evaluate the family caregivers' knowledge about the condition.

Data collection techniques vary somewhat, depending on the child's age. Record vital and neurologic signs. Note any fever, abdominal or chest pain, presence of bowel sounds, pain or swelling and warmth in the joints, and muscle spasms. Observe the young child for dactylitis (hand–foot syndrome), which is often very painful. It results from soft tissue swelling caused by interference with circulation (Fig. 37-6). This swelling further impairs circulation.

Nursing Care Focus

When developing evidence-based nursing care focuses for the child with a sickle cell crisis (vaso-occlusive crisis), acute pain, risk for dehydration, altered skin integrity, activity intolerance, and keeping the child comfortable are included. Family coping impairment and reinforcing family teaching are important aspects of caring for the child and the family.

Outcome Identification and Planning

Maintaining comfort and relieving pain, increasing fluid intake, and conserving energy are major goals for the child with a sickle cell crisis. Other goals include improving physical mobility, maintaining skin integrity, and reducing the family caregivers' anxiety. Another important goal is decreasing the number of future episodes by increasing the caregiver's knowledge about the causes of crisis episodes. Plan individualized nursing care according to these goals.

Nursing Care Focus

- Acute pain related to disease condition affecting abdominal organs or joints and muscles

Goal

- The child's pain will be reduced or eliminated.

Implementations for Relieving Pain

The child in sickle cell crisis often has severe abdominal pain because of enlargement of the spleen (splenomegaly). Joint and muscle pain are also common because of poor perfusion of the tissues. Monitor the child's pain level, use nursing measures to relieve pain, and provide prompt administration of analgesic medications. The family caregivers can be involved in helping administer comfort measures to the child. Sometimes diversional activities and nonpharmacologic comfort interventions, such as heat, imagery, massage, repositioning, and biofeedback, can help alleviate pain.

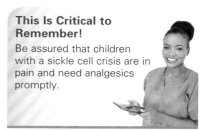

This Is Critical to Remember!

Be assured that children with a sickle cell crisis are in pain and need analgesics promptly.

Evaluation of Goal/Desired Outcome

- The child rests quietly and if possible, reports their comfort.

Nursing Care Focus

- Dehydration risk related to low fluid intake, impaired renal function, or both

Goal

- The child's fluid intake will improve.

Implementations for Maintaining Fluid Intake

Hydration helps prevent vaso-occlusive issues. The child is prone to dehydration due to decreased intake and because of the kidneys' inability to concentrate urine. Observe for signs of dehydration, such as dry mucous membranes, weight loss, or in the case of infants, sunken fontanels (fontanelles). Strict intake and output measurements and daily weights are necessary. Remind the family caregivers that fluid intake is important, and intake should be maintained at 1,500 to 2,000 mL when the child is not in crisis. Offer the child appealing fluids, such as juices, popsicles, noncaffeinated soda, and favorite flavored gelatins. Remind family caregivers that increasing fluid intake as the child ages will help avoid a crisis, especially during the child's activities such as hiking, swimming, and sports. The child needs increased fluids during episodes of infection or sickle cell crisis.

Evaluation of Goal/Desired Outcome

The child:

- shows no signs of dehydration.
- has an intake of 3,000 mL/day during crisis.

Nursing Care Focus

- Impaired comfort related to muscle and joint involvement

Goal

- The child's muscles and joints will remain flexible.

Implementations for Improving Physical Mobility

Sickling that affects the muscles and joints causes a great deal of pain and discomfort for the child. The child needs careful handling and should be moved slowly and gently. Joints can be supported with pillows. Warm soaks and massages may help relieve some of the discomfort by promoting vasodilation and increasing circulation. Administer analgesic medications before exercise and as needed. Passive exercises help prevent contractures and wasting of muscles.

Evaluation of Goal/Desired Outcome

- The child cooperates with daily passive exercises.

Nursing Care Focus

- Activity intolerance related to oxygen depletion and pain

Goal

- The child's energy will be conserved.

Implementations for Promoting Energy Conservation

The child may become dyspneic doing any kind of activity. Plan nursing care so that the child is disturbed as little as possible and can rest. Bed rest is necessary to decrease the demands of oxygen supply. Oxygen may be administered by mask or nasal cannula to improve tissue perfusion. Monitor oxygen saturation levels to maintain levels at 92% or higher.

Evaluation of Goal/Desired Outcome

The child's:

- activities are restricted to conserve energy.
- oxygen saturation is greater than 92%.

Nursing Care Focus

- Altered skin integrity risk related to decreased circulation

Goal

- The child's skin integrity will be maintained.

Implementations for Promoting Skin Integrity

Increased fluid intake and improved nutrition are important. Observe the child's skin regularly each shift, and provide good skin care consisting of lotion, massage, and skin-toughening agents, especially over bony prominences. Additional padding in the form of foam protectors and egg crate pads or mattresses may be helpful when there is irritation from bedding.

Evaluation of Goal/Desired Outcome

- The child's skin shows no signs of redness, irritation, or breakdown.

Nursing Care Focus

- Family coping impairment and anxiety related to child's condition

Goal

- The family caregivers' anxiety will be reduced.

Implementations for Promoting Family Coping

Guilt plays an important part in the anxiety that the family caregivers experience. Explain procedures, planned treatments, and care to help the family caregivers feel that they are being included in the care. Caregivers need to feel that they have some control over the disease.

Evaluation of Goal/Desired Outcome

The family caregivers:

- exhibit self-confidence.
- cooperate with nursing personnel.

Nursing Care Focus

- Knowledge deficiency of caregivers related to understanding of disorder and appropriate care measures

Goal

- The family caregivers will express understanding of the disease process.

Implementations for Reinforcing Family Teaching

Discuss measures that may help alleviate pain or encourage fluid intake. Also, emphasize the importance of protecting the child from situations that may cause overexhaustion or that may otherwise deplete the child's oxygen supplies or lead to dehydration. This knowledge may give the family caregivers a feeling of control. In addition, family caregivers may need more information concerning the disorder.

If the child's diagnosis is not new, the caregivers already have most likely had information presented to them. In this instance, determine their knowledge level and supplement and reinforce that information.

 C u l t u r a l   S n a p s h o t

In working with children and families of children who have disorders that are passed through genetics, it is important that genetic counseling be done in a sensitive, nonthreatening manner. Some cultures believe that the mother or the parents caused a hereditary disease because of certain behaviors or actions. The parents often feel guilty, so a sensitive, objective approach is essential.

Evaluation of Goal/Desired Outcome

The family caregivers:

- verbalize an understanding of the disease process.
- state ways to prevent a crisis from occurring.

> **TEST YOURSELF**
>
> ✔ What are some reasons iron-deficiency anemias might be seen in infants?
>
> ✔ Explain the shape of the RBC and how it affects the child with sickle cell disease.
>
> ✔ What is the most serious concern in the child with sickle cell disease?

THALASSEMIA

The thalassemia blood disorders are inherited mild-to-severe anemias in which the hemoglobin production is abnormal. There are two basic types of thalassemia, alpha and beta thalassemia. Beta thalassemia is further divided into three types—major, intermedia, and minor. Beta thalassemia major (Cooley anemia) presents in childhood, is the most common, and is discussed here. The disorder often occurs in people of Mediterranean descent, but may also be seen in other populations.

Clinical Manifestations

Anemia, fatigue, pallor, irritability, and failure to thrive are noted in children with thalassemia. Bone pain and fractures are seen. Many body systems can be affected, including enlargement of the spleen, overstimulation of bone marrow, and heart failure. The liver, gallbladder, and pancreas can also be involved. The skin may appear bronze colored or jaundiced. Skeletal changes occur, including deformities of the face and the skull. The forehead is prominent, upper teeth protrude, the nose is broad and flat, and the eyes are slanted.

Treatment and Nursing Care

Blood transfusions maintain the hemoglobin levels, diet and medications are used to prevent heart failure, and splenectomy or bone marrow transplants may be necessary. Frequent transfusions can lead to complications and additional concerns for the child, including the possibility of iron overload. For these children, iron-chelating drugs such as deferoxamine mesylate may be given. Slowed growth and delayed sexual maturation may cause the child to feel self-conscious. Child and family support is important because of the chronic nature and long-term treatment of this disease.

HEMOPHILIA

Hemophilia is one of the oldest known hereditary diseases. Hemophilia is a syndrome of several distinct inborn errors of metabolism; all result in the delayed coagulation of blood. Defects in protein synthesis lead to deficiencies in the factors in the blood plasma needed for thromboplastic activity. The principal factors involved are factors VIII, IX, and XI.

Mechanism of Clot Formation

The mechanism of clot formation is complex. In a simplified form, it can best be described as occurring in three stages:

1. Prothrombin is formed through plasma–platelet interaction.
2. Prothrombin is converted to thrombin.
3. Fibrinogen is converted into fibrin by thrombin.

Fibrin forms a mesh that traps RBCs and WBCs and platelets into a clot, closing the defect in the injured vessel. A deficiency in one of the thromboplastin precursors may lead to hemophilia. This progression of events is shown in Figure 37-7.

Refer to a specialized text on the circulatory system for a detailed discussion of the clot-forming mechanism.

Common Types of Hemophilia

The two most common types of hemophilia are factor VIII deficiency and factor IX deficiency. These two types are briefly presented in this chapter.

Hemophilia A

A deficiency of coagulation factor VIII, hemophilia A, or classic hemophilia is the most common type. It is inherited as a sex-linked recessive trait with transmission to affected males by carrier females. Hemophilia A occurs in about 1 in 4,000 to 1 in 5,000 male births and is the most severe.

Hemophilia B

A deficiency of coagulation factor IX hemophilia B is also called Christmas disease. Christmas disease was named after a 5-year-old boy who was one of the first clients diagnosed with a deficiency of factor IX. It is a sex-linked recessive trait appearing in male offspring of carrier females. Hemophilia B is indistinguishable from classic hemophilia in its clinical manifestations, particularly in its severe form. In either hemophilia A or B, 30% or more of the affected

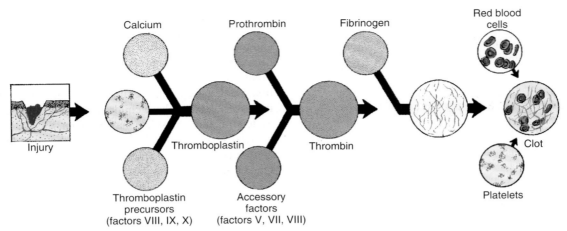

FIGURE 37-7 The mechanism of the formation of a blood clot is complex.

people can trace no family history of the disease; it is assumed that spontaneous mutations have occurred.

Clinical Manifestations

Hemophilia can be mild, moderate, or severe. All types of hemophilia are characterized by prolonged bleeding, with frequent hemorrhages externally and into the skin, the joint spaces, and the intramuscular tissues. Bleeding from tooth extractions, brain hemorrhages, and crippling disabilities are serious complications.

Sites of bleeding in the newborn include heel sticks, venipunctures, and circumcisions. An infant with hemophilia who is beginning to creep or walk bruises easily, and serious hemorrhages may result from minor lacerations. Bleeding often occurs from lip biting or from sharp objects put in the mouth. Tooth eruption seldom causes bleeding, but extractions require specialized handling and should be avoided by preventive care, if possible. However, family caregivers must avoid overprotecting the child. The pre-schooler is active and plays hard, and injuries are practically unavoidable. Common sites of bleeding in the older child include the forehead and joints. Clinical manifestations in any type of hemophilia are similar and are treated by admin-istration of the deficient factor and by measures to prevent or treat complications. In severe bleeding, the quantities of fresh blood or frozen plasma needed may easily overload the circulatory system. Administration of factor VIII con-centrate eliminates this problem.

Diagnosis

A careful examination of the family history and the type of bleeding present is conducted. Abnormal bleeding begin-ning in infancy when combined with a positive family his-tory suggests hemophilia. The activated partial prothrombin time (aPTT) is monitored and a markedly prolonged time and reduced hemophilia coagulation factors indicate a diag-nosis of hemophilia.

Treatment

Hemophilia treatment centers have been established and specialize in providing comprehensive care and treatment

with good success for the child with hemophilia (see www. hemophilia.org/Researchers-Healthcare-Providers). In treat-ing the child with hemophilia, factor replacement prepara-tions are available that supply high potency factors. Family caregivers and older children are taught how to reconstitute and administer the factor products at home in many cases. Children with severe hemophilia are given factor replace-ments prophylactically. Short-term use of prophylactic factor replacements may be used in certain situations where the child is at risk for bleeding, such as high-impact physical activities or surgical procedures. In less severe cases, factor replacements are given when an injury or bleeding epi-sode occurs. A synthetic preparation, desmopressin, which promotes the release of factor VIII, is used in individuals with mild hemophilia A. Desmopressin can be given by the intranasal route. Factor VIII and factor IX can be obtained from donor plasma which has been carefully screened. One of the problems with using blood products of any kind has been the risk of exposure to hepatitis B and human immuno-deficiency virus (HIV), the causative organism of acquired immunodeficiency syndrome (AIDS). Sophisticated screen-ing and purification processes have made these products much safer for the person who receives the product. Researchers continue to explore new ways to replace the missing factor while protecting the recipient from the threat of concerns or contracting an unknown illness.

Nursing Process and Care Plan *for the Child With Hemophilia*

Assessment (Data Collection)

Begin the data collection by reviewing the child's history with the family caregiver. Include previous episodes of bleeding, the usual treatment, medications the child takes, and the current episode of bleeding. Include the child in the interview if they are old enough to answer questions. Carefully observe the child for any signs of bleeding. Inspect the mucous membranes, examine the joints for tenderness and swelling, and check the skin for evidence of bruising. Question the child or family caregiver about hematuria, hematemesis, headache, or black tarry stools.

Nursing Care Focus

The nursing care focuses for the child with hemophilia include treating and managing pain and increasing the child's physical mobility. Preventing injury and bleeding episodes must be included. Recognize the need for helping the family develop coping skills and reinforcing family teaching about the condition, treatments, and hazards.

Outcome Identification and Planning

Use the information gathered to set goals with the cooperation and input of the family caregiver and the child. The major goals for the child include decreasing pain, increasing mobility, and preventing injury and bleeding. The family caregiver goals include increasing knowledge about the child's condition and care and helping the family learn to cope with the disease condition.

Nursing Care Focus

- Acute pain related to joint swelling and limitations secondary to hemarthrosis

Goal

- The child will experience diminished pain.

Implementations for Relieving Pain

Bleeding into the joint cavities often occurs after some slight injury and seems nearly unavoidable if the child is allowed to lead a normal life. Extreme pain is caused by the pressure of the confined fluid in the narrow joint spaces and requires the use of sedative or narcotic medications. Promptly immobilize the involved extremity to prevent contractures of soft tissues and the destruction of the bone and joint tissues. Immobilization helps relieve pain and decrease bleeding. A cast may be applied in the hospital to immobilize the affected part.

Aspirin and most nonsteroidal anti-inflammatory drugs (NSAIDs) are not given to children with hemophilia. Use of cold packs to stop bleeding is acceptable. The affected limb may be elevated above the level of the heart to slow blood flow. Use age-appropriate diversionary activities to help the child deal with the pain. Handle the affected joints carefully to prevent additional pain.

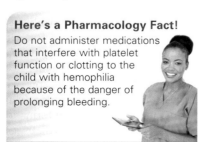

Here's a Pharmacology Fact!
Do not administer medications that interfere with platelet function or clotting to the child with hemophilia because of the danger of prolonging bleeding.

Evaluation of Goal/Desired Outcome

- The child rests quietly with minimal pain as evidenced by the child using a pain scale to report decreased pain.

Nursing Care Focus

- Altered physical mobility related to pain and tenderness of joints

Goal

- The child will move freely with minimal pain.

Implementations for Preventing Joint Contractures

Passive range-of-motion exercises help prevent the development of joint contractures. Do not use them, however, after an acute episode because stretching of the joint capsule may cause bleeding. Encourage the child to do active range-of-motion exercises because they can recognize their own pain tolerance. Encourage activities that are age-appropriate, fun, and increase range of motion to help motivate the child to participate in their treatment. Many clients who have had repeated episodes of **hemarthrosis** (bleeding into the joints) develop functional impairment of the joints, despite careful treatment. Use devices to position the limb in a functional position. Physical therapy is helpful after the bleeding episode is under control. Joint contractures are a serious risk, so make every effort to avoid them.

Evaluation of Goal/Desired Outcome

The child:

- is free from evidence of new joint contractures.
- maintains range of motion.

Nursing Care Focus

- Injury and bleeding risk related to trauma and secondary hemorrhage

Goal

- The child will be protected from any new injuries and bleeding episodes.

Implementations for Preventing Injury and Bleeding Episodes

The child with hemophilia is continuously at risk for additional injury. Protect the child from trauma caused by necessary procedures. Limit invasive procedures as much as possible; if possible, collect blood samples by a finger stick. Avoid intramuscular and other injections. Use the smallest gauge needle when injections must be given. When an invasive procedure must be done, compress the site for 5 minutes or longer after the procedure and apply cold compresses.

Remove any sharp objects from the child's environment. If the child is young, pad the crib sides to prevent bumping and bruising. Examine toys for sharp edges and hard surfaces. Soft toys are best for the young child. For mouth care, use a soft toothbrush or sponge-type brush to decrease the danger of bleeding gums. During daily hygiene, trim the nails to prevent scratching, and give adequate skin care to prevent irritation.

● The child is free from injuries or bleeding episodes caused as a result of procedures, treatments, or an unsafe environment.

Nursing Care Focus

● Knowledge deficiency of family caregivers related to condition, treatments, and hazards

Goal

● The family caregivers will verbalize an understanding of the disease, injury prevention, and care of the child.

Implementations for Reinforcing Family Teaching

Reinforce information and explanations the family has been given about hemophilia. Review the family's knowledge about the disease, and give additional information when needed. A child with hemophilia is healthy between bleeding episodes, but the fact that bleeding may occur as the result of slight trauma or often without any known injury causes considerable anxiety. Some evidence indicates that emotional stress can initiate bleeding episodes.

Topical fluoride applications to the teeth are particularly important in these children. Pay particular attention to proper oral hygiene, a well-balanced diet, and proper dental treatment, and reinforce teaching with the family about these considerations. Advise the family to select a dentist who understands the problems presented and who will set up an appropriate program of preventive dentistry.

Discuss safety measures for the home and the child's lifestyle. When possible, carpeting in the home helps soften the falls of a toddler just learning to walk. An older child may need to wear protective devices when playing outdoors and participating in sports activities. Playground areas can be treacherous for these children, but the child should participate in normal play activities, always being mindful of safety concerns.

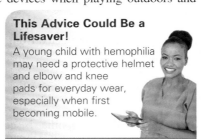

This Advice Could Be a Lifesaver!

A young child with hemophilia may need a protective helmet and elbow and knee pads for everyday wear, especially when first becoming mobile.

Reinforce teaching with the family about medications, signs that may indicate bleeding, emergency measures to stop or limit bleeding, range-of-motion exercises, and all aspects of the child's care. Ice packs should be available for instant use. When bleeding occurs, the child should rest the affected area, ice is applied, and the area should be raised above the level of the heart if possible. Before leaving for the healthcare facility, the caregiver should give factor replacement according to the protocol established with the child's health care provider.

The family experiences continuous anxiety over how much activity to allow their child, how to keep from overprotecting them, and how to help the child achieve a healthy mental attitude, while preventing mishaps that may cause serious bleeding episodes. Remind the family that it is essential to guide the child toward autonomy and independence within the framework of necessary limitations. At times, the emotional effects of social deprivation and restrained activity must be weighed against possible physical harm.

The financial strain on the family is considerable, as it is with most families with a child who has a chronic condition. Children who have had several episodes of hemarthrosis may be disabled to the extent of needing crutches and braces or wheelchairs. Measures toward rehabilitation require hospitalization, with possible surgery, casts, and other orthopedic appliances.

A child with hemophilia may miss a lot of school. Any child who must frequently interrupt schooling, for whatever reason, experiences considerable setbacks. Each child should be considered individually and provided with as normal an environment as possible.

The family caregivers:

● list safety measures to decrease the possibilities of injury to the child.
● explain the disease and the child's home care and ask and answer appropriate questions.

Nursing Care Focus

● Family coping impairment related to treatment and care of the child

Goal

● The family caregivers will develop appropriate coping mechanisms.

Implementations for Promoting Family Coping

Both the child and the family must accept the limitations and yet realize the importance of having normal social experiences. School, health, and community agencies can offer the family counseling, encouragement, and recommendations on how to raise the child in a healthy manner, both emotionally and physically. The National Hemophilia Foundation is a resource for services and publications (www.hemophilia.org). Give the family information about other available support systems.

Review all these concerns with the family. Through discussion, questions, and demonstrations, confirm that the family understands the information provided. Encourage family members to express their feelings about the effect the disease has on their lifestyle. The family may fear that the child will die of hemorrhaging. Guilt may play an important part in the family's reactions to the child. Recognizing and validating these feelings are important aspects of active listening. During hospitalization, involve the family in the child's care so that they can learn how to help the child without causing additional pain.

Evaluation of Goal/Desired Outcome

● The family members express their feelings and demonstrate good coping mechanisms, such as seeking help from appropriate support systems.

 A Personal Glimpse

My 6-year-old son Samuel has hemophilia. When he had a circumcision after he was born, he just kept bleeding. They asked us if anyone in our family had a bleeding disorder; we told them we didn't think so. We found out later my grandfather did have a bleeding problem, but we just had never known that. When Sam was little, he had bruises a lot, and finally they told us he had hemophilia. I felt so guilty because it came from my side of the family. We were so afraid and tried to protect him from any little accident, but he was such an active boy, it was so hard. I would get so nervous and upset whenever he got any kind of cut or even a little scratch. Now that he is a little older, he understands better, but he is disappointed when he has to be more careful when he plays or can't ride a bike like his friends do. We had to learn all about how to stop the bleeding and giving him factor VIII. I still always worry that he could get AIDS—they say it would be unlikely, but I know it has happened. Sam's sister is only 2 years older than he is; she loves her little brother so much and always tries to protect him. I have learned to relax a little more, and he really handles it well, but every day, I still worry that someday he will have something serious happen to him and we won't be able to stop the bleeding.

Theresa

Learning Opportunity: What are some resources and information you could offer to this mother? What would you say in response to the mother's statement regarding her child getting AIDS?

TEST YOURSELF

✔ Give examples of where bleeding might be seen in the child with hemophilia.

✔ Discuss how hemophilia is treated.

✔ What areas should be covered when reinforcing teaching with a family who has a child with hemophilia?

IMMUNE THROMBOCYTOPENIA

Purpura is a blood disorder associated with a deficit of platelets in the circulatory system causing hemorrhages into the skin or mucous membranes. The most common type of purpura is immune thrombocytopenia (ITP), formerly called idiopathic thrombocytopenic purpura (ITP). Purpura is preceded by a viral infection in about 60% of the diagnosed cases.

Clinical Manifestations and Diagnosis

The onset of ITP is often acute. Bruising and a generalized petechial rash occur. In severe cases, hemorrhage may occur in the mucous membranes; hematuria or difficult-to-control **epistaxis** (nosebleed) may be present. Rarely, the serious complication of intracranial hemorrhage occurs. In most cases, symptoms disappear in a few weeks without serious hemorrhage. A few cases may continue in a chronic form of the disease.

In ITP, the platelet count may be as low as $20,000/mm^3$ (normal, 150,000 to $400,000/mm^3$) or lower. The WBC count remains normal, and anemia is not present unless excessive bleeding has occurred.

Treatment and Nursing Care

If the platelet count is greater than $20,000/mm^3$, treatment may be delayed to see if a spontaneous remission will occur. Intravenous immunoglobulin has been used to increase the production of platelets until recovery occurs spontaneously. Corticosteroids may be used short term to reduce the severity and duration of the disease in some cases of ITP.

Nursing care consists of protecting the child from falls and trauma, observing for signs of external or internal bleeding, and providing a regular diet and general supportive care.

ACUTE LEUKEMIA

Leukemia, the most common type of cancer in children, accounts for about 25% of all the childhood cancers. Acute lymphoblastic leukemia (ALL) is responsible for the majority of the childhood leukemias, and acute myelogenous leukemia (AML) is responsible for almost all the rest. Fortunately, ALL is also the most curable of all major forms of leukemia. The incidence of ALL is greatest between the ages of 1 and 4 years and is higher in boys; ALL is more common in Hispanic and White children than in Black American children. This discussion focuses on ALL.

Pathophysiology

Leukemia is the uncontrolled reproduction of deformed WBCs. Despite intensive research, its cause is unknown. Mature leukocytes (WBCs) are made up of three types of cells.

● **Monocytes** (5% to 10% of WBCs) defend the body against infection.
● **Granulocytes** are divided into eosinophils, basophils, and neutrophils. Neutrophils (60% of the WBCs) can pass through capillary walls to surround and destroy bacteria.
● **Lymphocytes** (30% of WBCs) are divided into T cells, which attack and destroy virus-infected cells, foreign tissue, cancer cells, and B cells, which produce antibodies (proteins that help destroy foreign matter). An immature lymphocyte is called a **lymphoblast**.

Leukemia occurs when lymphocytes reproduce so quickly that they are mostly in the blast, or immature, stage. This rapid increase in lymphocytes causes crowding, which in turn decreases the production of RBCs and platelets. The decrease in RBCs, platelets, and normal WBCs causes the child to become easily fatigued and susceptible to infection and increased bleeding.

Clinical Manifestations

Clinical manifestations of leukemia appear with surprising abruptness in many affected children with few, if any, warning signs. The symptoms result from the proliferation of lymphoblasts. Presenting manifestations are often fatigue and pallor, caused by anemia, and low-grade or recurrent fever. Other early or presenting symptoms are bone and joint pain caused by invasion of the periosteum by lymphocytes, widespread **petechiae** (pinpoint hemorrhages beneath the skin), and purpura (hemorrhages into the skin or mucous membranes) as a result of a low thrombocyte count. The lymph nodes are often enlarged.

Although they are seldom presenting signs, anorexia, weight loss, abdominal pain, and distension often occur during the course of the disease, as a result of enlargement of the liver and spleen. Headache, vomiting, lethargy, and nuchal rigidity are symptoms related to increased intracranial pressure, caused by central nervous system involvement. Easy bruising is a constant problem. Anemia becomes increasingly severe.

Diagnosis

In addition to the history, symptoms, laboratory blood studies, and lumbar puncture, a bone marrow aspiration and biopsy must be done to confirm the diagnosis of leukemia.

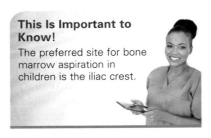

This Is Important to Know!

The preferred site for bone marrow aspiration in children is the iliac crest.

Treatment

The advances in the treatment of ALL have dramatically improved long-term survival. For children who have relapses or long-term complications of treatment, survival rates are greatly reduced.

The treatment therapy plan for leukemia is divided into three phases:

- Induction therapy—geared to achieving a complete remission with no leukemia cells.
- Consolidation therapy—given to prevent the regrowth of leukemic cells.
- Maintenance therapy—maintaining the remission.

Given periodically throughout each of the phases of treatment is:

- CNS preventive therapy—preventing invasion of the central nervous system by leukemia cells.

A combination of drugs is used during the induction phase to bring about remission. This phase takes 4 to 6 weeks to complete. Among the drugs used are vincristine, prednisone, daunorubicin. and L-asparaginase. During the consolidation phase, usually lasting several months, high-dose chemotherapeutic drugs are given, During the maintenance phase, which may last 2 or 3 years, a less intensive regimen of medications is given. During CNS preventive therapy, **intrathecal administration** (drugs injected into the cerebrospinal fluid by lumbar puncture) of methotrexate is used to eradicate leukemia cells in the central nervous system.

Nursing Process and Care Plan *for the Child With Leukemia*

Assessment (Data Collection)

The process of collecting data on the child with leukemia varies according to the stage of the illness. Conduct the admission interview with both the family caregiver and the child. Do not allow the caregiver to monopolize the interview; give the child an opportunity to express feelings and fears, and answer the questions. The physical examination should include observing for **adenopathy** (enlarged lymph glands), abnormal vital signs (especially a low-grade fever), signs of bruising, petechiae, bleeding from or ulcerations of mucous membranes, abdominal pain or tenderness, and bone or joint pain. Observe the child for lethargic behavior, and question the family caregiver about this. Note signs of local infection, including edema, redness, and swelling, or any indication of systemic infection. The diagnosis of leukemia is devastating. Observe and note the child and family's emotional states so that the nursing care plan can include helping them discuss and resolve their feelings and fears.

Nursing Care Focus

When developing evidence-based nursing care focuses for the child with leukemia, include the risk for infection, risk for injury and bleeding, acute pain, and managing fatigue. The child may have delayed growth and development and feelings related to an altered body image because of the disease and treatment process. The family needs support to deal with their issues of potential grief and loss.

Outcome Identification and Planning

Goals for the child with leukemia vary depending on individual circumstances. Preventing infection, preventing injury and bleeding, relieving pain, and reducing fatigue are major goals. Other important goals for the child may be promoting normal growth and development and improving body image. The goal for the family may be to verbalize feelings and to increase coping abilities.

Nursing Care Focus

- Infection risk related to increased susceptibility secondary to leukemic process and side effects of chemotherapy

Goal

- The child will remain free of signs and symptoms of infection.

Implementations for Preventing Infection

The immune system is weakened by the uncontrolled growth of lymphoblasts that overpower the normal production of granulocytes (particularly neutrophils) and monocytes. In addition, the chemotherapy necessary to inhibit this proliferation of lymphoblasts causes immunosuppression. Thus, these children are susceptible to infection, especially during chemotherapy. Infections are a frequent complication of treatment. To protect the child from infectious organisms, follow standard and transmission-based precautions. Carefully screen staff, family, and visitors to eliminate any known infection. Enforce handwashing and use of personal protective equipment as required. If the child is in reverse isolation to prevent infection exposure, this can be difficult for the child to understand and tolerate, so spend additional time with the child beyond that necessary for direct care. Playing games, coloring, reading stories, and doing puzzles are all good activities the child will enjoy.

Evaluation of Goal/Desired Outcome

The child:

- maintains a temperature that does not exceed 100°F (37.9°C).
- is free from inflammation, drainage, or other signs of infection.

Nursing Care Focus

- Injury and bleeding risk related to decreased platelet count

Goal

- The child will remain free from injury and excess bleeding.

Implementations for Preventing Injury and Bleeding

The mucous membranes bleed easily, so be gentle when doing oral hygiene. Use a soft, sponge-type brush, or gauze strips wrapped around your finger. Mouthwash composed of one part hydrogen peroxide to four parts saline solution or normal saline solution may be used. Epistaxis (nosebleed) is a common problem that can usually be handled by applying external pressure to the nose. Apply pressure to sites of injections or venipunctures to prevent excessive bleeding. Avoid

rectal medication and taking a rectal temperature. At least every 4 hours, monitor the child for any signs of bleeding such as petechiae, ecchymosis, hematemesis (bloody emesis), tarry stools, and swelling and tenderness of the joints. Protect the child from injury by external forces to prevent the possibility of hemorrhage from the injury. Take extra caution when the child's platelet count is especially low.

Evaluation of Goal/Desired Outcome

- The child has no signs of bleeding, including petechiae, ecchymosis, hematemesis, tarry stools, or swelling and tenderness of the joints.

Nursing Care Focus

- Acute pain related to the effects of chemotherapy and the disease process

Goal

- The child will show signs of being comfortable.

Implementations for Reducing Pain

Pain from the invasion of lymphoblasts into the periosteum and bleeding into the joints can be excruciating. Use gentle handling; place sheepskin pads under bony prominences and position the child to help relieve discomfort and skin breakdown. Many times painful procedures must be done that add to the child's discomfort. Explain to the child that these procedures are necessary to help and are not in any way a form of punishment. Provide a pain scale to help the child rate the pain and communicate its intensity. The numeric and the faces pain rating scales are useful with children 3 years of age and older (see Fig. 29-9). Administer analgesic medications as ordered to achieve maximum comfort.

Evaluation of Goal/Desired Outcome

The child:

- rests quietly.
- uses a pain scale to indicate that the pain is at a tolerable level.

Nursing Care Focus

- Fatigue related to disease, decreased energy, and anxiety

Goal

- The child's energy level will be maintained or will increase.

Implementations for Promoting Energy Conservation and Relieving Anxiety

As a result of anemia, the child is fatigued. Plan care and procedures so that the child has as much uninterrupted rest as possible. Stress adds to the child's feelings of exhaustion; to decrease fatigue, help the child deal with the stress caused by the illness and treatments. To help relieve anxiety, encourage the child to talk about feelings, and acknowledge the child's feelings as valid.

Evaluation of Goal/Desired Outcome

The child:

- participates in activities and procedures paced so that the child has adequate rest periods.
- expresses anxieties and feelings of stress related to illness.

Nursing Care Focus

- Risk for delayed growth and development related to impaired ability to achieve developmental tasks secondary to limitations of disease and treatment

Goal

- The child will accomplish appropriate growth and development milestones within the limits of the condition.

Implementations for Promoting Normal Growth and Development

During treatment, the child frequently may be prevented from participating in normal activity. The social isolation that accompanies reverse isolation often interferes with normal development. Physical activities are often limited simply because of the child's lack of energy. Knowledge of normal growth and development expectations is important to consider when planning developmental activities. Stimulate growth and development within the child's physical capabilities.

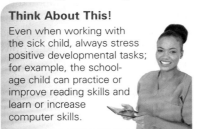

Think About This!

Even when working with the sick child, always stress positive developmental tasks; for example, the school-age child can practice or improve reading skills and learn or increase computer skills.

Encourage the family to help the child return to normal activities as much as possible during the treatment's maintenance phase in particular.

Evaluation of Goal/Desired Outcome

- The child is involved in age-appropriate activities provided by staff and family.

Nursing Care Focus

- Altered body image perception related to alopecia and weight loss

Goal

- The child will accept changes in physical appearance.

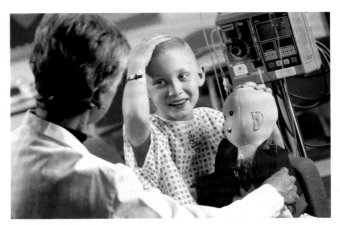

FIGURE 37-8 The child with alopecia needs support and encouragement.

Implementations for Promoting a Positive Body Image

The drugs administered in chemotherapy cause **alopecia** (loss of hair) (Fig. 37-8). Prepare the child and the family psychologically for this change in appearance. The child may want to wear a wig, especially when returning to school. Encourage the family caregiver to choose the wig before chemotherapy is started so that it matches the child's hair and the child has time to get used to it. A cap, hat, or scarf is often appealing to a child, particularly if it carries a special meaning for them. Reassure the child and the family that the hair will grow back in about 3 to 6 months. Wash the scalp regularly to avoid scaling. Prednisone therapy may cause the child to have a moon-faced appearance, which may be upsetting to the child or the family. Reassure them that this is temporary and will disappear when the drug is no longer needed. The child may be hesitant for peers to see these changes. Encourage visits from peers before discharge, if possible, so that the child can be prepared to handle their reactions and questions.

Acceptance Is Not as Hard as You Think!

A school teacher can be invaluable in preparing classmates to welcome the child with leukemia back to school with minimal reaction to the child's physical changes.

Encourage the family to enlist the assistance of the child's teacher, school nurse, and health care provider to ease the transition. Meeting other children who are undergoing chemotherapy and are in various stages of recovery is often helpful to the child and helps relieve the feeling that no one else has ever looked like this. Provide the child and the family opportunities to express their feelings and apprehensions.

Evaluation of Goal/Desired Outcome

The child:

- shows pride and adjustment in changes in body image.
- shares feelings about body image changes.

Nursing Care Focus

- Grief of the family related to the potential prognosis

Goal

- The family will verbalize feelings and develop coping mechanisms.

Implementations for Promoting Family Coping

Family members are often devastated when they first learn that their child has leukemia. Provide support from the moment of the first diagnosis, through the hospitalization, and continuing through the maintenance phase. Family members live one day at a time, hoping that the remission will not end and that their child will be the one who does not have a relapse and is finally considered cured. Provide opportunities for family members to freely express their feelings about the illness and treatment. The family will find comfort and stability in having one nurse caring for the child consistently. Involve the family caregivers in the care of the child during hospitalization, and give them complete information about what to expect when caring for the child at home during the maintenance phase. Identify a contact person for the family to call to answer questions during this phase. Help the family work through feelings of over-protectiveness toward the child so that the child can lead as normal a life as possible. Encourage the family caregiver to consider how siblings can fit into the child's return home. Siblings may have many questions about the seriousness of the illness and about the possible death of their brother or sister. Provide support for families to deal with these concerns. Most hospitals that provide care for pediatric oncology clients have family caregiver support groups that meet regularly. The American Childhood Cancer Organization, formerly known as Candlelighters, is a national organization for young cancer clients and their parents and families (www.acco.org).

Evaluation of Goal/Desired Outcome

The family:

- expresses feelings and fears about the child's prognosis.
- accepts counseling and support as needed.

TEST YOURSELF

✔ What symptoms are usually seen in the child with leukemia?

✔ Give some examples of how infection can be prevented in the child with leukemia.

✔ Define alopecia and discuss ways you can support the child who has alopecia.

After reading this chapter, what treatment and nursing care do you think you will be providing in caring for **Amalia?** Are there any long-term concerns Amalia might have because of her diagnosis? What teaching will you reinforce with Amalia's father?

KEY POINTS

- The cardiovascular system carries needed chemicals to and from the cells in the body so they can function properly. The major organ is the heart. The hematologic system includes the blood and blood-forming tissues. The cardiovascular and hematologic systems work together to remove the waste products from the cells so that they can be excreted from the body.

- By the time a child is a few months of age, the left ventricle is about two times the size of the right, about the same proportion as an adult. The infant's heart rate is higher than the older child's or adult's. By the time the child is 5 years old, the heart has matured, developed, and functions just as the adult's.

- The signs and symptoms seen in the child with congestive heart failure (CHF) often include fatigue; feeding problems; failure to gain weight; abdominal pain; nausea; vomiting; pale, mottled, or cyanotic color; tachycardia; rapid respiration; dyspnea; flaring of the nares; and use of accessory muscles with retractions. Such children may also have edema, heart enlargement, and liver enlargement.

- Treatment of CHF includes improving the cardiac function, removing excess fluids, decreasing the workload on the heart, and improving tissue oxygenation. Nursing care is focused on improving cardiac output and oxygenation, relieving inadequate respirations, maintaining adequate nutritional intake, and conserving energy.

- Group A *Streptococcus* is the bacterium usually responsible for acute rheumatic fever. Major manifestations include carditis (inflammation of the heart), polyarthritis (migratory arthritis), and Sydenham chorea (disorder characterized by emotional instability, involuntary movements, and muscular weakness). Other major manifestations include subcutaneous nodules and erythema marginatum (a pink-red rash on the trunk).

- Nursing care for the child with acute rheumatic fever is focused on reducing pain, providing diversional activities and sensory stimulation, conserving energy, and preventing injury. In addition, reinforcing teaching with the family caregiver to comply with drug therapy and the long-term care of the child is included.

- Kawasaki disease is an acute, febrile disease. The disease appears to be caused by an infectious agent. Intravenous immunoglobulin (IVIG) therapy is given to relieve the symptoms and prevent coronary artery abnormalities. Aspirin is used to control inflammation and fever. The most serious concern for a child with Kawasaki disease is development of cardiac involvement, which may not be seen for a period of time after the child's recovery.

- Iron-deficiency anemia is a common nutritional deficiency in children. It is difficult to get enough iron from food the child eats, and if the iron intake is inadequate, anemia quickly results.

- If the sickle cell trait is inherited from one parent, a child can inherit the trait and carry the sickle cell trait. If both parents carry the trait, the child can inherit the trait from each parent and have sickle cell disease.

- In sickle cell disease, the abnormal hemoglobin causes the red blood cells to assume a sickle shape. When sickling occurs, the affected red blood cells become crescent-shaped and the blood viscosity increases (blood becomes thicker), causing slowdown and sludging of the red blood cells. The impaired circulation results in decreased oxygen to the tissues; and ischemia, occlusion, and infarction occur.

- Nursing care for the child with sickle cell crisis is focused on maintaining comfort and relieving pain, increasing fluid intake, conserving energy, improving physical mobility, and maintaining skin integrity. Work closely with the family caregivers to decrease anxiety and increase their knowledge about the causes of crisis episodes.

- Common complications of thalassemia include enlargement of the spleen, overstimulation of bone marrow, and heart failure. Blood transfusions maintain the hemoglobin levels, diet and medications prevent heart failure, and splenectomy or bone marrow transplants may be necessary.

- Hemophilia is characterized by prolonged bleeding, with frequent hemorrhages externally and into the skin, the joint spaces, and the intramuscular tissues. The most common types of hemophilia are factor VIII deficiency and factor IX deficiency, which are inherited as a sex-linked recessive trait with transmission to male offspring by carrier females.

- Hemophilia is treated with factor replacement preparations. A synthetic preparation, desmopressin, is used in mild factor VIII deficiencies. Nursing care is focused on stopping the bleeding, decreasing pain, increasing mobility, and preventing injury. Work with the caregiver to increase knowledge about the child's condition and care and to help the family learn to cope.

- Symptoms of immune thrombocytopenia (ITP) formerly called idiopathic thrombocytopenic purpura include bruising, a generalized rash, and in severe cases, hemorrhage in the mucous membranes, hematuria, or difficult-to-control epistaxis. Rarely the serious complication of intracranial hemorrhage is seen.

- The child with leukemia often has fatigue, pallor, low-grade or recurrent fever, bone and joint pain, petechiae (pinpoint hemorrhages beneath the skin), and purpura (hemorrhages into the skin or mucous membranes). The lymph nodes may be enlarged and bruising is a constant problem.

- Drugs commonly used in the treatment of acute lymphatic leukemia are methotrexate, vincristine, prednisone, daunorubicin, and L-asparaginase. Nursing care is focused on preventing infection, preventing injury and bleeding, relieving pain, and reducing fatigue. Work with the child to help promote normal growth and development and improve body image. Encourage caregivers to verbalize feelings and help them to increase their coping abilities.

INTERNET RESOURCES

Kawasaki Disease
www.kdfoundation.org

Sickle Cell Disease
www.sicklecelldisease.org

Hemophilia
www.hemophilia.org

Leukemia
www.clf4kids.org
www.acco.org

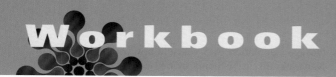

NCLEX-STYLE REVIEW QUESTIONS

1. When caring for a child with rheumatic fever, the nurse would anticipate that the child's history would *most* likely indicate which situation?
   a. A sibling diagnosed with the disease
   b. A recent strep throat infection
   c. The child bruises easily
   d. An increased urinary output

2. When developing a plan of care for a child with sickle cell crisis, which nursing intervention would be the *highest priority* to include?
   a. Provide support for family caregivers.
   b. Observe skin for any breakdown.
   c. Move the extremities gently.
   d. Administer analgesic medications promptly.

3. After discussing measures used to stop bleeding with the family caregiver of a child diagnosed with hemophilia, the caregiver makes the following statements. Which statement indicates a need for further teaching?
   a. "I always have ice and cold packs in our freezer."
   b. "Keeping pressure on an injury usually helps stop the bleeding."
   c. "Whenever my child gets hurt, I have him sit up with his head elevated and his feet down."
   d. "I know how to keep his arm from moving by using splints."

4. A nurse admits a child with a diagnosis of possible leukemia. Of the following signs and symptoms, which would *most* likely be seen in the child with leukemia?
   a. Low-grade fever, bone and joint pain
   b. High fever, sore throat
   c. Swelling around eyes, ankles, and abdomen
   d. Upward and outward slanted eyes

5. In planning care for a child with leukemia, which goal would be *most* important for this child?
   a. The child will remain free of signs and symptoms of infection.
   b. The child will participate in age-appropriate activities.
   c. The child will eat at least 60% of each meal.
   d. The child will share feelings about changes in body image.

6. The nurse is caring for a client who has leukemia. Which nursing interventions should the nurse implement to decrease the likelihood of injury or bleeding? Select all that apply.
   a. Use a soft, sponge-type brush or gauze strips to give oral care.
   b. Maintain reverse isolation.
   c. Use mouthwash composed of hydrogen peroxide and saline solution.
   d. Wear gloves when delivering the client's meal tray.
   e. Have the child wear a cap or a scarf.
   f. Apply pressure to sites of injections or venipunctures.

STUDY ACTIVITIES

1. Using the table below, make a list of safety measures to help protect the child with hemophilia. Include measures to be taken at home, school, and in the hospital settings. Explain the reasons that these measures are important.

Setting	Safety Measure	Reasons Measures are Important
Home		
School		
Hospital		

2. Missy is a 6-year-old girl with leukemia. Her single mother is unable to be away from her job to stay with Missy. Because of Missy's increased risk for infection, she has been placed in reverse isolation. Create an age-appropriate game or list of activities that could be used in caring for Missy.

3. Go to http://www.scinfo.org. This is a site for the Sickle Cell Information Center. As you search this site think about the following:
   a. What are some of the resources available that you might share with your peers?
   b. What are some of the resources available that you might suggest to a family who has a child with sickle cell disease?

CRITICAL THINKING: WHAT WOULD YOU DO?

1. The family of Sean, a 3-year-old boy with hemophilia, has heard and is concerned that Sean might get AIDS from his treatments.
   a. What is the likelihood of Sean being HIV-positive or of contracting AIDS from his treatments?
   b. What explanation will you give this family to reassure them?
   c. What teaching will you reinforce with this family regarding the methods used to treat a bleeding episode in the child who has hemophilia?

2. Andrew is an 18-month-old boy who has been admitted in a sickle cell crisis. His mother Jessica is 4 months pregnant with the family's second child. Tyrone, Andrew's father, tells you that they do not know much about sickle cell disease, but they have heard their second child may also have the disease.
   a. What information would you share with this family about sickle cell disease and the genetic factors related to sickle cell disease?
   b. What is the likelihood that their second child will also have the disease?
   c. What organizations would you refer this family to?

3. Dosage calculation: The nurse is caring for a newborn who has symptoms of congestive heart failure and is being treated with digoxin. The child weighs 6.5 lb. The usual dosage range of this medication is 4 to 8 μg/kg/day in divided doses, every 12 hours. Answer the following.
   a. How many micrograms (μg) are in a milligram (mg)?
   b. How many kilograms (kg) does the child weigh?
   c. What is the lowest dose of digoxin (in μg) that this child could be given in a 24-hour time period?
   d. What is the highest dose of digoxin (in μg) that this child could be given in a 24-hour time period?
   e. How many doses will the child receive in a day?

4. Dosage calculation: A 5-year-old boy with a diagnosis of Kawasaki disease is being treated with aspirin. His initial dose is 90 mg/kg in divided doses every 6 hours. After his symptoms have subsided, he will be given a dose of 4.5 mg/kg/day for the antiplatelet effect of the drug. The child weighs 39.6 lb. The medication comes in 81-mg tablets. Answer the following.
   a. How many kilograms (kg) does the child weigh?
   b. How many milligrams (mg) per day will be given for the initial dose?
   c. How many milligrams (mg) per dose will be given for the initial dose?
   d. How many tablets will be given for each of the initial doses?
   e. How many milligrams (mg) per day will be given for the antiplatelet dose?

The Child With a Gastrointestinal/Endocrine Disorder

Learning Objectives

At the conclusion of this chapter, you will:

1. Discuss ways the child's gastrointestinal system differs from the adult's system.
2. Discuss ways the child's endocrine system differs from the adult's system.
3. Describe conditions related to nutritional deficiencies and food allergies, and discuss nursing care.
4. Explain the diagnosis of celiac disease.
5. Discuss the diagnosis of gastroesophageal reflux disease, including the cause, symptoms, treatment, and nursing care.
6. Describe the symptoms noted in the child with colic.
7. Discuss the symptoms, treatment, and nursing care for the child with diarrhea or gastroenteritis.
8. Identify the symptoms, treatment, and nursing care for the child with pyloric stenosis.
9. State another name for congenital megacolon, and discuss the diagnosis, including symptoms, treatment, and nursing care.
10. Describe the diagnosis and treatment of intussusception.
11. List the symptoms, treatment, and nursing care of appendicitis; differentiate symptoms of the older child and the younger child.
12. Identify intestinal parasites common to children, and state the routes of entry, symptoms, and treatments for each.
13. Discuss ingestion of toxic substances in children.
14. List sources of lead that may cause chronic lead poisoning, and describe the symptoms, diagnosis, treatment, and prognosis.
15. Describe the treatment of a child who has swallowed a foreign object.
16. Discuss type 1 diabetes mellitus, including symptoms, diagnosis, treatment, nursing care, and teaching to be reinforced.
17. Explain type 2 diabetes mellitus.

Jackson Edwards has just turned 6 years old and is in the first grade. Recently, his mother noticed that although he is hungry and his food intake has increased, rather than gaining weight, he seems to be losing weight and also seems to have no energy. Jackson tells his mother that he is thirsty all the time, and she has noticed that he voids frequently. Jackson is now in the pediatric clinic, and you are his nurse. As you read this chapter, consider what might be causing the symptoms Jackson is exhibiting and what you would anticipate will need to be done for Jackson.

The gastrointestinal (GI) system is responsible for taking in and processing nutrients that nourish all parts of the body. As a result, any problem of the GI system, whether a lack of nutrients, an infectious disease, or a congenital disorder, can quickly affect other parts of the body and ultimately affect general health, growth, and development. The endocrine system consists of a number of ductless glands throughout the body that secrete hormones. All of the body systems overlap with the working of the endocrine glands.

GROWTH AND DEVELOPMENT OF THE GASTROINTESTINAL AND ENDOCRINE SYSTEMS

Gastrointestinal System

The main organs of the GI or digestive system are the mouth, pharynx (throat), esophagus, stomach, small intestine, large intestine, rectum, and anal canal. Other organs, called accessory organs, include structures that aid in the digestive process, as well as glands that secrete substances that further aid in digestion. These accessory organs include the teeth, tongue, gallbladder, appendix, the salivary glands, liver, and pancreas. Each of these organs and accessory organs plays a part in the process of digestion (Fig. 38-1).

The child takes in food and fluids through the GI tract, where they are broken down and absorbed to promote growth and maintain life. Food enters the mouth, and the digestive process begins. Digestion takes place by mechanical and chemical mechanisms. Chewing, muscular action, and peristalsis are physical or mechanical actions that break down food. Chemicals secreted along the GI tract by accessory organs further help the breakdown of food so that absorption can take place. As food is processed, nutrients are absorbed and distributed to the body cells. The large intestine is the organ of elimination that collects wastes and pushes them to the anus so the waste materials can be excreted.

The functioning of the GI system begins at birth. The GI tract of the newborn works in the same manner as that of the adult but with some limitations. For example, the enzymes secreted by the liver and pancreas are reduced. Thus, the infant cannot break down and use complex carbohydrates. As a result, the newborn diet must be adjusted to allow for this immaturity. By the age of 4 to 6 months, the needed enzymes are usually sufficient in amount.

The smaller capacity of the infant's stomach and the increased speed at which food moves through the GI tract require feeding smaller amounts at more frequent intervals. In addition, the small capacity of the colon leads to a bowel movement after each feeding. Reflexes are present in infants that allow for swallowing and prevention of aspiration when swallowing. The cardiac sphincter at the end of the esophagus may be lax in the infant, and food may be regurgitated from the stomach back into the esophagus. As the child grows, the muscles of the sphincter work more effectively and prevent food from going back into the esophagus. With continued growth, the GI tract matures, and the capacity of

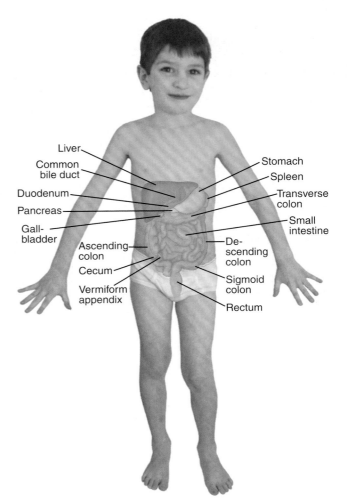

FIGURE 38-1 Anatomy of a child's gastrointestinal system.

the GI tract increases, but the digestive functioning throughout childhood into adulthood is the same.

Disorders and disruptions in the GI tract can cause changes in the functioning of the system. Most of these disorders stem from congenital defects, diseases, or infections in the GI tract. If any of these occur and the body does not get the needed nutrients to the cells, health and normal growth and development can be altered in children.

Endocrine System and Hormonal Function

The hormones secreted by the endocrine system are circulated through the bloodstream to control and regulate most of the activities and functions in the body. Regulating metabolism, growth, development, and reproduction are all functions of hormones. The endocrine system of the infant is adequately developed, although the functions are immature. As the child grows, the endocrine system matures in function.

Various disorders are caused by decreases, increases, or the absence of hormone secretions by the endocrine glands. The pancreas is the gland that secretes the hormone insulin.

Type 1 diabetes mellitus occurs in children when an insufficient amount of insulin is produced.

GASTROINTESTINAL DISORDERS

Malnutrition and Nutritional Problems

The World Health Organization has widely publicized that malnutrition and hunger affect more than half the world's population. In the United States food insecurity and malnutrition often occurs in low-income households. Malnourished children grow at a slower rate, have a higher rate of illness and infection, and have more difficulty concentrating and achieving in school. Appendix B lists foods that are good sources of the nutrients that a child needs for healthy growth.

Protein Malnutrition

Protein malnutrition results from an insufficient intake of high-quality protein or from conditions in which protein absorption is impaired or a loss of protein increases. Clinical evidence of protein malnutrition may not be apparent until the condition is well advanced.

Kwashiorkor

Kwashiorkor results from severe deficiency of protein with an adequate caloric intake. It accounts for most of the malnutrition in the world's children today. The highest incidence is in children of 4 months to 5 years of age. The affected child develops a swollen abdomen, edema, and GI changes; the hair is thin and dry with patchy alopecia; and the child becomes apathetic and irritable and has lagging growth with muscle wasting. In untreated clients, mortality rates are 30% or higher. Although strenuous efforts are being made around the world to prevent this condition, its causes are complex.

Traditionally, these babies have been breastfed until the age of 2 or 3 years. The child is weaned abruptly when the next child in the family is born. The older child then receives the regular family diet, which consists mostly of starchy foods with little meat or vegetable protein. Cow's milk is generally unavailable; in many places where goats are kept, their milk is not considered fit for human consumption (Fig. 38-2).

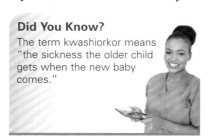

Did You Know?
The term kwashiorkor means "the sickness the older child gets when the new baby comes."

Marasmus

Marasmus is a deficiency in calories as well as protein and other nutrients. The child with marasmus is seriously ill. The condition is common in children in third world countries because of severe drought conditions. Not enough food is available to supply everyone in these countries, and the children are not fed until adults are fed. The child is severely malnourished and highly susceptible to disease. This syndrome may be seen in the child with nonorganic failure to thrive.

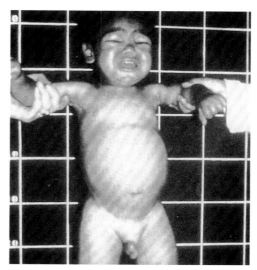

FIGURE 38-2 A child with kwashiorkor often has been abruptly weaned and may have a distended abdomen and muscle wasting.

Vitamin Deficiency Diseases
Vitamin D Deficiency

Rickets, a disease affecting the growth and calcification of bones, is caused by a lack of vitamin D. The absorption of calcium and phosphorus is diminished because of this lack of vitamin D, which is needed to regulate the use of these minerals. Early manifestations include **craniotabes** (softening of the occipital bones) and delayed closure of the fontanels. There is delayed dentition with defects in tooth enamel and a tendency to develop caries. As the disease advances, thoracic deformities, softening of the shafts of long bones, and spinal and pelvic bone deformities develop. The muscles are poorly developed and lacking in tone, so standing and walking are delayed. Deformities occur during periods of rapid growth. Although rickets itself is not a fatal disease, complications such as tetany, pneumonia, and enteritis are more likely to cause death in children with rickets than in healthy children.

Infants and children require an estimated 400 to 600 IU of vitamin D daily to prevent rickets. Because a child living in a temperate climate may not receive sufficient exposure to ultraviolet light, vitamin D is administered orally in the form of cod liver oil or synthetic vitamin. Whole milk and evaporated milk fortified with 400 Units of vitamin D per quart are available throughout the United States. Breastfed infants should receive vitamin D supplements, especially if the mother's intake of vitamin D is poor.

Vitamin C Deficiency

Scurvy is caused by inadequate dietary intake of vitamin C (ascorbic acid). Early inclusion of vitamin C in the diet, in the form of orange or tomato juice or a vitamin preparation, prevents the development of this disease. Febrile diseases seem to increase the need for vitamin C. A variety of fresh vegetables and fruits supply vitamin C for the older infant and child. Because much of the vitamin C content is destroyed by boiling or by exposure to air for long periods, the family caregivers should be taught to cook vegetables with minimal water in a covered pot and to store juices in a tightly covered opaque container. Vegetables cooked in a microwave oven retain more vitamin C because little water is added in the cooking process.

Early clinical manifestations of scurvy are irritability, loss of appetite, and digestive disturbances. A general tenderness in the legs severe enough to cause a pseudoparalysis develops. The child is apprehensive about being handled and assumes a frog position, with the hips and knees semiflexed and the feet rotated outward. The gums become red and swollen, and hemorrhage occurs in various tissues. Characteristic hemorrhages in the long bones are subperiosteal, especially at the ends of the femur and tibia.

Recovery is rapid with adequate treatment, but death may occur from malnutrition or exhaustion in untreated cases. Treatment consists of therapeutic daily doses of ascorbic acid.

Thiamine Deficiency

Thiamine is one of the major components of the vitamin B complex. Children whose diets are deficient in thiamine exhibit irritability, listlessness, loss of appetite, and vomiting. A severe lack of thiamine in the diet causes beriberi, a disease characterized by cardiac and neurologic symptoms. Beriberi does not occur when balanced diets that include whole grains are eaten.

Riboflavin Deficiency

Riboflavin deficiency usually occurs in association with thiamine and niacin deficiencies. A deficiency in riboflavin is mainly manifested by skin lesions. The primary source of riboflavin is milk. Riboflavin is destroyed by ultraviolet light; thus, opaque milk cartons are best for storage. Whole grains are also a good source of riboflavin.

Niacin Insufficiency

Niacin insufficiency in the diet causes a disease known as pellagra, which presents with GI and neurologic symptoms. Pellagra does not occur in children who ingest adequate whole milk or who eat a well-balanced diet.

Mineral Insufficiencies

Iron deficiency results in anemia. This condition is the most common cause of nutritional deficiency in children older than 4 to 6 months whose diets lack iron-rich foods. In the United States, anemia is often found in children younger than 6 years who are from low-income families. Iron-deficiency anemia is discussed in more detail in Chapter 37.

Calcium is necessary for bone and tooth formation and is also needed for proper nerve and muscle function. Hypocalcemia (insufficient calcium) causes neurologic damage, including intellectual disability. Rich sources of calcium include milk and milk products. Children with milk allergies are at an increased risk for hypocalcemia.

Food Allergies

The symptoms of food allergies vary from one child to another. Common symptoms are **urticaria** (hives), **angioedema** (swelling of the face, lips), **pruritus** (itching), nausea, abdominal pain and cramping, and respiratory symptoms. Some of the symptoms may appear quickly after the child has eaten the offending food, but other foods may cause a delayed reaction. Thus, the investigation to find the cause can be challenging.

Foods should be introduced to the child one at a time, with an interval of 4 or 5 days between each new food. If any GI or respiratory reaction occurs, the food should be eliminated. Among the foods most likely to cause allergic reactions are milk, eggs, wheat, corn, legumes (including peanuts and soybeans), oranges, strawberries, and chocolate (Table 38-1). If a food has been eliminated because of a suspected allergy or reaction, it can be reintroduced at a later time in small amounts to test again for the child's response. This testing should be done in a carefully controlled manner to avoid serious or life-threatening reactions. Many allergies disappear as the child's GI tract matures.

Milk Allergy

Milk allergy is the most common food allergy in the young child. Symptoms that may indicate an allergy to milk are diarrhea, vomiting, colic, irritability, respiratory symptoms, or eczema. Infants who are breastfed for the first 6 months or more may avoid developing milk allergies entirely unless a strong family history of allergies exists. Children with severe allergic reactions to milk are given commercial formulas that are soybean- or meat-based and formulated to be similar in nutrients to other infant formulas.

TABLE 38-1 Some Foods That May Cause Allergies and Possible Sources

FOOD	SOURCES
Milk	Yogurt, cheese, ice cream, puddings, butter, hot dogs, foods made with nonfat dry milk, lunch meat, chocolate candies
Eggs	Baked goods, ice cream, puddings, meringues, candies, mayonnaise, salad dressings, custards
Wheat	Breads, baked goods, hot dogs, lunch meats, cereals, cream soups. Oat, rye, and cornmeal products may have wheat added
Corn	Products made with cornstarch, corn syrup, or vegetable starch; many children's juices; popcorn; cornbreads or muffins; tortillas
Legumes	Soybean products, peanut butter, and peanut products
Citrus fruits	Oranges, lemons, limes, grapefruit, gelatins, children's juices, some pediatric suspensions (medications)
Strawberries	Gelatins, some pediatric suspensions
Chocolate	Cocoa, candies, chocolate drinks or desserts, colas

Lactose Intolerance

Children with **lactose intolerance** cannot digest **lactose**, the primary carbohydrate in milk, because of an inborn deficiency of the enzyme lactase. Congenital lactose intolerance is seen in some children of African-American, Hispanic, Native American, Eskimo, Asian, and Mediterranean heritage. Symptoms include abdominal cramping and distention, flatus, nausea, and diarrhea after ingesting milk.

Commercially available lactose-free formulas are made from soybean, meat-based, or protein mixtures. The child needs supplemental vitamin D. Yogurt is tolerated by these children.

Here's a Teaching Tip for You

If the child has a severe milk allergy, the family caregiver must learn to carefully read the labels on prepared foods to avoid lactose or lactic acid ingredients.

Nursing Process and Care Plan for the Child With Malnutrition and Nutritional Problems

Assessment (Data Collection)

Carefully interview the family caregiver to determine the underlying cause. If the difficulty lies in the caregiver's inability to provide for the child, try to determine if this can be attributed to lack of information, financial problems, indifference, or other reasons. Do not make assumptions. Cases of malnutrition have been reported in children of families who believed it was better for their child to eat only certain foods such as vegetables which would severely limit the protein and fat intake the child needs. If food allergies are suspected as the cause of malnourishment, include a careful history of food intake. Obtain a history of stools and voiding from the family caregiver.

The physical examination of the child includes observing skin turgor and skin condition, the anterior fontanel, signs of emaciation, weight, temperature, apical pulse, respirations, responsiveness, listlessness, and irritability.

Nursing Care Focus

The nursing care focuses for the child with malnutrition and nutritional problems include the risk for malnutrition, dehydration, and hypovolemia, often because of inadequate intake. Constipation and altered skin integrity also are concerns. Recognize the need for reinforcing family teaching related to the nutritional needs of the child.

Outcome Identification and Planning

The major nursing goals for the nutritionally deprived child focus on increasing nutritional intake, improving hydration, monitoring elimination, and maintaining skin integrity. Other goals concentrate on improving family caregiver knowledge and understanding of nutrition. Even with focused and individualized goals, developing a plan of care for the malnourished child may be challenging. It may be necessary to try a variety of tactics to feed the child successfully. Include the family caregiver in the plan of care because this is in the best interest of both the child and the caregiver.

Nursing Care Focus

- Malnutrition risk related to inadequate intake of nutrients secondary to poor sucking ability, lack of interest in food, lack of adequate food sources, or lack of knowledge of family caregiver

Goal

- The child will show interest in feedings.
- The child's nutritional intake will be adequate for normal growth.

Implementations for Promoting Adequate Nutrition

One primary nursing care concern may be persuading the child to take more nourishment than they want. Do not become discouraged if you find it difficult to persuade the uninterested child to take formula or food. Sometimes you can unknowingly communicate your insecurity and uncertainty to the child through impatience and a hurried attitude, and this will affect the amount of food you can persuade the child to eat. Instead, try wrapping and holding the infant snuggly while rocking the infant gently to promote relaxation and encourage a little more feeding. Also, you will find that as you and the child become accustomed to each other, you will both relax and feeding will become easier. Never prop the bottle in the crib.

In addition to having a lack of interest, the child is often weak and debilitated with little strength to suck. It is important for the child to develop an interest in food and in the process of sucking. A hard or small-holed nipple may completely discourage and frustrate the infant, who then no longer attempts to suck. The nipple should be soft with holes large enough to allow the formula to drip without pressure. However, it should not be so soft that it offers no resistance and collapses when sucked on. The holes should not be so large that milk pours out, causing the child to choke. Gavage feedings or intravenous (IV) fluids may be needed to improve the child's nutritional status.

Scheduling feedings every 2 or 3 hours is best because most weak babies can handle frequent, small feedings better than feedings every 4 hours. With more frequent feedings, promptness is important. Feedings should be limited to 20 to 30 minutes so that the child does not tire. Demand schedules are not wise because the child has probably lost the power to regulate the supply-and-demand schedule.

Evaluation of Goal/Desired Outcome

The child:

- shows evidence of adequate sucking.
- demonstrates ability to extend the amount of time feeding without showing signs of tiring.

- eats meals and snacks (older child).
- gains 0.75 to 1 oz (22 to 30 g) per day if younger than 6 months.
- gains 0.5 to 0.75 oz (13 to 22 g) per day if older than 6 months.

Nursing Care Focus

- Dehydration and hypovolemia related to insufficient fluid intake

Goal

- The child's fluid intake will improve, and the child will show signs of being hydrated.

Implementations for Monitoring and Improving Hydration Status

Improved nutritional status is evidenced by improved hydration, which is noted by monitoring skin turgor and fontanel tension. Accurately document intake and output. Check the fontanels each shift, and weigh the child daily in the early morning. Oral mucous membranes should be moist and pink. IV fluids may be needed initially to build up the child's energy so that they can take more oral nourishment to correct the fluid and electrolyte imbalance. During IV therapy, restraints should be adequate but kept to a minimum. At least every 2 hours, monitor the patency of the IV infusion and the insertion site for redness and induration. Report any unusual signs immediately.

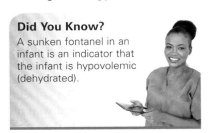

Did You Know?
A sunken fontanel in an infant is an indicator that the infant is hypovolemic (dehydrated).

Evaluation of Goal/Desired Outcome

The child's:

- fontanels are of normal tension.
- skin turgor is good.
- mucous membranes are pink and moist.

Nursing Care Focus

- Constipation related to insufficient fluid and dietary intake

Goal

- The child's urine and bowel outputs will be normal for their age.

Implementations for Monitoring Elimination Patterns

Carefully document intake and output, as well as the character, frequency, and amount of stools. Report any unusual characteristics of the stools or urine at once.

Evaluation of Goal/Desired Outcome

The child's:

- hourly urine output is 0.5 to 1 mL/kg.
- stool is soft and of normal character.

Nursing Care Focus

- Altered skin integrity related to malnourishment

Goal

- The child's skin will remain intact.

Implementations for Promoting Skin Integrity

Closely observe the skin condition. Use A+D ointment or lanolin for dry or reddened skin, and promptly change soiled diapers to prevent skin breakdown in the weakened child.

Evaluation of Goal/Desired Outcome

The child's:

- skin shows no signs of redness or breakdown.

Nursing Care Focus

- Knowledge deficiency of caregivers related to understanding of the child's nutritional requirements

Goal

- The family caregivers will verbalize a beginning knowledge of appropriate nutrition for a growing child.

Implementations for Reinforcing Family Teaching

If malnutrition is related to economic factors or inadequate caregiver knowledge of the child's needs, reinforce teaching with the family caregivers about the essential facts of infant and child nutrition, and make referrals for social services. Be alert to the possibility that the family caregiver cannot read or understand English, and be certain that the materials used are understood. Simply asking the family caregivers if they have questions is not sufficient to determine if the material has been understood.

Family caregivers may need information regarding assistance in obtaining nutritious food for the child. Infant formulas and baby food can be expensive, and economic factors may be the actual cause of the child's malnutrition. A referral to social services or the Women, Infants, and Children program may be appropriate (see Chapter 23).

Evaluation of Goal/Desired Outcome

- The family caregivers state essential facts about child nutrition.

Celiac Disease

Celiac disease is also known as gluten-sensitive enteropathy. Celiac disease is a basic defect of metabolism precipitated by the ingestion of dietary gluten, including wheat, barley, and rye, which leads to malabsorption, gastrointestinal symptoms, and impaired fat absorption. It is an autoimmune inflammatory disorder of the small intestine, caused by sensitivity to the gliadin fraction of gluten (a protein factor in grains). In many instances there is a genetic factor involved, and children who have other autoimmune disorders often have celiac disease.

Celiac disease is a chronic, common condition occurring in about 3 to 13 per 1,000 children in the United States (Hill, 2021). However, severe manifestations of the disorder have become rare in the United States and in Western Europe.

Clinical Manifestations

Signs generally do not appear before the age of 6 months and may be delayed until age 1 year or later, often after the introduction of gluten into the diet. The onset is generally insidious with manifestations including chronic diarrhea with foul, bulky, greasy, fatty stools (steatorrhea); abdominal distention and pain; and progressive malnutrition with failure to thrive. Some children have vomiting. Anorexia and a fretful, unhappy disposition are typical. If the condition becomes severe, the effects of malnutrition are prominent. Delayed growth and development; a distended abdomen; and thin, wasted buttocks and legs are characteristic signs (Fig. 38-3).

Diagnosis

Screening is done for children who exhibit symptoms that suggest celiac disease and for children who are at high risk for having the disorder. One way to determine if a small child's failure to thrive is caused by celiac disease is to initiate a trial gluten-free diet and observe the results.

Improvement in the nature of the stools and general well-being with a gain in weight should follow, although several weeks may elapse before clear-cut manifestations can be confirmed. Conclusive diagnosis can be made by a biopsy of the intestine through endoscopy that shows changes in the villi. Serum screening of immunoglobulin G and immunoglobulin A antigliadin antibodies shows the presence of the condition and also aids in monitoring the progress of therapy.

Treatment

Dietary and nutritional counseling is given to help determine the dietary needs of the child are being met. The child is started on a lifelong gluten-free diet. Wheat, rye, barley, and sometimes oats are completely eliminated from the diet. The child can usually be maintained on a regular diet with the exception of the eliminated products. Rice, corn, potato, buckwheat, and quinoa products are usually tolerated well. Food labels on prepared foods in particular must be carefully read to determine that no hidden sources of gluten are present. Although following a lifelong gluten-free diet is challenging, the response to the gluten-free diet most often has a good outcome for the child.

Nursing Care

The primary focus of nursing care is to help family caregivers maintain a restrictive diet for the child. Reinforcement of family teaching should include information regarding the disease and the need for long-term management, as well as guidelines for a gluten-free diet. Family caregivers must learn to read the list of ingredients on packaged foods carefully before purchasing anything. The diet of the young child may be monitored fairly easily, but when the child goes to school, monitoring becomes a much greater challenge. As the child grows, family caregivers and children might need additional nursing support to help them make dietary modifications.

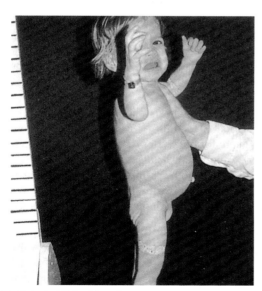

FIGURE 38-3 A child with celiac disease. Notice the protruding abdomen and wasted buttocks.

TEST YOURSELF

✔ Give some examples of vitamin and mineral deficiencies that can cause malnutrition in children.

✔ What are some common symptoms of food and milk allergies?

✔ List foods that may cause allergies, and name some sources of these foods.

✔ How is celiac disease diagnosed and treated?

Gastroesophageal Reflux Disease

Gastroesophageal reflux (GER) occurs when the sphincter in the lower portion of the esophagus, which leads into the stomach, is relaxed and allows gastric contents to be regurgitated back into the esophagus. GER is usually noted within the first week of the infant's life and is resolved within the first 18 months. The condition may correct itself as the esophageal sphincter matures, the child eats solid foods, and the child is more often in a sitting or standing position. Premature infants and children with neurologic conditions frequently have diagnoses of GER. GER is common, but if the child has complications such as esophagitis, poor weight gain, or respiratory issues related to the reflux, it is referred to as gastroesophageal reflux disease (GERD), which is a more serious concern.

Clinical Manifestations

The child with GER usually gains weight and feeds well. It must be determined if there are underlying symptoms or complications that might suggest GERD. In the child with GERD, almost immediately after feeding, the child vomits the contents of the stomach. The vomiting is effortless, not projectile in nature. The child with GERD is irritable and hungry, but may refuse to eat. Aspiration after vomiting may lead to respiratory concerns, such as apnea, wheezing, cough, and pneumonia. Failure to thrive and lack of normal weight gain occurs. Symptoms seen in the older child may include heartburn, nausea, epigastric pain, and difficulty swallowing.

Diagnosis and Treatment

A complete history will offer information regarding feeding, vomiting, and weight patterns. Esophageal pH monitoring may be done. An endoscopy will confirm the relaxed esophageal sphincter and any esophageal concerns, but is not routinely done. Correcting the nutritional status of the child includes giving formula thickened with rice cereal, placing the child in an upright position during and after feeding, and nasogastric (NG) or gastrostomy feedings, if necessary. A histamine-2 (H2) receptor antagonist, such as ranitidine or famotidine, may be given to reduce the acid secretion, which lessens the complications gastric acid may have on the esophageal tissue. Other medications, proton pump inhibitors such as esomeprazole and lansoprazole, may also be given to reduce the gastric acid. In severe cases, a surgical procedure known as Nissen fundoplication may be done. In this procedure, a part of the upper portion of the stomach is wrapped around the lower part of the esophagus to create a valvelike structure to prevent the regurgitation of stomach contents (Fig. 38-4).

Nursing Care

For the child with GERD, thicken feedings with rice cereal to decrease the likelihood of aspiration. Immediately report any signs of respiratory distress. Offer small, frequent feedings and burp the child frequently. Positioning after feedings continues to be a topic of debate. Holding the infant in an upright position after feedings for a period of time is recommended. In the past, an infant car seat was used to keep the child positioned after feedings, but studies suggest this position may increase the gastroesophageal reflux in the infant and should not be used. The child is then put in a supine position for sleeping. Monitor and document intake and output, daily weight, and emesis for amount and character. If an NG or gastrostomy tube is inserted, provide good

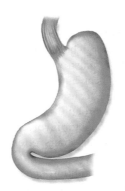
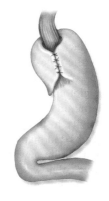

FIGURE 38-4 In the Nissen fundoplication procedure, the upper portion of the stomach is wrapped around the lower part of the esophagus.

skin care to help maintain skin integrity. It is important that you work with the family caregivers to reinforce teaching with them regarding feeding, positioning, and medication administration in order to decrease their anxiety.

Colic

Colic is described as episodes of crying in the infant, lasting up to several hours a day and recurring several times a week for several weeks. These episodes are often associated with recurrent gastrointestinal disturbances and are fairly common in young infants. Although many theories have been proposed, none has been accepted as the causative factor.

Clinical Manifestations and Diagnosis

Attacks occur suddenly, usually late in the day or evening. The infant cries loudly and continuously. The infant appears to be in considerable discomfort but otherwise seems healthy, breastfeeds or takes formula well, and gains weight as expected. The infant may be momentarily soothed by rocking or holding and eventually falls asleep, exhausted from crying. The infant with colic is often considered a "difficult" baby.

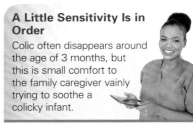

A Little Sensitivity Is in Order

Colic often disappears around the age of 3 months, but this is small comfort to the family caregiver vainly trying to soothe a colicky infant.

Differential diagnosis should be made to rule out an allergic reaction to milk or certain foods. Changing to a nonallergenic formula helps determine if there is an allergic factor or if the infant has lactose intolerance. If the infant is breastfed, the mother's diet should be studied to determine if anything she is eating might be affecting the infant. Intestinal obstruction or infection must also be ruled out.

Treatment and Nursing Care

No single treatment is consistently successful. A number of measures may be employed, one or more of which might work. Medications such as sedatives, antispasmodics, and antiflatulents are sometimes prescribed, but their effectiveness is inconsistent. The family must remember that the condition will pass, even though at the time it seems it will last forever. Family caregivers need to be reassured that their parenting skills are not inadequate. You can support the family and promote coping skills by reinforcing family teaching. See Tips for Reinforcing Family Teaching: Colic.

Diarrhea and Gastroenteritis

Diarrhea in children is a fairly common symptom of a variety of conditions. It may be mild, accompanied by slight dehydration, or it may be extremely severe, requiring prompt and effective treatment. Simple diarrhea that does not respond to treatment can quickly turn into severe, life-threatening diarrhea.

Chronically malnourished children with diarrheal symptoms are a common problem in many areas of the world. This condition is prevalent in areas lacking adequate clean water and sanitary facilities. Certain metabolic diseases, such as cystic fibrosis, have diarrhea as a symptom. Diarrhea may also be caused by antibiotic therapy.

Some conditions that cause diarrhea require readjustment of the child's diet. Allergic reactions to food are not uncommon and can be controlled by avoiding the offending food. Adjusting the child's diet by reducing sugars, fruit juices, bulk, or fat may be necessary.

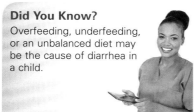

Did You Know?
Overfeeding, underfeeding, or an unbalanced diet may be the cause of diarrhea in a child.

Many diarrheal disturbances in children are caused by contaminated food or human or animal fecal waste through the oral–fecal route. Infectious diarrhea is commonly referred to as **gastroenteritis**. The infectious organisms may be *Salmonella*, *Escherichia coli*, *Shigella*, and various viruses, most notably rotaviruses. It is difficult to determine the causative factor in many instances. Because of the seriousness of infectious diarrhea in children and the danger of spreading diarrhea, the child with moderate or severe diarrhea is often isolated until the causative factor has been proved to be noninfectious.

Clinical Manifestations

Mild diarrhea may present as little more than loose stools; the frequency of defecation may be 2 to 12 per day. The child may be irritable and have a loss of appetite. Vomiting and gastric distention are not significant factors, and dehydration is minimal.

 Cultural Snapshot

Diarrhea, constipation, and vomiting are symptoms that may be embarrassing to the child and family. In some cultures, the embarrassment of discussing these symptoms may lead to attempts to control or manage the symptom by using home remedies. Sometimes serious concerns may be missed or ignored. Exploration of these symptoms with the family caregiver and child during the interview and ongoing data collection process is necessary.

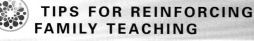

TIPS FOR REINFORCING FAMILY TEACHING

Colic

- Pick up and rock the baby in a rocker or with the baby's torso down across your knees, swinging your legs side to side. Be sure the baby's head is supported.
- Walk around the room while rocking the baby in your arms or in a front carrier. Hum or sing to the baby.
- Try a bottle, but do not overfeed. Give a pacifier if the baby has eaten well within 2 hours.
- The baby may like the rhythmic movements of a baby swing.
- Try taking the baby outside or for a car ride.
- When feeding the baby, try methods to decrease gas formation like frequent burping, giving smaller feedings more frequently, and positioning the baby in an infant seat after eating.
- Try doing something to entertain but not overexcite the baby.
- Gently rub the baby's abdomen if it is rigid.
- Sit with the baby resting on your lap with legs toward you; gently move the baby's legs in a pumping motion.
- Try putting the baby down to sleep in a darkened room.
- Keep remembering that it is temporary. Try to stay as calm and relaxed as possible.

Mild or moderate diarrhea can quickly become severe diarrhea in a child. Vomiting usually accompanies the diarrhea; together, they cause large losses of body water and electrolytes. The skin becomes extremely dry and loses its turgor. The fontanel becomes sunken, and the pulse is weak and rapid. The stools become greenish liquid and may be tinged with blood.

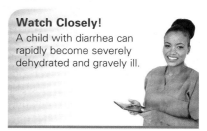

Watch Closely!
A child with diarrhea can rapidly become severely dehydrated and gravely ill.

Diagnosis

Stool specimens may be collected for culture and sensitivity testing to determine the causative infectious organism, if there is one. Subsequently, effective antibiotics can be prescribed as indicated.

 Concept Mastery Alert

Parents should be advised to first take their child's temperature and call their health care provider if their child develops diarrhea. Diarrhea can be infectious in nature, so it is important to monitor and consult the health care provider.

Treatment

Treatment to stop the potential complications of diarrhea must be initiated immediately. Establishing normal fluid and electrolyte balance is the primary concern in treating gastroenteritis. The child with acute dehydration may be given oral feedings of commercial electrolyte solutions, such as Pedialyte, Rehydralyte, and Infalyte, unless there is shock or severe dehydration. This treatment is called oral rehydration therapy (ORT). As the diarrhea clears, food may be offered. Salty broths and beverages with high sugar content should be avoided. Infants can return to breast-feeding if they have been NPO; formula-fed infants are given their formula.

Foods can be added as the child's condition improves, returning to a regular diet. Early return to the usual diet has been shown to reduce the number of stools and to decrease weight loss and the length of the illness.

Did You Know This?

Once commonly used, the BRAT diet (ripe banana, rice cereal, applesauce, and toast) is no longer used for the child with diarrhea because it is high in calories, low in protein, and does not provide adequate nutrition.

In severe diarrhea with shock and severe dehydration, oral feedings are discontinued completely. Fluids to be given IV must be carefully calculated to replace the lost electrolytes. Frequent laboratory determinations of the child's blood chemistries are necessary to guide the health care provider in this replacement therapy. For the child who has had a serious bout of diarrhea, the health care provider may prescribe soybean formula for a few weeks to avoid a possible reaction to milk proteins.

Nursing Process and Care Plan *for the Child With Diarrhea and Gastroenteritis*

Assessment (Data Collection)

In addition to basic information about the child, the interview with the family caregiver must include specific information about the history of bowel patterns and the onset of diarrheal stools with details on number and type of stools per day. Suggest terms to describe the color and odor of stools to assist the family caregiver with descriptions. Inquire about recent feeding patterns, nausea, and vomiting. Ask the family caregiver about fever and other signs of illness in the child and signs of illness in any other family members.

The physical examination of the child includes observation of skin turgor and condition, including excoriated diaper area; temperature; anterior fontanel (depressed, normal, or bulging); apical pulse rate (observing for weak pulse); stools (character, frequency, amount, color, and presence of blood); irritability; lethargy; vomiting; urine (amount and concentration); lips and mucous membranes of the mouth (dry, cracked); eyes (bright, glassy, sunken, dark circles); and any other notable physical signs.

Nursing Care Focus

A primary nursing focus in many instances is "diarrhea related to (whatever the cause is)." Other nursing focuses vary with the intensity of the diarrhea (mild or severe), as determined by the physical examination and family caregiver interview. These may include infection risk and altered skin integrity. In addition, the risk for dehydration and hyperthermia are concerns. The family caregivers may have anxiety and a knowledge deficiency related to understanding the condition and treatment for the child.

Outcome Identification and Planning

The major goal for the ill child is to control and stop the diarrhea while minimizing the risk for infection transmission. Other important goals for the ill child include maintaining good skin condition, improving hydration and nutritional intake, and satisfying sucking needs in the infant. A major goal for the family with a child who has diarrhea or gastroenteritis is eliminating the risk of infection transmission. The family should also be supported and should have teaching reinforced regarding the disease and treatment for the child. Plan individualized nursing care according to these goals.

Nursing Care Focus

- Infection risk related to inadequate measures to prevent or insufficient knowledge to avoid exposure to pathogens

Goal

- The family caregivers will follow infection control measures.

Implementations for Reducing the Risk of Infection Transmission

To prevent the spread of possibly infectious organisms to others, follow standard and transmission-based precautions issued by the Centers for Disease Control and Prevention (CDC) (see Appendix A). All healthcare staff, family caregivers, and visitors must follow precautions. The child will likely be on contact transmission precautions, so gowns should be worn. Gloves are used, especially when handling articles contaminated with feces. Place contaminated linens and clothing in specially marked containers to be processed according to the policy of the healthcare facility. Place disposable diapers and other disposable items in specially marked bags and dispose of them according to policy. Visitors are limited to family only.

Reinforce teaching with the family caregivers about the principles of infection control and observe them to ensure understanding and compliance. Careful handwashing is necessary and must be reinforced with family caregivers.

Evaluation of Goal/Desired Outcome

The family caregivers:

- verbalize standard and transmission-based precautions for infection control.
- follow measures and precautions to decrease and prevent spread of infection.

Nursing Care Focus

- Altered skin integrity related to constant presence of diarrheal stools

Goal

- The child's skin integrity will be maintained.

Implementations for Promoting Skin Integrity

Change diapers as quickly as possible after soiling. To reduce irritation and excoriation of the buttocks and genital area, cleanse those areas with plain water or mild soap. Avoid diaper wipes that contain alcohol or fragrance. Apply a soothing protective preparation, such as lanolin or A+D ointment. Some infants may be sensitive to disposable diapers, and others may be sensitive to cloth diapers, so it may be necessary to try both types. Leaving the diaper off and exposing the buttocks and genital area to the air may help decrease skin irritation and excoriation of the diaper area. Placing disposable pads under the infant can facilitate easy and frequent changing.

Evaluation of Goal/Desired Outcome

The child's:

- diaper area shows no evidence of redness or excoriation (infant).
- skin is clean and dry with no redness or irritation.

Nursing Care Focus

- Dehydration related to diarrheal stools and fluid loss due to vomiting

Goal

- The child will be well hydrated.
- The child's bowel elimination will return to pre-illness pattern.

Implementations for Monitoring for and Preventing Dehydration

A child can dehydrate quickly and can get into serious trouble after fewer than 3 days of diarrhea. Institute measures to control and stop the diarrhea and vomiting as ordered. Monitor vital signs, skin turgor, mucous membranes, and presence of tears, which indicate hydration status. Strictly monitor intake and output. Carefully count diapers and weigh them to determine the infant's output accurately. Measure each voiding in the older child. Closely observe all stools. Document the number and character of the stools, as well as the amount and character of any vomitus.

In severe dehydration, IV fluids are given to rest the GI tract, restore hydration, and maintain nutritional requirements. Monitor the placement, patency, and site of the IV infusion at least every 2 hours. The use of restraints, with relevant nursing interventions, may be necessary. Good mouth care is essential while the child is NPO. The infant who is NPO needs to have their sucking needs fulfilled. To accomplish this, offer the infant a pacifier. When oral fluids are started, the infant is given oral replacement solutions, such as those listed earlier. After the infant tolerates these solutions, half-strength formula may be introduced. After the infant tolerates this formula for several days, full-strength formula is given (possibly lactose-free or soy formula to avoid disaccharide intolerance or reaction to milk proteins). The breastfed infant can continue breast-feeding. Give the mother of a breastfed infant access to a breast pump if her infant is NPO. Breast milk may be frozen for later use, if desired. The older child may also be kept NPO and IV fluids and nutrition administered. As soon as symptoms of diarrhea and nausea lessen, oral rehydration therapy (ORT) is started and the child can usually soon return to a regular diet as tolerated.

Weigh the child daily on the same scale. Take measurements in the early morning before the child has fluids or food. Maintain precautions to prevent contamination of equipment while weighing the child.

Evaluation of Goal/Desired Outcome

The child's:

- intake is sufficient to produce hourly urine output of 0.5 to 1 mL/kg.
- skin turgor is good, mucous membranes are moist and pink, and fontanels in the infant exhibit normal tension.
- number of stools decreases in frequency and the stool consistency is appropriate for age.

Nursing Care Focus

- Hyperthermia risk related to dehydration

Goal

- The child will maintain a temperature within normal limits.

Implementations for Maintaining Body Temperature

Monitor vital signs at least every 2 hours if there is fever. Do not take the temperature rectally because insertion of a thermometer into the rectum can cause stimulation of stools, as well as trauma and tissue injury to sensitive mucosa. Follow the appropriate procedures for fever reduction, and administer antipyretics and antibiotics as prescribed. Take the temperature with a thermometer that is used only for that child.

Evaluation of Goal/Desired Outcome

● The child's temperature is 98.6°F to 100°F (37°C to 37.8°C).

Nursing Care Focus

● Acute family anxiety related to the seriousness of the child's illness

Goal

● The family caregivers' anxiety will be reduced.

Implementations for Supporting Family and Decreasing Anxiety

Being the family caregiver of a child who has become so ill in such a short time is frightening. Meeting the child's emotional needs is difficult but very important. Suggest to the family caregiver ways that the child might be consoled without interfering with care. Soothing, gentle stroking of the head, and speaking softly help the child bear the frustrations of the illness and its treatment. The child can be picked up and rocked, as long as this can be done without jeopardizing the IV infusion site. Help fulfill the child's emotional needs, and encourage the family caregiver to have some time away from the child's room without feeling guilty about leaving.

Evaluation of Goal/Desired Outcome

● The family caregivers will verbalize an understanding of the child's treatment.

Nursing Care Focus

● Knowledge deficiency of family caregivers related to understanding of and treatment for diarrhea

Goal

● The family caregivers verbalize an understanding of the child's condition and treatment.

Implementations for Reinforcing Family Teaching

Explain to the family caregivers the importance of GI rest for the child. The family caregivers may not understand the necessity for NPO status. Cooperation of the caregiver is improved with increased understanding. See Tips for Reinforcing Family Teaching: Diarrhea and Tips for Reinforcing Family Teaching: Vomiting.

Evaluation of Goal/Desired Outcome

The family caregivers:

● describe methods to increase hydration.
● list the warning signs of dehydration.

 ## TIPS FOR REINFORCING FAMILY TEACHING

Diarrhea

The danger in diarrhea is dehydration (drying out). If the child becomes dehydrated, they can become very sick. Increasing the amount of liquid the child drinks is helpful. Solid foods may need to be decreased so the child will drink more.

Suggestions

• Give liquids in small amounts (3 or 4 tbsp) about every half hour. If this goes well, increase the amount a little each half hour. Do not force the child to drink, because they may vomit.
• Give solid foods in small amounts. Do not give milk for a day or two, because this can make diarrhea worse.
• Give only nonsalty soups or broths.
• Liquids recommended for vomiting may also be given for diarrhea. Avoid beverages high in sugar content.
• Soft foods to give in small amounts: applesauce, finely chopped or scraped apple without peel, bananas, toast, rice cereal, plain unsalted crackers, rice, potatoes, or lean meats.

Call the Health Care Provider If ...

• The child develops sudden high fever.
• Stomach pain becomes severe.
• Diarrhea becomes bloody (more than a streak of blood).
• Diarrhea becomes more frequent or severe.
• The child becomes dehydrated (dried out).

Signs of Dehydration

• The child:
• has not urinated for 6 hours or more.
• has no tears when crying.
• mouth is dry or sticky to touch.
• eyes are sunken.
• is less active than usual.
• has dark circles under eyes.

Warning

Do not use medicines to stop diarrhea for children younger than 6 years unless specifically directed by the health care provider. These medicines can be dangerous if not used properly.

Diaper Area Skin Care

• Change diaper as soon as it is soiled.
• Wash area with plain water or mild soap, rinse, and dry well.
• Use soothing, protective lotion recommended by your health care provider.
• Do not use waterproof diapers or diaper covers; they increase diaper area irritation.
• Wash hands with soap and water after changing diapers or wiping the child.

TIPS FOR REINFORCING FAMILY TEACHING

Vomiting

Vomiting will usually stop in a couple days and can be treated at home as long as the child is getting some fluids.

Warning

Some medications used to stop vomiting in older children or adults are dangerous in infants or young children. DO NOT use any medicine unless your health care provider has told you to use it for this child. Give the child clear liquids to drink in small amounts.

Suggestions

• Pedialyte, Lytren, Rehydralyte, Infalyte
• Flat soda (no fizz). Use caffeine-free type; do not use diet soda.

• Jell-O water. Double the amount of water, let stand to room temperature.
• Ice popsicles
• Gatorade
• Tea
• Solid Jell-O
• Broth (not salty)

How to Give

Give small amounts often. One tbsp every 20 minutes for the first few hours is a good rule of thumb. If this is kept down without vomiting, increase to 2 tbsp every 20 minutes for the next couple of hours. If there is no vomiting, increase the amount the child may have. If the child vomits, wait for 1 hour before offering more liquids.

TEST YOURSELF

✔ What is the major concern in the child who has diarrhea and/or vomiting?

✔ How is the child with diarrhea treated? What is this treatment called?

✔ What precautions are followed when caring for a child with diarrhea to prevent the spread of infection from the child to other people?

Pyloric Stenosis

The pylorus is the muscle that controls the flow of food from the stomach to the duodenum. Pyloric stenosis (sometimes called hypertrophic pyloric stenosis) is characterized by hypertrophy of the circular muscle fibers of the pylorus with a severe narrowing of its lumen. The pylorus is thickened to as much as twice its size, is elongated, and has a consistency resembling cartilage. As a result of this obstruction at the distal end of the stomach, the stomach becomes dilated (Fig. 38-5A).

Pyloric stenosis is rarely symptomatic during the first days of life. It has occasionally been recognized shortly after birth, but the average affected infant does not show symptoms until about the third week of life. Symptoms rarely appear after the third month. Although symptoms appear late, pyloric stenosis is classified as a congenital defect. Its cause is unknown, but it occurs more frequently in males and has a familial tendency. Maternal smoking during pregnancy and administration of erythromycin to the infant appear to increase the risk of pyloric stenosis.

Clinical Manifestations

During the first weeks of life, the infant with pyloric stenosis often eats well, gains weight, and then starts vomiting occasionally after meals. Within a few days, the vomiting increases in frequency and force, becoming projectile. The vomited material is sour, undigested food; it may contain mucus but never bile because it has not progressed beyond the stomach.

Because the obstruction is a mechanical one, the infant does not feel ill, is ravenously hungry, and is eager to try again and again, but the food invariably comes back. As the condition progresses, the infant becomes irritable, loses weight rapidly, and becomes dehydrated. Alkalosis develops from the loss of potassium and hydrochloric acid, and the infant becomes seriously ill.

Constipation becomes progressive because little food gets into the intestine, and urine is scanty. Gastric peristaltic waves passing from left to right across the abdomen can usually be seen during or after feedings.

Diagnosis

Diagnosis is usually made on the clinical evidence. The nature, type, and times of vomiting are documented. When the infant

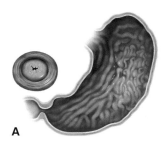

A

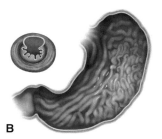

B

FIGURE 38-5 A. Hypertrophied pylorus muscle and narrowed stomach outlet. **B.** In pyloromyotomy, the pylorus is incised, thus increasing the diameter of the pyloric outlet.

drinks, gastric peristaltic waves are observed. The infant may have a history of weight loss with hunger and irritability.

Ultrasound or upper GI studies further clarify the diagnosis.

Treatment

A surgical procedure called a pyloromyotomy is the treatment of choice. This procedure simply splits the hypertrophic pyloric muscle down to the submucosa, allowing the pylorus to expand so that food may pass. Prognosis is excellent if surgery is performed before the infant is severely dehydrated (Fig. 38-5B).

Nursing Process and Care Plan *for the Infant With Pyloric Stenosis*

Assessment (Data Collection)

When the infant of 1 or 2 months of age has a history of projectile vomiting, pyloric stenosis is suspected. Carefully interview the family caregivers. Ask when the vomiting started, and determine the character of the vomiting (undigested formula with no bile, vomitus progressively more projectile). The family caregiver will relate a story of an infant who is an eager eater but cannot retain food. Ask the family caregiver about constipation and scanty urine.

Physical examination reveals an infant who may show signs of dehydration. Obtain the infant's weight and observe skin turgor and skin condition (including diaper area); anterior fontanel (depressed, normal, or bulging); temperature; apical pulse rate (observing for weak pulse and tachycardia); irritability; lethargy; urine (amount and concentration); lips and mucous membranes of the mouth (dry, cracked); and eyes (bright, glassy, sunken, dark circles). Observe for visible gastric peristalsis when the infant is eating. Document and report signs of dehydration to help determine the need for fluid and electrolyte replacement.

Do You Know Why?

An experienced practitioner often can feel an olive-sized mass through deep palpation in the right upper quadrants in the infant with pyloric stenosis.

Nursing Care Focus: Preoperative Phase

The nursing care focuses for the infant with pyloric stenosis during the preoperative phase include the risk for dehydration and malnutrition. The infant is kept NPO so the concerns of altered skin and tissue (mucous membranes) integrity are addressed. Family coping impairment in the preoperative time is an important aspect of caring for the child and the family.

Outcome Identification and Planning: Preoperative Phase

Before surgery, the major goals for the infant with pyloric stenosis include improving hydration and nutrition, maintaining mouth and skin integrity, and relieving family anxiety. Plan individualized nursing care according to these goals, including interventions to prepare the infant for surgery.

Nursing Care Focus

- Dehydration risk related to frequent vomiting
- Malnutrition risk related to inability to retain food

Goal

- The infant will be hydrated.
- The infant's nutritional status will be adequate for normal growth.

Implementations for Maintaining Adequate Fluid and Nutrition Intake

Hypertrophy of the pylorus narrows the passage from the stomach into the duodenum. As a result, food (breast milk or formula) cannot pass. The infant loses weight and becomes dehydrated. If the infant is severely dehydrated and malnourished, rehydration with IV fluids and electrolytes is necessary to correct hypokalemia and alkalosis and prepare the infant for surgery. Carefully monitor the IV site for redness and induration. Improved skin turgor, weight gain, correction of hypokalemia and alkalosis, adequate intake of fluids, and no evidence of gastric distention are signs of improved nutrition and hydration. Record the frequency and type of emesis.

In preparation for surgery, fluid and electrolyte balance must be restored, and the stomach must be empty. Typically, before surgery the infant is kept NPO and the infant receives IV fluids, electrolytes, and nutrition if needed.

Evaluation of Goal/Desired Outcome

- The infant maintains weight.

The infant's:

- skin turgor improves.
- mucous membranes are moist and pink.
- hourly urine output is 0.5 to 1 mL/kg.

Nursing Care Focus

- Altered skin and tissue (mucous membranes) integrity related to NPO status

Goal

- The infant's skin integrity will be maintained.

Implementations for Providing Mouth Care and Promoting Skin Integrity

The infant needs good mouth care as the mucous membranes of the mouth may be dry because of dehydration and the omission of oral fluids before surgery. A pacifier can satisfy the infant's need for sucking because of the interruption in normal feeding and sucking habits.

Depending on the severity of dehydration, the skin may easily crack or break down and become irritated. The infant is repositioned, the diaper is changed, and lanolin or A+D ointment is applied to dry skin areas. IV therapy may also affect skin integrity. Monitor the IV insertion site for redness and inflammation. Closely observe and document the infant's skin condition.

Evaluation of Goal/Desired Outcome

The infant:

- has mucous membranes that are moist and pink, and saliva is sufficient as evidenced by typical drooling.
- uses a pacifier sufficiently to meet sucking needs.
- shows no signs of skin irritation or breakdown.

Nursing Care Focus

- Family coping impairment related to seriousness of illness and impending surgery

Goal

- The family caregivers' anxiety will be reduced.

Implementations for Promoting Family Coping

The family caregivers are anxious because their infant is obviously seriously ill, and when they learn that the infant is to undergo surgery, their apprehensions increase. Include the family caregivers in the preparation for surgery. Reinforce teaching regarding the importance of the IV fluids preoperatively to improve electrolyte balance and rehydrate the infant and the reason for ultrasonography and upper GI studies.

Reinforce teaching about the location of the pylorus (at the distal end of the stomach) and what happens when the circular muscle fibers hypertrophy. You can compare it to a doughnut that thickens, so that the opening closes and very little food gets through. Clarify their understanding of the surgical procedure to be performed. During the procedure, the muscle is simply split down to, but not through, the submucosa, allowing it to balloon and let food pass.

Direct the family caregivers to the appropriate waiting area during surgery so that the surgeon can find them immediately after surgery. Explain to the family caregivers what to expect and about how long the surgery will last. Describe the procedure for the postanesthesia care unit so that the family caregivers know the infant will be under close observation after surgery until fully recovered.

Evaluation of Goal/Desired Outcome

The family caregivers:

- verbalize an understanding of the procedures and treatments.
- cooperate with the nursing staff.

- ask appropriate questions.
- express confidence in the treatment plan.

Nursing Care Focus: Postoperative Phase

The nursing care focuses for the infant with pyloric stenosis during the postoperative phase include the risk for aspiration and malnutrition. Managing the infant's pain, preventing infection, and promoting skin integrity are addressed. Acknowledging family anxiety and coping impairment in the postoperative time is an important aspect of caring for the child and the family.

Outcome Identification and Planning: Postoperative Phase

After surgery, the major goals for the infant include keeping the airway clear, improving nutrition status, maintaining comfort, preventing infection, preserving skin integrity, and reducing family anxiety. Individualize the nursing plan of care according to these goals.

Nursing Care Focus

- Aspiration and ineffective airway clearance risk related to postoperative vomiting

Goal

- The infant will not aspirate vomitus or mucus.

Implementations for Preventing Aspiration and Maintaining a Patent Airway

After surgery, position the infant on their side to prevent aspiration of mucus or vomitus, particularly during the anesthesia recovery period. After fully waking from surgery, the infant may be held by a family caregiver. Help the caregiver find a position that does not interfere with IV infusions and that is comfortable for both the family caregiver and infant.

Evaluation of Goal/Desired Outcome

- The infant rests quietly in a side-lying position without choking or coughing.

Nursing Care Focus

- Acute pain related to surgical procedure

Goal

- The infant will show signs of being comfortable.

Implementations for Promoting Comfort

Observe the infant's behavior to evaluate discomfort and pain. Excessive crying, restlessness, listlessness, resistance to being held and cuddled, rigidity, and increased pulse and respiratory rates can indicate pain. Administer analgesics as ordered. Nursing interventions that may provide comfort include rocking, holding, cuddling, and offering a pacifier. Include the family caregivers in helping to comfort the infant.

Evaluation of Goal/Desired Outcome

The infant:

- sleeps and rests in a relaxed manner.
- cuddles with family caregivers and nurses.
- does not cry excessively.

Nursing Care Focus

- Malnutrition risk related to postoperative condition

Goal

- The infant's nutrition status and fluid intake will improve.

Implementations for Providing Nutrition

The first feeding, given 4 to 6 hours after surgery, is usually an electrolyte replacement solution, such as Lytren or Pedialyte. Give feedings slowly in small amounts with frequent burping. Hold the infant in an upright position during and after the feeding. Vomiting may be noted after surgery, but small amounts of emesis are not concerning. IV fluid is necessary until the infant is taking sufficient oral feedings. Continue to use all nursing measures for IV care that were followed before surgery. Accurate intake, output, and daily weight determinations are required.

Evaluation of Goal/Desired Outcome

The infant's:

- daily weight gain is 0.75 to 1 oz (22 to 30 g).
- oral fluids are retained with minimal vomiting.
- hourly urine output is 0.5 to 1 mL/kg.

Nursing Care Focus

- Infection and altered skin integrity risk related to surgery and surgical incision

Goal

- The infant will remain free of signs and symptoms of infection
- The infant's skin integrity will be maintained.

Implementations for Monitoring for Infection and Promoting Skin Integrity

Monitor the infant's vital signs; document and report any abnormal readings. Closely observe the surgical site for blood, drainage, redness, or swelling. Record and report any odor. Make observations at least every 4 hours. Care for the incision and dressings as ordered by the health care provider.

Evaluation of Goal/Desired Outcome

The infant's:

- temperature is maintained within a normal range.
- surgical site shows no signs of infection, as evidenced by absence of redness, foul odor, or drainage.

Nursing Care Focus

- Family caregiver anxiety and coping impairment related to postoperative condition

Goal

- The family caregivers' anxiety will be reduced.

Implementations for Promoting Family Coping

The family caregivers will be anxious if the infant vomits after surgery; reassure them that this is not uncommon during the first 24 hours after surgery. The family caregivers should be involved in postoperative care. Reassure them that the care they gave at home did not cause the condition. Offer them support and understanding, and encourage them in feeding and providing for the infant's needs. Remind them that there is excellent likelihood of a satisfactory recovery in a few weeks with steady progression to complete recovery.

Evaluation of Goal/Desired Outcome

- The family caregivers' anxiety is reduced.
- The family caregivers are involved in the postoperative care and feeding of the infant.
- They demonstrate an understanding of feeding technique.

TEST YOURSELF

✔ What type of vomiting is seen in the infant with pyloric stenosis?
✔ What is done to treat an infant with pyloric stenosis?
✔ Explain the reason it is important to monitor accurate intake and output in the infant with pyloric stenosis.

Congenital Aganglionic Megacolon

Congenital aganglionic megacolon, also called Hirschsprung disease, is characterized by persistent constipation resulting from partial or complete intestinal obstruction of mechanical origin. In many cases, the condition may be severe enough to be recognized during the neonatal period; in other cases, the blockage may not be diagnosed until later infancy or early childhood.

Parasympathetic nerve cells regulate peristalsis in the intestine. The name aganglionic megacolon actually describes the condition because there is an absence of parasympathetic ganglion cells within the muscular wall of the distal colon and the rectum. As a result, the affected portion of the lower bowel has no peristaltic action. Thus, it narrows, and the portion directly proximal to (above) the affected area becomes greatly dilated and filled with feces and gas (Fig. 38-6).

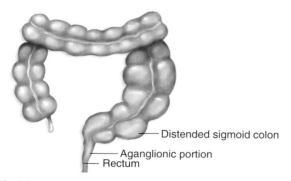

Distended sigmoid colon

Aganglionic portion

Rectum

FIGURE 38-6 Enlarged megacolon of Hirschsprung disease.

Clinical Manifestations

Accurate reporting of the first meconium stool in the newborn is vital. Failure of the newborn to have a stool in the first 24 hours may indicate a number of conditions, one of which is megacolon. The majority of children with Hirschsprung disease are diagnosed as neonates.

Other neonatal symptoms are suggestive of complete or partial intestinal obstruction, such as bile-stained emesis and generalized abdominal distention. Gastroenteritis with diarrheal stools may be present, and ulceration of the colon may occur.

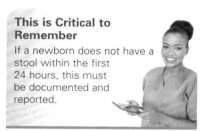

This is Critical to Remember

If a newborn does not have a stool within the first 24 hours, this must be documented and reported.

The affected older infant or child has obstinate, severe constipation dating back to early infancy. Stools are ribbon-like or consist of hard pellets. Formed bowel movements do not occur, except with the use of enemas, and soiling does not occur. The rectum is usually empty because the impaction occurs above the aganglionic segment.

As the child grows older, the abdomen becomes progressively enlarged and hard. General debilitation and chronic anemia are usually present. Differentiation must be made between this condition and psychogenic megacolon because of coercive toileting or other emotional problems. The child with aganglionic megacolon does not withhold stools or defecate in inappropriate places, and no soiling occurs.

Diagnosis

In the newborn, the absence of a meconium stool within the first 24 hours requires evaluation; in the older infant or child, a history of obstinate, severe constipation may indicate the need for further evaluation. Definitive diagnosis is made through barium studies and must be confirmed by rectal biopsy.

Treatment

Treatment involves surgery with the ultimate resection of the aganglionic portion of the bowel. The procedure may be done in one stage, but often a colostomy is placed during the surgery and a second procedure is done at a later time to reverse the colostomy. This allows the child to regain any weight lost and also gives the bowel a period of rest to return to a more normal state. Resection may be deferred until later in infancy.

Nursing Process and Care Plan *for the Child Undergoing Surgery for Congenital Aganglionic Megacolon*

Assessment (Data Collection)

Carefully gather a history from the family caregivers, noting especially the history of stooling. Ask about the onset of constipation; the character and odor of stools; the frequency of bowel movements; and the presence of poor feeding habits, anorexia, and irritability.

During the physical examination, observe for a distended abdomen and signs of poor nutrition (see Nursing Process and Care Plan for the Child with Malnutrition and Nutritional Problems). Record the child's weight and vital signs. Observe the child for developmental milestones.

Nursing Care Focus: Preoperative Phase

The nursing care focuses for the infant with congenital aganglionic megacolon during the preoperative phase include concerns related to constipation and malnutrition. In the older child the fear of having surgery is addressed. Family coping impairment in the preoperative time is an important aspect of caring for the child and the family.

Outcome Identification and Planning: Preoperative Phase

The preoperative goals for the child undergoing surgery for congenital aganglionic megacolon include preventing constipation, improving nutritional status, and relieving fear (in the older child). The major goal for the family is reducing anxiety. Base the preoperative nursing plan of care on these goals. Plan interventions that prepare the child for surgery.

Nursing Care Focus

● Constipation related to decreased bowel motility

Goal

● The child will have adequate bowel elimination without episodes of constipation.

Implementations for Preventing Constipation

Decreased bowel motility may lead to constipation, which in turn may result in injury. Enemas may be given to achieve bowel elimination. They may also be ordered before diagnostic and surgical procedures are performed. Administer colonic irrigations with saline solutions. Neomycin or other antibiotic solutions are used to cleanse the bowel and prepare the GI tract.

Don't!

Never administer soapsuds or tap water enemas to a child with Hirschsprung disease. The lack of peristaltic action causes the enemas to be retained and absorbed into the tissues, causing water intoxication. This could cause syncope, shock, or even death after only one or two irrigations.

Evaluation of Goal/Desired Outcome

The child's:

- bowel eliminations occur daily.
- colon is clean and well prepared for surgery.

Nursing Care Focus

- Malnutrition risk related to anorexia

Goal

- The child's nutritional status will be maintained preoperatively.

Implementations for Maintaining Adequate Nutrition

Parenteral nutrition may be needed to improve nutritional status because the constipation and distended abdomen cause loss of appetite. IV fluid therapy may be necessary. The child does not want to eat and has a poor nutritional status. In older children, a low-residue diet is given.

Evaluation of Goal/Desired Outcome

- The child's nutritional intake is adequate to maintain weight and promote growth.

Nursing Care Focus

- Fear (in the older child) related to impending surgery

Goal

- The older child will display minimal fear of bodily injury.

Implementations for Reducing Fear

Children who are preschool age or older are more aware of the approaching surgery and have a number of fears reflective of their developmental stage. Preschoolers are still in the age of magical thinking. They may overhear a word or two that they misinterpret and exaggerate; this can lead to imagined pain and danger. Careful explanations must be provided for the preschool-aged child to reduce any fears about mutilation. Talk about the surgery; reassure the child that their "insides won't come out," and answer questions seriously and sincerely. Encourage family caregivers to stay with the child, if possible, to increase the child's feelings of security.

The older school-aged child may have a more realistic view of what is going to happen but may still fear the impending surgery. Peer contact may help comfort the school-aged child. For more information on reducing preoperative fears and anxiety, see Chapter 29.

Evaluation of Goal/Desired Outcome

The older child:

- realistically describes what will happen in surgery.
- interacts with family, peers, and nursing staff in a positive manner.

Nursing Care Focus

- Family coping impairment related to the serious condition of the child and a knowledge deficiency about impending surgery

Goal

- The family caregivers will demonstrate an understanding of preoperative procedures.

Implementations for Promoting Family Coping and Understanding

Family caregivers are apprehensive about the preliminary procedures and the impending surgery. Explain all aspects of the preoperative care, including examinations, colonic irrigations, and IV fluid therapy. As with other surgical procedures, inform the family caregivers about the waiting area, the postanesthesia care unit, and the approximate length of the surgery; answer any questions. Building good rapport before surgery is an essential aspect of good nursing care. Answer the family caregivers' questions about the later resection of the aganglionic portion. With successful surgery, these children will grow and develop normally.

Evaluation of Goal/Desired Outcome

The family caregivers:

- cooperate with care.
- ask relevant questions.
- accurately explain procedures when asked to repeat information.

Nursing Care Focus: Postoperative Phase

The nursing care focuses for the infant with congenital aganglionic megacolon during the postoperative phase include the risk for altered skin and tissue (oral mucous membranes), management of pain, monitoring for complications, and the concern for hypovolemia in the child. Recognize the need for reinforcing family teaching related to the postoperative care of the child.

Outcome Identification and Planning: Postoperative Phase

The major postoperative goals for the child include maintaining skin and tissue integrity (oral mucous membranes), promoting comfort, monitoring for complications, and maintaining fluid balance. Goals for the family include reducing caregiver anxiety and preparing for home care of the child. Develop the individualized nursing plan of care according to these goals.

Nursing Care Focus

- Altered tissue integrity of oral mucous membranes related to NPO status
- Altered skin integrity risk related to irritation from the colostomy

Goal

- The child's oral mucous membranes are moist and pink.
- The child's skin integrity will be maintained.

Implementations for Providing Oral Care and Promoting Skin Integrity

Perform good mouth care at least every 4 hours. For the infant, sucking needs can be satisfied with a pacifier.

Maintaining skin integrity of the surgical site, especially around the colostomy stoma, is very important. When performing routine colostomy care, give careful attention to the area around the colostomy. Record and report redness, irritation, and rashy appearances of the skin around the stoma. Prepare the skin with skin-toughening preparations that strengthen it and provide better adhesion of the appliance.

Evaluation of Goal/Desired Outcome

The child:

- has moist, pink, and intact oral mucous membranes.
- has no skin irritation at the colostomy site.
- has no redness, foul odor, or purulent drainage at the surgical site.

Nursing Care Focus

- Acute pain related to the surgical procedure or possible complications

Goal

- The child's behavior will indicate minimal pain.

Implementations for Promoting Comfort and Monitoring for Complications

The child may have abdominal pain after surgery. Observe for signs of pain such as crying, pulse and respiration rate increases; restlessness; guarding of the abdomen; or drawing up the legs. Administer analgesics promptly; as ordered. Additional nursing measures that can be used are changing the child's position, holding the child when possible, stroking, cuddling, and engaging in age-appropriate activities.

Observe for signs of enterocolitis (inflammation of the intestines), a severe complication of Hirschsprung disease, such as abdominal pain and distention. Other signs that may indicate enterocolitis include fever, vomiting, explosive foul-smelling diarrhea, and rectal bleeding. Document and report any of these symptoms promptly.

Evaluation of Goal/Desired Outcome

The child:

- rests quietly without signs of restlessness.
- verbalizes comfort if old enough to communicate verbally.
- shows no signs or symptoms of complications.

Nursing Care Focus

- Hypovolemia related to postoperative condition

Goal

- The child's fluid intake will be adequate.

Implementations for Maintaining Fluid Balance

An NG tube may be in place after surgery; to keep the stomach decompressed, and IV fluids are given until bowel function is established. Accurate intake and output determinations and reporting the character, amount, and consistency of stools help determine when the child may have oral feedings. To monitor fluid loss, record and report the drainage from the NG tube every 8 hours. Immediately report any unusual drainage, such as bright red bleeding.

Evaluation of Goal/Desired Outcome

- The child's hourly urine output is 0.5 to 1 mL/kg, indicating adequate hydration.

Nursing Care Focus

- Knowledge deficiency of family caregivers related to understanding of postoperative care of the colostomy

Goal

- The family caregivers will demonstrate skill and knowledge in caring for the colostomy.

Implementations for Reinforcing Family Teaching

Show the family caregiver how to care for the colostomy at home. If available, a wound, ostomy, and continence nurse (WOCN) may be consulted to help teach the family caregivers. Discuss topics such as devices and their use, daily irrigation, and skin care. The caregivers should demonstrate their understanding by caring for the colostomy under the supervision of nursing personnel several days before discharge. Family caregivers also need referrals to support personnel.

Evaluation of Goal/Desired Outcome

- The family caregivers irrigate the colostomy and clean the surrounding skin under the supervision of nursing personnel.

 A Personal Glimpse

When our son was born, my wife and I were thrilled; we were so happy to be parents. My wife was breast-feeding, and I would get up at night and bring him to her so she could feed him; it was just like we had thought it would be. He started growing and getting bigger, so at first we weren't worried about his big belly. It was my job to change the "dirty" diapers when I was home. We started noticing the baby seemed constipated at times and had little hard stools but then had diarrhea. The pediatrician used the word "obstruction," and that was hard for us to really understand. They did a barium test and other tests; we felt so bad for our baby. My wife was so upset, she cried all the time. He had to have IVs and TPN, and then they told us he would have to have surgery and a colostomy. Seeing him with all those tubes and bags after surgery was heartbreaking. We took him home with the colostomy, and my job was still the "diaper" duty, but now it was taking care of the colostomy. I have gotten so good, now I can change the colostomy bag pretty fast. We know he has to go back for more surgery, but for now we are just glad we can take care of him at home and love and enjoy him.

David

Learning Opportunity: In what ways do you think this father was supportive of his wife and his son? What teaching would be important to reinforce with these parents about care of the colostomy? What community support might be available for this family?

Intussusception

Intussusception is the **invagination**, or telescoping, of one portion of the bowel into a distal portion. It occurs most commonly at the juncture of the ileum and the colon, although it can appear elsewhere in the intestinal tract. The invagination is from above downward; the upper portion slips over the lower portion and pulls the mesentery along with it (Fig. 38-7).

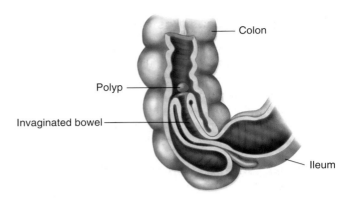

FIGURE 38-7 In this drawing of intussusception, note the telescoping of a portion of the bowel into the distal portion.

This condition occurs more often in boys than in girls and is the most common cause of intestinal obstruction in childhood. The highest incidence occurs in infants between the ages of 6 and 24 months. The condition usually appears in healthy babies without any demonstrable cause. Possible contributing factors may be the hyperperistalsis and unusual mobility of the cecum and ileum normally present in early life. Correlation has been made with respiratory viral illness, In particular, a recent or concurrent adenovirus infection. Occasionally a lesion such as Meckel diverticulum or a polyp is present.

Clinical Manifestations and Diagnosis

The infant who previously appeared healthy and happy has a sudden onset of severe, crampy abdominal pain; draws their legs up toward the abdomen; and cries inconsolably. The episode may last for several minutes, after which the infant relaxes and appears well until the next episode, which usually occurs 15 to 20 minutes later. The episodes become more frequent and more severe, and the child often becomes lethargic.

Most of these infants start vomiting just after the first episode of pain. Vomiting becomes progressively more severe and is eventually bile-stained. The infant strains with

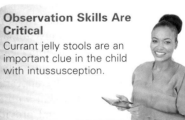

Observation Skills Are Critical

Currant jelly stools are an important clue in the child with intussusception.

each paroxysm, emptying the bowels of fecal contents. The stools consist of blood and mucus, thereby earning the name **currant jelly stools.** A sausage-shaped mass can often be felt through the right side of the abdominal wall.

Signs of shock can appear quickly and characteristically include a rapid, weak pulse; increased temperature; shallow, grunting respirations; pallor; and marked sweating. Shock, vomiting, and currant jelly stools are the cardinal symptoms of this condition. Because these signs coupled with the paroxysmal pain are quite severe, professional healthcare is often initiated early.

The initial symptoms seen with intussusception may be confused with other conditions such as gastroenteritis. Be aware that on occasions a more chronic form of the condition appears, particularly during an episode of severe diarrhea. The onset is more gradual and may be seen in an older child, and the infant or child may not show all the classic symptoms; the danger of sudden, complete strangulation of the bowel is present.

The health care provider can often make a diagnosis from the classic clinical symptoms, but the diagnosis is usually made using abdominal ultrasound and radiography.

Treatment and Nursing Care

This condition is an emergency in the sense that prolonged delay is dangerous. The telescoped bowel rapidly becomes gangrenous, thus markedly reducing the possibility of a simple reduction. Adequate treatment during the first 12 to 24 hours should have a good outcome with complete recovery. The outcome becomes more uncertain as the bowel deteriorates, making resection necessary.

Immediate treatment consists of IV fluids; NPO status; insertion of a nasogastric (NG) tube for gastric decompression; and a diagnostic air, saline, or contrast enema. The enema, done using fluoroscopy, can often reduce the invagination, simply by the pressure pushing against the telescoped portion. The enema should not be done if signs of bowel perforation or peritonitis are evident. Abdominal surgery, often laparoscopic, is performed if the enema does not correct the problem. Surgery may consist of manual reduction of the invagination, resection with anastomosis, or possible colostomy if the intestine is gangrenous.

If the invagination was reduced, the infant is returned to normal feedings within 24 hours and discharged in about 48 hours. Carefully observe for recurrence during this period. Preoperative and postoperative nursing focuses used for the child with congenital aganglionic megacolon also can be used when surgery is required for this condition.

TEST YOURSELF

✔ Explain what happens in the GI tract of the child who has congenital aganglionic megacolon (Hirschsprung disease).

✔ Explain what occurs with intussusception and describe the symptoms seen in the child with the diagnosis.

Appendicitis

Appendicitis refers to an inflammation of the appendix. The appendix is a blind pouch located in the cecum near the ileocecal junction. Obstruction of the lumen of the appendix is the primary cause of appendicitis. The obstruction is usually caused by undigested food, hardened fecal matter, or a foreign body. This obstruction causes circulation to be slowed or interrupted, resulting in pain and necrosis of the appendix. The necrotic area can rupture, causing escape of fecal matter and bacteria into the peritoneal cavity and resulting

in the complication of peritonitis. Most cases of appendicitis in childhood occur in the school-aged child.

Clinical Manifestations and Diagnosis

In young children, the symptoms may be difficult to evaluate. Symptoms in the older child may be the same as in an adult—pain and tenderness in the right lower quadrant of the abdomen, anorexia, nausea and vomiting, fever, and rebound tenderness. However, these symptoms are uncommon in young children; many children already have a ruptured appendix when first seen by the health care provider. The young child has difficulty localizing the pain, may act restless and irritable, and may have a fever, vomiting, and anorexia. The diagnosis is determined by the child's history, laboratory values (usually the white blood cell count is slightly elevated), and an abdominal ultrasound or CT scan.

> **Do You Know the Why?**
>
> When appendicitis is suspected, laxatives and enemas are contraindicated because they increase peristalsis, which increases the possibility of rupturing an inflamed appendix.

Treatment

Surgical removal of the appendix is necessary and should be performed as soon as possible after diagnosis. If the appendix has not ruptured before surgery, a laparoscopic procedure is often done with minimal operative risk. Even after perforation has occurred, the mortality rate is extremely low.

Food and fluids by mouth are withheld before surgery. IV fluids are administered to maintain hydration and electrolyte balance. If fever is present, measures are implemented to keep the temperature within normal limits. Antibiotics may be administered preoperatively as well as postoperatively.

Recovery is rapid and usually uneventful. If peritonitis or a localized abscess occurs, gastric suction for decompression, parenteral fluids, and antibiotics may be ordered.

Nursing Process and Care Plan *for the Child With Appendicitis*

Assessment (Data Collection)

When a child is admitted with a diagnosis of possible appendicitis, an emergency situation exists. The family caregiver who brings the child to the hospital is often upset and anxious. The admission examination and data collection must be performed quickly and skillfully. Obtain information about the child's condition for the last several days to formulate a picture of how the condition has developed. Emphasize GI complaints, appetite, bowel movements for the last few days, and general activity level. During the physical examination, include vital signs, especially noting any elevation of temperature, presence of bowel sounds, abdominal guarding, and nausea or vomiting. Immediately report diminished or absent bowel sounds. Provide the child and family caregiver with careful explanations about all procedures to be performed. Use special empathy and understanding to alleviate the child's and family's anxieties.

Nursing Care Focus

When determining nursing care focuses applicable to the child with appendicitis, the family's and child's fear are important to address. Pain and dehydration are also concerns for the child. The family caregivers need reinforcement of teaching related to the home care of the child.

Outcome Identification and Planning

Because of the urgent nature of the child's admission and preparation for surgery, great efforts must be taken to provide calm, reassuring care to both the child and the family caregivers. A major goal for both the child and the caregivers is relieving fear. Additional goals for the child are relieving pain and maintaining fluid balance. Another goal for the family is increasing knowledge of the postoperative and home care needs of the child.

Nursing Care Focus

- Fear of the child and family caregiver related to emergency surgery

Goal

- The child and family caregivers will have reduced or alleviated fear.

Implementations for Reducing Fear

Although procedures must be performed quickly, consider both the child's and the family's fear. The child may be extremely frightened by the sudden change of events and may also be in considerable pain. The family caregiver may be apprehensive about impending surgery. Introduce various healthcare team members by name and title as they come into the child's room to perform procedures. Explain to the child and the family what is happening and why. Explain the postanesthesia care unit (recovery room) to the child and the family caregiver. Encourage the family and child to verbalize fears, and try to allay these fears as much as possible. Let family members know where to wait during surgery, how long the surgery will last, where dining facilities are located, and where the surgeon will expect to find them after surgery. Throughout the preoperative care, be sensitive to verbalized or nonverbalized fears and provide understanding care.

What a Difference This Can Make

Before the child goes to surgery, if possible, demonstrate deep breathing, coughing, and abdominal splinting to the child, and have them practice it.

Evaluation of Goal/Desired Outcome

The child and family:

- verbalize fears.
- ask questions before surgery.
- cooperate with healthcare personnel.

Nursing Care Focus

- Acute pain related to necrosis of appendix and surgical procedure

Goal

- The child's pain will be controlled.

Implementations for Promoting Comfort

Analgesics are not given before surgery because they may conceal signs of tenderness that are important for diagnosis. Provide comfort through positioning and gentle care while performing preoperative procedures. Heat to the abdomen is contraindicated because of the danger of rupture of the appendix. After surgery, observe the child hourly for indications of pain, and administer analgesics as ordered. Provide quiet activities to help divert the child's attention from the pain. The child may fear postoperative ambulation because of pain. Many children are worried that the stitches will pull out. Reassure the child that this worry is understood, but that the sutures (or staples) are designed to withstand the strain of walking and moving. Activity is essential to the child's recovery but should be as pain free as possible. Help the child understand that as activity increases, the pain will decrease. The child whose appendix ruptured before surgery may also have pain related to the NG tube, abdominal distention, or constipation.

Evaluation of Goal/Desired Outcome

- The child's pain is at an acceptable level, as evidenced by the child's verbalization of pain according to a pain scale.

Nursing Care Focus

- Dehydration risk related to decreased intake

Goal

- The child will have adequate fluid intake.

Implementations for Monitoring Fluid Balance

Dehydration can be a concern, especially if the child has had preoperative nausea and vomiting. On admission to the hospital, the child is maintained NPO until after surgery. The child may have a nasogastric (NG) tube after surgery. Accurately measure and record all intake and output, including output from the NG tube. If the NG tube is irrigated, be sure to subtract the amount irrigated in from the output of the NG tube to get an accurate output. IV fluids are administered as ordered. After surgery, check dressings to detect evidence of excessive drainage or bleeding that indicates loss of fluids. After the bowel sounds return and the NG tube is removed, clear oral fluids are ordered. After the child takes and retains fluids successfully, a progressive diet is ordered. Monitor, record, and report bowel sounds at least every 4 hours because the health care provider may use this as a gauge to determine when the child can have solid food.

Evaluation of Goal/Desired Outcome

The child's:

- skin turgor is good.
- vital signs are within normal limits.
- hourly urine output is at least 0.5 to 1 mL/kg.

Nursing Care Focus

- Knowledge deficiency of family caregiver related to postoperative and home care needs

Goal

- The family caregivers will verbalize an understanding of postoperative and home care needs of the child.

Implementations for Reinforcing Family Teaching

The child who has had an uncomplicated appendectomy usually convalesces quickly and can return to school within a short period of time. Instruct the caregiver to keep the incision clean and dry. Activities are limited according to the health care provider's recommendations. The child whose appendix has ruptured may be hospitalized for a longer period of time and is more limited in activities after surgery. Instruct the family caregiver to observe for signs and symptoms of postoperative complications, including fever, abdominal distention, and pain. Emphasize the need for making and keeping follow-up appointments.

Evaluation of Goal/Desired Outcome

The family caregivers:

- discuss recovery expectations.
- demonstrate wound care as needed.
- list signs and symptoms to report.

Intestinal Parasites

A few intestinal parasites are common in the United States, especially in young and school-aged children. Hand-to-mouth practices contribute to infestations.

Enterobiasis (Pinworm Infection)

The pinworm (*Enterobius vermicularis*) is a white threadlike worm that invades the cecum and may enter the appendix. Articles contaminated with pinworm eggs spread pinworms from person to person. The infestation is common in children and occurs when a child unknowingly swallows the pinworm eggs. The eggs hatch in the intestinal tract and grow to maturity in the cecum. The female worm, when ready to lay her eggs, crawls out of the anus and lays the eggs on the perineum.

Itching around the anus causes the child to scratch and trap new eggs under the fingernails, which often causes reinfection when the child's fingers go into the mouth. Clothing, bedding, food, toilet seats, and other articles become infected, and the infestation spreads to other members of the family. Pinworm eggs can also float in the air and be inhaled.

The life cycle of these worms is 6 to 8 weeks, after which reinfestation commonly occurs without treatment. The incidence is highest in school-aged children and next highest in preschool-aged children. All members of the family are susceptible.

Clinical Manifestations and Diagnosis

Intense perianal itching is the primary symptom of pinworms. Young children who cannot clearly verbalize their feelings may be restless, irritable, sleep poorly, or have episodes of bed-wetting.

The usual method of diagnosis is to use cellophane tape to capture the eggs from around the anus and to examine them under a microscope. Adult worms may also be seen as they emerge from the anus when the child is lying quietly or sleeping. The cellophane tape test for identifying worms is performed in the early morning, just before or as soon as the child wakens. The test is performed in the following manner:

1. Wind clear cellophane tape around the end of a tongue blade, sticky side outward.
2. Spread the child's buttocks, and press the tape against the anus, rolling the tape from side to side.
3. Transfer the tape to a microscope slide, and cover with a clean slide to send to the laboratory. If the caregiver does not have slides or a commercially prepared kit, the caregiver should place the tongue blade in a plastic bag and bring it to the healthcare facility. The tape is then examined microscopically for eggs in the laboratory.

Treatment and Nursing Care

Treatment consists of the use of an **anthelmintic** (or vermifugal, a medication that expels intestinal worms). Pyrantel pamoate is a frequently used medication in the United States. It is available over the counter and is highly effective. Mebendazole or albendazole may also be given. The medication should be repeated in 2 or 3 weeks to eliminate any parasites that hatch after the initial treatment. Because pinworms are easily transmitted, encourage all family members to be treated.

It is often disturbing to children and family caregivers for the child to be found to have pinworms. Reassure them that pinworm infestation is as common as an infection or a cold. This support is important when caring for a child with any type of intestinal parasite.

As a preventive measure, teach the child to wash their hands after bowel movements and before eating. Encourage the child to observe other hygiene measures, such as regular bathing and daily change of underclothing. Reinforce teaching with the family caregivers to keep the child's fingernails short and clean. Caregivers also need to know that bedding should be changed frequently to avoid reinfestation. All bedding and clothing, especially underclothing, should be washed in hot water.

Roundworms

Ascaris lumbricoides is a large intestinal worm found only in humans. Infestation occurs through contact with the feces of people with infestation. It is usually found in areas where sanitary facilities are lacking and human excreta are deposited on the ground.

The adult worm is pink and 9 to 12 inches long. The eggs come from contaminated food or soil and are ingested. The eggs hatch in the intestinal tract, and the larvae migrate to the liver and lungs. The larvae reaching the lungs ascend up through the bronchi, get swallowed, and reach the intestine, where they grow to maturity and mate. Eggs are then discharged into the feces. Full development requires about 2 months. In tropical countries where infestation may be heavy, bowel obstructions may present serious problems.

Generally, no symptoms are present in ordinary infestations, but the child may show signs of malnutrition and weight loss. Identification is made by means of microscopic examination of feces for eggs. Mebendazole, albendazole, or ivermectin are the medications commonly used. Family caregivers require education about improved hygiene practices with sanitary disposal of feces, including diapers, as necessary to prevent infestation.

Hookworms

The hookworm lives in the human intestinal tract, where it attaches itself to the wall of the small intestine. Eggs are discharged in the feces of the host. These parasites are prevalent in areas where infected human excreta are deposited on the ground and where the soil, moisture, and temperature are favorable for the development of infective larvae of the worm. In the southeastern United States and tropical West Africa, the prevailing species is *Necator americanus.*

Clinical Manifestations and Diagnosis

After feces containing eggs are deposited on the ground, larvae hatch. They can survive there as long as 6 weeks and usually penetrate the skin of barefoot people. They produce an itching dermatitis on the feet (ground itch). The larvae pass through the bloodstream to the lungs and into the pharynx, where they are swallowed and reach the small intestine. In the small intestine, they attach themselves to the intestinal wall, where they feed on blood. Heavy infestation may cause anemia through loss of blood. Chronic infestation produces listlessness, fatigue, and malnutrition. Identification is made by examination of the stool under the microscope.

Treatment and Nursing Care

Pyrantel pamoate or albendazole may be used in the treatment of hookworms. Stress the need for the affected child to receive a well-balanced diet with additional protein and iron. Transfusions are rarely necessary. To prevent hookworm infestation, instruct family caregivers to keep children from running barefoot where there is any possibility of ground contamination with feces.

Giardiasis

Giardiasis is not caused by a worm, but by the protozoan parasite *Giardia duodenalis.* It is a common cause of diarrhea in world travelers and is also prevalent in children who attend day care centers and other types of residential facilities; it may be found in contaminated mountain streams or pools frequented by diapered infants. The child ingests the cyst containing the protozoa. The cyst is activated by stomach acid and passes into the duodenum where it matures and causes signs and symptoms.

Clinical Manifestations and Treatment

Maturation of the cyst leads to diarrhea, with foul smelling, fatty stools, weight loss, and abdominal cramps. Identification and diagnosis are made through examination of stool under the microscope. Tinidazole, nitazoxanide, and metronidazole are effective in treating the infestation.

Nursing Care

Alert the family caregiver that tinidazole and metronidazole have a metallic taste and that GI side effects such as nausea and vomiting can occur. To prevent infestations, stress to family caregivers the importance of careful handling of soiled diapers, especially in a childcare facility. Handwashing, avoiding pools and streams used by diapered infants, and avoiding contact with infected persons are also important.

TEST YOURSELF

✔ What is the appendix and where is it located?

✔ What is contraindicated if a diagnosis of appendicitis is suspected?

✔ What are common ways pinworm infections are spread?

Ingestion of Toxic Substances

One way in which toddlers find out about their environment is to taste the world around them. Toddlers and preschool-aged children are developing autonomy and initiative and refining their gross and fine motor skills, which adds to the tendency to examine their environments on their own. Because their senses of taste and smell are not yet refined, these age groups are prime targets for ingestion of poisonous substances.

The ordinary household has an abundance of poisonous substances in almost every room. The kitchen, bathroom, bedroom, and garage are the most common sites harboring substances that are poisonous when ingested. Although most poisonings occur in the child's home, grandparents' homes offer many temptations to the young child as well. Grandparents tend to be less concerned about placing dangerous substances out of children's reach simply because the children are not part of the household, or the grandparents may place supplies where they are convenient, while never considering the young grandchild's developmental stage and exploratory nature (see Tips for Reinforcing Family Teaching: Poison Prevention in the Home).

When a child is found with a container whose contents they have obviously sampled, action should be taken immediately. When a child manifests symptoms that are difficult to pinpoint or that do not appear to relate specifically to any known cause, the possibility of poisoning should be suspected. Ingestion of a poisonous substance can produce symptoms that simulate an attack of an acute disease: vomiting, abdominal pain, diarrhea, shock, cyanosis, coma, and convulsions. If evidence of such a disease is lacking, acute poisoning should be suspected.

Be Careful!
Young children ingest substances with tastes or smells that would repel an adult.

Stay Alert!
Batteries, especially button batteries (found in hearing aids, games and toys, watches, calculators, flashlights, and remote control devices), can be a cause of poisoning as well as a choking hazard in children.

In instances of apparent poisoning when the substance is unknown, family caregivers are asked to consider all medications in their home. Is it possible that any medication could have been available to the child, or did an older child or any other person possibly give the child the container to play with? Is it possible that a parent inadvertently gave a wrong dose or wrong medication to a child? All such possibilities need to be considered. In the meantime, the most important priority is treatment for the child who shows symptoms of poisoning.

The rate of deaths caused by poisoning has dramatically decreased because of the use of child-resistant closures, safer products, education, public awareness, poison control centers, and antidotes available.

Emergency Treatment

If the child has collapsed or is not breathing, 911 should be called for emergency help. In cases in which the child is conscious and alert and the caregiver suspects poison ingestion, the Poison Control Center (also called the Poison Help Line) should be called. The universal telephone number in the United States is (800) 222-1222. All homes with young children should have the Poison Control Center number posted

Now Recommended
In many cases of poisoning, the accepted treatment for years was to administer syrup of ipecac to induce vomiting. The American Academy of Pediatrics (AAP) now believes that using ipecac and inducing vomiting should no longer be recommended. In addition, the AAP further suggests that, because of the potential of misuse, existing ipecac in homes should be disposed of safely.

TIPS FOR REINFORCING FAMILY TEACHING

Poison Prevention in the Home

- Keep harmful products and household cleaning products locked up and out of a child's sight and reach. Be especially aware of highly concentrated laundry and dishwashing detergent packets, often called "pods."
- Keep hand sanitizers, wipes, and antibacterial cleaning materials out of children's reach and dispose of these carefully after use.
- Use safety latches or locks on drawers and cabinets.
- Read labels with care before using any product.
- Replace child-resistant closures and safety caps immediately after using product.
- Never leave alcohol or electronic cigarettes/nicotine refill cartridges within a child's reach.
- Keep products in their original containers; never put nonfood products in food or drink containers.
- Teach children not to drink or eat anything unless it is given to them by a trusted adult.
- Do not take medicine in front of small children; children tend to copy adult behavior.

- Do not refer to medicine as candy; call medicine by its correct name.
- Check your home often for old medications and get rid of them following the U.S. FDA drug disposal guidelines (U.S. FDA, 2021).
- Keep "button" battery compartments on household products taped and secured, store batteries out of reach and sight of children, and do not allow children to play with batteries.
- Keep plants off floor and out of children's reach.
- Keep lotion, cream, powder, cosmetics, and insect repellent out of children's reach.
- Post the Poison Control Center number near each telephone: (800) 222-1222.
- Program the Poison Control Center number into your and your children's cell phones and into your home phone.
- Seek help if your child swallows a substance that is not food, and call the Poison Help Line. Do not make your child vomit.

Adapted from Kelly (2021).

by every telephone for quick reference. The caregiver should remove any obvious poison from the child's mouth before calling. The poison control center evaluates the situation and tells the caller whether the child can be treated at home or needs to be transported to a hospital or treatment center.

In the emergency care setting, GI decontamination using activated charcoal, which absorbs many types of materials, may be used to reduce the dangers of ingested substances. The charcoal is a black, fine powder that is mixed with water. A dose of 10 grams per gram of ingested poison is given by mouth in 6 to 8 oz of water or may be given through an NG tube, if necessary.

If the substance the child has swallowed is known, the ingredients can be found on the label and the Poison Control Center can suggest an antidote. If the substance is a prescription drug, the pharmacist who filled the prescription or who is familiar with the drug can also be contacted for information. In some instances, it is necessary to analyze the stomach contents.

Specific antidotes are available for certain poisons, but not for all. Some antidotes react chemically with the poison to render it harmless, whereas others prevent absorption of the poison.

Treatment Steps in Order of Importance

The treatment steps in order of importance are as follows:

1. Remove the obvious remnants of the poison.
2. Call 911 for emergency help if child has collapsed or stopped breathing.
3. Call the Poison Control Center if child is conscious and alert. The universal poison control number is (800) 222-1222.
4. Follow instructions given by the Poison Control Center personnel.
5. Administer appropriate antidote if recommended.
6. Administer general supportive and symptomatic care.

Further specific treatment is given according to the kind and amount of the toxic substance ingested.

Common types of poisoning and general treatment are described in Table 38-2. Complete listings of poisonous substances with the specific treatment for each are available from the Poison Control Center, clinics, and pharmacies.

Lead Poisoning (Plumbism)

Chronic lead poisoning has been a serious problem among children for many years. It is responsible for neurologic handicaps, including intellectual disability, because of its effect on the central nervous system. Infants and toddlers are potential victims because of their tendency to put any object within their reach into their mouths. In some children, this habit leads to **pica** (the ingestion of nonfood substances such as clay, paper, and paint). The unborn fetus of a pregnant mother who is exposed to lead (such as lead dust from renovation of an older home) can also be affected by lead contamination. Screening for lead poisoning is part of a complete well-child checkup between ages 6 months and 6 years.

Sources of Chronic Lead Poisoning

The most common sources of lead poisoning are the following:

- Lead-containing paint used on the outside or the inside of older houses
- Furniture and toys painted with lead-containing paint; vinyl mini blinds
- Drinking water contaminated by lead pipes or copper pipes with lead-soldered joints
- Dust containing lead salts from lead paint; emission from lead smelters
- Storage of fruit juices or other food in improperly glazed earthenware
- Inhalation of fumes from engines containing lead or from burning batteries
- Exposure to industrial areas with smelteries or chemical plants
- Exposure to hobby materials containing lead (e.g., stained glass, solder, fishing sinkers, bullets)

Lead poisoning has other causes, but the most common cause has been the lead in paint. Children tend to nibble on fallen plaster, painted wooden furniture (including cribs), and painted toys because they have a sweet taste. Fine dust that results from removing lead paint in remodeling can also cause harm to the children in the household, without family caregivers being aware of exposure. When the danger of lead poisoning became apparent, the sale of paint containing lead was banned. However, this has not eliminated the problem because many older homes were painted with lead-based paint, and they still exist in inner-city areas, as well as in small towns and suburbs. Older mansions where upper-income families may live also may have lead paint because of the building's age. Only contractors experienced in lead-based paint removal should do renovations.

Clinical Manifestations

The onset of chronic lead poisoning is insidious. Some early indications may be irritability, hyperactivity, aggression, impulsiveness, or disinterest in play. Short attention span, lethargy, learning difficulties, and distractibility are also signs of poisoning.

The condition may progress to **encephalopathy** (degenerative disease of the brain) because of intracranial pressure. Manifestations may include convulsions, intellectual disability, blindness, paralysis, coma, and death. Acute episodes sometimes develop sporadically and early in the condition.

Diagnosis

The nonspecific nature of the presenting symptoms makes it important to examine the child's environmental history. Screening questionnaires and testing blood lead levels are used as screening methods. Target screening is done in areas where the risk of lead poisoning is high. Fingersticks, heelsticks, or venous blood can be used to collect samples for lead-level screening.

TABLE 38-2 Commonly Ingested Toxic Substances

AGENT	SYMPTOMS	TREATMENT
Acetaminophen	Under 6 years—vomiting is the earliest sign. Adolescents—vomiting, diaphoresis, general malaise. Liver damage can result in 48–96 hours if not treated.	Activated charcoal for GI decontamination. Administer N-acetylcysteine diluted with cola, fruit juice, or water. N-acetylcysteine can be administered IV.
Acetylsalicylic acid (aspirin)	Hyperpnea (abnormal increase in depth and rate of breathing), metabolic acidosis, tachypnea, tinnitus, vertigo, nausea, vomiting, and diarrhea are initial symptoms. Fever, altered mental status, coma, and death follow untreated heavy dosage.	Activated charcoal may be administered. IV fluids, sodium bicarbonate to combat acidosis, and hemodialysis for renal failure may be necessary when large amounts are ingested.
Ibuprofen	Nausea, vomiting, abdominal pain, headache, metabolic acidosis, seizures, renal damage.	Activated charcoal is administered in emergency department. Electrolyte determination is done to detect acidosis. IV fluids are given.
Ferrous sulfate (iron)	Vomiting, lethargy, diarrhea, weak rapid pulse, hypotension are common symptoms. Massive dose may produce shock; erosion of small intestine; black, tarry stools; bronchial pneumonia.	Deferoxamine, a chelating agent that combines with iron, may be used when child has ingested a toxic dose.
Barbiturates	Respiratory, circulatory, and renal depression may occur. Child may become comatose.	Establish airway; administer oxygen if needed; GI decontamination with activated charcoal; close observation of level of consciousness is needed.
Corrosives Alkali: lye, bleaches Acid: drain cleaners, toilet bowel cleaners, iodine, silver nitrate	Intense burning and pain with first mouthful; severe burns and injury to mouth and esophageal tract; shock, possible death.	*Never have child vomit.* *Do not give neutralizing or diluting agents (milk, water)* *Activated charcoal NOT given* Supportive care and close observation Continuing treatment may include enteral feedings and specialized care. A tracheostomy may be needed.
Hydrocarbons: kerosene, gasoline, furniture polish, lighter fluid, turpentine	Damage to the respiratory system is the primary concern. Vomiting often occurs spontaneously, possibly causing additional damage to the respiratory system. Pneumonia, bronchopneumonia, or lipoid pneumonia may occur.	Emergency treatment and assessment are necessary. Vital signs are monitored; oxygen is administered as needed. GI decontamination is performed only if the ingested substance contains other toxic chemicals that may threaten another body system or organs such as the liver, kidneys, or cardiovascular system.

Treatment and Nursing Care

The most important aspect of treatment of a child with lead poisoning is to remove the lead from the child's system and environment. The use of a **chelating agent** (an agent that binds with metal) increases the urinary excretion of lead. Several chelating agents are available. The drugs used are Edetate calcium disodium, known as EDTA, dimercaprol, also known as BAL, and succimer.

All the chelating drugs may have toxic side effects, and children being treated must be carefully monitored with frequent urinalysis, blood cell counts, and renal function tests. Adequate hydration is important with any of the drugs to decrease kidney concerns.

Prognosis

The prognosis after lead poisoning is uncertain. Emphasis is on primary prevention and screening. Early detection of the condition and removal of the child from the lead-containing surroundings offer the best hope. Follow-up should include routine examinations to prevent recurrence and to observe for signs of any residual brain damage not immediately apparent.

Although the incidence of lead poisoning has decreased, it is still prevalent. Measures to educate the public on the importance of preventing this disorder are essential if the problem is to be eliminated. Education of the family caregivers is an essential aspect of the treatment (see Tips for Reinforcing Family Teaching: Preventing Lead Poisoning). The National Lead Information Center (1-800-424-LEAD [5323]) is another resource for information regarding lead poisoning.

Ingestion of Foreign Objects

Young children are apt to put any small objects into their mouths; they often swallow these objects. Normally many of these objects pass smoothly through the digestive tract and

TIPS FOR REINFORCING FAMILY TEACHING

Preventing Lead Poisoning

- If you live in an older home, make sure your child does not have access to any chips of paint or chew any surface painted with lead-based paint. Look for paint dust on window sills, and clean with a high-phosphate sodium cleaner (the phosphate content of automatic dishwashing detergent is usually high enough).
- Wet-mop hard-surfaced floors and woodwork with cleaner at least once a week. Vacuuming hard surfaces scatters dust.
- Wash child's hands and face before eating.
- Wash toys and pacifiers frequently.

- Prevent child from playing in dust near an old lead-painted house.
- Prevent child from playing in soil or dust near a major highway.
- If your water supply has a high lead content, fully flush faucets before using for cooking, drinking, or making formula.
- Avoid contamination from hobbies or work.
- Make sure your child eats regular meals. Food slows absorption of lead.
- Encourage your child to eat foods high in iron and calcium.

Adapted from Sample (2021).

---

are expelled in the feces. Occasionally, however, something such as an open safety pin, a coin, a button, magnet, or a marble may lodge in the esophagus and need to be extracted. Foods such as hot dogs, peanuts, carrots, popcorn kernels, apple pieces, grapes, and round candy are frequent offenders. Batteries, especially button batteries (found in hearing aids, games and toys, watches, calculators, flashlights, and remote control devices), can be a choking hazard as well as a cause of poisoning.

Unless symptoms of choking, gagging, or pain are present, waiting and watching the feces carefully for 3 or 4 days is usually safe. Any object, however, may pass safely through the esophagus and stomach only to become fixed in one of the curves of the intestine, causing an obstruction or fever because of infection. Sharp objects also present the danger of perforation somewhere in the digestive tract.

Diagnosis of a swallowed solid object is often, but not always, made from the history. If a foreign object in the digestive tract is suspected, fluoroscopic and x-ray studies may be required.

Treatment and Nursing Care

If a family caregiver has seen a child swallow an object and begin choking, the caregiver should hold the child along the rescuer's forearm with the child's head lower than his chest and give the child several back blows. After delivering the back blows, the caregiver should support the child's back and head and turn the child over onto the opposite thigh. The caregiver should deliver as many as five quick downward chest thrusts and remove the foreign body if visualized. A child older than 1 year can be encouraged to continue to cough, as long as the cough remains forceful. If the cough becomes ineffective (no sound with cough) or respirations become more difficult and stridor is present, the caregiver can attempt the Heimlich maneuver (Fig. 38-8).

If the child is not having respiratory problems but coughing has not expelled the object, the child needs to be transported to an emergency department to be assessed by a health care provider. Objects in the esophagus are removed by direct vision through an esophagoscope. Attempts to push the object down into the stomach or to extract it blindly can be dangerous. Some objects may need to be removed surgically. If the object is small and the health care provider believes there is little danger to the GI tract, the family caregiver may be advised to take the child home and watch the child's bowel movements over the next several days to confirm that the object has passed through the system.

Increasing respiratory difficulties indicate that the object has been aspirated rather than swallowed. Foreign objects aspirated into the larynx or bronchial tree may become lodged in the trachea or larynx. Back blows and chest thrusts or the Heimlich maneuver should be delivered, as described. The child's airway should be opened and rescue breathing attempted. If the child's chest does not rise, the child should be repositioned and rescue breathing tried again. If the airway is still obstructed, these steps should be repeated until the object is removed and respirations are established. The child should be transported to the emergency department as quickly as possible. The family caregiver should get emergency assistance while continuing to try to remove the offending object.

Adults must be aware of the power of example. A child who sees an adult holding pins or nails in their mouth may follow this example with disastrous and often fatal results.

> ### TEST YOURSELF
> ✔ What are the steps that should be taken if a child has ingested a toxic substance?
> ✔ What are some indications that a child may have lead poisoning?
> ✔ How is lead poisoning treated?

ENDOCRINE DISORDERS

Diabetes mellitus is classified into two major types: type 1 diabetes mellitus and type 2 diabetes mellitus (Table 38-3). Type 1 diabetes mellitus is one of the most common chronic

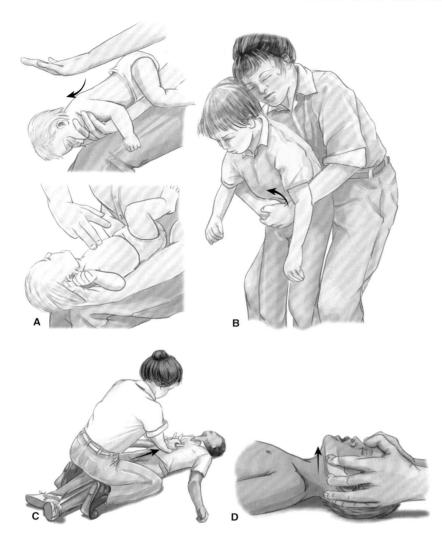

FIGURE 38-8 A., The Heimlich maneuver. Back blows (*top*) and chest thrusts (*bottom*) to relieve foreign-body airway obstruction in infant. Hold infant over arm as illustrated, supporting head by firmly holding jaw. Deliver up to five back blows. Turn infant over while supporting head, neck, jaw, and chest with one hand and back with other hand. Keep head lower than trunk. Give five quick chest thrusts with one finger below the intermammary line. If the foreign body is not removed and the airway remains obstructed, attempt rescue breathing. Repeat these two steps until successful. **B.** Abdominal thrusts with the child standing or sitting can be performed when the child is conscious. Standing behind the child, place the thumb side of one fist against the child's abdomen in midline, slightly above the navel and well below the xiphoid process. Grab your fist with the other hand and deliver five quick upward thrusts. Continue until successful or the child loses consciousness. **C.** Abdominal thrusts with the child lying can be performed on a conscious or unconscious child. Place heel of your hand on the child's abdomen, slightly above the navel and below the xiphoid process and rib cage. Place your other hand on top of the first hand. Deliver five separate, distinct thrusts. Open airway and attempt rescue breathing if object is not removed. Repeat until successful. **D.** Combined jaw thrust–spine stabilization maneuver for a child trauma victim with possible head or neck injury. To protect from damage to cervical spine, the neck is maintained in a neutral position, and traction on or movement of neck is avoided.

diseases in children and the most significant endocrine disorder that affects children. However, in recent years, type 2 diabetes mellitus, previously seen primarily in adults, has been seen more commonly in children.

Other endocrine conditions that may affect children are disorders of the pituitary gland, which alter growth, and diabetes insipidus. The incidence of these latter conditions is low.

Type 1 Diabetes Mellitus

Millions of Americans have been diagnosed with diabetes. Diabetes is often considered an adult disease, but a significant number of the diagnoses are children. Type 1 diabetes mellitus may begin in childhood and is usually diagnosed between the ages of 4 and 15 years. The incidence of this condition continues to increase. Management of diabetes in children is different from that in adults and requires conscientious care geared to the child's developmental stage.

Pathogenesis

The disease is caused as the result of an autoimmune destruction of the beta (insulin-secreting) cells of the islets of Langerhans in the pancreas. Genetics appears to be a

contributing factor. Some researchers believe that the presence of an acute infection during childhood may trigger a mechanism in genetically susceptible children, activating beta-cell dysfunction and disrupting insulin secretion.

Normally, the sugar derived from digestion and assimilation of foods is burned to provide energy for the body's activities. Excess sugar is converted into fat or glycogen and stored in the body tissues. Insulin, a hormone secreted by the pancreas, is responsible for the burning and storage of sugar. In diabetes, the secretion of insulin is inadequate or nonexistent, allowing sugar to accumulate in the bloodstream and spill over into the urine. In children, type 1 diabetes mellitus causes an abrupt pronounced decrease in insulin production, resulting in decreased ability to derive energy from the food eaten. Large amounts of protein and fat are used to supply the child's energy needs, causing loss of weight and slowed growth. This combination of failure to gain weight and lack of energy may be the initial reason the child is brought to the health care provider's attention. However, a health care provider may not see the child until symptoms of ketoacidosis are evident.

TABLE 38-3 Comparison of Type 1 and Type 2 Diabetes Mellitus

ASSESSMENT	TYPE 1 DIABETES MELLITIS	TYPE 2 DIABETES MELLITIS
Age at onset	4–6 years or at puberty	Increasingly occurring in younger children
Type of onset	Abrupt	Gradual
Weight changes	Marked weight loss is often initial sign	Associated with obesity
Other symptoms	Polydipsia	Polydipsia
	Polyuria (often begins as bed-wetting)	Polyuria
	Fatigue (marks fall in school)	Fatigue
	Blurred vision (marks fall in school)	Blurred vision
	Glycosuria	Glycosuria
	Polyphagia	Pruritus
	Pruritus	Mood changes
	Mood changes (may cause behavior problems in school)	
Therapy	Hypoglycemic agents never effective; insulin needed	Managed by diet, oral hypoglycemic agents, or insulin
	Diet only moderately restricted; no dietary foods used	Diet tends to be strict
	Common-sense foot care for growing children	Good skin and foot care necessary
Period of remission	Period of remission for 1–12 months generally follows initial diagnosis	Not demonstrable

Clinical Manifestations

Classic symptoms of type 1 diabetes mellitus are **polyuria** (dramatic increase in urinary output, probably with enuresis), **polydipsia** (increased thirst), and **polyphagia** (increased hunger and food consumption). These symptoms are usually accompanied by weight loss or failure to gain weight and lack of energy, even though the child has increased food consumption. Symptoms of diabetes in children often have an abrupt onset.

If the child's symptoms are not noted and referred for diagnosis, the disorder is likely to progress to diabetic ketoacidosis. Because of inadequate insulin production, carbohydrates are not converted into fuel for energy production. Fats are then mobilized for energy, but are incompletely oxidized in the absence of glucose. Ketone bodies (acetone, diacetic acid, and oxybutyric acid) accumulate. They are readily excreted in the urine, but the acid–base balance of body fluids excreted is upset and results in acidosis. **Diabetic ketoacidosis** is characterized by drowsiness, lethargy, dry skin, flushed cheeks and cherry-red lips, acetone breath with a fruity smell, and **Kussmaul breathing** (abnormal increase in the depth and rate of the respiratory movements). Nausea and vomiting may occur. If untreated, the child lapses into coma and exhibits dehydration, electrolyte imbalance, rapid pulse, and subnormal temperature and blood pressure.

Diagnosis

Early detection and control are critical in postponing or minimizing later complications of diabetes. Carefully observe for any signs or symptoms in all members of a family with a history of diabetes. The family should also be taught to observe the children for frequent thirst, urination, and weight loss. All relatives of people with diabetes are considered a high-risk group and should have periodic testing.

At each visit to a health care provider, children with a family history of diabetes should be monitored for glucose using a fingerstick glucose test and for ketones in the urine using a urine dipstick test. If the blood glucose level is elevated or ketonuria is present, a fasting blood sugar is performed. A fasting blood sugar result 200 mg/dL or more almost certainly is diagnostic for diabetes when other signs, such as polyuria and weight loss despite polyphagia, are present.

Although glucose tolerance tests are performed in adults to confirm diabetes, they are not commonly used in children. The traditional oral glucose tolerance test is often unsuccessful in children because they may vomit the concentrated glucose that must be swallowed.

Treatment

Management of type 1 diabetes mellitus in children includes insulin therapy and a meal and exercise plan. Treatment of the child with diabetes involves the family; child; and a number of health team members such as the nurse, the health care provider, the dietitian, and the diabetic nurse educator. After diabetes is diagnosed, the child may be hospitalized for a period of time, especially if they have been admitted with diabetic ketoacidosis. This allows the condition to be stabilized under supervision. This is a trying time, so you must plan care with an understanding of the emotional impact of the diagnosis. Outpatient settings work well with good results for many children newly diagnosed. Inform those who supervise the child during daily activities of the diagnosis, including the child's teacher and the school nurse.

Insulin Therapy

Insulin therapy is an essential part of the treatment of diabetes in children. The goal of insulin therapy is to keep the A1C (indicator of long-term control, usually checked every 3 months) less than 7.5% and the blood glucose level between 80 and 130 mg/dL. The dosage of insulin is adjusted according to blood glucose levels so that the levels are maintained near normal. Two kinds of insulin are often combined for the best results. Insulin can be grouped into rapid-acting, short-acting, intermediate-acting, and long-acting insulins (Table 38-4).

The introduction of rapid-acting insulin, such as lispro and aspart, has greatly changed insulin administration in children. The onset of action of rapid-acting insulin is less than 15 minutes and is typically given just before meals. Rapid-acting insulin can even be used right after a meal in children with unpredictable eating habits (Levitsky & Misra, 2021).

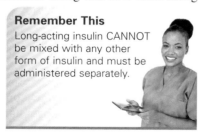

Good News

Lispro or aspart insulin can be administered immediately *after* the child has eaten, so the amount of food eaten can be taken into consideration when determining the dosage.

Two insulin types are often given in conjunction to give the child steady insulin coverage. Long-acting insulin preparations may be given once or twice a day to maintain glucose levels, and a rapid-acting insulin is given at meals and snack times. An intermediate-acting and a short-acting insulin may be given together. Some preparations come in a premixed proportion of 70% intermediate-acting and 30% short-acting insulin, eliminating the need for mixing. Children's insulin doses need to be individually regulated to keep their blood glucose levels as close to normal as possible.

Remember This

Long-acting insulin CANNOT be mixed with any other form of insulin and must be administered separately.

Hypoglycemic Reaction. Hypoglycemia is caused by an insulin overload, resulting in metabolism of the body's glucose that is too rapid. This may be attributable to a change in the body's requirement, carelessness in diet (such as failure to eat proper amounts of food), an error in insulin measurement, or increased exercise. Because diabetes in children is very labile (unstable, fluctuating), the child is subject to hypoglycemic reactions.

Some symptoms of impending hypoglycemia in children include tremors, pallor, sweating, and rapid heart rate. The child may have fatigue, lethargy, headache, seizures, or coma. Changes noted in the child's behavior may include irritability, agitation, erratic behavior, or tantrums in the young child. Children often have hypoglycemic reactions in the early morning. When hospitalized, observe the child at least every 2 hours during the night. Note tossed bedding, which would indicate restlessness, and any excessive perspiration. If necessary, try to rouse the child. As the child becomes regulated and observes a careful diet at home, parents do not need to watch so closely, but should have a thorough understanding of all aspects of this condition. Blood glucose monitoring often is scheduled for an early morning time in an effort to detect abnormal glucose levels.

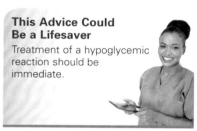

This Advice Could Be a Lifesaver

Treatment of a hypoglycemic reaction should be immediate.

To treat a hypoglycemic reaction, give the child 10 to 15 grams of concentrated simple carbohydrates such as sweetened fruit juice or glucose paste or tablets. This should be followed by giving the child a snack containing fat and protein such as a peanut butter sandwich or bagel and cream cheese. Repeated or impending reactions require consultation with the health care provider.

If the child cannot take a carbohydrate source orally, glucagon should be administered subcutaneously or intramuscularly to bring about a prompt increase in the blood glucose level. Glucagon can now also be administered by the intranasal route. Every adult responsible for a child with diabetes should clearly understand the procedure for administering this drug and should have easy access to it. Glucagon is a hormone produced by alpha cells of the pancreatic islets. An elevation in the blood glucose level

TABLE 38-4 Types of Insulin: Onset, Peak, and Duration

ACTION	PREPARATION	ONSET (HRS)	PEAK (HRS)	DURATION (HRS)
Rapid-acting	Lispro Aspart	0.25	0.5–1.5	3–5
Short-acting	Regular	0.5–1.5	2–4	5–8
Intermediate-acting	NPH	2–4	4–12	12–24
Long-acting	Glargine Detemir	1–2	No peak Continuous, steady	20–24

References may vary slightly on all figures.

results in insulin release in a normal person, but a decrease in the blood glucose level stimulates glucagon release. The released glucagon in the bloodstream acts on the liver to promote glycogen breakdown and glucose release. Glucagon is available as a pharmaceutical product and is packaged in prefilled syringes for immediate use. Glucagon acts within minutes to restore consciousness, after which the child should be given concentrated carbohydrates by mouth to maintain glucose level and decrease any nausea or vomiting. After a severe hypoglycemic episode, the child should be seen by a health care provider for evaluation.

Insulin Administration Methods. Insulin is often administered subcutaneously using an insulin syringe or a prefilled insulin pen or it may be administered continuously via an insulin pump.

The child may not be able to take over management of the insulin injection as early as blood glucose monitoring, but they can watch the preparation of the syringe and learn the technique for drawing up the dosage. It may be helpful to encourage the child to watch the process until it becomes routine. By 8 or 9 years of age, the child should be encouraged to talk with the family caregiver about the dose and to practice working with the syringe. The child may also draw up the dose and prepare for self-administration. The age at which this is possible varies. No two children mature at the same rate; some may be able to do this much earlier than others. Automatic injection devices can help the child self-administer insulin at a younger age (Fig. 38-9). The child should be encouraged to take over the management of the therapy when ready. If included in decision making, the child can learn the importance of the routine and accept the restrictions the disease imposes.

The insulin pump is a method of continuous insulin administration useful for some children with diabetes (Fig. 38-10). The pump is about the size of a cell phone and can be worn strapped to the waist or on a shoulder strap. It delivers a steady low dose of rapid-acting insulin into the subcutaneous tissue in the abdomen through a small needle attached to the pump by a small tubing. Extra insulin is released at mealtimes and other times when needed by pressing a button. Careful

blood glucose monitoring at least four times a day is necessary to adjust the dosage as needed. The pump must be removed to bathe, swim, or shower. The child may want to wear loose clothing to hide the pump. The needle site must be regularly observed for redness and irritation. The site is changed every 24 to 48 hours using an aseptic technique. Some insulin pumps also incorporate continuous glucose monitoring into the device. These devices are highly sophisticated and require skilled management of the child or adolescent's diabetes.

Unique Needs of the Adolescent

As it is for other young people, adolescence is an extremely trying period for many teenagers with diabetes. Like healthy adolescents, they must work from dependence to independence. Even when an adolescent has accepted responsibility for self-care, it is not unusual for them to rebel against the control that this condition demands, become impatient, and appear to ignore future health. The adolescent may skip meals, drop diet controls, or neglect glucose monitoring. Going barefoot and neglecting proper foot care can also cause problems for the adolescent with diabetes. It can be a difficult time for both the family caregiver and the adolescent. The caregivers naturally become concerned and are apt to give the adolescent more controls to rebel against.

The adolescent who completely understands all aspects of the condition (especially if allowed to assume control of treatment previously) should be allowed to continue managing their own treatment. An adolescent clinic can be of great value; the adolescent can discuss problems with understanding people who respond with care and provide dignity and attentive listening.

Treatment of Diabetic Ketoacidosis

Hyperglycemia results in diabetic ketoacidosis. Treatment for ketoacidosis requires skilled nursing care, and the child may be admitted to a pediatric intensive care unit. Regular insulin is administered intravenously. IV fluids are given to treat dehydration and to correct electrolyte imbalances. Glucose levels are monitored closely to prevent the levels from falling too rapidly.

Did you determine that **Jackson Edwards**, from the beginning of the chapter, has been diagnosed with type 1 diabetes mellitus? How will Jackson be treated to control his diabetes? What medications would you anticipate Jackson will be given, and how will these be administered? What signs and symptoms do you think Jackson's caregivers will be encouraged to watch for?

Nursing Process and Care Plan *for the Child With Type 1 Diabetes Mellitus*

Assessment (Data Collection)

When collecting data, ask the family caregiver about the child's symptoms leading up to the present illness. Ask

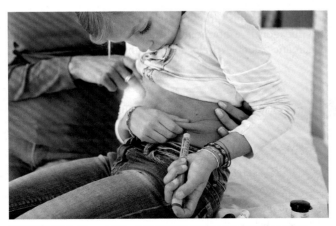

FIGURE 38-9 The child administers their own insulin using an insulin pen. (Reprinted with permission from Tagher C., & Knapp L. (2020). *Pediatric nursing a case-based approach* (UnFig. Patient Teaching 10-4, p. 122). Wolters Kluwer.)

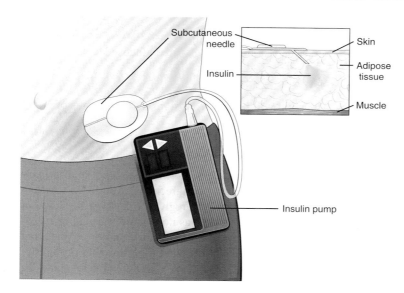

FIGURE 38-10 An insulin pump is programmed to administer a continuous insulin dose into the subcutaneous tissue. (Reprinted with permission from Tagher C., & Knapp L. (2020). *Pediatric nursing a case-based approach* (Fig. 10-2, p. 123). Wolters Kluwer.)

about the child's appetite, weight loss or gain, evidence of polyuria or enuresis in a previously toilet-trained child, polydipsia, dehydration (which may include constipation), irritability, and fatigue. Include the child in the interview and encourage them to contribute information. Observe for evidence of the child's developmental stage to help determine appropriate nursing focuses and plan effective care. If the child is first seen in diabetic ketoacidosis, adjust the initial nursing interview accordingly.

In the physical examination, measure the height and weight, and examine the skin for evidence of dryness or slowly healing sores. Note signs of hyperglycemia, record vital signs, and collect a urine specimen. Perform a blood glucose level determination using a glucose monitor.

Nursing Care Focus

When developing evidence-based nursing care focuses applicable to the child with type 1 diabetes mellitus, the risk for malnutrition and monitoring and regulating glucose levels are important to consider. The risk for altered skin integrity and infection is included. The child and family caregivers have the need for reinforcement of teaching related to complications of hypoglycemia and hyperglycemia, insulin administration, and appropriate exercise and activity. The family caregiver anxiety, impaired coping, and needs related to caring for a child with a chronic condition must be addressed along with the child's need for self-acceptance.

Outcome Identification and Planning

The major goals for the child include maintaining adequate nutrition, promoting skin integrity, preventing infection, monitoring and regulating glucose levels, and learning to adjust to having a chronic condition. Goals for the child and family include learning about and managing hypoglycemia and hyperglycemia, insulin administration, and exercise needs for the child. An additional goal is for family members to express their concerns about coping with the child's condition and for the child to show self-acceptance.

Nursing Care Focus

- Malnutrition risk related to insufficient caloric intake to meet growth and development needs and the inability of the body to use nutrients

Goal

- The child's caloric intake will be adequate to meet nutritional needs and to maintain appropriate growth.

Implementations for Ensuring Adequate and Appropriate Nutrition

The child with diabetes needs a sound nutritional program that provides adequate nutrition for normal growth while it maintains the blood glucose at near-normal levels. The food plan should be well balanced with foods that accommodate the child's food preferences, cultural customs, and lifestyle (see Tips for Reinforcing Family Teaching: Child's Diabetic Food Plan).

Help the child and family caregiver understand the importance of eating regularly scheduled meals. Special occasions can be planned so that the child does not feel left out of celebrations. If a particular meal is going to be late, the child should have a complex carbohydrate and protein snack. Children should be included in meal planning when possible to learn what is permissible and what is not. In this way, they can handle eating when they are on their own in school and in social situations.

Evaluation of Goal/Desired Outcome

The child:

- eats food at meals and snack times and maintains normal weight for age and height.
- demonstrates (along with family caregiver) understanding of meal planning by making appropriate menu choices.

TIPS FOR REINFORCING FAMILY TEACHING

Child's Diabetic Food Plan

- Plan well-balanced meals that are appealing to the child.
- Be positive with the child when talking about foods that they can eat; downplay the negatives.
- Space three meals and three snacks throughout the day. Daily caloric intake is divided to provide 20% at breakfast, 20% at lunch, 30% at dinner, and 10% at each of the snacks.
- Calories should be made up of 50% to 60% carbohydrates, 15% to 20% protein, and no more than 30% fat.
- Avoid concentrated sweets such as jelly, syrup, pie, candy bars, and soda pop.
- Artificial sweeteners may be used.
- The child must not skip meals. Make every effort to plan meals with foods that the child likes.
- Include foods that contain dietary fiber such as whole grains, cereals, fruits and vegetables, nuts, seeds, and legumes. Fiber helps prevent hyperglycemia.
- Dietetic food is expensive and unnecessary.
- Keep complex carbohydrates available to be eaten before exercise and sports activities to provide sustained carbohydrate energy sources.
- Teach the child day by day about the food plan to encourage independence in food selections when at school or away from home.

Nursing Care Focus

- Altered skin integrity related to slow healing process and decreased circulation

Goal

- The child's skin integrity will be maintained.

Implementations for Preventing Skin Breakdown

Skin breakdowns, such as blisters and minor cuts, can become major problems for the child with diabetes. Remind the family caregiver and child to inspect the skin daily and promptly treat even small breaks in the skin. Encourage daily bathing. Remind the child and family caregiver to dry the skin well after bathing, and give careful attention to any area where skin touches skin, such as the groin, axilla, or other skin folds. Emphasize good foot care. This includes wearing well-fitting shoes, inspecting between toes for cracks, trimming nails straight across, wearing clean socks, and not going barefoot. Establishing these habits early helps the child prepare for life-long care of diabetes.

Evaluation of Goal/Desired Outcome

The child:

- exhibits skin that is intact with no signs of breakdown.
- describes (along with family caregiver) methods for skin inspection and care.

Nursing Care Focus

- Infection risk related to elevated glucose levels

Goal

- The child will be free from signs and symptoms of infection.

Implementations for Preventing Infection

Children with diabetes may be more susceptible to urinary tract and upper respiratory infections. Reinforce teaching with the child and family caregiver to be alert for signs of urinary tract infection, such as itching and burning on urination. Instruct them to report signs of urinary tract or upper respiratory infections to the health care provider promptly.

Many children are subject to minor infections and illnesses during the school years, with little long-term effect. However, the child with diabetes is more susceptible to long-term complications. When this child has an infection and fever, the temperature and metabolic rate increase, and the body needs more sugar and therefore more insulin to make the sugar available to the body. Although the child may not be eating because of vomiting or anorexia, the body still needs insulin. Insulin should never be skipped during illness. Blood glucose levels should be checked every 2 to 4 hours during this time. Fluids need to be increased. Instruct the family caregivers to contact the health care provider when the child becomes ill, especially if the child is vomiting, cannot eat, or has diarrhea, so that close supervision can be maintained. Give the family caregiver guidelines for care of an ill child when reinforcing initial diabetic instructions.

It is extremely important for the child to wear a MedicAlert identification bracelet with information about diabetic status. Identification cards, such as those carried by many adults with diabetes, are seldom practical for a child.

Evaluation of Goal/Desired Outcome

The child:

- shows no signs of infection.
- has a temperature within normal range.
- discusses (along with family caregiver) the importance of promptly reporting infections.

Nursing Care Focus

- Altered health maintenance risk related to unstable glucose levels

Goal

- The child will maintain normal glucose levels.

Implementations for Monitoring and Regulating Glucose Levels

The child who is seen in the healthcare facility with diabetes may have a new diagnosis or may be experiencing an unstable episode as a result of illness or changing needs. The child's blood glucose level must be monitored to maintain it within normal limits. Determine the blood glucose level at least twice a day, before breakfast and before the evening meal, by means of bedside glucose monitoring.

On initial diagnosis of diabetes, the blood glucose level should be checked as often as every 4 hours until some stability is achieved. After the child is discharged, frequent blood glucose monitoring is done to avoid hypoglycemic episodes and to improve blood glucose control. Children and family caregivers often are not able to recognize symptoms of high or low blood glucose levels, so frequent and regular monitoring of blood glucose is essential. Reinforce teaching with the child and the family caregiver about how to perform blood glucose monitoring (Fig. 38-11).

Because this procedure involves a fingerstick, the child may object and resist it. Offer encouragement and support, helping the child to express fears and acknowledging that the fingerstick does hurt and that it is acceptable to dislike it. Consider the child's developmental stage when performing the testing. Table 38-5 provides some guidelines for diabetic care and teaching based on developmental stage. School-aged children can be involved in most of the process. Encourage the child to choose the finger to be used and clean it with soap and water. Automatic-release instruments make it easier for the child to do the fingerstick. Show the child how to read the results and explain the desired level. School-aged children, in the stage of industry versus inferiority, are usually interested in learning new information. Appeal to this developmental characteristic to gain the cooperation of a child this age.

Continuous glucose monitoring using a subcutaneous glucose sensor is sometimes used in children. There are several different types of continuous blood glucose monitoring devices. Some of these give current or real-time feedback, whereas others do not. Other types of continuous blood glucose monitors are used together with an insulin pump. While these devices have great potential for use in the child with diabetes, they are in the early stages of usage. These devices are expensive, have some reliability concerns, and require

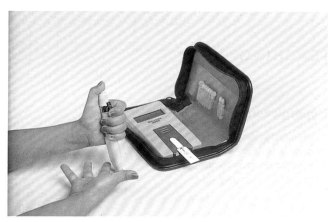

FIGURE 38-11 The child uses an automatic lancet to get a blood sample (*left*) and blood glucose monitor to determine blood glucose level (*right*).

the child or family caregiver to be motivated and have good skills to manage the diabetes.

Evaluation of Goal/Desired Outcome

The child:

- maintains blood glucose level of 80 to 130 mg/dL.
- has urine that is negative for ketones.
- does not show signs of hypoglycemia or hyperglycemia.

Nursing Care Focus

- Knowledge deficiency related to managing hypoglycemia and hyperglycemia

Goal

- The child and family caregiver will verbalize an understanding of the signs, symptoms, and management of hypoglycemia and hyperglycemia.

Implementations for Reinforcing Child and Family Teaching in the Management of Hypoglycemia and Hyperglycemia

The child is monitored closely for signs of hypoglycemia or hyperglycemia. If the blood glucose level is greater than 240 mg/dL, the urine may be tested for ketones. In addition, during an illness, the urine ketones are monitored. Be aware of the most likely times for an increase or decrease in the blood glucose level in relation to the insulin the child is receiving. Reinforce teaching with the child and family about the signs of both hypoglycemia and hyperglycemia (see Tips for Reinforcing Family Teaching: Signs of Hypoglycemia and Hyperglycemia) and how to be prepared to take the appropriate action if necessary. They must be alert to signs of hypoglycemia, especially when insulin is at peak action (Table 38-4).

Reinforce teaching with them about treating blood glucose levels less than 80 mg/dL with juice, sugar, or nondiet soda. If the blood glucose level cannot be checked promptly, the child should still consume a simple carbohydrate if there are any signs of hypoglycemia.

If the child cannot swallow, glucagon or dextrose should be administered, following the health care provider's orders. Glucagon is commercially available and can be administered intramuscularly or subcutaneously. Reinforce teaching with the family caregiver about how to mix and administer it.

Instruct the child to get help immediately when signs of hypoglycemia occur and to carry and take sugar cubes, Lifesavers, gumdrops, or a small tube of cake frosting. The reaction should be followed with a snack of a complex carbohydrate, such as crackers, and a protein such as cheese, peanut butter, or half of a meat sandwich. The snack is needed to maintain the increase in blood glucose level created by the simple carbohydrates and to prevent another hypoglycemic reaction.

Reassure the family caregiver and the child that hypoglycemia is much more likely to occur than hyperglycemia.

TABLE 38-5 Developmental Guidelines of Responsibilities for Children With Diabetes[a]

ISSUE	UNDER 4 YEARS	4–5 YEARS	6–7 YEARS	8–10 YEARS	11–13 YEARS	14+ YEARS
Food	Teaching focuses on parents.	Knows likes and dislikes.	Can begin to tell sugar content of food and know foods they should not have.	Has more ability to select foods according to criteria like exchange lists.	Knows if foods fit own diet plan.	Helps plan meals and snacks.
Insulin	Parents take responsibility for care.	Can tell where injection should be. Can pinch the skin.	Can begin to help with aspects of injections.	Gives own injections with supervision.	Can learn to measure insulin.	Can mix two insulins.
Testing		Can choose finger for fingerstick. Can wash finger with soap and water. Collects urine; should watch caregiver do testing; helps with recording.	Can do own fingerstick using automatic puncture device. Can help with some aspects of blood test. Can do own urine test and record results.	Can do blood tests with supervision.	Can see test results forming a pattern.	Can begin to use test results to adjust insulin.
Psychological		Identifies with being "bad" or "good"; these words should be avoided. A child this age may think they are bad if the test is said to be "bad."	Needs many reminders and supervision.	Needs reminders and supervision. Understands only immediate consequences, not long-term consequences, of diabetes control. "Scientific" mind developing; intrigued by tests.	May be somewhat rebellious. Concerned with being "different."	Understands long-term consequences of actions including diabetes control. Independence and self-image are important. Rebellion continues, and some supervision and continued support are still needed.

[a]These are only guidelines. Each child is an individual. Talk to your health care provider about any concerns you may have.

If there is any doubt as to whether the child is having a hypoglycemic or a hyperglycemic reaction, treat it like hypoglycemia. Instruct family caregivers to keep a record of the hypoglycemic reactions to determine if there is a pattern and if the insulin schedule or food plan needs to be adjusted.

Evaluation of Goal/Desired Outcome

The child and family caregiver:

- list the signs of hypoglycemia and hyperglycemia and discuss how to handle each.
- ask questions to clarify information.

 TIPS FOR REINFORCING FAMILY TEACHING

Signs of Hypoglycemia and Hyperglycemia

Hypoglycemia

- Shaking
- Irritability
- Nausea
- Diaphoresis
- Dizziness
- Drowsiness
- Pallor
- Changed level of consciousness
- Feeling "strange"

Hyperglycemia

- Polyphagia (excessive hunger)
- Polyuria (excessive urination)
- Dry mucous membranes
- Poor skin turgor, dry skin
- Lethargy
- Blurred vision
- Change in level of consciousness
- Ketones in urine
- Fruity smell to breath

Nursing Care Focus

- Knowledge deficiency related to insulin administration

Goal

- The child and family caregiver will verbalize an understanding of insulin administration.

Implementations for Reinforcing Child and Family Teaching on Insulin Administration

Clarify with the family caregiver and the child the correct way to give insulin. Disposable syringes and insulin pens make caring for equipment relatively easy. A doll may be used to practice the actual administration until the family caregiver (and child, if old enough) is comfortable and confident. Provide direct supervision until proficiency is demonstrated (Fig. 38-12).

Insulin administration is probably the most threatening aspect of the illness. Remember your feelings when you gave your first injection in nursing school. The child and family need a great deal of empathy and warm support. Increasing their confidence and skills of insulin administration will reduce their fear.

Reinforce instructions concerning the importance of rotating injection sites. A site that is used too frequently is likely to become indurated and eventually fibrosed, which hinders proper insulin absorption. The atrophic hollows in the skin, or the lumps of hypertrophied tissue, are unsightly as well. Some people appear to have greater skin sensitivity than others. Areas on the upper arms, upper thighs, abdomen, and buttocks can be used (Fig. 38-13).

Use of a careful plan allows several weeks to elapse before a site is used again. Usually, four to six injections are given in one area before going on to the next area. Starting from the inner upper corner of the area, each injection is given 0.5 in. below the preceding one, going down in a vertical line. The next series of injections in this area would start 0.5 in. outward at the upper level. If there is any sign of induration, the local site should be avoided for a few weeks

until all signs of irritation have disappeared. A chart recording the sites used and the rotation schedule is recommended.

Evaluation of Goal/Desired Outcome

The child and family caregiver:

- demonstrate insulin injection.
- describe various types of insulin and their reaction and peak times.
- develop a site rotation schedule.

Nursing Care Focus

- Knowledge deficiency related to appropriate exercise and activity

Goal

- The child and family caregiver will verbalize an understanding of exercise and activity for a child with diabetes.

Implementations for Reinforcing Child and Family Teaching About Exercise and Activity

Exercise decreases the blood glucose level because carbohydrates are being burned for energy. The therapeutic program should be adjusted to allow for this increase in energy requirements to avoid hypoglycemia. Adjustments may also be needed in the child's school schedule. For instance, physical education should never be scheduled right before lunch for a child with diabetes. Also, the child should not be scheduled for a late lunch period.

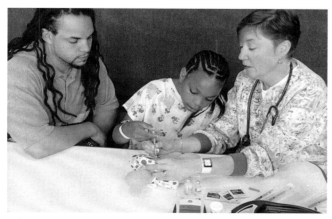

FIGURE 38-12 The school-aged child may first practice insulin injections on a doll.

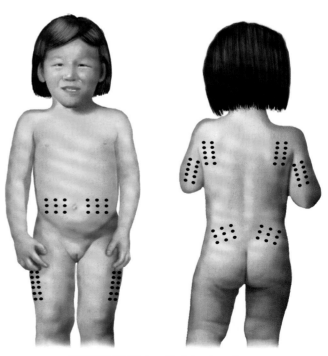

FIGURE 38-13 Insulin injection sites.

Evaluation of Goal/Desired Outcome

- The child and caregiver describe the effects of exercise on the blood glucose levels.

Nursing Care Focus

- Family anxiety and coping impairment related to the effect of the disease on child's and family's life

Goal

- The child and family caregiver will express their anxiety and concerns about coping with the child's illness.

Implementations for Decreasing Anxiety and Promoting Family Coping

When the diagnosis of diabetes is confirmed, the family caregiver may feel devastated. A young child will not understand the implications, but the school-aged or adolescent child will experience a great amount of fear and anxiety. The family caregiver may have feelings of guilt, resentment, or denial. Other family members may also experience strong feelings about the illness. All these feelings and concerns must be recognized and resolved to work successfully with the child with diabetes. Encourage the family to express these feelings and fears. To help them deal with feelings, involve the family caregiver in the child's care during hospitalization. Carefully listen to questions, and answer them completely and honestly. Many written materials are available to give to the caregiver, but be sure the caregiver can read and understand them. Videos are also available that are helpful in educating the child with diabetes and the family. Recommend available community support groups. Cover home care in detail. Provide the family caregiver with a support person to contact when questions arise after discharge.

Because so much information must be absorbed in a brief time, the caregivers may seem forgetful or confused. Careful, patient repetition of all aspects of diabetes and the child's care is necessary. When anxiety levels are high, information is often heard but not digested. Provide written material in an understandable form. Have caregivers repeat information, and question them to confirm that they understand. Demonstrate warmth and caring throughout the instruction process to increase the family's comfort; this also develops their confidence in nursing responses to their questions and apprehensions.

Evaluation of Goal/Desired Outcome

- As appropriate for age, the child discusses necessary adjustments to the daily schedule and activities and names several people to inform about the diabetic condition.
- The family caregiver demonstrates support of the child in managing daily and long-term care of diabetes.

Nursing Care Focus

- Low self-esteem risk

Goal

- The child will show adjustment and have a positive attitude about the condition.

Implementations for Promoting Self-Care and Positive Self-Esteem

The school-aged or older child may experience some strong feelings of inadequacy or being "sick." These feelings must be expressed and handled. To help allay fear, give the child as much information as is appropriate for their age. Tell the child about athletes and other famous people who have diabetes. When possible, another child who has diabetes may visit so that the child does not feel so alone. Encourage the child to become active in helping with self-care. Answer questions about how diabetes will affect the child's activities. Summer camps for children with diabetes are available in many areas and can help develop the child's self-assurance.

The child with diabetes can participate in normal activities. However, at least one friend should be told about the diabetic condition, and the child should not go swimming or hiking without a responsible person nearby who knows what to look for and what to do if the child has a reaction.

Some children are sensitive about their condition and fear they seem different from their friends. Even with the best instruction and preparation, they may feel this way and wish to keep their condition secret. They must understand that a teacher or some other adult in their environment must be acquainted with their condition. Classroom teachers need to know which of their students have such a condition and should understand the signs of an impending reaction.

Children with diabetes who have their glucose levels under good control do not need to be kept from activities such as camp-outs, overnight trips with the school band, or other similar activities away from home. Of course, these children must first be capable of measuring their insulin and giving their own injections. Some young people may find that a desire to participate in such an activity can be the factor that helps them overcome reluctance to measure and administer their own insulin.

Evaluation of Goal/Desired Outcome

The child:

- expresses feelings about having diabetes.
- participates in age-appropriate activities and realistic goal planning.

TEST YOURSELF

✔ What do the terms polyuria, polydipsia, and polyphagia mean?

✔ What causes diabetic ketoacidosis to occur?

✔ How is type 1 diabetes mellitus in the child treated?

✔ Describe the symptoms of hypoglycemia and hyperglycemia.

Type 2 Diabetes Mellitus

Type 2 diabetes mellitus, also referred to as noninsulin-dependent diabetes, is a condition in which the body does not use insulin properly. Previously, type 2 diabetes mellitus was primarily diagnosed only in adults, usually over 45 years of age and overweight. More recently, this type of diabetes has been diagnosed in children and adolescents. In particular, children who are overweight; have a family history of type 2 diabetes mellitus; or are of Native American, African, Hispanic, or Asian origin are at the greatest risk of developing type 2 diabetes mellitus.

Clinical Manifestations and Diagnosis

Many of the symptoms of type 2 diabetes are similar to those of type 1 diabetes—polydipsia, polyuria, and polyphagia (see Table 38-3 for a comparison between type 1 and type 2 diabetes). The child is usually overweight or obese. Symptoms are often present for months before a diagnosis is made. Many times, type 2 diabetes is diagnosed when a urine screening test is performed for some other reason and glucosuria is found. In addition, these children have high blood glucose levels. Although diabetic ketoacidosis is not common in adults diagnosed with type 2 diabetes, the condition may be seen in children with the diagnosis.

Treatment

One goal of treatment is to achieve normal or close to normal blood glucose levels. A second goal of treatment is to prevent or decrease the occurrence of long-term complications such as neurologic, kidney, and eye conditions. If the child presents with diabetic ketoacidosis, initial treatment is insulin administration, but then oral hypoglycemic agents, such as metformin, are often effective for controlling blood glucose levels. Lifestyle changes, such as weight loss and increased exercise, are important aspects of treatment for the child.

Nursing Care

Recognizing the child who is at high risk for type 2 diabetes mellitus is critical in changing the lifestyle behaviors that increase the child's risk. Work with both the child and the family caregivers to change patterns. Promote lifestyle changes such as healthy eating habits and dietary modifications, and increased physical activity and exercise to help manage the disease. Monitoring blood glucose levels, insulin administration, treatment of hypoglycemia and hyperglycemia, diabetic food plans, and reinforcing family teaching for type 2 diabetes are the same as with type 1 diabetes.

What are some of the topics about which **Jackson**'s parents will need reinforcement teaching? Considering Jackson's age and diagnosis, what are some of the things he will have to adjust to now and as he grows older?

KEY POINTS

- The GI tract of the newborn works in the same manner as that of the adult, but with some limitations. For example, the enzymes secreted by the liver and pancreas are reduced. The smaller capacity of the infant's stomach and the increased speed at which food moves through the GI tract require feeding smaller amounts at more frequent intervals. In addition, the small capacity of the colon leads to a bowel movement after each feeding.
- The endocrine system of the infant is adequately developed, although the functions are immature. As the child grows, the endocrine system matures in function.
- Nutritional deficiencies can cause children to grow at a slower rate, have a higher rate of illness and infection, and have more difficulty concentrating and achieving in school. Kwashiorkor is caused by a severe deficiency of protein. Marasmus is a deficiency of calories as well as protein. A lack of vitamin D causes rickets. Inadequate intake of vitamin C causes scurvy. An iron deficiency may result in anemia, and calcium deficiency can cause bone, teeth, and neurologic concerns. Foods most likely to cause allergic reactions are milk, eggs, wheat, corn, legumes (including peanuts and soybeans), oranges, strawberries, and chocolate.
- Celiac disease is a defect of metabolism precipitated by ingestion of wheat, barley, and rye, which leads to malabsorption, GI symptoms, and impaired fat absorption. It is often caused by an allergic reaction to the gliadin fraction of gluten (a protein factor in wheat). Treatment includes a restricted gluten-free diet.
- Gastroesophageal reflux (GER) occurs when the sphincter in the lower portion of the esophagus, which leads into the stomach, is relaxed and allows gastric contents to be regurgitated back into the esophagus. In gastroesophageal reflux disease (GERD), after feeding, the child vomits the contents of the stomach, which can cause failure to thrive or aspiration with respiratory concerns. A histamine-2 (H2) receptor antagonist or a proton pump inhibitor may be given to reduce the acid secretion. In severe cases, a surgical procedure known as Nissen fundoplication may be done.
- Colic consists of episodes of crying in the infant that can last for hours and recur frequently. The episodes are associated with recurrent gastrointestinal disturbances in which the infant appears to be in considerable discomfort. Attacks occur suddenly, usually late in the day or evening. The infant cries loudly and continuously and appears to be in pain but otherwise seems healthy. No single treatment is consistently successful.
- Mild diarrhea is loose stools, with the frequency of defecation 2 to 12 times per day. Severe diarrhea is usually accompanied by vomiting, and together they cause large losses of body water and electrolytes. The child is severely dehydrated and gravely ill. Infectious diarrhea is commonly referred to as gastroenteritis. Establishing normal fluid and electrolyte balance is the primary concern in treating gastroenteritis.
- The child with pyloric stenosis eats initially but then starts vomiting after meals. The vomiting increases in frequency and force, becoming projectile. The child is irritable, loses

weight rapidly, and becomes dehydrated. A surgical procedure called a pyloromyotomy is the treatment of choice.

- Congenital aganglionic megacolon is also called Hirschsprung disease. The common symptoms include failure of the newborn to have a stool in the first 24 hours, bile-stained emesis, and generalized abdominal distention. Gastroenteritis with diarrheal stools, ulceration of the colon, and severe constipation with ribbonlike or hard pellet stools are also seen. Treatment involves surgery with the resection of the aganglionic portion of the bowel.

- Intussusception is the invagination, or telescoping, of one portion of the bowel into a distal portion. It occurs most commonly at the juncture of the ileum and the colon. Immediate treatment consists of an air, saline, or contrast enema to attempt to correct the telescoping or abdominal surgery if the enema does not correct the problem.

- Symptoms of appendicitis in the older child may be pain and tenderness in the right lower quadrant of the abdomen, anorexia, nausea and vomiting, fever, and rebound tenderness. The young child has difficulty localizing the pain; may act restless and irritable; and may have a fever, vomiting, and anorexia. Usually the white blood cell count is slightly elevated. Surgical removal of the appendix is the treatment.

- Intestinal parasites common to the child include pinworm, roundworm, hookworm, and giardiasis. Pinworms invade the cecum and may enter the appendix. The infestation occurs when the pinworm eggs are swallowed. Roundworms are spread from the feces of infested people. They are usually found in areas where sanitary facilities are lacking and human excreta are deposited on the ground. The hookworm lives in the human intestinal tract and is prevalent in areas where infected human excreta are deposited on the ground; the hookworms penetrate the skin of barefoot people. Giardiasis is caused by the protozoan parasite *Giardia lamblia*. It is a common cause of diarrhea.

- Toddler and preschool-aged children often find out about their environments by tasting the world around them. Because their senses of taste and smell are not yet refined, young children ingest substances that would repel an adult because of their taste or smell and are often poisoned by the substance. Common substances children ingest include drugs such as acetaminophen, acetylsalicylic acid (aspirin), ibuprofen, ferrous sulfate, and barbiturates. They also ingest corrosives such as lye, bleach, and other cleaners and hydrocarbons such as gasoline and kerosene. Batteries, especially button batteries, can cause a choking as well as a poison hazard in children.

- Chronic lead poisoning may be caused when children ingest lead from lead-containing paint, furniture, toys, and vinyl mini blinds. Drinking water contaminated by lead pipes; storage of food in improperly glazed earthenware;

inhalation of engine fumes; and exposure to industrial areas and materials such as stained glass, solder, fishing sinkers, and bullets can also cause lead poisoning.

- Children with lead poisoning may have irritability, hyperactivity, aggression, impulsiveness, or disinterest in play. Short attention span, lethargy, learning difficulties, and distractibility are also signs of poisoning. Acute manifestations include convulsions, intellectual disability, blindness, paralysis, coma, and death. Blood lead levels are used to diagnose lead poisoning; the best treatment for lead poisoning is to remove the lead from the child's system by using chelating agents. Early detection of the condition and removal of the child from the lead-containing surroundings offer the best prognosis.

- If a child who has swallowed a foreign object is having respiratory distress, the Heimlich maneuver should be used and cardiopulmonary resuscitation started if necessary. If the child is not having respiratory problems and coughing has not resulted in removal of the object, the child should be taken to an emergency department to be assessed.

- In children, type 1 diabetes mellitus causes an abrupt pronounced decrease in insulin production, resulting in decreased ability to derive energy from the food eaten. Large amounts of protein and fat are used to supply the child's energy needs, causing weight loss and slowed growth. Management of type 1 diabetes in children includes insulin therapy and a meal and exercise plan. Reinforcement teaching for the child and family includes diet, skin concerns, preventing infection, regulating glucose levels, insulin administration, exercise, and learning to adjust to having a chronic condition.

- Type 2 diabetes mellitus is a condition in which the body does not use insulin properly. This type of diabetes has been diagnosed in children and adolescents, in particular, children who are overweight, have a family history of type 2 diabetes, or are from a race or country of origin with high incidence of type 2 diabetes. Healthy eating habits, dietary modifications, physical activity, and exercise help with management of the disease.

INTERNET RESOURCES

Food Allergies
www.foodallergy.org

Allergies
www.allergicchild.com

Celiac Disease
www.celiac.com

Diabetes
www.diabetes.org
www.childrenwithdiabetes.com

Poisoning
www.aapcc.org
www.poison.org/battery/guideline

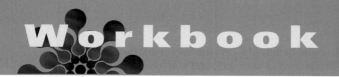

NCLEX-STYLE REVIEW QUESTIONS

1. If an infant has a diagnosis of pyloric stenosis, the child will likely have a history of which symptom?
   a. Iron deficiency
   b. Projectile vomiting
   c. Muscle spasms
   d. Nasal congestion

2. A nurse admits a child with a diagnosis of possible appendicitis. What signs and symptoms would *most* likely be seen in the child with appendicitis?
   a. Sore throat, bone and joint pain
   b. Itching, swelling around eyes and ankles
   c. Convulsions, weight gain or loss
   d. Fever, nausea, and vomiting

3. The nurse is reinforcing teaching with a group of parents of toddlers about what to do in cases of poisoning. If a toddler has swallowed an unknown substance, what should be the *first* action of the caregiver?
   a. Administer a recommended antidote.
   b. Call the Poison Control Center.
   c. Encourage the child to drink water.
   d. Place the child on a flat surface.

4. The nurse is working with a 12-year-old child with type 1 diabetes mellitus. The child asks the nurse why she cannot take pills instead of shots like her grandmother does. What would be the *best* response by the nurse?
   a. "The pills correct a different type of diabetes than you have."
   b. "When your blood glucose levels are better controlled, you can take the pills too."
   c. "Your body does not make its own insulin, so the insulin injections help replace it."
   d. "The pills only work for adults who have diabetes. Maybe when you are older, you can take the pills."

5. A child with a diagnosis of failure to thrive because of malnutrition has had an inadequate intake of calories. In planning care, all of the following goals would be appropriate for this child. What goal would be the *highest* priority for the child?
   a. The child will maintain good mouth and skin integrity.
   b. The child will increase amount of daily exercise.
   c. The child will increase daily fluid intake.
   d. The child will increase intake for appropriate weight gain.

STUDY ACTIVITIES

1. Develop a teaching aid or poster to use in instructing children with diabetes how to administer their own insulin injections. Include how you will help the children make an insulin site rotation chart. Present your project to your peers.

2. Survey your house (or a house you select), and list the hazards for ingestion of poisonous substances and objects that a child might find and ingest. After the hazards are identified, formulate a plan to correct or lessen the hazards.

3. Carmella has celiac disease. Using the table below, identify the foods that would be recommended and those that would not be recommended in her meal plan. With the help of a nutrition text or by reading labels, state why each of those foods is either recommended or not recommended.

Food	Recommended	Not Recommended	Explanation of Why Food Would or Would Not Be Recommended
Ice cream			
Corn flakes			
Grits			
Rice pudding			
Whole-wheat bread			
Baked beans			
Hamburger			
Hot dog			
French fries			
Fresh vegetables			
Yogurt			
Oatmeal			
Rice Krispies			
Orange juice			
Graham crackers			
Corn chips			
Peanut butter			
Baked potato			
Tuna salad			
Pizza			

4. Do a web search on "managing diabetes at school."
   a. What are some of the sites that you found?
   b. What would be important for the child with diabetes to be allowed to do at school in order to follow their diabetic plan?
   c. What are some ideas suggested to prevent discrimination of a child with diabetes?

CRITICAL THINKING: WHAT WOULD YOU DO?

1. Five-year-old Malcolm has been sent home from kindergarten with a note advising his caregiver of an outbreak of pinworms. There are five children between 2 and 8 years of age in the household where he lives, including cousins. Malcolm's aunt is the person who cares for the children.
   a. What would you explain to Malcolm's aunt when she asks you what pinworms are and how children get them?
   b. What symptoms will you clarify with her to observe for in the children?
   c. How will the diagnosis of pinworms be made?
   d. What is the treatment for pinworms?

2. Your next-door neighbor has found their 18-month-old child with an empty bottle of children's acetaminophen. She brings the child to your house.
   a. What immediate actions should you take?
   b. What is the specific antidote used in acetaminophen overdose? (Use a drug reference.)
   c. What organ can be damaged with an overdose of acetaminophen?

3. Nine-month-old Tina has severe diarrhea. She has been admitted to your unit, and you have been assigned to be her nurse.
   a. What symptoms would you expect Tina to exhibit?
   b. What physical characteristics will you observe her for?
   c. What documentation is especially important in her care?

4. Dosage calculation: After an appendectomy, an 8-year-old child is being medicated with meperidine (Demerol) for postoperative pain. The dosage range for this child is 1 to 1.8 mg/kg. The child weighs 55 lb. The Demerol comes in a prefilled syringe with 50 mg/mL. Answer the following.
   a. How many kilograms (kg) does the child weigh?
   b. What is the low dose for this child?
   c. What is the high dose for this child?
   d. How many milliliters (mL) will be given for the low dose of the medication?
   e. How many milliliters (mL) will be given for the high dose of the medication?

39

The Child With a Genitourinary Disorder

Key Terms

amenorrhea
anasarca
ascites
diurnal enuresis
dysmenorrhea
enuresis
hyperlipidemia
intercurrent infections
leukopenia
menarche
mittelschmerz
nocturnal enuresis
oliguria
orchiopexy
premenstrual syndrome (PMS)
pyelonephritis
striae
vaginitis

Learning Objectives

At the conclusion of this chapter, you will:

1. Discuss ways the child's genitourinary system differs from the adult's system.
2. Identify the symptoms, treatment, and nursing care of the child with a urinary tract infection.
3. Explain enuresis, including the possible physiologic and psychological causes.
4. Discuss the diagnosis of acute poststreptococcal glomerulonephritis, including the cause, symptoms, treatment, and nursing care.
5. Discuss the diagnosis of nephrotic syndrome, including the symptoms, treatment, and nursing care.
6. Compare acute poststreptococcal glomerulonephritis with nephrotic syndrome.
7. Explain the diagnosis of Wilms tumor.
8. Describe the structural defects that occur with hydrocele and cryptorchidism.
9. Compare premenstrual syndrome, dysmenorrhea, and amenorrhea.

The mother of 7-year-old **Christian Davis** calls the clinic concerned that her son's urine looks "smoke-colored" and bloody. Christian comes to the clinic, and in addition to the bloody urine, you note that he has periorbital edema and an elevated temperature. As you collect data from his mother, you learn that he was in the clinic 3 weeks ago with strep throat and an ear infection. As you read this chapter, consider what questions you will ask Christian about other symptoms he may be experiencing. Think about what these symptoms might indicate is going on with Christian.

Adequate functioning of the genitourinary (urinary and reproductive) system is affected by structural problems or defects, infections, disorders, and conditions. Although the symptoms seen in these conditions may be vague or seemingly not serious, they can be chronic, long term, or serious in their effects on the genitourinary system.

GROWTH AND DEVELOPMENT OF THE GENITOURINARY SYSTEM

The genitourinary system is made up of the kidneys, ureters, urinary bladder, and the urethra (Fig. 39-1). There are two kidneys and two ureters located on each side of the body, just above the waistline. Functions of the kidney include excreting excess water and waste products and

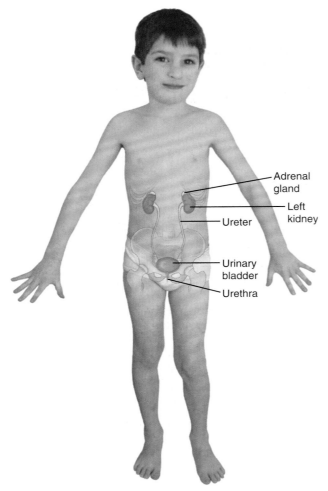

FIGURE 39-1 The urinary tract.

TABLE 39-1 Child's Average Urine Output in 24 Hours

AGE	AMOUNT OF URINE (mL)
6 months–2 years	540–600
2–5 years	500–780
5–8 years	600–1,200
8–14 years	1,000–1,500
>14 years	1,500

The kidneys in children are located lower in relationship to the ribs than in adults. This placement and the fact that the child has less of a fat cushion around the kidneys cause the child to be at greater risk for trauma to the kidneys. As the child grows, the kidneys also grow, especially during the first 2 years of life. The kidneys reach their full size and function by the time the child is an adolescent.

The reproductive portion of the genitourinary system in males and females matures at the time of puberty. The systems are made up of organs with the primary function of producing cells necessary for reproduction. The organs also provide the mechanism for conception to occur. Males and females have different structures in the reproductive systems. In the male, the reproductive structures include the testes, located in the scrotum, which produce sperm; the ducts that aid in the passage of sperm; the glands that secrete necessary fluids; and the external genitalia, including the penis. In the female, the reproductive organs include the ovaries, fallopian tubes, uterus, vagina, and the external genitalia. The genitals gradually increase in size during childhood. The hormonal changes in both males and females during puberty cause the reproductive system to more fully develop during adolescence.

URINARY TRACT INFECTIONS

UTIs are fairly common in the "diaper age," in infancy, and again between the ages of 2 and 6. The condition is more common in girls than in boys, except in the first 4 months of life, when it is more common in boys, especially if they are not circumcised. The sexually active female adolescent is at risk for development of UTIs. Although many different bacteria may infect the urinary tract, intestinal bacteria, particularly *Escherichia coli*, account for about 80% of acute episodes. The female urethra is shorter and straighter than the male urethra, so it is more easily contaminated with feces. Inflammation may extend into the bladder, ureters, and kidneys.

Clinical Manifestations

In children, the symptoms may be fever, irritability, vomiting, foul-smelling urine, poor feeding, weight loss, abdominal pain, urgency, and increased urination. Occasionally there is little or no fever. In children who are toilet-trained, incontinence or bed-wetting may be a symptom. In acute **pyelonephritis** (inflammation of the kidney and renal pelvis), the onset is abrupt, with a high fever for 1 or 2 days.

maintaining a balance of electrolytes and acid–base. Other functions of the kidney are regulating blood pressure by making the enzyme renin and making erythropoietin, which helps stimulate the production of red blood cells. Waste products are removed from the blood and excreted from the body through the urinary system.

The urine formed in the kidneys travels down the ureters and collects in the urinary bladder. When the bladder fills, there is an urge to empty the bladder. Urine passes through the urethra to be excreted from the body. In infants and children, emptying the bladder is a reflex action. Between ages 2 and 3, the child is able to hold the urine in the bladder and learns to urinate voluntarily, thus developing the control of urination.

In the newborn, the bladder empties when only about 15 mL of urine is present, so the newborn voids as many as 20 times a day. As the child gets older, the bladder has more capacity to hold larger amounts of urine before the child feels the urge to void. The child at different ages voids average amounts, depending on fluid intake and kidney health (Table 39-1). The urethra in females is much shorter than in males at all ages, making the female more susceptible to urinary tract infections (UTIs).

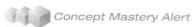

Concept Mastery Alert

Urination often increases as a result of a urinary tract infection and does not decrease. Passing small amounts of urine is frequent, and vomiting is common.

Diagnosis

Diagnosis is based on the finding of pus (white blood cells) and bacteria in the urine under microscopic examination. The urine specimen must be fresh and uncontaminated. A "clean catch" voided urine, properly performed, is essential for microscopic examination (see Chapter 30). If a culture is needed, the child may be catheterized, but this is usually avoided if possible. A suprapubic aspiration may also be done to obtain a sterile specimen. In the cooperative, toilet-trained child, clean midstream urine may be used successfully.

Treatment

Simple UTIs may be treated with anti-infectives (usually trimethoprim-sulfamethoxazole, amoxicillin, nitrofurantoin or cephalosporins) at home. A 7- to 14-day course is prescribed. The child with acute pyelonephritis is hospitalized and intravenous antibiotics are given. Fluids are given freely. The symptoms usually subside within a few days after antibiotic therapy has been initiated, but this is not an indication that the infection is completely cleared. Medication must be continued for the entire course of treatment, even after symptoms disappear. A renal and bladder ultrasound may be performed to assess the possibility of structural defects if the child has recurring infections.

Nursing Process and Care Plan *for the Child With a Urinary Tract Infection*

Assessment (Data Collection)

During the interview with the family caregiver, collect basic information about the child, such as feeding and sleeping patterns and history of other illnesses. Gather information about the current illness: when the fever started and its course thus far; signs of pain or discomfort on voiding; recent change in feeding pattern; presence of vomiting; irritability; lethargy; abdominal pain; unusual odor to urine; chronic diaper rash; and signs of febrile seizures. If the child is toilet-trained, ask the family caregivers about toileting habits (How does the child wipe? Does the child wash the hands when toileting?). Also, ask about the use of bubble baths and the type of soap used, especially for girls. Interview the adolescent alone to gather accurate information regarding their sexual history.

Data to collect regarding the child include temperature; pulse (be alert for tachycardia) and respiration rates; weight and height; observation of a wet diaper or the urine in an older child; inspection of the perineal area for rash; presence of irritability and lethargy; and general skin condition, color, and turgor. A urine specimen is needed on admission. A midstream urine collection method is desirable, and catheterization is avoided if possible. Record and report any indications of urinary burning, frequency, urgency, or pain.

Pay Attention!

Bruising, bleeding, or lacerations on the external genitalia, especially in the child who is withdrawn or appears frightened, may be a sign of child abuse and should be further explored.

In the child who has repeated UTIs, observe the interaction between the child and the family caregivers to detect any indications that the infection may be caused by sexual abuse. Look for possible physical indications of sexual abuse as well.

Nursing Care Focus

The nursing care focuses applicable for the child with a urinary tract infection include managing hyperthermia and urinary retention. Recognize the need for reinforcing family teaching related to the understanding of urinary tract infections.

Outcome Identification and Planning

Major goals for the child with a UTI include reducing temperature, maintaining normal urinary elimination, relieving pain, and increasing fluid intake. An important family goal is improving knowledge about infection control and ways to help prevent recurrent infections. Base the nursing plan of care on these goals with adjustments appropriate for the child's age.

Nursing Care Focus

- Hyperthermia related to infection

Goal

- The child will maintain a temperature within normal limits.

Implementations for Monitoring and Maintaining Body Temperature

Monitor the child's temperature frequently, at least every 2 hours if it is higher than 101.3°F (38.5°C). If the child has a fever, follow the procedures to reduce elevated temperatures (see Tips for Reinforcing Family Teaching: Reducing Fever, Chapter 30). Administer anti-infectives as ordered, and observe the child for signs of any reactions to the anti-infective agents. Antipyretic medications may be ordered. Increasing oral fluids will also help reduce body temperature.

Evaluation of Goal/Desired Outcome

● The child's temperature is 98.6°F to 100°F (37°C to 37.8°C).

Nursing Care Focus

● Urinary retention related to pain and burning on urination and decreased fluid intake

Goal

● The child's normal urinary elimination will be maintained.

Implementations for Decreasing Pain and Promoting Normal Elimination

Because of pain and burning on urination, the toilet-trained child may try to hold urine and not void. Encourage the child to void every 3 or 4 hours to prevent recurrent infection. Observe the child for signs of burning and pain when urinating. In addition, observe the voiding pattern to note urgency, frequency of urination, trickling, or other signs that the bladder is not being emptied completely. Carefully monitor and measure urine output. An infant's diaper should be weighed for accuracy (see Intake and Output Measurements, Chapter 30). Accurate intake and output measurements are important.

Increasing the child's fluid intake is necessary to help dilute the urine and flush the bladder. An increase in fluid intake also helps decrease the pain experienced on urination. Although getting the child to accept fluids is often difficult, frequent small amounts of glucose water or liquid gelatin may be accepted. Enlisting the aid of the family caregivers may be helpful. Most infants and children like apple juice, which helps acidify the urine. Cranberry juice is a good choice for the older child if they tolerate it. Administer analgesics and antispasmodics as ordered.

Evaluation of Goal/Desired Outcome

The child:

● voids every 3 to 4 hours, emptying the bladder each time without apprehension.
● produces 0.5 to 1 mL/kg of urine per hour.

Nursing Care Focus

● Knowledge deficiency of the family caregivers related to understanding of UTIs

Goal

● The family caregivers will verbalize an understanding of the genitourinary system and good hygiene habits.

Implementations for Reinforcing Family Teaching

The family caregivers are the key people in helping prevent recurring infections. See Tips for Reinforcing Family Teaching: Preventing Urinary Tract Infection. Prepare the family caregivers and the child for any procedures that may be ordered and give appropriate explanations.

TIPS FOR REINFORCING FAMILY TEACHING

Preventing Urinary Tract Infection

- Change infant's diaper when soiled, and clean baby with mild soap and water. Dry completely.
- Teach girls to wipe from front to back.
- Teach child to wash hands before and after going to the toilet.
- Avoid using bubble baths, which create a climate that encourages bacteria to grow, especially in young girls.
- Encourage young girls to take showers. Avoid using water softeners in tub baths.
- Encourage child to try to urinate every 3 or 4 hours and to empty the bladder.
- Watch for signs the child may need to urinate (crossing legs, holding genital area, doing the "potty dance").
- Have child wear cotton underwear to provide air circulation to perineal area.
- Have child avoid wearing tight jeans or pants.
- Encourage child to drink fluids, especially cranberry juice.
- Have older girls avoid whirlpools or hot tubs.

Evaluation of Goal/Desired Outcome

The family caregivers:

● list signs and symptoms of a UTI and methods to prevent recurrence.
● state when to contact a health care provider.

TEST YOURSELF

✔ What bacterium is the most common cause of urinary tract infections (UTI's)?
✔ How are UTI's detected and treated?
✔ Explain the reason a child with a UTI may try to hold their urine.

ENURESIS

Enuresis is continued incontinence of urine beyond the age when control of urination is commonly acquired. Daytime loss of urinary control is **diurnal enuresis** and nighttime bed-wetting is **nocturnal enuresis**. Many children do not acquire complete nighttime control before 5 to 7 years of age, and occasional bed-wetting may be seen in children as late as 9 or 10 years of age. Boys have more difficulty than do girls, and in some instances, enuresis may persist into the adult years.

Enuresis may have a physiologic or psychological cause and may indicate a need for additional exploration and treatment. Sometimes enuresis may occur because of a physical disorder or condition, such as diabetes or sickle cell anemia. Physiologic causes may include a small bladder capacity, UTI, constipation, or lack of awareness of the signal to empty the bladder because of sleeping too soundly. Persistent bed-wetting in a 5- or 6-year-old child may be a result of rigorous toilet training before the child was physically or psychologically ready. Enuresis in the older child may express resentment toward the family caregivers or a desire to regress to an earlier level of development to receive more care and attention. Emotional stress can be a precipitating factor. The healthcare team also needs to consider the possibility that enuresis can be a symptom of sexual abuse.

If a physiologic cause has been ruled out, efforts should be made to discover possible psychological causes, including emotional stress. If the child is interested in achieving control, waking the child during the night to go to the toilet, limiting fluids before retiring, and use of an enuresis alarm may be helpful. However, these measures should not be used as a replacement for searching for the cause. Help from a pediatric mental health professional may be needed.

Here's a Tip for You to Share!
An upcoming event the child is excited about attending, such as going to camp or visiting friends overnight, might be a motivator in helping the child with enuresis to achieve bladder control.

The family caregiver may become extremely frustrated about having to deal with smelly wet clothing and bedding. The child may go to great efforts to hide the fact that their clothing or bed is wet. Healthcare personnel must take a supportive understanding attitude toward the concerns of the family caregiver and the child, allowing each of them to ventilate feelings and providing a place where emotions can be freely expressed.

A Personal Glimpse

My 9-year-old daughter was potty trained when she was just barely 2 years old. I was so proud of her and happy that she was out of diapers and so quickly been trained. When she was almost 4, I had her little brother. She occasionally had an accident and wet pants, but I wasn't concerned. I just thought she wanted some attention. It was quite upsetting to me when shortly after she started the second grade she started wetting the bed. At first she was wet a few times a week, then every night. One day I got a call from the school saying I needed to bring her some dry clothes because she had wet her pants at school. That is when the worst part began. Now at 9 years, she wets her pants every day. She takes dry clothes to school, but sometimes she just stays in her wet ones. She smells like urine all the time. It is so upsetting to me. I feel frustrated and sometimes angry. Most of all I just feel so bad for my daughter. Her friends make fun of her; she never wants to spend the night anywhere except at home, and now she doesn't even seem to care. About 3 weeks ago I started taking her to a counselor the school nurse recommended. I hope she can help my daughter and me understand and change what is going on for her. It is painful to watch this happen.

Angela

Learning Opportunity: *What are some of the possible causes of this child's enuresis? What could you suggest to this mother to help her deal with her feelings regarding her child's situation?*

ACUTE POSTSTREPTOCOCCAL GLOMERULONEPHRITIS

Acute poststreptococcal glomerulonephritis is a condition that appears to be an inflammatory reaction to a specific bacterium, most often group A beta-hemolytic streptococcal infection, such as an upper respiratory or skin infection. The antigen–antibody reaction causes a response that injures and blocks the glomeruli, permitting red blood cells and protein to escape into the urine. Acute poststreptococcal glomerulonephritis has a peak incidence in children 5 to 12 years of age and occurs twice as often in boys. The disease is similar in some ways to nephrotic syndrome, which is discussed later in this chapter and in Table 39-2. The prognosis is usually excellent, but a few children develop chronic nephritis.

Clinical Manifestations
Presenting symptoms appear 1 to 3 weeks after the onset of a streptococcal infection such as strep throat, otitis media, tonsillitis, or impetigo. Usually the presenting symptom is grossly bloody urine. The family caregiver may describe the urine as smoky, tea or cola colored, or bloody. Edema may accompany or precede hematuria. Hypertension appears in 50% to 90% of clients during the first 4 or 5 days. Fever may be 103°F to 104°F (39.4°C to 40°C) at the onset of the condition but decreases in a few days to about 100°F (37.8°C). Slight headache and lethargy are usual, and vomiting may occur. Both hematuria and hypertension disappear within 3 weeks.

Oliguria (production of a subnormal volume of urine) may occur. Hematuria and proteinuria are noted in the urinalysis. The blood urea nitrogen, serum creatinine level, and the erythrocyte sedimentation rate may be normal or elevated. Cerebral symptoms such as headache, drowsiness, seizures, and vomiting occur in connection with hypertension in some cases. When the blood pressure is reduced, these symptoms disappear. Cardiopulmonary congestion may increase work of breathing or cause a cough.

Remember **Christian Davis**? With what do you think Christian might have been diagnosed? Is there anything in Christian's history that helped you think about what his diagnosis might be? What other symptoms would you anticipate might be noted in this child?

Treatment
Although the child usually feels better in a few days, activities should be limited until the clinical manifestations subside, generally 2 to 4 weeks after the onset. Antibiotics may be given during the acute stage to eradicate any existing infection; however, it does not affect the recovery from the disease because the condition is an immunologic response. Antihypertensives or diuretics may be given to control blood

TABLE 39-2 Comparison of Features of Acute Poststreptococcal Glomerulonephritis and Nephrotic Syndrome

ASSESSMENT FACTOR	ACUTE POSTSTREPTOCOCCAL GLOMERULONEPHRITIS	NEPHROTIC SYNDROME
Cause	Immune reaction to group A beta-hemolytic streptococcal infection	Idiopathic; possibly a hypersensitivity reaction
Onset	Abrupt	Insidious
Hematuria	Grossly bloody	Rare
Proteinuria	Mild to moderate	Extreme
Edema	Mild	Extreme
Hypertension	Marked	Mild
Hyperlipidemia	Rare or mild	Marked
Peak age frequency	5–12 years	2–3 years
Interventions	Limited activity; antihypertensives as needed; symptomatic therapy	Bed rest during edema stage Corticosteroid administration Immunosuppressant therapy if needed
Diet	Normal for age; no added salt if child is hypertensive	High protein, low sodium
Prevention	Prevention through treatment of group A beta-hemolytic streptococcal infections	None known

pressure. The diet is generally not restricted, but additional salt may be limited if edema is excessive. Treatment of complications is symptomatic.

Nursing Care

Bed rest is maintained until acute symptoms and gross hematuria disappear. The child should avoid contact with people with infections. When the child is allowed out of bed, they must not become fatigued.

Fluid intake and urinary output are carefully monitored and recorded. Special attention is needed to keep the intake within prescribed limits. The amount of fluid the child is allowed may be based on output, as well as on evidence of continued hypertension and oliguria. Blood pressure should be monitored regularly using the same arm and a properly fitting cuff.

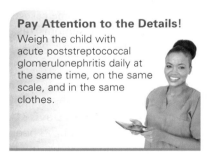

Pay Attention to the Details!
Weigh the child with acute poststreptococcal glomerulonephritis daily at the same time, on the same scale, and in the same clothes.

The urine must be tested regularly for protein and hematuria using dipstick tests. Traces of protein in the urine may persist for months after the acute symptoms disappear. Red blood cells in the urine may persist as well. Family caregivers must learn to test for urinary protein routinely. If the urinary signs persist for more than 1 year, the disease has probably assumed a chronic form.

NEPHROTIC SYNDROME

Several different types of nephrosis have been identified in nephrotic syndrome. The most common type in children is called idiopathic nephrotic syndrome, most commonly referred to as minimal change nephrotic syndrome (MCNS). All forms of nephrosis have early characteristics of edema and proteinuria; therefore, definite clinical differentiation cannot be made early in the disease. Minimal change nephrotic syndrome (MCNS) will be the focus of this discussion.

MCNS has an insidious onset in comparison to acute poststreptococcal glomerulonephritis, which has an abrupt onset (see Table 39-2 for a comparison of the two disorders). MCNS has a course of remissions and exacerbations that usually lasts for months. The recovery rate is generally good with the use of intensive corticosteroid therapy and protection against infection. The cause of MCNS is unknown. In rare cases, it is associated with other specific diseases. MCNS is most commonly seen in children younger than 6 years.

Clinical Manifestations

Edema is usually the presenting symptom, appearing first around the eyes and face, often when the child awakens (Fig. 39-2), resolving during the day as the fluid shifts and the edema is noted in the abdomen, lower extremities, and ankles. As the swelling advances, the edema becomes generalized and **anasarca** (massive edema) may result. Respiratory difficulty may be severe, and edema of the scrotum on the male is characteristic. The edema shifts when the child changes position when lying quietly or walking about. Loss of appetite, fatigue, and irritability develop. Malnutrition may become severe. However, the generalized edema masks the loss of body tissue, causing the child to present a chubby appearance. After diuresis,

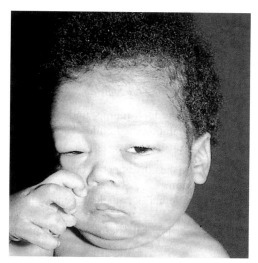

FIGURE 39-2 A child with nephrotic syndrome. Note the edema around the eyes.

the malnutrition becomes quite apparent. These children are usually susceptible to infection, and repeated acute respiratory conditions are the usual pattern. The administration of corticosteroids causes immunosuppression that intensifies the susceptibility to infection.

Diagnosis

Laboratory findings include marked proteinuria, especially albumin. Hematuria is not usually present, although a few red blood cells may appear in the urine. The blood serum protein and albumin level is reduced, and there is an increase in the level of lipoproteins in the blood (**hyperlipidemia**).

Treatment

The management of nephrotic syndrome is a long process with remissions and recurrence of symptoms common. In most cases, the use of corticosteroids has induced remissions and has reduced recurrences. Corticosteroid therapy usually produces diuresis in about 7 to 14 days, but use of the drug is continued until a remission occurs. Prednisone is the drug most commonly used. Daily urine testing for protein is continued whether the child is at home or in the hospital. It is important that accurate documentation be kept to track patterns of protein loss in the child.

Loop diuretics (e.g., furosemide) may be administered to promote diuresis, especially if the edema is severe or causes respiratory compromise. Intravenous albumin may be used if the serum albumin level is extremely low.

Immunosuppressant therapy may be used to reduce symptoms and prevent further relapses in children who do not respond adequately to corticosteroids. Cyclophosphamide and cyclosporine are commonly used. **Leukopenia** (leukocyte count is less than 5,000/mm³) can be expected, as well as the other common side effects of immunosuppressant therapy.

A general diet is recommended that appeals to the child's poor appetite with frequent, small feedings if necessary. The addition of salt is discouraged, and sometimes the child is put on a low-sodium diet. In addition, the child may be placed on a high-protein diet. Family caregivers need encouragement and support for the long months ahead. Relapses usually become less frequent as the child gets older.

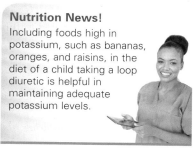

Nutrition News!

Including foods high in potassium, such as bananas, oranges, and raisins, in the diet of a child taking a loop diuretic is helpful in maintaining adequate potassium levels.

As the name implies, minimal change nephrotic syndrome (MCNS) causes few changes in the kidneys; these children have a good prognosis. Complications from kidney damage alter the course of treatment. Failure to achieve satisfactory diuresis or the need to discontinue corticosteroids because of adverse reactions requires a reevaluation of treatment. The presence of gross hematuria suggests renal damage. A child who has frequent relapses lasting into adolescence or adulthood may develop renal failure.

Nursing Process and Care Plan *for the Child With Nephrotic Syndrome*

Assessment (Data Collection)

Observe for edema when performing the physical examination of the child with nephrotic syndrome. Weigh the child, and record the abdominal measurements to serve as a baseline. Obtain vital signs including blood pressure. Note any swelling around the eyes, abdomen, ankles, and other dependent parts, and record the degree of pitting. Inspect the skin for pallor, irritation, or breakdown. Examine the scrotal area of the male child for swelling, redness, and irritation. Ask the family caregiver about the onset of symptoms, the child's appetite, urine output, and signs of fatigue or irritability.

Nursing Care Focus

When developing evidence-based nursing care focuses for the child with nephrotic syndrome, include the risk for fluid overload, malnutrition, and altered skin integrity. Fatigue and infection must also be addressed as nursing care focuses. The family caregivers may have a knowledge deficiency and coping impairment related to understanding the disease process, treatment, and home care for the child with a chronic condition.

Outcome Identification and Planning

The major goals for the child with nephrotic syndrome are relieving edema, improving nutritional status, maintaining skin integrity, conserving energy, and preventing infection.

The family caregiver goals include learning about the disease and treatments, as well as learning ways to cope with the child's long-term care.

Nursing Care Focus

- Fluid overload risk related to fluid accumulation in tissues and third spaces

Goal

- The child's edema will be decreased.

Implementations for Monitoring Fluid Intake and Output

Accurately monitor and document intake and output. Weigh the child at the same time every day on the same scale in the same clothing. Measure the child's abdominal girth daily at the level of the umbilicus (Fig. 39-3) and make certain that all healthcare personnel measure at the same level. The abdomen may be greatly enlarged with **ascites** (edema in the peritoneal cavity). The abdomen can even become marked with **striae** (stretch marks).

> **This Advice Will Be Useful!**
>
> Note the desired location for measuring the abdomen of the child with nephrotic syndrome on the nursing care plan so that everyone follows the same practice.

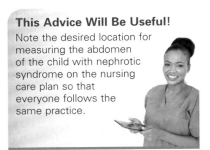

Test the urine regularly for protein (albumin). Albumin can be tested with reagent strips dipped into the urine and read by comparison with a color chart on the container.

Evaluation of Goal/Desired Outcome

- The child has appropriate weight loss and decreased abdominal girth.

Nursing Care Focus

- Risk for malnutrition related to anorexia

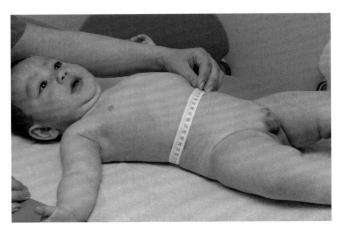

FIGURE 39-3 Measure the child's abdominal girth at the umbilicus.

Goal

- The child will have an adequate nutritional intake to meet normal growth needs.

Implementations for Improving Nutritional Intake

Although the child may look plump, underneath the edema is a thin, possibly malnourished child. The child's appetite is poor for several reasons:

- The ascites diminishes the appetite because of the full feeling in the abdomen.
- The child may be lethargic, apathetic, and simply not interested in eating.
- A no-added-salt or low-salt diet may be unappealing to the child.
- Corticosteroid therapy may decrease the appetite.

Offer a visually appealing and nutritious diet. Consult the child and the family caregiver to learn which foods are appealing to the child. Cater to the child's wishes as much as possible to perk up a lagging appetite. A dietitian can help plan appealing meals for the child. Serving six small snacks and meals may help increase the child's total intake better than the customary three meals a day.

Evaluation of Goal/Desired Outcome

- The child eats 80% or more of their snacks and meals.

Nursing Care Focus

- Risk for altered skin integrity related to edema

Goal

- The child's skin integrity will be maintained.

Implementations for Maintaining Skin Integrity

The child's skin is stretched with edema and becomes thin and fragile. Inspect all skin surfaces regularly for breakdown. Because the child is lethargic, turn and reposition the child frequently. Protect skin surfaces from pressure by means of pillows and padding. Protect overlapping skin surfaces from rubbing. Use air mattresses and alternating pressure mattresses to reduce the risk of skin concerns. Bathe the child regularly. Thoroughly wash the skin surfaces that touch each other with soap and water and dry them completely. If the scrotum is edematous, use a soft cotton support to provide comfort.

Evaluation of Goal/Desired Outcome

- The child's skin remains free of breakdown with no redness or irritation.

Nursing Care Focus

- Fatigue related to edema and disease process

Goal

- The child's energy will be conserved.

Implementations for Promoting Energy Conservation

Bed rest is common during the edema stage of the condition. The child rarely protests because of their fatigue. The sheer bulk of the edema makes movement difficult. When diuresis occurs several days after beginning corticosteroids, the child may be allowed more activity, but balance the activity with rest periods and encourage the child to rest when fatigued. Plan quiet, age-appropriate activities that interest the child. Most children love having someone read to them. Coloring books, puzzles, and some kinds of electronic and board games are quiet activities that many children enjoy. Involve the family in providing some of these activities. Avoid using television or electronic devices excessively as a diversion.

Evaluation of Goal/Desired Outcome

The child:

- rests as needed.
- engages in quiet diversional activities.

Nursing Care Focus

- Infection risk related to immunosuppression

Goal

- The child will be free from signs and symptoms of infection.

Implementations for Preventing Infection

The child with nephrotic syndrome is especially at risk for respiratory infections because the edema and the corticosteroid therapy lower the body's defenses. Protect the child from anyone with an infection: staff, family, visitors, and other children. Good handwashing and following standard transmission precautions are essential. Monitor vital signs every 4 hours and observe for any early signs of infection.

Evaluation of Goal/Desired Outcome

- The child has normal vital signs with no respiratory, gastrointestinal, or other signs and symptoms of infection.

Nursing Care Focus

- Knowledge deficiency of the family caregiver related to disease process, treatment, and home care

Goal

- The family caregivers will verbalize an understanding of the disease process, treatment, and the child's home care needs.

Implementations for Reinforcing Family Teaching

Children with nephrotic syndrome are usually hospitalized for diagnosis, thorough evaluation of their general health and specific condition, and institution of therapy. If the child has an infection, a course of anti-infective therapy may be given; unless unforeseen complications develop, the child is discharged with complete instructions for management at home. Provide a written plan to help the family caregivers follow the program successfully. They must keep a careful record of home treatment for the health care provider to review at regular intervals.

Reinforce teaching with the family caregivers about reactions that may occur with the use of corticosteroids and the adverse effects of abruptly discontinuing use of these drugs. If the family understands these aspects well, the incidence of forgetting to give the medication or of neglecting to refill the prescription may be reduced or eliminated. Encourage the family caregivers to promptly report any symptoms that they think are caused by medications. Reinforce teaching with the family about how important it is to keep the child in optimum health and that **intercurrent infections** (those occurring during the course of an already existing disease) must be reported promptly. Also, remind the family that exacerbations are common and that they need to understand these will probably occur. Stress the information that they should report, including rapidly increasing weight, increased proteinuria, or signs of infections. Any of these may be a reason for altering the therapeutic regimen or changing the specific antibiotic agents used.

Here's a Hint!

Help the family caregivers of the child with nephrotic syndrome develop a method for keeping accurate records—charts or calendars might work well.

Provide the family caregivers with home care information appropriate for any chronically ill child. Bed rest is indicated during an intercurrent illness. Activity is restricted only by edema, which may slow the child down considerably; otherwise, normal activity is beneficial. Sufficient food intake may be a problem, as in other chronic conditions. Fortunately, there are usually few or no food restrictions, and the appetite can be tempted by attractive, appealing foods.

Evaluation of Goal/Desired Outcome

The family:

- explains nephrotic syndrome.
- describes aspects of medications given.
- states signs and symptoms of infection.
- discusses home care.
- asks and answers appropriate questions.

Nursing Care Focus

- Impaired family caregiver coping related to care of a child with chronic condition

Goal

- The family caregivers will verbalize feelings and concerns.

Implementations for Providing Family Support

The family of the child who has nephrotic syndrome is faced with caring for a child with a chronic condition. Give the family and the child opportunities to voice concerns and anxieties. Respond with active listening techniques to help authenticate their feelings. Provide emotional support throughout the entire hospital stay. Demonstrate an interest and willingness to talk to the family; do not make family members feel as though they are intruding on time needed to do other things. As the nurse, you are the person who can best provide overall support.

Evaluation of Goal/Desired Outcome

The family:

- verbalizes feelings and concerns related to caring for a child with a chronic condition.
- receives adequate support.

TEST YOURSELF

✔ Give examples of physiologic and psychological causes of enuresis.

✔ Acute poststreptococcal glomerulonephritis may be an inflammatory reaction to what bacterium?

✔ What is the presenting symptom in the child with nephrotic syndrome, and where is this symptom noted?

✔ Why is the abdomen measured daily for the child with nephrotic syndrome? What might be detected with this measurement?

WILMS TUMOR (NEPHROBLASTOMA)

Wilms tumor is the most common renal malignancy in children and one of the most common abdominal tumors of early childhood. The tumor arises from bits of embryonic tissue that remain after birth. This tissue can spark rapid cancerous growth in the area of the kidney. The tumor is rarely discovered until it is large enough to be palpated through the abdominal wall. Often the family caregiver notes an abdominal mass or swelling. The child may have no other signs or symptoms. As the tumor grows, it invades the kidney or the renal vein and disseminates to other parts of the body. When the child is being evaluated and treated, a sign must be visibly posted stating that abdominal palpation should be avoided because cells may break loose and spread the tumor. Treatment consists of surgical removal of the tumor and the affected kidney as soon as possible after the growth is discovered, combined with radiation and chemotherapy.

Pay Attention!

DO NOT palpate the abdomen of a child with a Wilms tumor; doing so could rupture the tumor and cause metastasis of the cells. Handle the child carefully when diapering or bathing.

Prognosis depends of the staging of the tumor when it is diagnosed and the extent of metastasis, but the survival rate for these children is good. Follow-up consists of regular evaluation for metastasis to the lungs or other sites. All long-term implications for chemotherapy apply to this child.

HYDROCELE

Hydrocele is a collection of peritoneal fluid that accumulates in the scrotum through a small passage called the processus vaginalis. This processus is a fingerlike projection in the inguinal canal through which the testes descend. Usually the processus closes soon after birth; if the processus does not close, fluid from the peritoneal cavity passes through, causing hydrocele. This is the same passage through which intestines may slip, causing an inguinal hernia. If the hydrocele remains by the end of the first year, corrective surgery is performed.

CRYPTORCHIDISM

Shortly before or soon after birth, the male gonads (testes) descend from the abdominal cavity into their normal position in the scrotum. Occasionally one or both of the testes do not descend, which is a condition called cryptorchidism. The testes are usually normal in size; the cause for failure to descend is not clearly understood.

In most infants with cryptorchidism, the testes descend by the time the infant is 1 year old. If one or both testes have not descended by this age, treatment is recommended. If both testes remain undescended, the male will be sterile and at risk for testicular cancer.

A surgical procedure called **orchiopexy** is used to bring the testes down into the scrotum and anchor them there. Surgery is usually performed when the child is 1 to 2 years of age. Prognosis for a normal functioning testicle is good when the surgery is performed at this young age and no degenerative action has taken place before treatment.

MENSTRUAL DISORDERS

The beginning of menstruation, called **menarche**, normally occurs between the ages of 9 and 16. For many girls, this is a joyous affirmation of their womanhood, but others may have negative feelings about the event, depending on how they have been prepared for menarche and for their roles as women. Irregular menstruation is common during the first year until a regular cycle is established.

Some adolescent girls experience **mittelschmerz**, a dull, aching abdominal pain at the time of ovulation (hence the name, which means "midcycle"). The cause is not completely understood, but the discomfort usually lasts only a few hours and is relieved by analgesics, a heating pad, or a warm bath.

Premenstrual Syndrome

Women of all ages are subject to the discomfort of **premenstrual syndrome (PMS)**, but the symptoms may be alarming to the adolescent. Symptoms include edema (resulting in weight gain), headache, increased anxiety, mild depression, and mood swings. The exact causes of PMS are unknown. One possible cause of PMS is thought to be due to hormone level changes when progesterone production increases after ovulation (see Fig. 3-11 in Chapter 3).

Generally, the discomforts of PMS are minor and can be relieved by lifestyle changes such as regular exercise, a well-balanced diet, and stress reduction. Some women find dietary supplements, vitamins, and herbal preparations helpful. Taking mild analgesics and applying local heat may also help relieve symptoms. When symptoms are more severe, the health care provider may prescribe a mild diuretic to be taken the week before menstruation to relieve edema; oral contraceptive pills are also sometimes prescribed to prevent ovulation.

Dysmenorrhea

Dysmenorrhea (painful menstruation) is classified as primary or secondary. Many adolescent girls experience pain associated with menstruation, including cramping abdominal pain, leg pain, and backache. Primary dysmenorrhea occurs as part of the normal menstrual cycle without any associated pelvic disease. The increased secretion of prostaglandins, which occurs in the last few days of the ovulatory cycle and the first 2 days of menses, is thought to be a contributing factor in primary dysmenorrhea. Nonsteroidal anti-inflammatory drugs (NSAID's), such as ibuprofen, inhibit prostaglandins and are the treatment of choice for primary dysmenorrhea. These drugs are most effective when taken before cramps become too severe. Because nonsteroidal anti-inflammatory drugs are irritating to the gastric mucosa, they should always be taken with food and discontinued if epigastric burning occurs.

Secondary dysmenorrhea is the result of pelvic pathologic changes, most often pelvic inflammatory disease, fibroids, or endometriosis. The adolescent girl who has severe menstrual pain should be examined by a health care provider to determine if any pelvic pathologic changes are present. Treatment of the underlying condition helps relieve severe dysmenorrhea.

Amenorrhea

The absence of menstruation, or **amenorrhea**, can be primary (no previous menstruation) or secondary (missing three or more periods after menstrual flow has begun). Primary amenorrhea after 16 years of age warrants a diagnostic survey for genetic abnormalities, tumors, or other problems. Secondary amenorrhea can be the result of discontinuing contraceptives, a sign of pregnancy, the result of physical or emotional stressors, or a symptom of an underlying medical condition. A complete physical examination, including gynecologic screening, is necessary to help determine the cause.

VAGINITIS

Vaginitis (inflammation of the vagina) can occur for a number of reasons, such as diaphragms or tampons left in place too long, irritating douches or sprays, estrogen changes caused by birth control pills, and antibiotic therapy. These factors provide an opportunity for the infecting organisms to become active. The most common causes of vaginitis are *Candida albicans*, *Gardnerella vaginalis*, *Trichomonas*, and other organisms that cause bacterial vaginosis. *Trichomonas* is the only one of these organisms transmitted solely by sexual contact (Table 39-3).

TEST YOURSELF

✔ If the testes remain undescended, what is the long-term complication for the male?

✔ How do premenstrual syndrome (PMS), dysmenorrhea, and amenorrhea differ?

Did you determine that **Christian** was diagnosed with acute poststreptococcal glomerulonephritis? What treatments do you think he will have? In prioritizing nursing care for Christian, what nursing implementations do you think will be the most important for you as his nurse to do? What teaching will you reinforce with this child's family caregiver?

TABLE 39-3 Infectious Causes of Vaginitis

ORGANISM/INCIDENCE	SYMPTOMS	SEXUAL TRANSMISSION	TREATMENT
Candida albicans			
First episodes occur in adolescence, especially in sexually active girls	Severe itching, exacerbated just before menstruation Odor not present Milky "cottage cheese"–like discharge may be noted on examination	Normally present in vagina; most often results from anti-infective therapy, oral contraceptive medications, steroid therapy, or other factors that alter normal pH of vagina May result from oral–genital sex	Miconazole, clotrimazole, terconazole vaginal suppositories or creams
Bacterial Vaginosis (Multiple Organisms)			
Common among adolescent girls; sexual partner will probably also be infected	About half of patients have no symptoms Fishy odor after intercourse Discharge, if present, grayish and thin	Sexually transmitted	Metronidazole[a] or clindamycin
Trichomoniasis			
Most frequently diagnosed STI	Itching with severe infection, especially after menstruation Discharge has foul odor and may be frothy, gray, or yellow/green	Sexually transmitted	Metronidazole[a], tinidazole; sexual partners also should be treated

[a]Metronidazole is not ordered for the pregnant client because of possible danger to fetus.

KEY POINTS

- The kidneys in children are located lower in relationship to the ribs than in adults. This placement and the fact that the child has less of a fat cushion around the kidneys cause the child to be at greater risk for trauma to the kidneys. In infants and children, emptying the bladder is a reflex action. Between ages 2 and 3, the child develops control of urination. The reproductive portion of the genitourinary system in males and females matures at the time of puberty.

- Urinary tract infections (UTI's) are usually treated with anti-infectives such as trimethoprim-sulfamethoxazole, amoxicillin, nitrofurantoin, or cephalosporins. The entire course of the medication should be taken, even if the symptoms subside after a few days. Goals for the child with a UTI include reducing temperature, maintaining normal urinary elimination, relieving pain, and increasing fluid intake.

- Physiologic causes of enuresis may include a small bladder capacity, UTI, constipation, or lack of awareness of the signal to empty the bladder because of sleeping too soundly. If a physiologic cause has been ruled out, psychological causes, including emotional stress, may be the cause of the enuresis.

- Acute poststreptococcal glomerulonephritis is a condition that appears to be an inflammatory reaction to a specific bacterium—most often group A beta-hemolytic streptococcal infections, such as an upper respiratory or skin infection. Presenting symptoms of acute poststreptococcal glomerulonephritis appear 1 to 3 weeks after the onset of a streptococcal infection, with the most common symptom being grossly bloody urine, which may be described as smoky, tea or cola colored, or bloody. Edema may accompany or precede hematuria. Nursing care includes encouraging bed rest and preventing fatigue, protecting from infection, and monitoring vital signs, intake and output, and urine for protein and hematuria.

- Edema is usually the presenting symptom in nephrotic syndrome, appearing first around the eyes and face. The edema becomes generalized and anasarca (massive edema) may result. Respiratory problems and edema of the scrotum on the male are characteristics. Anorexia, fatigue, and irritability develop. The goals for the child with nephrotic syndrome are relieving edema, improving nutritional status, maintaining skin integrity, conserving energy, and preventing infection.

- Acute poststreptococcal glomerulonephritis has an abrupt onset and usually lasts for 2 to 3 weeks. Nephrotic syndrome has an insidious onset and a course of remissions and exacerbations that usually last for months.

- Wilms tumor is the most common renal malignancy in children and one of the most common abdominal tumors of early childhood. The tumor arises from bits of embryonic tissue that cause cancerous growth in the area of the kidney. Abdominal palpation should be avoided because cells may break loose and spread the tumor.

- Hydrocele is a collection of peritoneal fluid that accumulates in the scrotum through a small fingerlike projection in the inguinal canal through which the testes descend. Usually the processus closes soon after birth; if the processus does not close, fluid from the peritoneal cavity passes through, causing hydrocele.

- The condition called cryptorchidism occurs when the male gonads (testes) do not descend from the abdominal cavity into their normal position in the scrotum.

- Premenstrual syndrome (PMS) symptoms include edema (resulting in weight gain), headache, increased anxiety, mild depression, and mood swings. One possible cause of PMS is thought to be due to hormone level changes. Dysmenorrhea (painful menstruation) has symptoms of pain associated with menstruation, including cramping abdominal pain, leg pain, and backache. The absence of menstruation is called amenorrhea.

INTERNET RESOURCES

Kidney Disorders
www.kidney.org

Enuresis
www.nafc.org/pediatric-bedwetting/

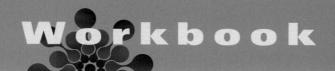

NCLEX-STYLE REVIEW QUESTIONS

1. After discussing ways to lower a fever with the family caregiver of an infant who has a urinary tract infection (UTI), the caregiver makes the following statements. Which statement indicates an understanding of appropriate ways to lower an infant's temperature?
   a. "I will give my child baby aspirin when she has a fever."
   b. "I know I need to dress my baby lightly if she has a fever."
   c. "When my baby has a fever, I will sponge her in cold water for 20 minutes."
   d. "I need to recheck my baby's temperature until it is below 97°F (36.1°C)."

2. In caring for a child with nephrotic syndrome, what intervention will be included in the child's plan of care?
   a. Ambulating three to four times a day
   b. Weighing on the same scale each day
   c. Increasing fluid intake by 50 mL an hour
   d. Testing the urine for glucose levels regularly

3. What situation will most likely be noted in the history for a child diagnosed with acute poststreptococcal glomerulonephritis?
   a. Sibling diagnosed with the same disease
   b. Recent illness, such as strep throat
   c. Hemorrhage or history of bruising easily
   d. Hearing loss with impaired speech development

4. The nurse is reinforcing teaching with the family caregiver of a 5-year-old child diagnosed with nephrotic syndrome regarding the no-added-salt diet the child has been placed on. In addition to not adding salt to foods, the nurse has discussed with the caregiver that helping the child avoid foods high in sodium is also recommended. The family caregiver marks the following foods on the child's menu selection for the next day. The nurse recognizes the family caregiver needs reinforcement of teaching regarding foods high in sodium when which of the following foods were selected? Select all that apply.
   a. Scrambled eggs with ham
   b. Apple juice
   c. Macaroni and cheese
   d. Hot dog in bun
   e. Fresh green beans
   f. Canned peaches

5. In caring for a child with a urinary tract infection (UTI), the nurse would perform the following nursing interventions. What intervention would be the highest priority for this child?
   a. The nurse will collect a "clean catch" voided urine.
   b. The nurse will observe for possible indications of sexual abuse.
   c. The nurse will instruct the caregivers to avoid bubble baths, especially in young girls.
   d. The nurse will remind girls to wipe from front to back.

STUDY ACTIVITIES

1. Create a poster to use as an aid when reinforcing teaching with a group of family caregivers of children with nephrotic syndrome. Include information regarding the use of corticosteroids and the adverse effects of abruptly discontinuing use of the drug, as well as symptoms that might be caused by the medication.

2. Develop a method to help the family caregivers of a child with nephrotic syndrome record information to be shared with their health care provider. Include information such as the child's weight, protein in the urine, and signs of infection.

3. Do an internet search on "pediatric nephrotic syndrome." What are some of the sites you discovered? After reading about nephrotic syndrome, answer the following questions.
   a. What organ is involved in nephrotic syndrome?
   b. How is the child with nephrotic syndrome monitored?
   c. What precautions should the family caregivers of a child with nephrotic syndrome take for their child?

CRITICAL THINKING: WHAT WOULD YOU DO?

1. Bradley is a 6-year-old boy who is in a playgroup with your child. Bradley's mother is talking with you and tells you she is concerned about Bradley because he has been potty trained, but now he is wetting the bed every night and sometimes has accidents during the day. She asks you if you think she should take her child to see their pediatrician.
   a. What would you suggest to Bradley's mother about seeing his pediatrician?
   b. What questions do you think the pediatrician might ask Bradley's mother?
   c. What are the possible physiologic causes of enuresis in children?
   d. What are frequent psychological causes of enuresis in children?

2. A classmate of yours has asked you to help give a presentation to a group of 12-year-old girls. The topic is human reproduction and sexuality. During the discussion, one of the girls tells you she has heard of PMS but does not know what it means.
   a. What will you explain to this group of girls regarding what PMS is?
   b. What is the physiologic cause of PMS?
   c. What symptoms might be seen when a woman is experiencing PMS?
   d. What will you explain to this group regarding the treatments that may be done when a woman experiences PMS?

3. Dosage calculation: A preschool child with a diagnosis of nephrotic syndrome is being treated with prednisolone. The child is being given a dose of 40 mg/day. The child weighs 44 lb. Answer the following:

  a. How many kilograms (kg) does the child weigh?
  b. How many milligrams (mg) per kilogram is this child's dose?
  c. If the dose is decreased to 30 mg/day, how many milligrams per kilogram will this dose be?

40

The Child With a Musculoskeletal Disorder

Key Terms

ankylosis
compartment syndrome
epiphysis
halo traction device
kyphosis
lordosis
metaphysis
scoliosis
skeletal traction
skin traction
synovitis
traction
uveitis

Learning Objectives

At the conclusion of this chapter, you will:

1. Discuss ways the child's musculoskeletal system differs from the adult's system.
2. Discuss types of fractures seen in children, and explain the treatment.
3. Describe the purpose of doing neurovascular checks in a child with a musculoskeletal disorder.
4. List and define the five P's to observe, record, and report when caring for a child in a cast.
5. Identify and explain different types of traction.
6. Discuss osteomyelitis, including the bacterium that usually causes it, the treatment, and nursing care.
7. Identify the most common form of muscular dystrophy (MD), and describe its characteristics.
8. Explain slipped capital femoral ephiphysis, including the age group it is commonly diagnosed, symptoms, and treatment.
9. Describe Legg–Calvé–Perthes disease.
10. Identify the treatment for the child with osteosarcoma and Ewing sarcoma.
11. Discuss juvenile idiopathic arthritis (JIA), including the classifications of the drugs used in the treatment.
12. Describe scoliosis, and identify methods of correction and nursing care.

Tyrone Williams, age 9, plays football in the local children's football league. During a game, he incurred a closed fracture of his right radius. As you read this chapter, think about what signs and symptoms you anticipate Tyrone may have.

As children explore the environments around them, they often cause injury to their musculoskeletal system. Physical activities including play and team sports create situations in which minor skeletal injuries, such as sprains and minor fractures, occur. However, some disorders of the musculoskeletal system can have lifelong effects.

GROWTH AND DEVELOPMENT OF THE MUSCULOSKELETAL SYSTEM

The musculoskeletal system provides the structure and framework to support, protect, and permit movement of the body. Bones are attached to each other by connecting links called joints, which allow for movement of the body parts. Skeletal muscles attach to the bones with moveable joints between them. Tendons and ligaments hold the muscles and bones together. Contraction of the muscles causes movement to take place. The heat produced as the muscles contract maintains the body temperature at a stable level. Minerals such as calcium, phosphorus, magnesium, and fluoride are stored in the bones. Blood cells are produced in the bone marrow.

The skeletal system is made up of four types of bone, each having a different function. Each of these types of bones has a specific shape—long, short, flat, irregular. During fetal life, tissue called cartilage, a type of connective tissue consisting of cells implanted in a gel-like substance, gradually calcifies and becomes bone. This calcification process develops the cartilage tissue into the major bones of the body.

Long bones grow from the long central shaft of the bone, called the diaphysis, to the rounded end of the bone, called the **epiphysis**. Cartilage makes up the epiphyseal plate that is between the epiphysis and the diaphysis. As long as cartilage remains, the child's bones continue to grow. Bones grow in width at the same time they are growing in length. When the epiphyseal plate becomes an epiphyseal line and cartilage is no longer present, this marks the end of the growth of that bone in the child.

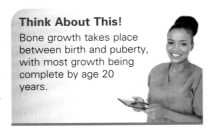

Think About This!

Bone growth takes place between birth and puberty, with most growth being complete by age 20 years.

During childhood, the bones are more spongelike and can bend and break more easily than in adults. In addition, because the bones are still in the process of growing, breaks in the bone heal more quickly than do breaks in adults.

The bones of the skull give shape to the head. The areas where these bones meet are called suture lines. These suture lines do not ossify or harden into bone during fetal life. Because these suture lines are not fused, during delivery the bones of the skull can move and overlap, allowing for the head to pass through the birth canal. Within the first 2 years of life, these suture lines or fontanels (fontanelles) fuse together.

The spine or vertebral column is made up of a series of separate bones connected in a way that allows for flexibility. There are four distinct curves in the adult spine. At birth, the spine is a continuous rounded convex curve. As the infant learns to hold up the head, the neck develops into a reverse curve. When the child begins to stand, another reverse curve is formed in the lower part of the back. The curves in the spine give support, strength, and balance to the body.

As the child grows, the muscles become stronger, and the child has more muscle tone, strength, and coordination (Fig. 40-1).

FRACTURES

A fracture, a break in a bone that is usually accompanied by vascular and soft tissue damage, is characterized by pain, swelling, and tenderness. Decreased function of the extremity is characteristic of a fracture. Children's fractures differ

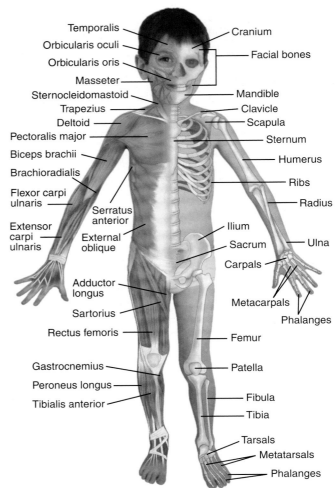

FIGURE 40-1 Bones and muscles of the body.

from those of adults in that they are generally less complicated, heal more quickly, and usually occur from different causes. The child has an urge to explore the environment but lacks the experience and judgment to recognize possible hazards. In some instances, family caregivers may be negligent in their supervision, but often the child uses immature judgment or is simply too fast for them.

The bones most commonly fractured in childhood are the forearm, wrist, clavicle, humerus, femur, tibia, and fingers. The classification of a fracture reflects the kind of bone injury sustained. If the fragments of fractured bone are separated and the break is across the entire section of the bone, the fracture is said to be complete (Fig. 40-2A). If fragments remain partially joined, the fracture is termed incomplete. Incomplete fractures often occur in children. Because children's bones are more porous, they often bow (a bowing deformity occurs) or buckle with an injury rather than

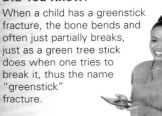

Did You Know?

When a child has a greenstick fracture, the bone bends and often just partially breaks, just as a green tree stick does when one tries to break it, thus the name "greenstick" fracture.

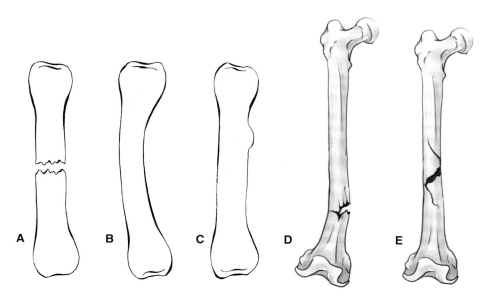

FIGURE 40-2 Types of fractures seen in children. **A.** Complete. **B.** Bowing (deformity). **C.** Buckle. **D.** Greenstick. **E.** Spiral. (A, B, C Reprinted with permission from Ricci, S., Kyle, T., & Carman, S. (2021). *Maternity and pediatric nursing* (Table 44-8 D, A, B, p. 1639). Wolters Kluwer.)

completely break (Fig. 40-2B, C). Greenstick fractures are another type of incomplete fracture, caused by incomplete ossification, also common in children (Fig. 40-2D). Spiral fractures, which twist around the bone, are frequently associated with child abuse and are caused by a wrenching force (Fig. 40-2E).

A closed fracture is a single break in the bone without penetration of the skin (Fig. 40-3A). When a broken bone penetrates the skin, the fracture is called an open fracture (Fig. 40-3B).

The epiphyses (rounded ends of the long bones) are where the primary growth of the bone takes place.

Be Aware!

Fractures occurring in the epiphyseal plate (growth plate) can cause permanent damage and severely impair growth.

This area is weak and easily susceptible to fractures. Force applied to this area during an injury may result in a serious fracture (Fig. 40-4).

Treatment and Nursing Care

Most childhood fractures are treated by realignment and immobilization using either traction or closed manipulation and casting. A few clients with severe fractures or additional injuries, such as burns and other soft tissue damage, may require surgical reduction, internal or external fixation, or both. Internal fixation devices include rods, pins, screws, and plates made of inert materials that do not trigger immune reactions. They allow early mobilization of the child to a wheelchair, crutches, or a walker.

What signs and symptoms do you think **Tyrone** exhibited? What treatment do you think will be required for his care? Would you anticipate he will need surgery as part of his treatment? Also consider Tyrone's age and how this injury might impact Tyrone at his stage of growth and development.

External fixation devices are used primarily in complex fractures often with other injuries or complications. These devices are applied under sterile conditions in the operating room and may be augmented by soft dressings and elevated by means of an overhead traction rope. External fixation devices are rarely used on young children.

Management of pain and assessment (data collection) of neurovascular status are priorities in nursing care (see Chapter 29 for discussion of pain management). The child with a fracture may be given nonsteroidal anti-inflammatory drugs (NSAIDs) to control the pain. For

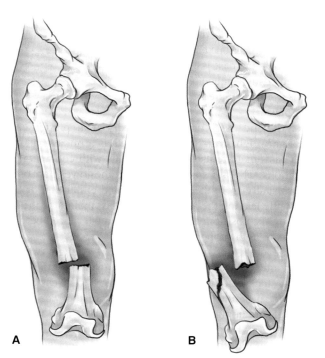

FIGURE 40-3 A. Closed fracture has no penetration of the skin. **B.** Open fracture penetrates through the skin.

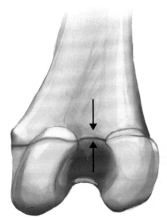

FIGURE 40-4 One form of epiphyseal injury; a crushing injury (as might occur in a fall from a height) can destroy the layer of germinal cells of the epiphysis, resulting in disturbance of growth.

severe pain, opioid analgesics may be given. After the fracture has been immobilized, the pain is most often significantly less.

Casts

The kind of cast used is determined by the age of the child, the severity of the fracture, the type of bone involved, and the amount of weight the child is allowed to bear on the extremity. Most casts are formed using synthetic material, such as fiberglass or polyurethane resin, which is pliable when wet but hardens when dry. Synthetic materials are light in weight and present a cleaner appearance because they can be sponged with water when soiled. Sometimes the cast is formed using gauze strips impregnated with plaster.

> **Have Some Fun With This!**
>
> Casts made of synthetic material are available in many colors. Children enjoy choosing a favorite color, a school color, or a color associated with a specific holiday, such as red for Valentine's Day.

Synthetic casts dry more rapidly than plaster casts. The lightweight casts tend to be used as arm casts and hip spica casts that are used to treat infants with congenital hip conditions. The hip spica cast covers the lower part of the body, usually from the waist down, and either one or both legs while leaving the feet open. The cast maintains the legs in a froglike position. Usually, there is a bar placed between the legs to help support the cast.

The child and the family should be taught what to expect after the cast is applied and how to care for the casted area. A stockinette is applied over the area to be casted, and the bony prominences are padded before the wet casting materials are applied. Although the materials may feel cool on the skin when applied, evaporation soon causes a temporary sensation of warmth. The cast may feel heavy and cumbersome (Fig. 40-5).

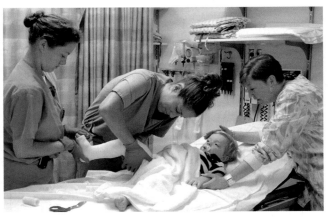

FIGURE 40-5 Encourage and support the child having a cast applied. Following cast application check the circulation in the extremity.

A wet plaster cast should be handled only with open palms because fingertips can cause indentations and result in pressure points. If the cast has no protective edge, it should be petaled (Fig. 40-6) with adhesive tape strips. If the cast is near the genital area, plastic should be taped around the edge to prevent wetting and soiling of the cast.

After the fracture has been immobilized, any reports of pain may signal possible complications, such as compartment syndrome, and should be recorded and reported immediately. **Compartment syndrome** is a serious neurovascular concern that occurs when increasing pressure within the muscle compartment causes decreased circulation. It is important that you monitor the child's neurovascular status frequently because of the risk of tissue and nerve damage.

> **This Is Critical to Remember!**
>
> *Any* complaint of pain in a child with a new cast or immobilized extremity needs to be explored and monitored closely for the possibility of compartment syndrome.

Performing neurovascular checks is sometimes referred to as CMS (circulation, movement, sensation) checks and these checks are done to monitor for and detect impaired

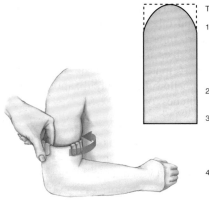

To petal a cast.

1. Cut several strips of adhesive tape or moleskin 3–4 in. in length. Use 1-in. tape for smaller areas (e.g., infant's foot) and 2-in. tape for larger areas (e.g., adolescent's waist).

2. Round one end of each strip to keep the corners from rolling.

3. Apply the first strip by tucking the straight end inside the cast and by bringing the rounded end over the cast edge to the outside.

4. Repeat the procedure, overlapping each additional strip, until all rough edges are completely covered.

FIGURE 40-6 Petaling the cast.

neurovascular function. These include observing, documenting, and reporting the five P's:

- Pain: Any sign of pain should be noted and the exact area determined.
- Pulse: If an upper extremity is involved, check brachial, radial, ulnar, and digital pulses. If a lower extremity is involved, monitor femoral, popliteal, posterior tibial, and dorsalis pedis pulses.
- Paresthesia: Check for any diminished or absent sensation or for numbness or tingling.
- Paralysis: Check hand function by having the child try to hyperextend the thumb or wrist, oppose the thumb and little finger, and adduct all fingers. Check function of the foot by having the child try to dorsiflex and plantarflex the ankles and flex and extend the toes.
- Pallor: Check the extremity and the nail beds distal to the site of the fracture for color. Paleness, discoloration, and coldness indicate circulatory impairment. Check for capillary refill.

In addition to the five P's, any foul odor or drainage on or under the cast; "hot spots" on the cast (areas warm to touch); looseness or tightness; or any elevation of temperature must be noted, documented, and reported. Family caregivers should be instructed to watch carefully for these same danger signals.

The child can return home after application of a cast, in most instances. The family caregivers and child should be provided with information about care of the cast at home and concerns that need to be observed for and reported to the health care provider (see Tips for Reinforcing Family Teaching: Cast Care).

When the fracture has healed, the cast is removed with a cast cutter. This can be frightening for the child unless the person using the cast cutter explains and demonstrates that the device will not cut flesh, but only the hard surface of the cast. The child should be told that there will be vibration from the cast cutter, but it will not burn.

After cast removal, the casted area will be tender and pale with flaky skin. Care must be taken to protect the new skin in the area (see Tips for Reinforcing Family Teaching: Cast Care, After cast is removed).

 A Personal Glimpse

One day I was jumping on my bed, trying to do a flip, but instead I fell on my arm. It hurt really bad, and I cried. I told my mom, and she put ice on it. But then I went to soccer camp the next day, and I fell on it again. It hurt even worse. My mom took me to the doctor's office. I could wiggle my fingers, but it only kind of hurt at the doctor's. So they took an x-ray. It was fun to see the picture of my arm. The next day I fell again at soccer camp; I was standing on my ball. This time my mom was sure it was broken. We went to get a cast. I chose a blue cast. My arm felt better, but I felt bad because it was my big sister's birthday. Everyone signed it. I had my cast on for 4 weeks. I couldn't wait to get it off. I finally got my cast off. I was excited! The girl used a saw to take it off. I wasn't scared. My arm really smelled bad! They took another x-ray to make sure my arm was better. It was! Then we left, and my mom washed my arm and put sunscreen on it. After that, everyone had trouble telling me and my twin apart.

Cassey, age 8 years

Learning Opportunity: What explanations would you give this child regarding the reason the x-rays were taken, the process of putting the cast on, and what to expect when the cast was removed? Which actions carried out by this mother would be important for the nurse to reinforce as appropriate actions for this situation?

 TIPS FOR REINFORCING FAMILY TEACHING

Cast Care

- Elevate the extremity at or above the level of the heart for the first 2 days as much as possible.
- Apply ice packs over the cast for 20 to 30 minutes every few hours when your child is awake for the first 2 days.
- Continue to apply ice packs as above if there is swelling or discomfort.
- Keep the cast dry, cover with plastic wrap or a plastic bag when bathing, do not put cast in water even if covered.
- Dry cast with hair dryer on low setting, if cast gets wet.
- Cover cast when child is eating or drinking.
- Clean soiled cast with slightly damp cloth.
- NEVER put anything inside the cast or let your child put anything inside the cast, no matter how much the casted area itches.
- Keep small toys and sticks or sticklike objects out of reach until the cast has been removed.
- Do not put powders or deodorants or let dirt or sand get inside cast.

- Blow cool air from a hair dryer or fan into cast to help relieve itching.
- Observe closely for any of the following and report these immediately to your child's health care provider:
  - Pain
  - Cool, discolored (bluish), pale, red or irritated skin
  - Numbness or tingling or swelling
  - Inability to wiggle fingers or toes
  - Foul smell from under cast
  - Increased temperature

After cast is removed:

- Soak, gently clean and pat dry skin; do not rub, scrap, or peel excess skin.
- Apply lotion or oil to area.
- Apply sunscreen when your child will have sun exposure to the previously casted area.

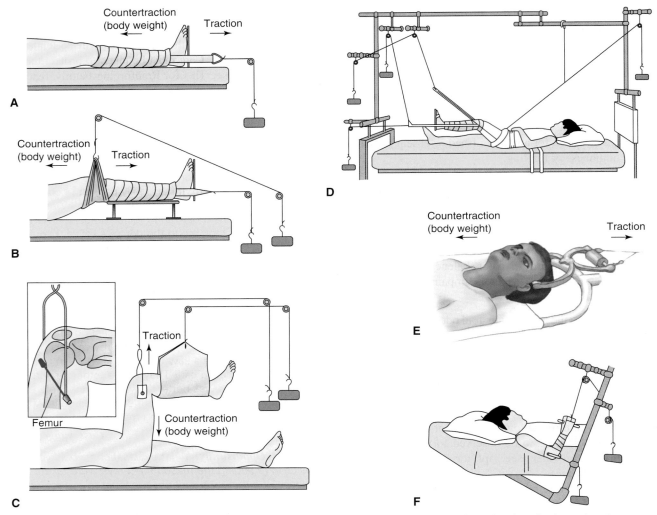

FIGURE 40-7 Types of traction. **A.** Buck (skin) traction. **B.** Russell (skin) traction. Two lines of traction (one horizontal and one vertical) allow for good bone alignment for healing. **C.** 90–90-degree (skeletal) traction; a wire pin is inserted into the distal femur. **D.** Balanced suspension (skeletal) traction. **E.** Cervical (skeletal) tongs traction. **F.** Dunlop (skeletal) traction. (Part A, B, C, D, F from Hatfield 4e. E, From Ricci, S., Kyle, T., & Carman, S. (2021). *Maternity and pediatric nursing* (Table 44.1, p. 1605). Wolters Kluwer.)

Traction

Traction is a pulling force applied to an extremity or other part of the body. A body part is pulled in one direction against a counterpull, or countertraction, exerted in the opposite direction. A system of weights, ropes, and pulleys is used to realign and immobilize fractures, reduce or eliminate muscle spasm, and prevent deformity and joint contractures.

Two basic types of traction are used: skin traction and skeletal traction. **Skin traction** applies pull on tape, rubber, or a plastic material attached to the skin, which indirectly exerts pull on the musculoskeletal system. Examples of skin traction are Bryant traction, Buck traction, and Russell traction. **Skeletal traction** exerts pull directly on skeletal structures by means of a pin, wire, tongs, or other device surgically inserted through a bone. Examples of skeletal traction are 90–90-degree traction, balanced suspension traction, and cervical skeletal tongs traction. Dunlop traction, sometimes used for fractures of the humerus or the elbow, can be either skin or skeletal traction. It is skeletal

traction if a pin is inserted into the bone to immobilize the extremity (Fig. 40-7).

Bryant traction (Fig. 40-8) may be used to treat the infant with developmental dysplasia of the hip or for

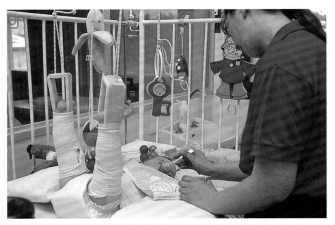

FIGURE 40-8 An infant in Bryant traction is being fed.

treatment of a fractured femur in children younger than 2 years. These fractures are often transverse (crosswise to the long axis of the bone) or spiral fractures. The child's legs are wrapped with elastic bandages that should be removed at least daily to observe the skin and then rewrapped. Skin temperature and the color of the legs and feet must be checked frequently to detect any circulatory impairment. The use of Bryant traction entails some risk of compromised circulation and may result in contractures of the foot and lower leg, particularly in an older child. Severe pain may indicate circulatory difficulty and should be reported immediately. When a child is in Bryant traction, the hips should not rest on the bed; a hand should be able to pass between the child's buttocks and the sheet.

Buck traction, in which the child's body provides the countertraction to the weights, is used for short-term immobilization. It is used to correct contractures and bone deformities, such as Legg–Calvé–Perthes disease, discussed shortly. For older children, Russell traction seems to be more effective.

Cervical skeletal tongs traction (Fig. 40-7E) is used for fractures, dislocations, or instability of the cervical vertebrae. Traction is achieved by using stainless steel pins inserted into the skull and then attached to the weights, while countertraction is attained by the gentle pull against the child's body weight.

A child in either skin or skeletal traction tends to slide down until the weights rest on the bed or the floor. The child should be pulled up to keep the weights free, the ropes must be in alignment with the pulleys, and the alignment should be checked frequently. An older child may try to coax a roommate to remove the weights or the sandbags used as weights.

Children in any kind of traction must be carefully monitored to detect any signs of neurovascular complications. Skin temperature and color; presence, or absence of edema; and peripheral pulse, sensation, and movement must be monitored every hour for the first 24 hours after traction has been applied, and every 4 hours after the first 24 hours, unless ordered otherwise. Skin care must be meticulous. Skin preparation (Skin-Prep) should be used to toughen the skin rather than lotions or oils, which softens the skin and contributes to tissue breakdown.

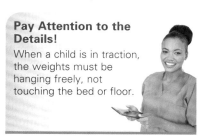

Pay Attention to the Details!

When a child is in traction, the weights must be hanging freely, not touching the bed or floor.

Children in skeletal traction require special attention to pin sites. Healthcare facilities and health care providers have individual policies and procedures regarding pin site care. Pin sites should be observed closely and pin care performed as ordered to prevent infection. Standard precautions and aseptic technique reduce the risk for infection. Any sign of infection (odor, local inflammation, or elevated temperature) must be recorded and reported at once.

Nursing Process and Care Plan *for the Child in Traction*

The child in traction has often experienced some type of incident in which a bone has been fractured, or they have a disorder being treated by the use of traction. The history related to the reason the child is in traction needs to be explored with the child and family caregiver. Information gathered regarding the child's situation helps to better anticipate what nursing care needs the child might have. After the application of the traction, observe the apparatus itself to be sure the ropes, weights, pulleys, and other parts of the traction are hanging and functioning correctly. The weights should not be touching the bed or the floor.

Assessment (Data Collection)

Data collected related to the physical examination of the child in traction include complaints of pain, vital signs, skin condition, and neurovascular status. Check for range of motion, mobility, and body alignment. If the child is in skeletal traction, observe the pin sites closely. Because the child may be in traction for a period of time, asking questions related to the child's everyday life and usual activities will be helpful in promoting normal growth and development. It is important to explore the child and family caregiver's understanding of the traction and treatment.

Nursing Care Focus

When developing evidence-based nursing care focuses for the child in traction, include the risk for altered tissue perfusion and integrity as well as the risk for altered skin integrity. Because of restricted mobility and the length of time the traction may be in place, it is important to encourage movement and activity within the limits of the traction and to meet the growth and development needs of the child. The child and family caregivers may have a knowledge deficiency related to the traction and how it is managed.

Outcome Identification and Planning

The goals for the child in traction include monitoring and maintaining adequate circulation and preventing neurovascular problems. In addition, maintaining skin integrity and range of motion, promoting growth and development, and increasing child and family caregiver knowledge are important goals.

Nursing Care Focus

- Altered tissue perfusion related to decreased circulation due to fracture and traction
- Altered tissue integrity related to possible neurovascular dysfunction

Goal

- The child will maintain adequate circulation and normal neurovascular status in extremities.

Implementations for Monitoring and Maintaining Circulation and Neurovascular Status

Monitor pulses in affected extremity and compare to pulses in other extremity. Comparison helps to determine if circulation is adequate in affected extremity. Monitor skin for color, temperature, sensation, and movement. Getting baseline data of the child's neurovascular status is important so that changes can be noted. Any change in neurovascular status could indicate impaired nerve function. Maintain proper body alignment with traction weights and pulleys hanging free of bed and off the floor. Body alignment must be maintained to prevent permanent injury or misalignment and decreased range of motion in affected extremity. Record and report any change in vital signs or neurovascular status. Immediate reporting leads to rapid treatment and decreases likelihood of long-term damage.

Evaluation of Goal/Desired Outcome

- The child's pulse rate is within a normal range with adequate pulses and capillary refill in all extremities.
- The child has good skin color, temperature, appropriate movement, and sensation in all extremities.

Nursing Care Focus

- Risk for altered skin integrity related to immobility

Goal

- The child will exhibit no skin breakdown.

Implementations for Maintaining Skin Integrity

Wash and thoroughly dry skin every day to stimulate circulation and keep skin clean.

Inspect skin at least every 4 hours for evidence of redness or broken skin. Early detection and treatment of skin breakdown can prevent long-term complications. Change position every 2 hours within restraints of traction to relieve pressure and decrease likelihood of skin breakdown and decreased circulation. Clean pin sites as prescribed following standard precautions to decrease risk of infection. Monitor temperature and observe for redness, drainage, and foul odor at pin sites. Record and report any signs and symptoms which might be indicative of possible infection.

Evaluation of Goal/Desired Outcome

- The child's skin remains intact without redness or irritation.
- The child will not show signs or symptoms of infection.

Nursing Care Focus

- Activity intolerance related to skeletal traction and bed rest

Goal

- The child will maintain adequate range of motion.

Implementations for Increasing Activity and Maintaining Mobility

Teach child active and passive range-of-motion exercises to maintain joint function and to increase muscle tone and circulation. Exercising the unaffected extremities increases circulation as well as decreases concerns of muscle atrophy and skin impairment. Encourage child to become active in self-care. Normal muscle function is increased by using the parts of the body not immobilized. If permitted, promote the use of a trapeze so child can assist with movement and repositioning. Participating in their own care also promotes a feeling of control over hospitalization.

Evaluation of Goal/Desired Outcome

- The child performs range of motion within limits of traction.
- The child does own self-care activities.

Nursing Care Focus

- Psychosocial needs related to risk for delayed growth and development secondary to being in traction and hospitalization

Goal

- The child will achieve developmental tasks appropriate for age.

Implementations for Promoting Growth and Development

Provide age-appropriate games, supplies, and activities that the child can do while in traction, such as books, puzzles, music, and electronic games and devices. Age-appropriate activities help the child develop and achieve milestones of growth and development. Encourage the child to communicate with peers by phone, letter, or electronic devices. Communication with peers allows for normal growth and development opportunities. Providing school work for the school-aged child helps decrease boredom and allows child to stay academically on level with their peers. Move the child's bed to a hallway or playroom to enable participation in activities to increase interaction with other children. Encourage family members to stay with child.

Evaluation of Goal/Desired Outcome

- The child selects and participates in age-appropriate activities and play.
- The child shows enjoyment in participating in activities.
- The child communicates and interacts with peers.

External Fixation Devices

In children who have severe fractures or conditions, such as having one extremity shorter than the other, external fixation devices are used to correct the condition (Fig. 40-9A, B). Another type of external fixation, a **halo traction device**, is used to treat cervical fractures or for immobilization following a cervical fusion, such as in the child with severe scoliosis (see discussion of scoliosis later in this chapter) (Fig. 40-9C). When an external fixation device is used, special skin care at the pin sites is necessary. The sites are left open to the air and should be inspected and kept clean. The appearance of the pins puncturing the skin and the unusual appearance of the device can be upsetting to the child, so be sensitive to any anxiety the child expresses.

As early as possible, the child (if old enough) or family caregivers should be taught to care for the pin sites. External fixation devices are sometimes left in place for long periods of time; therefore, it is important that the child accepts this temporary change in body image and learns to care for the affected site. Children with these devices will probably work with a physical therapist during the rehabilitation period and will have specific exercises to perform. Before discharge from the hospital, the child should feel comfortable moving about and should be able to recognize the signs of infection at the pin sites.

Crutches

Children with fractures of the lower extremities and other lower leg injuries often must learn to use crutches to avoid weight bearing on the injured area. Several types of crutches are available. The most common are axillary crutches, which are principally used for temporary situations. Forearm, or Canadian, crutches are usually recommended for children who need crutches permanently, such as paraplegic children with braces. Trough, or platform, crutches are more suitable for children with limited strength, or limited function, in the arms and hands.

A physical therapist teaches the use of crutches, and the nurse reinforces this teaching. The type of crutch gait taught is determined by the amount of weight bearing permitted, the child's degree of stability, whether or not the knees can be flexed, and the specific treatment goal.

OSTEOMYELITIS

Osteomyelitis is an infection of the bone usually caused by *Staphylococcus aureus*. Acute osteomyelitis is twice as common in boys and results from a primary infection, such as a staphylococcal skin infection (impetigo), burns, a furuncle (boil), a penetrating wound, or a fracture. The bacteria enter the bloodstream and are carried to the **metaphysis**, the growing portion of the bone, where an abscess forms, ruptures, and spreads the infection along the bone under the periosteum.

Clinical Manifestations and Diagnosis

Symptoms usually begin abruptly with fever, malaise, pain, irritability, and localized tenderness over the metaphysis of the affected bone. Joint motion is limited; the child may refuse to crawl, walk, or use the extremity. Diagnosis is based on laboratory findings with an increased erythrocyte sedimentation rate, elevated C-reactive protein and white blood cell count, and positive blood cultures. X-ray examination, ultrasound, CT scan, and MRI abnormalities help diagnose the condition.

Treatment

Treatment for acute osteomyelitis must be immediate. Intravenous (IV) antibiotic therapy is started at once and followed by administration of oral antibiotics to complete treatment. Surgical drainage of the involved metaphysis may be performed. If the abscess has ruptured into the subperiosteal space, chronic osteomyelitis follows.

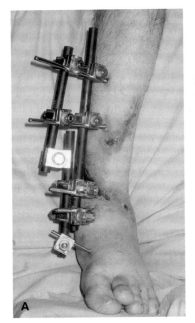

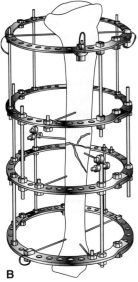

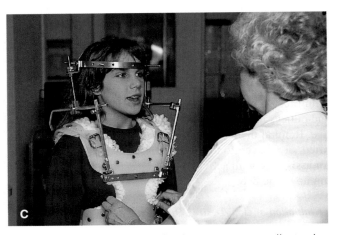

FIGURE 40-9 A. External fixation is required for complicated fractures. **B.** The Ilizarov fixator is a circular apparatus usually used for complicated lower extremity fractures. The pins are smaller in diameter, more like wires, than those used in other fixators. **C.** The halo traction device is used to treat cervical issues. (C, Reprinted with permission from Rosdahl, C., & Kowalski, M. (2017). *Textbook of basic nursing* (Figure 77-6B, p. 1328). Wolters Kluwer.)

If prompt specific antibiotic treatment is vigorously used, acute osteomyelitis may be brought under control rapidly, and the extensive bone destruction of chronic osteomyelitis is prevented. If extensive destruction of bone has occurred before treatment, surgical removal of necrotic bone becomes necessary.

Nursing Care

During the acute stage, nursing care includes reducing pain by positioning the affected limb, minimizing movement of the limb, and administering antipyretic and anti-infective medications. The usual procedure for IV antibiotic therapy is followed, including careful observance of the venipuncture site and monitoring of the rate, dosage, and time of antibiotic administration. An intermittent infusion device or peripherally inserted central catheter may be used for long-term IV therapy.

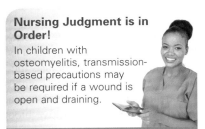

Nursing Judgment is in Order!

In children with osteomyelitis, transmission-based precautions may be required if a wound is open and draining.

Monitor oral nutrition and fluids because the child's appetite may be poor during the acute phase. Weight bearing on the affected limb must be avoided until healing has occurred because pathologic fractures occur very easily in the weakened stage. Physical therapy helps restore limb function.

MUSCULAR DYSTROPHY

Muscular dystrophy (MD) is a hereditary, progressive, degenerative disease of the muscles. The most common form of MD is Duchenne (pseudohypertrophic) muscular dystrophy. Duchenne MD, an X-linked recessive hereditary disease, occurs almost exclusively in males. Females are usually carriers of the disease. When MD has been diagnosed in a child, the mother and the siblings should be tested to see whether they have the disease, or are carriers of the disease.

Clinical Manifestations and Diagnosis

The first signs are noted in infancy or childhood, usually within the first 3 to 4 years of life. The child has difficulty standing and walking. Trunk muscle weakness develops and the child has trouble climbing stairs and running. The child cannot rise easily to an upright position from a sitting or squatting position on the floor; instead, they develop Gowers sign, a method where the child rises from the floor by "walking up" the lower extremities with the hands (Fig. 40-10). Weakness of leg, arm, and shoulder muscles progresses gradually. Increasing abnormalities in gait and posture appear by school age, with **lordosis** (forward curvature of the lumbar spine or swayback), walking on the toes or balls of feet with a pelvic waddling, and frequent falling (Fig. 40-11). Mild intellectual disability often accompanies this disease. The child becomes progressively weaker, usually becoming wheelchair-bound

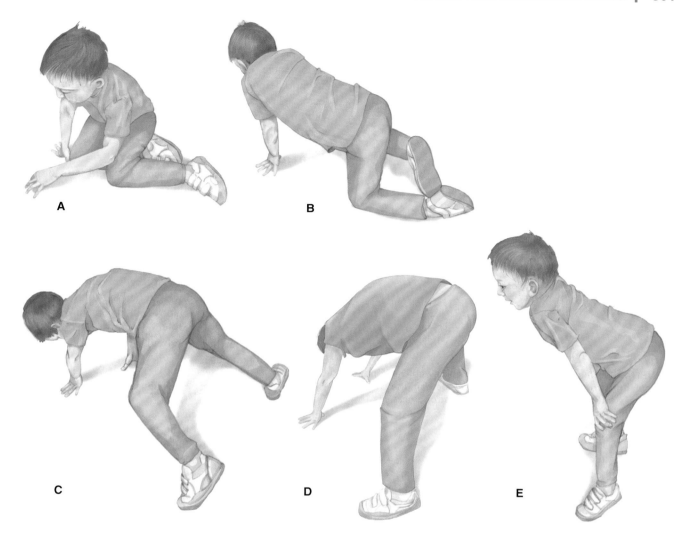

FIGURE 40-10 Gowers sign is used to rise from the floor. **A.** First the child must roll onto his hands and knees. **B.** Then he must bear weight by using his hands to support some of his weight, while raising his posterior. **C–E.** The boy then uses his hands to "walk" up his legs to assume an upright position.

by 10 to 12 years of age (middle school or junior high school age). The disease continues into adolescence and adulthood. With improved management of respiratory and cardiac complications, the lifespan of the client with MD has increased significantly.

In addition to symptoms in the first years of life, highly increased serum creatinine phosphokinase levels, as well as a decrease in muscle fibers seen in a muscle biopsy, can confirm the diagnosis.

Treatment and Nursing Care

No effective treatment for the disease has been found, but research continues with genetic identification and the use of medications to slow the progression of the disease as hopeful treatment in the future. The child is encouraged to be as active as possible to delay muscle atrophy and contractures. The use of orthopedic supports, devices, and adaptive equipment helps in this effort. To help keep the child active, promote physical therapy appropriate, diet (to avoid obesity), and family caregiver support. Encourage the child to participate in activities, within their intellectual and physical capabilities, that will provide stimulation and promote development. Even though sometimes difficult, participating in activities increases the child's self-esteem and positive feelings about themselves.

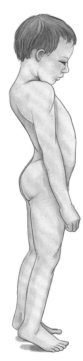

FIGURE 40-11 Characteristic posture of a child with Duchenne muscular dystrophy. Along with the typical toe gait, the child develops a lordotic posture as Duchenne dystrophy causes further deterioration.

When a child becomes wheelchair-bound, **kyphosis** (hunchback) develops and causes a decrease in respiratory function and an increase in the incidence of infections. Respiratory status and signs and symptoms of infection are monitored closely. Deep breathing exercises, encouraging coughing, and chest physiotherapy are a daily necessity for these children. Cardiac status is also monitored closely.

Advise the family to keep the child's life as normal as possible, which may be difficult. This disease can drain the emotional and financial reserves of the entire family. Suggest assistance through the Muscular Dystrophy Association—USA (800-572-1717; www.mda.org), through local chapters of this organization, and by talking with other family caregivers who face the same concerns.

SLIPPED CAPITAL FEMORAL EPIPHYSIS

Slipped capital femoral epiphysis is a common hip condition seen in adolescents. It can happen gradually over a period of time and occurs when the femoral head dislocates from the neck of the femur at the growth plate and slips down and backward. The condition commonly develops during an adolescent growth spurt or in the child who is overweight or obese. The slip may be classified as stable or unstable depending on if the child can or cannot walk. It is further classified according to the severity. It may be mild, moderate, or a severe slip.

Clinical Manifestations and Diagnosis

The child complains of a dull, aching pain in the hip, groin, thigh, or knee. Physical activity increases the pain and it can be acute, chronic, or intermittent. The pain results in the child being unable to bear weight on that leg and having decreased range of motion. A limp is present when walking with an external rotation of the toes. The diagnosis is made with radiologic studies.

Treatment and Nursing Care

When acute symptoms are present, the child is made non–weight bearing, put on bedrest, sometimes using crutches for bathroom privileges, or put in traction to stabilize the hip, until they receive treatment. Early detection and surgical intervention help prevent the risk of long-term deformity and complications due to the decreased blood supply to the area caused by the slip. Surgery is done to stabilize the slip, usually pinning with a screw placed. Following surgery, there is a period of limited weight bearing until healing has occurred. Nursing care includes reinforcement of teaching about the importance of following bedrest, weight bearing limits set by the health care provider, and reinforcing correct crutch walking and use.

LEGG–CALVÉ–PERTHES DISEASE

Legg–Calvé–Perthes disease is an aseptic necrosis, which affects the development of the femur. It occurs four to five times more often in boys than in girls and more often in White children than in other origin. It can be caused by trauma to the hip or genetic factors, but generally the cause is unknown.

Clinical Manifestations and Diagnosis

Symptoms first noticed are pain in the hip, thigh, knee, or groin and a limp accompanied by muscle spasms and limitation of motion. These symptoms mimic **synovitis** (inflammation of a joint, which is most commonly the hip in children), which makes immediate diagnosis difficult. X-ray examination may need to be repeated several weeks after the initial visit to demonstrate vascular necrosis for a definitive diagnosis. Bone scan and MRI are also used in the diagnostic process.

There are four stages of the disease; each lasts several months to years. In the first stage, x-ray studies show opacity of the epiphysis. Interruption of the blood supply to the femoral head causes bone growth to stop. In the second stage, which is called revascularization, the epiphysis becomes mottled and fragmented and new blood vessels increase the circulation to the area; during the third stage, reossification, or new bone growth, occurs. In the fourth stage, healing, bone regrowth is complete and the head of the femur is reshaped.

Treatment and Nursing Care

Treatment focuses on containing the femoral head within the acetabulum during the revascularization process so that the new femoral head will form to make a smoothly functioning joint and normal hip function will be restored. Bracing, traction, or casts may be used to hold the necrotic portions of the femoral head in place during healing. Activities are limited and non–weight bearing, so low-risk activities which maintain range of motion and mobility are recommended. Maintaining mobility helps in decreasing the complications that immobility can cause, such as skin breakdown, muscle weakness, and atrophy. Anti-inflammatory medications are used to relieve pain and muscle spasms. Surgery may be done in rare situations.

The prognosis for complete recovery without difficulty later in life depends on the child's age at the time of onset and the amount of involvement. Younger children usually have a better outcome with fewer long-term complications because they heal faster and have a longer time in which bone regrowth can occur.

Nursing care focuses on helping the child and family caregivers manage the corrective devices and reinforcing teaching about the importance of compliance to promote healing and to avoid long-term disability.

OSTEOSARCOMA

Osteosarcoma is a malignant tumor seen in the long bones, such as the femur, thigh, and humerus. It is more frequently seen in boys than in girls. Children who have had exposure to radiation or retinoblastoma are more prone to the malignancy.

Clinical Manifestations and Diagnosis

An injury, such as a sports injury, may draw attention to the pain and swelling at the sight of the tumor, but the injury itself did not cause the tumor. It is important to explain this to the child and family caregiver to decrease their possible feelings of guilt. Pathologic fractures of the bone can occur.

A biopsy, as well as radiography, bone scan, computed tomography, and magnetic resonance imaging confirm the diagnosis. Metastasis to the lungs can occur.

Treatment and Nursing Care

Surgical removal of the bone or the limb followed by chemotherapy is the treatment for the tumor. A prosthesis is fitted, often soon after the surgery.

A cancer diagnosis is frightening to the child and family, and honest answers and support are helpful. After an amputation, phantom pain in the amputated extremity can be relentless. Learning to live with a prosthesis may be a long and challenging process. Support groups with other children living with a prosthetic device can be helpful. With early diagnosis and treatment, many children survive this diagnosis and live into adulthood.

EWING SARCOMA

Ewing sarcoma is a malignant tumor found in the bone marrow of the long bones. It is often seen in older school-aged or adolescent boys.

Clinical Manifestations and Diagnosis

As with osteosarcoma, many times an injury draws attention to the pain at the site of the tumor. The pain may be sporadic for a period of time, but continues and becomes severe enough to keep the child awake at night. Metastasis to the lung and other bones may have already taken place by the time of diagnosis. A biopsy, bone scan, and bone marrow aspiration are done to further diagnose the tumor.

Treatment and Nursing Care

The tumor is removed and radiation, as well as chemotherapy, is given. In many cases, the limb does not have to be amputated, although this may be part of the treatment.

It is important that you offer support and encouragement while the child adjusts to the difficult course and effects of chemotherapy, such as hair loss, nausea, and vomiting.

JUVENILE IDIOPATHIC ARTHRITIS

Juvenile idiopathic arthritis (JIA), formerly called juvenile rheumatoid arthritis (JRA), is an autoimmune disorder which primarily affects the joints. It is the most common connective tissue disease of childhood. The occurrence of JIA appears to peak at two age levels: 1 to 3 years and 8 to 10 years. This disease has a long duration, but most of children with JIA reach adulthood without serious disability.

Clinical Manifestations and Diagnosis

Joint inflammation occurs first causing pain, joint stiffness (usually worse in the morning), redness, swelling, and warmth. If untreated, inflammation leads to irreversible changes in joint cartilage, ligaments, and menisci (the crescent-shaped fibrocartilage in the knee joints), eventually causing complete immobility, so early treatment is critical. In some forms of the disease, the eyes and other organs can be affected. The inflammation can be subdivided into three different types: systemic; oligoarticular (pauciarticular), involving four or fewer joints, most often the wrists, knees, and ankles; and polyarticular, involving five or more joints (Table 40-1).

JIA is diagnosed by physical findings and symptoms most often. Laboratory testing results may be normal or may show signs of mild anemia, an elevated erythrocyte sedimentation rate (ESR), a positive antinuclear antibody (ANA), an elevated C-reactive protein (CRP), or a positive result for the rheumatoid factor (RF) depending on the type of JIA.

Treatment and Nursing Care

The treatment goals are to suppress inflammation, maintain mobility, and preserve joint function. Treatment can include drugs and physical therapy. Early diagnosis and drug therapy to control inflammation and other systemic changes can reduce the need for other types of treatment. Early detection of visual changes and prevention of blindness is important.

Drug Therapy

Enteric-coated aspirin had long been the drug of choice for JIA, but because of the concern of aspirin therapy and Reye syndrome (see Chapter 35), NSAIDs such as naproxen, indomethacin, and ibuprofen are used in the treatment of

TABLE 40-1 Characteristics of Different Types of Juvenile Idiopathic Arthritis (JIA)

TYPE OF JIA	SYSTEMIC	OLIGOARTICULAR (PAUCIARTICULAR)	POLYARTICULAR
Frequency of cases	10%–20%	Most common	20%–30%
Number of joints involved	Variable May be in hips	Four or fewer Often knee Rarely hips	Five or more Small joints Rarely starts in hips
Nonjoint manifestations	Fever, rash Lymphadenopathy Anemia	Eye inflammation Malaise Poor appetite	Lymphadenopathy Fatigue Poor growth
Uveitis[a]	Rare	20%–25%	14%
Laboratory Findings			
Erythrocyte sedimentation rate (ESR)	Highly elevated	Normal or mildly elevated	Elevated
Antinuclear antibodies (ANA)	Negative	Positive	Positive
Rheumatoid factors (RF)	Negative		Rare
C-reactive protein (CRP)	Highly elevated		

[a]Uveitis—an inflammation of the middle (vascular) tunic of the eye; includes the iris, ciliary body, and choroid.

JIA. These drugs may cause gastrointestinal irritation and bleeding.

Reinforce teaching with family caregivers about the importance of regular administration of the medications, even when the child is not experiencing pain. The primary purpose of NSAIDs is not to relieve pain, but to decrease joint inflammation.

In addition to NSAIDs, disease-modifying antirheumatic drugs (DMARDs), such as methotrexate, are given to slow the progression of the disease. These drugs have many serious side effects and their use must be closely monitored. Corticosteroids are given to suppress the inflammatory symptoms of JIA, but do not cure the disease or prevent joint damage.

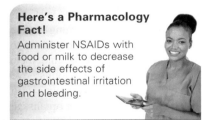

Here's a Pharmacology Fact!
Administer NSAIDs with food or milk to decrease the side effects of gastrointestinal irritation and bleeding.

Pay Close Attention!!
Disease-modifying antirheumatic drugs (DMARDs) have immunosuppressive actions and can mask signs of infection. Watch closely for any signs that might indicate infection.

Physical Therapy

Physical therapy is used to improve strength and flexibility, especially when the large joints of the lower extremities are involved. Exercise, heat–cold therapy, massage, and electrical stimulation may be used. Gentle daily exercise is necessary to prevent **ankylosis** (immobility of a joint). Stress to the family caregivers the importance of encouraging the child to perform independent activities of daily living to maintain function and independence.

Depending on the degree of disease, activity, range-of-motion exercises, isometric exercises, swimming, and riding a tricycle or bicycle may be part of the treatment plan. Inform family caregivers that these exercises should not increase pain; if exercise does trigger increased pain, the amount of exercise should be decreased.

TEST YOURSELF

✔ What is the cause of osteomyelitis, and how is it treated?

✔ What is the most common form of muscular dystrophy (MD), and what signs are usually noted in the child with MD?

✔ Why is it important to treat the joint inflammation in the child with juvenile idiopathic arthritis (JIA)?

✔ What are the common medications given to the child with JIA?

SCOLIOSIS

Scoliosis, a lateral curvature of the spine, occurs in two forms: structural and functional (postural). Structural scoliosis involves rotated and malformed vertebrae. Functional scoliosis, the more common type, can have several causes: poor posture, muscle spasm caused by trauma, or unequal length of legs. When the primary problem is corrected, elimination of the functional scoliosis begins.

Most cases of structural scoliosis are idiopathic (no cause is known); a few are caused by congenital deformities or infection. Idiopathic scoliosis is seen in school-aged children at 10 years of age and older. Although mild curves occur as often in boys as in girls, idiopathic scoliosis requiring treatment occurs 10 times more frequently in girls than in boys (Scherl, 2021).

Diagnosis

Diagnosis is based on a screening examination. Many states require regular examination of students for scoliosis beginning in the fifth or sixth grade. Scoliosis screening should last through at least eighth grade. Nurses play an important role in screening for this disorder. School nurses and others who work in healthcare settings with children aged 10 years and older should conduct or assist with screening programs. A school nurse often does the initial screening (see Fig. 26-7 in Chapter 26). Nurses in other healthcare settings are responsible for further screening of these children during regular well-child visits.

During examination, observe the undressed child from the back and note any lateral curvature of the spinal column; asymmetry of the shoulders, shoulder blades, or hips; and an unequal distance between the arms and waist (Fig. 40-12). The examiner then asks the child to bend at the hips (touch the toes) and observes for prominence of the scapula on one side and curvature of the spinal column.

Treatment

Treatment depends on many factors and is either nonsurgical or surgical. Treatment is long term and often lasts through the rest of the child's growth cycle.

Curvatures of less than 25 degrees are observed, but not usually treated. Transcutaneous electrical muscle stimulation (TENS) and exercise may be used as a nonsurgical treatment for mild curvatures. Curvatures between 25 and 40 degrees are usually corrected with a brace.

Curvatures of more than 40 degrees are usually corrected surgically. Surgical treatment includes the use of rods, screws, hooks, and spinal fusion.

Braces

The Milwaukee brace was the first type of brace used for scoliosis, but is now more commonly used to treat kyphosis, an abnormal rounded curvature of the spine that is also called humpback. Either the Boston brace or the TLSO (thoraco-lumbo-sacral-orthosis) brace is more commonly used to treat scoliosis (Fig. 40-13). The Boston brace and the TLSO brace are made of plastic and are customized to fit the child.

The brace should be worn constantly except during bathing or swimming to achieve the greatest benefit. It is worn over a T-shirt or undershirt to protect the skin. The fit of the device is monitored closely, and the child and family caregiver should be taught to notify the health care provider if there is any rubbing. During the first couple of weeks of wearing the brace, the child can be given a mild analgesic for discomfort and aching. The child's health care provider may also prescribe certain exercises to be done several times a day. These are taught before the brace is applied, but are done while the brace is in place.

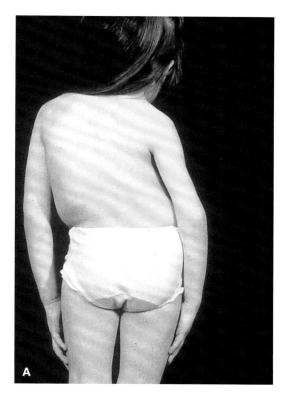

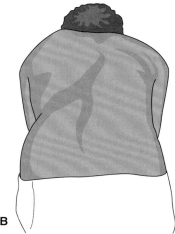

FIGURE 40-12 A. Posterior view of child's back with lateral curvature. **B.** View of child bending over with prominence of scapular area and asymmetry of flank demonstrated.

Surgical Treatment

Various types of instruments, such as rods, screws, and hooks, may be placed along the spinal column to realign the spine, and then spinal fusion is performed to maintain the corrected position. This procedure, which is done in cases of severe curvatures, is frightening to the child and family. It is major surgery, and the child and family caregiver must be well prepared for it. Because this is an elective procedure, thorough preoperative teaching can be carried out for the

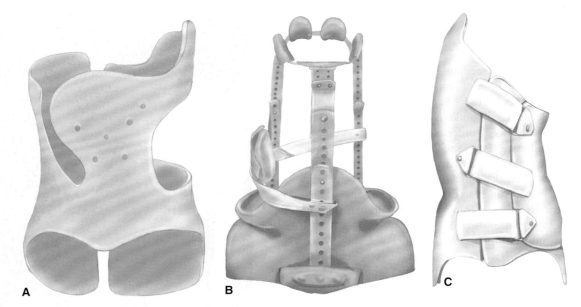

FIGURE 40-13 **A**. Boston brace. **B**. Milwaukee brace. **C**. Nighttime bending brace.

child and the family. The child can expect to have postoperative pain and will have to endure days of remaining flat in bed, being turned only in a logrolling fashion (Fig. 40-14). After surgery, the neurovascular status of the extremities is monitored closely. The child may be given a patient-controlled analgesia pump to control pain. An indwelling urinary (Foley) catheter is usually inserted because of the need for the client to remain flat. The rods remain in place permanently. In some cases, the child may be placed in a body cast for a period of time to ensure fusion of the spine. About 6 months after surgery, the child can take part in most activities, except contact sports (such as tackle football, gymnastics, and wrestling). Because the bones are fused and rods are implanted, this procedure arrests the child's growth in height, which contributes to the emotional adjustment that the child and family must make.

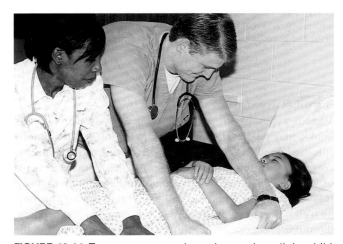

FIGURE 40-14 Two nurses use a draw-sheet to logroll the child to a side-lying position.

Nursing Process and Care Plan *for the Child With Scoliosis Requiring a Brace*

Assessment (Data Collection)

The child with scoliosis must be reassessed every 4 to 6 months. Document the degree of curvature and related impairments. Scoliosis is often diagnosed in late school age or early adolescence. This is a sensitive age for children, when privacy and the importance of being like everyone else are top priorities. Keep this in mind when interviewing and during examination of the child. Provide privacy and protect the child's modesty.

The child who is admitted to a healthcare facility for application of a brace, or other instrumentation, may be carrying a lot of unseen emotional baggage. Be sensitive to this emotional state. The family caregivers may also be upset, but are trying to hide it for the child's sake. In addition to routine observations, look for clues to the emotional states of both the child and family caregivers.

Nursing Care Focus

The nursing care focuses for the child with scoliosis requiring a brace include recognizing the child has an activity intolerance and decreased physical mobility because of their restricted movement. The risk for injury and altered skin integrity must be addressed. Because the child must wear the brace for a long period of time, dealing with the child's altered body image perception and possible nonadherence related to long-term treatment are important focuses for nursing care.

Outcome Identification and Planning

Consult the child and family caregiver when establishing client goals. Be especially sensitive to the child's needs.

Goals for the child may include minimizing the disruption of activities, preventing injury, and maintaining skin integrity and self-image. Goals for the child and family caregiver include complying with long-term care.

Nursing Care Focus

- Activity intolerance and decreased physical mobility related to restricted movement

Goal

- The child will move effectively within the limits of the brace.

Implementations for Promoting Mobility

Prescribed exercises help increase muscle strength and flexibility and help to prevent atrophy. They must be practiced and performed as directed. These can help minimize the risks of immobility. Encourage and support the child during these exercises to help promote self-esteem. The child may need to be in traction before the brace is applied which further causes decreased mobility.

Evaluation of Goal/Desired Outcome

The child:

- participates in prescribed exercise program.
- ambulates regularly.
- participates in daily activities.

Nursing Care Focus

- Injury risk related to decreased mobility

Goal

- The child will remain free from injury while in the brace.

Implementations for Preventing Injury

Evaluate the child's environment after the brace has been applied and take precautions to prevent injury. Help the child practice moving about safely: going up and down-stairs; getting in and out of vehicles, chairs, and desks; and getting out of bed. Remind the child to avoid hazardous surfaces. Listen carefully to the child and the family caregiver to determine any other hazards in the home or school environment. Advise the family caregiver to contact school personnel to ensure that the child has comfortable, supportive seating at school, and that adjustments are made in the physical education program.

Evaluation of Goal/Desired Outcome

The child:

- demonstrates safe practices related to everyday activities at home and in the school environment.

- has no signs of injury while wearing brace.

Nursing Care Focus

- Altered skin integrity risk related to irritation of brace

Goal

- The child's skin will remain intact.

Implementations for Monitoring Skin Integrity and Preventing Skin Irritation

When the brace is first applied, check the child regularly to confirm proper fit. Observe for any areas of rubbing, discomfort, or skin irritation, and adjust the brace as necessary. Reinforce teaching with the child about how to inspect all areas under the brace daily. Instruct the child and family caregiver that reddened areas should be reported to the health care provider so that adjustments can be made. Skin under the pads should be massaged daily. Daily bathing is essential, and clean cotton underwear or a T-shirt should be worn under the brace to provide protection.

Evaluation of Goal/Desired Outcome

The child:

- uses methods to reduce skin irritation and bathes regularly.
- exhibits skin that is free from irritation and breakdown.

Nursing Care Focus

- Altered body image perception related to wearing a brace continuously

Goal

- The child will exhibit positive coping behaviors.

Implementations for Promoting Positive Body Image

The child should be involved in all aspects of care planning. Self-image and the need to be like others are very important at this age. Wearing a brace creates a distinct change in body image, especially in the older school-aged child or adolescent at a time when body consciousness is at an all-time high. Clothing choices are a challenge when wearing a brace.

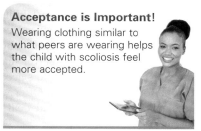

Acceptance is Important! Wearing clothing similar to what peers are wearing helps the child with scoliosis feel more accepted.

The need to wear the brace and deal with the limitations it involves may cause anger; the change in body image can cause a grief reaction. Handling these feelings successfully requires understanding support from the nurse, family, and peers. It is important for the child to have an opportunity to talk about their feelings. Sometimes it is helpful for the client in a brace to talk with other clients with scoliosis and learn how they have coped. Understanding the disorder itself and the important benefits of treatment can also ease the adjustment. Refer the child and family to the National Scoliosis Foundation (www.nsf@scoliosis.org) for support.

Learning to be confident enough to handle the comments of peers can be difficult for the child. Give the child frequent opportunities to ventilate feelings about being different and offer suggestions about how to explain the diagnosis and treatment to peers. Help the child select clothing that blends with current styles, but is loose enough to hide the brace. Encourage the child to find extracurricular activities with which the brace will not interfere. Active sports are not permitted, but many other activities are available. Help the child focus and enhance a positive attribute about characteristics, such as hair or complexion. Encourage the child and family caregiver to discuss accommodations with school personnel together.

Evaluation of Goal/Desired Outcome

The child:

- demonstrates self-confidence.
- has an attractive well-groomed appearance.
- verbalizes feelings about the need to wear the brace.

Nursing Care Focus

- Nonadherence related to long-term treatment

Goal

- The child will comply with therapy.

Implementations for Promoting Compliance With Therapy

The child may need to wear the brace for years until the spinal growth is completed. Then, the child needs to be weaned from it gradually by wearing it only at night. During this period, the family caregivers and the child need emotional support from healthcare personnel. Be certain that the child and family caregivers have a complete understanding of the importance of wearing the brace continually. To encourage compliance, reinforce teaching with them about possible complications of spinal instability and possible further deformity if correction is unsuccessful. Inform the family caregiver about the need to monitor the child for compliance. Help the family caregiver understand the importance of being empathic to the child's need to be like others during this period of development. Offer ways in which the family caregiver can help the child deal with adjustment to the therapy.

Evaluation of Goal/Desired Outcome

- The child wears the brace as directed, and their condition shows evidence of compliance.
- Family caregivers report compliance.

TEST YOURSELF

✔ Explain the difference between structural and functional scoliosis.

✔ When should screening for scoliosis be started? What is the procedure for scoliosis screening?

✔ What are the ways scoliosis can be treated?

Did you determine that **Tyrone** will likely have a closed reduction of the fracture and be placed in a cast? What nursing care will he need while he is in the cast? What will you monitor closely in Tyrone when the cast is applied as well as during his recovery process? What will you reinforce related to teaching for Tyrone and his family caregivers?

KEY POINTS

- Bone growth takes place between birth and puberty. During childhood, the bones are more spongelike and can bend and break more easily than in adults. Because the bones are still in the process of growing, breaks in the bone heal more quickly than do breaks in adults.

- In a complete fracture, the fragments of the bone are separated. In an incomplete fracture, the fragments remain partially joined. The types of fractures seen in children are often incomplete; the bone may buckle or bow rather than break. Greenstick fractures are caused by incomplete ossification and spiral fractures twist around the bone. A closed fracture is a single break in the bone without penetration of the skin; an open fracture is where the bone penetrates the skin. Most fractures are treated by realignment and immobilization using either traction or closed manipulation and casting.

- Neurovascular checks are done in a child with a musculoskeletal disorder to monitor the child's neurovascular status to detect and prevent tissue and nerve damage. Compartment syndrome is a serious neurovascular concern that occurs when increasing pressure within the muscle compartment causes decreased circulation.

- Monitoring the neurovascular status is sometimes referred to as CMS (circulation, movement, sensation) checks and includes observing, documenting, and reporting pain, pulses, paresthesia, paralysis, or pallor.

- The basic types of traction are skin traction and skeletal traction. Examples of skin traction are Bryant traction, Buck traction, and Russell traction. Examples of skeletal traction are 90–90-degree traction, balanced suspension traction, and cervical skeletal tongs traction. Dunlop traction can be either skin or skeletal.

- Osteomyelitis is an infection of the bone usually caused by *Staphylococcus aureus*. IV antibiotic medications are followed by administration of oral antibiotics for treatment. Nursing care includes reducing pain by positioning the affected limb, minimizing movement of the limb, and administering medication.

- The most common form of MD is Duchenne (pseudohypertrophic) muscular dystrophy. The characteristics include difficulty standing or walking, trunk muscle weakness, and mild intellectual disability. Weakness of leg, arm, and shoulder muscles progresses gradually with the child usually becoming wheelchair-bound.

- Slipped capital femoral epiphysis is a condition that occurs when the femoral head dislocates from the neck of the femur at the growth plate and slips down and backward. It commonly develops during an adolescent growth spurt or in an overweight or obese child. Pain and a limp are presenting symptoms. Bedrest is maintained until surgical correction is done to treat the condition.

- Legg–Calvé–Perthes disease is an aseptic necrosis of the head of the femur. The treatment includes use of a brace, traction, or cast to hold the head of the femur in place during healing.

- The treatment for osteosarcoma is to remove the bone or the limb where the tumor is found. For Ewing sarcoma, the tumor must be removed and radiation is done. In both disorders, chemotherapy is given.

- Juvenile idiopathic arthritis (JIA) is an autoimmune disorder which primarily affects the joints and connective tissue. Enteric-coated aspirin had long been the drug of choice for JIA, but because of the concern of aspirin therapy and Reye syndrome, nonsteroidal anti-inflammatory drugs (NSAIDs), such as naproxen and ibuprofen, are used. The primary benefit of using these drugs is their anti-inflammatory effects. To decrease the side effects, the drugs should be administered with food or milk. disease-modifying antirheumatic drugs (DMARDs) and glucocorticoids also are used in the treatment of JIA.

- Scoliosis is a lateral curvature of the spine, either structural or functional. Nonsurgical treatment may be transcutaneous electrical muscle stimulation (TENS) and exercise for mild curvatures. The most common treatment is the use of braces, such as the Boston brace or the TLSO brace. Surgical treatment includes the use of rods, screws, hooks, and spinal fusion. Goals include minimizing the disruption of activities, preventing injury, and maintaining skin integrity and self-image.

INTERNET RESOURCES

Muscular Dystrophy
www.mda.org

Juvenile Idiopathic Arthritis
www.arthritis.org

Scoliosis
www.nsf@scoliosis.org

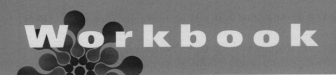

NCLEX-STYLE REVIEW QUESTIONS

1. The nurse is leading a discussion with a group of peers regarding different types of fractures. Which of the following best describes an open fracture?
   a. A fracture in which the fragments of the bone are separated
   b. A fracture in which the broken bone penetrates the skin
   c. A fracture in which there is a single break in the bone without penetration of the skin
   d. A fracture in which the fragments of the bone remain partially joined

2. In caring for a child in traction, of the following interventions, which is the *highest* priority for the nurse?
   a. The nurse should monitor for decreased circulation every 4 hours.
   b. The nurse should clean the pin sites at least once every 8 hours.
   c. The nurse should provide age-appropriate activities for the child.
   d. The nurse should record accurate intake and output.

3. The nurse is reinforcing client teaching with a child who has been placed in a brace to treat scoliosis. Which of the following statements made by the child indicates an understanding of the treatment?
   a. "I am so glad I can take this brace off for the school dance."
   b. "At least when I take a shower I have a few minutes out of this brace."
   c. "Wearing this brace only during the night won't be so embarrassing."
   d. "When I start feeling tired, I can just take my brace off for a few minutes."

4. The nurse is caring for a child after an accident in which the child fractured his arm. A cast has been applied to the child's right arm. Which of the following actions should the nurse implement? Select all that apply.
   a. Wear a protective gown when moving the child's arm.
   b. Document any signs of pain.
   c. Check radial pulse in both arms.
   d. Wear sterile gloves when removing or touching the cast.
   e. Monitor the color of the nail beds in the right hand.

STUDY ACTIVITIES

1. Using the table below, list the areas that must be checked and monitored when doing a neurovascular status check (CMS check) on a child with a fracture. Include the area to be monitored, the definition or explanation, observations, and documentation.

Area to be Monitored (the Five P's)	Definition or Explanation	Observations (What Signs to Look for)	Documentation

2. Develop a list of games and activities that would be appropriate to use for a 10-year-old girl in skeletal traction. Keep in mind the child's age and stage of growth and development. Share your list with your peers.

3. Call the Muscular Dystrophy Association national headquarters or your local Muscular Dystrophy Association chapter. Ask what is available in your community to help and support children and families of children with MD.

4. Do an internet search on "juvenile idiopathic arthritis." List the sites you found in this search. What are some of the topics you noted were discussed on these sites about this disorder. Share with your peers how you can use this information in working with children and families of children who have juvenile idiopathic arthritis.

CRITICAL THINKING: WHAT WOULD YOU DO?

1. Twelve-year-old Carrie has scoliosis and must wear a TLSO brace. She says she thinks it is really ugly. Carrie tells you she does not want to go to school because she cannot wear clothes similar to those of her friends.
   a. What feelings do you think Carrie might be going through in this situation?
   b. What would you say in response to Carrie?
   c. What are some ideas you could share with Carrie regarding clothing she might wear?

2. You are caring for 2-year-old Cole, who has muscular dystrophy (MD). Cole's family begins asking you questions about the disease. How would you answer the following questions?

   a. What caused Cole to have MD?
   b. What will happen to Cole physically as he gets older and the disease progresses?
   c. What is the long-term prognosis for Cole?
   d. Where can we find other families who have a child with MD?

3. Dosage calculation: After a course of IV antibiotic medications for treatment of osteomyelitis, a child has been prescribed a regimen of nafcillin by mouth. The child weighs 17.6 lb. The usual dosage range of this medication is 6.25 to 12.5 mg/kg every 6 hours. Answer the following.

   a. How many kilograms does the child weigh?
   b. What is the low dose of nafcillin for this child every 6 hours?
   c. What is the high dose of nafcillin for this child every 6 hours?
   d. If the child is given the high dose, how much nafcillin will be given in a 24-hour period?

41

The Child With an Integumentary Disorder/ Communicable Disease

Learning Objectives

At the conclusion of this chapter, you will:

1. Discuss ways the child's integumentary and immune systems differ from the adult's systems.
2. Explain integumentary disorders, including seborrheic dermatitis, miliaria rubra, diaper dermatitis, candidiasis, staphylococcal infections, and impetigo.
3. Discuss acne vulgaris, including the causes, treatment, and nursing care.
4. Explain fungal infections seen in children.
5. Describe pediculosis and scabies, and discuss the treatment and nursing concerns when treating a child with these conditions in the hospital.
6. Discuss allergic disorders and how allergens that produce positive reactions on skin testing are commonly treated.
7. Describe the causes, manifestations, treatment, and nursing care of the child diagnosed with atopic dermatitis (eczema).
8. Describe contact dermatitis, and discuss the causes, manifestations, and treatment.
9. Compare various types of bites often seen in children, including animal, spider, tick, snake, and insect bites.
10. Differentiate among superficial, partial-thickness, and full-thickness burns.
11. Describe emergency treatment of a minor burn and of a moderate or severe burn.
12. State the major causes of burns in small children, and discuss the nursing care of the child with a burn.
13. List the organisms that cause HPV, gonorrhea, chlamydia, genital herpes, and syphilis, and the drug of choice to treat them.
14. Discuss human immunodeficiency virus (HIV) and acquired immunodeficiency syndrome (AIDS), including how the virus is transmitted, treatment, and nursing care.
15. Describe infectious mononucleosis.
16. Discuss communicable diseases, including modes of transmission; ways to prevent them; active, natural, and passive immunity; and nursing care.

Charlotte Dey is now 9 months old. When Charlotte was 7 months old, her mother noticed reddened areas on her cheeks, which eventually seemed to spread to her arms and legs. Charlotte was fussy and scratched the areas as if they were itching. A diagnosis of atopic dermatitis (eczema) was made. As you read this chapter, think about what might be some possible causes of atopic dermatitis in Charlotte.

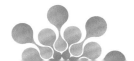

GROWTH AND DEVELOPMENT OF THE INTEGUMENTARY AND IMMUNE SYSTEMS

The skin is the major organ of the integumentary system and is the largest organ of the body. Accessory structures, such as the hair and nails, also make up the integumentary system. The major role of the skin is to protect the organs and structures of the body against bacteria, chemicals, and injury. The skin helps regulate the body temperature by heating and cooling. Excretion in the form of perspiration is also a function of the skin glands, called the sweat glands. Sebaceous glands in the skin secrete oils to lubricate the skin and hair. These oils help prevent dryness of the skin. As a sensory organ, the skin has nerve endings that respond to pain, pressure, heat, and cold. When the skin is exposed to sunlight (ultraviolet light), synthesis of vitamin D occurs.

The integumentary system, including the accessory structures, is in place at birth but the system is immature. The newborn's skin is thin and has less subcutaneous fat beneath the layer of skin. Regulating temperature is more difficult in the newborn because of these factors. As the child grows, the sweat glands mature and increase the capability of the skin to help in the regulation of temperature. The sebaceous secretions in the infant and young child are less than those in the older child and adult, causing the skin of children to dry and crack more easily. In addition, the infant is more susceptible to skin irritants and bacteria, which might cause infection. Injury and some disorders can cause bruising to the skin, especially in the child.

Protecting the body from attacks from microorganisms and helping the body get rid of or resist invasion by foreign materials are the major roles of the immune system. Unlike other systems in the body that are made up of organs, the immune system is made up of cells and tissues that work to protect the body. Protective barriers, such as the skin and mucous membranes, help prevent pathogens from entering the body. When a pathogen enters the body, the immune system works to destroy the pathogen. This occurs when white blood cells known as macrophages surround, ingest, or neutralize the pathogen. The inflammatory process further helps get rid of the foreign substances. Another process of the immune system occurs when substances called antibodies destroy antigens, which are foreign protein substances. When the body is exposed to certain bacteria or viruses, the immune system fights to destroy the substance. In addition, the body develops immunity to that disease, so if the person has an exposure in the future, the immune system immediately responds, and symptoms do not occur. Immunizations work by creating artificial exposure to a certain agent that helps the body create immunity to that agent.

During fetal life, the mother's antibodies cross the placenta, giving the fetus temporary immunity against certain diseases. This immunity is present at birth and decreases during the first year of life. In the meantime, the infant begins developing antibodies to fight against pathogens and disease. In addition, during the first year of life, immunizations are started to help the infant develop protection against certain diseases. As the child grows and develops, the immune system also develops. The antibodies in the child increase as the child progresses through childhood.

INTEGUMENTARY DISORDERS

Integumentary disorders occur often in children. These disorders can be mild and resolve quickly, or they can be chronic and severe and can be difficult for the child and family caregivers to cope with.

Seborrheic Dermatitis

Seborrheic dermatitis is commonly known as cradle cap. Washing the child's hair and scalp every day can usually prevent it. Characterized by yellowish, greasy, scaly, or crusted patches on the scalp, it occurs in newborns and older infants, possibly as a result of excessive sebaceous gland activity. Family caregivers may be afraid to vigorously wash over the "soft spot." However, they need to understand that this is where cradle cap often begins and that careful but vigorous washing of the area with a washcloth can prevent this disorder. Using a fine-toothed baby comb after shampooing is also a helpful preventive measure. These principles are included in reinforcement of teaching about care of the newborn.

Once the condition exists, daily application of mineral oil helps loosen the crust. However, no attempt should be made to loosen it all at once because the delicate skin on the scalp may break and bleed and can easily become infected.

Miliaria Rubra

Miliaria rubra, often called prickly heat, is common in children who are exposed to summer heat or are overdressed. It also may appear in febrile illnesses and may be mistaken for the rash of one of the communicable diseases.

Clinical Manifestations

The rash appears as pinhead-sized erythematous (reddened) papules. It is most noticeable in areas where sweat glands are concentrated, such as folds of the skin, the axilla, and around the neck. It usually causes itching, making the child uncomfortable and fretful.

Treatment and Nursing Care

Treatment should be primarily preventive. The infant should be dressed in clothing that can breathe (such as cotton), or a diaper might be all the child needs to wear.

Tepid baths without soap help control the itching. A small amount of baking soda may be added to the bath water to help relieve discomfort.

Here's a Tip to Share

Family caregivers are often concerned that their baby is going to be cold; it is important they avoid bundling their child in layers of clothing in hot weather.

Diaper Dermatitis

Diaper dermatitis (diaper rash) is common in infancy, causing the baby discomfort and fretfulness. Some children seem to be more susceptible than others, possibly because of inherited sensitive skin.

Clinical Manifestations

Bacterial decomposition of urine produces ammonia, which is irritating to a child's tender skin. Diarrheal stools also produce a burning erythematous area in the anal region. Prolonged exposure to wet or soiled diapers, infrequently changed disposable diapers, inadequate cleansing of the diaper area (especially after bowel movements), sensitivity to some soaps or disposable diaper perfumes, and the use of strong laundry detergents without thorough rinsing are considered to be the causes. Yeast infections, notably candidiasis, are also causative factors.

Treatment and Nursing Care

Family caregivers should be reminded that the primary treatment is prevention. Diapers must be changed frequently without waiting for obvious leaking. Regular checking is necessary. Manufacturers of disposable diapers are constantly trying to improve the ability of disposable diapers to wick the wetness away from the child's skin. Diapers washed at commercial laundries are sterilized, preventing the growth of ammonia-forming bacteria. Many cloth diaper types are available and are presoaked, washed at home in hot water with a mild soap, and rinsed thoroughly, which decreases the potential skin irritants. Drying diapers in the sun or in a dryer also helps destroy bacteria. Exposing the diaper area to the air helps clear up the dermatitis.

Cleaning the diaper area from front to back with warm water and drying thoroughly with each diaper change helps improve or prevent the condition. If soap is necessary when cleaning stool from the child's buttocks and rectal area, be certain that the soap is completely rinsed before diapering. The use of commercial wet wipes may aggravate the condition. If the area becomes excoriated and sore, the health care provider may prescribe using a topical barrier ointment or paste, often containing petrolatum or zinc oxide. See Tips for Reinforcing Family Teaching: Preventing and Treating Diaper Rash.

Did You Know?

The use of baby powder when diapering is discouraged because caked powder helps create an environment in which organisms thrive.

Candidiasis

Candidiasis is caused by *Candida albicans*, the organism responsible for thrush and some cases of diaper rash.

Clinical Manifestations

Newborns can be exposed to a candidiasis vaginal infection in the mother during delivery. Thrush appears in the child's mouth as a white coating that looks like milk curds. Poor handwashing practices and inadequate washing of bottles

TIPS FOR REINFORCING FAMILY TEACHING

Preventing and Treating Diaper Rash

- Change diapers as soon as they are wet or soiled.
- Wash the baby's bottom with lukewarm water (a small amount of a mild cleansing product may be used but is not necessary), using wet cotton balls or by pouring water over area using a plastic squeeze bottle or washcloth soaked in water. Thoroughly dry diaper area by patting with a soft cloth before rediapering.
- Avoid using commercial baby wipes if skin is irritated. If used as an alternative to water, they must be fragrance- and alcohol-free.
- Expose the baby's bottom to air without diapers as much as possible to help the rash heal.
- Do not rub the rash. A cool, wet cloth can be soothing when placed over the area for 5 minutes three or four times a day.
- Use ointment or paste as recommended by the health care provider. Apply a very thin layer only. Wash off at each diaper change, using mineral oil on a cotton ball if needed.
- Avoid using powder, corn starch, or baking soda; these can cause respiratory problems.
- Rinse cloth diapers in clear water after presoaking and washing in hot water.
- Do not use fabric softeners because they can cause a skin reaction.
- Avoid fastening the diaper too tightly, which irritates the baby's skin.
- Rinse all of the baby's clothes thoroughly to eliminate soap or detergent residue that may irritate the baby's skin.
- Do not overdress or overcover the baby. Sweating makes the rash worse.

and nipples are contributing factors. In addition, infants and toddlers may experience episodes of thrush or diaper rash after antibiotic therapy, which may upset the balance of normal intestinal flora, leading to candidal overgrowth.

Treatment and Nursing Care

Treatment for diaper rash caused by *C. albicans* (Fig. 41-1) is the application of nystatin ointment or cream to the affected

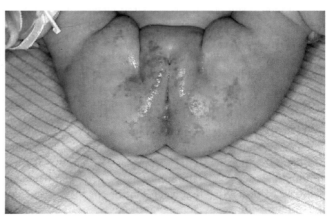

FIGURE 41-1 A bright red rash occurs with diaper rash caused by *C. albicans*.

area. Application of nystatin to the oral lesions every 6 hours is an effective treatment. In all cases, good hygiene practices should be reinforced.

TEST YOURSELF

✔ How can seborrheic dermatitis (cradle cap) be prevented?

✔ What causes diaper dermatitis?

✔ What is the causative agent for thrush? How might a newborn be exposed to this, and how is it treated?

Staphylococcal Infection

Staphylococcal infections are most often caused by the bacterium *Staphylococcus aureus*. These infections can range from mild to severe and may be seen in various parts of the body, but often they are skin infections. The staphylococci bacterium may be found in the nose or on the skin; when the skin is broken or injured, the bacterium may cause infection.

The skin lesions look like pimples and may be red, swollen, painful, and may have pus or drainage. Staph infections are contagious, and direct contact with the infected area is commonly how the infection is spread. Contact with personal items, such as hair brushes, towels, and sports equipment, may also spread the infection. Good handwashing and keeping the injured area clean decrease the spread. Transmission-based precautions are followed to prevent spreading the bacterium, and antibiotics are used to treat the skin infection.

Methicillin-resistant *S. aureus* (MRSA) is a strain of the bacteria that is resistant to the antibiotics normally used for treatment, thus making the skin infection much harder to treat. If the child gets an MRSA infection while in the hospital, it is called **nosocomial**, or hospital- or healthcare-associated infection. In recent years, cases of MRSA acquired outside the hospital, known as community-associated infection, have been seen more frequently. Cases have been noted in day care centers and among children who participate with athletic teams in contact sports. The difficulty of treating these infections increases the severity of the infection and may cause serious concerns.

Impetigo

Impetigo is a superficial bacterial skin infection (Fig. 41-2). In the newborn, the primary causative organism is *S. aureus*. In the older child, the most common causative organism is group A beta-hemolytic streptococci. Impetigo in the newborn is usually bullous (blisterlike, fluid filled); in the older child, the lesions are nonbullous and have a honey-colored, crusted appearance.

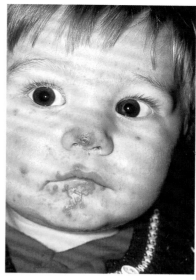

FIGURE 41-2 Typical lesions of impetigo. Note the honey-colored crusting appearance.

Treatment

Treatment for impetigo includes the use of topical antibiotic therapy, such as mupirocin. Oral antibiotics may be administered for a 7- to 10-day course. Daily washing of the crusts helps speed the healing process. Because impetigo is commonly a streptococcal infection in the older child, rheumatic fever or acute glomerulonephritis is a possible concern. Reinforcement of teaching with family caregivers should include following the treatment guidelines and watching for symptoms that might indicate a concern.

> **Warning!**
> Impetigo is highly contagious and can spread quickly. Impetigo in the newborn nursery is cause for immediate concern.

Nursing Care

When caring for a young child who has impetigo and is hospitalized, you must follow contact (skin and wound) transmission precautions, including wearing a cover gown and gloves. The child should be separated from other children to deter spread of the disease. Crusts can be soaked off with warm water, followed by an application of topical antibiotics. Cover the child's hands or apply elbow restraints to prevent scratching of lesions. Careful handwashing by nursing personnel and family members is essential.

The older child with impetigo is treated at home. The family caregivers must follow good hygiene practices to prevent the spread of impetigo to other children in the household or other contacts of the child in the day care center, preschool, or elementary school. Lesions occur primarily on the face but may spread to any part of the body. The crusts and drainage are contagious. Because the lesions are pruritic (itchy), the child must learn to keep their fingers and hands away from the lesions. Nails should be trimmed to prevent scratching of lesions. Family members should be reminded not to share towels and washcloths.

Acne Vulgaris

Acne may be only a mild case of oily skin and a few blackheads, or it may be a severe type with ropelike cystic lesions that leave deep scars, both physical and emotional. To adolescents who want to be attractive and popular, even a mild case of acne (often called "zits") can cause great anxiety, shyness, and social withdrawal.

Clinical Manifestations

Characterized by the appearance of **comedones** (blackheads and whiteheads), papules, and pustules on the face, the back, and to some extent the chest, acne is caused by a variety of factors, including the following:

- Increased hormonal levels, especially androgens
- Hereditary factors
- Irritation and irritating substances, such as vigorous scrubbing and cosmetics with greasy bases
- Growth of anaerobic bacteria

Each hair follicle has an associated sebaceous gland that in adolescents produces increased **sebum** (oily secretion). The sebum is blocked by epithelial cells and becomes trapped in the follicle. When anaerobic organisms infect this collection, inflammation occurs, which causes papules, pustules, and nodules (Fig. 41-3). Several types of acne lesions are often present at one time.

Treatment and Nursing Care

The topical medications may be a combination of benzoyl peroxide, salicylic acid, and retinoids and come in a variety of forms, such as topical cleansers, lotions, creams, sticks, pads, gels, and bars. The usual treatment plan for mild acne is topical application of one of these medications once or twice a day. These medications should not be applied to normal skin or allowed to get into the eyes or nose or on other mucous membranes. Antibiotics may be administered for inflammatory acne. Antibiotic therapy may require an extended treatment course followed by tapering of the dosage.

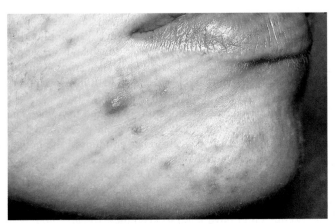

FIGURE 41-3 Acne vulgaris.

Isotretinoin may be used for severe inflammatory acne. There has been controversy over the use of this medication because of the concern over the potential side effects of depression, suicide, and the danger to the fetus if a woman becomes pregnant while taking isotretinoin. This potent, effective oral medication is used for hard-to-treat cystic acne. Side effects are common but often diminish when the drug dosage is reduced. Warn the adolescent about some of the side effects, including dry lips and skin, eye irritation, temporary worsening of acne, epistaxis (nosebleed), bleeding and inflammation of the gums, itching, photosensitivity (sensitivity to the sun), and joint and muscle pain.

> **This Is Critical to Remember**
>
> Isotretinoin is a pregnancy category X drug; it must not be used at all during pregnancy because of serious risk of fetal abnormalities. The FDA developed a restricted distribution program called iPLEDGE for prescribing and administration of isotretinoin. Prescribers, clients, and pharmacies must be registered and follow strict adherence to the iPLEDGE requirements (the female client must commit to two forms of contraception a month before, during, and 1 month after therapy, and she must have two negative blood or urine pregnancy tests before beginning) in order for the medication to be given to an individual. A pregnancy test is done once a month while on the medication.

Although the adolescent's perception of the disfigurement caused by acne may seem out of proportion to the actual severity of the condition, acknowledge and accept their feelings. Reinforce teaching with the adolescent and the family caregiver to wash the lesions gently with soap and water; do not scrub vigorously. Comedones should be removed gently by following the health care provider's recommendations and using careful aseptic techniques. Careful removal produces no scarring—a goal for every teen.

Your and the family caregiver's understanding and support are the most important aspects of caring for the adolescent with acne. Reassure the teen that eating chocolate and fatty foods does not cause acne, but a well-balanced, nutritious diet does promote healing.

FUNGAL INFECTIONS

Fungi that live in the outer (dead) layers of the skin, hair, and nails can develop into superficial infections. **Tinea**, also called ringworm, is the term commonly applied to these fungal infections, which are further differentiated by the part of the body infected.

Tinea Capitis (Ringworm of the Scalp)

A fungal infection of the scalp is called tinea capitis. The most common cause is infection with *Microsporum audouinii*, which is transmitted from person to person through combs, towels, hats, barber scissors, or direct contact.

A less common type, *Microsporum canis*, is transmitted from animal to child.

Clinical Manifestations

Tinea capitis begins as a small papule, sometimes appearing like a black dot, on the scalp and spreads, leaving scaly patches of baldness. There may be severe itching. The hairs become brittle and break off easily.

Treatment and Nursing Care

Griseofulvin, an oral antifungal, is the medication of choice. Because treatment may be prolonged (3 months or more), compliance must be reinforced. Be sure that family caregivers and children understand the medication therapy. Children who are properly treated may attend school. Assure the child and family caregiver that hair loss is not permanent.

Tinea Corporis (Ringworm of the Body)

Tinea corporis is ringworm of the body that affects the epidermal skin layer. The child usually contracts tinea corporis from direct contact with an infected person or with an infected puppy or kitten.

The lesions appear as an itchy, scaly ring with clearing in the center, occurring on any part of the body. They resemble the lesions of scalp ringworm. Topical antifungal agents, such as terbinafine, clotrimazole, tolnaftate, and griseofulvin, are used to treat this condition.

Tinea Pedis

Tinea pedis, ringworm of the feet, is more commonly known as athlete's foot. It is evidenced by the scaling or cracking of the skin between the toes. The area itches, is tender to touch, and sometimes has a foul odor. Transmission is by direct or indirect contact with skin lesions from infected people. Contaminated sidewalks, floors, pool decks, and shower stalls spread the condition to those who walk barefoot. Tinea pedis, usually found in adolescents and adults, is becoming more prevalent among school-age children. Examination under a microscope of scrapings from the lesions is necessary for definite diagnosis.

Care includes washing the feet with soap and water and then gently removing scabs and crusts and applying a topical agent, such as tolnaftate or butenafine. Griseofulvin by mouth is also useful. During the chronic phase, the use of ointment, scrupulous foot hygiene, and frequent changing of white cotton socks are helpful. Application of a topical agent for as long as 6 weeks is recommended.

Tinea Cruris

Tinea cruris, more commonly known as jock itch or ringworm of the inner thighs and inguinal area, is caused by the same organisms that cause tinea corporis. It is more common in athletes and is uncommon in preadolescent children. Tinea cruris is pruritic and localized to the area. Treatment is the same as for tinea corporis. Cotton underwear is recommended. Sitz baths may also be soothing.

> ### TEST YOURSELF
> ✔ Why is impetigo a concern in the newborn nursery? What procedures should you follow when caring for a child with impetigo?
> ✔ Why should comedones, seen in acne vulgaris, be removed carefully?
> ✔ How is ringworm of the scalp, tinea capitis, usually transmitted?
> ✔ Which classification of medication is given to treat ringworm?

PARASITIC INFECTIONS

Parasites are organisms that live on or within another living organism, from which they obtain their food supply. Lice and the scabies mite live by sucking the blood of the host.

Pediculosis

Pediculosis (lice infestation) may be caused by *Pediculus humanus capitis* (head lice), *Pediculus humanus corporis* (body lice), or *Pthirus pubis* (pubic lice). Head lice are the most common infestation in children. Animal lice are not transferred to humans.

Head lice are passed from child to child by direct contact or indirectly by contact with combs, headgear, or bed linen.

Clinical Manifestations

Lice, which are rarely seen, lay their eggs, called nits, on the head where they attach to hair strands. The nits can be seen as tiny pearly white flecks attached to the hair shafts. They look much like dandruff, but dandruff flakes can be flicked off easily, whereas the nits are tightly attached and not easily removed. The nits hatch in about 1 week, and the lice become sexually mature in about 2 weeks.

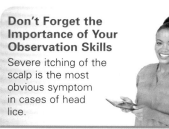

Don't Forget the Importance of Your Observation Skills
Severe itching of the scalp is the most obvious symptom in cases of head lice.

Treatment and Nursing Care

Nonprescription medications, topical pediculicides, are available to treat cases of head lice. These include pyrethrins and permethrin, which are extracts from the chrysanthemum flower. These medications are safe and usually effective in killing the lice. A second treatment is suggested in 7 to 9 days to kill the nits after they have hatched. If over-the-counter preparations do not effectively kill the lice, prescription medications may be used. Malathion is effective in treating lice and nits. Few side effects have been reported, but if used on open sores, it may cause the skin to sting, so it should not be used if the head has been scratched. Lindane shampoo has been one of the most commonly used treatments for many years and is usually safe. Overuse, misuse, or accidental swallowing of lindane can be toxic to the brain and nervous system, so its use is suggested only in cases that do not respond to other treatments.

After the hair is wet with warm water, the medication is applied like any ordinary shampoo—about 1 oz is used. The head should be lathered for several minutes, following the directions on the label for each specific medication, and then rinsed thoroughly and dried. After the hair is dry, it should be combed with a combing tool or a fine-toothed comb dipped in warm white vinegar to remove remaining nits and nit shells. Shampooing is repeated according to the product instructions to remove any lice that may have been missed as nits and since hatched. Avoid getting medication into the eyes or on mucous membranes. When treating a child in the hospital for pediculosis, wear a disposable gown, gloves, and head cover for protection.

Family caregivers are often embarrassed when the school nurse sends word that the child has head lice. They can be reassured that lice infestation is common and can happen to any child; it is not a reflection on the caregiver's housekeeping. All family members should be inspected and treated as needed. See Tips for Reinforcing Family Teaching: Eliminating Pediculi Infestations for other useful information.

TIPS FOR REINFORCING FAMILY TEACHING

Eliminating Pediculi Infestations

- Wash all of the child's bedding and clothing in hot water, and dry in a hot dryer.
- Vacuum carpets, car seats, mattresses, and upholstered furniture very thoroughly. Discard vacuum dust bag.
- Wash pillows, stuffed animals, and other washable items the same way clothing is washed.
- Dry clean nonwashable items.
- If items cannot be washed or dry cleaned, seal in plastic bag for at least 5 to 6 days to break the reproductive cycle of lice.
- Wash combs, brushes, and other hair items (rollers, curlers, barrettes, etc.) in shampoo and soak for 1 hour.
- Remind children not to share hats and combs.
- If you discover the infestation, report it to the child's school or day care.
- Have school personnel disinfect headphones.

 Concept Mastery Alert

It is important to explain that the treatment for head lice must be repeated in 7 to 9 days so that lice that were nits during the first treatment can be now treated.

Scabies

Scabies is a skin infestation caused by the scabies mite *Sarcoptes scabiei*. The female mite burrows in areas between the fingers and toes and in warm folds of the body, such as the axilla, buttocks, and groin, to lay eggs. Transmission occurs through close personal skin-to-skin contact.

Clinical Manifestations

Burrows are visible as dark lines, and the mite is seen as a black dot at the end of the burrow. Severe itching occurs, causing scratching with resulting secondary infection.

Treatment and Nursing Care

The body, except for the face, is treated with permethrin cream. The directions for the medication should be followed closely. The body is first cleaned with soap and water, and then the lotion is applied on all areas of the body except the face. It is usually left on the skin for 8 to 14 hours and then washed off with warm water. The treatment is repeated in 1 to 2 weeks.

Family caregivers should follow the tips recommended for pediculosis. All who had close contact with the child within a 30- to 60-day period should be treated. The rash and itch may continue for several weeks even though the mites have been successfully eliminated.

TEST YOURSELF

✔ Explain what pediculosis is and at what sites it is frequently found in children.

✔ How is pediculosis treated?

✔ Why is it important for the child with scabies to avoid scratching involved areas?

ALLERGIC DISORDERS

Millions of Americans have allergic disorders, many of which begin in childhood. Children with allergies are hampered because of poor appetites, poor sleep, and restricted physical activity in play and at school, all of which often result in altered physical and personality development. Children whose parents or grandparents have allergies are more likely to become allergic than are other children. An allergic condition is caused by sensitivity to a substance called an **allergen** (an antigen that causes an allergy). Thousands of allergens exist.

Allergens may enter the body through various routes, the most common being the nose, throat, eyes, skin, digestive tract, and bronchial tissues in the lungs. The first time the child comes in contact with an allergen, no reaction may be evident, but an immune response is stimulated—helper lymphocytes stimulate B lymphocytes to make immunoglobulin E antibody. The immunoglobulin E antibody attaches to mast cells and macrophages. When contacted again, the allergen attaches to the immunoglobulin E receptor sites, and a response occurs in which certain substances, such as histamine, are released; these substances produce the symptoms known as allergy.

Anaphylaxis is an acute hypersensitive response to an allergen and can occur with exposure to any allergen, but in particular is seen with reactions to drug, food, insect stings, radiopaque dye, and latex sensitivities. Anaphylaxis may be life-threatening; can involve many body systems; and include severe symptoms of dyspnea, airway obstruction, and shock. The condition can occur within seconds or minutes of exposure to the allergen, is a medical emergency, and is treated with lifesaving measures. Children with allergies who are at high risk for severe reactions and anaphylaxis are prescribed an epinephrine auto-injector (EpiPen). The child and family caregiver are educated about when and how to use it should the child have a reaction. They are encouraged to have it with them at all times.

Allergic rhinitis is an allergic disorder caused by sensitization to allergens in the environment such as animal dander, house dust, pollens, and molds. The allergic response often presents with nasal discharge, postnasal drip, sneezing and conjunctivitis (see Chapter 36 for discussion of allergic rhinitis). Asthma may be triggered by a hypersensitive response to allergens, including food allergies and irritants. Symptoms seen with these allergic responses include cough, wheezing, and difficulty breathing (see Chapter 36 for discussion of asthma).

Medications such as anti-inflammatory drugs (NSAIDs) and antibiotics (penicillin is the most common allergen of this group) can cause allergic reactions. Sometimes the response with a drug allergy is an anaphylactic reaction.

Food allergies or a hypersensitivity to certain foods or food additives occurs with ingestion of or sometimes contact with these foods. Common food allergies include milk, eggs, nuts, shellfish, wheat, soy, and chocolate. Responses to these allergens may include hives; flushing; swelling of the mouth, lip, face, and/or tongue; urticaria; gastrointestinal symptoms such as nausea, abdominal pain and cramping, vomiting, and diarrhea; and sometimes respiratory symptoms. The food allergen must be identified and removed from the child's diet. Some children have a food intolerance in which they have a negative physiological response to a food. These have to be differentiated from being a true food allergy.

Diagnosis of an allergy requires a careful history and physical examination and possibly skin and blood tests. Skin testing is generally done when removal of obvious allergens is impossible or has not brought relief. If a food allergy is suspected, an elimination diet may help identify the allergen. Eliminating the food suspected is sometimes difficult because there are often "hidden" ingredients in food products.

Be Careful!
The family caregivers of a child allergic to peanuts must always read labels of food products. They will find many unexpected products contain peanuts or peanut oil.

When specific allergens have been identified, clients can either avoid them or, if impossible, undergo immunization therapy by injection. This process is called **hyposensitization** or immunotherapy.

Hyposensitization is performed for the allergens that produce a positive reaction on skin testing. The allergist sets up a schedule for injections in gradually increasing doses until a maintenance dose is reached. The client should remain in the health care provider's office for 20 to 30 minutes after the injection in case any reaction occurs. Reactions are treated with epinephrine. Severe reactions in children are uncommon, and hyposensitization is considered a safe procedure with considerable benefit for some children.

Atopic Dermatitis (Eczema)

Atopic dermatitis or eczema is considered, at least in part, an allergic reaction to an irritant. It is fairly common during the first year of life after the age of 3 months. It is uncommon in breast-fed babies before they are given additional foods.

Eczema is characterized by three factors:

- Hereditary predisposition
- Hypersensitivity of the deeper layers of the skin to protein or proteinlike allergens
- Allergens to which the child is sensitive that may be inhaled, ingested, or absorbed through direct contact

Infants who have eczema tend to have allergic rhinitis or asthma later in life.

Clinical Manifestations

Atopic dermatitis usually starts on the cheeks and spreads to the extensor surfaces of the arms and legs (Fig. 41-4). Eventually the entire trunk may become affected. The skin is severely dry with initial reddening quickly followed by papule and vesicle formation. Itching is intense, and the child's scratching makes the skin weep and crust. The areas easily become infected by *S. aureus* or herpes simplex.

Diagnosis

The most common allergens involved in eczema are as follows:

- Foods: egg white, cow's milk, wheat products, orange juice, tomato juice
- Inhalants: house dust, pollens, animal dander
- Materials: wool, nylon, plastic

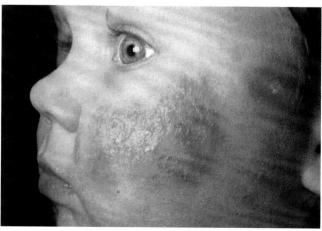

FIGURE 41-4 Infant with atopic dermatitis (eczema).

However, diagnosis is not simple. Often, trial by elimination is as effective as any other diagnostic tool. Skin testing on a young child generally is not considered valid, so it is discouraged as a means of diagnosis.

An elimination diet may be helpful in ruling out offending foods. The child is fed a hypoallergenic diet consisting of a milk substitute, such as soy formula; vitamin supplements; and other foods known to be hypoallergenic. If the skin condition shows improvement, other foods are added one at a time at an interval of about 1 week; the effects are noted, and any foods that cause a reaction are eliminated. The protein of egg white is such a common offender that most health care providers advise against feeding whole eggs to infants until late in the first year of life (see Table 38-1 for a list of foods that may cause allergies).

Great care must be taken to prevent the child from becoming undernourished. An elimination program must always be initiated under the supervision of a nutritionist or health care provider.

Treatment

Oral antihistamines may help relieve the itching and allow rest. Oral antibiotics may be ordered for a coexistent infection, such as a staphylococcal infection. If no infection exists, topical corticosteroid ointments may be used to relieve inflammation.

Wet soaks or colloidal baths may also be prescribed for their soothing effects. The water should be tepid for further soothing, and soap may not be recommended because of its drying effect. Some health care providers recommend the use of a mild soap, such as Dove or Neutrogena, or a soap substitute. Lubrication is essential to retain moisture and prevent evaporation after the bath. Emollients containing lanolin or petrolatum, such as Aquaphor or Eucerin, may be prescribed.

Inhalant and contact allergens should be avoided as much as possible. In the child's bedroom, window drapes or curtains, dresser scarves, and rugs should be removed or made of washable fabric that can be frequently laundered. Furniture should be washed frequently. The crib mattress should have a nonallergenic covering and be washed frequently with careful cleaning along the binding. Feather pillows must be eliminated, and stuffed toys should be washable. It may be necessary to provide new homes for household pets. However, dander from the pets can remain in carpets, crevices, and overstuffed furniture for a long time. Carpets and area rugs may need to be removed. A home, especially an older one with a damp basement, may be harboring molds that shed allergenic spores. Bathrooms are also places for molds and mildews to hide, especially in warm, humid climates.

Take Note, This Could Be Serious

Smallpox vaccinations are not given routinely but are sometimes given to persons preparing to travel. Smallpox vaccinations are contraindicated for the child with eczema, and the child must be kept away from anyone who has recently been vaccinated. As well, the child should be kept away from anyone with a herpes simplex infection (cold sore).

Nursing Process and Care Plan *for the Child With Atopic Dermatitis (Eczema)*

Assessment (Data Collection)

The family caregivers of the child with eczema are often frustrated and exhausted. Although the caregiver can be assured that most cases of eczema clear up by the age of 2 years, this does little to relieve the current situation. Hospitalization is avoided unless intensive treatment is necessary because these children are highly susceptible to infections.

During the interview with the family caregivers, cover the history of the condition, including treatments that have been tried and foods that have been ruled out as allergens. Include a thorough review of the home environment. Evaluate the family caregivers' knowledge of the condition.

The data collection about the child includes obtaining vital signs, observing general nutritional state, and doing a complete examination of all body parts with careful documentation of the eruptions and their location and size. Unaffected areas as well as those that are weeping and crusted should be noted.

Nursing Care Focus

When developing evidence-based nursing care focuses for the child with atopic dermatitis (eczema), altered skin integrity, impaired comfort, and sleep deprivation must be considered. The child is at risk for malnutrition and infection; prevention of these concerns is important. Reinforcing family teaching is a key aspect of caring for the child and the family.

Outcome Identification and Planning

The major goals for the child with atopic dermatitis are preserving skin integrity, maintaining comfort, improving sleep patterns, maintaining good nutrition (within the constraints of allergens), and preventing infection of skin lesions. A family caregiver goal is increasing knowledge about the disease process. Base the nursing plan of care on these goals.

Nursing Care Focus

- Altered skin integrity related to lesions and inflammatory process

Goal

- The child's skin integrity will be maintained or will improve.

Implementations for Maintaining Skin Integrity

Cover the lesions with light clothing. The child's nails must be kept closely cut, and mittenlike hand coverings can be used. Use restraints only if necessary. Elbow restraints may sometimes be used. Remove restraints at least every hour—more often, if feasible—but do not allow the child to rub or scratch while the restraints are off. If ointments or wet dressings must be kept in place on the child's face to maintain skin hydration, a mask may be made by cutting holes into a cotton stockinette-type material to correspond to eyes, nose, and mouth. Wet dressings on the rest of the body can be kept in place by wrapping the child in a "mummy" fashion. Dressings may be left on for an extended period, but they should not be allowed to dry because that can create open areas when they are removed.

Check Out This Tip

"Onesies," one-piece, loose-fitting terry cloth or cotton outfits for children, come in many colors, patterns, and designs and can be helpful in keeping a child from scratching.

Evaluation of Goal/Desired Outcome

The child:

- has decreased scratching.
- exhibits skin with fewer breakdowns.

Nursing Care Focus

- Impaired comfort and sleep deprivation related to intense itching and irritation

Goal

- The child will have less itching and adequate sleep.

Implementations for Providing Comfort and Promoting Sleep

Plan soothing baths, such as a colloidal bath (Aveeno), just before naptime or bedtime, to help promote sleep. Keep the skin hydrated using topical ointments and fragrance-free creams and moisturizers. Time medications, such as antihistamines, so that they will be effective immediately after the bath when the child is most relaxed.

Evaluation of Goal/Desired Outcome

- The child has less itching and sleeps more comfortably.

Nursing Care Focus

- Malnutrition risk related to elimination diet

Goal

- The child's nutritional intake will meet the needs for growth and development.

Implementations for Maintaining Adequate Nutrition

Weigh the child on admission and daily thereafter. This procedure gives some indication of weight gain. If an elimination diet is being used, the diet should be carefully balanced within the framework of the foods permitted and supplemented with vitamin and mineral preparations as needed. Encourage drinking of fluids to prevent dehydration.

Evaluation of Goal/Desired Outcome

The child:

- has no weight loss.
- has weight gain appropriate for age.

Nursing Care Focus

- Infection risk related to broken skin and lesions

Goal

- The child will be free of infected skin lesions.

Implementations for Preventing Infection

As stated, usually these children are kept out of the healthcare facility because of the concern about infection. However, they can also become infected at home. Whether in the healthcare facility or at home, the child should be placed in a room alone or in a room where there is no other child with any type of infection. Administer antibiotics as ordered. For open lesions, good handwashing and aseptic techniques are necessary to prevent infection.

Evaluation of Goal/Desired Outcome

The child:

- does not scratch lesions.
- shows no signs of infection related to lesions.

Nursing Care Focus

- Knowledge deficiency of family caregivers related to disease condition and treatment

Goal

- The family caregivers understand the disease and its treatment.

Implementations for Reinforcing Family Teaching

Help the family caregivers understand the condition and possible food, contact, or inhalant allergens. Reinforce teaching with them about ways to soothe the child. They should avoid overdressing and overheating the child because perspiration causes itching. Explain that they should use a mild detergent to launder the child's clothing and bedding. Help them determine ways to encourage normal growth and development. Reinforce teaching with them to read labels of prepared foods, watching carefully for hidden allergens. Family caregivers may feel apprehensive or repulsed by this unsightly child. Support them in expressing their feelings, and help them view this as a distressing but temporary skin condition.

Children with eczema are frequently active and "behaviorally itchy." Assist family caregivers in handling challenging behavior. Help caregivers develop a strong self-image in the child to protect against strangers' openly negative reactions.

Evaluation of Goal/Desired Outcome

● The family caregivers demonstrate an acceptance of the child and the condition by interacting in a positive fashion with the child.

In caring for **Charlotte**, how do think her age and stage of growth and development will contribute to her nursing care? What symptoms do you think she may be exhibiting? What issues and concerns do you think her parents may be dealing with?

Contact Dermatitis

Contact dermatitis is inflammation of the skin as the result of a hypersensitive reaction to direct contact with a substance. It can be caused by an irritant in which the reaction is immediate or an allergen in which the reaction may be delayed. Irritant contact occurs with diaper dermatitis (discussed in this chapter) and with dry skin dermatitis, which can be caused by excess use or inadequate rinsing of soap, licking lips, or thumbsucking.

Allergic contact dermatitis can occur with exposure to allergens such as soaps, creams, dyes used in clothing, metals found in jewelry, fragrances, products made with latex, or plants like poison ivy and poison oak. With an allergic dermatitis, two phases occur. The sensitization phase occurs with the initial exposure to the allergen. The immune system then goes through a process and builds antibodies, which then are able to recognize the offending allergen. With another exposure to the allergen, the elicitation phase causes the allergic response to occur.

Clinical Manifestations and Diagnosis

A rash appears in the area of the exposure to the skin. It is often bright red and swollen with blisterlike vesicles. These vesicles may weep or rupture and form a crust. Intense itching (pruritus) is common. The location of the rash helps potentially identify the allergen (Fig. 41-5). Often the allergen can be identified through history, but patch testing is sometimes done to identify the specific allergen in order be able to help the child avoid exposure in the future.

Treatment

Avoiding the allergen is important to preventing recurrence. If the allergen can be identified, it can be removed from the child's environment. Treatment is aimed at reducing and controlling the symptoms. Topical corticosteroids are used to decrease the swelling and relieve the itching. Oral corticosteroids may be

> **Pay Close Attention**
>
> Poison ivy is a common cause of contact dermatitis, particularly during the summer. The source of the allergy is the extremely potent oil, urushiol, which is present in all parts of the plant—leaves, stem and root.

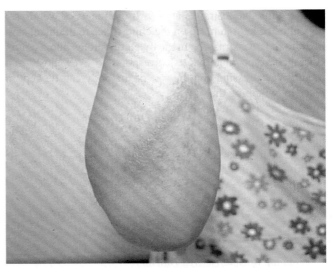

FIGURE 41-5 Poison ivy on a child's arm. Note characteristic vesicular rash in linear formation.

indicated for severe cases. Antihistamine drugs (topical or systemic) are used to relieve itching, reduce swelling, and allow the child to sleep at night. The itching must be relieved as much as possible because scratching can introduce additional pathogens to the affected area. Cool wet dressings are soothing, reduce redness, and also help relieve itching. Fingernails should be kept short and clean. The child should be taught to recognize and avoid poisonous plants. The plants should also be removed from the environment when possible. Children at high risk for latex allergies, such as the child with spina bifida, should be closely monitored for potential exposure to any product which may contain latex.

BITES

Because children are active, inquisitive, and not completely inhibited in their actions, they commonly experience animal and human bites as well as insect stings and bites. Many of these are minor, particularly if the skin is not broken.

Animal Bites

Children enjoy pets, but often they are not alert to possibly dangerous encounters with pets or wild animals. Dog and cat bites are common. Fortunately, because of rabies vaccination programs for dogs, few dog bites cause rabies; in fact, cats are the domestic animal most likely to carry rabies.

> **Pay Attention**
>
> Some bites can have life-threatening implications if proper care is not given.

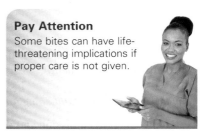

Any pet that bites should be held until it can be determined if the animal has been vaccinated against rabies. If not, the child must undergo a series of injections to prevent this potentially fatal disease. The series consists of both active and passive immunizations.

All animal and human bites have the risk of becoming infected and should be thoroughly washed with soap and water and irrigated if necessary. An antiseptic, such as 70% alcohol or povidone-iodine, should be applied after the wound has been thoroughly rinsed. Most bite wounds are left open to heal rather than being sutured. The wound must be observed for signs of infection until it is well healed. Antibiotics may be given, and tetanus immunizations need to be current. Animal bites should be promptly reported to the proper authorities.

Children should be taught at an early age about the danger of animal bites, particularly of strange or wild animals, such as skunks, raccoons, bats, and squirrels.

Spider Bites

Spider bites can cause serious illness if untreated. Bites of black widow spiders, brown recluse spiders, and scorpions demand medical attention. Applying ice to the affected area until medical care is obtained can slow absorption of the poison. Most spider bites have a local reaction with symptoms of itching, redness, swelling, and sometimes pain, which usually last for less than 24 hours. Scratching the area can lead to a secondary infection and should be avoided. Cold compresses are applied to decrease symptoms and relieve itching.

Tick Bites

Wood ticks carried by chipmunks, ground squirrels, weasels, and wood rats can cause Rocky Mountain spotted fever. Most cases are found in the south Atlantic, south central, and southeastern United States. Dogs are often the carriers to humans. People living in areas where ticks are common can be immunized against this disease.

Deer ticks, carried by white-footed mice and white-tailed deer, can carry the organism that causes Lyme disease. Most cases of Lyme disease in the United States have been seen in northeastern, mid-Atlantic, and upper north central regions and in some northwestern counties of California. The first stage of the disease begins with a lesion at the site of the bite. The lesion appears as a macule with a clear center. The second stage occurs several weeks to months later if the client is not treated. The symptoms of this stage may affect the central nervous system and the heart. If untreated, the third stage may occur months to years later, causing arthritis, neurologic disorders, and bone and joint disease.

Children and adults should wear long pants, long-sleeved shirts, and insect repellent when walking in the woods. Pant legs should be tucked into socks. If a tick is found on the body, the tick should be carefully removed with tweezers. To prevent the release of pathogenic organisms, care should be taken not to crush the tick. A health care provider must be consulted if there is any suspicion that a deer tick has bitten a child or an adult.

Snake Bites

Snake bites demand immediate medical intervention. The wound should be washed, ice applied, and the involved body part immobilized. Prompt transport to the nearest medical facility is essential.

Insect Stings or Bites

Insect stings or bites can prove fatal to children who are sensitized. Swelling may be localized or may include an entire extremity. Circulatory collapse, airway obstruction, and anaphylactic shock can cause death within 30 minutes if the child is untreated. Immediate treatment is necessary and may include injection of epinephrine, antihistamines, or corticosteroids. These children should wear a MedicAlert bracelet and carry an anaphylaxis kit that includes an epinephrine auto injector (EpiPen) and an antihistamine. The teacher, school nurse, and anyone who cares for the child should be alerted to the child's allergy and should know where the anaphylaxis kit is and how to use it when necessary.

BURNS

Among the many accidents that occur in children's lives, burns are the most frightening. Most burn accidents in children happen to those younger than 5 years. Nearly all childhood burns are preventable, and this causes considerable guilt for families and the child. Adult carelessness, the child's exploring and curious nature, and failure to supervise the child adequately all contribute to the high incidence of burns in children. In addition, burns are a common form of child abuse.

Burns may result from various causes including the following:

- Thermal or heat burns occur when contact is made with a heat source. Scalds from hot liquids are common in small children, often resulting from situations such as pans of hot liquid left on the stove with handles turned out, cups of hot tea or coffee, bowls of soup or other hot liquids, or small children left alone in bathtubs. Hot objects such as irons, ovens, stoves, barbecue grills, and curling irons can cause thermal burns. Dangerous, sometimes fatal, burns can occur from these conditions.
- Thermal burns from fire are the second most common kind of burn, resulting from children playing with matches, fireworks, or being left alone in buildings that catch fire. Careless use of smoking materials is a common cause of house fires. Even if cigarette lighters contain a "child-safe" lighting mechanism, they should still be kept away from children.
- Electricity can cause severe facial or mouth burns in infants and toddlers who bite on electrical cords plugged into a socket; such burns may require extensive plastic surgery. These burns may be more serious than they first appear because of the damage to underlying tissues.

• Chemical burns occur when chemicals such as those found in household drain, oven, and toilet bowl cleaners come in contact with the skin. If a child swallows a caustic substance, a chemical burn can occur.

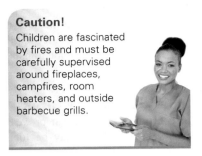

Caution!
Children are fascinated by fires and must be carefully supervised around fireplaces, campfires, room heaters, and outside barbecue grills.

Types of Burns

Burns are divided into types according to the depth of tissue involvement: superficial, partial thickness (either superficial or deep), or full thickness (Fig. 41-6; Table 41-1).

Superficial

The epidermis is injured, but there is no destruction of tissue or nerve endings. Thus, there is erythema, edema, and pain but prompt regeneration (Fig. 41-7).

Partial-Thickness (Formerly Called Second-Degree Burns)

The epidermis and the underlying dermis are both injured and devitalized or destroyed. Regeneration of the skin occurs from the remaining viable epithelial cells in the dermis (Fig. 41-8). With superficial partial-thickness burns, blistering and weeping occurs, and they are red and very painful. In the deep partial-thickness burn, the area blisters and varies in color, from a patchy white to red color. These burns take longer to heal than the superficial partial-thickness burn and often scar.

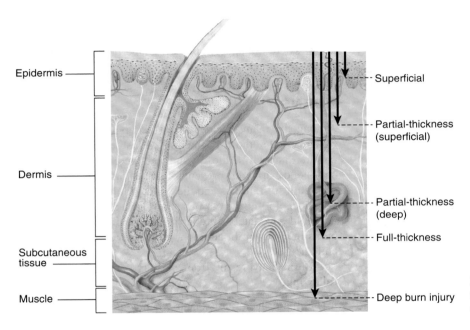

FIGURE 41-6 Cross section of the skin showing the relative depths of the types of burn injuries.

TABLE 41-1 Characteristics of Burn Types

CHARACTERISTIC	SUPERFICIAL	PARTIAL-THICKNESS SUPERFICIAL	PARTIAL-THICKNESS DEEP	FULL-THICKNESS
Layers of skin involved	Epidermis	Epidermis, papillary (top layer) of dermis	Deep into dermis, reticular layer	Into subcutaneous tissue
Appearance	Dry	Moist, weeping	Moist or waxy dry	Dry
Color	Red, blanches with pressure	Red, blanches with pressure	Patchy white to red, does not blanch with pressure	Mixed—white (waxy or pearly), gray to black (charred) Does not blanch
Sensation	Intact	Intact	Reduced	Absent
Blisters	Absent	Present	Present, broken	Absent
Pain Level	Mild to moderate	Extreme	Pain with pressure	None
Healing Time	7 days or less	7–21 days	21 days or more	Small areas, weeks Large areas grafted, months
Other			Scarring	Scarring Grafting common

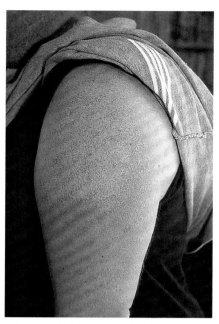

FIGURE 41-7 Superficial burn—painful but without blisters.

Full-Thickness (Formerly Called Third-Degree Burns)

The epidermis, dermis, and nerve endings are all destroyed and the injury can go into the subcutaneous tissue (Fig. 41-9).

Pain is minimal and the skin varies from a waxy white to a gray to a black charred color. There is no longer any barrier to infection or any remaining viable epithelial cells. Deep burn injuries, known as fourth-degree burns are extensions of full-thickness burns with involvement of soft tissue, fat, muscle, and bone and are potentially life-threatening.

Emergency Treatment

Removing the heat source and stopping the burning for a thermal burn is necessary. If the source is electrical, caution must be taken to ensure electricity is turned off to prevent further injury to the child or rescuer. A priority is to determine if the child's situation is emergent and if so provide emergency care. Cool water is an excellent emergency treatment for burns involving small areas. The immediate application of cool compresses or cool water to burn areas inhibits capillary

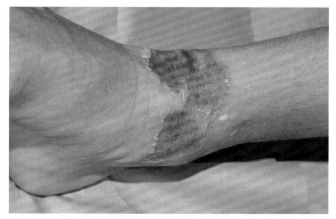

FIGURE 41-8 Partial-thickness burn—very painful with blistering.

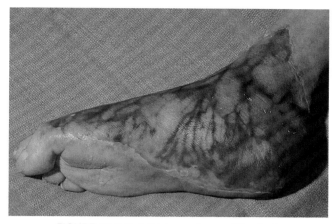

FIGURE 41-9 Full-thickness burn of the foot.

permeability and thus suppresses edema, blister formation, and tissue destruction. Ice water or ice packs must not be used because of the danger of increased tissue damage. Immersing a burned extremity in cool water alleviates pain and may prevent further thermal injury. This can be done after the airway, breathing, and circulation have been observed and restored if necessary. This action should not be done when large areas are involved because of the danger of hypothermia.

In the case of a fire victim, special attention should be given to the airway to observe for signs of smoke inhalation and respiratory passage burns. Clothing should be removed to inspect the whole body for burned areas; in addition, clothing may retain heat, which can cause additional tissue damage. The child should be transported to a medical facility for assessment. If transported to a special burn unit, the child may be wrapped in a sterile sheet and the burn treated on arrival.

Superficial Burns

Superficial burns can usually be treated on an outpatient basis because they heal readily unless infected. The area is cleaned, an antimicrobial ointment or cream such as bacitracin or sulfadiazine is applied, and the burn is covered with a sterile gauze bandage or dressing. An analgesic may be needed to relieve pain. Blisters should not be intentionally broken because of the risk of infection, but blisters that are already broken may be débrided (cut away). The child is seen again in 2 days to inspect for infection. The family caregiver is instructed to keep the area clean and dry until the burn is healed, usually in about a week.

Partial- and Full-Thickness Burns

Distinguishing between partial- and full-thickness burns is not always possible. In the presence of infection, a partial-thickness burn may be converted into a full-thickness one, and with extensive burns, a greater amount of full-thickness burn often exists than had been estimated.

Partial-thickness burns may have biosynthetic dressings, such as Mepilex Ag or Biobrane, applied, which remain in place for several days without needing to be changed. These dressings help prevent infection, reduce the pain of dressing changes, and promote healing.

Full-thickness burns require intense management. Specific criteria are used to determine if a child needs admission to a hospital or burn center. Many factors are considered including the percent of total body surface area involved and location of burn, depth of burn, cause of injury, suspicion of child abuse, or the presence of additional injuries or a chronic disease or disorder.

Treatment of Moderate-to-Severe Burns: First Phase—48 to 72 Hours

Hypovolemic shock is the major manifestation in the first 48 hours in massive burns. As extracellular fluid pours into the burned area, it collects in enormous quantities, which dehydrates the body. Edema becomes noticeable, and symptoms of severe shock appear. Intense pain is seldom a major factor. Symptoms of shock are low blood pressure, rapid pulse, pallor, and considerable apprehension.

Airway

The adequacy of the airway must be determined in case an endotracheal tube needs to be inserted or (rarely) a tracheostomy performed. Inhalation injury is a leading cause of complications in burns. If there are burns around the face and neck or if the burns occurred in a small enclosed space, inhalation injury should be suspected. In fires, toxic substances and the heat produced can cause damage to the respiratory tract. All these possibilities must be considered, and the child should be observed for them.

Intravenous Fluids

The primary concern is to replace body fluids that have been lost or immobilized at the burn areas. Because there is a distinct relationship between the extent of the surface area burned and the amount of fluid lost, the percentage of affected skin area as well as the classification of the burns must be estimated to determine the medical treatment. The "rule of nines" may be used to calculate the percentage of **total body surface area (TBSA)** burned, but the Lund-Browder chart is most accurate for determining TBSA in children. This method takes into account the growth factors noted in children. Children have proportionally larger heads and smaller extremities than do adults (Fig. 41-10).

Using the Lund-Browder chart, the child's age and the percentage of areas affected by either partial-thickness (second-degree) or full-thickness (third-degree) burns are used to calculate the TBSA. An intravenous (IV) infusion site must be selected and fluids started; most often lactated Ringer solution for the first 24 hours is used to administer replacement fluids. IV fluids for maintenance and replacement of lost body fluids are estimated for the first 24 hours, with half of this calculated requirement given during the first 8 hours. The Parkland formula uses the child's weight in kilograms and the TBSA burned to determine the fluid replacement needed.

However, the client's needs may change rapidly, necessitating a change in the rate of flow or the amount or type of fluid. The client's urinary output, vital signs, and general appearance are all part of the information that the health care provider needs to determine the fluid requirements.

Nutritional Support

Adequate nutrition is important for the healing process. The child's caloric and nutritional requirements are two or three times those needed for normal growth. To meet the nutritional needs, enteral nutrition is often started within the first 24 hours. IV fluids should relieve the child's thirst, which is usually severe, and sips of water may be allowed. Oral feedings can be started when tolerated, but enteral feedings may be continued for a period of time to supplement intake.

Urine Output and Diuresis

Urinary output, which may be decreased because of the decrease in blood volume, must be monitored closely. Renal shutdown may be a threat. An output of 1 to 2 mL/kg/hr for children weighing 30 kg (66 lb) or less, or 30 to 50 mL/hr for those weighing more than 30 kg, is desirable. An indwelling catheter facilitates the accurate measurement of urine and specific gravity. After the first hour, the volume of urine should be relatively constant. Any change in volume or specific gravity should be reported.

After the initial fluid therapy brings the burn shock under control and compensates for the extracellular fluid deficit, the client faces another hazard with the onset of the diuretic phase. This occurs within 24 to 96 hours after the injury. The plasmalike fluid is picked up and reabsorbed from the third space in the burn areas, and the client may rapidly become **hypervolemic** (exhibit an abnormal increase in the blood volume in the circulatory system), even to the point of pulmonary edema. This is the principal reason for the extremely close check on all vital signs and for the close monitoring of IV fluids that must now be slowed or stopped entirely.

Notifying the health care provider immediately is necessary if any of the following signs of the onset of this phase occurs:

• Rapid rise in urinary output; may increase to 250 mL/hr or higher
• Tachypnea followed by dyspnea
• Increase in pulse pressure; mean blood pressure may also increase. Central venous pressure, if measured, is elevated

Infection Control

The child has lost a portion of the integumentary system, which is a primary defense against infection. For this reason, measures must be taken to protect the child from infection. Antibiotics are not considered very effective in controlling infection of this type, most likely because the injured capillaries cannot carry the antibiotic to the site. A tetanus vaccine should be ordered according to the status of the child's previous immunization. If immunizations are up to date, a booster dose of tetanus toxoid may be all that is required.

To protect the child from infection introduced into the burn, sterile equipment and aseptic technique must be used in the child's care. Wear a gown, mask, head cover, and gloves when performing dressing changes. Visitors are also required to meticulously scrub and wear a gown and mask.

Burn units are designed to be self-contained with treatment and operating areas, hydrotherapy units, and client

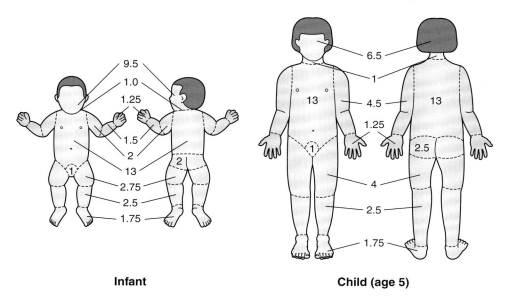

Infant

Child (age 5)

Area	Birth 1 yr	1–4 yrs	5–9 yrs	10–14 yrs	15 yrs	Adult	2°	3°	Total
Head	19	17	13	11	9	7			
Neck	2	2	2	2	2	2			
Ant. Trunk	13	13	13	13	13	13			
Post. Trunk	13	13	13	13	13	13			
R. Buttock	2 1/2	2 1/2	2 1/2	2 1/2	2 1/2	2 1/2			
L. Buttock	2 1/2	2 1/2	2 1/2	2 1/2	2 1/2	2 1/2			
Genitalia	1	1	1	1	1	1			
R.U. Arm	4	4	4	4	4	4			
L.U. Arm	4	4	4	4	4	4			
R.L. Arm	3	3	3	3	3	3			
L.L. Arm	3	3	3	3	3	3			
R. Hand	2 1/2	2 1/2	2 1/2	2 1/2	2 1/2	2 1/2			
L. Hand	2 1/2	2 1/2	2 1/2	2 1/2	2 1/2	2 1/2			
R. Thigh	5 1/2	6 1/2	8	8 1/2	9	9 1/2			
L. Thigh	5 1/2	6 1/2	8	8 1/2	9	9 1/2			
R. Leg	5	5	5 1/2	6	6 1/2	7			
L. Leg	5	5	5 1/2	6	6 1/2	7			
R. Foot	3 1/2	3 1/2	3 1/2	3 1/2	3 1/2	3 1/2			
L. Foot	3 1/2	3 1/2	3 1/2	3 1/2	3 1/2	3 1/2			
						Total			

FIGURE 41-10 The Lund-Browder chart uses the child's age and the affected areas of partial-thickness (second-degree) and full-thickness (third-degree) burns to calculate the total body surface area (TBSA) of the burn.

care areas. In hospitals where there is no specific burn unit, a private room with a door that can be closed should be set up as a burn unit. The strictest aseptic technique must be observed.

Wound Care

Two types of burn care are generally used: the open method and the closed method. The open method of burn care is most often used for superficial burns, burns of the face, and burns of the perineum. In open burn care, the wound is not covered, but antimicrobial ointment is applied topically. This type of care requires strict aseptic technique.

In the closed burn method of burn care, nonadherent materials are used to cover the burn. The child can be moved more easily, and the danger of added injury or pain is decreased. Dressing changes are very painful, and infection may occur under the dressings. Occlusive dressings help minimize pain because of the reduced exposure to air.

In both methods, daily **débridement** (removal of necrotic tissue) usually preceded by **hydrotherapy** (use of water in treatment) is performed. Débridement is extremely painful, and the child must have an analgesic administered before the therapy. The child is placed in the tub of water to soak the dressings; this helps to remove any sloughing tissue, **eschar** (hard crust or scab), exudate, and old medication. Often, the tissue is trapped in the mesh gauze of the dressing, so soaking eases necrotic tissue removal. Loose tissue is trimmed before the burn is redressed. Hosing

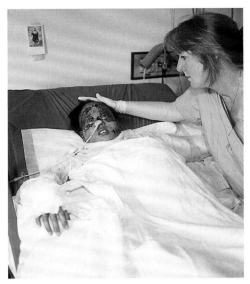

FIGURE 41-11 The nurse gives support to the child during débridement.

instead of tub soaking is used in some centers to reduce the risk of infection. Débridement is difficult emotionally for both the child and the nurse (Fig. 41-11).

Diversionary activities may be used to help distract the child. Researchers have also found that children who are encouraged to participate actively in their burn care, even to help change dressings, experience healthy control over their situation and often experience less anxiety than those who are completely dependent on the nurse. The child should never be scolded or reprimanded for uncooperative behavior.

Topical medications that may be used to reduce invading organisms include antimicrobial ointments, silver sulfadiazine, mafenide acetate, chlorhexidine, and bacitracin. Each of these agents has advantages and disadvantages. The choice of agent is made by the health care provider and is determined, at least partially, by the organisms found in cultures of the burn area.

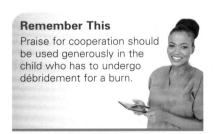

Remember This

Praise for cooperation should be used generously in the child who has to undergo débridement for a burn.

Grafting

Grafts may be **homograft**, **heterograft** (xenograft), or **autograft**. Homografts and heterografts are short-term grafts which provide a temporary dressing after débridement and have proven to be lifesaving measures for children with extensive burns. A homograft consists of skin taken from another person, which is eventually rejected by the recipient tissue and sloughed off after 3 to 6 weeks, but has great value for immediate covering. Skin from cadavers is often used as a homograft in a procedure called an **allograft**; this skin can be stored and used up to several weeks. A heterograft is skin obtained from animals, often porcine (pigs).

An autograft, consisting of skin taken from the child's own body, is the only kind of skin accepted permanently by recipient tissues. Obtaining enough healthy skin to cover a large area is usually impossible. If the donor site is kept free from infection and grafts of sufficient thinness are taken, the site should be ready for use again in 10 to 12 days. After grafting, the donor and the graft sites are kept covered with sterile dressings.

Complications

The healthcare team must guard carefully against the complication of **contractures**. If the burn extends over a movable body part, fibrous scarring that forms in the healing process can cause serious deformities and limit movement. Joints must be positioned, possibly in overextension, so that maximal flexibility is maintained. Splinting, exercise, and pressure are also used to prevent contractures. When burns are severe, pressure garments may be used. These garments help decrease hypertrophy of scar tissue. However, they may need to be worn for 12 to 18 months. The child must wear these garments continuously, except when bathing.

Long-Term Care

The rehabilitative phase of care for the child is often long and difficult. Even after discharge from the healthcare facility, the child needs to return for additional treatment or plastic surgery to release contractures and revise scar tissue. The emotional scars of the family and the child must be evaluated, and therapy must be initiated or continued. The impact of scarring and disfigurement may need to be resolved by both the child and members of the family.

Nursing Process and Care Plan *for the Child With a Burn*

Assessment (Data Collection)

Assessment of the child with a burn is complex and varies with the extent and depth of the burn, the stage of healing, and the age and general condition of the child. Initially, the primary concerns are the cardiac and respiratory state, the assessment of shock, and an evaluation of the burns.

After the first phase (the first 24 to 48 hours), the healing of the child's burns must be evaluated and the child's nutrition, signs of infection, and pain level must be monitored. The emotional conditions of the child and the family must also be evaluated.

Nursing Care Focus

When developing evidence-based nursing care focuses for the child with a burn, the risk for infection, malnutrition, activity intolerance, and decreased mobility must be addressed. Helping the child deal with pain and anxiety are important aspects of caring for the child. Family coping impairment and reinforcing family teaching are included in working with the child and the family.

Outcome Identification and Planning

During the first phase of care, the major goals relate to cardiopulmonary stabilization, fluid and electrolyte balance, and infection control. After the first 72 hours, more long-term goals are developed. The child's goals are limited by their age and ability to communicate. Goals related to the child include preventing infection, maintaining adequate nutrition, reducing pain, increasing mobility, and relieving anxiety. The family caregiver's goals include concerns about stress on the family related to the child's injury. Other goals relate to reinforcing family teaching to optimize healing, decrease the risk of complications to minimize permanent disability, and gaining an understanding of the long-term implications of care.

Nursing Care Focus

- Infection risk related to the loss of the protective layer (skin) secondary to burn injury

Goal

- The child will be free from signs or symptoms of infection.

Implementations for Preventing and Monitoring for Infection

The immaturity of the child's immune system, the destruction of the skin layer, and the presence of necrotic tissue (an ideal medium for bacterial growth) contribute to a significant danger of infection. Conscientious handwashing is necessary for anyone who has contact with the child. Observe rigid infection control precautions, and use only sterile equipment and supplies. Monitor vital signs, including temperature, on a 1-, 2-, or 4-hour schedule. Screen all people who have any contact with the child, including visitors, family, or staff for any signs of upper respiratory or skin infection.

When caring for the burn, wear a sterile gown, mask, and head cover. Wear sterile gloves or use a sterile tongue blade to apply ointment to the burn. Maintain the room temperature at around 80°F because water evaporates quickly through the denuded areas and even through the leathery burn eschar, with thermal loss resulting. Note and document all drainage. Report immediately and document any unusual odor. Cultures are done regularly. Avoid injury to the eschar and the donor site if the child has a graft. Hair on the tissue adjacent to the burn area is often shaved.

Evaluation of Goal/Desired Outcome

The child:

- exhibits pulse and respirations within normal limits for age.
- has temperature of 98.6°F to 101°F (37°C to 38.4°C).
- is free from malodorous drainage.

Nursing Care Focus

- Malnutrition risk related to increased caloric needs secondary to burns and anorexia

Goal

- The child's caloric intake will be adequate to meet their needs for tissue repair and growth.

Implementations for Ensuring Adequate Nutrition

The child who has received extensive burns requires special attention regarding nutritional needs. The nutritional problem is much more complex than simply getting a seriously ill child to eat. The child is in negative caloric balance from a number of causes, including the following:

- Poor intake because of anorexia
- External loss caused by exudative losses of protein through the burn wound
- Hypermetabolism caused by fever and infection

A bland diet high in protein (for healing and replacement) and calories is an essential component of therapy for the child with a burn. It is important to use every effort possible to interest the child in foods essential for tissue building and repair. Find out the child's likes and dislikes and serve foods the child will enjoy. Do not serve large servings because the child often experiences anorexia. In addition, the child's physical condition often interferes with their ability to eat. Foods are of no value if the child refuses to eat them. Try using colorful trays, foods with visual appeal, and any special touches to spur a child's appetite. Allow the child to have some control to encourage cooperation.

Even with the best efforts the child with a burn seldom can eat enough food to meet the increased needs. Enteral feedings are often necessary to supplement the oral intake. Commercial high-calorie formulas are available for these feedings that meet the child's needs. Explain the need for the enteral feedings and make sure the child understands. Demonstrate the feeding process with a doll to help the child grasp the idea.

Weigh the child daily at the same time and with the child wearing the same amount of clothing or covering. Carefully monitor intake and output.

Evaluation of Goal/Desired Outcome

The child:

- consumes at least 80% of diet high in calories and protein.
- maintains weight or has weight gain appropriate for age.

A Little Nutrition News

Foods high in protein and calories that may appeal to and encourage the child to eat are flavored milk, ice cream, milk shakes, high-protein drinks, milk and egg desserts, and pureed meats and vegetables.

Nursing Care Focus

● Acute pain related to tissue destruction and painful procedures

Goal

● The child will show signs of being comfortable.

Implementations for Relieving Pain and Providing Comfort Measures

The pain of a thermal injury can be severe. As a result of the pain or the fear and anxiety that pain causes, the child may not sleep well, may experience anorexia, and may be apprehensive and uncooperative during treatments and care. Analgesics must be administered to provide the most relief possible. Administer analgesics at least 20 to 30 minutes before dressing changes and débridement. Avoid scheduling the administration of pain medications close to mealtimes; otherwise, the child may be too sedated to eat.

Monitor the child's physiologic response to the pain and analgesics. Document the child's pupil reaction, heart and respiratory rates, and behavior in response to pain and analgesics.

Provide support and comfort during painful procedures. Use diversionary activities to help the child focus on something other than the pain. Promising a favorite activity after a dreaded procedure is acceptable. Television may be helpful, but be cautious not to overuse it. The younger child may enjoy learning new songs, playing age-appropriate games, or listening to someone reading stories. The older child may enjoy video or computer games, books, and board or card games. Acknowledge the child's pain, give the child as much control as possible, and work with the child and the family caregivers to minimize the pain and bring about the greatest rewards for all involved.

Evaluation of Goal/Desired Outcome

The child:

● uses a pain scale appropriate for age to indicate decreased pain level.
● rests quietly and does not cry or moan excessively.
● has pulse and respiratory rates that are regular and normal for age.

Nursing Care Focus

● Activity intolerance and decreased mobility related to pain and scarring

Goal

● The child will have increased mobility, and contractures will be minimal.

Implementations for Promoting Mobility and Preventing Contractures

Care must be taken to avoid contractures and scarring that limit movement. Never permit two burned body surfaces, such as fingers, to touch. If the neck is involved, the child may have to be kept with the neck hyperextended, the arms may need to be placed in a brace to prevent underarm contractures, and joints of the knee or elbow must be extended to prevent scar formation from causing contractures that limit movement. Pressure dressings and pressure suits may be used for this purpose and may need to be worn for more than a year. Physical therapy may be needed, and splints may be used to position the body part to prevent contractures. All these measures can add to the child's discomfort.

Encourage range-of-motion, early ambulation, and self-help activities as additional means of promoting mobility and preventing contractures. Use creativity to devise ways to involve the child in enjoyable activities that encourage movement of the affected part.

Evaluation of Goal/Desired Outcome

The child:

● participates in range-of-motion and other physical activities.
● maintains splints, pressure dressings and suits, and positions.
● shows no evidence of contractures.

Nursing Care Focus

● Anxiety related to changes in body image caused by thermal injury

Goal

● The older child will express feelings related to changes associated with burns.

Implementations for Reducing Anxiety

The child's age and level of understanding influence the amount of anxiety that they have about scarring and disability related to the burn. If the child is in a burn unit with other children, seeing others may cause unrealistic fears. Encourage the child to explore their feelings about changes, especially those involving body image. Use therapeutic play with puppets or dolls if possible. Encourage both the family and the nursing staff to provide the child with continuous support.

Evaluation of Goal/Desired Outcome

The child:

● expresses feelings and fears about body image.
● demonstrates a positive attitude of acceptance.

Nursing Care Focus

- Coping impairment of family caregiver related to the effect of the injury on the child's and family's lives

Goal

- The family caregivers will verbalize feelings related to the child's injury and take steps to develop coping skills.

Implementations for Promoting Family Coping

The family may feel guilty about the injury; one member may feel especially responsible. These feelings affect the family's coping abilities. Give both the family and the child opportunities to discuss and express their feelings. Suggest counseling if necessary to help family members handle their feelings. Put the family in touch with support groups, if available, to help the family work through problems. Explain the child's care to family members, and involve them in the care when possible. Avoid saying anything that might add to the guilt or anxiety that the family members are feeling.

Evaluation of Goal/Desired Outcome

The family caregivers:

- verbalize fears, anxieties, and other feelings related to the child's injury.
- discuss the impact of the injury on the child and family's life.
- participate in counseling.
- become involved in support groups.

Nursing Care Focus

- Knowledge deficiency of family caregivers related to optimizing the child's healing process and to the long-term care required by the child

Goal

- The family caregivers will verbalize an understanding of the child's long-term home care management.

Implementations for Reinforcing Family Caregiver Teaching

Provide the family caregivers with explanations about the whole process of burns, the care, the healing process, and the long-term implications. Give information to the family caregiver as they are ready for it; do not thrust it on them all at once. To prepare for home care, reinforce teaching with the family caregiver about wound care; dressing changes; signs and symptoms to observe and report; and the importance of diet, rest, and activity. Help the family find resources for any necessary supplies and equipment. Make a referral to social services to assist them in home care planning.

Evaluation of Goal/Desired Outcome

Family caregivers:

- demonstrate wound care and dressing changes.
- list signs and symptoms to observe for and report.
- secure needed home care equipment.
- use social service assistance if appropriate.

> **TEST YOURSELF**
> ✔ What are the major causes of burns in children?
> ✔ Explain the differences among superficial, partial-thickness (second-degree), and full-thickness (third-degree) burns.
> ✔ Explain the process of débridement and how you can support the child during the care of a burn wound.

SEXUALLY TRANSMITTED INFECTIONS

The incidence of sexually transmitted infections (STIs) (sometimes referred to as sexually transmitted diseases [STDs]) is higher in adolescents than in any other age group. The diseases range from infections that can be easily treated to diseases that are life-threatening, such as infection with human immunodeficiency virus (HIV) (Table 41-2).

Infants infected with STIs are usually infected prenatally or during birth. Children infected after the neonatal period must be considered victims of sexual abuse until disproved. Severe or repeated cases of pelvic inflammatory disease (PID) or severe genital warts are warning signs that a girl should be tested for HIV.

Prevention is the most effective tool in the campaign against STIs. The only certain way to avoid contracting an STI is sexual abstinence. However, sexual activity in adolescents indicates that this is often not a practical solution. Condoms with spermicide (discussed in Chapter 4) provide protection, but they are not fail-safe. Adolescents must be educated about all aspects of the consequences of sexual activity.

Human Papillomavirus

Human papillomavirus (HPV) is the most common STI seen in the adolescent. A group of many related viruses are included in the group called HPV. Many times the HPV is asymptomatic and goes away on its own, but if it does not, some of the viruses cause genital warts and some cause cancers, cervical cancer in particular. It is recommended that all males and females be immunized at age 11 or 12 years to prevent HPV.

Gonorrhea

Gonorrhea is one of the most commonly reported communicable diseases in the United States. Slang names for gonorrhea are sometimes used to refer to the disease, such as "the clap," "the drips," or "the dose." Gonorrhea has mild primary symptoms, particularly in females, and often goes undetected and thus untreated until it progresses to a serious pelvic disorder. This disease can cause sterility in males.

TABLE 41-2 Major Sexually Transmitted Infections

INFECTION AND AGENT	TRANSMISSION	SYMPTOMS	POSSIBLE COMPLICATIONS	PREVENTION
Human papillomaviruses (HPV)	Sexual contact	Often asymptomatic; genital warts	Genital warts; cervical cancer	Immunization of males and females age 11 or 12
Gonorrhea—bacteria: *Neisseria gonorrhoeae*	Sexual contact; mother to fetus during vaginal delivery	Yellow mucopurulent discharge of the genital area, painful or frequent urination, pain in the genital area; may be asymptomatic. Frequent cause of PID	Sterility, cystitis, arthritis, endocarditis	Public should be educated on safe sex practices; mother should be tested before delivery. Newborn's eyes should be treated with tetracycline ointment or erythromycin ointment. All contacts should be treated with antibiotics
Chlamydia—bacteria: *Chlamydia trachomatis*	Sexual contact; mother to fetus during vaginal delivery	Mucopurulent genital discharge, genital pain, dysuria. Frequent cause of PID, often in combination with gonorrhea	Sterility	Public should be educated about safe sex practices. Sexual contact should be avoided when lesions are present. Infected mothers should have cesarean deliveries
Genital herpes virus: herpes simplex virus type 1 and type 2	Sexual contact; mother to fetus during vaginal delivery	Genital soreness, pruritus, and erythema; vesicles appear that usually last for about 10 days during which time transmission of virus is likely		Public should be educated about safe sex practices. Sexual contact should be avoided when lesions are present. Infected mother should have a cesarean delivery
Syphilis—spirochete bacterium: *Treponema pallidum*	Sexual contact; mother to fetus via placenta	Primary stage: genital or body lesion (chancre), enlarged lymph nodes. Secondary stage (6 weeks later): lesions of skin and mucous membrane with generalized symptoms of headache and fever	Tertiary stage: central nervous system and cardiovascular damage, paralysis, psychosis	Public should be educated about safe sex practices. Serologic testing before and during pregnancy. Contact with body secretions from infected clients should be avoided
Acquired immunodeficiency syndrome (AIDS)—virus: human immunodeficiency virus (HIV)	Sexual contact; sharing needles; mother to fetus or infant	Primary infection: rash, fever, malaise, lymphadenopathy. Mildly symptomatic: HIV-positive, enlarged lymph nodes, liver, spleen, persistent infections. Moderately symptomatic: HIV-positive, oral candidiasis, HIV encephalopathy, pneumonia, sepsis, herpes infections. Severely symptomatic: HIV-positive, serious infections, opportunistic infections	Neurologic impairment	Public, especially high-risk groups, should be educated about safe sex practices. Administration of daily preexposure prophylaxis (PrEP) in high-risk individuals. IV drug users should not share needles. Standard precautions should be used consistently in all healthcare settings. Measures to avoid needlesticks among healthcare workers should be instituted

Several drugs may be used to treat gonorrhea, including ceftriaxone, azithromycin, and doxycycline to prevent an accompanying chlamydial infection. Adolescents are asked to name their sexual contacts so that they may also be treated. Adolescents must learn that their bodies will not develop immunity to the organism, and they might become infected again if they continue to expose themselves by engaging in sexual activity, especially high-risk sexual behavior.

Chlamydia Infection

Chlamydia infections have replaced gonorrhea as the most common and fastest spreading bacterial STI in the United States. Symptoms may be mild or the individual may be asymptomatic, causing a delay in diagnosis and treatment until serious complications and transmission to others has occurred.

Adolescents must be made aware of the seriousness of PID, a common result of a chlamydia infection. PID can cause sterility in the female, primarily by causing scarring in the fallopian tubes that prohibits the passage of the fertilized ovum into the uterus. A tubal pregnancy may be the consequence of a chlamydial infection. In the male, sterility may result from epididymitis caused by a chlamydial infection.

Doxycycline or azithromycin is used to treat chlamydial infection. In the pregnant adolescent, erythromycin or amoxicillin can be used to avoid the teratogenic effects of these drugs. All sexual partners must be treated.

Genital Herpes

Genital herpes has reached epidemic proportions in the United States. The disease begins as a vesicle that ruptures to form a painful ulcer on the genitalia. The initial ulcer lasts 10 to 12 days. Recurrent episodes occur intermittently and last 4 to 5 days. No cure is available, but acyclovir is useful in relieving or suppressing the symptoms.

Genital herpes is associated with a much higher than average risk for cervical cancer; therefore, the female client who has genital herpes should have an annual Pap smear. Genital herpes is not transmitted to the fetus in utero. However, if the mother has an active case of genital herpes at the time of delivery, cesarean birth is indicated to reduce the risk of infection as the fetus passes through the vagina. In newborns, the infection can become systemic and cause death.

Syphilis

Caused by the spirochete *Treponema pallidum*, syphilis is a destructive disease that can involve every part of the body. Untreated, it can have devastating long-term effects. Infected mothers are highly likely to transmit the infection to their unborn infants.

Syphilis is spread primarily by sexual contact. Symptoms of the primary stage usually appear about 3 weeks after exposure. If allowed to progress without treatment, syphilis has a secondary stage, a latent stage, and a tertiary stage.

Clinical Manifestations

The cardinal sign of the primary stage is the **chancre**, which is a hard, red, painless lesion at the point of entry of the spirochete. This lesion can appear on the penis, the vulva, or the cervix. It can also appear on the mouth, the lips, or the rectal area as a result of oral–genital or anal–genital contact. The secondary stage, marked by rash, sore throat, and fever, appears 2 to 6 months after the original infection. Signs of both the first and second stages disappear without treatment, but the spirochete remains in the body. The latent period can persist for as long as 20 years without symptoms; however, blood tests are still positive. In the tertiary stage, syphilis causes severe neurologic and cardiovascular damage, mental illness, and gastrointestinal disorders.

Treatment

Syphilis responds to one intramuscular injection of benzathine penicillin G; if the child is sensitive to penicillin, oral doxycycline can be administered as alternative treatment. If treatment is not obtained before the tertiary stage, the neurologic and cardiovascular complications can lead to death.

Human Immunodeficiency Virus

The human immunodeficiency virus (HIV) is the virus that causes acquired immunodeficiency syndrome (AIDS). The HIV replicates, attacks, and destroys the CD4 (T-helper) cells, causing a decrease in the CD4 cell count. The T-helper lymphocytes are cells that direct the immune response to viral, bacterial, and fungal infections and remove some malignant cells from the body. As the virus continues to replicate, the CD4 count continues to drop and puts the child at risk for developing life-threatening infections, known as opportunistic infections. If this occurs, they are then diagnosed with acquired immunodeficiency syndrome (AIDS).

Transmission of HIV occurs through sharing of infected needles (IV drug use, tattooing), exposure to infected body secretions through sexual contact, as well as from an HIV-positive woman to her unborn fetus or newborn infant. The virus cannot be transmitted through casual contact. The diagnosis of any STI increases the risk of HIV infection. Transmission of HIV from contaminated blood products is a very rare concern.

Infants are usually infected through the placenta during prenatal life, in the birth process when contaminated by the mother's blood, or through breast-feeding. Children and teens can also be infected through sexual abuse. Adolescents are most often infected through intimate heterosexual or homosexual relations and through IV drug use. Adolescents' attitude of **impunity** (the belief that nothing can hurt them) and the increasing rate of sexual activity in this age group, often involving multiple partners, contribute to the infection rate in adolescents. The incubation period for HIV can vary from 3 to 12 years; thus, many who contract the disease in adolescence will not have symptoms until they are in their 20s when they are at their reproductive peak.

Clinical Manifestations and Treatment

Infants and children with HIV are often asymptomatic. Failure to thrive, oral candidiasis, chronic diarrhea, and developmental delays may be seen. Flu-like symptoms such as fever, rash, sore throat, enlarged spleen, and lymphadenopathy also may be present. Following this acute stage, the child may have no symptoms, but often has recurrent bacterial infections. During this time, the child is infectious and the CD4 count continues to drop. The immune system becomes more suppressed, and symptoms of opportunistic infections are seen. *Pneumocystis* pneumonia, wasting syndrome, HIV encephalopathy, or cytomegalovirus often develops.

Treatment with highly active antiretroviral drug therapy (HAART) does not cure HIV infection, but using these drugs, especially beginning with early signs of infection, has greatly decreased the incidence of opportunistic infections and improved survival rates. Compliance with the lifelong treatment is difficult. Many of the drugs have unpleasant side effects, but adherence to the treatment is important.

Prevention

Reinforcement of teaching, in particular about behaviors that put an individual at high risk for contracting HIV, is an essential part of preventing HIV and AIDS. The proper use of a condom with spermicide (see Chapter 4) during any type of sexual contact is reinforced. Adolescents may have sexual experiences with older partners who have had many previous sexual partners. This increases the risk for the Adolescent females and in turn can increase the risk for any partner with whom they are sexually intimate. Administration of daily preexposure prophylaxis (PrEP) in high-risk individuals helps reduce the incidence of HIV.

 Cultural Snapshot

Cultural influences may play an important role in the spread of HIV. The adolescent often finds it difficult to insist that the partner use a condom. If the partner refuses and claims to be "safe" (uninfected) or protests that the condom decreases pleasure, the adolescent might give in for fear of breaking up the relationship. In addition, in some cultures, the more sexual conquests a male has, the more manly he is considered.

Nursing Process and Care Plan *for the Child With HIV/AIDS*

Assessment (Data Collection)

When collecting data from the child with HIV/AIDS, gather a complete history, including chief complaint, presenting symptoms, past medical history, immunization status, family history, and social history. Interview the family caregiver if present, but be certain to provide the adolescent with a private interview. The adolescent may be extremely reluctant to reveal either social or sexual history, especially in the presence of a family member. Carefully review the adolescent's history of vaginal candidiasis, PID, sexual activity and partners, and IV drug use. The adolescent may have various emotions, including anger, denial, guilt, and rebelliousness; it is important that you accept these emotions and reactions to the illness.

During the physical examination, maintain strict standard precautions. Include vital signs and especially observe for fever, which may indicate infection, and perform a thorough survey of all body systems. Observe for poor skin turgor, rashes or lesions, alopecia, mucous membrane lesions or thrush, weight loss, mental or neurologic changes, respiratory infections, diarrhea or abdominal pain, vaginal discharge, perineal lesions, or genital warts. Help prepare the child for diagnostic tests that must be performed.

Nursing Care Focus

The nursing care focuses for the child for with HIV/AIDS include the risk of infection for the child and the risk of transmitting the virus to others. Managing acute pain, preventing malnutrition, and encouraging compliance with medication routine are important. Recognizing psychosocial needs and promoting normal growth and development are essential.

Family coping impairment and reinforcing family teaching are included in working with the child and the family.

Outcome Identification and Planning

Planning the nursing care of a child with HIV/AIDS can be challenging. The child needs support to accept the diagnosis and move in a positive direction to follow the treatment plan to the best of their ability. You can play a critical role in helping the child understand the treatment and prognosis and their impact on the child's life. Major goals for the child include maintaining the highest level of wellness possible by preventing infection and the spread of the infection, minimizing pain, improving nutrition, complying with medication regimen, alleviating social isolation, and diminishing a feeling of hopelessness. The primary goal for the family caregiver is improving coping skills, helping the child cope with the illness, and increasing knowledge about the diagnosis and treatment.

Nursing Care Focus

- Infection risk related to increased susceptibility secondary to a compromised immune system

Goal

- The child will experience minimal risk of infection.

Implementations for Preventing Infection

In the healthcare facility, strict adherence to appropriate infection control measures is extremely important. A primary goal is to reinforce teaching with the child to prevent infections. Review good handwashing technique; the client should take care to wash between the fingers and under rings and should use a pump-type soap. Encourage the child to keep nails trimmed to avoid harboring microorganisms under the nails. Reinforce that skin care includes showering (not a tub bath) with a mild soap (no strong, perfumed soaps), using an emollient cream, and patting the skin dry while avoiding vigorous rubbing. Instruct the child to brush the teeth at least three times a day using a soft toothbrush and nonabrasive toothpaste. Routine dental care is vital.

Reinforce with the child that someone else should care for pets. Cleaning an aquarium or birdcage or emptying a cat's litter box can expose the child to opportunistic organisms that will attack the compromised immune system. Help the child learn to avoid people who have any infectious disease. Advise them that prompt attention to an apparently minor infection helps avoid more serious illness. The child with HIV/AIDS should receive immunizations as indicated. If the child is immunosuppressed, live vaccine immunizations may be withheld.

Evaluation of Goal/Desired Outcome

The child:

- practices good hygiene measures.
- identifies ways to prevent infection and ways to protect their health at home.

Nursing Care Focus

● Infection risk related to possibility of transmitting virus to others

Goal

● The child will not spread the disease to others.

Implementations for Preventing Infection Transmission

The good hygienic practices necessary to protect the child from an acquired or opportunistic infection also help prevent transmission of the virus to others. The household where the child lives must be cleaned carefully and regularly. A household bleach solution of 1 part bleach to 10 parts of water is a good solution to use. Particular attention should be paid to the refrigerator, the stove, the oven, and the microwave to prevent contamination of foods during preparation or storage. Household items that may be contaminated should be discarded in double plastic bags to prevent spread to others. Laundry bleach should be used when washing the child's clothing, especially underwear.

In addition, the adolescent needs counseling about sexual practices. One of the most emotionally difficult tasks for the adolescent may be to list sexual contacts. This is a delicate matter that must be approached in a nonjudgmental, sympathetic manner, but the teen needs to understand that anyone with whom they have been sexually intimate may be infected and must be identified. The teen may find that the sexual partner from whom they contracted the virus already knew that they were infected. Infection with HIV does not necessarily mean that the child was promiscuous. The adolescent may have been sexually intimate with only one person, and that person may have assured the teen that they were not infected. The adolescent may be extremely angry about exposure by a trusted person.

Reinforce teaching with the adolescent about safe sex practices. The adolescent needs to understand that they are protecting not only future sexual partners from contracting the disease, but also themselves from contracting other strains of the virus. Both males and females need to have complete instructions on the use of condoms and spermicide (see Chapter 4). The adolescent must not be sexually intimate with anyone without using a condom, no matter what kind of argument the other person uses. Also the teen needs to learn how HIV is transmitted, including vaginal intercourse, oral–genital contact, anal intercourse, or any contact with blood or body fluids, including menstrual discharge. The teen who practices oral–genital sex must learn to use a dental dam (a square of latex worn in the mouth to prevent contact of body fluids with mucous membranes of the mouth).

The adolescent female needs to be counseled about pregnancy. The probability of transmitting the virus to her unborn child is high. She must consider that even if her child is not infected, there is a possibility that she may not live to see the child reach adulthood. All these considerations are overwhelming, and the adolescent needs continuous support to understand, accept, and deal with them.

A discussion of the use of injectable drugs is important. Counsel the child and adolescent about the importance of stopping drug use. However, the reality is that they may not quit, so explain the importance of using sterile needles. Many communities have needle exchange programs that provide access to sterile needles.

Evaluation of Goal/Desired Outcome

The child:

● practices infection transmission precaution measures.
● identifies sexual partners and safer sexual practices.

Nursing Care Focus

● Acute pain related to symptoms of the disease

Goal

● The child will experience minimal pain from complications of the disease.

Implementations for Promoting Comfort

Pain is caused by several manifestations of HIV/AIDS. Skin and mucous membrane lesions may be very painful. Topical anesthetic solutions, such as viscous lidocaine, and meticulous mouth care can relieve pain caused by oral mucous membrane infections. Smoking, alcohol, and spicy or acidic foods irritate the oral mucous membranes and often cause additional pain. PID, a common complication of STIs, is usually accompanied by abdominal pain. The child with respiratory complications also has bouts of chest pain. Administer analgesics to relieve pain, and use all appropriate nursing measures to help the child feel more comfortable. As the disease develops, the pain may be greater, so every effort must be made to provide comfort.

Evaluation of Goal/Desired Outcome

The child:

● learns to manage pain.
● rests comfortably with minimal discomfort.

Nursing Care Focus

● Malnutrition related to anorexia, oral or esophageal lesions, or diarrhea

Goal

● The child's food intake will meet their nutritional needs.

Implementations for Improving Nutrition

Anorexia, or a poor appetite, is a common problem of the client with HIV/AIDS. Dehydration, diarrhea, infection, malabsorption, oral candidiasis, and some drugs also can contribute to the child's poor state of nutrition. Malnutrition can cause additional problems with increased and more serious infections. The child's diet must be nutritious and often higher in calories than normal. Several small meals supplemented by high-calorie, high-protein snacks may be desirable. Dietary supplements, such as Ensure, may also be useful. Explore the child's food likes and dislikes, and develop a meal plan using this information. If malnutrition becomes severe, the child may need enteral feedings or parenteral nutrition.

Evaluation of Goal/Desired Outcome

The child:

- eats nutritionally sound meals.
- includes frequent small meals in the food plan.
- maintains an appropriate weight for their age.

A Little Nutrition News

To help decrease the possibility of infection, raw fruits and vegetables should be washed and peeled or cooked to avoid the danger of bacteria; meats must be well cooked. The child must avoid unpasteurized dairy products and foods grown in organic fertilizer.

Nursing Care Focus

- Nonadherence to medication regimen

Goal

- The child will follow daily medication regime.

Implementations for Promoting Adherence to Medication Regimen

Compliance with taking daily medications may be a challenge. Many of the drugs have uncomfortable side effects. Explain the ways the drugs work and the importance of taking the medications. Support the child by listening to their concerns and feelings.

Evaluation of Goal/Desired Outcome

- The child complies with medication regimen as prescribed.

Nursing Care Focus

- Psychosocial needs related to social isolation, possible rejection by others, and hopelessness secondary to the diagnosis of HIV/AIDS

Goal

- The child will not experience social isolation and will make adjustments to their future expectations.

Implementations for Easing Social Isolation and Hopelessness

The child may fear having others know about the illness because they anticipate a negative reaction from peers and family. Provide the child with supportive counseling and guidance to help them deal with these fears. The child may not feel that they can tell the family for fear of rejection. In fact, many families have rejected their children who have HIV/AIDS. Many others have risen to the challenge; although family members

may tell the adolescent they do not like their behavior, they continue to offer love and support. The child may need support to help tell social acquaintances as well. Refer the child or adolescent to an HIV/AIDS support group if one is available through the hospital or community. Adolescents often find that adult support groups are not as helpful because the adults' needs are different from those of adolescents.

Because the child is facing life with a serious, chronic illness that requires frequent treatment and lifelong medication and has an unknown outcome, the child may feel a special sense of purpose to "spread the word" to others. The child needs support and guidance to set priorities. School officials may need to be told, but families have the legal right to decide whether or not they share the diagnosis with others. If the family is not supportive, the child needs even more support from members of the healthcare team.

Evaluation of Goal/Desired Outcome

The child:

- voices fears and feelings about social isolation and their future.
- makes and carries out plans to maintain relationships.
- seeks support from others.
- begins to make realistic future plans.

This Approach is Important to Remember

The adolescent has the right to decide how to conduct their life; you must remain nonjudgmental through all contacts with the teen.

Nursing Care Focus

- Family caregiver coping impairment and knowledge deficiency related to the diagnosis of HIV/AIDS

Goal

- The family will show evidence of coping with and understanding the illness and supporting the child.

Implementations for Promoting Family Coping and Reinforcing Teaching

The adolescent must be involved in telling family members about the diagnosis if they do not already know. The sexual activity of adolescent children is a topic with which many families find difficult to deal, especially if the activity is homosexual or promiscuous.

The family caregivers usually need support as much as the child does. They are often devastated by the prospect of the child's illness. If the adolescent is pregnant or has a child, the family must also consider the future of that child. For the family who plays a supportive role in the child's life, the period after diagnosis is a difficult one.

Give the family as much information about the disease as possible. They must learn how to prevent the spread of the virus among family members, as well as how to prevent opportunistic infections in the child who is HIV-positive. It is important to reinforce teaching with the family about treatments, medications, nutrition guidelines, and signs and symptoms of opportunistic infections. Stress the importance of reporting even minor complications to the health care provider, and suggest ways to help support the child. See Tips for Reinforcing Family Teaching: Supporting the Child or Adolescent with HIV/AIDS.

Although reinforcing teaching with the child and the family is necessary, remember that a person can absorb only so much detail at one time. Do not present too much in one setting, rather offer information over a period of time. Give the family caregiver and the child written materials that repeat the information, and review it verbally with them by asking questions and clarifying material until they show evidence of clear understanding of the concepts they need to know. It is important to provide the entire family with the best possible support and information.

Evaluation of Goal/Desired Outcome

The family:

- expresses anxieties.
- voices understanding of the illness and treatment.
- supports the child in future plans.

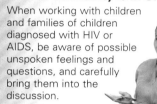

A Little Sensitivity Is In Order
When working with children and families of children diagnosed with HIV or AIDS, be aware of possible unspoken feelings and questions, and carefully bring them into the discussion.

INFECTIOUS MONONUCLEOSIS

Common in the adolescent population and sometimes called the "kissing disease," infectious mononucleosis ("mono") is caused by the Epstein–Barr virus, one of the herpes virus groups. The organism is transmitted through saliva. No immunization is available, and treatment is symptomatic. Adolescents and young adults seem to be most susceptible to this disorder, although sometimes it is also seen in younger children.

Clinical Manifestations

Infectious mononucleosis can present a variety of symptoms, ranging from mild to severe. Symptoms include fever; sore throat with enlarged tonsils; thick, white membrane covering the tonsils (Fig. 41-12); palatine petechiae (red spots on the soft palate); swollen lymph nodes; and enlargement of the spleen accompanied by extreme fatigue and lack of energy. In some instances, headache, abdominal pain, and epistaxis are also present.

Diagnosis

Diagnosis of infectious mononucleosis is based on clinical symptoms, laboratory evidence of lymphocytes in the peripheral blood smear, and a positive heterophil agglutination test. Monospot is a valuable diagnostic test—rapid, sensitive, inexpensive, and simple to perform. Monospot can detect significant agglutinins at lower levels, thus allowing earlier diagnosis. Infectious mononucleosis is often confused with streptococcal infections because of the fever and the appearance of the throat and tonsils.

Treatment and Nursing Care

No cure exists for infectious mononucleosis; treatment is based on symptoms. An analgesic–antipyretic, such as acetaminophen or an NSAID, is usually recommended for the fever and headaches. Fluids and a soft, bland diet are encouraged to reduce throat irritation. Corticosteroids are sometimes used to decrease the inflammation. Bed rest is suggested to relieve fatigue but is not imposed for a specific amount of time. If the spleen is enlarged, the child is cautioned to avoid contact sports that might cause a ruptured spleen. Because the immune system is weakened, the child must take precautions to avoid secondary infections.

The course of mononucleosis is usually uncomplicated. Fever and sore throat may last from 1 week to 10 days. Fatigue generally disappears 2 to 4 weeks after the appearance of acute symptoms but may last longer. The limitations that this disorder imposes on the adolescent's school and social life may cause depression. However, in most

 TIPS FOR REINFORCING FAMILY TEACHING

Supporting the Child or Adolescent With HIV/AIDS

- Assist in learning about and accepting diagnosis.
- Provide educational literature on HIV/AIDS.
- Explain the difference between being HIV-positive and having AIDS.
- Encourage them to verbalize feelings (anger, fear, hopelessness, etc.).
- Encourage participation in local support groups.
- Promote eating an adequate diet, exercising regularly, and sleeping 8 to 10 hours/night.
- Encourage small, frequent meals or suggest nutritional supplements, such as Ensure, to prevent weight loss.
- Discuss prescribed drugs: indications, schedules, doses, and how to recognize and manage side effects.
- Make a schedule for medicines and daily eating times that will work for you and your child.
- Use reminders, such as a timer or a watch with an alarm, calendars, and a check-off list of when a dose is due or has been taken.

- Color-code the bottles of liquid medicines with matching oral syringes. This makes giving the right dose easier. Put the same color for the medicine on the calendar or checklist.
- Explain how HIV is spread (by direct contact with infected body fluids, usually through sex, sharing needles, or blood transfusion).
- Talk about how to avoid transmitting the virus to others or contracting yet another strain.
- Discuss safer sex strategies, such as using condoms.
- Discuss why and how to notify sex partners of infection; explain that partners need counseling, testing, and if HIV-positive, referral for treatment; offer to help with the notification process if necessary.
- Discuss the importance of primary healthcare.
- Encourage adolescent girls to have regular gynecologic examinations and Pap smears.

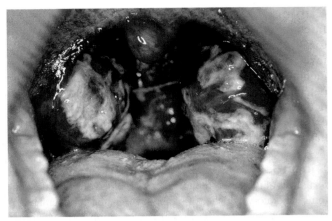

FIGURE 41-12 Tonsils of an adolescent who has infectious mononucleosis; note the red, enlarged tonsils with the thick white covering. (©Dr. P. Marazzi/Science Source.)

instances, the child can resume normal activities within 1 month after symptoms present.

Nursing care includes encouraging the child to express feelings about the interruptions the illness is causing in school, social, and work plans. Long-term effects are rarely seen.

TEST YOURSELF

✔ List the most common STIs in adolescents, and explain how each of these is treated.

✔ Discuss what you would say to an adolescent about STIs.

✔ How is mononucleosis treated?

COMMUNICABLE DISEASES OF CHILDHOOD

Half a century ago, growing up meant being able to survive measles, mumps, whooping cough, diphtheria, and often poliomyelitis. These diseases were expected almost as routinely as the loss of the deciduous teeth. Immunization has changed that outcome so drastically that some family caregivers have become less conscientious about having their children immunized until the immunization is required for entrance to school. The incidence of childhood diseases has decreased with only an occasional outbreak in certain communities where many children are not immunized.

Understanding the various communicable diseases and their preventions, symptoms, and treatments (Table 41-3) requires knowledge of specific terms (Box 41-1). Some communicable diseases require specific precautions to prevent spreading of the infection. Follow the guidelines recommended by the CDC regarding standard and transmission-based precautions (see Appendix A). Specific transmission protocol and procedures can be found in the procedure manuals of individual institutions.

Prevention

The Centers for Disease Control and Prevention (CDC) recommends appropriate vaccinations throughout childhood, and family caregivers are encouraged to follow the current recommended immunization schedule (www.cdc.gov/vaccines). During routine well-child visits and in community-based clinics, the child's immunization record is reviewed and immunizations are administered to keep the child current. Family caregivers of children whose immunizations are incomplete must be urged to have the immunizations brought up to date. For families of limited means, free immunizations are usually available at clinics.

Nursing Care

Many times the child who develops a communicable disease is at home. However, in some cases, the child may develop the disease while hospitalized. For the child who develops a communicable disease and is hospitalized, explain to the child and the family caregivers the reason for the transmission-based precautions. Precautions are done to protect the child from the threat of infection or to protect others from the infection the child has. Otherwise, the child may feel that the precautions are a form of punishment. Families are more likely to follow the correct procedures if they understand the need for them. Transmission-based precautions may intensify the normal loneliness of being ill, so the child needs extra attention and stimulation during this time.

 A Personal Glimpse

One time last year when I was in kindergarten, I felt so sick. I had a red spot on my face, and when I woke up my tummy was covered with spots. I was so hot, and I itched all over. My mom called the nurse at my doctor's office to see if she should take me and they said, "No way. She's got the chickenpox." It was like Halloween at school, but it was really called the Fall Fiesta. I was going to be Bruce the shark from "Finding Nemo" because I watch it all the time on video. My sister and all my friends walked to school in their costumes, but I couldn't go, and I itched a lot. I was so sad. To keep me from being sad, my mom said I could draw pictures, and I drew pictures of me making a soccer goal and of my slingshot. I decided when I was better I could use my costume to play Shark Attack. I would pretend I was swimming in the ocean and if I catch other people, they turn into friendly sharks. I was crying, and I was so itchy, and my mom put lotion on, but it didn't help. My mom said she could give me a bath in oatmeal, and it would feel better. I was kind of grossed out because I don't usually take a bath in food, but she said we could put it in a special cloth instead of a bowl. She was right; I stopped itching a little. When my sister came home with candy and treats, I felt a little better, but I still had the chickenpox.

Jocie, age 6 years

Learning Opportunity: *What questions do you think the nurse in the health care provider's office asked to determine this child should be cared for at home, rather than be seen in the office? For what reason would this mother give her child an "oatmeal" bath?*

Think back to **Charlotte Dey**, the 9-month-old diagnosed with atopic dermatitis. What are some of the possible causes of her diagnosis? Describe the nursing care you think would be important for Charlotte. What will you do to support both Charlotte and her parents?

TABLE 41-3 Communicable Diseases of Childhood

DISEASE	PERIOD OF COMMUNICABILITY WHEN/HOW LONG CONTAGIOUS	PREVENTION, IMMUNIZATION, IMMUNITY	CLINICAL MANIFESTATIONS	TREATMENT NURSING CARE IMPLEMENTATION	COMPLICATIONS
Hepatitis B					
Causative agent: *A Hepadnavirus; hepatitis B virus* Mode of transmission: body fluids, transfusion of contaminated blood, use of contaminated needle, to fetus via mother Incubation period: average 60–90 days	End of incubation time and during acute stage	Use of standard precautions Vaccine for hepatitis B After exposure— HBIG (hepatitis B immune globulin)	Anorexia, abdominal discomfort, nausea, vomiting, jaundice	Rest, nutrition with good caloric intake	Possibly fatal, liver problems, in some cases possibly leads to chronic hepatitis
Diphtheria					
Causative agent: *Corynebacterium diphtheriae* Mode of transmission: droplet, direct contact with infected person, carrier, or contaminated article Incubation period: 2–7 days	2–4 weeks in untreated person 1–2 days with antibiotic therapy	Active immunity from diphtheria toxin in DTaP vaccine Passive immunity with diphtheria antitoxin	Mucous membranes of nose and throat covered by gray membrane, purulent nasal discharge, brassy cough, toxin from organism passes through bloodstream to heart and nervous system	Strict droplet transmission precautions, IV antitoxin and antibiotics, bed rest, liquid to soft diet, analgesics for throat pain, immunization for nonimmunized contacts	Neuritis, carditis, heart failure, respiratory failure
Tetanus (Lockjaw)					
Causative agent: *Clostridium tetani* Mode of transmission: direct or indirect contamination of a closed wound Incubation period: 3–21 days	None—not transmitted from person to person	Active immunity from tetanus toxoid in DTaP vaccine	Stiffness of neck and jaw, muscle rigidity of trunk and extremities, arched back, abdominal muscle stiffness, unusual facial appearance, pain because of muscle spasms	Quiet room, wound cleaning and débridement, penicillin G or erythromycin, muscle relaxants	Serious, fatal if untreated, possible respiratory complications
Pertussis (Whooping Cough)					
Causative agent: *Bordetella pertussis* Mode of transmission: droplet, direct contact with respiratory discharges Incubation period: 5–21 days	About 4–6 weeks, greatest in respiratory stage	Active immunity from pertussis vaccine in DTaP vaccine Disease gives natural immunity	Begins with mild upper respiratory symptoms; in second week progresses to severe paroxysmal cough with inspiratory whoop, sometimes followed by vomiting; especially dangerous for young infants, may last 4–6 weeks	Bed rest, infants hospitalized, oxygen therapy possible, observation for airway obstruction, provision of high humidity, protection from secondary infections, increased fluid intake, refeeding if vomiting occurs	Pneumonia (can cause death of infant), otitis media, hemorrhage, convulsions

(Continued)

TABLE 41-3 Communicable Diseases of Childhood (Continued)

DISEASE	PERIOD OF COMMUNICABILITY WHEN/HOW LONG CONTAGIOUS	PREVENTION, IMMUNIZATION, IMMUNITY	CLINICAL MANIFESTATIONS	TREATMENT NURSING CARE IMPLEMENTATION	COMPLICATIONS
Haemophilus influenzae Type B					
Causative agent: Coccobacilli H. influenzae bacteria Mode of transmission: droplet, discharge from nose and throat Incubation period: 2–4 days	As long as organisms are present; non-communicable after antibiotic therapy for 24–48 hours	Vaccine H. influenzae type B (HIB)	Fever, vomiting, lethargy, meningeal irritation with bulging fontanel or stiff neck and back, stupor, coma	Antibiotics	Meningitis, epiglottitis, pneumonia
Poliomyelitis (Infantile Paralysis)					
Causative agent: poliovirus Mode of transmission: direct and indirect contact, fecal–oral route Incubation period: 7–14 days	Greatest just before onset and just after onset of symptoms, when virus is present in throat and feces, 1–6 weeks	Inactivated polio vaccine (IPV) Disease causes active immunity against specific strain	Fever, headache, nausea, vomiting, abdominal pain, stiff neck, pain, and tenderness in lower extremities that proceed to paralysis	Bed rest, moist hot packs to extremities, range-of-motion exercises, supportive care, long-term ventilation if respiratory muscles involved	Permanent paralysis, respiratory arrest
Rubeola (Measles)					
Causative agent: measles virus Mode of transmission: direct or indirect contact with droplets, nasal, and throat secretions Incubation period: 10–12 days	Fifth incubation day through first few days after rash erupts	Attenuated live vaccine (part of MMR vaccine) Disease gives lasting natural immunity	High fever, sore throat, coryza (runny nose), cough, enlarged lymph nodes (head and neck), Koplik spots (small red spots with blue-white centers on oral mucosa, specific to rubeola), conjunctivitis, photophobia, maculopapular rash starts at hairline and spreads to entire body	Antipyretics; comfort measures for rash including tepid baths, soothing lotion, maintenance of dry skin; dimly lighted room for comfort; fluids	Otitis media, pneumonia, encephalitis, airway obstruction
Parotitis (Mumps)					
Causative agent: Paramyxovirus Mode of transmission: airborne, droplet, direct contact with saliva of infected person Incubation period: 14–21 days	Shortly before swelling appears until after it disappears	Attenuated live mumps vaccine (part of MMR vaccine) Disease gives natural immunity	Parotid glands swollen, unilaterally or bilaterally; may have fever, headache, malaise, and complain of earache before swelling appears; angle of jaw obliterated on affected side	Liquids and soft foods because chewing is painful; avoidance of sour foods, which cause discomfort; analgesics for pain; antipyretics for fever; local compresses of heat or cold	In males past puberty, orchitis (inflammation of the testes); meningoencephalitis; possible severe hearing impairment (rare)

(Continued)

TABLE 41-3 Communicable Diseases of Childhood (Continued)

DISEASE	PERIOD OF COMMUNICABILITY WHEN/HOW LONG CONTAGIOUS	PREVENTION, IMMUNIZATION, IMMUNITY	CLINICAL MANIFESTATIONS	TREATMENT NURSING CARE IMPLEMENTATION	COMPLICATIONS
Rubella (German Measles)					
Causative agent: Rubella virus Mode of transmission: direct or indirect contact with droplets, nasopharyngeal secretions Incubation period: 14–21 days	5–7 days before until about 5 days after rash appears	Attenuated live vaccine (part of MMR vaccine) Disease gives lasting natural immunity Immune serum globulin may be given to pregnant women	Low-grade fever; headache; malaise; anorexia; sore throat; lymph glands of neck and head enlarged; pink-red rash begins on face, spreads downward, disappears in 3 days; may have joint pain	Comfort measures for rash, antipyretics for fever and joint pain	Severe birth defects possible if mother is exposed and nonimmunized (especially in first trimester)
Varicella (Chickenpox)					
Causative agent: *Varicella zoster* virus Mode of transmission: airborne, direct or indirect contact with saliva or uncrusted vesicles Incubation period: 10–21 days	One day before rash appears to about 5–6 days after it appears (until all vesicles crusted)	Attenuated live varicella virus vaccine gives active immunity Disease causes lasting natural immunity; may reactivate in adult as herpes zoster	Low-grade fever; malaise; successive crops of macules, papules, vesicles, and crusts, all present at the same time; itching is intense; scarring may occur when scabs are removed before ready to fall off	Antihistamines, soothing baths, and lotions to reduce itching; prevention of scratching with short fingernails or use of mittens; acyclovir to shorten the course of the disease; *no aspirin* should be given	Reye syndrome possible if child has had aspirin during illness, secondary infection of lesions if scratched, pneumonia, encephalitis
Hepatitis A					
Causative agent: *A picornavirus; hepatitis A virus* Mode of transmission: ingestion of fecal-contaminated food or water or contaminated surfaces Incubation period: average 25–30 days	Highest during 2 weeks before onset of symptoms	Good handwashing, sanitary disposal of feces Vaccine for hepatitis A After exposure— immune globulin	Fever, malaise, anorexia, nausea, abdominal discomfort, jaundice	Enteric precautions, rest, nutritious diet	
Erythema Infectiosum (Fifth Disease)					
Causative agent: *Human parvovirus B19* Mode of transmission: droplet, contact with respiratory secretions Incubation period: 6–14 days	Uncertain; child may return to school when rash appears, no longer infectious at that point	No immunity	Fever, headache, malaise; a week later, red rash appears on face, called a "slapped face" rash; rash appears on extremities, then on trunk; rash can reappear with heat, sunlight, cold	Supportive treatment with antipyretics, analgesics, droplet transmission precautions (when hospitalized)	Arthritis possible, dangerous for fetus (keep infected child away from pregnant women)

(Continued)

TABLE 41-3 Communicable Diseases of Childhood (Continued)

DISEASE	PERIOD OF COMMUNICABILITY WHEN/HOW LONG CONTAGIOUS	PREVENTION, IMMUNIZATION, IMMUNITY	CLINICAL MANIFESTATIONS	TREATMENT NURSING CARE IMPLEMENTATION	COMPLICATIONS
Roseola (Exanthema subitum)					
Causative agent: Human herpes virus type 6 Mode of transmission: unknown Incubation period: about 10 days	During febrile period	Contracting disease gives lasting immunity	High fever; irritability; anorexia; lymph nodes enlarged; decreased WBC; rash appears just after sharp decline in temperature; rash is rose-pink, mostly on trunk, lasts 1–2 days	Symptomatic for rash and fever, standard precautions (if hospitalized)	
Lyme Disease					
Causative agent: *Borrelia burgdorferi* Mode of transmission: deer tick bite Incubation period: 3–30 days	Not communicable from one person to another	Avoid tick-infected areas; inspect skin after being in wooded areas Active immunity from Lyme disease vaccine	Starts as a red papule that spreads and becomes a large, round red ring; fever; malaise; headache; mild neck stiffness with rash; leads to systemic symptoms and chronic problems	Antibiotics	Cardiac, musculoskeletal, and neurologic involvement
Scarlet Fever					
Causative agent: *Beta-hemolytic streptococci group A* Mode of transmission: direct contact, droplet Incubation period: 2–5 days	During acute respiratory phase, 1–7 days	Lasting immunity after having disease	Begins abruptly; fever; sore throat; headache; chills; malaise; red rash on skin and mucous membranes; tonsils inflamed; enlarged; white exudate; tongue—differentiates from other rashes, by day 4–5, "red strawberry" appearance	Soft or liquid diet, antipyretics, analgesics, comfort measures for itching rash, penicillin for streptococcal infection	Glomerulonephritis or rheumatic fever if untreated

BOX 41-1 Common Terms in Communicable Disease Nursing

Active immunity: stimulates development of antibodies to destroy infective agent without causing disease; occurs when vaccine is given

Antibody: a protective substance in the body produced in response to the introduction of an antigen

Antigen: a foreign protein that stimulates the formation of antibodies

Antitoxin: an antibody that unites with and neutralizes a specific toxin

Carrier: a person in apparently good health whose body harbors the specific organisms of a disease

Causative agent: pathogen that causes disease

Enanthem: an eruption on a mucous surface

Endemic: habitual presence of a disease within a given area

Epidemic: an outbreak in a community of a group of illnesses of similar nature in excess of the normal expectancy

Erythema: redness of the skin produced by congestion of the capillaries

Exanthem: an eruption appearing on the skin during an eruptive disease

Host: a human, animal, or plant that harbors or nourishes another organism

Incubation period: the time interval between the infection and the appearance of the first symptoms of the disease

Macule: a discolored skin spot not elevated above the surface

Mode of transmission: mechanism by which an infectious agent is spread or transferred to humans

Natural immunity: resistance to pathogen or infection, genetically determined

Pandemic: a worldwide epidemic

Papule: a small, circumscribed, solid elevation of the skin

Passive immunity: antibodies obtained from an immune person, given to someone exposed to disease to prevent them from getting disease

Period of communicability: time that infectious agent can be transmitted or passed from an infected person or animal to another person

Pustule: a small elevation of epidermis filled with pus

Toxin: a poisonous substance produced by certain organisms, such as bacteria

Toxoid: a toxin that has been treated to destroy its toxicity but that retains its antigenic properties

Vaccine: a suspension of attenuated or killed microorganisms administered for the prevention of a specific infection

Vesicle: a small blister containing clear fluid

KEY POINTS

- The integumentary system, including the accessory structures, is in place at birth and matures as the child grows. Protecting the body from attacks from microorganisms and helping the body get rid of or resist invasion by foreign materials are the major roles of the immune system. The immune system matures and develops as the child progresses through childhood.

- Seborrheic dermatitis is known as cradle cap. It appears as yellowish, scaly crusted patches on the scalp and can usually be prevented by daily washing of hair and scalp. In the child with miliaria rubra, a rash appears as pinhead-sized erythematous (reddened) papules and usually causes itching. Treatment is primarily preventive by not overdressing, especially in warm weather. *C. albicans* is the causative agent for thrush and some cases of diaper rash. It appears as a white coating in the child's mouth and is treated with nystatin. Skin infections caused by *S. aureus* are prevented by using good handwashing and following transmission precautions. MRSA is resistant to the antibiotics used to kill the bacterium, making it harder to treat. Impetigo is a bacterial skin infection characterized by a honey-colored, crusted appearance.

- Acne vulgaris is caused by a variety of factors, including increased hormonal levels, hereditary factors, irritation and irritating substances, and growth of anaerobic bacteria. Treatment for mild acne is application of a topical medication, such as benzoyl peroxide or retinoids, once or twice a day. Antibiotics may be administered for inflammatory acne. Isotretinoin, a pregnancy category X drug, may be used for severe inflammatory acne.

- Tinea (ringworm) is the term commonly applied to fungal infections. These occur in various parts of the body and are treated by antifungal medications.

- Pediculosis of the scalp is treated using nonprescription medications and topical pediculicides, such as pyrethrins and permethrin. After the hair is shampooed thoroughly and dried, it is combed with a fine-toothed comb dipped in warm white vinegar to remove remaining nits and nit shells. For protection when treating a child in the hospital, wear a disposable gown, gloves, and head cover. Scabies is a skin infestation and is treated with permethrin cream.

- Anaphylaxis is an acute hypersensitive response to an allergen, can occur with exposure to any allergen, and may be life-threatening. Hyposensitization is performed for the allergens that produce a positive reaction on skin testing. The allergist sets up a schedule for injections in gradually increasing doses until a maintenance dose is reached.

- Atopic dermatitis or eczema is considered, at least in part, an allergic reaction to an irritant. Common allergens involved in eczema are foods, inhalants, and materials. Goals when caring for the child include preserving skin integrity, maintaining comfort, improving sleep patterns, maintaining good nutrition, and preventing infection of skin lesions.

- Contact dermatitis is inflammation of the skin as the result of a hypersensitive reaction to direct contact with a substance. It can be caused by an irritant or by an allergy. A bright red rash, swelling, blisterlike vesicles, and intense itching (pruritus) are common. Avoiding the allergen by removing it from the child's environment is important. Treatment is aimed at reducing and controlling the symptoms.

- All animal and human bites should be thoroughly cleaned and observed for signs of infection. Spider bites can cause serious illness if untreated. Tick bites can be prevented by wearing long pants and long-sleeved shirts, and using insect repellent when walking in the woods. Snakebites demand immediate medical intervention. Insect stings or bites can prove fatal to children who are sensitized, so immediate treatment is required if a child with sensitivity is bitten.

- Superficial burns occur when the epidermis is injured but there is no destruction of tissue or nerve endings. Partial-thickness (second-degree) burns occur when the epidermis and underlying dermis are both injured and devitalized or destroyed. Blistering usually occurs, as does an escape of body plasma. With full-thickness (third-degree) burns, the epidermis, dermis, and nerve endings are all destroyed. Pain is minimal, and there is no longer any barrier to infection or any remaining viable epithelial cells.

- Emergency treatment in the case of a burn involves first removing the heat source and providing emergency care. For burns involving small areas, immediate application of cool compresses or cool water to burn areas inhibits capillary permeability and thus suppresses edema, blister formation, and tissue destruction. For moderate burns, immersing a burned extremity in cool water alleviates pain and may prevent additional thermal injury. In severe burns, the airway, breathing, and circulation must be observed and restored if necessary, and the child is transported to a medical facility for assessment. Hypovolemic shock is the major manifestation in the first 48 hours in massive burns. As extracellular fluid pours into the burned area, it collects in enormous quantities, which dehydrates the body and causes the symptoms of shock to occur.

- Major causes of burns in children include thermal or heat burns, electricity, and chemicals. Nursing care for the child with a burn focuses on preventing infection, maintaining adequate nutrition, reducing pain, increasing mobility, and relieving anxiety as well as optimizing healing and decreasing complications to minimize permanent disability.

- Human papillomavirus (HPV) is the most common sexually transmitted infection (STI) seen in the adolescent. Immunizations are given to males and females at age 11 or 12 to prevent HPV.

- Gonorrhea is caused by the organism *Neisseria gonorrhoeae*. Chlamydia is caused by *Chlamydia trachomatis*. Genital herpes is caused by herpes simplex type 2. Syphilis is caused by *T. pallidum*.

- The drugs of choice to treat gonorrhea are ceftriaxone, azithromycin, and doxycycline to prevent an accompanying chlamydial infection. Doxycycline or azithromycin is used to treat chlamydial infection. Acyclovir is useful in relieving or suppressing the symptoms of genital herpes. Syphilis responds to one intramuscular injection of benzathine penicillin G; if the individual is sensitive to penicillin, oral doxycycline can be administered.

- The human immunodeficiency virus (HIV) is transmitted by sexual contact with an infected person, by sharing infected needles, and from an HIV-positive woman to her fetus or infant. Nursing care focuses on maintaining the highest level of wellness possible by preventing infection and the spread of the infection, minimizing pain, improving nutrition, promoting adherence to the medication regimen, alleviating social isolation, and diminishing a feeling of hopelessness.

- Infectious mononucleosis ("mono") is caused by the Epstein–Barr virus, which is one of the herpes virus groups. The organism is transmitted through saliva, and treatment is symptomatic.

- Modes of transmission of communicable diseases include droplet; direct or indirect contact with body fluids and discharges; and contaminated blood, food, or water. Many communicable diseases can be prevented by immunization with vaccinations and the use of standard transmission precautions.

- Active immunity occurs when antibodies are formed after immunization with a vaccine. Natural immunity is often genetically determined and gives a person a resistance to a pathogen. Passive immunity occurs when a person who has been exposed to a certain disease is given antibodies that have been obtained from an immune person.

- Nursing interventions for the child with a communicable disease are usually supportive. Depending on the disease symptoms, the implementations might include providing rest, adequate nutrition and fluids, following transmission precautions, giving medications as appropriate, and offering comfort measures.

INTERNET RESOURCES

Burns
www.ameriburn.org

Sexually Transmitted Infections
www.ashasexualhealth.org

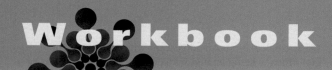

NCLEX-STYLE REVIEW QUESTIONS

1. In caring for a 3.5-year-old child admitted after being severely burned, the nurse collects the following data. Which of the following would be *most* important for the nurse to report immediately?

  a. The child's respiratory rate is 32 breaths/min.
  b. The child's temperature is 38.4°C.
  c. The child's hourly urinary output is 150 mL.
  d. The child's pain level is an 8 on the pain scale.

2. The nurse is discussing STIs with a group of adolescents. If the adolescents make the following statements, which statement indicates a need for reinforcement of teaching?

  a. "Even though guys don't like to use condoms, at least they protect a person from most STIs."
  b. "My girlfriend has never had sex with anyone except me, so I don't have to worry about STIs."
  c. "It is a relief to know that other than HIV, most STIs can be treated with antibiotics."
  d. "My girlfriend is pregnant, but since she does not have an STI, our baby most likely won't either."

3. In caring for a child with atopic dermatitis (eczema), which of the following nursing interventions would be included in this child's care? Select all that apply.

  a. The nurse will keep child's fingernails cut short.
  b. The nurse will dress the child in several layers of clothing at all times.
  c. The nurse will monitor for symptoms of infection.
  d. The nurse will give soothing baths just before bedtime.
  e. The nurse will encourage the child to drink fluids frequently.
  f. The nurse will use a bleach solution to launder the child's clothing.

4. After an outbreak of pediculosis in the school, the nurse is reinforcing teaching with a group of parents and teachers about ways to help prevent the spread of head lice in the classroom and at home. Which of the following actions would the nurse recommend to this group? Select all that apply.

  a. Wash all bedding and clothing in hot water, and dry in a hot dryer.
  b. Apply medicated lotion to all areas of the body except the face.
  c. Wash combs and brushes in medicated shampoo, and soak for at least an hour.
  d. Report any evidence of infestation immediately to the school officials.
  e. Vacuum carpets, car seats, mattresses, and upholstered furniture thoroughly.
  f. Wear gloves when preparing food or snacks.

STUDY ACTIVITIES

1. Using the table below, compare the six most common STIs seen in adolescents. Describe the symptoms, treatment, and complications or long-term concerns seen with these infections.

STI	Symptoms	Treatment	Complications or Long-Term Concerns

2. Using the table below, make a list of substances that may cause allergies in infants and children. List some sources of these substances that may cause allergies.

Substance That May Cause Allergies	Sources of Substances That May Cause Allergies

3. Identify the relation between *C. albicans* and some cases of diaper dermatitis. Detail the teaching that you would reinforce with a mother about diaper rash.

4. Do an Internet search on "treating burns in children."

  a. List some of the sites you discovered which you think would be helpful when working with a child who has suffered a burn.
  b. What are some of the suggestions and recommendations you found that might be helpful to share with your peers?

CRITICAL THINKING: WHAT WOULD YOU DO?

1. Brian is HIV-positive and lives with his family. The family is frightened that other members may get the virus.

  a. What will you tell the family to reassure them?
  b. What teaching will you reinforce with them in regard to prevention of the spread of the virus in their home?
  c. What guidelines will you give the family caregivers to help them protect Brian from infectious or opportunistic diseases?

2. Two-year-old Omar has partial- and full-thickness burns from a wood stove accident. You are helping develop a teaching plan covering the importance of infection control for Omar during his convalescence.

   a. What is the most important action that can be taken to prevent infection?
   b. Who should be included in reinforcement teaching regarding infection control?
   c. What are the signs that might indicate an infection?
   d. Why is it important to detect signs and symptoms of an infection early?

3. Dosage calculation: An adolescent with a diagnosis of gonorrhea is being treated with ceftriaxone. The dose to be given is 250-mg IM. The medication is available in a preparation of 1 g/10 mL. Answer the following.

   a. How many milligrams (mg) are in 1 gram (g)?
   b. How many milliliters will be given in this 250-mg dose to this adolescent? After the administration of ceftriaxone, the adolescent will be given doxycycline 100-mg BID by mouth for 7 days. Answer the following.
   c. How many milligrams (mg) will be given in a 24-hour period?
   d. How many total milligrams (mg) will be given in the 7 days?

The Child With a Cognitive, Behavioral, or Mental Health Disorder

Key Terms

anorexia nervosa
binging
bulimia nervosa
dependence
echolalia
encopresis
gynecomastia
obesity
overweight
polyphagia
refeeding syndrome
rumination
substance abuse
tolerance
withdrawal symptoms

Learning Objectives

At the conclusion of this chapter, you will:

1. Describe autism spectrum disorder (ASD), including the diagnosis, characteristics, treatment, and nursing care.
2. Identify characteristics that may be seen in a child with attention deficit hyperactivity disorder (ADHD) and discuss the treatment of the disorder.
3. Describe and compare oppositional defiant disorder and conduct disorder, including the characteristics seen in children with these disorders.
4. Discuss characteristics and behaviors seen in the child who bullies other children.
5. Describe and compare generalized anxiety disorder, separation anxiety, and phobias, including symptoms seen in children with these disorders.
6. Differentiate enuresis and encopresis.
7. Discuss the diagnosis of depression in the young child and the adolescent.
8. Discuss the warning signs seen in children who are considering suicide.
9. List substances commonly abused by children.
10. State the negative effects of commonly abused substances.
11. Describe the characteristics of the child with pica and nonorganic failure to thrive (NFTT).
12. Discuss the characteristics, signs, and symptoms seen in the child with anorexia nervosa and state goals of treatment for the hospitalized client with anorexia nervosa.
13. Describe the signs, symptoms, and nursing care for the child with bulimia nervosa.
14. Discuss binge eating disorder, obesity, and the goal of health care professionals who work with obese children.

The Gallegos family and their four children live in your neighborhood. **Jacob** is the oldest child in the family and just turned 16. His mother knows you are a nurse and confides in you that she is concerned that Jacob may have a substance abuse problem. As you read this chapter, think about what will be most helpful for you to say to Jacob's mother.

Cognitive, behavioral, or mental health disorders seen in children may have genetic, physiologic, or environmental causes. These disorders are sometimes difficult to diagnose in children, but early recognition of signs and symptoms and treatment may decrease the effects the disorder will have on the child's formative and growing years, as well as into adulthood.

AUTISM SPECTRUM DISORDER

Autism spectrum disorder (ASD) is a complex neurodevelopmental disorder characterized by deficits in social interaction and communication, and repetitive patterns, activities, and behaviors. The severity of the symptoms ranges from mild to severe. Children with ASD are often self-absorbed and unable to relate to others; they may exhibit unusual patterns in behaviors. The child has difficulty with understanding and processing input from around them. The cause of ASD appears to be genetic factors that lead to abnormal brain development, which impairs social and communication skills. Because the cause of ASD is not well understood and because some children have a few mild symptoms, whereas others have severe, disabling symptoms, treatment is difficult. Children with ASD experience the normal health problems of childhood in addition to those that result from their behaviors.

Clinical Manifestations

The characteristics of ASD are most often recognized during the second or third year of life, although present earlier. Impaired verbal and nonverbal communication including delays and deviations in language development, impaired social and emotional exchanges and relationships with others, and repetitive movements and obsessive behavior patterns are often seen in the child with ASD. The repetitive behaviors may include rocking, twirling, flapping arms and hands, walking on tiptoe, and twisting and turning fingers. In children with cognitive disabilities as well as ASD, self-injurious behaviors such as head-banging, face or body slapping, and self-biting may be seen. Children with ASD often prefer the same, identical routine each day and if that routine is disrupted it may cause distress.

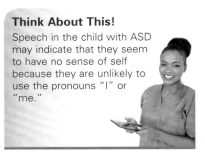

Think About This!

Speech in the child with ASD may indicate that they seem to have no sense of self because they are unlikely to use the pronouns "I" or "me."

The child with ASD is slow to develop speech, and speech that develops may be ineffective in its ability to communicate. **Echolalia** ("parrot speech") is typical of children with severe ASD; they echo words they have heard, such as those in a television commercial, but offer no indication that they understand the words. Atypical sensory perception is common and they may be overresponsive or underresponsive to stimuli such as noises, touch, odors, light, and tastes. Sleeping problems include resistance to going to bed, restlessness, or being unable to stay asleep.

Standard intelligence tests that count on verbal ability may indicate that these children test in the cognitively impaired range of intelligence. However, many of these children demonstrate unusual memory and mathematic, artistic, and musical abilities.

Diagnosis

The diagnosis of ASD is made based on the history, including family history, symptoms, examination, and observations of behavior of the child. Specific diagnostic criteria are found in the Diagnostic and Statistical Manual of Mental Disorders, Fifth Edition (DSM-5), developed by the American Psychiatric Association. The criteria include the use of diagnostic tools to determine abnormalities in social interaction, social communication, and restricted, repetitive patterns of behavior, interests, and activities.

Because the symptoms of ASD can suggest other disorders, a complete physical and neurologic examination is necessary. In addition, a complete prenatal, natal, and postnatal history, including development, nutrition, and family dynamics, is taken. Many members of the health team may be involved in the evaluation and treatment of the child with ASD, including audiologists, psychiatrists, psychologists, special education teachers, speech and language therapists, and social workers.

Treatment

The treatment of a child with ASD is extremely challenging. The condition is chronic and the right treatment for ASD depends on the age of the child, how severe the symptoms of the disorder are, and whether the child has any other medical problems. There is no cure for ASD, but children are often able to overcome many of the issues it causes. A treatment goal is for the child to have their highest level of functioning within the limitations of the disorder. The American Academy of Pediatrics recommends a plan that provides structure, direction, and organization for the child. Treatment for ASD focuses on behavioral and educational interventions that target the core symptoms of ASD. Early intervention is important to improve outcomes for children with ASD. Pharmacologic interventions may be used to address medical or psychiatric concerns or provide control of symptoms such as hyperactivity, inattention, aggression, anxiety, depression, and repetitive behaviors. In addition, many families seek complementary or alternative therapies. Treatments must be individually planned and highly structured. Mixed results occur, and no one technique has met with resounding success. The family needs help and support to understand and work with their child in managing the symptoms of the disorder.

Nursing Care

Caring for the child with ASD requires recognizing that ASD creates great stresses for the entire family. The problems that cause family caregivers to seek diagnosis may be difficult to live with, diagnosis itself is usually a lengthy and expensive process, and successful treatment is not certain. Many family caregivers of children with ASD feel guilty, despite the fact that current theories accept organic, rather than psychological, causes for this disorder. The possibility of genetic factors adds to this guilt. Often other children in the family who are normal suffer from a lack of attention because the family caregivers' energies are directed toward dealing with the concerns of the child with ASD.

Family caregivers are your most valuable source of information about the child's habits and communication skills. To gain the child's cooperation, learn which techniques the family caregivers use to communicate with the child. It is essential to establish a relationship of trust and to provide consistency for the child. In the hospital setting, a private or semiprivate room is generally preferred; visual and auditory stimulation should be minimized. Familiar toys or other valued objects from home reduce the child's anxiety about the strange environment.

TEST YOURSELF

✔ What are the common characteristics of the child who has autism spectrum disorder (ASD)?

✔ When a child with ASD is said to have echolalia, what does this mean?

✔ Explain the goal of treatment for the child with ASD.

ATTENTION DEFICIT HYPERACTIVITY DISORDER

Attention deficit hyperactivity disorder (ADHD) is characterized by degrees of inattention, impulsive behavior, and hyperactivity. About 8% to 10% of school-aged children have ADHD; boys are more commonly affected than are girls. The cause of the disorder is unclear but genetic, environmental, and dietary factors all may play a role. The disorder affects every part of the child's life.

Clinical Manifestations

The child with ADHD may have these characteristics:

- Impulsiveness
- Easy distractibility
- Excessive fidgeting or squirming
- Difficulty sitting still
- Difficulty playing quietly
- Problems following through on instructions, despite being able to understand them
- Inattentiveness when being spoken to
- Frequently losing things, lack of organization
- Going from one uncompleted activity to another
- Difficulty taking turns, interrupting
- Frequent excessive talking, blurting out
- Engaging in dangerous activities without considering the consequences

Although these children may have poor success in the classroom because of their inability to pay attention, they are not intellectually impaired. The child's poor impulse control contributes to disciplinary problems in the classroom. Some children with ADHD may have learning disorders, such as dyslexia and perceptual deficits. Social skills may be impaired and the child may have trouble making and keeping friends and participating in team sports. The child's self-confidence can suffer from feeling inferior to the other children. Special arrangements can be made to provide an educational atmosphere that is supportive for the child without the need for the child to leave the classroom.

Diagnosis

Diagnosis can be made after the child is 3 years of age, but it is often not made until the child reaches school age and has trouble settling into the routine of being in the classroom setting. Diagnosis can be difficult and may also be controversial because many of the symptoms are subjective. A multidisciplinary approach is most effective for diagnosis involving pediatric and education specialists, a psychologist, the preschool or classroom teacher, and family caregivers. The symptoms may be a result of environmental factors that can include strained family relationships and stress. A careful detailed history, including school and social functioning, psychological testing, and physical and neurologic examinations, can help in making the diagnosis.

Treatment and Nursing Care

Treatment is also multidisciplinary. Behavioral therapy and environmental changes that can be used by the family caregivers and the teacher are helpful for the child. Daily schedules, organization tools, small realistic goals with rewards, minimal distractions, and helping the child find activities they can succeed in doing are important aspects of treatment. Medication is used for some children. Short-, intermediate-, and long-acting stimulant medications, such as methylphenidate, dexmethylphenidate, and dextroamphetamine, have been used. Common side effects of these medications include anorexia, weight loss, nervousness, and sleep disturbances. Using stimulants for a hyperactive child seems paradoxical, but these drugs stimulate the area of the child's brain that aids in concentration, thus enabling the child to have better control. Atomoxetine is also sometimes used, especially in the adolescent who has a substance abuse concern.

Maintain a calm, patient attitude toward the child with ADHD. The child should be given only one simple instruction at a time. Limiting distractions, using consistency, and offering praise for accomplishments are invaluable methods of working with these children. The families of children with ADHD need a great deal of support. Primary family caregivers in particular can become frustrated and upset by the constant challenge of dealing with a child with ADHD. Building the child's self-esteem, confidence, and academic success must be the primary goal of all who work with these children.

 A Personal Glimpse

I don't really mind it. When I don't take my meds, I go crazy or bonkers (sometimes). I'm on my pills [be]cause of my behavior. And also to control the ways I talk (like so I won't blurt out in class). I was taught to control my actions, don't let my actions control me.

Eddie, a 9-year-old who takes medication for ADHD

Learning Opportunity: *What feelings do you think this child experiences in those times when he is not able to control his behavior? What would you say to this child to encourage him to talk about his disorder and his feelings?*

OPPOSITIONAL DEFIANT DISORDER

The child with oppositional defiant disorder (ODD) exhibits a pattern of angry, irritable, argumentative, defiant, hostile, and sometimes vindictive behavior, which is excessive compared to other children of the same age. A traumatic or dysfunctional family situation, maltreatment, inconsistent or harsh discipline, bullying, or a stressful life event may be risk factors noted in the child's environment. The behaviors are often directed at family members and teachers.

Clinical Manifestations

Children with ODD are easily annoyed, frustrated, and lose their temper frequently. Arguing and refusing to follow rules or comply with requests from authority figures is common. They may be angry and resentful and blame others for their mistakes and difficulties, often doing things to annoy others. The child may see their behavior as justifiable and be vindictive with their behaviors. The frequency of these behaviors helps in determining if these behaviors are symptoms or a part of the child's normal development process.

Treatment

Because the child with ODD does not see their behavior as unacceptable, they frequently cause distress in the family. Professional intervention and help is often necessary. Working with family caregivers and reinforcing teaching related to parenting strategies and appropriate discipline is important. A collaborative approach with the family, health care professionals, and school authorities is most effective in treating the child with ODD.

CONDUCT DISORDER

The child with a conduct disorder exhibits a repetitive and continual pattern of behavior that goes against the rules of society and societal norms appropriate for the child's age. The behaviors often violate the rights of other people. The onset of these behaviors may be noted in early childhood. A negative or dysfunctional family situation, maltreatment, neglect, harsh discipline, bullying, or a stressful life event may be risk factors.

Clinical Manifestations

Children with conduct disorders have aggressive behavior that can result in physical harm to people or animals, including hitting, fighting, and cruelty to animals. The behaviors might not be aggressive, but may cause damage to property, such as vandalism and starting fires. Stealing, lying, breaking rules and laws, not attending school, and running away from home commonly occur. As the child gets older, the aggressive behaviors in social relationships may be bullying and verbal in nature, causing hurt, alienation, and impaired peer relationships.

Treatment

Because of the aggressive behavior seen in the child with a conduct disorder, referrals and early professional intervention are important. The safety of the child and the individuals around the child are priorities. Any evidence of maltreatment or neglect must be addressed to determine the child is in a safe living situation. Working with family caregivers and reinforcing teaching related to parenting strategies and appropriate discipline is important. A collaborative approach with the family, health care professionals, and school authorities is critical.

BULLYING

Bullying is a form of aggressive behavior which is deliberate and repeated, usually toward a person who is physically weaker, shy, or less able to defend themselves from the abuser. One person is the victim of the bully (see Chapter 33 for discussion of the child who is a victim), and the individual who acts as the offender is known as the bully. The bully may have been a victim of abuse or may have witnessed violence as a normal behavior in their life. The bully acts to have power or control over a person, often someone who is in some way different or perceived as different or does not seem to "fit in" with others. The behavior of the bully is vicious and may lead to more violent or even criminal behavior as the child gets older. They may lack social skills, break rules, be impulsive and easily frustrated, and lack a caring attitude toward others. The child who bullies may have a psychosocial disorder and needs professional help to deal with the issues underlying the bullying behavior.

TEST YOURSELF

✔ What characteristics are seen in the child with attention deficit hyperactivity disorder (ADHD)?

✔ How is ADHD treated?

✔ In what ways are oppositional defiant disorder, conduct disorder, and bullying similar?

ENURESIS AND ENCOPRESIS

Enuresis is continued incontinence of urine beyond the age when control of urination is commonly acquired. Enuresis may have a physiologic or psychological cause and may indicate a need for further exploration and treatment (see Chapter 39 for further discussion).

Encopresis is chronic involuntary fecal soiling beyond the age when control is expected (about 3 years of age). Speech and learning disabilities may accompany this problem. If no organic causes (e.g., worms, megacolon) exist, encopresis indicates the possibility of a serious psychological concern and a need for counseling for the child and the family caregivers. Some experts believe that overcontrol or undercontrol by a family caregiver can cause encopresis. Recommendations for treatment differ; however, the most important goal is recognition of the problem and referral for treatment and counseling.

ANXIETY DISORDERS

Anxiety disorders in children are a common diagnosis. Children have normal fears and worries throughout each stage of development. Infants fear loud noises and being startled; toddlers fear separation from their family caregiver and are afraid of the dark. The preschool-aged child worries about imaginary beings, school-age children are afraid of imaginary events, and the adolescent has fears related to being socially accepted and successful in school. If these and other concerns become excessive, out of proportion to the situation, or persistent and cause distress to the child, an anxiety disorder is suspected. The child's family history often includes individuals with anxiety disorders or a stressful event or situation.

There are several classifications of anxiety disorders noted in children. Generalized anxiety disorder, separation anxiety, and phobias are discussed here.

Generalized Anxiety Disorder

The child with generalized anxiety disorder (GAD) usually has a variety of things they worry about or are concerned about. Often school performance and the feeling they need to perform perfectly, or they are no good, cause the child to worry and focus on their mistakes. Other fears include concerns about their safety and health or the safety and health of the people they love. They may not be able to sleep out of fear that something of concern will happen during the night. The child may show signs of being restless, fatigued, and irritable, having muscle tension and difficulty concentrating, as well as sleep disturbances.

Separation Anxiety Disorder

Normal separation anxiety occurs at about 8 months of age and continues for a period of time. When the child has excessive anxiety related to being separated from their home or family caregiver, they are often diagnosed with a separation anxiety disorder. When the child is seen in the health care setting, they cannot separate themselves from their family caregiver, and the caregiver may as well show signs of not wanting to separate from their child. The child may fear something bad will happen if they are not with their parent. They may refuse to go anywhere without the family caregiver.

Phobias

The child with a phobia may have a dread and preoccupation or fear of an object or being in a particular situation or environment. Crowded or small enclosed spaces may create the fear that they are unable to get away or out of a situation. School-phobic children may have a separation anxiety because of a strong attachment to one parent, usually the mother, and they fear separation from that family caregiver, perhaps because of anxiety about losing them while away from home or at school. School phobia may be the child's unconscious reaction to a seemingly overwhelming problem at school. The family caregiver can unwittingly reinforce school phobia by permitting the child to stay home. The child may have symptoms—vomiting, diarrhea, abdominal or other pain, and even a low-grade fever—which are genuine and are caused by anxiety that may approach panic. They disappear with relief of the immediate anxiety after the child has been given permission to stay home.

Treatment

Treatment of anxiety disorders includes a complete medical examination to rule out any organic cause for the symptoms the child shows. The goal of treatment is to reduce the anxiety and help the child find a sense of security. Cognitive behavioral therapy helps the child recognize the fear and anxiety and gives them tools to cope with those feelings. Psychotherapy often includes the child and family working together. The use of therapeutic play may be incorporated. Medications may be used when needed.

DEPRESSION AND SUICIDE

Depression is a mood disorder in which the child may have persistent sadness or unhappiness which interferes with doing the activities they normally enjoy. Depression in children may be difficult to recognize because often the signs that indicate depression are hard to distinguish from the emotions seen in normal development. Depression can be seen in children of any age, but it is noted more frequently in the adolescent than in the younger child. Risk factors for depression include a family history of depression, family dysfunction, loss (e.g., loss of a parent, sibling, or something important in the child's life), traumatic life events, injury or chronic conditions, and emotional, physical, or sexual abuse. It is common for the child with depression to have additional mental health disorders such as anxiety disorders, behavior disorders, eating disorders, and substance abuse issues.

Clinical Manifestations

A key symptom is the overwhelming feeling of being low, down, gloomy, or sad much of the time. Infants and toddlers can show signs which indicate depression. Withdrawal, poor attachment, delayed development, clingy behavior, low energy, and lack of enjoyment in play activities may be symptoms. Younger children may show symptoms of anger, irritability, changes in appetite and sleep patterns, physical complaints, inattention, and difficulty concentrating. The school-aged child may as well be grouchy, annoyed, show a lack of interest in school and in participating in activities with friends. Often family caregivers and teachers recognize and report these behaviors as concerning. Symptoms in the adolescent may be similar to those in the child, but may be more like those seen in adults. In addition, behavioral changes such as missing curfews, extreme defiance, shoplifting, dropping grades, spending more time alone, self-hatred, talking about death or suicide, and the use of drugs and alcohol may indicate depression in the adolescent.

In children of any age who suffer depression, suicide is a major concern. Monitoring closely for signs that may indicate the child is suicidal is the priority in caring for the depressed child. Suicide is one of the leading causes of death in children 10 to 19 years of age. Because some deaths reported as accidents, particularly one-car accidents, are thought to be suicides, the rate actually may be higher. Adolescent boys commit suicide more often than adolescent girls do, but girls attempt suicide more often than boys do. Boys use more lethal means of committing suicide (firearms, hanging) than girls do (overdose, cutting) and thus are successful more often.

Children who have attempted suicide once have a high risk of attempting it again, perhaps more effectively. Attempted suicide rarely occurs without warning and is usually preceded by a long history of emotional problems, difficulty forming relationships, feelings of rejection, and low self-esteem. Loss of one or both parents through death or divorce, a family history that includes suicide of one or more members, and lack of success in academic or athletic performance are other common contributing factors. To this history is added one or more of the normal developmental crises of adolescence:

- Difficulty establishing independence
- Identity crisis

- Lack of intimate relationships
- Breakdown in family communication
- A sense of alienation
- A conflict that interferes with problem solving

The child's situation may be further complicated by an unwanted or unplanned pregnancy, alcohol or drug addiction, or physical or sexual abuse that leads to depression and a feeling of total hopelessness.

Health care professionals involved with children and family caregivers must be aware of factors that place a child at risk for suicide, as well as hints that signal an impending suicide attempt (see Tips for Reinforcing Family Teaching: Suicide Warning Signs for Caregivers). Some of these desperate young people will verbalize their hopelessness with statements such as "I won't be around much longer" or "After Monday, it won't matter anyhow." They may begin giving away prized possessions or appear suddenly elated after a long period of acting dejected.

Never, Never!

Don't ignore behaviors or statements of hopelessness in children and teenagers. Make an effort to ensure the child's safety until counseling and treatment resources are in place.

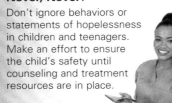

 Cultural Snapshot

Depression and other psychological concerns in some cultures may be disregarded or not expressed because of the fear of social stigma or shame. A confidential and compassionate approach by the nurse may encourage the child to express their feelings or the family caregiver to share the worry they have about symptoms in their child.

During the initial interview with the child, include questions that draw out feelings of alienation, depression, and hopelessness. If any of these indications are present, report and document these findings immediately. Question the family caregiver about any such signs and follow through with seeking additional help for the child.

Treatment and Nursing Care

Early recognition of symptoms and the use of depression screening tools are valuable in the child getting treatment. It is important that counseling and treatment resources be found to help these children. For the child with moderate to severe depression, therapy combined with pharmacologic treatment with antidepressants may be used. Strive to help the child understand that although suicide is an option in problem solving, it is a final option, and other options exist that are not so final. Be aware of the community resources such as hotlines and counselors that specialize in working with people who are contemplating or have attempted suicide. The child's safety and suicide prevention is the priority for any child with depression. In the inpatient setting, often the child is put on a

 TIPS FOR REINFORCING FAMILY TEACHING

Suicide Warning Signs for Caregivers

Warning Signs in Children's Behavior

- Previous suicide attempt
- Thoughts of wishing to kill self
- Plans for self-destructive acts
- Feeling "down in the dumps"
- Withdrawal from social activities
- Loss of pleasure in daily activities
- Change in activity—increase or decrease
- Poor concentration
- Complaints of headaches, upset stomach, joint pains, frequent colds
- Change in eating or sleeping patterns
- Strong feelings of guilt, inadequacy, hopelessness
- Preoccupation with thoughts of people dying, getting sick, or being injured
- Substance abuse
- Violence, truancy, stealing, or lying
- Lack of judgment
- Poor impulse control
- Rapid swing in appropriateness of expressed emotions, sudden lift in mood
- Pessimistic view of self and world
- Saying goodbye
- Giving things away

Changes in Child's Interpersonal Relationships

- Conflicts with peers
- Loss of boyfriend or girlfriend
- School problems—behavioral or academic
- Feelings of great frustration, being misunderstood, or not being part of the group
- Lack of positive support from family, peers, or other
- Earlier suicide of a family member, friend, or classmate
- Separations, deaths, births, moves, or serious illnesses in the family

one-to-one status with constant observation and anything that could be used to harm themselves is removed from the child's access.

TEST YOURSELF

✔ What are some characteristics seen in the child with anxiety disorders?
✔ What symptoms might be seen in children who have depression?
✔ What warning signs are often seen in children who are contemplating committing suicide?

SUBSTANCE ABUSE

Substance abuse is the misuse of an addictive substance that changes the user's mental state. Regular use of substances increases the risk of developing substance use disorder.

The addictive substances commonly abused are tobacco, alcohol, and controlled or illicit drugs. Children are influenced by peers, and in some instances, adults in the family use drugs and alcohol to avoid facing their problems, escape and forget the pain of life as they see it, add excitement to social events, or bow to peer pressure. Throughout history, people have used alcohol and other mood-altering drugs as a means of relieving the tensions and pressures of their lives. Many cultures still sanction use of some of these substances but object to their abuse (i.e., excessive use or use in a way that is medically, socially, or culturally unacceptable).

Use or abuse of these substances can lead to addiction or **dependence** (a compulsive need to use a substance for its satisfying or pleasurable effects). Dependence may be psychological, physical, or both. Psychological dependence means that the substance is desired for the effects or sensations it produces: alertness, euphoria, relaxation, a sense of well-being, and a false sense of control over problems. Physical dependence results from drug-induced changes in body tissue functions that require the drug for normal activity. The magnitude of physical dependence determines the severity of **withdrawal symptoms** (physical and psychological symptoms that occur when the drug is no longer being used) such as vomiting, chills, tremors, seizures, and hallucinations. The symptoms vary with the amount, type, frequency, and duration of drug use. Continued use of an addictive substance can result in **tolerance** (the ability of body tissues to endure and adapt to continued or increased use of a substance); this dynamic means the drug user requires larger doses of the drug to produce the desired effect.

Four stages of use have been identified that help describe the progression of substance abuse (Table 42-1). Use the clues from these stages when you are working in any capacity with children in order to be more alert to signs of possible substance abuse.

The children at greatest risk of becoming substance abusers are those who:

- have families in which alcohol or drug abuse is or has been present.
- suffer from abuse, neglect, or loss, or have no close relationships.
- are in a dysfunctional/distressed family environment.
- have behavioral problems, or are aggressive, impulsive, or rebellious.
- are slow learners, have learning disabilities or cognitive impairments, or have problems with depression and low self-esteem.

In some instances, early identification of these factors by family, teachers, counselors, or other caregivers and prompt referral for treatment can help avoid the potential tragedy of substance abuse. Screening questions and tools are used to identify children who have a substance abuse concern. One tool used commonly with adolescents is the CRAFFT questionnaire (Box 42-2).

TABLE 42-1   Progression of Substance Abuse in Children

STAGE	PREDISPOSITION	BEHAVIOR	FAMILY REACTION
Stage 1. Experimentation, Learning the Mood Swing			
Infrequent use of alcohol/marijuana No consequences Some fear of use Low tolerance	Curiosity Peer pressure Attempt to assume adult role	Learning the mood Feels good Positive reinforcement Can return to normal	Often unaware Denial
Stage 2. Seeking the Mood Swing			

Increasing frequency in use of various
    drugs
Minimal defensiveness
Tolerance
	Impress others
	Social function
	Modeling adult
	    behavior
		Using to get high
		Pride in amount consumed
		Using to relieve feelings (i.e., anxieties of dating)
		Denial of problem
			Attempts at elimination
			Blaming others

Stage 3. Preoccupation With the Mood Swing			

Peer group activities revolve around use
Steady supply
Possible dealing
Few or no straight friends
Consequences frequent
	Using to get
	    loaded, not just
	    high
		Begins to violate values and rules
		Use before and during school
		Use despite consequences
		Solitary use
		Trouble with school
		Overdoses, "bad trips," blackouts
		Promises to cut down or attempts to quit
		Protection of supply, hides use from peers
		Deterioration in physical condition
			Conspiracy of silence
			Confrontation
			Reorganization with
			    or without affected
			    person

Stage 4. Using to Feel Normal			

Continue to use despite adverse
    outcomes
Loss of control
Inability to stop
Compulsion
	Use to feel normal	Daily use
		Failure to meet expectations
		Loss of control
		Paranoia
		Suicide gestures, self-hate
		Physical deterioration (poor eating and sleep
		    habits)
			Frustration
			Anger
			May give up

Adger, H. (1999). Adolescent drug abuse. In McMillan, J. A., DeAngelis, C. D., Feigin, R. D., & Warshaw, J. W. (Eds.). *Oski's pediatrics: Principles and practice* (3rd ed.). Lippincott Williams & Wilkins.

BOX 42-1   CRAFFT Screening Tool for Substance Use

The six CRAFFT screening questions are asked if the adolescent endorses drinking alcohol, smoking marijuana or hashish, or using any other substance to get high during the previous 12 months. Two or more positive answers indicate a positive screen:
- C—Have you ever ridden in a Car driven by someone (including self) who was high, drunk, or had been using drugs?
- R—Have you ever used drugs or alcohol to Relax?
- A—Do you ever use Alone?
- F—Do you ever Forget things that you did while using?
- F—Do Family or Friends tell you to cut down?
- T—Have you ever gotten into Trouble when using?

Bukstein, O. (2021). Substance use disorder in adolescents: Epidemiology, pathogenesis, clinical manifestations and consequences, course, assessment, and diagnosis. *UpToDate*. https://www.uptodate.com/contents/substance-use-disorder-in-adolescents-epidemiology-pathogenesis-clinical-manifestations-and-consequences-course-assessment-and-diagnosis.

Prevention and Treatment

The most effective and least expensive treatment for substance abuse is prevention, beginning with education in the early school years. Information about drugs and using problem-solving skills to cope with issues rather than using drugs should be provided.

Educational programs may have less impact if the child comes from a home in which alcohol or other drugs are used by family caregivers.

When prevention is ineffective, emergency care and long-term treatment become necessary. An overdose or a "bad trip" may force the child to seek treatment. Emergency measures may even require artificial ventilation and oxygenation to restore normal respiration.

Balance is the Order of the Day!

"Scare" techniques are completely ineffective in trying to persuade children to refrain from using substances. These techniques arouse disbelief and often add the tempting thrill of danger.

Long-term treatment involves a team of health care professionals, including nurses, psychologists or psychiatrists, social workers, and drug rehabilitation counselors. The child is an important member of the treatment team and must admit the problem and the need for help and be willing to take an active part in treatment. Both outpatient and inpatient treatment programs are available. Many of these programs are geared specifically to adolescents. The earlier the child can be identified and treatment begun, the better the prognosis (see Tips for Reinforcing Family Teaching: Resources for Information and Help With Drug and Alcohol Problems).

Alcohol Abuse

In many parts of American culture, drinking alcoholic beverages is considered acceptable and desirable social behavior. Although the purchase of alcohol is legally restricted to adults 21 years of age and older, alcohol is available in many homes and consequently is the first drug most children try. It is also the most commonly abused drug among children and adolescents. Alcohol abuse occurs when a person ingests a quantity sufficient to cause intoxication (drunkenness). Alcoholism (chronic alcohol abuse or dependence) has reached epidemic proportions in America.

TIPS FOR REINFORCING FAMILY TEACHING

Resources for Information and Help With Drug and Alcohol Problems

If you suspect your child may be using alcohol or drugs, a number of helpful national organizations offer valuable information on their websites or can be contacted by phone.

Adult Children of Alcoholics/Dysfunctional Families: Call 310-534-1815. Website: www.adultchildren.org

Al-Anon/Alateen Family Group Headquarters, Inc.: Call 757-563-1600. Website: www.al-anon.org

Alcoholics Anonymous World Services: Check the phone directory for your local AA chapter or call 212-870-3400. Website: www.aa.org

Community Anti-Drug Coalitions of America: For information on current issues or legislation, call 1-800-54 CADCA (22322). Website: www.cadca.org

Nar-Anon Family Group Headquarters, Inc.: Call 1-800-477-6291. Website: www.nar-anon.org

National Criminal Justice Reference Service: Call 1-800-851-3420. Website: www.ncjrs.gov

National Family Partnership: Call 1-888-474-0008. Website: www.nfp.org

Substance Abuse and Mental Health Services Administration: Call 1-877-726-4727. Website: www.samhsa.gov

Partnership to End Addiction: Text CONNECT to 55753. Email contact@toendaddiction.org Website: www.drugfree.org

Drinking often begins in the preadolescent years and increases in frequency throughout adolescence. Some children use alcohol in combination with marijuana and other drugs, potentiating the effects of both substances and increasing the probability of intoxication.

Alcoholism is a major chronic, progressive, and potentially fatal disease process that affects every organ of the body, mental health, and social competence. Alcoholism tendencies appear to be inherited, so children with family histories of alcoholism may be prone to problems with alcohol. It is costly in dollars and in damage to the lives of alcohol abusers and their families. During adolescence, alcohol abuse is closely linked to automobile accidents.

Most states determine charges of driving under the influence using a standard percentage of blood alcohol content. In many states, the limit is up to 0.08%. Many children do not realize that fine motor control and judgment are affected at even lower levels, driving ability may be decreased, and fatality rates are high.

Children and adolescents who receive treatment and counseling for problem drinking are more likely to recover than are adults who have been problem drinkers for a long time. However, children, especially adolescents, are difficult to treat because of their feelings of immortality and the rapid progression of the disease in adolescents.

Treatment begins with detoxification ("drying out") and management of withdrawal symptoms. After that, a well-balanced diet, high-potency vitamins (especially vitamin B), and plenty of rest help eliminate the disease's harmful side effects.

Counseling to identify and address the problems that led to compulsive drinking is an essential part of treatment. Many counselors who work with alcoholic clients are people who are recovering from drinking problems themselves, which gives the counselor additional insight and empathy for the problem.

Alcoholics Anonymous (AA), the best known of all self-help groups, offers fellowship and understanding to the compulsive drinker (www.aa.org). Chapters are available in every sizable community and many have special programs for children as well as for families of alcoholics (Alateen, Al-Anon, ACA—Adult Children of Alcoholics). Anyone who has a desire to stop drinking is welcomed into AA and is helped to stay sober by taking it "one day at a time." Recovery from alcoholism is a lifetime matter. The earlier the problem is diagnosed, the better the person's chances to respond to treatment. Ongoing support from health professionals, peers, family, and community is essential to successful treatment.

Tobacco Abuse

Tobacco is a commonly abused drug among preadolescents and adolescents. Any use of tobacco is abuse. Nicotine is highly addictive and nicotine dependence can occur rapidly with use. A high percentage of young people try tobacco by smoking or chewing. Children may smoke because it gives them a feeling of maturity. Children whose family caregivers smoke are at increased risk for smoking because they have difficulty accepting that they are seriously endangering themselves by smoking. Many elementary and secondary schools have developed programs that warn children of the dangers of smoking, but threats of long-term physical illnesses are far enough in the future that the child tends to ignore them and they believe they can quit any time they want to.

The use of "smokeless tobacco" (snuff or chewing tobacco) has increased among adolescents. These children believe they are not damaging their lungs. However, this type of tobacco use can cause teeth and gum issues and mouth, lip, and throat cancers that are disfiguring and life-threatening.

The use of electronic (e-cigarettes) cigarettes has become increasingly popular among adolescents, especially newer devices that resemble a USB flash drive, which are easy to conceal and go unnoticed. The battery-operated devices heat a liquid usually containing nicotine, often flavorings, and other components, producing a vapor that the user inhales. The term "vaping" is used to describe this process to differentiate it from smoking a cigarette. Inhaling the vapor may be less harmful than inhaling cigarette smoke, but there are many negative health effects of e-cigarettes. The nicotine exposure from the e-cigarettes increases the heart rate and the blood levels of nicotine. There is an increased risk for chronic bronchitis, pneumonia and severe pulmonary disease, sleep disturbances, and cancer. An additional concern with the use of e-cigarettes is that they may be a gateway to nicotine dependence and conventional cigarette smoking in the adolescent in particular. Public health authorities have recommended restricting e-cigarette marketing and advertising to youth, much in the same way that conventional cigarette smoking advertising is restricted.

Marijuana/Cannabis Abuse

The most frequently used illicit drug among adolescents is marijuana/cannabis. The reported use of marijuana among children has decreased somewhat, but smoking marijuana at a younger age appears to be a current trend. Many children believe marijuana smoking is not risky.

The effects of marijuana are mostly behavioral. It affects judgment, sense of time, short-term memory, and motivation. These effects make driving hazardous and may even cause hallucinations at higher doses. In addition, marijuana smoke is three to five times more carcinogenic than cigarette smoke. Although recreational marijuana use is now legal in some states, it is still illegal in most states. Even where it is legal, there are no manufacturing controls over it, and the user has no idea regarding the potency, where it came from, or what additives may have been used. As a nurse, you must make every effort to inform children about the dangers of marijuana and discourage them from using it.

Cocaine Abuse

Although cocaine may not rank among the first three drugs most commonly used by children, it is an extremely dangerous drug. Use of cocaine and its derivative, "crack," can be found everywhere from inner cities to rural neighborhoods.

Cocaine is a fine, white, powdery substance that directly affects the brain cells and causes physical and psychological effects. It is snorted, injected, or smoked and is absorbed through the mucous membranes and into the bloodstream. The physical results are an increase in pulse, respirations, blood pressure, and temperature. The psychological effect is a feeling of euphoria and increased sociability. The high is reached in about 20 minutes and lasts 20 to 30 minutes. In contrast, crack enters the bloodstream in about 30 seconds with a fast and powerful but short high that lasts only about 5 minutes. As a result of the rapid, short high from crack, users tend to seek repeated highs over short periods, decreasing the time it takes to become addicted. Because of the rapid absorption of crack, immediate cardiac arrest can occur from its use. After smoking crack, the user may experience a "crash" that causes depression. To relieve this depression, crack users turn to alcohol and marijuana. This multiple use further complicates the drug's effects. Some cocaine users inject cocaine to obtain a faster high, which adds to their risk of contracting HIV from contaminated needles.

It is important to stress to children the danger of using cocaine and crack. School education programs should start at the elementary level. You can perform a community service by volunteering to present programs to local school children. Children and adolescents must be alerted to the dangers of these drugs and taught ways to refuse offers of drugs.

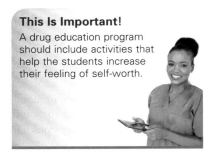

This Is Important!

A drug education program should include activities that help the students increase their feeling of self-worth.

Narcotic Abuse

The most commonly abused narcotics are morphine and heroin. These drugs decrease anger, sex drive, and hunger by producing a dreamlike, euphoric state. Narcotics are highly addictive and extremely expensive, and narcotic abuse results in teenage prostitution, pushing (selling) drugs, and robbery as a means to support the drug habit. Any drugs that are injected subject adolescents to the added risk of contracting HIV from using contaminated needles.

Other Abused Drugs

Other mood-altering drugs commonly abused by children include hallucinogens (psychedelic drugs), depressants, amphetamines/methamphetamines, and analgesics. Anabolic steroids, although not mood-altering, are also abused by adolescents.

Hallucinogens (psychedelic drugs), although not addictive in a physical sense, can create a psychological dependence from the resulting hallucinations. This category of drugs includes LSD, PCP ("angel dust"), psilocybin (derived from mushrooms), mescaline, DMT (derived from plants), and airplane glue. These drugs cause distortions in vision, smell, or hearing. Effects can include intoxication, "bad trips," and flashbacks, and overdoses are common.

The drug known as ecstasy is similar to amphetamines in chemical makeup but has the effect of elevating mood and increasing tactile sensations similar to the use of hallucinogens. The drug releases large amounts of serotonin, the neurotransmitter that regulates mood and emotion. The drug is used in party and club settings, where the users dance and party for extended periods of time; the drug suppresses their needs to eat, drink, or sleep. The drug can cause increased heart rate and blood pressure, muscle tension, teeth clenching, nausea, blurred vision, chills, and sweating. The drug is harmful to the brain and can cause confusion, depression, and anxiety, even days and weeks after use.

Depressants, sometimes referred to as hypnotics, are as addictive as narcotics, and withdrawal from them must be carefully controlled to prevent delirium, seizures, or death. Barbiturates, glutethimide, ethchlorvynol, and methaqualone are the most commonly abused drugs in this group; they are sometimes used with alcohol, which increases the intoxicating effects, such as sleepiness, slurred speech, and impaired cognitive and motor functions.

Amphetamines/methamphetamines ("uppers" or "speed") produce increased alertness, wakefulness, reduced awareness of fatigue, and increased confidence and energy. Although not physically addicting, they encourage psychological dependence and are abused by millions of Americans, many of whom become trapped in a destructive cycle of uppers and "downers" (barbiturates). The amphetamines are often manufactured in methamphetamine ("meth") laboratories in people's homes, which increase the potential dangers to the child who uses these substances.

Children abuse analgesics, particularly those that are combinations of narcotic and nonnarcotics, such as oxycodone. Chronic abuse can result in blood and kidney disorders. These drugs may be prescribed to a family member, which makes them easy for the child to obtain.

Anabolic steroids are not mood-altering drugs, but their abuse among athletes is a cause for great concern. Adolescent athletes take anabolic steroids to build up muscle mass in the belief that the drug will increase their athletic ability. Other adolescents may take them to build muscles and to achieve a "manly" appearance that they believe will make them more attractive. The side effects of euphoria and decreased fatigue make these drugs even more inviting to adolescents.

The use of excessively large doses of anabolic steroids may cause **gynecomastia** (excessive development of mammary glands in the male) or premature fusion of the long bones, which stunts growth in the adolescent who has not yet completed growth. Liver damage, including liver tumors and cancer; predisposition to atherosclerosis; hypertension; aggression; and psychotic and manic symptoms may also result. School programs about drug abuse should include the topic of anabolic steroid abuse.

TEST YOURSELF

✔ What are the reasons children use alcohol and other substances?

✔ Explain the difference between psychological and physical dependence in substance use.

✔ Name common substances children might use.

What is substance abuse? What behaviors do you think **Jacob's** mother has seen that makes her concerned that her son has a substance abuse problem? When Jacob is seen by the health care provider, he admits that he has been using substances. What questions would you anticipate the health care provider will ask Jacob to screen for his use of substances?

EATING DISORDERS

An eating disorder can impair health as well as cause psychological concerns. These disorders include pica, nonorganic failure to thrive, rumination disorder, anorexia nervosa, bulimia nervosa and binge-eating disorder.

Pica is repeated eating of nonfood substances such as chalk, clay, dirt, paper, or paint chips. It may be seen during pregnancy or sometimes in children. Pica may be a symptom of iron deficiency anemia. Pica may occur in children with mental health disorders such as autism or intellectual disability.

Nonorganic Failure to Thrive/Rumination Disorder

Rumination is regurgitation of food, which may be spit out, or rechewed and reswallowed. This is a characteristic noted in infants with a rumination disorder or nonorganic failure to thrive (NFTT). A medical condition such as gastroesophageal reflux or pyloric stenosis (see Chapter 38 for discussion of these disorders), which is the cause of organic failure to thrive, is not the cause of the rumination. Often in the child with NFTT, there is a disrupted family relationship, in particular a lack of mother–child attachment. There may be an environmental issue, such as a knowledge deficit of what to expect as a parent, a marriage problem, stress, or poverty. In addition, the family caregiver may have a mental health disorder such as depression or drug or alcohol abuse. The father may be absent or emotionally unavailable, adding to the mother's feelings of isolation and inadequacy and leading to an atmosphere of additional stress and conflict.

Children with NFTT often fall into the classification of "difficult" or irritable babies, but others may be listless and passive and do not seem to care about feedings. The problem is not with the family caregiver or with the child alone, but instead with their interaction and mutual lack of responsiveness. They are not in harmony. The family caregiver does not stimulate the child; therefore, the child has no one to respond to. Infants with NFTT are often seriously below average weight and height, have poor muscle tone, are emaciated with loss of subcutaneous fat, and are immobile for long periods of time (Fig. 42-1). These infants may smell "sour" because of frequent vomiting. They may be unresponsive to (or actually try to avoid) cuddling and vocalization. Long-term care is necessary to treat the physical and psychological aspects of nonorganic failure to thrive. Avoid judgmental, stereotyped feelings when dealing with the family caregivers of such a child.

Anorexia Nervosa

Preoccupation with reducing diets and the quest for the "perfect" (i.e., thin) figure sometimes leads to **anorexia nervosa**, or self-inflicted starvation. This disorder occurs most commonly in adolescent females, although there are reported cases among adolescent males as well. The onset of the disorder is typically during adolescence and is the result of psychological and physiologic factors. A family history of anorexia and eating disorders is commonly noted.

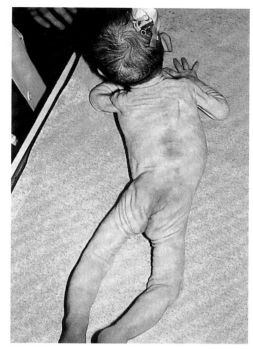

FIGURE 42-1 The child with failure to thrive is often seriously below average weight.

Characteristics

Children with anorexia are often described as successful students who tend to be perfectionists and are always trying to please parents, teachers, and other adults. The families of these children may be overly involved in the child's life (which tends to be overwhelming to the adolescent in particular), but display no evidence of conflict within the family. An adolescent in a controlled family environment may try to establish independence and identity by controlling their own appetite and body weight. Depression and anxiety disorders are common in these adolescents. People with anorexia deny weight loss and, because of their disturbed body image, actually see themselves as fat, even when they look skeletal to others. They often adhere to a rigid program of exercise to further their efforts in weight reduction. They may make demands on themselves for cleanliness and order in their environment, often showing obsessive–compulsive traits. They may engage in rigid schedules for studying and other ritualistic behavior. These adolescents deny hunger but often suffer from fatigue.

Clinical Manifestations and Diagnosis

People with anorexia are visibly emaciated, with an almost skeletonlike appearance. They appear sexually immature, have dry skin and brittle nails, and often have lanugo (downy hair) over their backs and extremities. Other symptoms include amenorrhea (absence of menstruation), constipation, intolerance to cold, bradycardia, arrhythmias, low blood pressure, and anemia. Malnutrition, dehydration, and electrolyte imbalances are often significant. The person with anorexia often eats only small amounts of food, overexercises, and has a significantly lower body weight than would be normal. Even though they have a low body weight, they are preoccupied with a fear gaining weight or becoming fat and do not recognize the serious concerns they may be creating in their bodies. Complications stemming from the low body weight, accompanying malnutrition, and electrolyte imbalances can affect every body system and organ. Serious cardiac involvement is a major concern with anorexia, often leading to hospitalization. Even after successful treatment of anorexia, cardiac damage and conditions remain.

Treatment and Nursing Care

After medical stabilization of the child with anorexia nervosa, hospitalization is aimed at achieving two goals of treatment: correction of malnutrition and identification and treatment of the psychological cause. An approach involving several disciplines is necessary. Therapy is required to help the child gain insight into the problem. In addition, family therapy, nutritional therapy, and behavior modification are used. Treatment options include inpatient, partial hospitalization (day treatment), and outpatient.

Adolescents with anorexia have become experts in manipulating others and their environments. Once treatment begins, they may try to avoid gaining weight by ordering only low-calorie foods; by disposing of their meals in plants, trash, toilets, or dirty linen; or by exercising in the hall or jogging in place in their rooms. In some instances, nasogastric tube feedings or total parenteral nutrition (TPN) is necessary to provide nutritional support. A potential fatal complication that can occur with aggressive nutritional rehabilitation and weight gain in cases of severe malnutrition is called **refeeding syndrome**. To keep this syndrome from occurring, calorie intake and weight gain is closely monitored. Daily monitoring of electrolytes and other blood levels is necessary.

Treatment based on behavior modification may deprive the client of all privileges, such as visitors, electronics, television, and phone, until the child begins to gain weight. Privileges are then gradually restored. These techniques are effective only when the client and the family caregivers understand the program and its purpose and have agreed on individualized goals and rewards.

Group therapy may be used to provide peer support and the opportunity to associate with other clients with the same diagnosis in a nonthreatening setting.

The long-term outlook for the child with anorexia is unclear. Some children recover completely, others have eating problems into adulthood, and still others have problems with social adjustment that are not related to eating. Predicting the outcome is difficult (Fig. 42-2).

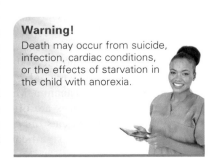

Warning!

Death may occur from suicide, infection, cardiac conditions, or the effects of starvation in the child with anorexia.

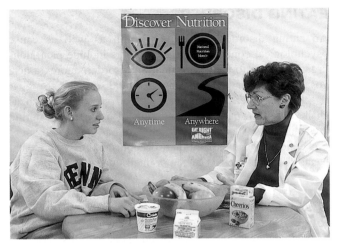

FIGURE 42-2 This anorexic teen, who is in the later stages of treatment, continues to meet with the counselor to discuss her food choices, exercise program, and overall well-being.

Bulimia Nervosa

Bulimia nervosa is characterized by binge eating followed by purging, with these episodes occurring over a period of time. The typical person with bulimia is in late adolescence or early adulthood and is of normal weight or slightly overweight. Those who are underweight usually fulfill the criteria for anorexia nervosa, although some people with anorexia periodically practice binging and purging. Inadequate social skills, low self-esteem, depression, and other mental health issues may be noted in the child's history.

Binging, eating a large amount of food in a short time period (usually 1 to 2 hours, often in secrecy), episodes occur. The amount of food is much more than would normally be eaten in that time frame and frequently occurs late in the day when the child is alone. This binging is followed by guilt, fear, shame, and self-condemnation. To relieve the uncomfortable physical sensation, emotional distress, and to avoid weight gain from the food eaten, the child follows the binging with purging by means of self-induced vomiting, laxatives, diuretics, and excessive exercise.

Clinical Manifestations and Diagnosis

The person with bulimia consumes a large amount of food in a distinct time period with an inability to stop or to control eating. Ritualistic eating behaviors may be seen. The manifestations noted in bulimia nervosa include dental caries and erosion from frequent exposure to stomach acid, throat irritation, and endocrine and electrolyte imbalances that may cause cardiac irregularities and menstrual problems. Calluses or abrasions may be noted on the back of the hand from frequent contact with the teeth while inducing vomiting and the child's breath is foul smelling. Possible complications are esophageal tears and acute gastric dilation. Hypokalemia may also occur, especially if the child abuses diuretics to prevent weight gain. Behaviors noted include immediately going to the restroom after eating, not eating in social settings, chewing gum or breath mints. Other behavior problems seen in many persons with bulimia include drug abuse, alcoholism, stealing (especially food and money), promiscuity, and other impulsive activities.

Treatment

Treatment of bulimia nervosa is varied. Many aspects of the treatment are similar to treatment for the child with anorexia. Food diaries are often used as a tool to evaluate the child's eating patterns. In some instances, antidepressant drugs (SSRIs) may be useful. A support group may prove helpful.

Nursing Process and Care Plan *for the Child With Anorexia Nervosa or Bulimia Nervosa*

Assessment (Data Collection)

Data collection of the child with an eating disorder begins with a complete interview and history, including previous illnesses, allergies, a dietary history, and a description of eating habits. The child may not give an accurate dietary history or description of eating habits. Question the family caregiver in a separate interview to gain added information. In the physical examination, include height, weight, blood pressure, temperature, pulse, and respirations. Carefully inspect and observe the skin, mucous membranes, state of nutrition, and state of alertness and cooperation. Complete documentation of findings is necessary.

Nursing Care Focus

When developing evidence-based nursing care focuses for the child with anorexia nervosa or bulimia nervosa, the risk for malnutrition is a priority focus. Recognizing the child may have an altered body image perception and activity intolerance is important. When developing a plan of care, include managing constipation, diarrhea, and maintaining skin integrity. Encouraging compliance with the treatment regimen must be addressed. Family coping impairment and reinforcing family teaching are included in working the child and the family.

Outcome Identification and Planning

The evaluation of a child with anorexia nervosa or bulimia nervosa is an ongoing process that continues throughout the hospital stay as well as in outpatient settings. The major goals for the child with an eating disorder relate to meeting nutritional needs and improving body image, self-concept, and self-esteem. Other goals include establishing appropriate activity levels, maintaining normal bowel activity, maintaining skin integrity, and complying with the treatment program. The goals for the family include understanding the condition, learning how to manage the condition and its treatment, reinforcing the child's self-esteem, and developing coping strategies.

Nursing Care Focus

- Malnutrition related to minimal food intake, self-induced vomiting, and use of laxatives or diuretics

Goal

- The child will gain a predetermined amount of weight per week.

Implementations for Improving Nutritional Status

The child with anorexia nervosa or bulimia nervosa does not receive the nutrients needed to achieve adequate growth during this period of development. Supervise food intake. Weigh the child at the same time each day but do not make an issue of weight fluctuation. Be observant when weighing the client; the child may try to add weight by putting heavy objects in pockets, shoes, or other hiding places. While being weighed, the client should wear minimal clothing (preferably a patient gown with no pockets) and have bare feet.

The health care provider and a dietitian work with the child to devise a food plan to meet the child's nutrition requirements. The goal of the food plan is not a sudden weight gain, but a slow, steady gain with an established goal that has been agreed upon by the health care team and the child. Often the child keeps a food diary that is reviewed daily with the health team.

Clients with eating disorders are often manipulative and deceptive. Observe the client during and after eating to make certain the child eats the required food and does not get rid of it after apparently consuming it.

Contract agreements are often recommended for clients with eating disorders. These agreements, which are usually part of a behavioral modification plan, specify the child's and the staff's responsibilities for the diet, activity expectations for the child, and other aspects of the child's behavior. The contract may also spell out specific privileges that can be gained by meeting the contract goals. This places the child in greater control of the outcome.

In addition to daily weights, test urine for ketones and regularly evaluate the skin turgor and mucous membranes to gather further information about nutritional status. Immediately report and document any evidence of deteriorating physical condition. If weight loss continues, nasogastric tube feedings may need to be implemented. This possibility can also be included in the contract.

If the child's condition is at a critical stage with fluid and electrolyte deficiencies, parenteral fluids are necessary immediately to hydrate the client before additional treatment can be implemented. Observe the child continuously to prevent any attempt to remove intravenous lines or otherwise disrupt the treatment. Closely monitor serum electrolytes, cardiac and respiratory status, and renal complications. During administration of parenteral fluids, continue to encourage the child to maintain an oral intake.

Evaluation of Goal/Desired Outcome

The child:

- eats at least 80% of each meal.
- gains 1 to 2 lb (450 to 900 grams) a week.
- keeps a food diary.
- signs a contract agreement.

Nursing Care Focus

- Altered body image perception related to fear of obesity and potential rejection

Goal

- The child will show evidence of improved self-esteem.

Implementations for Reinforcing Positive Body Image and Self-Concept

Consistent assignment of the same nursing personnel to care for the child helps establish a climate in which the child can relate to the nurse and begin to build a positive self-concept. It is important that you function as an active, nonjudgmental listener to the child. Report and document any signs of depression without delay. Also, report and document any negative feelings expressed by the child. Do not minimize or ignore these feelings. Reinforce positive behavior. Psychotherapy and counseling groups are necessary to help the child work through feelings of negative self-worth. Encourage the child to express fears, anger, and frustrations, and help the client recognize that everyone has these feelings from time to time. Never ridicule or belittle these feelings. Encourage the child to explore ways in which destructive feelings may be changed. These are feelings that can be dealt with in counseling sessions; therefore, report and document them carefully.

Evaluation of Goal/Desired Outcome

The child:

- verbally expresses positive attitudes.
- expresses insight into reasons behind eating pattern.
- expresses feelings about food, exercise, and weight loss.
- maintains peer relationships and is groomed.

Nursing Care Focus

- Activity intolerance related to fatigue secondary to malnutrition

Goal

- The child will pace activity to avoid fatigue.

Implementations for Balancing Rest and Activity

Exercise and activity are important parts of the contract negotiated with the child. Explain to the child that fatigue is a result of the extreme depletion of energy reserves related to nutritional deficits. Encourage the child to become involved in all activities of daily living. Provide ample rest periods when the child's energy reserves are depleted. Discourage the child from pushing beyond endurance, and closely observe for secretive excessive activity.

Evaluation of Goal/Desired Outcome

The child:

- is involved in activity as prescribed in a contract.
- does not exhibit any signs of excessive exercise or activity.

Nursing Care Focus

- Constipation and diarrhea risk related to decreased food, fluid intake, and laxative use

Goal

- The child's bowel elimination will be normal.

Implementations for Monitoring Bowel Habits

Make a careful record of bowel movements. The child may not be reliable as a reporter of bowel habits, so devise methods to prevent the child from using the bathroom without supervision. Report at once and document constipation or diarrhea. Watch carefully to prevent the child from obtaining and taking a laxative. The child may go to great lengths to obtain a laxative to purge themselves of food. Immediately report any evidence or suspicions of this type of behavior. Monitor fluid intake and output as well as electrolyte levels.

Evaluation of Goal/Desired Outcome

The child:

- experiences no episodes of diarrhea or constipation.
- does not attempt deceit to obtain laxatives.

Nursing Care Focus

- Altered skin integrity related to loss of subcutaneous fat and dry skin secondary to malnutrition

Goal

- The child's skin will show no evidence of breakdown.

Implementations for Maintaining Skin Integrity

Good skin care is essential in the care of the child with a severely restricted nutritional intake. The skin may be dry and tend to break down easily because of the lack of a subcutaneous fat cushion. Inspect daily for redness, irritation, or signs of decubitus ulcer formation. Specifically observe the bony prominences. Encourage the child to be out of bed most of the day. When the child is in bed, encourage regular position changes so that no pressure areas develop.

Evaluation of Goal/Desired Outcome

The child's:

- skin is intact with no signs of redness, irritation, or excessive pressure.
- skin turgor is good.

Nursing Care Focus

- Nonadherence to treatment regimen related to unresolved conflicts over food and eating

Goal

- The child will comply with treatment regimen.

Implementations for Promoting Compliance

The long-term outcome for children with eating disorders is precarious. Children with severe eating disorders often have multiple inpatient admissions. During inpatient treatment, goals should be set and plans made for discharge. Specific consequences must be established for noncompliance. Counseling must continue after discharge. A support group referral may be helpful in encouraging compliance. Family involvement is necessary. The child must recognize that discharge from the health care facility does not mean that they are "cured."

Evaluation of Goal/Desired Outcome

The child:

- agrees to, signs, and adheres to a contract agreement.
- keeps counseling appointments.
- joins a support group.
- continues to gain or maintain weight as per contract agreement.

Nursing Care Focus

- Family caregiver coping impairment and knowledge deficiency related to eating disorders, treatment regimen, and dangers associated with an eating disorder

Goal

- The family will show evidence of improved coping and understanding of disorder.

Implementations for Improving Family Coping and Reinforcing Family Teaching

The family of the child needs counseling along with the child. Some families may deny that the child has a problem or that the problem is as severe as perceived by health care team members. Family therapy meets with varied success. Usually, the earlier the family therapy is initiated, the better the results. Family members must be able to identify behaviors of their own that contribute to the child's condition. Family members must also learn to cooperate with behavior modification programs and, with guidance, carry them out at home when necessary. Ongoing contact between the family, the child, and consistent health team members is essential.

Evaluation of Goal/Desired Outcome

The family caregiver:

- attends counseling sessions.
- identifies behaviors that aggravate the child's condition.
- explains the disorder, treatment, and possible complications.

> ## TEST YOURSELF
> ✔ What symptoms are seen in the child with nonorganic failure to thrive (NFTT)?
> ✔ Explain the difference between anorexia nervosa and bulimia nervosa.
> ✔ What are the goals of treatment for a child with an eating disorder?

BINGE-EATING DISORDER/OBESITY

Binge-eating occurs in a variety of different ways, but there is an ingestion of a larger amount of food than needed. The individual loses control of their eating and feels they cannot stop. Unlike with bulimia nervosa, there is no purging behavior. Following the binge eating, guilt and shame may create a cycle of binge eating in an effort to relieve the anxiety and distress. The person is usually overweight and often has obesity.

Obesity is generally defined as an excessive accumulation of fat that increases body weight by 20% or more over ideal weight (see Appendix E). **Overweight** means that a person's weight is more than average for height and body build.

Obesity is a national problem in the United States, largely as a result of an overabundance of food and too little exercise. The thin figure, particularly for women, has become so idealized that being overweight can handicap a person socially and professionally and severely damage self-esteem.

Factors that may indicate the child is high risk for obesity include genetics, environment, culture, intake of high glycemic foods, decreased intake of high-fiber foods, and psychological issues. Children of obese parents are likely to share this problem not only because of some inherited predisposition toward obesity, but also because of family eating patterns and the emotional climate surrounding food. Certain cultures equate obesity with being loved and being prosperous. The child who struggles with being overweight or obese is at high risk for developing a binge-eating disorder.

Clinical Manifestations and Diagnosis

Obesity often begins in childhood and if not treated successfully, leads to chronic obesity and potentially binge-eating disorder in adult life. The obese child often feels isolated from the peer group that is normally a source of support and friendship. Because of the obesity, the child is often embarrassed to participate in sports, thus eliminating one method of burning excess calories. In addition, type 2 diabetes mellitus, which was formerly seen almost exclusively in adults and is associated with being overweight, is now being diagnosed in childhood with long-range health concerns.

Many children use food as a means of satisfying emotional needs, which establishes a vicious cycle. Children's eating habits include skipping meals, especially breakfast, and indulging in late-night eating. This behavior compounds the problem because calories consumed before a person goes to bed are not used for energy but are stored as fat. Snacking, often on foods high in calories and low in nutrients while watching television, also contributes to an overindulgent caloric intake.

Decreased physical activity and increased time spent doing sedentary activities have increased the incidence of childhood obesity. Time spent on using electronic devices and watching television often replaces physical activities and adds to the sedentary lifestyle.

Some children experience **polyphagia** (compulsive overeating), which may lead to binge-eating disorder. They lack control of their food intake, cannot postpone their urge to eat, hide food for later secret consumption, eat when not hungry or to escape from worries, and expend a great deal of energy thinking about securing and eating food.

Treatment

Obesity is difficult to treat in any age group, but is especially difficult in adolescence. Much of teenage life centers on food: after-school snacks, the ice cream shop, late-night diners, the pizza parlor, and fast-food restaurants serving high-fat, high-calorie foods with little nutritional value. Diets that emphasize nutritionally sound meals and reduced caloric intake produce results too slowly for impatient teenagers. Thus, the many quick weight-loss programs, diet pills, and diet books find a ready market among children.

Treatment must include a thorough exploration of the obese child's food attitudes. A team approach is often useful in developing a complete treatment plan. Summer camps that center on weight reduction with nutritious, calorie-controlled food; exercise; and activity are successful for some children but are too costly for many families. In addition, many children may fall back into old habits after summer camp is over unless there is a continuing support system.

Caregivers who work with obese children need to stress that obesity does not make them unacceptable. Finding the support of a caring adult who will help the child gain control of this aspect of their life can help give the necessary incentive to lose weight (see Tips for Reinforcing Family Teaching: Tips for Caregivers of Obese Children).

TIPS FOR REINFORCING FAMILY TEACHING

Tips for Caregivers of Obese Children

- Have the child keep a food diary for a week. Include food eaten, time eaten, what the child was doing, and how the child felt before and after eating; identify what stimulates urge to eat.
- Study diary with the child to look for eating triggers.
- Set a reasonable goal of no more than 1 or 2 lb of weight loss a week, or perhaps maintaining weight with no gain.
- Advise the child to eat only at specific, regular mealtimes.
- Recommend that the child eat only at dining or kitchen table (not in front of TV or on the run).
- Have the child use small plates to make amount of food seem larger.
- Teach the child to eat slowly. Count and chew each bite (25 to 30 is a good goal).
- Suggest that the child try to leave a little on the plate when done.
- Have the child survey home and get rid of tempting high-calorie foods.
- Stock up on low-calorie snacks: carrot sticks, celery sticks, and other raw vegetables.
- Help the child get involved in an active project that occupies time and also helps burn calories: any active team sport; bicycling, walking, hiking, swimming, skating.
- Promote walking instead of riding whenever possible.
- Encourage the child to attend a support group or develop a buddy system for support.
- Weigh only once a week on the same scale at the same time of day in the same clothing.
- Make a chart to keep track of the child's weight.
- Help the child to focus on a positive asset and make the most of it to help build self-concept.
- Encourage good grooming. A group could put on a "mini" fashion show, choosing with guidance clothes that help maximize best features or simply using magazine illustrations if actual clothing is not available.
- Reward each small success with positive reinforcement.
- Enlist cooperation of all family members to support the child with encouragement and a positive atmosphere.

Think back to Jacob Gallegos from the beginning of the chapter. What are some of the substances Jacob may be abusing? What are some of the forms of treatment used to help the adolescent with a substance abuse problem?

KEY POINTS

- Autism spectrum disorder (ASD) is characterized by abnormal or impaired social interaction and impaired verbal and nonverbal communication. Repetitive patterns and behaviors may be seen. The cause of ASD appears to be genetic factors that lead to abnormal brain development, which impairs social and communication skills. Treatment of ASD is extremely challenging and a goal of treatment is for the child to have their highest level of functioning within the limitations of the disorder. Treatment focuses on behavioral and educational interventions that target the core symptoms of ASD. Pharmacologic interventions may be used. The family needs support to help relieve guilt and help them understand this child.

- Characteristics seen in the child with ADHD include impulsive behavior, ease in being distracted, fidgeting or squirming, difficulty sitting still, problems following through on instructions despite being able to understand them, inattentiveness when spoken to, losing of things, going from one uncompleted activity to another, difficulty taking turns, interrupting, and talking excessively. The child often engages in dangerous activities without considering the consequences. Treatment is multidisciplinary, and stimulant medications such as methylphenidate are often used.

- The child with oppositional defiant disorder (ODD) exhibits a pattern of angry, irritable, argumentative, defiant, hostile, and sometimes vindictive behavior, which is excessive compared to other children of the same age. Working with family caregivers and getting professional help is usually necessary.

- The child with a conduct disorder exhibits a repetitive and continual pattern of behavior that goes against the rules of society and societal norms appropriate for the child's age. The behaviors often violate the rights of other people. Aggressive behavior that can result in physical harm to people or animals, damage to property, stealing, lying, breaking rules and laws, not attending school, and running away from home are common behaviors.

- The child who bullies other children attempts to have power or control over the other person, often a child who is in some way different. The bully may lack social skills, break rules, be impulsive and easily frustrated, and lack a caring attitude toward others. The child who bullies needs professional help to deal with the issues underlying the bullying behavior.

- Enuresis is continued incontinence of urine beyond the age when control of urination is commonly acquired. Enuresis may have a physiologic or psychological cause. Encopresis is chronic involuntary fecal soiling beyond the age when control is expected. If no organic causes (e.g., worms, megacolon) exist, encopresis may indicate a serious psychological concern.

- Anxiety disorders noted in children, generalized anxiety disorder, separation anxiety, and phobias often manifest as concerns of the child that are excessive, out of proportion to the situation, or persistent and cause distress to the child. Some of those concerns include fears of safety or health, fears of being away from their family caregiver, or a dread or fear of an object or situation. The goal of treatment is to reduce the anxiety and help the child find a sense of security.

- The depressed child may have persistent sadness or unhappiness which interferes with the activities they normally enjoy. Younger children often show symptoms of anger, irritability, changes in appetite and sleep patterns, physical complaints, and difficulty concentrating. School-aged children may be grouchy, annoyed, or show lack of interest in school and friends. Symptoms in the adolescent may also include behaviors such as missing curfews, extreme defiance, shoplifting, grades dropping, spending more time alone, self-hatred, and talking about death or suicide, and the use of drugs and alcohol may indicate depression in the adolescent. Suicide is a major concern in the depressed child.

- Children who are considering suicide often have previous suicide attempts, withdraw from or change participation in activities, have physical complaints and a preoccupation with dying, change moods, say goodbye, or give away personal items.

- Substances commonly abused by children include alcohol, tobacco, marijuana, cocaine, morphine, heroin, hallucinogens, depressants, amphetamines, analgesics, anabolic steroids, hallucinogens, and ecstasy.

- The use of substances can lead to addiction or dependence, which may be psychological, physical, or both. Alcohol abuse can lead to potentially fatal consequences. Tobacco or smokeless tobacco damages the lungs and can cause mouth, lip, and throat cancers. Marijuana affects judgment, sense of time, and motivation. The physical results of using cocaine are an increase in pulse, respirations, blood pressure, and temperature. Narcotics are highly addictive and extremely expensive, which can result in teenage prostitution, pushing (selling) drugs, and robbery as a means to support the drug habit. Hallucinogens (psychedelic drugs), although not addictive in a physical sense, can create a psychological dependence, as well as the effects of intoxication, "bad trips," and flashbacks, and are often associated with overdoses. Withdrawal from barbiturates must be carefully controlled to prevent delirium, seizures, or death.

- Eating disorders can impair health as well as cause psychological concerns. Pica may be a symptom of iron deficiency anemia. Children with nonorganic failure to thrive (NFTT) are often listless and below average in weight and height; have poor muscle tone and a loss of subcutaneous fat; and are immobile for long periods of time. They may be unresponsive or try to avoid cuddling and vocalization. A common characteristic is rumination (voluntary regurgitation), perhaps as a means of self-satisfaction.

- The child with anorexia nervosa may be a perfectionist, be depressed, deny weight loss, and actually see themselves as fat. They often follow rigid programs of exercise. People with anorexia are visibly emaciated, with an almost skeletonlike appearance. Two goals of treatment for the hospitalized client with anorexia are correction of malnutrition and identification and treatment of the psychological cause. Serious cardiac involvement is a major concern with anorexia even after successful treatment of the anorexia.

- The child with bulimia nervosa has episodes of binging followed by purging behavior with vomiting or use of laxatives. They may have dental caries and erosion from frequent exposure to stomach acid, throat irritation, endocrine and electrolyte imbalances, cardiac irregularities, and menstrual problems. Calluses or abrasions may be noted on the back of the hand from frequent contact with the teeth while inducing vomiting. Possible complications are esophageal tears, acute gastric dilation, and hypokalemia. Goals of treatment for the child with an eating disorder relate to meeting nutritional needs and improving body image, self-concept, and self-esteem.

- The child who is overweight or obese may develop a binge-eating disorder. Nutrition habits and deficiencies, decreased physical activity, sedentary life style, and lack of exercise lead to obesity concerns. Professionals who work with obese children need to stress that obesity does not make them unacceptable. Finding the support of a caring adult who will help the child gain control of this aspect of their life can help give the necessary incentive to lose weight.

INTERNET RESOURCES

Alcohol and Drugs
www.samhsa.gov

ADHD
www.add.org

Suicide
www.suicidology.org

Substance Abuse
www.drugabuse.gov

Tobacco
www.tobaccofreekids.org

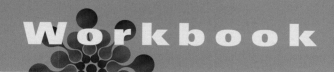

NCLEX-STYLE REVIEW QUESTIONS

1. A nurse admits an adolescent girl with a diagnosis of possible anorexia nervosa. Of the following characteristics, which would *most* likely be seen in the adolescent with anorexia?

   a. The adolescent gets low grades in school.
   b. The adolescent has a sedentary lifestyle.
   c. The adolescent freely expresses emotions.
   d. The adolescent follows a strict routine.

2. The nurse is assisting with a physical examination on an adolescent with bulimia nervosa. Of the following signs and symptoms, which would *most* likely be seen in the adolescent with bulimia?

   a. Dry skin
   b. Dental caries
   c. Low body weight
   d. Amenorrhea

3. In planning care for an adolescent with an eating disorder, which goal would be *most* important for the adolescent?

   a. The adolescent will verbally express positive attitudes and feelings.
   b. The adolescent will plan and participate in age-appropriate activities.
   c. The adolescent will maintain a fluid and electrolyte balance.
   d. The adolescent will have normal bowel and bladder patterns.

4. The nurse is discussing teenage depression and suicide with a group of family caregivers of adolescent-aged children. Which statement made by the family caregiver would require further data collection?

   a. "My child has so many ideas about how she can fix all the problems in the world."
   b. "She told me she is happy that she broke up with her long-time boyfriend."
   c. "My son enjoys spending all his time alone in his room listening to his music."
   d. "My child eats all the time but never seems to want to go to sleep."

5. The nurse is caring for an infant with failure to thrive. The infant took in 2 oz of formula every 2 hours during the 12-hour shift, with the first 2 oz at 7 AM and the last feeding at 7 PM. She vomited three times: 20 mL the first time, 36 mL the second time, and 28 mL the third time. The infant had four wet diapers during the shift. After subtracting the dry weight of the diapers, the diapers weighed 20 grams, 18 grams, 25 grams, and 22 grams. She had one medium-sized stool during the shift. What was the infant's total intake and output during the 12-hour shift?

STUDY ACTIVITIES

1. A coworker says to you, "That Jeff in room 204 is bouncing off the walls." You are assigned to this child, who has a diagnosis of ADHD. Make a list of behavior techniques to use with the child who has ADHD. Develop a plan of care you could use to care for Jeff.

2. Do an internet search on "communicating with teens about drugs."

   a. List some of the sites you find.
   b. What are the some important communication methods suggested for parents to use in communicating with their teens?
   c. List barriers that parents should be aware of when communicating with their teenage children.

CRITICAL THINKING: WHAT WOULD YOU DO?

1. Tanya, 16 years old, is 65 inches (165 cm) tall and weighs 98 lb (44.5 kg). She moans about how fat her thighs are. You believe she is anorexic. A diagnosis of anorexia nervosa is confirmed and she is hospitalized.

   a. What symptoms will you observe for in addition to her weight loss?
   b. What are the characteristics often seen in the anorexic child's personality?
   c. What will be included in Tanya's nursing care plan?

2. Your best friend shares with you that she thinks her teenage son might have a problem with alcohol and drugs. She tells you that her son has behaviors that make her think he is drinking every day and using drugs every weekend.

   a. Why do you think alcohol is the most commonly abused drug among adolescents?
   b. What factors do you think put adolescents at the greatest risk for becoming substance abusers?
   c. What do you think could be helpful in reducing each of the above risk factors?

3. Dosage calculation: A child with a diagnosis of ADHD is being treated with methylphenidate. The child weighs 75 lb. The usual dosage of this medication is 0.3 mg/kg/dose to 2 mg/kg/day, not to exceed 60 mg/day. The medication is given two times a day (BID). Answer the following.

   a. How many kilograms (kg) does the child weigh?
   b. How many milligrams (mg) would be given for the low dose?
   c. How many milligrams (mg) would be given for the high dose?
   d. Would the high dose of the medication be an appropriate dose for this child? Explain your answer.

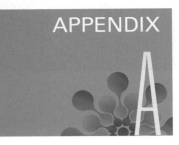

Standard and Transmission-Based Precautions

Use Standard Precautions, or the equivalent, for the care of all patients. *Category IB*[1]

    Note: The following precautions are from the CDC's *Guideline for isolation precautions: Preventing transmission of infectious agents in healthcare settings.*

Hand Hygiene

1. Wash hands after touching blood, body fluids, secretions, excretions, and contaminated items, whether or not gloves are worn. Wash hands immediately after gloves are removed, between patient contacts, and when otherwise indicated to avoid transfer of microorganisms to other patients or environments. It may be necessary to wash hands between tasks and procedures on the same patient to prevent cross-contamination of different body sites. *Category IB*
2. Use a plain (nonantimicrobial) or antiseptic-containing soap for routine handwashing. *Category IB*
3. Use an antimicrobial agent or an alcohol-based waterless antiseptic agent (gels, rinses, foams) in the absence of visible soiling and for specific circumstances (e.g., control of outbreaks or hyperendemic infections), as defined by the infection control program. *Category IB* (See contact precautions for additional recommendations on using antimicrobial and antiseptic agents.)

Gloves

Wear gloves (clean, nonsterile gloves are adequate) when touching blood, body fluids, secretions, excretions, and contaminated items. Put on clean gloves just before touching mucous membranes and nonintact skin. Change gloves between tasks and procedures on the same patient after contact with material that may contain a high concentration of microorganisms. Remove gloves promptly after use, before going to another patient or touching noncontaminated items and environmental surfaces, and wash hands immediately to avoid transfer of microorganisms to other patients or environments. *Category IB*

Mask, Eye Protection, Face Shield

Wear a mask and eye protection or a face shield to protect mucous membranes of the eyes, nose, and mouth during procedures and patient-care activities that are likely to generate splashes or sprays of blood, body fluids, secretions, and excretions. *Category IB*

Gown

Wear a gown (a clean, nonsterile gown is adequate) to protect skin and to prevent soiling of clothing during procedures and patient-care activities that are likely to generate splashes or sprays of blood, body fluids, secretions, or excretions. Select a gown that is appropriate for the activity and amount of fluid likely to be encountered. Remove a soiled gown as promptly as possible, and wash your hands to avoid transfer of microorganisms to other patients or environments. *Category IB*

---

[1]*Category IB*. Strongly recommended for all healthcare settings and reviewed as effective by experts in the field and a consensus of HICPAC members on the basis of strong rationale and suggestive evidence, even though definitive studies have not been done.

Patient-Care Equipment

Handle used patient-care equipment soiled with blood, body fluids, secretions, and excretions in a manner that prevents skin and mucous membrane exposures, contamination of clothing, and transfer of microorganisms to other patients and environments. Ensure that reusable equipment is not used for the care of another patient until it has been cleaned and reprocessed appropriately. Ensure that single-use items are discarded properly. *Category IB*

Environmental Control

Ensure that the hospital has adequate procedures for the routine care, cleaning, and disinfection of environmental surfaces, beds, bedrails, bedside equipment, and other frequently touched surfaces, and ensure that these procedures are being followed. *Category IB*

Linen

Handle, transport, and process used linen soiled with blood, body fluids, secretions, and excretions in a manner that prevents skin and mucous membrane exposures and contamination of clothing and that avoids transfer of microorganisms to other patients and environments. *Category IB*

Occupational Health and Blood-Borne Pathogens

1. Take care to prevent injuries when using needles, scalpels, and other sharp instruments or devices; when handling sharp instruments after procedures; when cleaning used instruments; and when disposing of used needles. Never recap used needles, or otherwise, manipulate them using both hands, or use any other technique that involves directing the point of a needle toward any part of the body; rather, use either a one-handed "scoop" technique or a mechanical device designed for holding the needle sheath. Do not remove used needles from disposable syringes by hand, and do not bend, break, or otherwise manipulate used needles by hand. Place used disposable syringes and needles, scalpel blades, and other sharp items in appropriate puncture-resistant containers, which are located as close as practical to the area in which the items were used, and place reusable syringes and needles in a puncture-resistant container for transport to the reprocessing area. *Category IB*
2. Use mouthpieces, resuscitation bags, or other ventilation devices as an alternative to mouth-to-mouth resuscitation methods in areas where the need for resuscitation is predictable. *Category IB*

Patient Placement

Place a patient who contaminates the environment or who does not (or cannot be expected to) assist in maintaining appropriate hygiene or environmental control in a private room. If a private room is not available, consult with infection control professionals regarding patient placement or other alternatives. *Category IB*

Respiratory Hygiene/Cough Etiquette

Instruct symptomatic persons to cover mouth/nose when sneezing/coughing; use tissues and dispose in no-touch receptacle; observe hand hygiene after soiling of hands with respiratory secretions; wear surgical masks if tolerated or maintain spatial separation greater than 3 ft if possible. *Category IB*

Note: The following precautions are recommended from UpToDate.

Standard Precautions

Perform hand hygiene before and after every patient contact:

Gloves, gowns, eye protection as required.

Safe disposal or cleaning of instruments and linen.

Cough etiquette: Patients and visitors should cover their nose or mouth when coughing, promptly dispose of used tissues, and practice hand hygiene after contact with respiratory secretions.

Contact Precautions

In addition to standard precautions:

Private room preferred; cohorting allowed if necessary.

Gloves required upon entering room.

Change gloves after contact with contaminated secretions.

Gown required if clothing may come into contact with the patient or environmental surfaces or if the patient has diarrhea.

Minimize risk of environmental contamination during patient transport (e.g., patient can be placed in a gown).

Noncritical items should be dedicated to use for a single patient if possible.

Droplet Precautions

In addition to standard precautions:

Private room preferred; cohorting allowed if necessary.

Wear a mask when within three feet of the patient.

Mask the patient during transport.

Cough etiquette: Patients and visitors should cover their nose or mouth when coughing, promptly dispose of used tissues, and practice hand hygiene after contact with respiratory secretions.

Airborne Precautions

In addition to standard precautions:

Place the patient in an AIIR (a monitored negative pressure room with at least 6 to 12 air exchanges per hour).

Room exhaust must be appropriately discharged outdoors or passed through a HEPA filter before recirculation within the hospital.

A certified respirator must be worn when entering the room of a patient with diagnosed or suspected tuberculosis.

Susceptible individuals should not enter the room of patients with confirmed or suspected measles or chickenpox.

Transport of the patient should be minimized; the patient should be masked if transport within the hospital is unavoidable.

Cough etiquette: Patients and visitors should cover their nose or mouth when coughing, promptly dispose of used tissues, and practice hand hygiene after contact with respiratory secretions.

Siegel, J. D., Rhinehart, E., Jackson, M., Chiarello, L., & The Healthcare Infection Control Practices Advisory Committee. (2007). *Guideline for isolation precautions: Preventing transmission of infectious agents in healthcare settings*. https://www.cdc.gov/infectioncontrol/pdf/guidelines/isolation-guidelines-H.pdf

Anderson, D. J. (2021). Infection prevention: Precautions for preventing transmission of infection. *UpToDate*. https://www.uptodate.com/contents/infection-prevention-precautions-for-preventing-transmission-of-infection

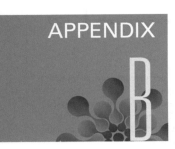

Good Sources of Essential Nutrients

Nutrient	Sources
Protein	Meat, poultry, fish, milk products, and eggs. Whole wheat grains, nuts, peanut butter, and legumes are also good sources of protein but need to be supplemented by some animal protein, such as meat, eggs, milk, cheese, cottage cheese, or yogurt.
Vitamin A	Green leafy vegetables, deep yellow vegetables and fruits, whole milk or whole milk products, egg yolk.
Vitamin B	
Thiamine	Meat, fish, poultry, eggs, whole grain, legumes, potatoes, green leafy vegetables.
Riboflavin	Milk (best source), meat, egg yolk, green vegetables.
Niacin	Meat, fish, poultry, peanut butter, wheat germ, brewer's yeast. Although the amount in milk is small, children whose intake of milk is adequate do not develop pellagra.
Vitamin C	Citrus fruits and fresh or frozen citrus fruit juices, tomatoes, strawberries, cantaloupe.
Vitamin D	Sunlight, fish liver oils, fortified milk, and synthetic vitamin D.
Minerals	
Calcium	Milk and milk products, squash, sweet potatoes, raisins, rhubarb, well-cooked dried beans, turnip greens, Swiss chard, mustard greens.
Iron	Green leafy vegetables, liver, meats and eggs, dried fruits, whole grain or enriched bread and cereals.
Iodine	Seafood, plants grown on soil near the sea, iodized salt.

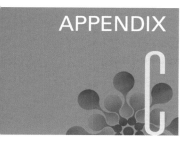

Breast-Feeding and Medication Use

General Considerations

- Most medications pass from the woman's bloodstream into the breast milk. The amount is usually very small and for most medications is unlikely to harm the baby; however, the woman should always check with her health care provider or lactation specialist before taking any medication, including over-the-counter and herbal products.
- Inform the woman who breast-feeds that she has the right to seek a second opinion if the health care provider does not perform a risk-versus-benefit assessment before prescribing medications or advising against breast-feeding.
- A preterm or other special needs neonate is more susceptible to the adverse effects of medications in breast milk. A woman who is taking medications and whose baby is in the neonatal intensive care unit or special care nursery should consult with the pediatrician or neonatologist before feeding her breast milk to the baby.
- The woman should take any medication just after breast-feeding. This practice helps ensure that the lowest possible dose of medication reaches the baby through the breast milk.
- Some medications can cause changes in the amount of milk the woman produces. Teach the woman to report any changes in milk production.

Lactation Risk Categories (LRC)[1]

Lactation		
Category	Risk	Rationale
L1	Safest	Clinical research or long-term observation of use in many breast-feeding women has not demonstrated risk to the infant.
L2	Safer	Limited clinical research has not demonstrated an increase in adverse effects in the infant.
L3	Moderately safe	There is possible risk to the infant; however, the risks are minimal or nonthreatening in nature. These medications should be given only when the potential benefit outweighs the risk to the infant.
L4	Possibly hazardous	There is positive evidence of risk to the infant; however, in life-threatening situations or for serious diseases, the benefit might outweigh the risk.
L5	Contraindicated	The risk of using the medication clearly outweighs any possible benefit from breast-feeding.

[1]As defined by Dr. Thomas W. Hale, PhD.

Potential Effects of Selected Medication Categories on the Breast-Fed Infant

Analgesics—Narcotic

- Codeine and hydrocodone appear to be safe in low doses. Rarely, the neonate may experience sedation and/or apnea. (LRC: L3)
- Meperidine can lead to sedation of the neonate. (LRC: L3)
- Morphine and fentanyl are found in human milk in small amounts. (LRC: L2) However, neonates are sensitive to narcotics and they should only be used in low doses in the immediate postpartum period. It is best to use nonnarcotics whenever possible.

Analgesics—Nonnarcotic and NSAIDs

- Acetaminophen and ibuprofen are approved for use. (LRC: L1)
- Naproxen may cause neonatal hemorrhage and anemia if used for prolonged periods. (LRC: L3 for short-term use and L4 for long-term use)
- Celecoxib appears to be safe for use. (LRC: L2)
- Aspirin should be avoided.

Antibiotics

- Levels in breast milk are usually very low.
- The penicillins and cephalosporins are generally considered safe to use. (LRC: L1 and L2)
- Tetracyclines can be safely used for short periods but are not suitable for long-term therapy (e.g., for treatment of acne). (LRC: L2)
- Sulfonamides should not be used during the neonatal stage (the first month of life). (LRC: L3)

Antidepressants

- The risk to the baby is often higher if the woman is depressed and remains untreated, rather than taking the medication.
- The selective serotonin uptake inhibitors (SSRIs) are considered to be safe and have a lower side effect profile, which makes them more palatable to the woman. (LRC: L2 and L3)
- If the woman has been taking an antidepressant during pregnancy, the risk of switching to a different medication for breast-feeding should be done cautiously and is often not advised.

Antihypertensives

- Some beta-blockers (e.g., propranolol, metoprolol, labetalol) can be used with caution.
- Methyldopa is considered to be safe but increases the risk for depression and should be avoided in the early postpartum period. (LRC: L2)

930

- ACE inhibitors are not recommended in the early postpartum period.
- Diuretics may be used but increase the risk for decreased milk volume.

Anxiolytics
- Most anxiolytics (e.g., alprazolam, buspirone, lorazepam) are (LRC: L3) except diazepam which is (LRC: L4) when used chronically.

Corticosteroids
- Corticosteroids do not pass into the milk in large quantities.
- Inhaled steroids are safe to use because they don't accumulate in the bloodstream.

Mood Stabilizers (Antimanic Medication)
- Lithium is found in breast milk and should not be used in the breast-feeding woman. (LRC: L3)
- Valproic acid seems to be a safe choice for the woman with bipolar disorder. The infant will need periodic laboratory studies to check platelets and liver function. (LRC: L2)

Sedatives and Hypnotics
- Lorazepam is safe but sedation is possible if repeated doses are taken.
- Promethazine is ok in prn doses.
- Chlorpromazine may lead to drowsiness.

Thyroid Medication
- Thyroid medications, such as levothyroxine, can be taken while breast-feeding.
- Most are in LRC category L1.

Medications That Are Usually Contraindicated for the Breast-Feeding Woman
- Amiodarone
- Antineoplastic agents
- Chloramphenicol
- Doxepin
- Ergotamine and other ergot derivatives
- Iodides
- Lithium
- Methotrexate and immunosuppressants
- Pseudoephedrine (found in many over-the-counter medications)
- Radiopharmaceuticals
- Ribavirin
- Tetracycline (prolonged use—more than 3 weeks)

Material in this Appendix was adapted from information found in:

August P. (2021). Treatment of hypertension in pregnant and postpartum women. UpToDate. https://www.uptodate.com/contents/treatment-of-hypertension-in-pregnant-and-postpartum-women

Kimmel M. C. & Meltzer-Brody S. (2020). Breastfeeding infants: Safety of exposure to antipsychotics, lithium, stimulants, and medications for substance use disorders. UpToDate. https://www.uptodate.com/contents/breastfeeding-infants-safety-of-exposure-to-antipsychotics-lithium-stimulants-and-medications-for-substance-use-disorders

Kimmel M. C. & Meltzer-Brody S. (2020). Safety of infant exposure to antidepressants and benzodiazepines through breastfeeding. UpToDate. https://www.uptodate.com/contents/safety-of-infant-exposure-to-antidepressants-and-benzodiazepines-through-breastfeeding

National Center for Biotechnology Information, U.S. National Library of Medicine. (2016). Drugs and Lactation Database (LactMed). https://www.ncbi.nlm.nih.gov/books/NBK501922/?report=classic

Newport D. J. (2021). Hale's Breastfeeding Safety Ratings: Part 1—Rating System. http://www.womensmentalhealth.emory.edu/Blog/indexBreastfeeding%202011.10.28.html

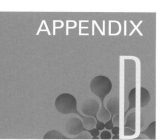

Cervical Dilation Chart

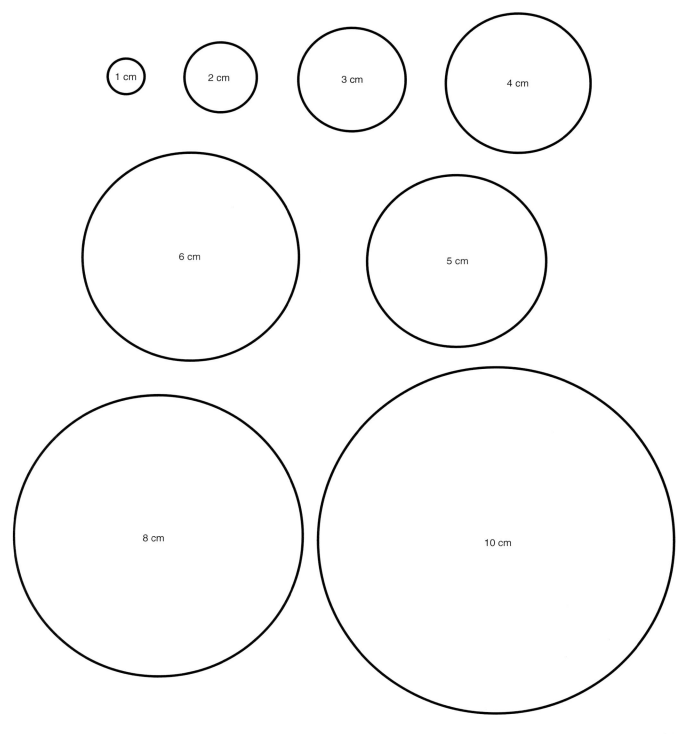

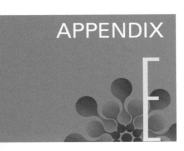
Growth Charts

Birth to 36 Months: Boys
Length-for-Age and Weight-for-Age Percentiles

NAME _____

RECORD no. _____

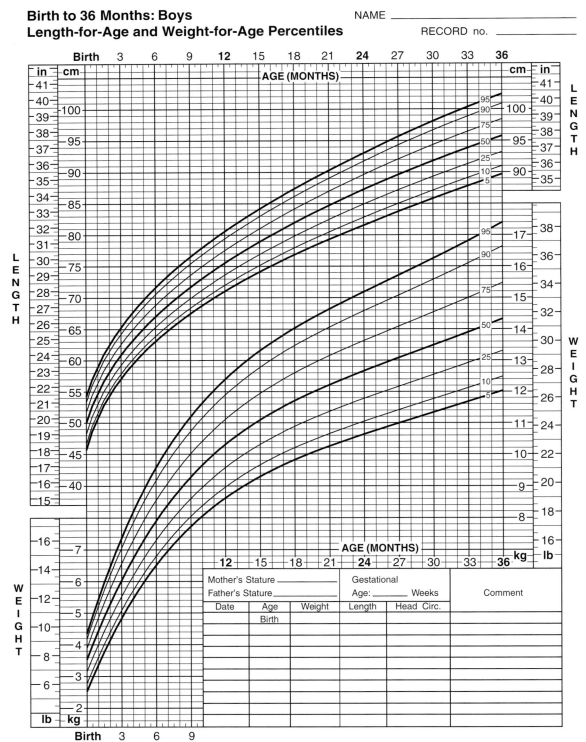

Published May 30, 2000 (modified 4/20/01).
SOURCE: Developed by the National Center for Health Statistics in collaboration with
the National Center for Chronic Disease Prevention and Health Promotion (2000).
http://www.cdc.gov/growthcharts

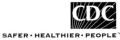

SAFER · HEALTHIER · PEOPLE™

Birth to 36 Months: Boys
Head Circumference-for-Age and
Weight-for-Length Percentiles

NAME _____

RECORD no. _____

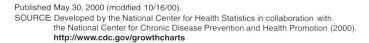

AGE (MONTHS)

Birth 3 6 9 **12** 15 18 21 **24** 27 30 33 **36**

HEAD CIRCUMFERENCE

Date	Age	Weight	Length	Head Circ.	Comment

LENGTH

WEIGHT

Published May 30, 2000 (modified 10/16/00).
SOURCE: Developed by the National Center for Health Statistics in collaboration with
the National Center for Chronic Disease Prevention and Health Promotion (2000).
http://www.cdc.gov/growthcharts

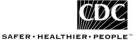

SAFER·HEALTHIER·PEOPLE™

Birth to 36 Months: Girls
Length-for-Age and Weight-for-Age Percentiles

NAME _____

RECORD no. _____

AGE (MONTHS)

| | | | | | | | | | | |
Birth 3 6 9 **12** 15 18 21 **24** 27 30 33 **36**

LENGTH

in cm — 41 40 100 39 95 38 37 90 36 35 34 85 33 32 80 31 30 75 29 28 70 27 26 65 25 24 60 23 22 55 21 20 50 19 18 45 17 16 40 15

95
90
75
50
25
10
5

WEIGHT

95
90
75
50
25
10
5

AGE (MONTHS)

12 15 18 21 **24** 27 30 33 **36** kg lb

Mother's Stature _____			Gestational		
Father's Stature _____			Age: _____ Weeks		Comment
Date	Age	Weight	Length	Head Circ.	
	Birth				

WEIGHT

lb kg 16 7 14 6 12 5 10 4 8 3 6 2 lb kg

Birth 3 6 9

Published May 30, 2000 (modified 4/20/01).
SOURCE: Developed by the National Center for Health Statistics in collaboration with
the National Center for Chronic Disease Prevention and Health Promotion (2000).
http://www.cdc.gov/growthcharts

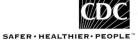

SAFER · HEALTHIER · PEOPLE™

Birth to 36 Months: Girls
Head Circumference-for-Age and
Weight-for-Length Percentiles

NAME _____

RECORD no. _____

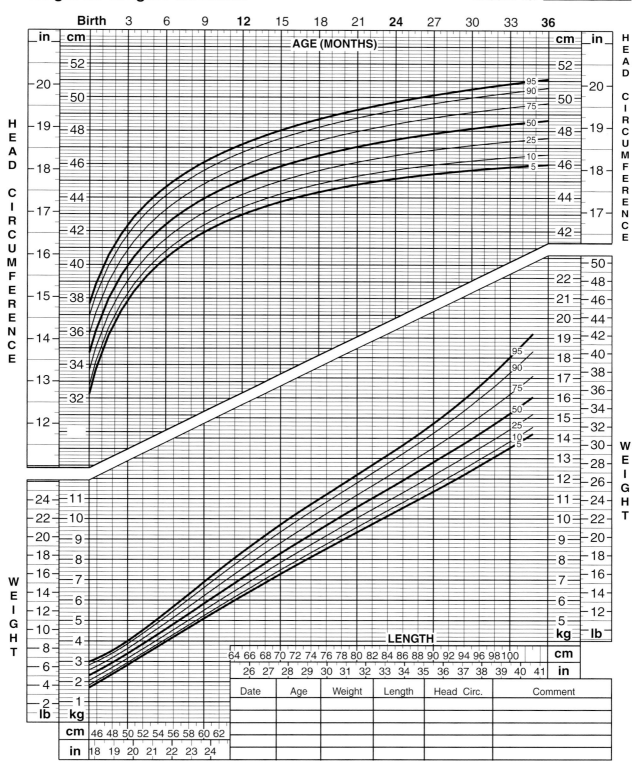

Date	Age	Weight	Length	Head Circ.	Comment

Published May 30, 2000 (modified 10/16/00).

SOURCE: Developed by the National Center for Health Statistics in collaboration with
the National Center for Chronic Disease Prevention and Health Promotion (2000).
http://www.cdc.gov/growthcharts

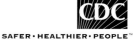

SAFER·HEALTHIER·PEOPLE™

2 to 20 Years: Boys
Stature-for-Age and Weight-for-Age Percentiles

NAME _____

RECORD no. _____

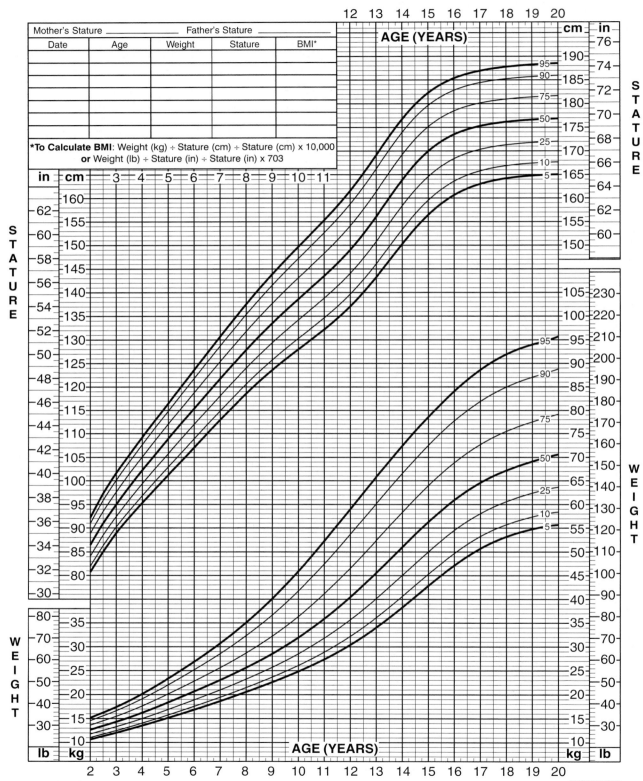

Published May 30, 2000 (modified 11/21/00).
SOURCE: Developed by the National Center for Health Statistics in collaboration with
the National Center for Chronic Disease Prevention and Health Promotion (2000).
http://www.cdc.gov/growthcharts

SAFER · HEALTHIER · PEOPLE™

2 to 20 Years: Girls
Stature-for-Age and Weight-for-Age Percentiles

NAME _____

RECORD no. _____

Mother's Stature _____		Father's Stature _____		
Date	Age	Weight	Stature	BMI*

*To Calculate BMI: Weight (kg) ÷ Stature (cm) ÷ Stature (cm) x 10,000
or Weight (lb) ÷ Stature (in) ÷ Stature (in) x 703

AGE (YEARS)

12 13 14 15 16 17 18 19 20

STATURE

Stature percentiles: 95, 90, 75, 50, 25, 10, 5

Weight percentiles: 95, 90, 75, 50, 25, 10, 5

WEIGHT

AGE (YEARS)

2 3 4 5 6 7 8 9 10 11 12 13 14 15 16 17 18 19 20

in cm   3 4 5 6 7 8 9 10 11

STATURE: cm 160 155 150 145 140 135 130 125 120 115 110 105 100 95 90 85 80 / in 62 60 58 56 54 52 50 48 46 44 42 40 38 36 34 32 30

WEIGHT: kg 35 30 25 20 15 10 / lb 80 70 60 50 40 30 10

Published May 30, 2000 (modified 11/21/00).
SOURCE: Developed by the National Center for Health Statistics in collaboration with
the National Center for Chronic Disease Prevention and Health Promotion (2000).
http://www.cdc.gov/growthcharts

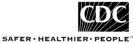

SAFER · HEALTHIER · PEOPLE™

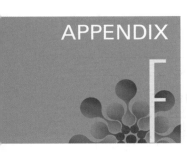
Pulse, Respiration, and Blood Pressure Values for Children

Normal Pulse Ranges in Children

Age	Normal Range (beats per minute)
Newborn	100–180
Infant	90–180
Toddler	80–140
Preschooler	65–120
School-age	60–110
Adolescent	55–95

Normal Respiration Ranges in Children

Age	Rate (breaths per minute)
Infant (birth to 12 months)	30–60
Toddler	24–40
Preschooler	22–34
School-age	18–30
Adolescent	12–16

Normal Blood Pressure Ranges in Children (mm Hg)

Age	Systolic (mm Hg)	Diastolic (mm Hg)
Newborn	60–80	40–45
Infant	72–104	37–56
Toddler	86–106	42–63
Preschooler	89–112	46–72
School-age	97–115	57–76
Adolescent	102–131	61–83

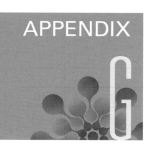

Temperature and Weight Conversion Charts

Conversion of Pounds to Kilograms

Pounds	0	1	2	3	4	5	6	7	8	9
0	—	0.45	0.90	1.36	1.81	2.26	2.72	3.17	3.62	4.08
10	4.53	4.98	5.44	5.89	6.35	6.80	7.25	7.71	8.16	8.61
20	9.07	9.52	9.97	10.43	10.88	11.34	11.79	12.24	12.70	13.15
30	13.60	14.06	14.51	14.96	15.42	15.87	16.32	16.78	17.23	17.69
40	18.14	18.59	19.05	19.50	19.95	20.41	20.86	21.31	21.77	22.22
50	22.68	23.13	23.58	24.04	24.49	24.94	25.40	25.85	26.30	26.76
60	27.21	27.66	28.12	28.57	29.03	29.48	29.93	30.39	30.84	31.29
70	31.75	32.20	32.65	33.11	33.56	34.02	34.47	34.92	35.38	35.83
80	36.28	36.74	37.19	37.64	38.10	38.55	39	39.46	39.91	40.37
90	40.82	41.27	41.73	42.18	42.63	43.09	43.54	43.99	44.45	44.90
100	45.36	45.81	46.26	46.72	47.17	47.62	48.08	48.53	48.98	49.44
110	49.89	50.34	50.80	51.25	51.71	52.16	52.61	53.07	53.52	53.97
120	54.43	54.88	55.33	55.79	56.24	56.70	57.15	57.60	58.06	58.51
130	58.96	59.42	59.87	60.32	60.78	61.23	61.68	62.14	62.59	63.05
140	63.50	63.95	64.41	64.86	65.31	65.77	66.22	66.67	67.13	67.58
150	68.04	68.49	68.94	69.40	69.85	70.30	70.76	71.21	71.66	72.12
160	72.57	73.02	73.48	73.93	74.39	74.84	75.29	75.75	76.20	76.65
170	77.11	77.56	78.01	78.47	78.92	79.38	79.83	80.28	80.74	81.19
180	81.64	82.10	82.55	83	83.46	83.91	84.36	84.82	85.27	85.73
190	86.18	86.68	87.09	87.54	87.99	88.45	88.90	89.35	89.81	90.26
200	90.72	91.17	91.62	92.08	92.53	92.98	93.44	93.89	94.34	94.80

Conversion of Pounds and Ounces to Grams for Newborn Weights

Pounds	\							Ounces								
	0	1	2	3	4	5	6	7	8	9	10	11	12	13	14	15
0	—	28	57	85	113	142	170	198	227	255	283	312	369	397	425	430
1	454	482	510	539	567	595	624	652	680	709	737	765	794	822	850	879
2	907	936	964	992	1,021	1,049	1,077	1,106	1,134	1,162	1,191	1,219	1,247	1,276	1,304	1,332
3	1,361	1,389	1,417	1,446	1,474	1,503	1,531	1,559	1,588	1,616	1,644	1,673	1,701	1,729	1,758	1,786
4	1,814	1,843	1,871	1,899	1,928	1,956	1,984	2,013	2,041	2,070	2,098	2,126	2,155	2,183	2,211	2,240
5	2,268	2,296	2,325	2,353	2,381	2,410	2,438	2,466	2,495	2,523	2,551	2,580	2,608	2,637	2,665	2,693
6	2,722	2,750	2,778	2,807	2,835	2,863	2,892	2,920	2,948	2,977	3,005	3,033	3,062	3,090	3,118	3,147
7	3,175	3,203	3,232	3,260	3,289	3,317	3,345	3,374	3,402	3,430	3,459	3,487	3,515	3,544	3,572	3,600
8	3,629	3,657	3,685	3,714	3,742	3,770	3,799	3,827	3,856	3,884	3,912	3,941	3,969	3,997	4,026	4,054
9	4,082	4,111	4,139	4,167	4,196	4,224	4,252	4,281	4,309	4,337	4,366	4,394	4,423	4,451	4,479	4,508
10	4,536	4,564	4,593	4,621	4,649	4,678	4,706	4,734	4,763	4,791	4,819	4,848	4,876	4,904	4,933	4,961
11	4,990	5,018	5,046	5,075	5,103	5,131	5,160	5,188	5,216	5,245	5,273	5,301	5,330	5,358	5,386	5,415
12	5,443	5,471	5,500	5,528	5,557	5,585	5,613	5,642	5,670	5,698	5,727	5,755	5,783	5,812	5,840	5,868
13	5,897	5,925	5,953	5,982	6,010	6,038	6,067	6,095	6,123	6,152	6,180	6,209	6,237	6,265	6,294	6,322
14	6,350	6,379	6,407	6,435	6,464	6,492	6,520	6,549	6,577	6,605	6,634	6,662	6,690	6,719	6,747	6,776
15	6,804	6,832	6,860	6,889	6,917	6,945	6,973	7,002	7,030	7,059	7,087	7,115	7,144	7,172	7,201	7,228

Conversion of Celsius to Fahrenheit

Celsius	Fahrenheit	Celsius	Fahrenheit	Celsius	Fahrenheit
34	93.2	37	98.6	40	104
34.2	93.6	37.2	99	40.2	104.4
34.4	93.9	37.4	99.3	40.4	104.7
34.6	94.3	37.6	99.7	40.6	105.2
34.8	94.6	37.8	100	40.8	105.4
35	95	38	100.4	41	105.9
35.2	95.4	38.2	100.8	41.2	106.1
35.4	95.7	38.4	101.1	41.4	106.5
35.6	96.1	38.6	101.5	41.6	106.8
35.8	96.4	38.8	101.8	41.8	107.2
36	96.8	39	102.2	42	107.6
36.2	97.2	39.2	102.6	42.2	108
36.4	97.5	39.4	102.9	42.4	108.3
36.6	97.9	39.6	103.3	42.6	108.7
36.8	98.2	39.8	103.6	42.8	109

$(°C) \times (9/5) + 32 = °F$

$(°F - 32) \times (5/9) = °C$

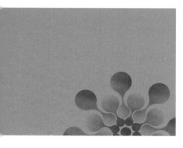

Glossary

A

abruptio placentae, or placental abruption the premature separation of a normally implanted placenta.

abstinence (as related to birth control) refraining from vaginal sexual intercourse.

accelerations spontaneous elevations of the fetal heart rate (FHR).

accommodation occurs when the pupils constrict in order to bring an object into focus. When a bright object is held at a distance and then quickly moved toward the face, the pupil will constrict.

achylia absence of pancreatic enzymes in gastric secretions.

acid–base balance state of equilibrium between the acidity and the alkalinity of body fluids.

acidosis excessive acidity of body fluids.

acrocyanosis blue hands and/or feet with a natural color trunk.

actual nursing focus focus of nursing care that identifies existing health problems.

acute bilirubin encephalopathy (kernicterus) neurologic disorder in which excess bilirubin can cause irreversible injury and death.

adenoids mass of lymphoid tissue in the nasal pharynx; extends from the roof of the nasal pharynx to the free edge of the soft palate.

adenopathy enlarged lymph glands.

afterpains uterine pain felt after delivery.

alcoholism chronic alcohol abuse.

alkalosis excessive alkalinity of body fluids.

allergen antigen that causes an allergic reaction.

allograft skin graft taken from a genetically different person for temporary coverage during burn healing. Skin from a cadaver sometimes is used.

alopecia loss of hair.

amblyopia dimness of vision from disuse of the eye; sometimes called "lazy eye."

amenorrhea absence of menstruation.

amniocentesis a diagnostic procedure whereby a needle is inserted into the amniotic sac and a small amount of fluid is withdrawn and used for biochemical, chromosomal, and genetic studies.

amnioinfusion infusion of sterile isotonic fluid into the uterine cavity during labor.

amnion a thick fibrous lining, made up of several layers, that helps to protect the fetus and forms the inner part of the sac in which the fetus grows.

amniotic fluid the specialized fluid that fills the amniotic cavity and serves to protect the fetus.

amniotomy also known as artificial rupture of membranes (AROM). The rupture of the woman's membranes (amniotic sac) with a medical instrument called an amniohook.

analgesia the use of medication to reduce the sensation of pain.

anasarca massive edema.

android pelvis heart-shaped pelvis.

anesthesia the use of medication to partially or totally block all sensation to an area of the body.

angioedema swelling of the face, lips.

ankylosis immobility of a joint.

anorexia nervosa eating disorder characterized by self inflicted starvation due to emotional causes (e.g., usually excessive fear of becoming [or being] fat).

anthelmintic medication that expels intestinal worms; vermifuge.

anthropoid pelvis pelvis that is elongated in its dimensions. The anterior–posterior diameter is roomy, but the transverse diameter is narrow.

anticipatory grief preparatory grieving that often helps caregivers mourn the loss of their child when death actually comes.

anticipatory guidance preparatory education that helps caregivers understand and prepare for what to expect at a stage of growth and development.

anuria absence of urine.

Apgar a scoring tool used as a means of quickly assessing the newborn's transition to extrauterine life based upon evaluation of five parameters: heart rate, respiratory effort, muscle tone, reflex irritability, and color.

apnea temporary interruption of the breathing impulse.

appropriate for gestational age (AGA) a newborn whose weight, length, and/or head circumference fall(s) between the 10th and 90th percentiles for gestational age.

archetypes predetermined patterns of human development that, according to Carl Jung, replace instinctive behavior of other animals; prototype.

areola darkened area around the nipple.

arthralgia painful joints.

artificial nutrition infant formula.

artificial rupture of membranes (AROM) also called an amniotomy, is the rupture of the woman's membranes (amniotic sac) with a medical instrument called an amniohook.

ascites edema in the peritoneal cavity.

associative play being engaged in a common activity without any sense of belonging or fixed rules.

astigmatism error in light refraction on the retina caused by unequal curvature in the eye's cornea; light rays bend in different directions to produce a blurred image.

ataxia lack of coordination caused by disturbances in the kinesthetic and balance senses.

atresia absence of a normal body opening or the abnormal closure of a body passage.

atrial septal defect an abnormal opening between the right and left atria.

attachment the enduring emotional bond that develops between the parent and infant.

augmentation something added to labor in order to improve it.

aura a sensation that signals an impending seizure; may involve sight, sound, taste, smell, touch, or emotions (e.g., a feeling of fear).

autograft skin taken from an individual's own body. Except for the skin of an identical twin, autograft is the only kind of skin accepted permanently by recipient tissues.

autonomy ability to function in an independent manner.

azotemia nitrogen-containing compounds in the blood.

B

ballottement a probable sign of pregnancy that occurs when the examiner pushes up on the uterine wall during a pelvic examination, then feels the fetus bounce back against the examiner's fingers.

bilateral pertaining to both sides (e.g., bilateral cleft lip involves both sides of the lip).

binging eating a large amount of food in a short time period, often in secrecy.

binocular vision normal vision maintained through the muscular coordination of eye movements of both eyes. A single vision results.

biophysical profile (BPP) a method to determine fetal well-being based upon five fetal biophysical variables: fetal heart rate acceleration observed from a nonstress test, fetal breathing, body movements, tone, and amniotic fluid volume observed from an ultrasound.

Bishop score one commonly used scoring method to determine cervical readiness that evaluates five factors: cervical consistency, position, dilation, effacement, and fetal station.

blastocyst the structure that forms about 5 days after fertilization when the dividing cell mass develops a hollow, fluid-filled core.

blended family both partners in a marriage bring children from a previous marriage into the household.

body surface area (BSA) formula used to calculate dosages. Using a West nomogram, the child's weight is marked on the right scale and the height is marked on the left scale. A straight edge is used to draw a line between the two marks. The point at which the line crosses the column labeled SA (surface area) is the BSA expressed in square meters (m^2).

body weight method for calculating dosages uses the child's weight as a basis for computing medication dosages.

boggy uterus a uterus in the postpartum period that is not contracted and feels soft and spongy, rather than firm and well contracted.

bolus feeding an intermittent enteral feeding in which a specific amount of feeding is given over a short period of time, usually 15 to 30 minutes, and then feedings are administered at specific time intervals.

bonding The initial component of healthy attachment begins with a predictable pattern of parental behavior. The way the new mother and partner become acquainted with their newborn.

brachycephaly shortness of the head.

bradycardia decreased pulse rate.

Braxton Hicks contractions the painless, intermittent, "practice" contractions of pregnancy.

breakthrough pain occurs when the basal dose of analgesia does not control the pain adequately.

brown fat a specialized form of heat-producing tissue found only in fetuses and newborns.

bulimia nervosa eating disorder characterized by episodes of binge eating, followed by purging by self-induced vomiting or use of laxatives.

C

caput succedaneum edematous swelling of the soft tissues of the scalp caused by prolonged pressure of the occiput against the cervix during labor and delivery. The edema disappears within a few days.

cardinal movements the seven turns and movements made by the fetus during birth. They are engagement, descent, flexion, internal rotation, extension, external rotation, and expulsion.

carditis inflammation of the heart.

case management a systematic process to ensure that a client's health and service needs are met.

cataract development of opacity in the crystalline lens that prevents light rays from entering the eye.

cephalhematoma (also cephalohematoma) collection of blood between the periosteum and the skull caused by excessive pressure on the head during birth.

cephalocaudal the pattern of growth of the child that follows an orderly pattern, starting with the head and moving downward.

cephalopelvic disproportion (CPD) the fetal head is too large to fit through the pelvis.

cerclage placement of a purse-string type suture in the cervix to keep it from dilating.

cervical insufficiency painless cervical dilatation with bulging of fetal membranes and sometimes fetal parts through the external os, formerly known as incompetent cervix.

cervix a tubular structure that connects the vagina and uterus. The external os (opening) dips into the vagina, and the internal os opens into the uterine isthmus, the lower portion of the uterus.

cesarean birth the delivery of a fetus through abdominal and uterine incisions, also called cesarean section.

Chadwick sign the bluish-purplish color of the cervix, vagina, and perineum during pregnancy.

chancre hard, red, painless primary lesion of syphilis at the point of entry of the spirochete.

chelating agent agent that binds with metal.

chief complaint the reason for the child's visit to the healthcare setting.

child abuse acts of commission which may result in harm or a threat of harm to the child.

child advocacy speaking or acting on behalf of a child to ensure that their needs are recognized.

child maltreatment term used to define all types of child abuse including physical, sexual, emotional, and any acts of negligence. Child maltreatment is usually committed by a person responsible for the care of the child.

child neglect acts of omission in which there is a failure to provide for the child's needs or to protect the child from harm.

child-life program program to make hospitalization less threatening for children and their parents. These programs are usually under the direction of a child-life specialist whose background is in psychology and early childhood development.

chloasma or mask of pregnancy; brown blotchy areas on the forehead, cheeks, and nose of the pregnant woman.

chordee chord-like anomaly that extends from the scrotum to the penis; pulls the penis downward in an arc.

chorea continuous, rapid, jerky involuntary movements.

chorioamnionitis bacterial or viral infection of the amniotic fluid and membranes.

choriocarcinoma malignancy of the uterine lining.

chorion a second layer of thick fibrous tissue that surrounds the amnion.

chorionic villi finger-like projections that extend out from the chorion, giving it a rough appearance.

chorionic villus sampling (CVS) a procedure similar to amniocentesis that can provide chromosomal studies of fetal cells.

chromosomes thread-like structures that occur in pairs and carry genetic information.

chronic condition condition of long duration or one that progresses slowly, shows little change, and often interferes with daily functioning.

circumcision surgical removal of the foreskin (prepuce) of the penis.

circumoral around the mouth.

circumoral pallor a white area around the mouth.

classification ability to group objects by rank, grade, or class.

cleavage the process of mitotic division performed by the zygote.

client advocacy speaking or acting on behalf of clients.

clonus rapid involuntary muscle contraction and relaxation.

clove hitch restraints restraints used to secure an arm or leg; used most often when a child is receiving an intravenous infusion. The restraint is made of soft cloth formed in a figure eight.

coarctation of the aorta is a constriction or narrowing of the aortic arch or the descending aorta usually adjacent to the ligamentum arteriosum.

codependent parent parent who supports, directly or indirectly, the other parent's addictive behavior.

cognitive development progressive change in the intellectual process, including perception, memory, and judgment.

cohabitation family a living situation in which a couple live together but are not married.

coitus interruptus or withdrawal; requires the man to pull the penis out of the vagina before ejaculation to avoid depositing sperm in or near the vagina.

cold stress a serious, potentially life-threatening condition, where exposure to temperatures cooler than normal body temperature results in the newborn using energy to maintain heat.

colic episodes of crying in the infant, often associated with recurrent gastrointestinal disturbances that are fairly common among young infants and that usually disappear around the age of 3 months.

colostomy a surgical procedure in which a part of the colon is brought through the abdominal wall to create an outlet for elimination of fecal material.

colostrum the antibody-rich breast secretion that is the precursor to breast milk, is normally excreted by the breasts in the last weeks of pregnancy and continues to be excreted in the first few postpartum days.

comedones collection of keratin and sebum in the hair follicle; blackhead; whitehead.

communal family a family where there is a large group of various couples and children that can include singles and elderly members, and where members share responsibility for homemaking and child-rearing. All children are the collective responsibility of adult members.

community-based nursing a type of nursing that focuses on prevention and is directed toward the individuals and families within a community and delivered outside the traditional hospital system.

compartment syndrome a serious neurovascular concern that occurs when increasing pressure within the muscle compartment causes decreased circulation.

congestive heart failure (CHF) result of impaired pumping capability of the heart. It may appear in the first year of life in infants with conditions such as large ventricular septal defects, coarctation of the aorta, and other defects that place an increased workload on the ventricles.

conjunctivitis acute inflammation of the conjunctiva that may be caused by a virus, bacteria, allergy, or foreign body.

conservation ability to recognize that change in shape does not necessarily mean change in amount or mass.

contracture fibrous scarring that forms over a burned movable body part. This part of the healing process can cause serious deformities and limit movement.

cooperative play children play with each other, as in team sports.

cordocentesis or percutaneous umbilical blood sampling (PUBS) a procedure similar to amniocentesis where fetal blood is withdrawn from the umbilical cord.

corpus luteum a yellow body that forms after ovulation from the remnants of the follicle.

coryza runny nose.

couplet care the healthy newborn remains in the same room with the mother following birth, if there is no medical indication for separation, and one nurse is responsible for the care of both the newborn and the mother.

couvade syndrome phenomenon in which some partners actually experience some of the physical symptoms of pregnancy, such as nausea and vomiting, along with the pregnant woman.

craniotabes softening of the occipital bones caused by a reduction of mineralization of the skull.

critical pathways standard plans of care used to organize and monitor the care provided.

croup general term that typically includes symptoms of a barking cough, hoarseness, and inspiratory stridor.

cultural competency the capacity to work effectively with people by integrating the elements of their culture into nursing care.

currant jelly stools stools that consist of blood and mucus.

cyanotic heart disease congenital heart disease that causes right-to-left shunting of blood in the heart; results in a depletion of oxygen to such an extent that the oxygen saturation of the peripheral arterial blood is 85% or less. Defects that permit right-to-left shunting may occur at the atrial, ventricular, or aortic level.

cystitis infection of the bladder.

D

dawdling wasting time; whiling away time; being idle.

debridement removal of necrotic tissue.

decentration ability to see several aspects of a problem at the same time and understand the relationships of various parts to the whole situation.

decidua the endometrium that has changed to support a pregnancy.

deciduous teeth primary teeth that usually erupt between 6 and 8 months of age.

deliriants inhalants that contain chemicals whose fumes can produce confusion, disorientation, excitement, and hallucinations.

denial defense mechanism in which the existence of unpleasant actions or ideas is unconsciously repressed; in the grieving process, one of the stages many people go through; also a type of response by caregivers when caring for chronically ill children in which the caregivers deny the condition's existence and encourage the child to overcompensate for any disabilities.

dependence compulsive need to use a substance for its satisfying or pleasurable effects.

dependent nursing actions nursing actions that the nurse performs as a result of a physician's orders, such as administering analgesics for pain.

deep vein thrombosis (DVT) formation of a blood clot (thrombus) in the deeper veins of the calf, thigh, or pelvis.

dermatome an area on the body surface supplied by a particular sensory nerve.

development progressive change in the child's maturation.

developmental tasks basic achievements associated with each stage of development. Basic tasks must be mastered to move on to the next developmental stage. To achieve maturity, a person must successfully complete developmental tasks at each stage.

diabetic ketoacidosis characterized by drowsiness, dry skin, flushed cheeks, cherry-red lips, and acetone breath with a fruity smell as a result of excessive ketones in the blood in uncontrolled diabetes.

diastasis recti abdominis also referred to as rectus abdominis diastasis, a condition in which the abdominal muscles separate during the pregnancy, leaving part of the abdominal wall without muscular support.

digitalization the use of large doses of digoxin, at the beginning of therapy, to build up the blood levels of the drug to a therapeutic level.

diplopia double vision.

discipline to train or instruct to produce self-control and a particular behavior pattern, especially moral or mental improvement.

diurnal enuresis daytime loss of urinary control.

dizygotic fraternal twins that develop from separate egg and sperm fertilizations.

doula a nonmedical support person who assists the pregnant, laboring, and postpartum woman.

dramatic play a type of play that allows a child to act out troubling situations and to control the solution to the problem.

ductus arteriosus a fetal shunt that links the pulmonary artery with the aorta and allows the oxygenated blood to flow to the body without having to reenter the heart; shunt closes within the first 3 or 4 days of life.

ductus venosus a fetal shunt between the umbilical vein and the inferior vena cava; does not achieve complete closure until the end of the second month of life.

duration the interval from the beginning of a contraction to its end.

dysarthria poor speech articulation.

dysfunctional family family that cannot resolve routine stresses in a positive, socially acceptable manner.

dysmenorrhea painful or difficult menses.

dyspareunia painful intercourse.

dysphagia difficulty swallowing.

E

early adolescence begins at about age 10 years in girls and about age 12 years in boys with a dramatic growth spurt that signals the advent of puberty; preadolescence; pubescence.

early childhood caries formerly referred to as bottle mouth (nursing bottle) caries, a condition caused by the erosion of enamel on the infant's deciduous teeth from sugar in formula or sweetened juice that coats the teeth for long periods. This condition also can occur in infants who sleep with their mothers and nurse intermittently throughout the night.

early deceleration the dip in the fetal heart rate (FHR) tracing that occurs in conjunction with, and mirrors, a uterine contraction.

echolalia "parrot speech" typical of autistic children. They echo words they hear, such as a television commercial, but do not appear to understand the words.

eclampsia the presence of seizure activity or coma in a woman with preeclampsia.

ectopic pregnancy a pregnancy that occurs outside of the uterus. The fertilized ovum implants in another location other than the uterus.

effacement shortening and thinning of the cervix during labor.

effleurage a form of touch that involves light circular fingertip movements on the abdomen; a technique a woman can use in early labor to block pain sensations.

ego in psychoanalytic theory, the conscious self that controls the pleasure principle of the id by delaying the instincts until an appropriate time.

egocentric concerned only with one's own activities or needs; unable to put oneself in another's place or to see another's point of view.

elbow restraint restraint made of muslin with two layers. Pockets wide enough to enclose tongue depressors are placed vertically along the width of the fabric. The restraint is wrapped around the arm to prevent the infant from bending the arm.

elective induction an induction of labor in which the health care provider and woman decide to induce labor in the absence of a medical reason to do so.

electrolytes chemical compounds (minerals) that break down into ions when placed in water.

electronic fetal monitoring (EFM) a monitoring device is placed on, and secured to, the woman's abdomen and is connected to a machine that makes a graph of the contraction intensity and length as well as the fetal heart rate.

embryo the developing conceptus, from weeks 2 to 8.

en face position the baby's face is in direct line of vision and full eye contact is made with the newborn.

encephalopathy degenerative disease of the brain.

encopresis chronic involuntary fecal soiling with no medical cause.

endometriosis a painful reproductive disorder in which endometrial tissue grows outside of the uterus, usually in the pelvic cavity.

endometritis an infection of the uterine lining.

endometrium the vascular mucosal inner layer of walls of the corpus and fundus that changes under hormonal influence every month in preparation for possible pregnancy.

engaged when the presenting part of the fetus has settled into the true pelvis at the level of the ischial spines.

engorgement swelling in the breasts that first occurs when they start producing milk. The breasts may become hard and warm to the touch and can be quite painful.

enteral tube feeding provides nourishment directly through a tube passed into the GI tract.

enuresis continued incontinence of urine beyond the age when control of urination is commonly acquired.

epidural pain medication given through a small catheter placed in the epidural space of the spinal column by an anesthesiologist or anesthetist.

epididymis an intricate network of coiled ducts on the posterior portion of each testis that is approximately 6 m (20 ft) in length.

epiphyses growth centers at the ends of long bones and at the wrists.

episiotomy a surgical incision made into the perineum to enlarge the posterior part of the vaginal opening just before the baby is born.

episodic changes variations in the fetal heart rate not associated with uterine contractions.

epispadias condition in which the opening of the urinary meatus is located abnormally on the dorsal (upper) surface of the glans penis.

epistaxis nosebleed.

Epstein pearls small white cysts found on the midline portion of the hard palate of some newborns.

Erb palsy a facial paralysis resulting from injury to the cervical nerves.

erythema marginatum a pink-red rash on the trunk seen in acute rheumatic fever.

eschar hard crust or scab.

esotropia eye deviation toward the other eye.

estimated date of delivery (EDD) the estimated date that the baby will be born, also called the "due date."

euglycemia normal blood glucose levels.

exotropia eye deviation away from the other eye.

extended family consists of one or more nuclear families plus other relatives; often crosses generations to include grandparents, aunts, uncles, and cousins. The needs of individual members are subordinate to the needs of the group, and the children are considered an economic asset.

external version a process of manipulating the position of the fetus while in utero, to try to turn the fetus to a cephalic presentation.

extracellular fluid fluid situated outside a cell or cells.

extravasation escape of fluid into surrounding tissue.

extremely low birth weight (ELBW) weight less than 1,000 g.

extrusion reflex the infant's way of taking food by thrusting the tongue forward as if to suck; has the effect of pushing solid food out of the mouth.

exudate drainage.

F

fallopian tubes are tiny, muscular corridors that arise from the superior surface of the uterus near the fundus and extend laterally on either side toward the ovaries.

false pelvis the flared upper portion of the bony pelvis; in lay terms, the "hips."

febrile seizure seizure occurring in infants and young children commonly associated with a fever of 102°F to 106°F (38.9°C to 41.1°C).

fertilization process by which the male's sperm unites with the female's ovum.

fetal alcohol spectrum disorder (FASD) a term used to describe the range of effects that can occur in an individual who was exposed to alcohol prenatally and who may have lifelong concerns from the alcohol exposure.

fetal attitude the relationship of the fetal parts to one another.

fetal lie describes the position of the long axis of the fetus in relation to the long axis of the pregnant woman.

fetal presentation refers to the foremost part of the fetus that enters the pelvic inlet.

fetus term for the developing human from the beginning of the ninth week after fertilization until birth.

focal (partial) seizure a type of seizure with manifestations that are limited to a particular area of the brain.

fontanel "soft spot" covered by a tough membrane at the junctures of the six bones of a newborn's skull. At birth, two fontanels can be detected—the anterior fontanel at the junction of the frontal and parietal bones and the posterior fontanel at the junction of the parietal and occipital bones. They are ossified (filled in by bone) during the normal growth process.

foramen ovale a hole that connects the right and left atria of the fetus and closes with the first breath.

forceps metal instruments with curved, blunted blades (somewhat like large flattened spoons) that are placed around the head of the fetus by the birth attendant to facilitate delivery.

forceps marks noticeable marks on the infant's face that may occur if delivery was assisted with forceps; usually disappear within a day or two.

foremilk the first milk the baby receives during the nursing session; milk is watery, thin and may have a bluish tint.

frequency how often contractions are occurring; measured by counting the time interval from the beginning of one contraction to the beginning of the next contraction.

frontal-occipital circumference (FOC) measurement of the widest circumference of the head (ie, from the occipital prominence around to just above the eyebrows).

G

gag reflex reaction to any stimulation of the posterior pharynx by food, suction, or passage of a tube that causes elevation of the soft palate and a strong involuntary effort to vomit; continues throughout life.

gametes sex cells.

gametogenesis the formation and development of gametes or germ cells by the process of meiosis.

gastric residual the amount of an enteral feeding remaining in the stomach, after a period of time following the feeding, which indicates absorption of feedings and gastric emptying.

gastroenteritis infectious diarrhea caused by infectious organisms, including *Salmonella*, *Escherichia coli*, dysentery bacilli, and various viruses, most notably rotaviruses.

gastrostomy tube tube usually surgically inserted through the abdominal wall into the stomach under general anesthesia. Used in children who have conditions that interfere with their ability to eat or drink.

gavage feeding nutrition provided through a tube passed directly into the stomach through the nose (nasogastric) or mouth (orogastric).

generalized seizure seizures that involve both hemispheres of the brain.

gestational age the length of time between fertilization of the egg and birth of the infant.

gestational diabetes mellitus (GDM) a type of diabetes mellitus (DM) that is unique to pregnancy but in many respects mimics type 2 DM.

gestational hypertension elevated blood pressure (systolic ≥140 mm Hg or diastolic ≥90 mm Hg) that develops for the first time during pregnancy, after 20 weeks gestation, without the presence of protein in the urine.

gestational surrogate or surrogate mother; a woman who donates the use of her uterus; she may also donate her ovum and agree to be inseminated with the male partner's sperm.

gestational trophoblastic neoplasia malignancy of the uterine lining.

glycosuria glucose in the urine.

goniotomy surgical opening into Schlemm canal that allows drainage of aqueous humor; performed to relieve intraocular pressure in glaucoma.

Goodell sign softening of the cervix during pregnancy.

gradual acceptance type of response by family caregivers when caring for a chronically ill child in which caregivers adopt a common sense approach to the child's condition and encourage the child to function within their capabilities.

grand multiparity five or more pregnancies.

granulocytes type of white blood cell; divided into eosinophils, basophils, and neutrophils.

gravida the number of pregnancies the woman has had, regardless of the outcome, including the present pregnancy.

growth result of cell division and marked by an increase in size and weight; physical increase in body size and appearance caused by increasing numbers of new cells.

gynecoid pelvis a pelvis that is rounded in shape, which allows the fetus room to pass through the dimensions of the bony passageway.

gynecomastia excessive growth of the mammary glands in the male.

H

halo traction device external fixation device used to treat cervical fractures or for immobilization following a cervical fusion.

Harlequin sign characterized by a clown suit-like appearance of the newborn. The newborn's skin is dark red on one side of the body while the other side of the body is pale. The dark red color is caused by dilation of blood vessels, and the pallor is caused by contraction of blood vessels.

Hegar sign softening of the uterine isthmus during pregnancy.

hemarthrosis bleeding into the joints.

hematoma a collection of blood within tissues; the blood loss is concealed.

hemolysis destruction of red blood cells with the release of hemoglobin into the plasma.

hernia abnormal protrusion of part of an organ through a weak spot or other abnormal opening in a body wall.

heterograft graft of tissue obtained from an animal. For burn patients, pig skin (porcine) is often used.

heterosexual intimate relationship between two people of the opposite sex.

hierarchical arrangement grouping by some common system such as rank, grade, or class.

hind milk breast milk that replaces foremilk in a nursing session and is thicker and whiter than foremilk. It contains a higher quantity of fat than foremilk and therefore has a higher caloric content than foremilk.

homeostasis uniform state; signifies biologically the dynamic equilibrium of the healthy organism.

homograft graft of tissue, including organs, from a member of one's own species.

homosexual intimate relationship between two people of the same sex.

hordeolum purulent infection of the follicle of an eyelash; generally caused by *Staphylococcus aureus*. Localized swelling, tenderness, and pain are present with a reddened lid edge; a stye.

hospice provides comforting and supportive care to terminally ill clients and their families. There are few hospice programs for children in the United States.

human trafficking a modern form of slavery in which people are deceived and misled and end up in a situation where one person exerts control over another person for the purpose of exploitation in some form.

hydatidiform mole also referred to as a molar pregnancy, benign growth of placental tissue.

hydramnios excessive amniotic fluid.

hydrotherapy use of water in a treatment.

hyperbilirubinemia high levels of unconjugated bilirubin in the bloodstream (serum levels of 4 to 6 mg/dL and greater).

hyperemesis gravidarum a disorder of early pregnancy that is characterized by severe nausea and vomiting that results in weight loss, nutritional deficiencies, and/or electrolyte and acid–base imbalance.

hyperglycemia elevated blood glucose levels.

hyperinsulinemia increased insulin levels.

hyperlipidemia increase in the level of cholesterol in the blood.

hyperopia refractive condition in which the person can see objects better at a distance; farsightedness.

hyperpnea increase in depth and rate of breathing.

hyperthermia overheating.

hypervolemia increased volume of circulating plasma.

hypochylia diminished flow of pancreatic enzymes.

hypoglycemia blood glucose levels lower than normal.

hyposensitization immunization therapy by injection; immunotherapy.

hypospadias condition that occurs when the opening to the urethra is on the ventral (under) surface of the glans.

hypothermia low body temperature; may be a symptom of a disease or dysfunction of the temperature-regulating mechanism of the body, or it may be deliberately induced, such as during open heart surgery, to reduce oxygen needs and provide a longer time for the surgeon to complete the operation without the client experiencing brain damage. When caring for the newborn, it is important to remember that heat loss can lead to hypothermia because of the infant's immature temperature-regulating system.

hypovolemia decreased volume of circulating plasma.

hypovolemic shock condition characterized by a weak, thready, rapid pulse; drop in blood pressure; cool, clammy skin; and changes in level of consciousness.

I

id in psychoanalytic theory, part of the personality that controls physical needs and instincts of the body; dominated by the pleasure principle.

ileostomy a surgical procedure in which a part of the ileum is brought through the abdominal wall to create an outlet to drain fecal material.

immediate family family structure that consists of only the father, the mother, and the children living in one household.

immunologic properties properties from the woman that help protect the newborn from infections and strengthen the newborn's immune system.

imperforate anus congenital disorder in which the rectal pouch ends blindly above the anus and there is no anal orifice.

impunity belief, common among adolescents, that nothing can hurt them.

incest sexually arousing physical contact between family members not married to each other.

independent nursing actions nursing actions that may be performed based on the nurse's own clinical judgment.

induced abortion the purposeful interruption of pregnancy before 20 weeks' gestation.

induration hardness.

infant mortality rate the number of deaths during the first 12 months of life, which includes neonatal mortality.

infertility the inability to conceive after a year or more of regular and unprotected intercourse, or the inability to carry a pregnancy to term.

infiltration fluid leaking into the surrounding tissues.

inhalant substance that may be taken into the body through inhaling; substance whose volatile vapors can be abused.

intensity the strength of the uterine contraction at the peak of the contraction; described as mild, moderate, or strong.

intercurrent infection infection that occurs during the course of an already existing disease.

interdependent nursing actions nursing actions that the nurse must work with other health team members to accomplish, such as meal planning with a dietary therapist and teaching breathing exercises with a respiratory therapist.

intermittent infusion device a type of device that is used for administering medications by the intravenous route and can be left in place and used at intervals.

interstitial fluid also called intracellular or tissue fluid; has a composition similar to plasma but contains almost no protein. This reservoir of fluid outside the body cells decreases or increases easily in response to disease.

intracellular fluid fluid contained within the cell membranes; constitutes about two-thirds of total body fluids.

intrathecal administration a one-time dose of medication placed into the spinal fluid (in the subarachnoid space), also known as a spinal block.

intrauterine growth restriction (IUGR) condition in which babies are small because of circumstances that occurred during the pregnancy, causing limited fetal growth.

intravascular fluid fluid situated within the blood vessels or blood plasma.

invagination telescoping; infolding of one part of a structure into another.

involution the process through which the uterus, cervix, and vagina return to the nonpregnant size and function.

isoimmunization development of antibodies against Rho(D)-positive blood in the pregnant woman.

J

jacket restraint used to secure the child from climbing out of bed or a chair or to keep the child in a horizontal position; must be the correct size for the child.

jaundice a yellow staining of the skin that occurs when a large amount of unconjugated bilirubin is present.

K

kangaroo care the newborn is skin-to-skin with the mother or father and both are covered with blankets; a way to maintain the newborn's temperature and promote bonding.

kernicterus (acute bilirubin encephalopathy) neurologic disorder in which excess bilican cause irreversible injury and death.

Kussmaul breathing abnormal increase in the depth and rate of the respiratory movements.

kwashiorkor syndrome occurring in infants and young children soon after weaning; results from severe deficiency of protein. Symptoms include a swollen abdomen, retarded growth with muscle wasting, edema, gastrointestinal changes, thin dry hair with patchy alopecia, apathy, and irritability.

kyphosis backward and lateral curvature of the cervical spine; hunchback.

L

labor dystocia an abnormally slow progression of labor.

lacrimation secretion of tears.

lactation production and secretion of milk from the breast.

lactation consultant a nurse or layperson who has received special training to assist and support the breast-feeding woman.

lactose a sugar found in milk that, when hydrolyzed, yields glucose and galactose.

lactose intolerance inability to digest lactose because of an inborn deficiency of the enzyme lactase.

laminaria cervical dilators that are used to soften and dilate the cervix.

lanugo fine downy hair that is present in abundance on the preterm infant and found in thinning patches on the shoulders, arms, and back of the term newborn.

large for gestational age (LGA) an infant whose weight, length, and/or head circumference is above the 90th percentile for gestational age.

latchkey child a child who comes home to an empty house after school each day because family caregivers are at work.

late decelerations a decrease in the fetal heart rate that begins late in the contraction and recovers to baseline after the contraction has ended.

lecithin major component of surfactant.

leukemia uncontrolled reproduction of deformed white blood cells.

leukopenia a leukocyte count <5,000 mm^3.

libido sexual drive.

linea nigra a darkened line that develops on the skin in the middle of the abdomen of pregnant women.

lochia vaginal discharge during the postpartum period that is composed of blood, mucus, tissue, and white blood cells.

lordosis increased curvature of the lumbar spine; swayback.

low birth weight (LBW) newborns that weigh <2,500 g.

lymphoblast a lymphocyte that has been changed by antigenic stimulation to a structurally immature lymphocyte.

lymphocytes single-nucleus, nonphagocytic leukocytes that are instrumental in the body's immune response.

M

macroglossia abnormally large tongue.

macrosomia condition that is diagnosed if the birth weight exceeds 4,500 g (9.9 lb) or the birth weight is greater than the 90th percentile for gestational age.

magical thinking child's belief that thoughts are powerful and can cause something to happen (e.g., illness or death of a loved one occurs because the child wished it in a moment of anger).

malattachment emotional distancing in the maternal–infant relationship.

malocclusion the improper alignment of the teeth.

marasmus deficiency in calories as well as protein. The child suffers growth retardation and wasting of subcutaneous fat and muscle.

mastitis infection of the connective tissue of the mammary gland (breast).

maternal mortality rate the number of maternal deaths per 100,000 live births caused by a pregnancy-related complication that occurs during pregnancy or during the 42 days after pregnancy.

maturation completed growth and development.

meconium the first stool of the newborn, a thick black tarry substance composed of dead cells, mucus, and bile that collects in the rectum of the fetus in utero.

menarche the first menstrual period signifying the beginning of menstruation.

menopause the time in a woman's life when reproductive capability ends.

menorrhagia heavy or prolonged uterine bleeding.

menstrual cycle or the female reproductive cycle, refers to the recurring changes that take place in a woman's reproductive tract associated with menstruation and the events that surround menstruation.

menstruation the casting away of blood, tissue, and debris from the uterus as the inner lining sheds.

metaphysis growing portion of the bone.

metered-dose inhaler (MDI) a handheld pressurized canister that delivers a premeasured dose of medication via an attached mouthpiece.

metrorrhagia menstrual bleeding that is normal in amount but occurs at irregular intervals between menstrual periods.

microcephaly a very small cranium.

micrognathia abnormal smallness of the lower jaw.

milia tiny white papules found on the face of the newborn; common skin manifestation.

mittelschmerz pain experienced midcycle in the menstrual cycle at the time of ovulation.

molding a temporary elongation of the fetal skull caused by the bones of the skull overlapping during labor, which reduces the diameter of the head.

monocytes 5% to 10% of white blood cells that defend the body against infection.

monozygotic identical twins that are derived from one zygote; one egg and one sperm which divide into two zygotes shortly after fertilization.

morbidity the number of persons afflicted with the same disease condition per a certain number.

morula the solid cell cluster that forms about 3 days after fertilization, when the total cell count has reached 32.

mottling a red and white lacy pattern sometimes seen on the skin of newborns who have fair complexions.

multigravida a woman who has had more than one pregnancy.

mummy restraint snug wraps used to restrain an infant or small child's body during a procedure that involve the head or neck.

mutation fundamental change that takes place in the structure of a gene; results in the transmission of a trait different from that normally carried by that particular gene.

myometrium the muscular middle layer of the walls of the corpus and fundus of the uterus that is responsible for the contractions of labor.

myopia ability to see objects clearly at close range but not at a distance; nearsightedness.

myringotomy incision of the eardrum performed to establish drainage and to insert tiny tubes into the tympanic membrane to facilitate drainage of serous or purulent fluid in the middle ear.

N

nadir the lowest point of the deceleration of the fetal heart rate (FHR).

Naegele rule a formula used to determine the pregnancy due date by adding 7 days to the date of the first day of the last menstrual period (LMP), then subtracting 3 months.

nebulizer medication administration device that turns liquid medication into a mist that can be more easily delivered into the lungs via an attached mouthpiece or facemask.

negativism opposition to suggestion or advice; associated with the toddler age group because the toddler, in search of autonomy, frequently responds "no" to almost everything.

neonate term used to describe a newborn in the first 28 days of life.

nocturnal emissions involuntary discharge of semen during sleep; also known as wet dreams.

nocturnal enuresis nighttime bedwetting.

noncommunicative language egocentric speech exhibited by children who talk to themselves, toys, or pets without any purpose other than the pleasure of using words.

nosocomial hospital- or healthcare-associated infection.

nuchal rigidity stiff neck.

nuclear family composed of a man, a woman, and their children (either biologic or adopted) who share a common household.

nulligravida a woman who has never been pregnant.

nursing process proven form of problem solving based on the scientific method. The nursing process consists of five components: assessment (data collection), nursing care focus (sometimes called nursing diagnosis), outcome identification and planning, implementation, and evaluation.

nutrition history information regarding the child's eating habits and preferences.

nystagmus involuntary, rhythmic movements of the eyes.

O

obesity excessive accumulation of fat that increases body weight by 20% or more over ideal weight.

object permanence the concept that just because an object cannot be seen does not mean it is gone.

objective data in the nursing assessment (data collection), the data gained by the nurse's direct observation.

oliguria decreased production of urine, especially in relation to fluid intake.

onlooker play interest in the observation of an activity without participation.

open-glottis pushing pushing with contractions using an open glottis so that air is released during the pushing effort.

opioids medications with opium-like properties (also known as narcotic analgesics); the most frequently administered medications to provide analgesia during labor.

opisthotonos arching of the back so that the head and the heels are bent backward and the body is forward.

ophthalmia neonatorum a severe eye infection contracted in the birth canal of a woman with gonorrhea or chlamydia.

orchiopexy surgical procedure used to bring an undescended testis down into the scrotum and anchor it there.

orthodontia a type of dentistry dealing with prevention and correction of incorrectly positioned or aligned teeth.

orthoptics therapeutic exercises to improve the quality of vision.

outcomes goals that are specific, stated in measurable terms, and have a time frame for accomplishment.

ovaries glands located on either side of the uterus.

overprotection type of response by family caregivers when caring for chronically ill children in which the caregivers protect the child at all costs, engage in hovering that prevents the child from achieving new skills, avoid the use of discipline, and use every means to prevent the child from suffering any frustration.

overriding aorta in tetralogy of Fallot, the aorta shifts to the right over the opening in the ventricular septum so that blood from both right and left ventricles is pumped into the aorta.

overweight more than 10% over ideal weight.

ovulation the process through which the ovaries release the mature ovum into the abdominal cavity, which occurs on day 14 of a 28-day cycle.

P

palpebral fissures opening between the eyes.

papilledema swelling of the optic disc.

papoose board commercial restraint board for use with toddlers or preschool-age children that uses canvas strips to secure the child's body and extremities. One extremity can be released to allow treatment to be performed on that extremity.

parallel play one child plays alongside another child or children involved in the same type of activity, but the children do not interact with each other.

parity or para, refers to the number of pregnancies (not fetuses) carried past the age of viability; each pregnancy is counted as one, even if the woman delivers twins or triplets. The current pregnancy is not counted in parity.

patient-controlled analgesia (PCA) programmed intravenous infusion of narcotic analgesia that the patient can control within set limits.

pedodontist dentist who specializes in the care and treatment of children's teeth.

pelvic rest a situation in which nothing is placed in the vagina (including tampons or the health care provider's fingers to perform a cervical examination); this includes sexual abstinence.

percutaneous umbilical blood sampling (PUBS) or cordocentesis a procedure similar to amniocentesis in which fetal blood is withdrawn from the umbilical cord.

perimenopause the time before menopause when vasomotor symptoms (hot flashes, night sweats) and irregular menses begin, also known as the climacteric.

perimetrium the tough outer layer of the walls of the corpus and fundus, which is made of connective tissues and supports the uterus.

perinatologist a maternal–fetal medicine specialist.

perineum a band of fibrous, muscular tissue that extends from the posterior portion of the labia majora to the anus.

periodic changes variations in the fetal heart rate (FHR) pattern that occur in conjunction with uterine contractions.

perioperative period the period of time encompassing the surgery that has three phases: preoperative, intraoperative, and postoperative.

personal history data collected about a client's personal habits, such as hygiene, sleeping, and elimination patterns, as well as activities, exercise, special interests, and favorite objects (toys).

petechiae a small hemorrhage appearing as a nonraised, purplish-red spot of the skin, nail beds, or mucous membranes.

philtrum vertical groove in the middle of the upper lip.

phimosis adherence of the foreskin to the glans penis.

photophobia intolerance to light.

photosensitivity sensitivity to sunlight.

physiologic jaundice icterus neonatorum; jaundice that occurs in a large number of newborns but has no medical significance; result of the breakdown of fetal red blood cells.

pica persistent ingestion of nonfood substances such as clay, laundry starch, freezer frost, or dirt.

pincer grasp using the thumb and index finger to pick up food or small objects.

pinna the upper, external, protruding part of the ear.

placenta previa a condition in which the placenta is implanted close to, or covers, the cervical os.

platypelloid pelvis a pelvis that has a very narrow anterior–posterior diameter and a wide transverse diameter.

play therapy technique of psychoanalysis that psychiatrists or psychiatric nurse clinicians use to uncover a disturbed child's underlying thoughts, feelings, and motivations, to better help them.

point of maximum impulse (PMI) the point over the heart on the chest wall where the heartbeat can be heard the best using a stethoscope.

polyarthritis inflammation of several joints.

polycythemia excess number of red blood cells.

polydipsia abnormal thirst.

polyhydramnios excess levels of amniotic fluid.

polyphagia increased food consumption.

polyuria dramatic increase in urinary output, often with enuresis.

postcoital test evaluates the interaction of the man's sperm with the woman's cervical mucus.

postpartum blues sometimes called the "baby blues," a temporary condition that usually begins about the third day after delivery, lasts for 2 or 3 days, and usually has resolved by 2 weeks postpartum in which the woman may be tearful, have difficulty sleeping and eating, and feel generally letdown.

postterm or postmature, a newborn born at 42 weeks or more gestation.

precipitous labor labor that lasts less than 3 hours from the start of uterine contractions to birth.

preeclampsia a serious condition of pregnancy in which the blood pressure in a woman who has had normal blood pressures rises to ≥140 mm Hg systolic or ≥90 mm Hg diastolic on two separate occasions and is accompanied by proteinuria.

pregestational diabetes condition in which a woman enters pregnancy with either type 1 or type 2 diabetes mellitus.

prelabor rupture of membranes (PROM) (formerly called premature rupture of membranes) the spontaneous rupture of the amniotic sac before the onset of labor. PROM is different from preterm PROM (PPROM), which refers to rupture of the amniotic sac before the onset of labor in a woman who is fewer than 37 weeks gestation.

premenstrual syndrome (PMS) symptoms occurring before menstruation, including edema (resulting in weight gain), headache, increased anxiety, mild depression or mood swings, premenstrual tension.

prepuce or foreskin; a layer of tissue that covers the glans of the penis.

preterm or premature, a newborn born at 37 weeks' gestation or fewer; commonly called premature.

priapism prolonged, abnormal erection of the penis.

primary circular reactions a stage of development named by Piaget in which infants explore objects by touching or putting them in their mouths; the infant is unaware of actions that they can cause.

primary prevention health-promoting activities to prevent the development of illness or injury, includes giving information regarding safety, diet, rest, exercise, and disease prevention through immunizations; emphasizes the nursing roles of educator and client advocate.

proteinuria the presence of protein in the urine.

proximodistal pattern of growth in which growth starts in the center and progresses toward the periphery or outside.

pruritus itching.

pseudomenstruation false menstruation; a slight red-tinged vaginal discharge in female infants resulting from a decline in the hormonal level after birth compared with the higher concentration in the maternal hormone environment before birth.

puberty period during which secondary sexual characteristics begin to develop and reproductive maturity is attained.

puerperal fever an illness marked by high fever caused by infection of the reproductive tract after the birth of a child.

puerperium the postpartum period, encompasses the 6 to 12 weeks after birth. This is sometimes referred to as "the fourth trimester."

pulmonary embolism occurs when a clot (thrombus), or part of the clot, breaks free from the vessel wall (becoming an embolus), travels to the heart, and then moves through the pulmonary circulation, where it lodges and interrupts the blood flow to the lungs.

pulmonary stenosis narrowing of the opening between the right ventricle and the pulmonary artery that decreases blood flow to the lungs.

punishment penalty given for wrongdoing.

purpura hemorrhages into the skin or mucous membranes.

purpuric rash rash consisting of ecchymoses (bruises) and petechiae caused by bleeding under the skin.

pyelonephritis infection of the kidneys.

pyrosis heartburn caused by acid reflux through the relaxed lower esophageal sphincter.

Q

quickening when the woman feels the fetus move for the first time, around 16 to 20 weeks gestation.

R

refeeding syndrome potentially fatal complication that can occur with aggressive nutritional rehabilitation and weight gain in cases of severe malnutrition.

refraction the way light rays bend as they pass through the lens of the eye to the retina.

regurgitation spitting up of small quantities of milk; occurs rather easily in the young infant.

rejection type of response by family caregivers when caring for a chronically ill child in which the caregivers distance themselves emotionally from the child and, although they provide physical care, tend to scold and correct the child continuously.

respite care care of the child by someone other than the usual caregiver so that the caregiver can get temporary relief and rest.

reversibility ability to think in either direction.

right ventricular hypertrophy increase in thickness of the myocardium of the right ventricle.

risk nursing focus focus of nursing care that identifies health problems to which the client is especially vulnerable.

ritualism practice employed by the young child to help develop security; consists of following a certain routine; makes rituals of simple tasks.

rooming-in arrangement in which the healthcare facility permits a family caregiver to stay with a child. A cot or sleeping chair is provided for the family caregiver.

ruddy dark red color seen in the palms of the hands and soles of the feet of the newborn.

rumination voluntary regurgitation.

S

salpingectomy removal of the fallopian tube.

salpingitis infection of the fallopian tube.

school history information regarding the child's grade level in school and their academic performance.

scoliosis lateral curvature of the spine.

seborrhea a scalp condition characterized by yellow, crusty patches; also called cradle cap.

sebum oily secretion of the sebaceous glands.

secondary circular reactions a stage of development named by Piaget in which the infant realizes that their actions cause pleasurable sensations.

secondary prevention health-screening activities that aid in early diagnosis and encourage prompt treatment before long-term negative effects arise.

seminiferous tubules tiny coils of tissue in the lobes of the testis in which spermatogenesis occurs.

sexual abuse sexual contact between a child and someone in a caregiving position such as a parent, babysitter, or teacher.

sexual assault sexual contact made by someone who is not functioning in the role of the child's caregiver.

simian crease a single straight palmar crease; a finding that is associated with Down syndrome.

single-parent family family that is headed by one adult and includes one or more children.

skeletal traction pull exerted directly on skeletal structures by means of pins, wire, tongs, or another device surgically inserted through the bone.

skin traction use of tape, rubber, or plastic materials attached to the skin that indirectly exerts pull on the musculoskeletal system.

small for gestational age (SGA) a newborn whose weight, length, and/or head circumference fall(s) below the 10th percentile for gestational age.

smegma the cheese-like secretion of the sebaceous glands found under the foreskin, or within the folds of the labia.

social history information about the environment in which the child lives.

socialization process through which the child learns the rules of the society and culture in which the family lives including language, values, ethics, and acceptable behaviors.

solitary independent play playing apart from others without making an effort to be part of the group or group activity.

sonogram a picture obtained with ultrasound.

spermatogenesis production of sperm.

spinnbarkeit an elastic quality of cervical mucus that allows it to be stretched 5 cm or more between the thumb and forefinger.

spontaneous abortion loss of a pregnancy before 20 weeks of gestation, which in lay terms is often called a miscarriage. It is referred to as early pregnancy loss.

spontaneous rupture of membranes (SROM) when the woman's membranes (amniotic sac) have ruptured without medical intervention, often indicated by reports from the woman of a gush or continual leaking of warm fluid from the vagina.

startle reflex follows any loud noise; similar to the Moro reflex, but the hands remain clenched. This reflex is never lost.

station the relationship of the presenting part of a fetus to the ischial spines of the woman's pelvis.

status asthmaticus a severe asthma attack that doesn't respond to treatment (such as bronchodilators), leads to hypoxemia (low O_2 levels in the blood), hypercapnia (increased CO_2 levels in the blood) and can lead to respiratory failure.

status epilepticus an emergency complication of epilepsy whereby seizure activity continues for 5 to 30 minutes or more or when three or more seizures occur without full recovery between seizures.

steatorrhea fatty stools.

stepfamily consists of custodial parent, children, and a new spouse.

stigma negative perception of a person because they are believed to be different from the general population; may cause embarrassment or shame in the person being stigmatized.

strabismus failure of the two eyes to direct their gaze at the same object simultaneously; squint; crossed eyes.

striae stretch marks.

stridor shrill, harsh respiratory sound, usually on inspiration.

subjective data in the nursing assessment (data collection), data spoken by the child or family.

sublimation process of directing a desire or impulse into more acceptable behaviors.

substance abuse the misuse of an addictive substance, such as alcohol or drugs, that changes the user's mental state.

superego in psychoanalytic theory, the conscience or parental value system; acts primarily as a monitor over the ego.

supernumerary excessive in number (e.g., more than the usual number of teeth).

supine hypotensive syndrome condition that occurs when the uterus and its contents compress the aorta and vena cava against the spine, which decreases the amount of blood returned to the heart, causing the cardiac output and the blood pressure to fall.

surfactant a substance found in the alveoli of mature fetuses that decreases the surface tension and keeps the alveoli from collapsing after they first expand after birth.

suture narrow band of connective tissue that divides the six non-united bones of a newborn's skull.

symmetry a balance in shape, size, and position from one side of the body to the other; a mirror image.

synovitis inflammation of a joint; most commonly in the hip in children.

T

tachypnea rapid respirations.

temper tantrums behaviors in children that spring from frustrations caused by their urge for independence; a violent display of temper. The child reacts with enthusiastic rebellion against the wishes of the caregiver.

temperament the combination of all of an individual's characteristics; the way the person thinks, behaves, and reacts.

teratogen from the Greek *terato*, meaning monster, and *genesis*, meaning birth; an agent or influence that causes a defect or disruption in the prenatal growth process. The effect of a teratogen depends on when it enters the fetal system and the stage of differentiation of the organs or organ systems at that time. Generally, the fetus is most vulnerable to teratogens during the first trimester.

term a newborn who is born between the beginning of week 38 and the end of week 41 of gestation.

tertiary prevention health-promoting activities that focus on rehabilitation and providing information to prevent further injury or illness.

tetralogy of Fallot a grouping of heart defects (tetralogy denotes four abnormal conditions): (1) pulmonary stenosis, (2) ventricular septal defect, (3) overriding aorta, and (4) right ventricular hypertrophy.

thanatologist person, sometimes a nurse, trained especially to work with the dying and their families.

therapeutic play play technique that may be used by play therapists, nurses, child-life specialists, and trained volunteers.

thermoneutral environment an environment in which heat is neither lost nor gained.

thermoregulation the process by which the body balances heat production with heat loss to maintain adequate body temperature.

thrush a fungal infection (caused by *Candida albicans*) in the oral cavity.

time out one part of the Universal Protocol developed to reduce the incidence of wrong site, wrong procedure, and wrong person surgery. Each member of the surgical team and the client stop right before the procedure to confirm agreement that the right procedure is being performed on the right client with documented informed consent.

tinea ringworm.

tissue perfusion circulation of blood through the capillaries carrying nutrients and oxygen to the cells.

tocolytic a substance that relaxes the uterine muscle.

tolerance in substance abuse, ability of body tissues to endure and adapt to continued or increased use of a substance.

tonsils two oval masses attached to the side walls of the back of the mouth between the anterior and posterior pillars (folds of mucous membranes at the sides of the passage from the mouth to the pharynx).

TORCH an acronym for a special group of infections that can be acquired during pregnancy and transmitted through the placenta to the fetus. The "T" stands for toxoplasmosis, the "O" for other infections (hepatitis B, syphilis, varicella, and herpes zoster), the "R" is for rubella, the "C" is for cytomegalovirus (CMV), and the "H" stands for herpes simplex virus (HSV).

total parenteral nutrition (TPN) the administration of dextrose, lipids, amino acids, electrolytes, vitamins, minerals, and trace elements into the circulatory system to meet the nutritional needs of the child whose needs cannot be met through the gastrointestinal tract.

tracheostomy surgical procedure in which an opening is made into the trachea and a tube is put in place to give the client a patent airway.

traction force applied to an extremity or other part of the body to maintain proper alignment and to facilitate healing of a fractured bone or dislocated joint.

transgender person born with male or female anatomy who has the internal sense that they are in the "wrong body" and who identifies as a person of the opposite sex.

transposition of the great arteries occurs when the aorta arises from the right ventricle instead of the left, and the pulmonary artery arises from the left ventricle instead of the right.

traumatic brain injury (TBI) head injury that affects the brain; can be mild, moderate, or severe in nature.

true pelvis the bony passageway through which the fetus must pass during delivery; the portion of the pelvis below the linea terminalis.

tympanic membrane sensor device used to determine the temperature of the tympanic membrane by rapidly sensing infrared radiation from the membrane. The tympanic thermometer offers the advantage of recording the temperature rapidly with little disturbance to the child.

U

unfinished business completing matters that will help ease the death of a loved one; saying the unsaid and doing the undone acts of love and caring that may seem difficult to express; recognizing time is limited and filling that time with the important issues that need to be addressed.

unilateral one side (e.g., in cleft lip, only one side of the lip is cleft).

unoccupied behavior daydreaming; fingering clothing or a toy without any apparent purpose.

urge-to-push method method of pushing during birth in which the woman bears down only when she feels the urge to do so using any technique that feels right for her.

urostomy a surgical opening created to help with the elimination of urine.

urticaria hives.

uterine atony inability of the uterus to contract effectively.

uterine subinvolution a condition in which the uterus returns to its prepregnancy shape and size at a rate that is slower than expected (usually the result of retained placental fragments or an infection).

uteroplacental insufficiency diminished or deficient blood flow to the uterus and placenta.

uterus (or womb) a hollow, pear-shaped, muscular structure located within the pelvic cavity between the bladder and the rectum.

uveitis an inflammation of the middle (vascular) tunic of the eye; includes the iris, ciliary body, and choroid.

V

vacuum extraction procedure used to assist delivery in which the birth attendant places a suction cup (usually a soft silicone cup) on the fetal head and applies suction.

vagina (or birth canal) a muscular tube that leads from the vulva to the uterus.

vaginal birth after cesarean (VBAC) delivery of infant vaginally when a previous delivery has been a cesarean birth.

vaginitis inflammation of the vagina.

variability fluctuations of the fetal heart rate (FHR) from the baseline rate.

variable deceleration a change in the FHR that may occur at any point during a contraction and has a jagged, erratic shape on the fetal monitor tracing.

vas deferens the muscular tube in which sperm begin their journey out of the man's body.

vasectomy male sterilization.

vasospasm spasm of the arteries.

venous thromboembolism the umbrella term for deep vein thrombosis (DVT) and pulmonary embolism.

ventricular septal defect abnormal opening in the septum of the heart between the ventricles; allows blood to pass directly from the left to the right side of the heart; the most common intracardiac defect.

ventriculoperitoneal shunting silicone tubing implanted into the cerebral ventricle passing under the skin to the peritoneal cavity, providing drainage for excessive cerebrospinal fluid. Excess tubing can be inserted to accommodate the child's growth.

vernix caseosa a white, cheese-like substance that covers the body of the fetus and protects the skin during fetal life; consists of sebum and desquamated epithelial cells.

very low birth weight (VLBW) newborns weighing <1,500 g.

viable able to live outside of the uterus (fetus).

vigorous pushing also called Valsalva pushing, a pushing technique during birth where the woman is told to take a deep breath, hold the breath, and push while counting to 10.

W

wellness nursing focus focus of nursing care that identifies the potential of an individual, family, or community to move to a higher level of wellness.

West nomogram graph with several scales arranged so that when two values are known, the third can be plotted by drawing a line with a straight edge; commonly used to calculate body surface area (BSA).

Wharton jelly a clear gelatinous substance that gives support to the cord and helps prevent compression of the cord, which could impair blood flow to the fetus.

wheezing high-pitched sound of expired air being pushed through narrowed or obstructed airways.

withdrawal symptoms in substance abuse, physical and psychological symptoms that occur when the drug is no longer being used.

Z

zygote (or conceptus) results when an ovum and a spermatozoon unite. The zygote has the full complement of 46 chromosomes, arranged in 23 pairs.

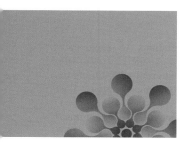

References and Selected Readings

Chapter 1

Centers for Disease Control and Prevention (CDC). (2021). Reproductive health: Pregnancy mortality surveillance system. https://www.cdc.gov/reproductivehealth/maternal-mortality/pregnancy-mortality-surveillance-system.htm?CDC_AA_refVal=https%3A%2F%2Fwww.cdc.gov%2Freproductivehealth%2Fmaternalinfanthealth%2Fpregnancy-mortality-surveillance-system.htm

Kochanek, K. D., Murphy, S. L., Xu, J., & Arias, E. (2019). Deaths: Final data for 2017. *National Vital Statistics Reports*, 68(9), 1–77. https://www.cdc.gov/nchs/data/nvsr/nvsr68/nvsr68_09-508.pdf

U.S. Department of Health & Human Services. (2020). *Office of disease prevention and health promotion*. Healthy People 2020. https://www.healthypeople.gov/2020/topics-objectives, Last updated October 8, 2020.

United States infant mortality rates from 1940 to 2017. (Redrawn from Kochanek, K. D., Murphy, S. L., Xu, J., & Arias, E. (2019). Deaths: Final data for 2017. *National Vital Statistics Reports*, 68(9), 1–77. https://www.cdc.gov/nchs/data/nvsr/nvsr68/nvsr68_09-508.pdf (This is citation for Fig. 1-4).

World Health Organization. (2019). *Maternal mortality*. https://www.who.int/news-room/fact-sheets/detail/maternal-mortality, Last updated September 19, 2019.

Xu, J., Murphy, S. L., Kochanek, K. D., & Arias, E. (2020). *Mortality on the United States, 2018*. National Center for Health Statistics. NCHS Data Brief No. 355, January 2020. https://www.cdc.gov/nchs/products/databriefs/db355.htm

Chapter 2

Betancourt, J. R., Green, A. R., & Carrillo, J. E. (2020). Cross-cultural care and communication. *UpToDate*. https://www.uptodate.com/contents/cross-cultural-care-and-communication, Last updated April 13, 2020.

McGinnis, S., Lee, E., Kirkland, K., Smith, C., Miranda-Julian, C., & Greene, R. (2019). Engaging at-risk fathers in home visiting services: Effects on program retention and father involvement. *Child and Adolescent Social Work Journal*, 36, 189–200. https://doi.org/10.1007/s10560-018-0562-4

Stapleton, S. (2019). Birth centers. *UpToDate*. https://www.uptodate.com/contents/birth-centers, Last updated June 25, 2019.

Chapter 3

Hiort, O. (2021). Typical sex development. *UpToDate*. https://www.uptodate.com/contents/typical-sex-development, Last updated January 19, 2021.

Matsumoto, A. M., & Anawalt, B. D. (2020). Male reproductive physiology. *UpToDate*. https://www.uptodate.com/contents/male-reproductive-physiology, Last updated June 28, 2020.

MedlinePlus, National Library of Medicine. (2015). *Male reproductive system*. https://medlineplus.gov/malereproductivesystem.html, Last updated August 19, 2015.

MedlinePlus, National Library of Medicine. (2018). *Female reproductive system*. https://medlineplus.gov/femalereproductivesystem.html, Last updated August 27, 2018.

MedlinePlus, National Library of Medicine. (2020). *Menstruation*. https://medlineplus.gov/menstruation.html, Last updated November 18, 2020.

Welt, C. K. (2019). Evaluation of the menstrual cycle and timing of ovulation. *UpToDate*. https://www.uptodate.com/contents/evaluation-of-the-menstrual-cycle-and-timing-of-ovulation, Last updated May 5, 2019.

Welt, C. K. (2021). Physiology of the normal menstrual cycle. *UpToDate*. https://www.uptodate.com/contents/physiology-of-the-normal-menstrual-cycle, Last updated January 11, 2021.

World Health Organization. (2020). *Female genital mutilation fact sheet*. http://www.who.int/mediacentre/factsheets/fs241/en/, Last updated February 3, 2020.

Chapter 4

American Cancer Society. (2020a). *About breast cancer*. https://www.cancer.org/content/dam/CRC/PDF/Public/8577.00.pdf, Last updated September 18, 2019.

American Cancer Society. (2020b). *American Cancer Society recommendations for the early detection of breast cancer*. https://www.cancer.org/cancer/breast-cancer/screening-tests-and-early-detection/american-cancer-society-recommendations-for-the-early-detection-of-breast-cancer.html, Last revised November 17, 2020.

American Cancer Society. (2020c). *Breast cancer early detection and diagnosis*. https://www.cancer.org/cancer/breast-cancer/screening-tests-and-early-detection.html

Center for Disease Control (CDC). (2020a). *Pelvic inflammatory disease (PID) - CDC fact sheet*. https://www.cdc.gov/std/pid/stdfact-pid-detailed.htm

CDC. (2020b). *Key findings: Folic acid fortification continues to prevent neural tube defect*. https://www.cdc.gov/ncbddd/folicacid/features/folicacid-prevents-ntds.html

CDC. (2020c). *Planning for pregnancy*. https://www.cdc.gov/preconception/planning.html, Last updated April 16, 2020.

CDC. (2020d). *Folic acid helps prevent neural tube defects*. National Center on Birth Defects and Developmental Disabilities, Centers for Disease Control and Prevention, Centers for Disease Control and Prevention. https://www.cdc.gov/ncbddd/folicacid/data.html, Last updated August 12, 2019.

Daniels, K., & Abma, J. C. (2018). *Current contraceptive status among women aged 15–49: United States, 2015–2017*. National Center for Health Statistics. NCHS Data Brief, No 327. https://www.cdc.gov/nchs/products/databriefs/db327.htm

Kaunitz, A. M. (2019). Hormonal contraception for suppression of menstruation. *UpToDate*. https://www.uptodate.com/contents/hormonal-contraception-for-suppression-of-menstruation, Last updated August 6, 2019.

National Cancer Institute. (2020a, April). *SEER cancer stat facts: Female breast cancer.* https://seer.cancer.gov/statfacts/html/breast.html

National Cancer Institute. (2020b, April). *SEER cancer stat facts: Cervical cancer.* https://seer.cancer.gov/statfacts/html/cervix.html

National Cancer Institute. (2020c). *HPV and Pap testing.* http://www.cancer.gov/types/cervical/pap-hpv-testing-fact-sheet#q4

Office on Women's Health. (2020). *Infertility.* https://www.womenshealth.gov/a-z-topics/infertility, Last updated April 1, 2019.

Sharp, H. T. (2019). An overview of endometrial ablation. *UpToDate.* https://www.uptodate.com/contents/an-overview-of-endometrial-ablation, Last updated October 17, 2019.

Smith, R. P., & Kaunitz, A. M. (2020). Dysmenorrhea in adult women: Clinical features and diagnosis. *UpToDate.* https://www.uptodate.com/contents/dysmenorrhea-in-adult-women-clinical-features-and-diagnosis, Last updated January 13, 2020.

Stewart, E. A., & Laughlin-Tommaso, S. K. (2020). Uterine fibroids (leiomyomas): Epidemiology, clinical features, diagnosis, and natural history. *UpToDate.* https://www.uptodate.com/contents/uterine-fibroids-leiomyomas-epidemiology-clinical-features-diagnosis-and-natural-history, Last updated November 18, 2020.

U.S. Department of Health & Human Services. (2020). *Office of disease prevention and health promotion.* Healthy People 2020. http://www.healthypeople.gov/2020/topics-objectives, Last updated October 8, 2020.

Welt, C. K., & Barbieri, R. L. (2020). Evaluation and management of secondary amenorrhea. *UpToDate.* https://www.uptodate.com/contents/evaluation-and-management-of-secondary-amenorrhea, Last updated June 28, 2020.

Yonkers, K. A., & Casper, R. F. (2019). Epidemiology and pathogenesis of premenstrual syndrome and premenstrual dysphoric disorder. *UpToDate.* https://www.uptodate.com/contents/epidemiology-and-pathogenesis-of-premenstrual-syndrome-and-premenstrual-dysphoric-disorder, Last updated October 22, 2019.

Chapter 5

Bacino, C. A. (2019). Birth defects: Causes. *UpToDate.* https://www.uptodate.com/contents/birth-defects-causes, Last updated June 11, 2019.

Fletcher, G. E. (2019). Multiple births: Epidemiology. In Nimavat, D. J. (Ed.), *eMedicine.* Medscape. http://emedicine.medscape.com/article/977234-overview#a6, Updated December 20, 2019.

Resnik, R., & Mari, G. (2020). Fetal growth restriction: Evaluation and management. *UpToDate.* https://www.uptodate.com/contents/fetal-growth-restriction-evaluation-and-management, Last updated September 2, 2020.

Tulandi, T. (2020). Ectopic pregnancy: Epidemiology, risk factors, and anatomic sites. *UpToDate.* https://www.uptodate.com/contents/ectopic-pregnancy-epidemiology-risk-factors-and-anatomic-sites, Last updated October 15, 2020.

Chapter 6

August, P., & Jeyabala, A. (2021). Preeclampsia: Prevention. *UpToDate.* https://www.uptodate.com/contents/preeclampsia-prevention, Last updated January 6, 2021.

Bauer, K. A. (2020). Maternal adaptations to pregnancy: Hematologic changes. *UpToDate.* https://www.uptodate.com/contents/maternal-adaptations-to-pregnancy-hematologic-changes, Last updated August 12, 2020.

Foley, M. R. (2020). Maternal adaptations to pregnancy: Cardiovascular and hemodynamic changes. *UpToDate.* https://www.uptodate.com/contents/maternal-adaptations-to-pregnancy-cardiovascular-and-hemodynamic-changes, Last updated February 25, 2020.

Garner, C. D. (2020). Nutrition in pregnancy. *UpToDate.* https://www.uptodate.com/contents/nutrition-in-pregnancy, Last updated October 6, 2020.

Sebastiani, G., Barbero, A. H., Borrás-Novell, C., Casanova, M. A., Aldecoa-Bilbao, V., Andreu-Fernández, V., Tutusaus, M. P., Martínez, S. F., Roig, M. D. G, & García-Algar, O. (2019). The effects of vegetarian and vegan diet during pregnancy on the health of mothers and offspring. *Nutrients, 11*(3), 557. https://doi.org/10.3390/nu11030557. PMCID: PMC6470702. PMID: 30845641.

Thadhani, R. I., & Maynard, S. E. (2020). Maternal adaptations to pregnancy: Renal and urinary tract physiology. *UpToDate.* https://www.uptodate.com/contents/maternal-adaptations-to-pregnancy-renal-and-urinary-tract-physiology, Last updated April 29, 2020.

U.S. Food and Drug Administration. (2020). *Advice about eating fish for women who are or might become pregnant, breastfeeding mothers, and young children.* https://www.fda.gov/food/consumers/advice-about-eating-fish

United States Department of Agriculture. https://www.myplate.gov

Weinberger, S. E. (2019). Maternal adaptations to pregnancy: Physiologic respiratory changes and dyspnea. *UpToDate.* https://www.uptodate.com/contents/maternal-adaptations-to-pregnancy-physiologic-respiratory-changes-and-dyspnea, Last updated March 14, 2019.

Young, S., & Cox, J. T. (2019). Pica in pregnancy. *UpToDate.* https://www.uptodate.com/contents/pica-in-pregnancy, Last updated February 19, 2019.

Chapter 7

Artal, R. (2021). Exercise during pregnancy and the postpartum period. *UpToDate.* https://www.uptodate.com/contents/exercise-during-pregnancy-and-the-postpartum-period, Last updated January 5, 2021.

Bermas, B. L. (2020). Maternal adaptations to pregnancy: Musculoskeletal changes and pain. *UpToDate.* https://www.uptodate.com/contents/maternal-adaptations-to-pregnancy-musculoskeletal-changes-and-pain, Last updated April 1, 2020.

Chang, G. (2020). Alcohol intake and pregnancy. *UpToDate.* https://www.uptodate.com/contents/alcohol-intake-and-pregnancy, Last updated September 29, 2020.

Chang, G. (2021). Substance use during pregnancy: Overview of selected drugs. *UpToDate.* https://www.uptodate.com/contents/substance-use-during-pregnancy-overview-of-selected-drugs, Last updated January 25, 2021.

Dukhovny, S., & Wilkins-Haug, L. (2021). Open neural tube defects: Risk factors, prenatal screening and diagnosis, and pregnancy management. *UpToDate.* https://www.uptodate.com/contents/open-neural-tube-defects-risk-factors-prenatal-screening-and-diagnosis-and-pregnancy-management, Last updated January 21, 2021.

Durnwald, C. (2020). Diabetes mellitus in pregnancy: Screening and diagnosis. *UpToDate.* https://www.uptodate.com/contents/diabetes-mellitus-in-pregnancy-screening-and-diagnosis?search=glucose%20tolerance%20test&source=search_result&selectedTitle=1~120&usage_type=default&display_rank=1, Last updated December 9, 2020.

Ghidini, A. (2019). Diagnostic amniocentesis. *UpToDate*. https://www.uptodate.com/contents/diagnostic-amniocentesis, Last updated October 10, 2019.

Ghidini, A. (2021). Chorionic villus sampling. *UpToDate*. https://www.uptodate.com/contents/chorionic-villus-sampling, Last updated January 20, 2021.

Lockwood, C. J., & Magriples, U. (2020). Prenatal care: Initial assessment. *UpToDate*. https://www.uptodate.com/contents/prenatal-care-initial-assessment?search=initial%20prenatal%20assessment&source=search_result&selectedTitle=1~150&usage_type=default&display_rank=1#H1, Last updated December 9, 2020.

Mackenzie, A. P., Stephenson, C. D., & Funai, E. F. (2020). Prenatal assessment of gestational age, date of delivery, and fetal weight. *UpToDate*. https://www.uptodate.com/contents/prenatal-assessment-of-gestational-age-date-of-delivery-and-fetal-weight?search=prenatal%20assessment%20of%20gestational%20age&source=search_result&selectedTitle=1~150&usage_type=default&display_rank=1, Last updated July 17, 2020.

Manning, F. A. (2019). Biophysical profile test for antepartum fetal assessment. *UpToDate*. https://www.uptodate.com/contents/biophysical-profile-test-for-antepartum-fetal-assessment, Last updated December 30, 2019.

March of Dimes. (2020a). *Caffeine in pregnancy*. http://www.marchofdimes.com/pregnancy/caffeine-in-pregnancy.aspx

March of Dimes. (2020b). *Marijuana and pregnancy*. https://www.marchofdimes.org/pregnancy/marijuana.aspx

Messerlian, G. M., & Palomaki, G. E. (2020). Down syndrome: Overview of prenatal screening. *UpToDate*. https://www.uptodate.com/contents/down-syndrome-overview-of-prenatal-screening?search=down%20syndrome%20prenatal%20screening&source=search_result&selectedTitle=1~150&usage_type=default&display_rank=1, Last updated September 14, 2020.

Miller, D. A. (2019). Nonstress test and contraction stress test. *UpToDate*. https://www.uptodate.com/contents/nonstress-test-and-contraction-stress-test, Last updated May 23, 2019.

Rodriguez, D. (2020). Cigarette and tobacco products in pregnancy: Impact on pregnancy and the neonate. *UpToDate*. https://www.uptodate.com/contents/cigarette-and-tobacco-products-in-pregnancy-impact-on-pregnancy-and-the-neonate, Last updated October 19, 2020.

Shipp, T. D. (2021). Overview of ultrasound examination in obstetrics and gynecology. *UpToDate*. https://www.uptodate.com/contents/overview-of-ultrasound-examination-in-obstetrics-and-gynecology, Last updated January 11, 2021.

Smith, J. A., Fox, K. A., & Clark, S. M. (2020). Nausea and vomiting of pregnancy: Treatment and outcome. *UpToDate*. https://www.uptodate.com/contents/nausea-and-vomiting-of-pregnancy-treatment-and-outcome, Last updated October 21, 2020.

U.S. Department of Health & Human Services. (2020). *Office of disease prevention and health promotion*. Healthy People 2020. https://www.healthypeople.gov/2020/topics-objectives, Last updated October 8, 2020.

Chapter 8

Cunningham, F. G., Leveno, K. J., Bloom, S. L., Spong, C. Y., Dashe, J. S., Hoffman, B. L., & Casey, B. M. (2018). *Williams obstetrics* (25th ed.). McGraw-Hill Education.

Gray, C. J., & Shanahan, M. M. (2020). *Breech presentation*. StatPearls; National Center for Biotechnology Information; U.S.

National Library of Medicine. https://www.ncbi.nlm.nih.gov/books/NBK448063/, Last updated August 11, 2020.

King, T. L., Brucker, M. C., Osborne, K., & Jevitt, C. M. (2019). *Varney's midwifery* (6th ed.). Jones & Barlett Learning

Norwitz, E. R. (2019). Physiology of parturition. *UpToDate*. https://www.uptodate.com/contents/physiology-of-parturition, Last updated April 16, 2019.

Chapter 9

Caughey, A. B. (2019). Nonpharmacological approaches to management of labor pain. *UpToDate*. https://www.uptodate.com/contents/nonpharmacologic-approaches-to-management-of-labor-pain, Last updated February 5, 2019.

Grant, G. J. (2020a). Adverse effects of neuraxial analgesia and anesthesia for obstetrics. *UpToDate*. http://www.uptodate.com/contents/adverse-effects-of-neuraxial-analgesia-and-anesthesia-for-obstetrics

Grant, G. J. (2020b). Pharmacologic management of pain during labor and delivery. *UpToDate*. https://www.uptodate.com/contents/pharmacologic-management-of-pain-during-labor-and-delivery

Chapter 10

Cunningham, F. G., Leveno, K. J., Bloom, S. L., Spong, C. Y., Dashe, J. S., Hoffman, B. L., & Casey, B. M. (2018). *Williams obstetrics* (25th ed.). McGraw-Hill Education.

Funai, E. F., & Norwitz, E. R. (2021). Management of normal labor and delivery. *UpToDate*. https://www.uptodate.com/contents/management-of-normal-labor-and-delivery, Last updated January 7, 2021.

Lee, S. M., Lee, J., Seong, H. S., Lee, S. E., Park, J. S., Romero, R., & Yoon, B. H. (2009). The clinical significance of a positive Amnisure Test™ in women with term labor with intact membranes. *Journal of Maternal and Fetal Neonatal Medicine*, 22(4), 305–310. https://www.ncbi.nlm.nih.gov/pmc/articles/PMC2744034/

Miller, D. A. (2020). Intrapartum fetal heart rate monitoring: Overview. *UpToDate*. https://www.uptodate.com/contents/intrapartum-fetal-heart-rate-monitoring-overview, Last updated May 1, 2020.

Stapleton, S. (2019). Birth centers. *UpToDate*. https://www.uptodate.com/contents/birth-centers, Last updated June 25, 2019.

Stuebe, A., & Barbieri, R. L. (2020). Continuous labor support by a doula. *UpToDate*. https://www.uptodate.com/contents/continuous-labor-support-by-a-doula, Last updated December 16, 2020.

Chapter 11

ACOG. (2017). Practice Bulletin No. 184: Vaginal birth after cesarean delivery. *Obstetrics and Gynecology*, 130(5), e217–e233. https://vbacfacts.com/wp-content/uploads/2018/05/ACOG-PB184-VBAC-2017.pdf

American College of Obstetricians and Gynecologists [ACOG]. (2019). ACOG Committee Opinion No. 766: Approaches to limit intervention during labor and birth. *Obstetrics and Gynecology*, 133(2), e164–e173. https://www.acog.org/clinical/clinical-guidance/committee-opinion/articles/2019/02/approaches-to-limit-intervention-during-labor-and-birth

Berghella, V. (2020a). Cesarean delivery: Surgical technique. *UpToDate*. https://www.uptodate.com/contents/cesarean-delivery-surgical-technique, Last updated May 1, 2020.

Berghella, V. (2020b). Cesarean delivery: Preoperative planning and patient preparation. *UpToDate*. https://www.uptodate.com/

contents/cesarean-delivery-preoperative-planning-and-patient-preparation, Last updated September 15, 2020.

Berghella, V. (2020c). Cesarean delivery: Postoperative issues. *UpToDate*. https://www.uptodate.com/contents/cesarean-delivery-postoperative-issues

Berkowitz, L. R., & Foust-Wright, C. E. (2020). Approach to episiotomy. *UpToDate*. https://www.uptodate.com/contents/approach-to episiotomy, Last updated April 1, 2020.

Caughey, A. B. (2018). Vaginal birth after cesarean delivery. In Smith, C. V. (Ed.), *eMedicine*. Medscape. https://emedicine.medscape.com/article/272187-overview, Last updated May 11, 2018.

Chodankar, R., Sood, A., & Gupta, J. (2017). An overview of the past, current and future trends for cervical ripening in induction of labour. *The Obstetrician & Gynaecologist*, 19(3), 219–226. https://obgyn.onlinelibrary.wiley.com/doi/10.1111/tog.12395

Grobman, W. (2020a). Induction of labor with oxytocin. *UpToDate*.https://www.uptodate.com/contents/induction-of-labor-with-oxytocin, Last updated August 20, 2020.

Grobman, W. (2020b). Techniques for ripening the unfavorable cervix prior to induction. *UpToDate*. https://www.uptodate.com/contents/techniques-for-ripening-the-unfavorable-cervix-prior-to-induction, Last updated April 27, 2020.

Landon, M. B., & Frey, H. (2020). Uterine rupture: After previous cesarean delivery. *UpToDate*. https://www.uptodate.com/contents/uterine-rupture-after-previous-cesarean-delivery, Last updated July 17, 2020.

Martin et al., 2019 Martin, J. A., Hamilton, B. E., Osterman, M. J. K., & Driscoll, A. K. (2019). Births: Final data for 2018. *National Vital Statistics Reports*, 68(13), 1–47. https://www.cdc.gov/nchs/data/nvsr/nvsr68/nvsr68_13-508.pdf

Wegner, E. K., & Bernstein, I. M. (2020). Operative vaginal delivery. *UpToDate*. https://www.uptodate.com/contents/operative-vaginal-delivery, Last updated August 25, 2020.

Chapter 12

Berens, P. (2020). Overview of the postpartum period: Normal physiology and routine maternal care. *UpToDate*. https://www.uptodate.com/contents/overview-of-the-postpartum-period-normal-physiology-and-routine-maternal-care?search=postpartum%20care&source=search_result&selectedTitle=1~118&usage_type=default&display_rank=1, Last updated May 29, 2020.

Berghella, V. (2020). Cesarean delivery: Postoperative issues. *UpToDate*. https://www.uptodate.com/contents/cesarean-delivery-postoperative-issues?search=Cesarean%20Delivery:%20Postoperative%20issues&source=search_result&selectedTitle=1~150&usage_type=default&display_rank=1, Last updated September 28, 2020.

Fowles, E. R., & Horowitz, J. A. (2006). Clinical assessment of mothering during infancy. *Journal of Obstetric, Gynecologic & Neonatal Nursing*, 35(5), 662–670.

Grant, G. J. (2020a). Adverse effects of neuraxial analgesia and anesthesia for obstetrics. *UpToDate*. https://www.uptodate.com/contents/adverse-effects-of-neuraxial-analgesia-and-anesthesia-for-obstetrics?search=Adverse%20effects%20of%20neuraxial%20analgesia%20and%20anesthesia%20for%20obstetrics&source=search_result&selectedTitle=1~150&usage_type=default&display_rank=1, Last updated February 28, 2020.

Grant, G. J. (2020b). Pharmacologic management of pain during labor and delivery. *UpToDate*. https://www.uptodate.com/contents/pharmacologic-management-of-pain-during-labor-and-delivery?search=anesthesia%20and%20analgesia%20in%20labor&source=search_result&selectedTitle=1~150&usage_type=default&display_rank=1, Last updated October 14, 2020.

Hockenberry, M. J., & Wilson, D. (2018). *Wong's nursing care of infants and children* (11th ed.). Mosby Elsevier.

Kendall-Tackett, K. (2017). *How cultures protect the new mother.* Praeclarus Press. https://womenshealthtoday.blog/2017/07/30/how-cultures-protect-the-new-mother/

Kim-Godwin, Y. S. (2003). Postpartum beliefs and practices among non-western cultures. *MCN, The American Journal of Maternal/Child Nursing*, 28(2), 74–78. https://journals.lww.com/mcnjournal/Abstract/2003/03000/Postpartum_Beliefs_and_Practices_Among_Non_Western.6.aspx

Mercer, R. T. (2006). Nursing support of the process of becoming a mother. *Journal of Obstetric, Gynecologic & Neonatal Nursing*, 35(5), 649–651.

Sonalkar, S., & Mody, S. K. (2020). Postpartum contraception: Counseling and methods. *UpToDate*. https://www.uptodate.com/contents/postpartum-contraception-counseling-and-methods, Last updated June 24, 2020.

Viguera, A. (2019). Postpartum blues. *UpToDate*. https://www.uptodate.com/contents/postpartum-blues?search=postpartum%20blues&source=search_result&selectedTitle=1~14&usage_type=default&display_rank=1, Last updated January 16, 2019.

Viguera, A. (2020). Postpartum unipolar major depression: Epidemiology, clinical features, assessment, and diagnosis. *UpToDate*. https://www.uptodate.com/contents/postpartum-unipolar-major-depression-epidemiology-clinical-features-assessment-and-diagnosis?search=postpartum%20depression&source=search_result&selectedTitle=1~120&usage_type=default&display_rank=1, Last updated October 13, 2020.

Chapter 13

American Academy of Pediatrics. (2020). States of consciousness in newborns. https://www.healthychildren.org/English/ages-stages/baby/Pages/States-of-Consciousness-in-Newborns.aspx

Boston Children's Hospital, Harvard Medical School. (2021). *The Newborn Behavioral Observations (NBO) system™*. https://www.childrenshospital.org/Research/Centers-Departmental-Programs/brazelton-institute/nbo

Hockenberry, M. J., & Wilson, D. (2018). *Wong's nursing care of infants and children* (11th ed.). Mosby Elsevier.

Karlsen, K. (2013). *The S.T.A.B.L.E. program: Post resuscitation/Pre-transport stabilization care of sick infants guidelines for neonatal healthcare providers learner manual* (6th ed.). S.T.A.B.L.E., Inc.

Ricci, S. S. (2017). *Essentials of maternity, newborn, and women's health nursing* (4th ed.). Wolters Kluwer.

Rozance, P. J. (2020). Management and outcome of neonatal hypoglycemia. *UpToDate*. https://www.uptodate.com/contents/management-and-outcome-of-neonatal-hypoglycemia#:~:text=For%20at%2Drisk%20neonates%20without,after%2048%20hours%20of%20life, Last updated February 13, 2020.

Chapter 14

American Academy of Pediatrics. (2012). Task force on circumcision. *Pediatrics*. http://pediatrics.aappublications.org/content/pediatrics/130/3/585.full.pdf

American Academy of Pediatrics. (2016). SIDS and other sleep-related infant deaths: Updated 2016 recommendations for a safe infant sleeping environment pediatrics. *Pediatrics*, 138(5), e20162938. https://doi.org/10.1542/peds.2016-2938; https://pediatrics.aappublications.org/content/138/5/e20162938

American Academy of Pediatrics and American Heart Association. (2016). *Textbook of neonatal resuscitation* (7th ed.).

National Center for Missing and Exploited Children. (2021). Infant abductions. https://www.missingkids.org/theissues/infantabductions, Last updated December 1, 2020.

National Institute of Health. (2020). Newborn screening. https://www.nichd.nih.gov/health/topics/newborn

Chapter 15

Center for Disease Control and Prevention (CDC). (2020). *Breastfeeding Report Card, 2020*. https://www.cdc.gov/breastfeeding/data/reportcard.htm

CDC. (2020). Proper storage and preparation of breastmilk. https://www.cdc.gov/breastfeeding/recommendations/handling_breastmilk.htm#:~:text=Freshly%20expressed%20or%20pumped%20milk,to%2012%20months%20is%20acceptable

Eidelman, A. I., & Schanler, R. J. (2012). American academy of pediatrics policy statement: Breastfeeding and the use of human milk. *Pediatrics*, 129(3), e827–e841. http://pediatrics.aappublications.org/content/129/3/e827.full

Hockenberry, M. J., & Wilson, D. (2018). *Wong's nursing care of infants and children* (11th ed.). Mosby Elsevier.

Meek, J. Y. (2020). Infant benefits of breastfeeding. *UpToDate*. https://www.uptodate.com/contents/infant-benefits-of-breastfeeding, Last updated November 19, 2020.

Perez-Escamilla, R., & Segura-Perez, S. (2019). Maternal and economic benefits of breastfeeding. *UpToDate*. https://www.uptodate.com/contents/maternal-and-economic-benefits-of-breastfeeding?search=maternal%20benefit%20of%20breastfeeding&source=search_result&selectedTitle=1~150&usage_type=default&display_rank=1, Last updated November 26, 2019.

Ricci, S. S. (2017). *Essentials of maternity, newborn, and women's health nursing* (4th ed.). Wolters Kluwer.

Spencer, J. (2020). Common problems of breastfeeding and weaning. *UpToDate*. https://www.uptodate.com/contents/common-problems-of-breastfeeding-and-weaning, Last updated June 18, 2020.

U.S. Department of Health & Human Services. (2020). *Office of disease prevention and health promotion*. Healthy People 2020. http://www.healthypeople.gov/2020/topics-objectives, Last updated October 8, 2020.

Chapter 16

Bauer, K. A. (2020). Maternal adaptations to pregnancy: Hematologic changes. *UpToDate*. https://www.uptodate.com/contents/maternal-adaptations-to-pregnancy-hematologic-changes, Last updated August 12, 2020.

Center for Disease Control and Prevention (CDC). (2020). Cytomegalovirus (CMV) and Congenital CMV Infection. http://www.cdc.gov/cmv/, Last updated August 18, 2020.

Center for Disease Control. (2020). Pregnancy Mortality Surveillance System. http://www.cdc.gov/reproductivehealth/maternalinfanthealth/pmss.html, Last updated November 25, 2020.

Center for Disease Control. (2020). STDs and HIV-CDC fact sheet. http://www.cdc.gov/std/hiv/stdfact-std-hiv-detailed.htm, Last updated March 30, 2020.

CDC. (2019). Pregnancy-Related Deaths: Data from 14 U.S. Maternal Mortality Review Committees, 2008-2017. https://www.cdc.gov/reproductivehealth/maternal-mortality/erase-mm/mmr-data-brief.html

Chacko, M. R. (2020). Pregnancy in adolescents. *UpToDate*. https://www.uptodate.com/contents/pregnancy-in-adolescents, Last updated December 3, 2020.

Cunningham, F. G., Leveno, K. J., Bloom, S. L., Spong, C. Y., Dashe, J. S., Hoffman, B. L., & Casey, B. M. (2018). *Williams obstetrics* (25th ed.). McGraw-Hill Education.

DeCara, J. M., Lang, R. M., & Foley, M. R. (2018). Management of heart failure in pregnancy. *UpToDate*. https://www.uptodate.com/contents/management-of-heart-failure-during-pregnancy, Last updated December 5, 2018.

Demmler-Harrison, G. J. (2020). Congenital cytomegalovirus infection: Clinical features and diagnosis. *UpToDate*. https://www.uptodate.com/contents/congenital-cytomegalovirus-infection-clinical-features-and-diagnosis, Last updated January 8, 2020.

Dobson, S. R. (2019). Congenital syphilis: Clinical features and diagnosis. *UpToDate*. https://www.uptodate.com/contents/congenital-syphilis-clinical-features-and-diagnosis, Last updated January 29, 2019.

Erikson, E. H. (1963). *Childhood and society* (2nd ed.). Norton.

Fretts, R. C. (2019). Management of pregnancy in women of advanced age. *UpToDate*. https://www.uptodate.com/contents/management-of-pregnancy-in-women-of-advanced-age, Last updated October 28, 2019.

Hammerschlag, M. R. (2018). Chlamydia trachomatis infections in the newborn. *UpToDate*. https://www.uptodate.com/contents/chlamydia-trachomatis-infections-in-the-newborn, Last updated November 15, 2018.

Hockenberry, M. J., & Wilson, D. (2018). *Wong's nursing care of infants and children* (11th ed.). Mosby Elsevier.

Iftikhar, S. F., & Biswa, M. (2020). Cardiac disease in pregnancy. https://www.ncbi.nlm.nih.gov/books/NBK537261, Last updated July 13, 2020.

Martin, J. A., Hamilton, B. E., Osterman, M. J. K., & Driscoll, A. K. (2019). Births: Final data for 2018. *National Vital Statistics Reports*, 68(13), 1–47. https://www.cdc.gov/nchs/data/nvsr/nvsr68/nvsr68_13-508.pdf

Moore, T. R. (2020). Diabetes mellitus and pregnancy. In Griffing, G. T. (Ed.), *eMedicine*. Medscape. http://emedicine.medscape.com/article/127547-overview, Last updated April 29, 2020.

Pennell, P. B., & McElrath, T. (2020). Management of epilepsy during preconception, pregnancy, and the postpartum period. *UpToDate*. https://www.uptodate.com/contents/management-of-epilepsy-during-preconception-pregnancy-and-the-postpartum-period, Last updated July 21, 2020.

Price, G. A., & Bash, M. C. (2019). Epidemiology and pathogenesis of *Neisseria gonorrhoeae* infection. *UpToDate*. https://www.uptodate.com/contents/epidemiology-and-pathogenesis-of-neisseria-gonorrhoeae-infection, Last updated October 10, 2019.

Ricci, S. S. (2017). *Essentials of maternity, newborn, and women's health nursing* (4th ed.). Wolters Kluwer.

Riley, L. E. (2019a). Rubella in pregnancy. *UpToDate*. https://www.uptodate.com/contents/rubella-in-pregnancy, Last updated October 24, 2019.

Riley, L. E. (2019b). Varicella-zoster virus infection in pregnancy. *UpToDate*. https://www.uptodate.com/contents/varicella-zoster-virus-infection-in-pregnancy, Last updated August 29, 2019.

Riley, L. E., & Wald, A. (2020). Genital herpes simplex virus infection and pregnancy. *UpToDate*. https://www.uptodate.com/

contents/genital-herpes-simplex-virus-infection-and-pregnancy, Last updated June 10, 2020.

Speer, M. E. (2019). Varicella-zoster infection in the newborn. *UpToDate.* https://www.uptodate.com/contents/varicella-zoster-infection-in-the-newborn, Last updated November 14, 2019.

Vichinsky, E. P. (2020). Sickle cell trait. *UpToDate.* https://www.uptodate.com/contents/sickle-cell-trait, Last updated December 2, 2020.

Waksmonski, C. A., & Foley, M. R.(2020). Pregnancy in women with congenital heart disease: General principles. *UpToDate.* https://www.uptodate.com/contents/pregnancy-in-women-with-congenital-heart-disease-general-principles, Last updated April 8, 2020.

Weil, A. (2020). Intimate partner violence: Diagnosis and screening. *UpToDate.* https://www.uptodate.com/contents/intimate-partner-violence-diagnosis-and-screening, Last updated September 28, 2020.

Weinberger, S. E., & Schatz, M. (2020). Asthma in pregnancy: Clinical course and physiologic changes. *UpToDate.* https://www.uptodate.com/contents/asthma-in-pregnancy-clinical-course-and-physiologic-changes, Last updated March 17, 2020.

Workowski, K. A., & Bolan, G. A. (2015). Sexually transmitted diseases treatment guidelines, 2015. *MMWR Recommendations and Reports,* 64(RR-03), 1–137. https://www.ncbi.nlm.nih.gov/pmc/articles/PMC5885289/

Chapter 17

Ananth, C. V., & Kinzler, W. L. (2020). Placental abruption: Clinical features and diagnosis. *UpToDate.* https://www.uptodate.com/contents/placental-abruption-pathophysiology-clinical-features-diagnosis-and-consequences, Last updated September 30, 2020.

August, P., & Jeyabalan, A. (2021). Preeclampsia: Prevention. *UpToDate.* https://www.uptodate.com/contents/preeclampsia-prevention, Last updated January 6, 2021.

August, P., & Sibai, B. M. (2021). Preeclampsia: Clinical features and diagnosis. *UpToDate.* https://www.uptodate.com/contents/preeclampsia-clinical-features-and-diagnosis, Last updated January 21, 2021.

Bakker, R. (2018). Placenta previa. In Smith, C. V. & Pierce, J. G. (Eds.), *eMedicine.* Medscape. http://emedicine.medscape.com/article/262063-overview, Updated January 8, 2018.

Berkowitz, R. S., & Horowitz, N. S. (2020). Hydatidiform mole: Epidemiology, clinical features, and diagnosis. *UpToDate.* https://www.uptodate.com/contents/hydatidiform-mole-epidemiology-clinical-features-and-diagnosis, Last updated December 16, 2020.

Chasen, S. T., & Chervenak, F. A. (2020). Twin pregnancy: Prenatal issues. *UpToDate.* https://www.uptodate.com/contents/twin-pregnancy-prenatal-issues, Last updated October 20, 2020.

Cunningham, F. G., Leveno, K. J., Bloom, S. L., Spong, C. Y., Dashe, J. S., Hoffman, B. L., & Casey, B. M. (2018). *Williams obstetrics* (25th ed.). McGraw-Hill Education.

Deering, S. H. (2018). Abruptio placenta. In Smith, C. V., Talavera, F., & Pierce, J. G. (Eds.), *eMedicine.* Medscape. http://emedicine.medscape.com/article/252810-overview, Last updated November 30, 2018.

Fletcher, G. E. (2019). Multiple births. In Nimavat, D. J. (Ed.), *eMedicine.* Medscape. http://emedicine.medscape.com/article/977234-overview#a6, Last updated December 20, 2019.

Hockenberry, M. J., & Wilson, D. (2018). *Wong's nursing care of infants and children* (11th ed.). Mosby Elsevier.

Lockwood, C. J., & Russo-Stieglitz, K. (2019). Placenta previa: Epidemiology, clinical features, diagnosis, morbidity and mortality. *UpToDate.* https://www.uptodate.com/contents/placenta-previa-epidemiology-clinical-features-diagnosis-morbidity-and-mortality, Last updated July 1, 2019.

Moise, K. J. (2020). RhD alloimmunization: Prevention in pregnant and postpartum patients. *UpToDate.* https://www.uptodate.com/contents/rhd-alloimmunization-prevention-in-pregnant-and-postpartum-patients, Last updated December 16, 2020.

Moore, L. E. (2018). Hydatidiform mole. In Huh, W. K., Talavera, F., & Barnes, A. D. (Eds.), *eMedicine.* Medscape. http://emedicine.medscape.com/article/254657-overview, Updated February 16, 2018.

Ogunyemi, D. A. (2017). Hyperemesis gravidarum. In Isaacs, C., Talavera, F., & Legro, R. S. (Eds.), *eMedicine.* Medscape. http://emedicine.medscape.com/article/254751-overview#a2, Last updated January 4, 2017.

Prager, S., Micks, E., & Dalton, V. K. (2021). Pregnancy loss (miscarriage): Risk factors, etiology, clinical manifestations, and diagnostic evaluation. *UpToDate.* https://www.uptodate.com/contents/pregnancy-loss-miscarriage-risk-factors-etiology-clinical-manifestations-and-diagnostic-evaluation, Last updated January 25, 2021.

Ricci, S. S. (2017). *Essentials of maternity, newborn, and women's health nursing* (4th ed.). Wolters Kluwer.

Sibai, B. M. (2020). HELLP syndrome (hemolysis, elevated liver enzymes, and low platelets). *UpToDate.* https://www.uptodate.com/contents/hellp-syndrome-hemolysis-elevated-liver-enzymes-and-low-platelets, Last updated August 25, 2020.

Smith, J. A., Fox, K. A., & Clark, S. M. (2020). Nausea and vomiting of pregnancy: Treatment and outcome. *UpToDate.* https://www.uptodate.com/contents/nausea-and-vomiting-of-pregnancy-treatment-and-outcome, Last updated October 21, 2020.

Tulandi, T. (2020). Ectopic pregnancy: Clinical manifestations and diagnosis. *UpToDate.* https://www.uptodate.com/contents/ectopic-pregnancy-clinical-manifestations-and-diagnosis, Last updated November 2, 2020.

Chapter 18

Argani, C. H., & Satin, A. J. (2020). Occiput posterior position. *UpToDate.* https://www.uptodate.com/contents/occiput-posterior-position, Last updated May 27, 2020.

Baldisseri, M. R. (2020). Amniotic fluid embolism. *UpToDate.* https://www.uptodate.com/contents/amniotic-fluid-embolism, Last updated April 2, 2020.

Center for Disease Control and Prevention. (2020). *Preterm birth.* http://www.cdc.gov/reproductivehealth/MaternalInfantHealth/PretermBirth.htm, Last updated October 30, 2020.

Cunningham, F. G., Leveno, K. J., Bloom, S. L., Spong, C. Y., Dashe, J. S., Hoffman, B. L., & Casey, B. M. (2018). *Williams obstetrics* (25th ed.). McGraw-Hill Education.

Duff, P. (2020). Preterm prelabor rupture of membranes: Clinical manifestations and diagnosis. *UpToDate.* https://www.uptodate.com/contents/preterm-prelabor-rupture-of-membranes-clinical-manifestations-and-diagnosis, Last updated May 29, 2020.

Goldfarb, I. T. (2020). Amnioinfusion. *UpToDate.* https://www.uptodate.com/contents/amnioinfusion, Last updated August 25, 2020.

Hockenberry, M. J., & Wilson, D. (2018). *Wong's nursing care of infants and children* (11th ed.). Mosby Elsevier.

Hofmeyr, G. J. (2019). Overview of breech presentation. *UpToDate.* https://www.uptodate.com/contents/overview-of-breech-presentation, Last updated December 16, 2019.

Hofmeyr, G. J. (2021a). Delivery of the singleton fetus in breech presentation. *UpToDate*. https://www.uptodate.com/contents/delivery-of-the-singleton-fetus-in-breech-presentation, Last updated January 7, 2021.

Hofmeyr, G. J. (2021b). External cephalic version. *UpToDate*. https://www.uptodate.com, Last updated January 22, 2021.

Jazayeri, A. (2018a). Premature rupture of membranes. In Talavera, F. & Smith, C. V., (Eds.), *eMedicine*. Medscape. http://emedicine.medscape.com/article/261137-overview#a2, Last updated October 5, 2018.

Jazayeri, A. (2018b). PPROM in the second trimester. In Talavera, F. & Smith, C. V., (Eds.), *eMedicine*. Medscape. http://emedicine.medscape.com/article/261137-overview#a5, Last updated October 5, 2018.

Landon, M. B., & Frey, H. (2020). Uterine rupture: After previous cesarean delivery. *UpToDate*. https://uptodate.com/contents/uterine-rupture-after-previous-cesarean-delivery, Last updated July 14, 2020.

Mattingly, P. J. (2016). Evaluation of fetal death. In Smith, C. V. & Talavera, F. (Eds.), *eMedicine*. Medscape. http://emedicine.medscape.com/article/259165-overview#a4, Last updated March 13, 2016.

Nahum, G. G. (2018). Uterine rupture in pregnancy. In Talavera, F. & Legro, R. S. (Eds.), *eMedicine*. Medscape. http://reference.medscape.com/article/275854-overview, Last updated July 5, 2018.

Norwitz, E. R. (2020). Progesterone supplementation to reduce the risk of spontaneous preterm birth. *UpToDate*. https://www.uptodate.com, Last updated August 17, 2020.

Norwitz, E. R. (2021). Postterm pregnancy. *UpToDate*. https://www.uptodate.com/contents/postterm-pregnancy, Last updated January 14, 2021.

Ricci, S. S. (2017). *Essentials of maternity, newborn, and women's health nursing* (4th ed.). Wolters Kluwer.

Ringer, S. (2020). Postterm infant. *UpToDate*. https://www.uptodate.com, Last updated July 15, 2020.

Rodis, J. F. (2019). Shoulder dystocia: Intrapartum diagnosis, management, and outcome. *UpToDate*. https://www.uptodate.com/contents/shoulder-dystocia-intrapartum-diagnosis-management-and-outcome, Last updated October 22, 2019.

Ross, M. G. (2018). Preterm labor. In Smith, C. V., Talavera, F., & Legro, R. S. (Eds.), *eMedicine*. Medscape. http://emedicine.medscape.com/article/260998-overview#a3, Last updated December 17, 2018.

Scorza, W. E. (2020). Management of prelabor rupture of the fetal membranes at term. *UpToDate*. https://www.uptodate.com/contents/management-of-prelabor-rupture-of-the-fetal-membranes-at-term, Last updated March 26, 2020.

Simhan, H. N., & Caritis, S. (2020). Inhibition of acute preterm labor. *UpToDate*. https://www.uptodate.com/contents/inhibition-of-acute-preterm-labor, Last updated October 26, 2020.

Strauss, R. A., & Herrera, C. A. (2021). Transverse fetal lie. *UpToDate*. https://www.uptodate.com/contents/transverse-fetal-lie, Last updated January 8, 2021.

Chapter 19

Belfort, M. A. (2021). Overview of postpartum hemorrhage. *UpToDate*. https://www.uptodate.com/contents/postpartum-blues?search=postpartum%20blues&source=search_result&selectedTitle=1~14&usage_type=default&display_rank=1, Last updated January 28, 2021.

Berens, P. (2021). Overview of the postpartum period: Normal physiology and routine maternal care. *UpToDate*. https://www.uptodate.com/contents/overview-of-the-postpartum-period-normal-physiology-and-routine-maternal-care?search=postpartum%20care&source=search_result&selectedTitle=1~118&usage_type=default&display_rank=1, Last updated January 25, 2021.

Center for Disease Control and Prevention, Division of Reproductive Health, National Center for Chronic Disease Prevention and Health Promotion. (2020). Depression among women: Postpartum depression. http://www.cdc.gov/reproductivehealth/Depression/#Postpartum, Last updated May 14, 2020.

Chaar, C. I. O. (2020). *Phlegmasia alba and cerulea dolens*. In Rowe, V. L. & Talavera, F. (Eds.), *eMedicine*. Medscape. https://emedicine.medscape.com/article/461809-overview#a4, Last updated July 27, 2020.

Chen, K. T. (2020). Postpartum endometritis. *UpToDate*. https://www.uptodate.com/contents/postpartum-blues?search=postpartum%20blues&source=search_result&selectedTitle=1~14&usage_type=default&display_rank=1, Last updated December 1, 2020.

Cox, J. L., Holden, J. M., & Sagovsky, R. (1987). Detection of postnatal depression: Development of the 10-item Edinburgh Postnatal Depression Scale. *British Journal of Psychiatry*, 150, 782–786. https://med.stanford.edu/content/dam/sm/ppc/documents/DBP/EDPS_text_added.pdf

Dixon, J. M. (2020). Lactational mastitis. *UpToDate*. https://www.uptodate.com/contents/postpartum-blues?search=postpartum%20blues&source=search_result&selectedTitle=1~14&usage_type=default&display_rank=1, Last updated January 15, 2020.

Hockenberry, M. J., & Wilson, D. (2018). *Wong's nursing care of infants and children* (11th ed.). Mosby Elsevier.

Kimmel, M. C., & Meltzer-Brody, S. (2020). Safety of infant exposure to antidepressants and benzodiazepines through breastfeeding. *UpToDate*. https://www.uptodate.com/contents/postpartum-blues?search=postpartum%20blues&source=search_result&selectedTitle=1~14&usage_type=default&display_rank=1, Last updated October 8, 2020.

Payne, P. (2018). Postpartum psychosis: Epidemiology, pathogenesis, clinical manifestations, course, assessment, and diagnosis. *UpToDate*. https://www.uptodate.com/contents/postpartum-blues?search=postpartum%20blues&source=search_result&selectedTitle=1~14&usage_type=default&display_rank=1, Last updated February 27, 2018.

Payne, J. (2019). Treatment of postpartum psychosis. *UpToDate*. https://www.uptodate.com/contents/postpartum-blues?search=postpartum%20blues&source=search_result&selectedTitle=1~14&usage_type=default&display_rank=1, Last updated April 11, 2019.

Ricci, S. S. (2017). *Essentials of maternity, newborn, and women's health nursing* (4th ed.). Wolters Kluwer.

Viguera, A. (2019). Postpartum blues. *UpToDate*. https://www.uptodate.com/contents/postpartum-blues?search=postpartum%20blues&source=search_result&selectedTitle=1~14&usage_type=default&display_rank=1, Last updated January 16, 2019.

Viguera, A. (2021). Postpartum unipolar major depression: Epidemiology, clinical features, assessment, and diagnosis. *UpToDate*. https://www.uptodate.com/contents/postpartum-unipolar-major-depression-epidemiology-clinical-features-assessment-and-diagnosis?search=postpartum%20depression&source=search_result&selectedTitle=1~120&usage_type=default&display_rank=1, Last updated January 28, 2021.

Chapter 20

Ballard, J. L. (1991). New Ballard score expanded to include extremely premature infants. *Journal of Pediatrics*, 119, 417–423.

Berger, K. S. (2020). *The developing person through the life span* (9th ed.). Worth Publishers.

Bowden, V. R., & Greenberg, C. S. (2016). *Pediatric nursing procedures* (4th ed.). Wolters Kluwer.

Calhoun, D. A. (2021). Postnatal diagnosis and management of hemolytic disease of the fetus and newborn. *UpToDate*. https://www.uptodate.com/contents/postnatal-diagnosis-and-management-of-hemolytic-disease-of-the-fetus-and-newborn

Corwin, M. J. (2021). Sudden infant death syndrome: Risk factors and risk reduction strategies. *UpToDate*. https://www.uptodate.com/contents/sudden-infant-death-syndrome-risk-factors-and-risk-reduction-strategies

Garcia-Prats, J. A. (2021). Meconium aspiration syndrome: Pathophysiology, clinical manifestations, and diagnosis. *UpToDate*. https://www.uptodate.com/contents/meconium-aspiration-syndrome-pathophysiology-clinical-manifestations-and-diagnosis

Garcia-Prats, J. A. (2021). Meconium aspiration syndrome: Prevention and management. *UpToDate*. https://www.uptodate.com/contents/meconium-aspiration-syndrome-prevention-and-management

Hockenberry, M., Rodgers, C., & Wilson, D. (2016). *Wong's essentials of pediatric nursing* (10th ed.). Mosby.

Jansson, L. M. (2021). Infants of mothers with substance use disorder. *UpToDate*. https://www.uptodate.com/contents/infants-of-mothers-with-substance-use-disorder

Kim, J. H. (2021). Neonatal necrotizing enterocolitis: Clinical features and diagnosis. *UpToDate*. https://www.uptodate.com/contents/neonatal-necrotizing-enterocolitis-clinical-features-and-diagnosis

Kyle, T., & Carman, S. (2020). *Essentials of pediatric nursing* (4th ed.). Wolters Kluwer.

Mandy, G. T. (2021a). Infants with fetal (intrauterine) growth restriction. *UpToDate*. https://www.uptodate.com/contents/infants-with-fetal-intrauterine-growth-restriction

Mandy, G. T. (2021b). Short-term complications of the preterm infant. *UpToDate*. https://www.uptodate.com/contents/short-term-complications-of-the-preterm-infant

Martin, R. (2021a). Pathophysiology, clinical manifestations, and diagnosis of respiratory distress syndrome in the newborn. *UpToDate*. https://www.uptodate.com/contents/pathophysiology-clinical-manifestations-and-diagnosis-of-respiratory-distress-syndrome-in-the-newborn

Martin, R. (2021b). Prevention and treatment of respiratory distress syndrome in preterm infants. *UpToDate*. https://www.uptodate.com/contents/prevention-and-treatment-of-respiratory-distress-syndrome-in-preterm-infants

McKee-Garrett, T. M. (2021). Postnatal assessment of gestational age. *UpToDate*. https://www.uptodate.com/contents/postnatal-assessment-of-gestational-age

Nichols, J. (2021). Normal growth patterns in infants and prepubertal children. *UpToDate*. https://www.uptodate.com/contents/normal-growth-patterns-in-infants-and-prepubertal-children

Resnik, R., & Mari, G. (2021). Fetal growth restriction: Evaluation and management. *UpToDate*. https://www.uptodate.com/contents/fetal-growth-restriction-evaluation-and-management

Ricci, S. (2021). *Essentials of maternity, newborn, and women's health nursing* (5th ed.). Wolters Kluwer

Ricci, S., Kyle, T., & Carman, S. (2021). *Maternity and pediatric nursing* (4th ed.). Wolters Kluwer.

Ringer, S. (2021). Postterm infant. *UpToDate*. https://www.uptodate.com/contents/postterm-infant

Tagher, C., & Knapp, L. (2020). *Pediatric nursing a case-based approach*. Wolters Kluwer.

Weitzman, C., & Rojmahamongkol, P. (2021). Fetal alcohol spectrum disorder: Management and prognosis. *UpToDate*. https://www.uptodate.com/contents/fetal-alcohol-spectrum-disorder-management-and-prognosis

Chapter 21

Altman, C. A. (2021). Identifying newborns with critical congenital heart disease. *UpToDate*. https://www.uptodate.com/contents/identifying-newborns-with-critical-congenital-heart-disease

Bacino, C. A. (2021). Birth defects: Epidemiology, types, and patterns. *UpToDate*. https://www.uptodate.com/contents/birth-defects-epidemiology-types-and-patterns

Berger, K. S. (2020). *The developing person through the life span* (9th ed.). Worth Publishers.

Bodamer, O. A. (2021). Overview of phenylketonuria. *UpToDate*. https://www.uptodate.com/contents/overview-of-phenylketonuria

Bowden, V. R., & Greenberg, C. S. (2016). *Pediatric nursing procedures* (4th ed.). Wolters Kluwer.

Bowman, R. M. (2021). Myelomeningocele (spina bifida): Anatomy, clinical manifestations, and complications. *UpToDate*. https://www.uptodate.com/contents/myelomeningocele-spina-bifida-anatomy-clinical-manifestations-and-complications

Doyle, T., & Kavanaugh-McHugh, A. (2021a). Clinical manifestations and diagnosis of patent ductus arteriosus in term infants, children, and adults. *UpToDate*. https://www.uptodate.com/contents/clinical-manifestations-and-diagnosis-of-patent-ductus-arteriosus-in-term-infants-children-and-adults

Doyle, T., & Kavanaugh-McHugh, A. (2021b). Pathophysiology, clinical features, and diagnosis of tetralogy of Fallot. *UpToDate*. https://www.uptodate.com/contents/pathophysiology-clinical-features-and-diagnosis-of-tetralogy-of-fallot

Doyle, T., Kavanaugh-McHugh, A., Soslow, J., & Hill, K. (2021). Management of patent ductus arteriosus in term infants, children, and adults. *UpToDate*. https://www.uptodate.com/contents/management-of-patent-ductus-arteriosus-in-term-infants-children-and-adults

Erikson, E. H. (1963). *Childhood and society* (2nd ed.). Norton.

Erikson, E. H., & Senn, M. J. (1958). *Symposium on the healthy personality*. Macy Foundation.

Haridas, A., & Tadanori, T. (2021a). Hydrocephalus in children: Clinical features and diagnosis. *UpToDate*. https://www.uptodate.com/contents/hydrocephalus-in-children-clinical-features-and-diagnosis

Haridas, A., & Tadanori, T. (2021b). Hydrocephalus in children: Management and prognosis. *UpToDate*. https://www.uptodate.com/contents/hydrocephalus-in-children-management-and-prognosis

Haridas, A., & Tadanori, T. (2021c). Hydrocephalus in children: Physiology, pathogenesis, and etiology. *UpToDate*. https://www.uptodate.com/contents/hydrocephalus-in-children-physiology-pathogenesis-and-etiology

Hedrick, H. L., & Adzick, N. S. (2021). Congenital diaphragmatic hernia in the neonate. *UpToDate*. https://www.uptodate.com/contents/congenital-diaphragmatic-hernia-in-the-neonate

Hockenberry, M., Rodgers, C., & Wilson, D. (2016). *Wong's essentials of pediatric nursing* (10th ed.). Mosby.

Kyle, T., & Carman, S. (2020). *Essentials of pediatric nursing* (4th ed.). Wolters Kluwer.

Magriples, U. (2021). Prenatal diagnosis of talipes equinovarus (clubfoot). *UpToDate*. https://www.uptodate.com/contents/prenatal-diagnosis-of-talipes-equinovarus-clubfoot

Messerlian, G. M., & Palomaki, G. E. (2021). Down syndrome: Overview of prenatal screening. *UpToDate*. https://www.uptodate.com/contents/down-syndrome-overview-of-prenatal-screening

Nichols, J. (2021). Normal growth patterns in infants and prepubertal children. *UpToDate*. https://www.uptodate.com/contents/normal-growth-patterns-in-infants-and-prepubertal-children

Oermann, C. M. (2021). Congenital anomalies of the intrathoracic airways and tracheoesophageal fistula. *UpToDate*. https://www.uptodate.com/contents/congenital-anomalies-of-the-intrathoracic-airways-and-tracheoesophageal-fistula

Ostermaier, K. K. (2021). Down syndrome: Clinical features and diagnosis. *UpToDate*. https://www.uptodate.com/contents/down-syndrome-clinical-features-and-diagnosis

Ricci, S. (2021). *Essentials of maternity, newborn, and women's health nursing* (5th ed.). Wolters Kluwer

Ricci, S., Kyle, T., & Carman, S. (2021). *Maternity and pediatric nursing* (4th ed.). Wolters Kluwer.

Sutton, V. R. (2021). Galactosemia: Clinical features and diagnosis. *UpToDate*. https://www.uptodate.com/contents/galactosemia-clinical-features-and-diagnosis

Tagher, C., & Knapp, L. (2020). *Pediatric nursing a case-based approach*. Wolters Kluwer.

Wilkins-Haug, L. (2021). Etiology, prenatal diagnosis, obstetric management, and recurrence of cleft lip and/or palate. *UpToDate*. https://www.uptodate.com/contents/etiology-prenatal-diagnosis-obstetric-management-and-recurrence-of-cleft-lip-and-or-palate

Chapter 22

Baggett, T. P., & Kertesz, S. G. (2021). Health care of people experiencing homelessness in the United States. *UpToDate*. https://www.uptodate.com/contents/health-care-of-people-experiencing-homelessness-in-the-united-states

Berger, K. S. (2020). *The developing person through the life span* (9th ed.). Worth Publishers.

Dudek, S. G. (2017). *Nutrition essentials for nursing practice* (8th ed.). Wolters Kluwer.

Duryea, T. K. (2021). Dietary recommendations for toddlers, preschool, and school-age children. *UpToDate*. https://www.uptodate.com/contents/dietary-recommendations-for-toddlers-preschool-and-school-age-children

Erikson, E. H. (1963). *Childhood and society* (2nd ed.). Norton.

Erikson, E. H., & Senn, M. J. (1958). *Symposium on the healthy personality*. Macy Foundation.

Hockenberry, M., Rodgers, C., & Wilson, D. (2016). *Wong's essentials of pediatric nursing* (10th ed.). Mosby.

Kyle, T., & Carman, S. (2020). *Essentials of pediatric nursing* (4th ed.). Wolters Kluwer.

Nichols, J. (2021). Normal growth patterns in infants and prepubertal children. *UpToDate*. https://www.uptodate.com/contents/normal-growth-patterns-in-infants-and-prepubertal-children

Piaget, J. (1967). *The language and thought of the child*. World Publishing.

Ricci, S. (2021). *Essentials of maternity, newborn, and women's health nursing* (5th ed.). Wolters Kluwer

Ricci, S., Kyle, T., & Carman, S. (2021). *Maternity and pediatric nursing* (4th ed.). Wolters Kluwer.

Tagher, C., & Knapp, L. (2020). *Pediatric nursing a case-based approach*. Wolters Kluwer.

Chapter 23

Berger, K. S. (2020). *The developing person through the life span* (9th ed.). Worth Publishers.

Dudek, S. G. (2017). *Nutrition essentials for nursing practice* (8th ed.). Wolters Kluwer.

Duryea, T. K. (2021a). Dietary recommendations for toddlers, preschool, and school-age children. *UpToDate*. https://www.uptodate.com/contents/dietary-recommendations-for-toddlers-preschool-and-school-age-children

Duryea, T. K. (2021b). Introducing solid foods and vitamin and mineral supplementation during infancy. *UpToDate*. https://www.uptodate.com/contents/introducing-solid-foods-and-vitamin-and-mineral-supplementation-during-infancy

Erikson, E. H. (1963). *Childhood and society* (2nd ed.). Norton.

Erikson, E. H., & Senn, M. J. (1958). *Symposium on the healthy personality*. Macy Foundation.

Hockenberry, M., Rodgers, C., & Wilson, D. (2016). *Wong's essentials of pediatric nursing* (10th ed.). Mosby.

Kyle, T., & Carman, S. (2020). *Essentials of pediatric nursing* (4th ed.). Wolters Kluwer.

Nichols, J. (2021). Normal growth patterns in infants and prepubertal children. *UpToDate*. https://www.uptodate.com/contents/normal-growth-patterns-in-infants-and-prepubertal-children

Nowak, A. J., & Warren, J. J. (2021). Preventive dental care and counseling for infants and young children. *UpToDate*. https://www.uptodate.com/contents/preventive-dental-care-and-counseling-for-infants-and-young-children

Phillips, S. M & Jensen, C. (2021). Dietary history and recommended dietary intake in children. *UpToDate*. https://www.uptodate.com/contents/dietary-history-and-recommended-dietary-intake-in-children

Piaget, J. (1967). *The language and thought of the child*. World Publishing.

Ricci, S. (2021). *Essentials of maternity, newborn, and women's health nursing* (5th ed.). Wolters Kluwer

Ricci, S., Kyle, T., & Carman, S. (2021). *Maternity and pediatric nursing* (4th ed.). Wolters Kluwer.

Tagher, C., & Knapp, L. (2020). *Pediatric nursing a case-based approach*. Wolters Kluwer.

Wright, J. T. (2021). Anatomy and development of the teeth. *UpToDate*. https://www.uptodate.com/contents/anatomy-and-development-of-the-teeth

Chapter 24

Berger, K. S. (2020). *The developing person through the life span* (9th ed.). Worth Publishers.

Burns, M. M. (2021a). Potentially toxic plant ingestions in children: Clinical manifestations and evaluation. *UpToDate*. https://www.uptodate.com/contents/potentially-toxic-plant-ingestions-in-children-clinical-manifestations-and-evaluation

Burns, M. M. (2021b). Toxic plant ingestions and nicotine poisoning in children: Management. *UpToDate*. https://www.uptodate.com/contents/toxic-plant-ingestions-and-nicotine-poisoning-in-children-management

Dudek, S. G. (2017). *Nutrition essentials for nursing practice* (8th ed.). Wolters Kluwer.

Duryea, T. K. (2021). Dietary recommendations for toddlers, preschool, and school-age children. *UpToDate*. https://www.

uptodate.com/contents/dietary-recommendations-for-toddlers-preschool-and-school-age-children

Erikson, E. H. (1963). *Childhood and society* (2nd ed.*)*. Norton.

Erikson, E. H., & Senn, M. J. (1958). *Symposium on the healthy personality*. Macy Foundation.

Gill, A. C., & Kelly, N. R. (2021). Pediatric injury prevention: Epidemiology, history, and application. *UpToDate*. https://www.uptodate.com/contents/pediatric-injury-prevention-epidemiology-history-and-application

Hockenberry, M., Rodgers, C., & Wilson, D. (2016). *Wong's essentials of pediatric nursing* (10th ed.). Mosby.

Kelly, N. R. (2021). Prevention of poisoning in children. *UpToDate*. https://www.uptodate.com/contents/prevention-of-poisoning-in-children

Kyle, T., & Carman, S. (2020). *Essentials of pediatric nursing* (4th ed.). Wolters Kluwer.

Nichols, J. (2021). Normal growth patterns in infants and prepubertal children. *UpToDate*. https://www.uptodate.com/contents/normal-growth-patterns-in-infants-and-prepubertal-children

Piaget, J. (1967). *The language and thought of the child*. World Publishing.

Ricci, S. (2021). *Essentials of maternity, newborn, and women's health nursing* (5th ed.). Wolters Kluwer

Ricci, S., Kyle, T., & Carman, S. (2021). *Maternity and pediatric nursing* (4th ed.). Wolters Kluwer.

Sinclair, K., & Hill, I. D. (2021). Button and cylindrical battery ingestion: Clinical features, diagnosis, and initial management. *UpToDate*. https://www.uptodate.com/contents/button-and-cylindrical-battery-ingestion-clinical-features-diagnosis-and-initial-management

Tagher, C., & Knapp, L. (2020). *Pediatric nursing a case-based approach*. Wolters Kluwer.

Chapter 25

Berger, K. S. (2020). *The developing person through the life span* (9th ed.). Worth Publishers.

Dudek, S. G. (2017). *Nutrition essentials for nursing practice* (8th ed.). Wolters Kluwer.

Duryea, T. K. (2021). Dietary recommendations for toddlers, preschool, and school-age children. *UpToDate*. https://www.uptodate.com/contents/dietary-recommendations-for-toddlers-preschool-and-school-age-children

Erikson, E. H. (1963). *Childhood and society* (2nd ed.). Norton.

Erikson, E. H., & Senn, M. J. (1958). *Symposium on the healthy personality*. Macy Foundation.

Hockenberry, M., Rodgers, C., & Wilson, D. (2016). *Wong's essentials of pediatric nursing* (10th ed.). Mosby.

Kyle, T., & Carman, S. (2020). *Essentials of pediatric nursing* (4th ed.). Wolters Kluwer.

Nichols, J. (2021). Normal growth patterns in infants and prepubertal children. *UpToDate*. https://www.uptodate.com/contents/normal-growth-patterns-in-infants-and-prepubertal-children

Piaget, J. (1967). *The language and thought of the child*. World Publishing.

Ricci, S. (2021). *Essentials of maternity, newborn, and women's health nursing* (5th ed.). Wolters Kluwer

Ricci, S., Kyle, T., & Carman, S. (2021). *Maternity and pediatric nursing* (4th ed.). Wolters Kluwer.

Tagher, C., & Knapp, L. (2020). *Pediatric nursing a case-based approach*. Wolters Kluwer.

Chapter 26

Berger, K. S. (2020). *The developing person through the life span* (9th ed.). Worth Publishers.

Dudek, S. G. (2017). *Nutrition essentials for nursing practice* (8th ed.). Wolters Kluwer.

Duryea, T. K. (2021). Dietary recommendations for toddlers, preschool, and school-age children. *UpToDate*. https://www.uptodate.com/contents/dietary-recommendations-for-toddlers-preschool-and-school-age-children

Erikson, E. H. (1963). *Childhood and society* (2nd ed.). Norton.

Erikson, E. H., & Senn, M. J. (1958). *Symposium on the healthy personality*. Macy Foundation.

Hockenberry, M., Rodgers, C., & Wilson, D. (2016). *Wong's essentials of pediatric nursing* (10th ed.). Mosby.

Kyle, T., & Carman, S. (2020). *Essentials of pediatric nursing* (4th ed.). Wolters Kluwer.

Perry, H. (2021). Inhalant abuse in children and adolescents. *UpToDate*. https://www.uptodate.com/contents/inhalant-abuse-in-children-and-adolescents

Piaget, J. (1967). *The language and thought of the child*. World Publishing.

Ricci, S. (2021). *Essentials of maternity, newborn, and women's health nursing* (5th ed.). Wolters Kluwer

Ricci, S., Kyle, T., & Carman, S. (2021). *Maternity and pediatric nursing* (4th ed.). Wolters Kluwer.

Tagher, C., & Knapp, L. (2020). *Pediatric nursing a case-based approach*. Wolters Kluwer.

Chapter 27

Berger, K. S. (2020). *The developing person through the life span* (9th ed.). Worth Publishers.

Demory-Luce, D., & Motil, J. K. (2021). Vegetarian diets for children. *UpToDate*. https://www.uptodate.com/contents/vegetarian-diets-for-children

Dudek, S. G. (2017). *Nutrition essentials for nursing practice* (8th ed.). Wolters Kluwer.

Duryea, T. K. (2021). Dietary recommendations for toddlers, preschool, and school-age children. *UpToDate*. https://www.uptodate.com/contents/dietary-recommendations-for-toddlers-preschool-and-school-age-children

Erikson, E. H. (1963). *Childhood and society* (2nd ed.). Norton.

Erikson, E. H., & Senn, M. J. (1958). *Symposium on the healthy personality*. Macy Foundation.

Hockenberry, M., Rodgers, C., & Wilson, D. (2016). *Wong's essentials of pediatric nursing* (10th ed.) Mosby.

Kyle, T., & Carman, S. (2020). *Essentials of pediatric nursing* (4th ed.). Wolters Kluwer.

Nichols, J. (2021). Normal growth patterns in infants and prepubertal children. *UpToDate*. https://www.uptodate.com/contents/normal-growth-patterns-in-infants-and-prepubertal-children

Piaget, J. (1967). *The language and thought of the child*. World Publishing.

Ricci, S. (2021). *Essentials of maternity, newborn, and women's health nursing* (5th ed.). Wolters Kluwer.

Ricci, S., Kyle, T., & Carman, S. (2021). *Maternity and pediatric nursing* (4th ed.). Wolters Kluwer.

Steele, G. S, Richie, J. P, Oh, W. K., & Michaelson, M. D. (2021). Clinical manifestations, diagnosis, and staging of testicular germ cell tumors. *UpToDate*. https://www.uptodate.com/contents/clinical-manifestations-diagnosis-and-staging-of-testicular-germ-cell-tumors

Tagher, C., & Knapp, L. (2020). *Pediatric nursing a case-based approach*. Wolters Kluwer.

Wiemann, C. M., & Miller, E. (2021). Date rape: Identification and management. *UpToDate*. https://www.uptodate.com/contents/date-rape-identification-and-management

Wiemann, C. M., & Miller, E. (2021). Date rape: Risk factors and prevention. *UpToDate*. https://www.uptodate.com/contents/date-rape-risk-factors-and-prevention

Chapter 28

Berger, K. S. (2020). *The developing person through the life span* (11th ed.). Worth Publishers.

Bowden, V. R., & Greenberg, C. S. (2016). *Pediatric nursing procedures* (4th ed.). Wolters Kluwer.

Corwin, M. J. (2021). Use of home cardiorespiratory monitors in infants. *UpToDate*. https://www.uptodate.com/contents/use-of-home-cardiorespiratory-monitors-in-infants

Drutz, J. E. (2021). The pediatric physical examination: General principles and standard measurements. *UpToDate*. https://www.uptodate.com/contents/the-pediatric-physical-examination-general-principles-and-standard-measurements

Hockenberry, M., Rodgers, C., & Wilson, D. (2016). *Wong's essentials of pediatric nursing* (10th ed.). Mosby.

Kotagal, S. (2021). Detailed neurologic assessment of infants and children. *UpToDate*. https://www.uptodate.com/contents/detailed-neurologic-assessment-of-infants-and-children

Kyle, T., & Carman, S. (2020). *Essentials of pediatric nursing* (4th ed.). Wolters Kluwer.

Lippincott. (2018). *Lippincott nursing procedures* (8th ed.). Wolters Kluwer.

Maaks, D., Starr, N., Brady, M., Gaylord, N., Driessnack, M., & Duderstadt, K. (2020). *Burns' pediatric primary care* (7th ed.). Elsevier.

Mattoo, T. K. (2021). Definition and diagnosis of hypertension in children and adolescents. *UpToDate*. https://www.uptodate.com/contents/definition-and-diagnosis-of-hypertension-in-children-and-adolescents

Mechem, C. C. (2021). Pulse oximetry. *UpToDate*. https://www.uptodate.com/contents/pulse-oximetry

Nichols, J. N. (2021). Normal growth patterns in infants and prepubertal children. *UpToDate*. https://www.uptodate.com/contents/normal-growth-patterns-in-infants-and-prepubertal-children

Piaget, J. (1967). *The language and thought of the child*. World Publishing.

Ricci, S. (2021). *Essentials of maternity, newborn, and women's health nursing* (5th ed.). Wolters Kluwer.

Ricci, S., Kyle, T., & Carman, S. (2021). *Maternity and pediatric nursing* (4th ed.). Wolters Kluwer.

Rosdahl, C., & Kowalsik, M. (2017). *Textbook of basic nursing* (11th ed.). Wolters Kluwer.

Ward, M. A. (2021). Fever in infants and children: Pathophysiology and management. *UpToDate*. https://www.uptodate.com/contents/fever-in-infants-and-children-pathophysiology-and-management

Chapter 29

Anderson, D. J. (2021). Infection prevention: Precautions for preventing transmission of infection. *UpToDate*. https://www.uptodate.com/contents/infection-prevention-precautions-for-preventing-transmission-of-infection

Berger, K. S. (2020). *The developing person through the life span* (11th ed.). Worth Publishers.

Bowden, V. R., & Greenberg, C. S. (2016). *Pediatric nursing procedures* (4th ed.). Wolters Kluwer.

Hauer, J., & Jones, B. L. (2021). Evaluation and management of pain in children. *UpToDate*. https://www.uptodate.com/contents/evaluation-and-management-of-pain-in-children

Hockenberry, M., Rodgers, C., & Wilson, D. (2016). *Wong's essentials of pediatric nursing* (10th ed.). Mosby.

Huang, P. P., & Durbin, D. R. (2021). Promoting safety in children with disabilities. *UpToDate*. https://www.uptodate.com/contents/promoting-safety-in-children-with-disabilities

Kyle, T., & Carman, S. (2020). *Essentials of pediatric nursing* (4th ed.). Wolters Kluwer.

Lee, L. K., & Fleisher, G. R. (2021). Trauma management: Approach to the unstable child. *UpToDate*. https://www.uptodate.com/contents/trauma-management-approach-to-the-unstable-child

Lippincott. (2018). *Lippincott nursing procedures* (8th ed.). Wolters Kluwer.

Maaks, D., Starr, N., Brady, M., Gaylord, N., Driessnack, M., & Duderstadt, K. (2020). *Burns' pediatric primary care* (7th ed.). Elsevier.

Piaget, J. (1967). *The language and thought of the child*. World Publishing.

Ricci, S. (2021). *Essentials of maternity, newborn, and women's health nursing* (5th ed.). Wolters Kluwer.

Ricci, S., Kyle, T., & Carman, S. (2021). *Maternity and pediatric nursing* (4th ed.). Wolters Kluwer.

Rosdahl, C., & Kowalsik, M. (2017). *Textbook of Basic nursing* (11th ed.). Wolters Kluwer.

Schechter, W. (2021. Approach to the management of acute perioperative pain in infants and children. *UpToDate*. https://www.uptodate.com/contents/approach-to-the-management-of-acute-perioperative-pain-in-infants-and-children

Srinivassan, S., & Schwartz, H. P. (2021). Pediatric considerations in prehospital care. *UpToDate*. https://www.uptodate.com/contents/pediatric-considerations-in-prehospital-care

Chapter 30

Berger, K. S. (2020). *The developing person through the life span* (11th ed.). Worth Publishers.

Bowden, V. R., & Greenberg, C. S. (2016). *Pediatric nursing procedures* (4th ed.). Wolters Kluwer.

DeLegge, M. H. (2021). Gastrostomy tubes: Placement and routine care. *UpToDate*. https://www.uptodate.com/contents/gastrostomy-tubes-placement-and-routine-care

Dudek, S. G. (2017). *Nutrition essentials for nursing practice* (8th ed.). Wolters Kluwer.

Fastle, R. K., & Bothner, J. (2021). Lumbar puncture: Indications, contraindications, technique, and complications in children. *UpToDate*. https://www.uptodate.com/contents/lumbar-puncture-indications-contraindications-technique-and-complications-in-children

Fleet, S. E., & Duggan, C. (2021). Overview of enteral nutrition in infants and children. *UpToDate*. https://www.uptodate.com/contents/overview-of-enteral-nutrition-in-infants-and-children

Hockenberry, M., Rodgers, C., & Wilson, D. (2016). *Wong's essentials of pediatric nursing* (10th ed.). Mosby.

Hyzy, R. C., & McSparron, J. I. (2021). Overview of tracheostomy. *UpToDate*. https://www.uptodate.com/contents/overview-of-tracheostomy

Kyle, T., & Carman, S. (2020). *Essentials of pediatric nursing* (4th ed.). Wolters Kluwer.

Lippincott. (2018). *Lippincott nursing procedures* (8th ed.). Wolters Kluwer.

Maaks, D., Starr, N., Brady, M., Gaylord, N., Driessnack, M., & Duderstadt, K. (2020). *Burns' pediatric primary care* (7th ed.). Elsevier.

Ricci, S. (2021). *Essentials of maternity, newborn, and women's health nursing* (5th ed.). Wolters Kluwer.

Ricci, S., Kyle, T., & Carman, S. (2021). *Maternity and pediatric nursing* (4th ed.). Wolters Kluwer.

Rosdahl, C., & Kowalsik, M. (2017). *Textbook of Basic nursing* (11th ed.). Wolters Kluwer.

Ward, M. A. (2021). Fever in infants and children: Pathophysiology and management. *UpToDate.* https://www.uptodate.com/contents/fever-in-infants-and-children-pathophysiology-and-management

Chapter 31

Baker, R. D., Baker, S. S., Briggs, J., & Bojczuk, G. (2021). Parenteral nutrition in infants and children. *UpToDate.* https://www.uptodate.com/contents/parenteral-nutrition-in-infants-and-children

Berger, K. S. (2020). *The developing person through the life span* (11th ed.). Worth Publishers.

Bowden, V. R., & Greenberg, C. S. (2016). *Pediatric nursing procedures* (4th ed.). Wolters Kluwer.

Cravero, J. P., & Roback, M. F. (2021). Pharmacologic agents for pediatric procedural sedation outside of the operating room. *UpToDate.* https://www.uptodate.com/contents/pharmacologic-agents-for-pediatric-procedural-sedation-outside-of-the-operating-room

Dudek, S. G. (2017). *Nutrition essentials for nursing practice* (8th ed.). Wolters Kluwer.

Hockenberry, M., Rodgers, C., & Wilson, D. (2016). *Wong's essentials of pediatric nursing* (10th ed.). Mosby.

Kyle, T., & Carman, S. (2020). *Essentials of pediatric nursing* (4th ed.). Wolters Kluwer.

Lippincott. (2018). *Lippincott nursing procedures* (8th ed.). Wolters Kluwer.

Lippincott, Williams & Wilkins. (2021). *Nursing 2021 drug handbook* (41st ed.). Wolters Kluwer.

Maaks, D., Starr, N., Brady, M., Gaylord, N., Driessnack, M., & Duderstadt, K. (2020). *Burns' pediatric primary care* (7th ed.). Elsevier.

Paulsen, A. W., & Ruskin, K. J. (2021). Intravenous infusion devices for perioperative use. *UpToDate.* https://www.uptodate.com/contents/intravenous-infusion-devices-for-perioperative-use

Ricci, S. (2021). *Essentials of maternity, newborn, and women's health nursing* (5th ed.). Wolters Kluwer.

Ricci, S., Kyle, T., & Carman, S. (2021). *Maternity and pediatric nursing* (4th ed.). Wolters Kluwer.

Rosdahl, C., & Kowalsik, M. (2017). *Textbook of Basic nursing* (11th ed.). Wolters Kluwer.

Smith, S. R. (2021). Vascular (venous) access for pediatric resuscitation and other pediatric emergencies. *UpToDate.* https://www.uptodate.com/contents/vascular-venous-access-for-pediatric-resuscitation-and-other-pediatric-emergencies

Tagher, C., & Knapp, L. (2020). *Pediatric nursing a case-based approach.* Wolters Kluwer.

Womble, D. M., & Kincheloe, C. A. (2020). *Introductory mental health nursing.* Wolters Kluwer.

Chapter 32

Berger, K. S. (2020). *The developing person through the life span* (11th ed.). Worth Publishers.

Gan, L. L., Lum, A., Wakefield, C. E., Nandakumar, B., & Fardell, J. E. (2017). School experiences of siblings of children with chronic illness: A systematic literature review. *Journal of Pediatric Nursing, 33*(2), 23–32.

Hockenberry, M., Rodgers, C., & Wilson, D. (2016). *Wong's essentials of pediatric nursing* (10th ed.). Mosby.

Kuo, D. Z., & Turchi, R. M. (2021). Children and youth with special health care needs. *UpToDate.* https://www.uptodate.com/contents/children-and-youth-with-special-health-care-needs

Kyle, T., & Carman, S. (2020). *Essentials of pediatric nursing* (4th ed.). Wolters Kluwer.

Maaks, D., Starr, N., Brady, M., Gaylord, N., Driessnack, M., & Duderstadt, K. (2020). *Burns' pediatric primary care* (7th ed.). Elsevier.

O'Meara, A. (2019). *Maternity, newborn, and women's health nursing a case-based approach.* Wolters Kluwer.

Ricci, S., Kyle, T., & Carman, S. (2021). *Maternity and pediatric nursing* (4th ed.). Wolters Kluwer.

Tagher, C., & Knapp, L. (2020). *Pediatric nursing a case-based approach.* Wolters Kluwer.

Chapter 33

Bechtel, K & Bennett, B. L. (2021). Evaluation of sexual abuse in children and adolescents. *UpToDate.* https://www.uptodate.com/contents/evaluation-of-sexual-abuse-in-children-and-adolescents

Bechtel, K & Bennett, B. L. (2021). Management and sequelae of sexual abuse in children and adolescents. *UpToDate.* https://www.uptodate.com/contents/management-and-sequelae-of-sexual-abuse-in-children-and-adolescents

Berger, K. S. (2020). *The developing person through the life span* (11th ed.). Worth Publishers.

Boos, S. C. (2021a). Physical child abuse: Diagnostic evaluation and management. *UpToDate.* https://www.uptodate.com/contents/physical-child-abuse-diagnostic-evaluation-and-management

Boos, S. C. (2021b). Physical child abuse: Recognition. *UpToDate.* https://www.uptodate.com/contents/physical-child-abuse-recognition

Child Welfare Information Gateway. (2019). *About CAPTA: A legislative history.* U.S. Department of Health and Human Services, Children's Bureau.

Franchek-Roa, K. M. (2021). Intimate partner violence: Childhood exposure. *UpToDate.* https://www.uptodate.com/contents/intimate-partner-violence-childhood-exposure

Harper, N. S., & Foell, R. (2021). Child neglect: Evaluation and management. *UpToDate.* https://www.uptodate.com/contents/child-neglect-evaluation-and-management

Hockenberry, M., Rodgers, C., & Wilson, D. (2016). *Wong's essentials of pediatric nursing* (10th ed.). Mosby.

Jee, S. H., & Szilagyi, M. A. (2021). Comprehensive health care for children in foster care. *UpToDate.* https://www.uptodate.com/contents/comprehensive-health-care-for-children-in-foster-care

Kyle, T., & Carman, S. (2020). *Essentials of pediatric nursing* (4th ed.). Wolters Kluwer.

Maaks, D., Starr, N., Brady, M., Gaylord, N., Driessnack, M., & Duderstadt, K. (2020). *Burns' pediatric primary care* (7th ed.). Elsevier.

Narang, S. K. (2021). Child abuse: Social and medicolegal issues. *UpToDate.* https://www.uptodate.com/contents/child-abuse-social-and-medicolegal-issues

O'Meara, A. (2019). *Maternity, newborn, and women's health nursing a case-based approach.* Wolters Kluwer.

Ricci, S., Kyle, T., & Carman, S. (2021). *Maternity and pediatric nursing* (4th ed.). Wolters Kluwer.

Roesler, T. A., & Jenny, C. (2021). Medical child abuse (Munchausen syndrome by proxy). *UpToDate.* https://www.uptodate.com/contents/medical-child-abuse-munchausen-syndrome-by-proxy

Scherl, S. A. (2021). Differential diagnosis of the orthopedic manifestations of child abuse. *UpToDate.* https://www.uptodate.com/contents/differential-diagnosis-of-the-orthopedic-manifestations-of-child-abuse

Sege, R. D. (2021). Peer violence and violence prevention. *UpToDate.* https://www.uptodate.com/contents/peer-violence-and-violence-prevention

Tagher, C., & Knapp, L. (2020). *Pediatric nursing a case-based approach.* Wolters Kluwer.

Tracy, E. E., & Macias-Konstantopoulos, W. (2021). Human trafficking: Identification and evaluation in the health care setting. *UpToDate.* https://www.uptodate.com/contents/human-trafficking-identification-and-evaluation-in-the-health-care-setting

Chapter 34

Berger, K. S. (2020). *The developing person through the life span* (11th ed.). Worth Publishers.

Hauer, J. (2021). Pediatric palliative care. *UpToDate.* https://www.uptodate.com/contents/pediatric-palliative-care

Hockenberry, M., Rodgers, C., & Wilson, D. (2016). *Wong's essentials of pediatric nursing* (10th ed.) Mosby.

Jefferies, J. L. (2021). Sudden cardiac arrest and death in children. *UpToDate.* https://www.uptodate.com/contents/sudden-cardiac-arrest-and-death-in-children

Kyle, T., & Carman, S. (2020). *Essentials of pediatric nursing* (4th ed.). Wolters Kluwer.

Maaks, D., Starr, N., Brady, M., Gaylord, N., Driessnack, M., & Duderstadt, K. (2020). *Burns' pediatric primary care* (7th ed.). Elsevier.

Middleman, A. B., & Olson, K. A. (2021). Confidentiality in adolescent health care. *UpToDate.* https://www.uptodate.com/contents/confidentiality-in-adolescent-health-care

Ricci, S., Kyle, T., & Carman, S. (2021). *Maternity and pediatric nursing* (4th ed.). Wolters Kluwer.

Tagher, C., & Knapp, L. (2020). *Pediatric nursing a case-based approach.* Wolters Kluwer.

Chapter 35

Barkoudah, E., & Glader, L. (2021). Cerebral palsy: Epidemiology, etiology, and prevention. *UpToDate.* https://www.uptodate.com/contents/cerebral-palsy-epidemiology-etiology-and-prevention

Barkoudah, E., & Glader, L. (2021). Cerebral palsy: Overview of management and prognosis. *UpToDate.* https://www.uptodate.com/contents/cerebral-palsy-overview-of-management-and-prognosis

Coats, D. K. (2021). Vision screening and assessment in infants and children. *UpToDate.* https://www.uptodate.com/contents/vision-screening-and-assessment-in-infants-and-children

Di Pentima, C. (2021). Viral meningitis: Management, prognosis, and prevention in children. *UpToDate.* https://www.uptodate.com/contents/viral-meningitis-management-prognosis-and-prevention-in-children

Di Pentima, C., & Kaplan, S. L. (2021). Viral meningitis: Clinical features and diagnosis in children. *UpToDate.* https://www.uptodate.com/contents/viral-meningitis-clinical-features-and-diagnosis-in-children

Glader, L., & Barkoudah, E. (2021). Cerebral palsy: Clinical features and classification. *UpToDate.* https://www.uptodate.com/contents/cerebral-palsy-clinical-features-and-classification

Hockenberry, M., Rodgers, C., & Wilson, D. (2016). *Wong's essentials of pediatric nursing* (10th ed.). Mosby.

Kaplan, S. L. (2021a). Bacterial meningitis in children older than one month: Clinical features and diagnosis. *UpToDate.* https://www.uptodate.com/contents/bacterial-meningitis-in-children-older-than-one-month-clinical-features-and-diagnosis

Kaplan, S. L. (2021b). Bacterial meningitis in children older than one month: Treatment and prognosis. *UpToDate.* https://www.uptodate.com/contents/bacterial-meningitis-in-children-older-than-one-month-treatment-and-prognosis

Kaplan, S. L. (2021c). Bacterial meningitis in children: Neurologic complications. *UpToDate.* https://www.uptodate.com/contents/bacterial-meningitis-in-children-neurologic-complications

Kyle, T., & Carman, S. (2020). *Essentials of pediatric nursing* (4th ed.). Wolters Kluwer.

Lau, C., & Teo, W. Y. (2021a). Clinical manifestations and diagnosis of central nervous system tumors in children. *UpToDate.* https://www.uptodate.com/contents/clinical-manifestations-and-diagnosis-of-central-nervous-system-tumors-in-children

Lau, C., & Teo, W. Y. (2021b). Overview of the management of central nervous system tumors in children. *UpToDate.* https://www.uptodate.com/contents/overview-of-the-management-of-central-nervous-system-tumors-in-children

Lippincott, Williams & Wilkins. (2021). *Nursing 2021 drug handbook* (41st ed.). Wolters Kluwer.

Maaks, D., Starr, N., Brady, M., Gaylord, N., Driessnack, M., & Duderstadt, K. (2020). *Burns' pediatric primary care* (7th ed.). Elsevier.

Meehan, W. P & O'Brien, M. J. (2021). Concussion in children and adolescents: Clinical manifestations and diagnosis. *UpToDate.* https://www.uptodate.com/contents/concussion-in-children-and-adolescents-clinical-manifestations-and-diagnosis

Millichap, J. J. (2021). Clinical features and evaluation of febrile seizures. *UpToDate.* https://www.uptodate.com/contents/clinical-features-and-evaluation-of-febrile-seizures

O'Meara, A. (2019). *Maternity, newborn, and women's health nursing a case-based approach.* Wolters Kluwer.

Pivalizza, P. (2021). Intellectual disability in children: Management, outcomes, and prevention. *UpToDate.* https://www.uptodate.com/contents/intellectual-disability-in-children-management-outcomes-and-prevention

Pivalizza, P., & Lalani, S. R. (2021). Intellectual disability in children: Definition, diagnosis, and assessment of needs. *UpToDate.* https://www.uptodate.com/contents/intellectual-disability-in-children-definition-diagnosis-and-assessment-of-needs

Rajajee, V. (2021). Traumatic brain injury: Epidemiology, classification, and pathophysiology. *UpToDate.* https://www.uptodate.com/contents/traumatic-brain-injury-epidemiology-classification-and-pathophysiology

Reynolds, J. D., & Reynolds, A. L. (2021). Overview of glaucoma in infants and children. *UpToDate.* https://www.uptodate.com/contents/overview-of-glaucoma-in-infants-and-children

Ricci, S. (2021). *Essentials of maternity, newborn, and women's health nursing* (5th ed.). Wolters Kluwer.

Ricci, S., Kyle, T., & Carman, S. (2021). *Maternity and pediatric nursing* (4th ed.). Wolters Kluwer.

Smith, R. J. H., & Gooi, A. (2021a). Hearing loss in children: Etiology. *UpToDate.* https://www.uptodate.com/contents/hearing-loss-in-children-etiology

Smith, R. J. H., & Gooi, A. (2021b). Hearing loss in children: Screening and evaluation. *UpToDate*. https://www.uptodate.com/contents/hearing-loss-in-children-screening-and-evaluation

Tagher, C., & Knapp, L. (2020). *Pediatric nursing a case-based approach*. Wolters Kluwer.

Wald, E. R. (2021). Acute otitis media in children: Clinical manifestations and diagnosis. *UpToDate*. https://www.uptodate.com/contents/acute-otitis-media-in-children-clinical-manifestations-and-diagnosis

Wilfong, A. (2021a). Seizures and epilepsy in children: Classification, etiology, and clinical features. *UpToDate*. https://www.uptodate.com/contents/seizures-and-epilepsy-in-children-classification-etiology-and-clinical-features

Wilfong, A. (2021b). Seizures and epilepsy in children: Initial treatment and monitoring. *UpToDate*. https://www.uptodate.com/contents/seizures-and-epilepsy-in-children-initial-treatment-and-monitoring

Chapter 36

Adams, L. V., & Starke, J. R. (2021). Tuberculosis disease in children. *UpToDate*. https://www.uptodate.com/contents/tuberculosis-disease-in-children

Baker, R. D., & Baker, S. S. (2021). Cystic fibrosis: Nutritional issues. *UpToDate*. https://www.uptodate.com/contents/cystic-fibrosis-nutritional-issues

Barr, F. E., & Graham, B. S. (2021a). Respiratory syncytial virus infection: Clinical features and diagnosis. *UpToDate*. https://www.uptodate.com/contents/respiratory-syncytial-virus-infection-clinical-features-and-diagnosis

Barr, F. E., & Graham, B. S. (2021b). Respiratory syncytial virus infection: Treatment. *UpToDate*. https://www.uptodate.com/contents/respiratory-syncytial-virus-infection-treatment

Barson, W. J. (2021). Pneumonia in children: Epidemiology, pathogenesis, and etiology. *UpToDate*. https://www.uptodate.com/contents/pneumonia-in-children-epidemiology-pathogenesis-and-etiology

deShazo, R. D., & Kemp, S. F. (2021). Allergic rhinitis: Clinical manifestations, epidemiology, and diagnosis. *UpToDate*. https://www.uptodate.com/contents/allergic-rhinitis-clinical-manifestations-epidemiology-and-diagnosis

Fanta, C. H. (2021). An overview of asthma management. *UpToDate*. https://www.uptodate.com/contents/an-overview-of-asthma-management

Gerald, L. B., & Carr, T. F. (2021). Peak expiratory flow monitoring in asthma. *UpToDate*. https://www.uptodate.com/contents/peak-expiratory-flow-monitoring-in-asthma

Hockenberry, M., Rodgers, C., & Wilson, D. (2016). *Wong's essentials of pediatric nursing* (10th ed.). Mosby.

Horburgh, C. R. (2021). Epidemiology of tuberculosis. *UpToDate*. https://www.uptodate.com/contents/epidemiology-of-tuberculosis

Katkin, J. P. (2021). Cystic fibrosis: Clinical manifestations and diagnosis. *UpToDate*. https://www.uptodate.com/contents/cystic-fibrosis-clinical-manifestations-and-diagnosis

Kyle, T., & Carman, S. (2020). *Essentials of pediatric nursing* (4th ed.). Wolters Kluwer.

Lippincott, Williams & Wilkins. (2021). *Nursing 2021 drug handbook* (41st ed.). Wolters Kluwer.

Maaks, D., Starr, N., Brady, M., Gaylord, N., Driessnack, M., & Duderstadt, K. (2020). *Burns' pediatric primary care* (7th ed.). Elsevier.

McIntosh, K. (2021). Coronaviruses. *UpToDate*. https://www.uptodate.com/contents/coronaviruses

O'Meara, A. (2019). *Maternity, newborn, and women's health nursing a case-based approach*. Wolters Kluwer.

Pappas, D. E. (2021). The common cold in children: Clinical features and diagnosis. *UpToDate*. https://www.uptodate.com/contents/the-common-cold-in-children-clinical-features-and-diagnosis

Paradise, J. L., & Wald, E. R. (2021). Tonsillectomy and/or adenoidectomy in children: Indications and contraindications. *UpToDate*. https://www.uptodate.com/contents/tonsillectomy-and-or-adenoidectomy-in-children-indications-and-contraindications

Ricci, S. (2021). *Essentials of maternity, newborn, and women's health nursing* (5th ed.). Wolters Kluwer.

Ricci, S., Kyle, T., & Carman, S. (2021). *Maternity and pediatric nursing* (4th ed.). Wolters Kluwer.

Sawicki, G, & Haver, K. (2021). Asthma in children younger than 12 years: Initial evaluation and diagnosis. *UpToDate*. https://www.uptodate.com/contents/asthma-in-children-younger-than-12-years-initial-evaluation-and-diagnosis

Sawicki, G, & Haver, K. (2021). Asthma in children younger than 12 years: Initiating therapy and monitoring control. *UpToDate*. https://www.uptodate.com/contents/asthma-in-children-younger-than-12-years-initiating-therapy-and-monitoring-control

Tagher, C., & Knapp, L. (2020). *Pediatric nursing a case-based approach*. Wolters Kluwer.

Tuomanen, E. I., & Kaplan, S. L. (2021). Pneumococcal pneumonia in children. *UpToDate*. https://www.uptodate.com/contents/pneumococcal-pneumonia-in-children

Woods, C. R. (2021a). Croup: Clinical features, evaluation, and diagnosis. *UpToDate*. https://www.uptodate.com/contents/croup-clinical-features-evaluation-and-diagnosis

Woods, C. R. (2021b). Epiglottitis (supraglottitis): Clinical features and diagnosis. *UpToDate*. https://www.uptodate.com/contents/epiglottitis-supraglottitis-clinical-features-and-diagnosis

Chapter 37

Benz, E. J., & Angelucci, E. (2021). Management and prognosis of the thalassemias. *UpToDate*. https://www.uptodate.com/contents/management-and-prognosis-of-the-thalassemias

Bussel, J. B. (2021). Immune thrombocytopenia (ITP) in children: Clinical features and diagnosis. *UpToDate*. https://www.uptodate.com/contents/immune-thrombocytopenia-itp-in-children-clinical-features-and-diagnosis

Field, J. J., & Vichinsky, E. P. (2021). Overview of the management and prognosis of sickle cell disease. *UpToDate*. https://www.uptodate.com/contents/overview-of-the-management-and-prognosis-of-sickle-cell-disease

Hockenberry, M., Rodgers, C., & Wilson, D. (2016). *Wong's essentials of pediatric nursing* (10th ed.). Mosby.

Hoots, W. K., & Shapiro, A. D. (2021). Clinical manifestations and diagnosis of hemophilia. *UpToDate*. https://www.uptodate.com/contents/clinical-manifestations-and-diagnosis-of-hemophilia

Horton, T. M., & Steuber, C. P. (2021). Overview of the treatment of acute lymphoblastic leukemia/lymphoma in children and adolescents. *UpToDate*. https://www.uptodate.com/contents/overview-of-the-treatment-of-acute-lymphoblastic-leukemia-lymphoma-in-children-and-adolescents

Kyle, T., & Carman, S. (2020). *Essentials of pediatric nursing* (4th ed.). Wolters Kluwer.

Lippincott, Williams & Wilkins. (2021). *Nursing 2021 drug handbook* (41st ed.). Wolters Kluwer.

Maaks, D., Starr, N., Brady, M., Gaylord, N., Driessnack, M., & Duderstadt, K. (2020). *Burns' pediatric primary care* (7th ed.). Elsevier.

O'Meara, A. (2019). *Maternity, newborn, and women's health nursing a case-based approach.* Wolters Kluwer.

Powers, J. M., & Mahoney, D. H. (2021). Iron deficiency in infants and children <12 years: Screening, prevention, clinical manifestations, and diagnosis. *UpToDate.* https://www.uptodate.com/contents/iron-deficiency-in-infants-and-children-less-than12-years-screening-prevention-clinical-manifestations-and-diagnosis

Ricci, S. (2021). *Essentials of maternity, newborn, and women's health nursing* (5th ed.). Wolters Kluwer.

Ricci, S., Kyle, T., & Carman, S. (2021). *Maternity and pediatric nursing* (4th ed.). Wolters Kluwer.

Singh, R. K., & Singh, T. P. (2021a). Heart failure in children: Etiology, clinical manifestations, and diagnosis. *UpToDate.* https://www.uptodate.com/contents/heart-failure-in-children-etiology-clinical-manifestations-and-diagnosis

Singh, R. K., & Singh, T. P. (2021b). Heart failure in children: Management. *UpToDate.* https://www.uptodate.com/contents/heart-failure-in-children-management

Steer, A., & Gibofsky, A. (2021a). Acute rheumatic fever: Clinical manifestations and diagnosis. *UpToDate.* https://www.uptodate.com/contents/acute-rheumatic-fever-clinical-manifestations-and-diagnosis

Steer, A., & Gibofsky, A. (2021b). Acute rheumatic fever: Treatment and prevention. *UpToDate.* https://www.uptodate.com/contents/acute-rheumatic-fever-treatment-and-prevention

Sundel, R. (2021a). Kawasaki disease: Clinical features and diagnosis. *UpToDate.* https://www.uptodate.com/contents/kawasaki-disease-clinical-features-and-diagnosis

Sundel, R. (2021b). Kawasaki disease: Initial treatment and prognosis. *UpToDate.* https://www.uptodate.com/contents/kawasaki-disease-initial-treatment-and-prognosis

Tagher, C., & Knapp, L. (2020). *Pediatric nursing a case-based approach.* Wolters Kluwer.

Vichinsky, E. P. (2021). Overview of the clinical manifestations of sickle cell disease. *UpToDate.* https://www.uptodate.com/contents/overview-of-the-clinical-manifestations-of-sickle-cell-disease

Chapter 38

Burks, W. (2021). Clinical manifestations of food allergy: An overview. *UpToDate.* https://www.uptodate.com/contents/clinical-manifestations-of-food-allergy-an-overview

Gilger, M. A. (2021). Foreign bodies of the esophagus and gastrointestinal tract in children. *UpToDate.* https://www.uptodate.com/contents/foreign-bodies-of-the-esophagus-and-gastrointestinal-tract-in-children

Goday, P. S. (2021). Malnutrition in children in resource-limited countries: Clinical assessment. *UpToDate.* https://www.uptodate.com/contents/malnutrition-in-children-in-resource-limited-countries-clinical-assessment

Hill, I. D. (2021). Epidemiology, pathogenesis, and clinical manifestations of celiac disease in children. *UpToDate.* https://www.uptodate.com/contents/epidemiology-pathogenesis-and-clinical-manifestations-of-celiac-disease-in-children

Hill, I. D. (2021). Management of celiac disease in children. *UpToDate.* https://www.uptodate.com/contents/management-of-celiac-disease-in-children

Hockenberry, M., Rodgers, C., & Wilson, D. (2016). *Wong's essentials of pediatric nursing* (10th ed.). Mosby.

Jarvinen-Seppo, K. (2021). Milk allergy: Clinical features and diagnosis. *UpToDate.* https://www.uptodate.com/contents/milk-allergy-clinical-features-and-diagnosis

Kelly, N. R. (2021). Prevention of poisoning in children. *UpToDate.* https://www.uptodate.com/contents/prevention-of-poisoning-in-children

Kyle, T., & Carman, S. (2020). *Essentials of pediatric nursing* (4th ed.). Wolters Kluwer.

Laffel, L., & Svoren, B. (2021). Epidemiology, presentation, and diagnosis of type 2 diabetes mellitus in children and adolescents. *UpToDate.* https://www.uptodate.com/contents/epidemiology-presentation-and-diagnosis-of-type-2-diabetes-mellitus-in-children-and-adolescents

Levitsky, L. L., & Misra, M. (2021). Epidemiology, presentation, and diagnosis of type 1 diabetes mellitus in children and adolescents. *UpToDate.* https://www.uptodate.com/contents/epidemiology-presentation-and-diagnosis-of-type-1-diabetes-mellitus-in-children-and-adolescents

Lippincott, Williams & Wilkins. (2021). *Nursing 2021 drug handbook* (41st ed.). Wolters Kluwer.

Maaks, D., Starr, N., Brady, M., Gaylord, N., Driessnack, M., & Duderstadt, K. (2020). *Burns' pediatric primary care* (7th ed.). Elsevier.

Misra, M. (2021). Vitamin D insufficiency and deficiency in children and adolescents. *UpToDate.* https://www.uptodate.com/contents/vitamin-d-insufficiency-and-deficiency-in-children-and-adolescents

Olive, A. P., & Endom, E. E. (2021). Infantile hypertrophic pyloric stenosis. *UpToDate.* https://www.uptodate.com/contents/infantile-hypertrophic-pyloric-stenosis

O'Meara, A. (2019). *Maternity, newborn, and women's health nursing a case-based approach.* Wolters Kluwer.

Phillips, S. M., & Jensen, C. (2021). Micronutrient deficiencies associated with malnutrition in children. *UpToDate.* https://www.uptodate.com/contents/micronutrient-deficiencies-associated-with-malnutrition-in-children

Powers, J. M., & Mahoney, D. H. (2021). Iron deficiency in infants and children <12 years: Screening, prevention, clinical manifestations, and diagnosis. *UpToDate.* https://www.uptodate.com/contents/iron-deficiency-in-infants-and-children-less-than12-years-screening-prevention-clinical-manifestations-and-diagnosis

Ricci, S. (2021). *Essentials of maternity, newborn, and women's health nursing* (5th ed.). Wolters Kluwer.

Ricci, S., Kyle, T., & Carman, S. (2021). *Maternity and pediatric nursing* (4th ed.). Wolters Kluwer.

Sample, J. A. (2021). Childhood lead poisoning: Exposure and prevention. *UpToDate.* https://www.uptodate.com/contents/childhood-lead-poisoning-exposure-and-prevention

Tagher, C., & Knapp, L. (2020). *Pediatric nursing a case-based approach.* Wolters Kluwer.

Turner, T. L., & Palamountain, S. (2021). Infantile colic: Clinical features and diagnosis. *UpToDate.* https://www.uptodate.com/contents/infantile-colic-clinical-features-and-diagnosis

Velez, L. I., Shepherd, J. G., & Goto, C. S. (2021). Approach to the child with occult toxic exposure. *UpToDate.* https://www.uptodate.com/contents/approach-to-the-child-with-occult-toxic-exposure

Vo, N. J., & Sato, T. T. (2021). Intussusception in children. *UpToDate.* https://www.uptodate.com/contents/intussusception-in-children

Wesson, D. E., & Brandt, M. L. (2021). Acute appendicitis in children: Clinical manifestations and diagnosis. *UpToDate*. https://www.uptodate.com/contents/acute-appendicitis-in-children-clinical-manifestations-and-diagnosis

Wesson, D. E., & Lopez, M. E. (2021). Congenital aganglionic megacolon (Hirschsprung disease). *UpToDate*. https://www.uptodate.com/contents/congenital-aganglionic-megacolon-hirschsprung-disease

Winter, H. S. (2021a). Gastroesophageal reflux in infants. *UpToDate*. https://www.uptodate.com/contents/gastroesophageal-reflux-in-infants

Winter, H. S. (2021b). Management of gastroesophageal reflux disease in children and adolescents. *UpToDate*. https://www.uptodate.com/contents/management-of-gastroesophageal-reflux-disease-in-children-and-adolescents

Chapter 39

Chintagumpala, M. (2021). Presentation, diagnosis, and staging of Wilms tumor. *UpToDate*. https://www.uptodate.com/contents/presentation-diagnosis-and-staging-of-wilms-tumor

Hockenberry, M., Rodgers, C., & Wilson, D. (2016). *Wong's essentials of pediatric nursing* (10th ed.). Mosby.

Kyle, T., & Carman, S. (2020). *Essentials of pediatric nursing* (4th ed.). Wolters Kluwer.

Lippincott, Williams & Wilkins. (2021). *Nursing 2021 drug handbook* (41st ed.). Wolters Kluwer.

Maaks, D., Starr, N., Brady, M., Gaylord, N., Driessnack, M., & Duderstadt, K. (2020). *Burns' pediatric primary care* (7th ed.). Elsevier.

Niaudet, P. (2021a). Etiology, clinical manifestations, and diagnosis of nephrotic syndrome in children. *UpToDate*. https://www.uptodate.com/contents/etiology-clinical-manifestations-and-diagnosis-of-nephrotic-syndrome-in-children

Niaudet, P. (2021b). Poststreptococcal glomerulonephritis. *UpToDate*. https://www.uptodate.com/contents/poststreptococcal-glomerulonephritis

Niaudet, P. (2021c). Treatment of idiopathic nephrotic syndrome in children. *UpToDate*. https://www.uptodate.com/contents/treatment-of-idiopathic-nephrotic-syndrome-in-children

O'Meara, A. (2019). *Maternity, newborn, and women's health nursing a case-based approach*. Wolters Kluwer.

Ricci, S. (2021). *Essentials of maternity, newborn, and women's health nursing* (5th ed.). Wolters Kluwer.

Ricci, S., Kyle, T., & Carman, S. (2021). *Maternity and pediatric nursing* (4th ed.). Wolters Kluwer.

Shaikh, N., & Hoberman, A. (2021a). Urinary tract infections in children: Epidemiology and risk factors. *UpToDate*. https://www.uptodate.com/contents/urinary-tract-infections-in-children-epidemiology-and-risk-factors

Shaikh, N., & Hoberman, A. (2021b). Urinary tract infections in infants and children older than one month: Clinical features and diagnosis. *UpToDate*. https://www.uptodate.com/contents/urinary-tract-infections-in-infants-and-children-older-than-one-month-clinical-features-and-diagnosis

Shaikh, N., & Hoberman, A. (2021c). Urinary tract infections in infants older than one month and young children: Acute management, imaging, and prognosis. *UpToDate*. https://www.uptodate.com/contents/urinary-tract-infections-in-infants-older-than-one-month-and-young-children-acute-management-imaging-and-prognosis

Tagher, C., & Knapp, L. (2020). *Pediatric nursing a case-based approach*. Wolters Kluwer.

Chapter 40

Darras, B. T. (2021a). Duchenne and Becker muscular dystrophy: Clinical features and diagnosis. *UpToDate*. https://www.uptodate.com/contents/duchenne-and-becker-muscular-dystrophy-clinical-features-and-diagnosis

Darras, B. T. (2021b). Duchenne and Becker muscular dystrophy: Management and prognosis. https://www.uptodate.com/contents/duchenne-and-becker-muscular-dystrophy-management-and-prognosis

Hockenberry, M., Rodgers, C., & Wilson, D. (2016). *Wong's essentials of pediatric nursing* (10th ed.). Mosby.

Kimura, Y. (2021). Systemic juvenile idiopathic arthritis: Clinical manifestations and diagnosis. *UpToDate*. https://www.uptodate.com/contents/systemic-juvenile-idiopathic-arthritis-clinical-manifestations-and-diagnosis

Krogstad, P. (2021a). Hematogenous osteomyelitis in children: Clinical features and complications. *UpToDate*. https://www.uptodate.com/contents/hematogenous-osteomyelitis-in-children-clinical-features-and-complications

Krogstad, P. (2021b). Hematogenous osteomyelitis in children: Management. *UpToDate*. https://www.uptodate.com/contents/hematogenous-osteomyelitis-in-children-management

Kyle, T., & Carman, S. (2020). *Essentials of pediatric nursing* (4th ed.). Wolters Kluwer.

Lippincott, Williams & Wilkins. (2021). *Nursing 2021 drug handbook* (41st ed.). Wolters Kluwer.

Maaks, D., Starr, N., Brady, M., Gaylord, N., Driessnack, M., & Duderstadt, K. (2020). *Burns' pediatric primary care* (7th ed.). Elsevier.

Mathison, D. J., & Agrawal, D. (2021). General principles of fracture management: Fracture patterns and description in children. *UpToDate*. https://www.uptodate.com/contents/general-principles-of-fracture-management-fracture-patterns-and-description-in-children

O'Meara, A. (2019). *Maternity, newborn, and women's health nursing a case-based approach*. Wolters Kluwer.

Ricci, S. (2021). *Essentials of maternity, newborn, and women's health nursing* (5th ed.). Wolters Kluwer.

Ricci, S., Kyle, T., & Carman, S. (2021). *Maternity and pediatric nursing* (4th ed.). Wolters Kluwer.

Scherl, S. A. (2021a). Adolescent idiopathic scoliosis: Clinical features, evaluation, and diagnosis. *UpToDate*. https://www.uptodate.com/contents/adolescent-idiopathic-scoliosis-clinical-features-evaluation-and-diagnosis

Scherl, S. A. (2021b). Adolescent idiopathic scoliosis: Management and prognosis. *UpToDate*. https://www.uptodate.com/contents/adolescent-idiopathic-scoliosis-management-and-prognosis

Schweich, P. (2021). Closed reduction and casting of distal forearm fractures in children. *UpToDate*. https://www.uptodate.com/contents/closed-reduction-and-casting-of-distal-forearm-fractures-in-children

Tagher, C., & Knapp, L. (2020). *Pediatric nursing a case-based approach*. Wolters Kluwer.

Chapters 41

Aronson, M. D., & Auwaerter, P. G. (2021). Infectious mononucleosis. *UpToDate*. https://www.uptodate.com/contents/infectious-mononucleosis

Baddour, L. M. (2021). Impetigo. *UpToDate*. https://www.uptodate.com/contents/impetigo

Baddour, L. M., & Harper, M. (2021). Animal bites (dogs, cats, and other animals): Evaluation and management. *UpToDate*.

https://www.uptodate.com/contents/animal-bites-dogs-cats-and-other-animals-evaluation-and-management

Cohen, M. S. (2021). HIV infection: Risk factors and prevention strategies. *UpToDate.* https://www.uptodate.com/contents/hiv-infection-risk-factors-and-prevention-strategies

Fortenberry, J. D. (2021). Sexually transmitted infections: Issues specific to adolescents. *UpToDate.* https://www.uptodate.com/contents/sexually-transmitted-infections-issues-specific-to-adolescents

Gauglitz, G. G., & Williams, F. N. (2021). Overview of the management of the severely burned patient. *UpToDate.* https://www.uptodate.com/contents/overview-of-the-management-of-the-severely-burned-patient

Gillespie, S. L. (2021). Pediatric HIV infection: Classification, clinical manifestations, and outcome. *UpToDate.* https://www.uptodate.com/contents/pediatric-hiv-infection-classification-clinical-manifestations-and-outcome

Goldstein, A. O., & Goldstein, B. G. (2021a). Dermatophyte (tinea) infections. *UpToDate.* https://www.uptodate.com/contents/dermatophyte-tinea-infections

Goldstein, A. O., & Goldstein, B. G. (2021b). Pediculosis capitis. *UpToDate.* https://www.uptodate.com/contents/pediculosis-capitis

Hockenberry, M., Rodgers, C., & Wilson, D. (2016). *Wong's essentials of pediatric nursing* (10th ed.). Mosby.

Horii, K. A. (2021). Diaper dermatitis. *UpToDate.* https://www.uptodate.com/contents/diaper-dermatitis

Hu, L. (2021). Evaluation of a tick bite for possible Lyme disease. *UpToDate.* https://www.uptodate.com/contents/evaluation-of-a-tick-bite-for-possible-lyme-disease

Joffe, M. D. (2021). Moderate and severe thermal burns in children: Emergency management. *UpToDate.* https://www.uptodate.com/contents/moderate-and-severe-thermal-burns-in-children-emergency-management

Kyle, T., & Carman, S. (2020). *Essentials of pediatric nursing* (4th ed.). Wolters Kluwer.

Lippincott, Williams & Wilkins. (2021). *Nursing 2021 drug handbook* (41st ed.). Wolters Kluwer.

Maaks, D., Starr, N., Brady, M., Gaylord, N., Driessnack, M., & Duderstadt, K. (2020). *Burns' pediatric primary care* (7th ed.). Elsevier.

Mayer, K. H., & Krakower, D. (2021). Administration of pre-exposure prophylaxis against HIV infection. *UpToDate.* https://www.uptodate.com/contents/administration-of-pre-exposure-prophylaxis-against-hiv-infection

Middleman, A. B., & Olson, K. A. (2021). Confidentiality in adolescent health care. *UpToDate.* https://www.uptodate.com/contents/confidentiality-in-adolescent-health-care

O'Meara, A. (2019). *Maternity, newborn, and women's health nursing a case-based approach.* Wolters Kluwer.

Ricci, S. (2021). *Essentials of maternity, newborn, and women's health nursing* (5th ed.). Wolters Kluwer.

Ricci, S., Kyle, T., & Carman, S. (2021). *Maternity and pediatric nursing* (4th ed.). Wolters Kluwer.

Rice, P. L., & Orgill, D. P. (2021). Assessment and classification of burn injury. *UpToDate.* https://www.uptodate.com/contents/assessment-and-classification-of-burn-injury

Romanowski, K. S. (2021). Overview of nutrition support in burn patients. *UpToDate.* https://www.uptodate.com/contents/overview-of-nutrition-support-in-burn-patients

Sasseville, D. (2021). Cradle cap and seborrheic dermatitis in infants. *UpToDate.* https://www.uptodate.com/contents/cradle-cap-and-seborrheic-dermatitis-in-infants

Sax, P. E. (2021). Acute and early HIV infection: Clinical manifestations and diagnosis. *UpToDate.* https://www.uptodate.com/contents/acute-and-early-hiv-infection-clinical-manifestations-and-diagnosis

Tagher, C., & Knapp, L. (2020). *Pediatric nursing a case-based approach.* Wolters Kluwer.

Thwaites, L. (2021). Tetanus. *UpToDate.* https://www.uptodate.com/contents/tetanus

Treat, J. R. (2021). Tinea capitis. *UpToDate.* https://www.uptodate.com/contents/tinea-capitis

Vetter, R. S., & Swanson, D. L. (2021). Approach to the patient with a suspected spider bite: An overview. *UpToDate.* https://www.uptodate.com/contents/approach-to-the-patient-with-a-suspected-spider-bite-an-overview

Wiktor, A., & Richards, D. (2021). Treatment of minor thermal burns. *UpToDate.* https://www.uptodate.com/contents/treatment-of-minor-thermal-burns

Chapter 42

Alvarez, E., Puliafico, A., Leonte, K. G., & Albano, A. M. (2021). Psychotherapy for anxiety disorders in children and adolescents. *UpToDate.* https://www.uptodate.com/contents/psychotherapy-for-anxiety-disorders-in-children-and-adolescents

American Psychiatric Association. (2013). *Diagnostic and statistical manual* (5th ed.). American Psychiatric Association.

Augustyn, M. (2021). Autism spectrum disorder: Terminology, epidemiology, and pathogenesis. *UpToDate.* https://www.uptodate.com/contents/autism-spectrum-disorder-terminology-epidemiology-and-pathogenesis

Augustyn, M., & von Hahn, L. E. (2021a). Autism spectrum disorder: Clinical features. *UpToDate.* https://www.uptodate.com/contents/autism-spectrum-disorder-clinical-feature

Augustyn, M., & von Hahn, L. E. (2021b). Autism spectrum disorder: Evaluation and diagnosis. *UpToDate.* https://www.uptodate.com/contents/autism-spectrum-disorder-evaluation-and-diagnosis

Bennett, S., & Walkup, J. T. (2021a). Anxiety disorders in children and adolescents: Assessment and diagnosis. *UpToDate.* https://www.uptodate.com/contents/anxiety-disorders-in-children-and-adolescents-assessment-and-diagnosis

Bennett, S., & Walkup, J. T. (2021b). Anxiety disorders in children and adolescents: Epidemiology, pathogenesis, clinical manifestations, and course. *UpToDate.* https://www.uptodate.com/contents/anxiety-disorders-in-children-and-adolescents-epidemiology-pathogenesis-clinical-manifestations-and-course

Bonin, L. (2021). Pediatric unipolar depression: Epidemiology, clinical features, assessment, and diagnosis. *UpToDate.* https://www.uptodate.com/contents/pediatric-unipolar-depression-epidemiology-clinical-features-assessment-and-diagnosis

Bonin, L., & Moreland, C. S. (2021). Overview of prevention and treatment for pediatric depression. *UpToDate.* https://www.uptodate.com/contents/overview-of-prevention-and-treatment-for-pediatric-depression

Bukstein, O. (2021a). Approach to treating substance use disorder in adolescents. *UpToDate.* https://www.uptodate.com/contents/approach-to-treating-substance-use-disorder-in-adolescents

Bukstein, O. (2021b). Substance use disorder in adolescents: Epidemiology, pathogenesis, clinical manifestations and consequences, course, assessment, and diagnosis. *UpToDate.* https://www.uptodate.com/contents/substance-use-disorder-in-adolescents-epidemiology-pathogenesis-clinical-manifestations-and-consequences-course-assessment-and-diagnosis

Dugosh, K. L., & Cacciola, J. S. (2021). Clinical assessment of substance use disorders. *UpToDate.* https://www.uptodate.com/contents/clinical-assessment-of-substance-use-disorders

Hockenberry, M., Rodgers, C., & Wilson, D. (2016). *Wong's essentials of pediatric nursing* (10th ed.). Mosby.

Hoffman, R. J. (2021). MDMA (ecstasy) intoxication. *UpToDate.* https://www.uptodate.com/contents/mdma-ecstasy-intoxication

Kennebeck, S., & Bonin, L. (2021a). Suicidal behavior in children and adolescents: Epidemiology and risk factors. *UpToDate.* https://www.uptodate.com/contents/suicidal-behavior-in-children-and-adolescents-epidemiology-and-risk-factors

Kennebeck, S., & Bonin, L. (2021b). Suicidal ideation and behavior in children and adolescents: Evaluation and management. *UpToDate.* https://www.uptodate.com/contents/suicidal-ideation-and-behavior-in-children-and-adolescents-evaluation-and-management

Klish, W. J., & Skelton, J. A. (2021a). Definition, epidemiology, and etiology of obesity in children and adolescents. *UpToDate.* https://www.uptodate.com/contents/definition-epidemiology-and-etiology-of-obesity-in-children-and-adolescents

Klish, W. J., & Skelton, J. A. (2021b). Overview of the health consequences of obesity in children and adolescents. *UpToDate.* https://www.uptodate.com/contents/overview-of-the-health-consequences-of-obesity-in-children-and-adolescents

Knull, K. R. (2021a). Attention deficit hyperactivity disorder in children and adolescents: Clinical features and diagnosis. *UpToDate.* https://www.uptodate.com/contents/attention-deficit-hyperactivity-disorder-in-children-and-adolescents-clinical-features-and-diagnosis

Knull, K. R. (2021b). Attention deficit hyperactivity disorder in children and adolescents: Epidemiology and pathogenesis. *UpToDate.* https://www.uptodate.com/contents/attention-deficit-hyperactivity-disorder-in-children-and-adolescents-epidemiology-and-pathogenesis

Knull, K. R. (2021c). Attention deficit hyperactivity disorder in children and adolescents: Overview of treatment and prognosis. *UpToDate.* https://www.uptodate.com/contents/attention-deficit-hyperactivity-disorder-in-children-and-adolescents-overview-of-treatment-and-prognosis

Kyle, T., & Carman, S. (2020). *Essentials of pediatric nursing* (4th ed.). Wolters Kluwer.

Lippincott, Williams and Wilkins. (2021). *Nursing 2021 drug handbook* (41st ed.). Wolters Kluwer.

Maaks, D., Starr, N., Brady, M., Gaylord, N., Driessnack, M., & Duderstadt, K. (2020). *Burns' pediatric primary care* (7th ed.). Elsevier.

Mehler, P. (2021a). Anorexia nervosa in adults and adolescents: Medical complications and their management. *UpToDate.* https://www.uptodate.com/contents/anorexia-nervosa-in-adults-and-adolescents-medical-complications-and-their-management

Mehler, P. (2021b). Anorexia nervosa in adults and adolescents: The refeeding syndrome. *UpToDate.* https://www.uptodate.com/contents/anorexia-nervosa-in-adults-and-adolescents-the-refeeding-syndrome

O'Meara, A. (2019). *Maternity, newborn, and women's health nursing a case-based approach.* Wolters Kluwer.

Ricci, S. (2021). *Essentials of maternity, newborn, and women's health nursing* (5th ed.). Wolters Kluwer.

Ricci, S., Kyle, T., & Carman, S. (2021). *Maternity and pediatric nursing* (4th ed.). Wolters Kluwer.

Rigotti, N. A. (2021). Vaping and e-cigarettes. *UpToDate.* https://www.uptodate.com/contents/vaping-and-e-cigarettes

Rosen, J. B., & Sockrider, M. (2021). Management of smoking and vaping cessation in adolescents. *UpToDate.* https://www.uptodate.com/contents/management-of-smoking-and-vaping-cessation-in-adolescents

Skelton, J. A., & Klish, W. J. (2021). Clinical evaluation of the child or adolescent with obesity. *UpToDate.* https://www.uptodate.com/contents/clinical-evaluation-of-the-child-or-adolescent-with-obesity

Snyder, P. J. (2021). Use of androgens and other hormones by athletes. *UpToDate.* https://www.uptodate.com/contents/use-of-androgens-and-other-hormones-by-athletes

Sockrider, M., & Rosen, J. B. (2021). Prevention of smoking and vaping initiation in children and adolescents. *UpToDate.* https://www.uptodate.com/contents/prevention-of-smoking-and-vaping-initiation-in-children-and-adolescents

Weissman, L. (2021). Autism spectrum disorder in children and adolescents: Overview of management. *UpToDate.* https://www.uptodate.com/contents/autism-spectrum-disorder-in-children-and-adolescents-overview-of-management

Womble, D. M., & Kincheloe, C. A. (2020). *Introductory mental health nursing.* Wolters Kluwer.

Yager, J. (2021). Eating disorders: Overview of epidemiology, clinical features, and diagnosis. *UpToDate.* https://www.uptodate.com/contents/eating-disorders-overview-of-epidemiology-clinical-features-and-diagnosis

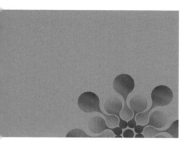

Index

Note: Page numbers followed by "f" indicate figures, "t" indicate tables, "b" indicate boxes.

A

AAIDD. *See* American Association on Intellectual and Development Disability (AAIDD)
AAP. *See* American Academy of Pediatrics (AAP)
Abdominal hysterectomy, 365
Abdominal incisions, 224, 225f
Abduction, infant, prevention of, 292
"Abductor" profile, 294b
ABO incompatibility, 447
Abortion, 74t
  complete, 362
  elective, 359
  habitual, 362t
  incomplete, 362t
  induced, 73
  inevitable, 362t
  missed, 362t
  postabortion teaching, 73
  spontaneous, 73
Abruptio placentae. *See* Placental abruption
Absence seizures, 719
Abstinence, 60–61
Abuse
  bullying, 687
  during pregnancy. *See* Intimate partner violence (IPV)
  examples of, 348b
  human trafficking, 686
  in family
    child, 680–686. *See also* Child abuse (maltreatment)
    domestic violence, 686–687. *See also* Domestic violence, in family
    dysfunctional family in, 679
    nursing care plan for abused child, 684–686
    nursing process for abused child, 684–686
    substance abuse, parental, 687–689
  signs of, 680–681
  substance abuse, parental, 687–689
  types of, 680–684
Abusive head trauma (shaken baby syndrome), 681
Accelerations, fetal heart rate, 194
Accident prevention
  in adolescent, 555
  in infants, 526
  in preschoolers, 555
  in school-aged child, 569–570
  in toddlers, 539–541
    burns, 540
    drowning, 540
    motor vehicle accidents, 540, 540f
    toxic ingestion, 540–541
Accommodation, 605
Acetaminophen, 821t
  childhood poisoning, 541
  in engorgement, 315
  for pain management, 296
  in pregnancy, 929
  for urinary tract infection (UTI), 415
Achylia, 759
Acne vulgaris, 876, 876f
Acquired immunodeficiency syndrome (AIDS), 345

Acrocyanosis, 274
Active alert state, newborn, 270
Active phase (active labor)
  assessment (data collection), 199–200, 200f
  breathing patterns, 200
  danger signs during labor, 199b
  fetal status assessment, 199
  maternal status assessment, 200–201
  pain management, 200
  preventing infection, 201
Acupressure, for relief of labor pain, 170t, 172
Acupuncture/acupressure
  for nausea and vomiting, 357
  for relief of labor pain, 170t, 172
Acute bronchiolitis
  clinical manifestations, 748
  diagnosis, 748
  nursing care, 748–749
  treatment, 748–749
Acute laryngotracheobronchitis
  clinical manifestations and diagnosis, 747
  treatment and nursing care, 747
Acute lymphoblastic leukemia (ALL)
  clinical manifestations, 788
  diagnosis of, 788
  nursing care plan, 788–791
  nursing process, 788–791
  pathophysiology of, 787–788
  treatment of, 788
Acute nasopharyngitis (common cold)
  clinical manifestations, 744
  diagnosis, 744
  nursing care, 744
  treatment, 744
Acute/nonrecurrent seizures
  clinical manifestations, 718
  diagnosis, 718
  nursing care plan, 721–723
  nursing process, 721–723
  treatment, 718
Acute poststreptococcal glomerulonephritis
  clinical manifestations, 841
  features, 842t
  nephrotic syndrome, 842t
  nursing care, 842
  treatment, 841–842
Adaptation, physiologic, of newborn, 267–270. *See also* Physiologic adaptation, of newborn
Adenoiditis
  clinical manifestations, 744–745
  diagnosis, 744–745
  nursing care, 745
  nursing care plan, 745–747
  nursing process, 745–747
  treatment, 745
Admission orders, 188–189
Admission to hospital, labor and
  additional assessments
    labor and birth preferences, 188
    labor status, 187–188, 189f
    maternal health history and physical assessment, 187, 187b
  admission orders, 188–189

immediate assessments
  birth imminence, 185
  fetal status, 185
  maternal status, 186
  precipitous delivery, 185, 186f
  risk assessment, 186
Adolescence/adolescents
  communication with, 505
  death and dying in, 695
  defined, 574
  developmental tasks of, 577t
  early, 574
  growth and development in. *See* Growth and development, 11-18 years
Adolescent development
  body image, 578–579
  developmental tasks in, 577t
  personality development, 577–578
  physical development, 576
  psychosocial development, 576–577
    body image in, 578–579
    overview of, 575
    personality in, 577–578
Adolescent pregnancy
  and birth rates, 351
  clinical manifestations, 351
  consequences of, 351
  diagnosis of, 351
  nursing care
    developmental needs, 352
    emotional/psychological needs and, 352
    physical needs, 352
  and nutrition, 351
  prevention of, 351
  and social support, 351
  treatment, 351–352
Adoptive family, 21
Afterpains, 241, 251
Airway care
  during burns, 886
  infants, 299–300
Alcohol abuse, 914–915
Alcohol intake
  by adolescents, 449
  preconception, 59
  in pregnancy, 139
Alkalosis, 660
Allergic contact dermatitis, 882
Allergic disorders
  allergens, 878
  atopic dermatitis
    clinical manifestations, 879
    diagnosis of, 879–880
    nursing care plan, 880–882
    nursing process, 880–882
    treatment of, 880
  diagnosis of, 879–880
Allergic rhinitis (hay fever), 879
  clinical manifestations, 744
  nursing care, 744
  treatment, 744
Allograft, 888
Alpha-fetoprotein (AFP), 127, 457
Ambiguous genitalia, 478